PERCUTANEOUS ANGIOGRAPHY

PERCUTANEOUS ANGIOGRAPHY

SWAMY

Siddalingappa Srikantaswamy, M.D.

Radiologist, Michael Reese Medical Center
Consultant, Cook County Hospital
Chicago Osteopathic School of Medicine
Chicago

SEGAL

Lewis Irwin Segal, M.D.

Radiologist, Louis A. Weiss Memorial Hospital
Clinical Assistant Professor of Medical Radiology
Abraham Lincoln School of Medicine
University of Illinois, Chicago

MOULI

Siddalingappa Chandramouli, M.D.

Fellow in Neuroradiology
Foster-McGaw Medical Center, Northwestern Memorial Hospital
Chicago

CHARLES C THOMAS · PUBLISHER

Springfield · Illinois · U.S.A.

Published and Distributed Throughout the World by

CHARLES C THOMAS • PUBLISHER
Bannerstone House
301-327 East Lawrence Avenue, Springfield, Illinois, U.S.A.

ISBN 0-398-03540-7

Library of Congress Catalog Card Number: 75-10374

With THOMAS BOOKS careful attention is given to all details of manufacturing and design. It is the Publisher's desire to present books that are satisfactory as to their physical qualities and artistic possibilities and appropriate for their particular use. THOMAS BOOKS will be true to those laws of quality that assure a good name and good will.

Library of Congress Cataloging in Publication Data

Srikantaswamy, Siddalingappa.
Percutaneous angiography.

Bibliography: p.
Includes index.
1. Angiography. I. Segal, Lewis Irwin, joint author. II. Chandramouli, Siddalingappa, joint author. III. Title. [DNLM: 1. Angiography. WG500 S774p]
RC691.6.A53S74 616.07'572 75-10374
ISBN 0-398-03540-7

Printed in the United States of America
C-1

Dedicated to
Our Wives

PREFACE

Unique are these footprints of the creatures, on the Sahara sand, Antarctica, or the Grecian island

IT IS TRUE THAT the distinctive footprints of different creatures were the same wherever and whenever they were discovered.

Our case material collected over the years revealed certain basic vascular patterns, irrespective of the organs. The patterns are best classified as (1) subtle but specific, (2) obvious and specific, (3) obvious and nonspecific.

The infiltrated vessels of a pancreatic malignancy are no different from the infiltrated vessels of a cholangiocarcinoma or mesenteric fibrosis. With a little stretch of imagination, "prune tree vessels" in the kidney resemble the "corkscrew vessels" of the liver, although the etiology and histology are dissimilar. Make your choice—prunes or corks.

The main intention of this book is to assist and guide an angiographer in training and one who is trained but uses one's skills occasionally. Numerous sketches help explain in detail basic angiographic techniques and the solutions for many common technical problems.

One section deals with the programming of standard studies (catheter, wire, amount of contrast, rate of filming, etc.), and a special recipe section is devoted entirely to the systematic method of studying common disease processes in its entirety.

Emphasis is placed on salient physiological points, along with the gross histological architecture of lesions and their meaningful angiographic representations.

The angiographic patterns have been classified pathologically rather than anatomically. This is attempted through the available examples with a special reference to common patterns. This is done with the intention of achieving a broad logical background, to assist in establishing a proper diagnosis whenever possible.

Certainly our experience would be incomplete without the cooperation and feedback of our colleagues, especially the surgeons and pathologists.

Most of the views expressed here are the authors', enriched by the experiences of others. *This experience has been classified both from learning from yesterday's mistakes and anticipating the suspense of tomorrow's problems.*

SWAMY, SEGAL, MOULI

ACKNOWLEDGMENTS

WE NUMBERED THREE when the writing of this book began. Now, several years later, three have become a group of many who gave unstintingly of their time and energy to help us convert our initial ideas into a finished product.

Specifically, we will always be grateful to Drs. Edwin Hirsh and Harry Sassoon who first implanted in us the idea of writing this book and were, thereafter, a constant source of encouragement and inspiration.

From the time of our first conversation, Mr. Peter Finley of Charles C Thomas, Publisher has been an enthusiastic supporter of this book. He has spared no effort toward helping us produce a book of high quality. Furthermore, his understanding, good nature and optimism have helped us through many of the difficulties we encountered while writing the manuscript.

Drs. Bertram Levin, Leon Bobrow and Sanford Rabushka have provided moral support, seasoned advice and wise counsel. Their supportive attitude and good humor were always there to encourage us during any decline in our enthusiasm.

Since the day we first entered the field of Radiology, Drs. Leon Love and Rogelio Moncada have always stood behind us; and their superb guidance and invaluable teachings throughout the years speak for themselves in these pages.

A special thanks must go to Angelito Jimenez, who drew the magnificent illustrations whose clarity simplifies the angiographic techniques.

Mr. William S. Cornwell of the Eastman Kodak Company and Editor Emeritus of *Medical Radiography* and his associate, Mr. Charles C. Heckman, spent their invaluable time teaching us their double masking technique to photograph roentgenograms.

Both Ms. Jackey Rappaport and Ms. Audrey Kaiser spent the better part of the last year and a half in the dark room converting the roentgenograms into photographs.

Mrs. Sara Loevy, with her meticulous attention to detail and knowledge of rhetoric, insures the reader that every sentence is concise and coherent.

Mrs. Evelyn Kaufman, Mrs. Lucille Kartun, Ms. Jacque Dempster and Ms. Patricia Hill spent innumerable hours converting our handwritten hieroglyphics into organized paragraphs.

A special note of thanks is reserved for all the radiologists throughout the world whose contributions to angiography made our work possible, and to our residents and technologists whose efforts too often go unacknowledged.

SWAMY, SEGAL, MOULI

CONTENTS

PART I—BASICS

PART II—TECHNIQUES

PART III—PATTERNS

PERCUTANEOUS ANGIOGRAPHY

PART I
BASICS

THE HISTORY

The glorious heritage of the vascular catheterization is indebted to an incomparable, lubricated, ureteral catheter. Losing its lubrication . . . Entering the field of diagnostic radiology, percutaneously . . . Traveling a long way in a short time . . . Yielding itself into curvaceous shapes . . . Bumping into a plastic world . . . Becoming energized by the dynamic power of the pigtail and headhunter . . . Searching for the cobra . . . Tunneling through obstacles . . . Plugging the leaks . . . Trespassing to sample the streams . . . thus the endless journey continues . . . *

---

* References 1 to 16.

CHAPTER 1
THE PATIENT

EACH PATIENT is a unique human and should be treated from that perspective. He is more than a collection of organs and should not be regarded as a kidney, a liver or a pancreas. Most often the person who needs an angiographic study is the one with diseased blood vessels, unstable cardiovascular status, fluid and electrolyte imbalance; this patient is highly susceptible to the adverse hemodynamic effects of a large bolus of hyperosmolar contrast material.

A patient is not a phantom with blood vessels and organs. A pretty picture is worthless if the patient succumbs to a serious complication. General care of the entire patient is as important to the patient as it is to the radiologist.

PREPARATION OF THE PATIENT

The Preangiogram Visit

A complete explanation in simple language of the procedure, the discomforts involved, and the occurrence of rare, but unpredictable, complications will usually gain the patient's cooperation and confidence. At this time any adverse reactions to previous use of contrast material or other drugs may come to light. In addition, information about the drugs the patient is taking will be obtained.

The greatest concern is whether or not the patient is on anticoagulants. This will avoid undesirable hematomas at the puncture site which may demand surgical drainage. The prothrombin time[52] gives an indication of the total amount of prothrombin in the blood. Depending upon the exact procedure used, the time required for coagulation to take place is normally about twelve seconds. A prothrombin time below 60 percent of normal may be a relative contraindication. If done with care, however, excessive bleeding may not occur even if the prothrombin time is 30 percent or below.

At the time of this visit, inspection of the regional anatomy pertinent to the angiographic procedure is performed. This inspection involves palpating the femoral pulses and those distal to it on both sides. The same applies to the axillary artery if it is anticipated that this approach will be necessary.

The Consent

"Fair treatment of the honest patient pays dividends through better rapport, and reduces the chances of unwarranted legal action."[17] *It is impractical to draft an informed consent form which is universally applicable and acceptable.* One should formulate an informed consent form after proper consultation with the legal authorities of the hospital. Small booklets are available which in simple language explain angiographic procedures in general and contain consent forms at their end.

We discuss the entire procedure with the patient or parents (if the patient is a minor) at the initial visit. We reveal the general complications involved with the use of contrast material, complications pertinent to the vessel catheterized and the organ involved, and possible local complications at the puncture site. Although emphasis is on the importance of the study, we do discuss our *inability to guarantee against unavoidable and unpredictable complications that may happen to somebody, somewhere, someday.*

In our experience the honest disclosure of the procedure and effects has resulted in only twelve out of 6700 patients refusing angiography. A questionnaire sent to 500 patients after angiography revealed the following responses:

"Wouldn't mind if I had to
come for a second time" ......35 percent
"An exciting experience" ......20 percent
"It was O.K." ....20 percent

"Not as bad as I thought it was going to be" ....15 percent
"No desire to ever see the angiographer's face again" ....10 percent

Orders

Dietary restriction is necessary, as it is the common observation that intravenous and occasionally aortic arch injections of contrast may cause nausea and vomiting. For *intravenous injections,* no solid foods are given eight hours prior to the injection and no oral fluids are given for the two hours prior to the exam. For the *intra-arterial injections,* no solid foods are given six hours prior to the injection and no fluids by mouth for the prior hour. If the clinical condition permits, small sips of fluid before the examination help combat the adverse effects of the hyperosmolar contrast.

Premedication

Routine premedication is felt by one of us to be unnecessary. It is administered only to very nervous individuals and routinely only to pediatric patients. If the patient's attending physician feels premedication is necessary, then preferably Valium®, 5 mg by mouth, is given the previous evening, and 5 mg is given intramuscularly one hour prior to the study. Pediatric patients, provided there are no contraindications, receive needed premedications from their physicians. In patients with suspected pheochromocytoma, extra efforts are made to see that they are adequately sedated.

Shaving

For all patients, both groins are shaved in the event that either spasm occurs in one artery or that the artery is occluded. It is preferable to do this just prior to the procedure, as shaving of the puncture sites during angiography is not hygienic. For elderly individuals the left axilla is also shaved if it is anticipated that obstruction due to severe tortuosity or atherosclerotic plaques may prevent the use of the femoral arteries. Both groins and the right axilla are shaved in patients suspected of dissecting aortic aneurysms.

CHAPTER 2

THE DOCTOR

IN THIS THREE-PRONG attack on an obscure lesion, the doctor and the technical equipment are as important as the patient. Whether trained or trainee, a thorough knowledge of the vascular anatomy and an awareness of the avoidable and unavoidable complications are mandatory. This knowledge and understanding help to prevent the avoidable and to combat the unavoidable complications.

The importance of reviewing the patient's clinical and laboratory findings and other studies can never be overemphasized. The clues obtained will direct the angiographer to the area of interest, thereby shortening the duration of the procedure and decreasing the morbidity. A substantial knowledge of the clinical manifestations and their meaning aids in proper selection of the needed study. Prior knowledge of the regional anatomy and the biological behavior of the lesion helps to explore the adjacent organs in the hope of determining whether a lesion is operable or inoperable.

An awareness of the angiographic patterns reminds one of the procedural limitations and expedites quick decisions regarding further steps to be taken during a procedure. Neglect-

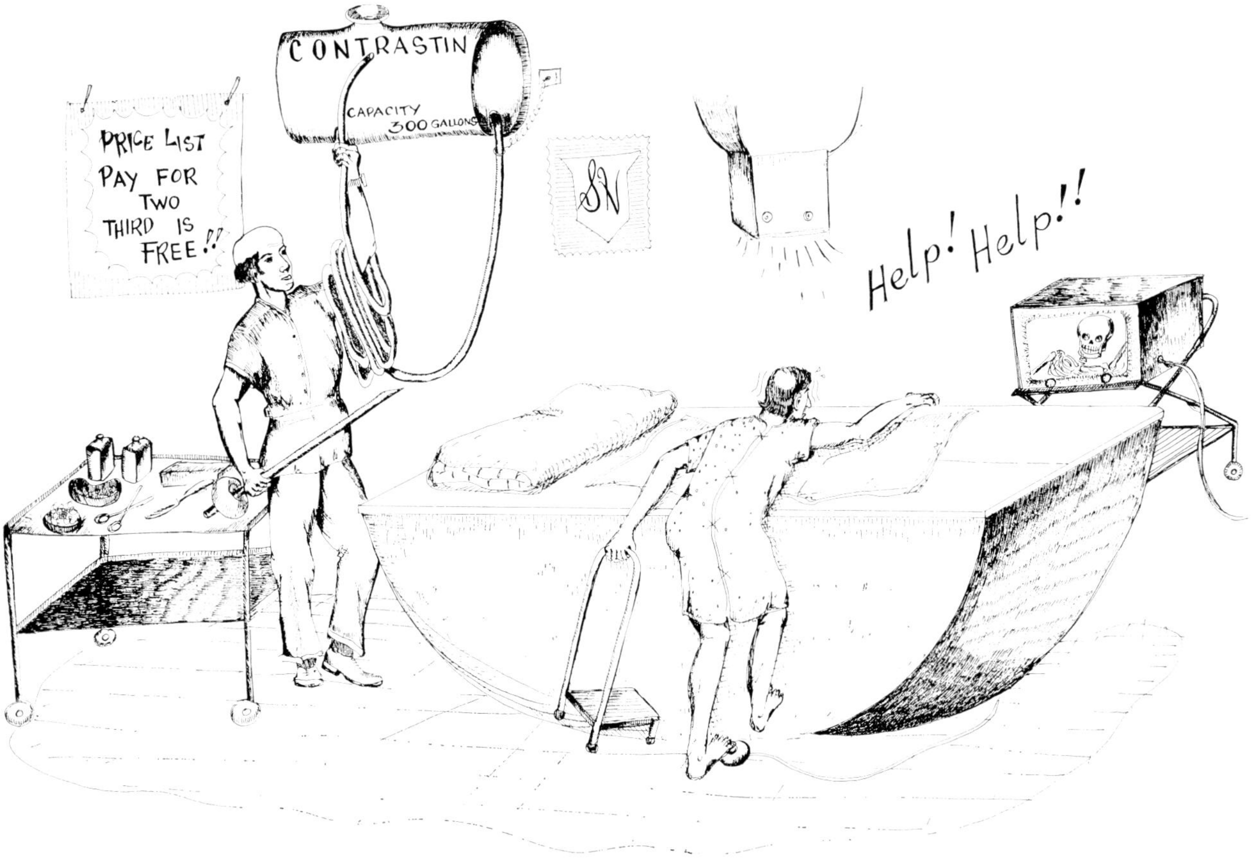

Figure 2.1

ing the proper approach or taking shortcuts only prolongs the duration of the study and increases the morbidity and mortality of the procedure. Meticulous technique and a conservative approach will always be rewarded. Thorough knowledge in the field of clinical radiology will achieve the same goal, thereby reducing the number of procedures indicated.

While performing a procedure, undue exclamatory expressions, discussion of other patients or their complications without reference, will only serve to increase the anxiety of an already apprehensive patient. While the atmosphere of the special procedures room need not be oppressive, neither should a circus-like atmosphere prevail.

The angiographer should be able to discontinue the examination immediately after obtaining the needed information. This will decrease complications from undue catheterization of lumbar, intercostal and thyrocervical arteries. A systematic approach and a proper protocol for evaluating different lesions will increase the efficiency of the available facility, decrease the duration of examination and the amount of contrast used, and will help to make angiography a pleasantly exciting experience for the patient.

CHAPTER 3
THE TOOLS

NEEDLES

To puncture the vessels percutaneously, a sharp needle with a short bevel and a thin wall[35] which admits the desired guide wire is essential. Needles with Teflon® sleeves[36] are also available and are useful for phlebograms and brachial or carotid arterial injections. Occasionally these needles may replace the regular percutaneous needle when the artery of entry cannot be properly fixed. The Teflon sleeve has the advantage of further introduction into the artery for additional security, which helps to avoid inadvertent subintimal injection. It can

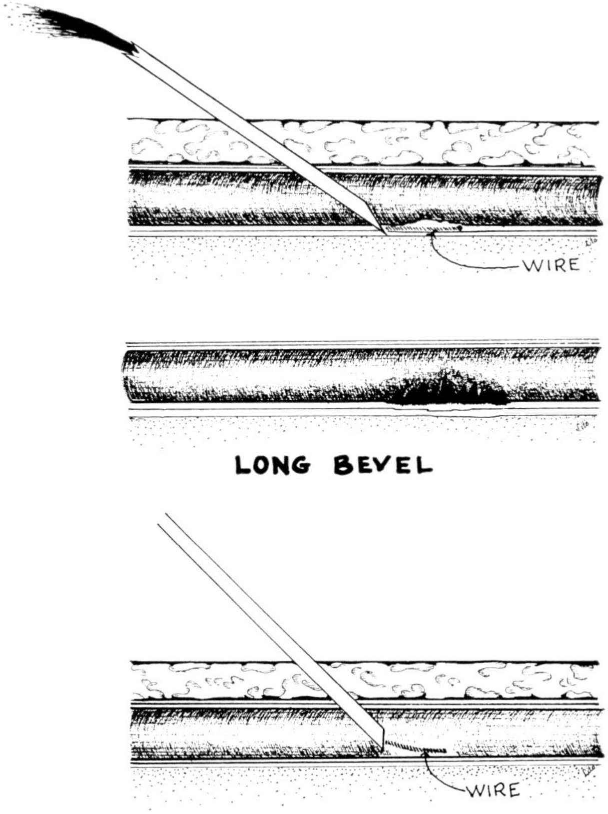

Figure 3.1. The disadvantages of a long bevel needle and the advantage of the short bevel one.

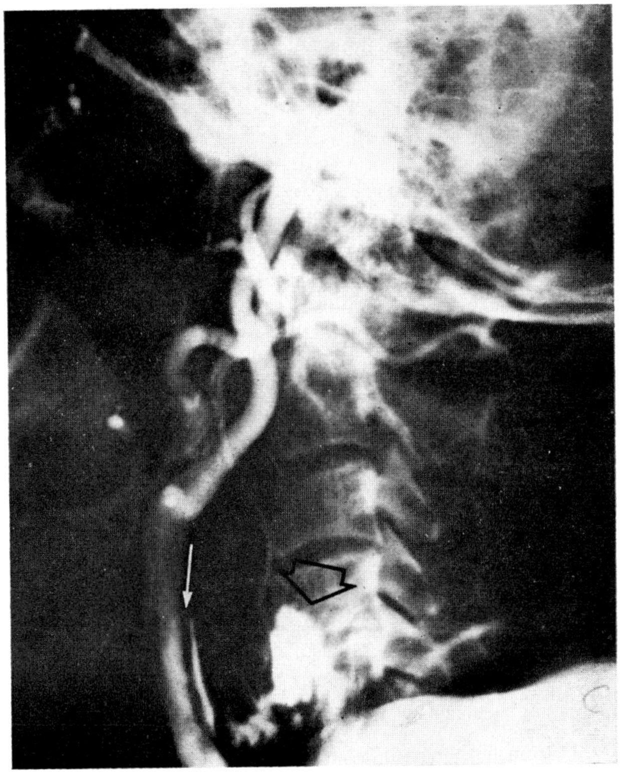

Figure 3.2. Needle Carotid Arteriogram. Reveals subintimal dissection (Arrow) and periarterial collection of contrast medium (Blank Arrow). *Comment:* Complication of a long bevel needle causing subintimal dissection and periarterial extravasation.

easily deliver 15 to 20 cc of contrast per second.

Needles with long bevels should be avoided, as they frequently cause long intimal lacerations, thereby increasing the risk of subintimal passage of the guide wire (Fig. 3-1). This is especially common in the small arteries of children and in those arteries which have undergone spasm (Figs. 3-2, 3-3).

WIRES

Safety guide wires are made of stainless steel cores which are bonded at both ends to an outer coiled layer of the same metal. The leading seg-

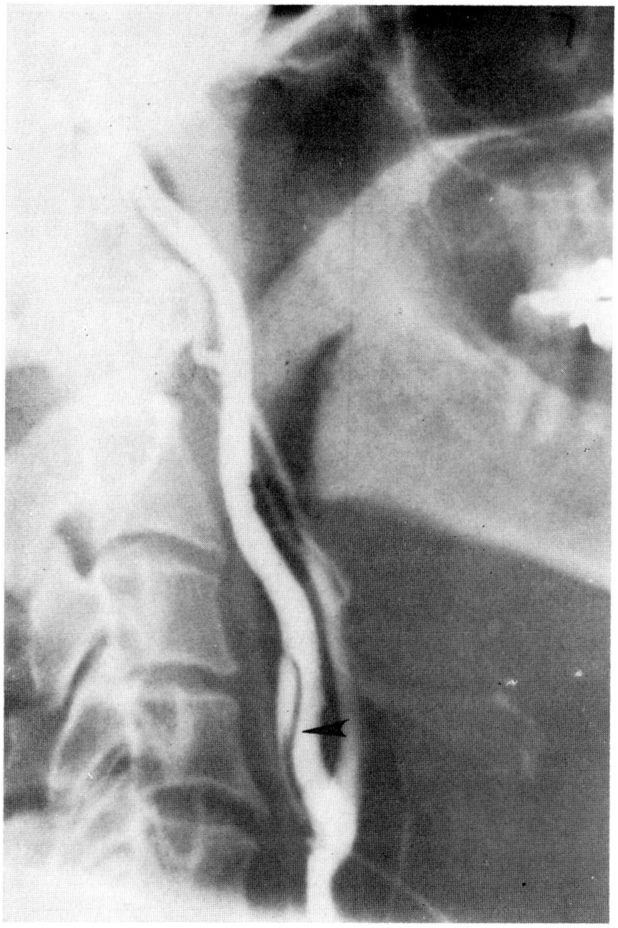

Figure 3.3. Carotid Arteriogram. Note the lucent defect in the internal carotid artery. *Diagnosis:* Intimal flap due to subintimal injection.

ment is flexible, while the trailing segment is rigid. *The flexible portion always enters the artery or vein first.*

A variety of guide wires are available which serve different purposes in clinical angiography. The *straight* wire has a short, straight flexible segment at the leading edge. *J wires* have curved segments; these curves are of varying radii. The *floppy* wire essentially has a long, straight flexible leading segment which can loop over on itself when an obstruction is met. Movable core[42] and deflector guide wires[35, 37] are also available.

The thickness of the guide wire varies to fit different French size catheters.[35, 37–39] Regardless of French size,[37, 38] the majority of available catheters easily admit a guide wire of .035 inches in diameter. On rare occasions, a wire thicker (.045 inches) or thinner (.025 inches) than the standard .035- or .038-inch guide wire is needed.

Guide wire lengths vary from 100 to 150 cm. It is safer to keep only one length of guide wire, preferably the longest, in supply. This will reduce the chance of accidental retraction of the guide wire from the vessel during a procedure while either wiping it off or threading a catheter over it. The selected guide wire should be at least 40 to 45 cm *longer* than the chosen catheter. The guide wire should *snugly* fit the tip of the catheter to enable smooth entry of the catheter through the subcutaneous tissues and into the arterial lumen. However, it should be easily maneuverable within the catheter to avoid adherence to the internal catheter wall. If it fits tightly, it tends to fracture more readily while being withdrawn from the catheter. Guide wires with kinks of any type should be discarded to avoid breaking in the vessel lumen.

Because of the difficulty in cleaning used guide wires, they should be discarded after each examination. Their reuse is not recommended. It is always advisable to have two or three of the desired guide wire types available to make provision for accidental contamination, bending, or the inevitable fall to the floor.

Types of Wires

Straight Wires

These have short, flexible leading segments, but are difficult to negotiate through tortuous curves or kinks of the vessel. *They have a higher incidence of dislodging atherosclerotic plaques and are not recommended for superselective studies.* They are, however, very good in younger-aged patients. Straight wires can be used to straighten catheters with loops or buckles, or those with reverse curved tips. They can also be used to provide torque to very soft straight catheters in tortuous vessels. If used for this purpose, the wire should be kept at least 1 cm proximal to the tip of the catheter

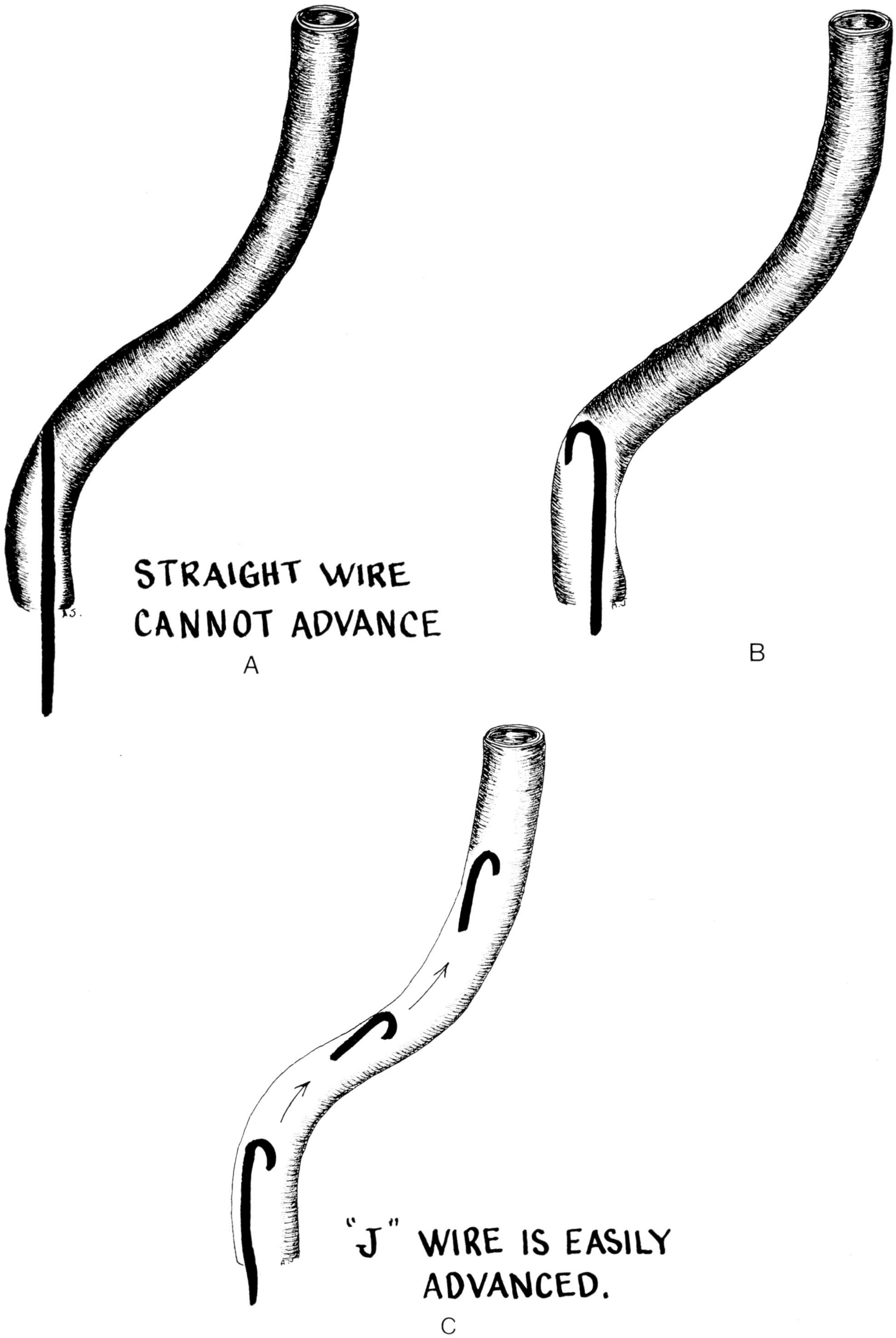

Figure 3.4. Advantages of a "J" wire.

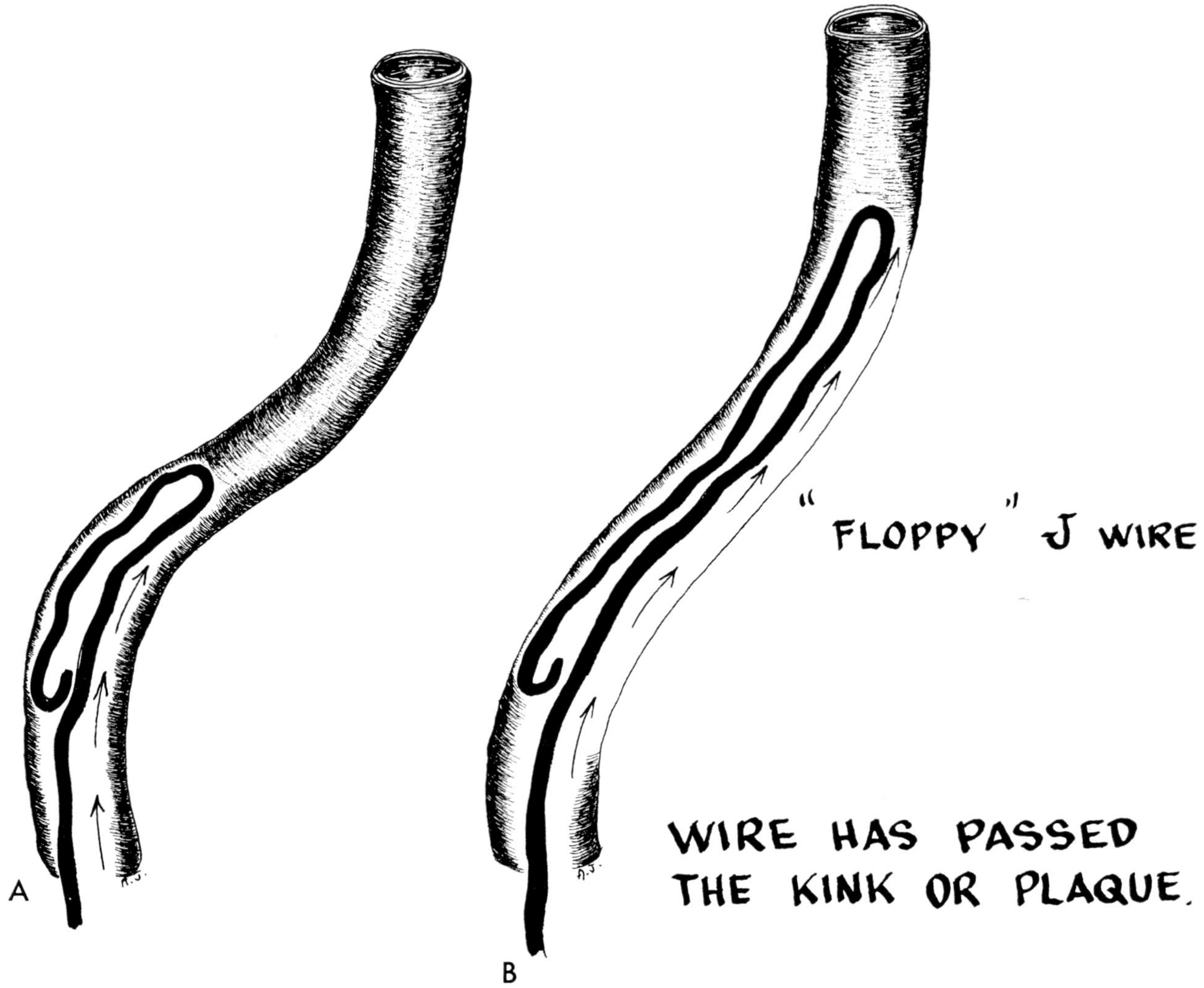

Figure 3.5. Advantages of a "J" wire.

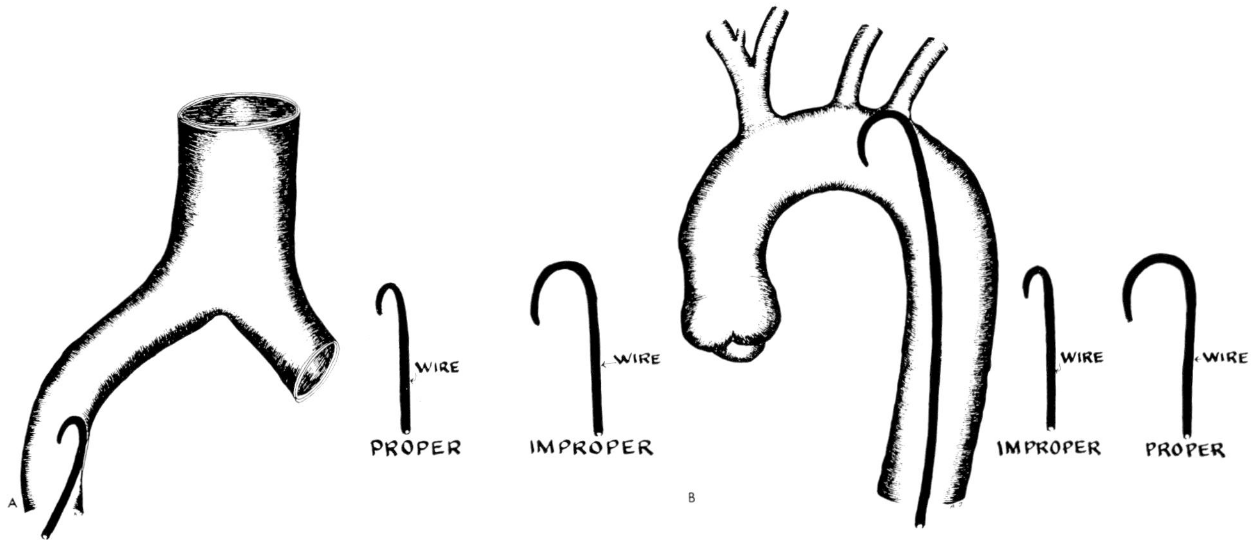

Figure 3.6. Selection of a proper "J" wire.

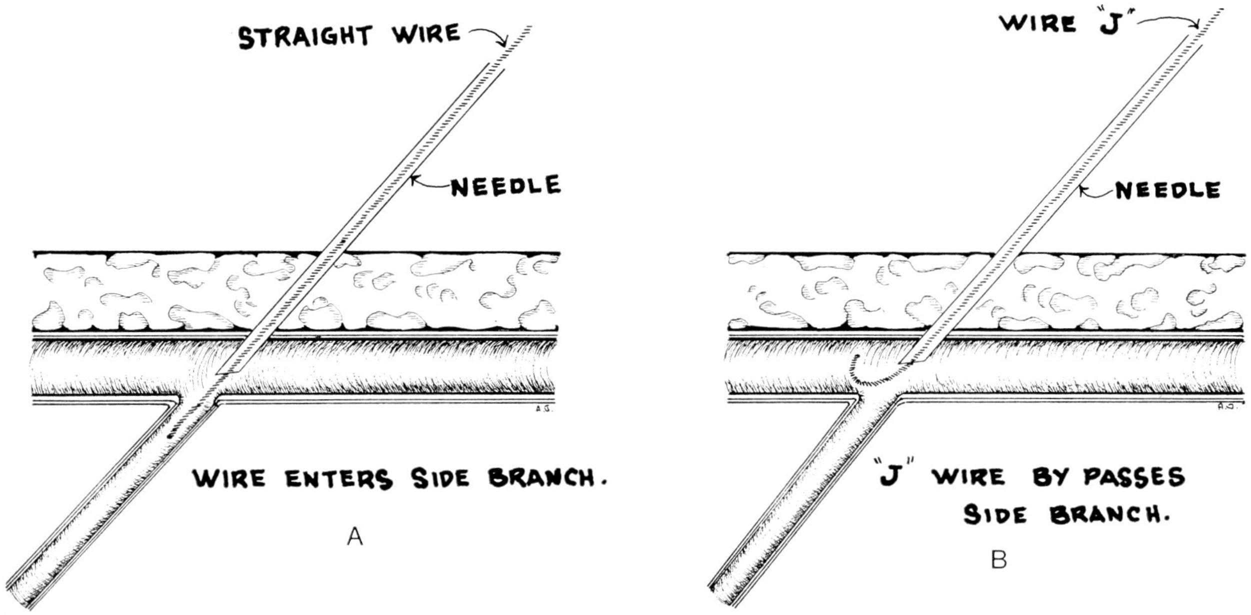

Figure 3.7

to avoid intimal damage. In this situation the wire should not be left too long in the catheter.

J Wires

J wires[40] with different radii are meant to easily *negotiate* tortuous curves or kinks in the vessels, to bypass orifices of side arterial branches, and to diminish the chance of dislodgement of atherosclerotic plaques. *During negotiation within a tortuous vessel, the width of the J radius should be smaller than the diameter of that vessel.* If it is not, the wire will not act in the J configuration. *When used to bypass the orifice of a side branch, the width of the J radius should be wider than the diameter of the orifice.* Otherwise, the guide wire will enter rather than bypass the orifice (Figs. 3-4 to 3-9). They are also very useful during catheterization of second and third order vessels. The smallest radius of the J available should be selected for these studies (Fig. 3-6).

Long, Floppy Guide Wires

The leading flexible segment of this wire[41] is appreciably longer than a standard straight guide wire. This enables it to smoothly negotiate tortuous arteries. It is useful in superselective studies, providing the trunk of the branch is longer than the floppy segment of the wire. If not, the wire and the catheter together will bounce back into the aortic lumen because a *catheter cannot be advanced over a floppy segment of wire.* It should also be remembered that when the catheter is advanced over the wire, *both of them move together as a single unit.* It is a unified movement rather than just the catheter sliding over the wire. This concept is extremely important to remember when manipulating the wire and catheter together (Fig. 3-5).

Short Guide Wires

These guide wires, 25 to 30 cm in length, are handy for further insertion of Teflon sleeve needles into veins or into the femoral, brachial or carotid arteries.[35]

DILATORS

The vessel dilator[35, 37] is a demi-catheter made from comparatively rigid plastic material. It is available in different French sizes and has a smooth, tapered tip with only an end hole. The dilator, when used over the existing guide wire, widens the hole in the subcutaneous tissues and

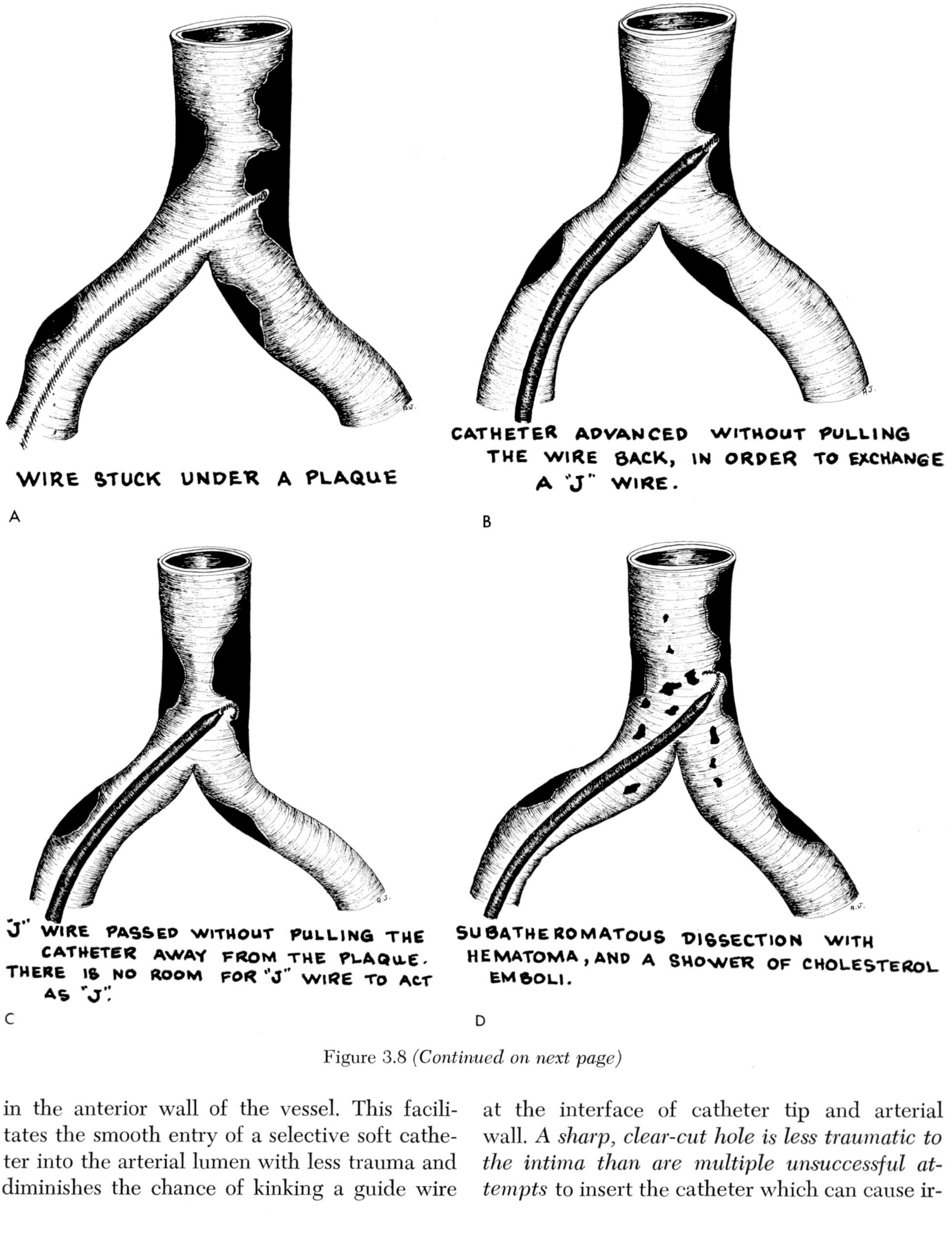

Figure 3.8 *(Continued on next page)*

in the anterior wall of the vessel. This facilitates the smooth entry of a selective soft catheter into the arterial lumen with less trauma and diminishes the chance of kinking a guide wire at the interface of catheter tip and arterial wall. *A sharp, clear-cut hole is less traumatic to the intima than are multiple unsuccessful attempts* to insert the catheter which can cause ir-

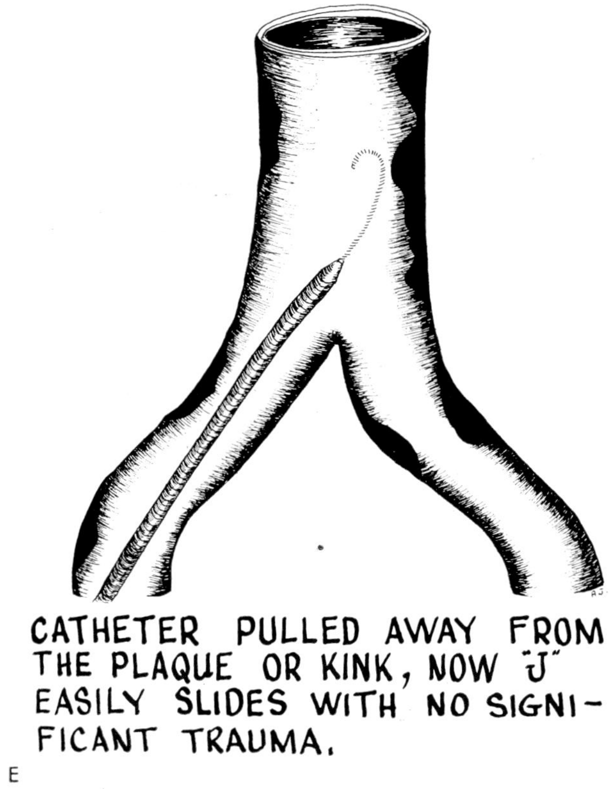

Figure 3.8. Precautions during introduction of a "J" wire.

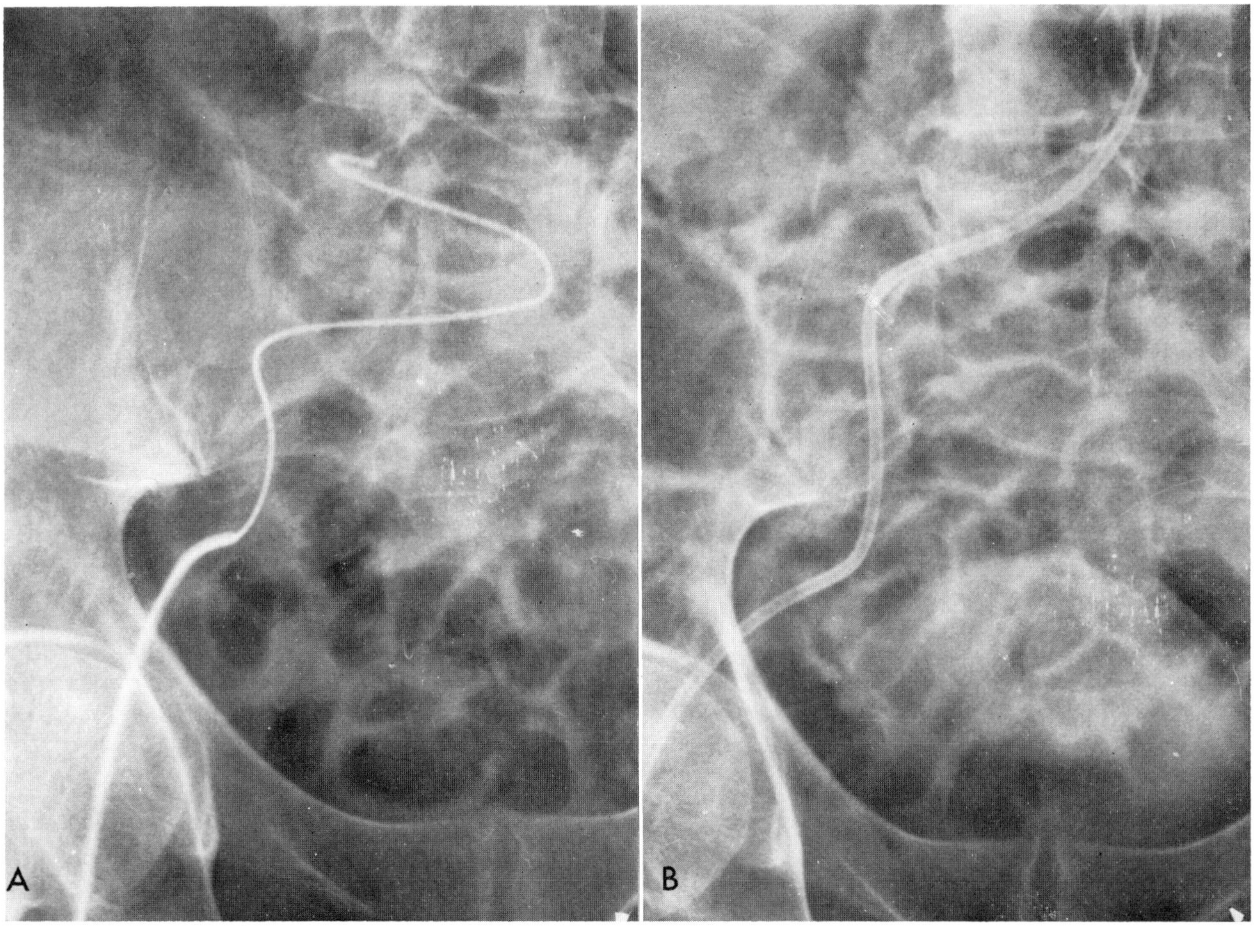

Figure 3.9. (A) Initially there was resistance for the passage of a straight wire which was overcome by using a "J" wire. (B) Catheter reaches its destination with the help of a "J" wire.

regular intimal lacerations. This is especially true in obese individuals and in patients with scar tissue at the puncture site.

A dilator of one French size smaller than that of the selected catheter is used in thin, but average patients and in patients with decreased prothrombin levels. In other words, if the desired catheter is French seven in size, then a dilator of French six size is used. In obese individuals or those with scar tissue at the puncture site, the same French size dilator is used as catheter. *Dilators wider than catheters are contraindicated* because the subsequent hole which is made in the arterial wall is larger than that of the catheter size which results in continuous oozing of blood about the catheter. In the course of a long procedure, this may represent a significant loss of blood. Dilators are not needed when catheters of rigid material with straight tips are used.

CATHETERS

Catheters are made of thermoplastic material with or without the reinforcement of a braided shaft. They are usually impregnated with radiopaque material for better fluoroscopic visibility. Teflon, polyethylene, polyurethane, dacron and nylon are all used to make catheter tubing. The *ideal catheter is nonthrombogenic and has good memory, good torque control, and sufficient strength to accommodate a high flow rate of contrast.*

Properties of a Catheter

Thrombogenicity

All available catheters are foreign bodies in the bloodstream. Because of this, thrombi form at the tip and on both the outer and inner surfaces of the catheter. A thin surface coating of benzalkonium heparin complex delays and decreases thrombus formation on the surface of the catheter and guide wire.[43, 44]

Memory

This is the inherent ability of the catheter to retain its given shape inside, as well as outside of, the lumen of the vessel.

Torque Control

This is the ability to deliver precisely the externally applied message to the tip of the catheter. That is, if the catheter is rotated in either a clockwise or counterclockwise manner along its longitudinal axis, the tip should rotate in the same direction and to the same degree. It should also be able to respond to a combination of movements such as propulsion and rotation. *Torque control is directly proportional to the stiffness of the material used.* Catheters with a braided shaft reinforcement are excellent conductors of a given message. At the same time, they accept a given curve.[37,45]

With each bend of a tortuous vessel, the delivered message is dampened. This may reach such a degree that a negative, or even a reverse, response to a given message may be obtained. For this reason, catheters with good torque control work well in tortuous vessels. These catheters are excellent for beginners until sufficient control of the catheter is learned (Fig. 16-15).

Thin wall catheters with no reinforcement have poor torque control, but with the assistance of a guide wire, perform well during superselective catheterization.

Strength

Catheters should be able to withstand high injection pressure of large amounts of contrast material per unit time. In aortography the rate of delivery may be from 25 to 35 cc per second. Only certain catheters, usually made of Teflon, with end and side holes can withstand such injection pressures without breaking near the hub.[35]

Sizes

Catheters are available in multiple French sizes ranging from three to eight. As the number increases, the catheter diameter increases. The internal diameter of the catheter and its tip determine the size of the guide wire and the amount of contrast the catheter will be able to deliver. The external diameter is as important to the catheter as is the internal diameter. *The external diameter must be considered important as it may approach the size of small vessels and occlude them.* Regional ischemia, spasm and thrombogenicity are directly proportional to the external diameter of a catheter. The internal diameter may be increased at the cost of the thickness of the catheter wall without increasing the external diameter. The product of such a compromise is a thin-walled catheter with poor torque control and increased susceptibility to kinks and tears. This is particularly true in untrained hands.

If different French size catheters are to be used, it is preferable to use ones with a uniform internal diameter which admits one particular size guide wire. This avoids the frustration of mismatching and the necessity of stocking different size guide wires and catheters.

Flow Rate

Within certain limitations the shorter the catheter, the wider the internal diameter, and the greater the number of side holes, the higher the flow rate for a given size catheter. But there is still no substitute for the angiographer's knowledge of the performance and the limitations of his tool *in vitro* before it is applied *in vivo. All newly introduced catheters should be subjected to different pressure injections in vitro to assess their limitations.*

Shapes and Holes

A catheter may be provided with an end hole or a blunt tip and side holes or both an end hole and side holes.

A catheter with both an end hole and side holes is used to obtain a uniform distribution of concentrated contrast material to all the right angled branches of the aorta. At the same time, the end hole creates turbulence and good mixing of the contrast with the blood pool. If the total bolus must be equally proportioned, the holes should be successively smaller distally, i.e. the middle hole smaller than the proximal and the distal hole smaller than the middle. Adding side holes to an end hole catheter diminishes jet effect injury and cavitation.[47] *The side holes, when punched out by the angiographer, should be at different positions and levels. They should not oppose each other, as this weakens the wall of the catheter.* Catheters with side holes may be straight or have a predeter-

TABLE 3-I

MAXIMUM INJECTION RATES

(For Both Renografin®-60 and Renografin-76)

Teflon catheter—straight—end hole and multiple side hole[35]		40 cc/sec
Polyethylene braided shaft catheters[37, 45]	French 7	20 cc/sec
	French 6	15 cc/sec
	French 5	8 cc/sec
Pigtail catheters[38]	French 7	20 cc/sec
	French 6	15 cc/sec
Teflon sleeve[36]	#16	20 cc/sec
	#18	12 cc/sec

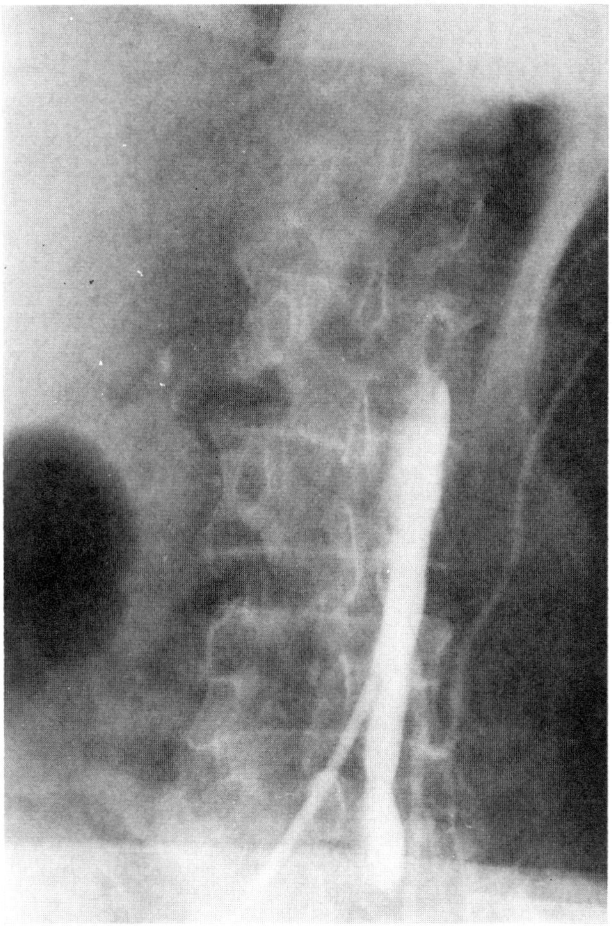

Figure 3.10. Abdominal Aortogram. There is a persistent collection of contrast which was not washed away by the blood. *Diagnosis:* A subintimal injection of contrast due to impaction of the catheter tip in the wall of the vessel. The catheter had both end and side holes.

mined shape. There are no advantages to more than three side holes.[46]

Straight Catheters with End and Side Holes

These are used for *aortography* or *inferior venacavography* to deliver a large bolus of contrast in a short time. This will opacify both a large vascular pool which is moving with great velocity as well as its multiple branches. They are useful in accessible straight course vessels such as the subclavian, femoral and axillary arteries. They are not, however, satisfactory for selective opacification of second or third order branches because of opacification of other arteries from the side holes.

When using one of these catheters, *aspiration of blood does not assure that one of the holes is not plugged by a clot which may later be dislodged* during pressure injection into a vital circulatory structure such as the brain. *Aspiration of blood does not guarantee that the tip is not impacted under an arteriosclerotic plaque or under the intima.* If the tip is in fact impacted, frank dissection may occur when contrast is injected. This problem can easily be avoided by testing with a hand injection of contrast under fluoroscopic control to make sure the tip is in the lumen of the artery (Fig. 3-10).

When used in capacious vessels with a uniform arch-like configuration, such as the aortic arch or a tortuous abdominal aorta, straight catheters are susceptible to whipping and backlash. During these types of movements, the tip may enter a side branch such as the innominate and deliver the entire bolus of contrast into that vessel with tragic outcome (Fig. 3-11). Subintimal hematomas or even frank dissection may also occur (Fig. 3-12). This is infrequent in vessels with a straight course such as the abdominal aorta or descending thoracic aorta.

Curved Catheters with End Hole and Side Holes

These are used to diminish the chance of recoil during injection. Right angled branches arising from a main trunk are well perfused. The addition of one or two holes on the superior surface of a curved catheter will assure good filling of right angled cephalad branches from a trunk, e.g. inferior adrenal from the renal, left gastric from the celiac, vertebral from the subclavians. An occasional *disad-*

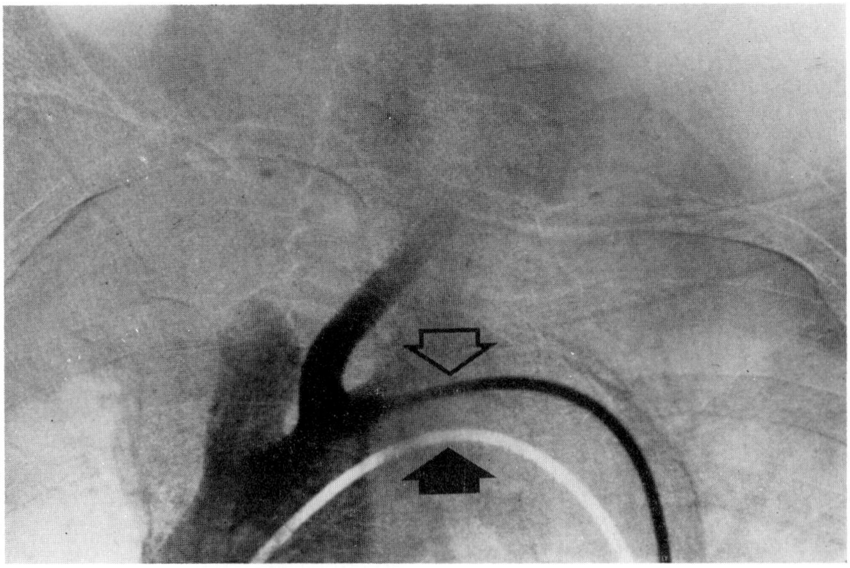

Figure 3.11. Aortic Arch Angiogram (left anterior oblique projection): A composite film using the subtraction technique graphically reveals how the catheter can recoil from the ascending aorta (Arrow) into the aortic arch (Blank Arrow) due to the pressure of injection.

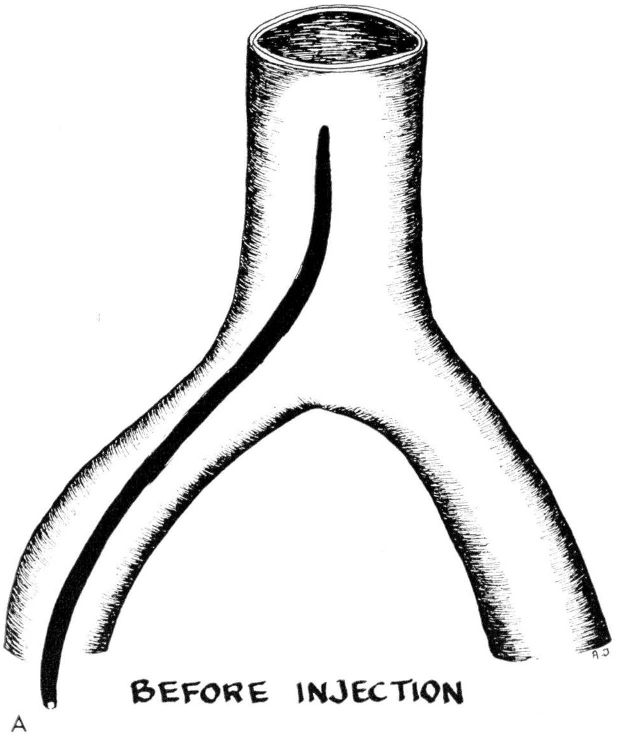

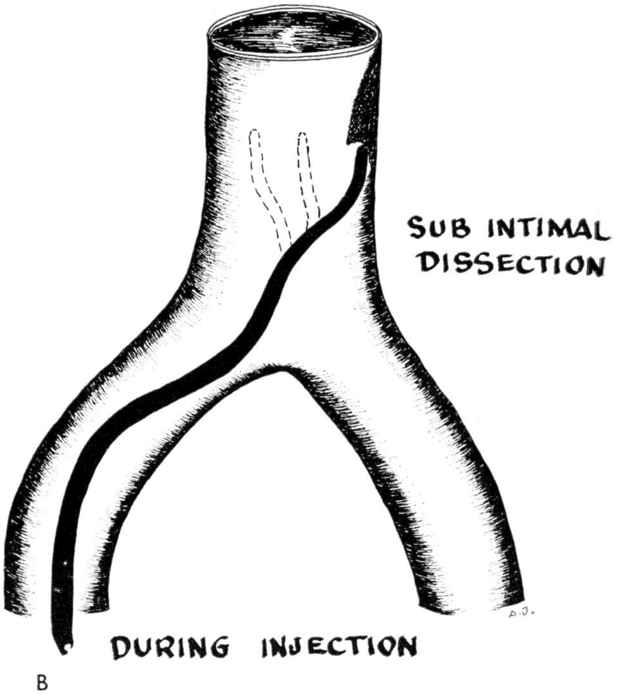

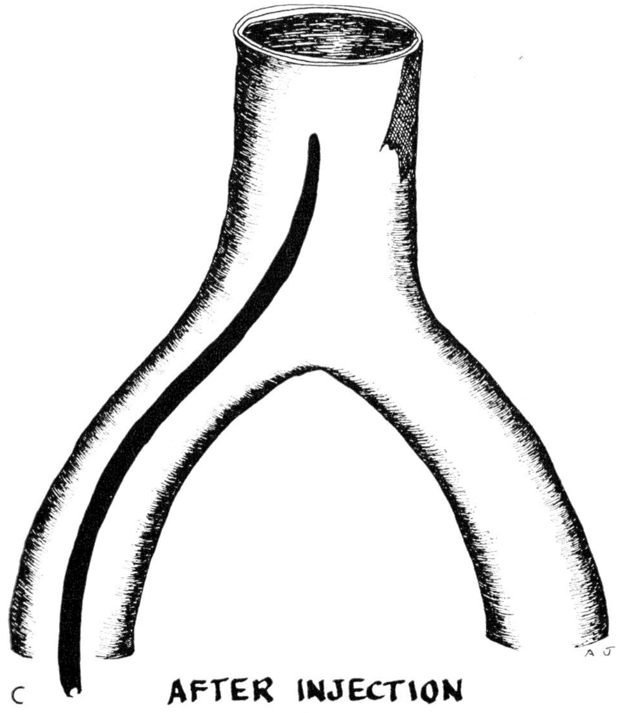

Figure 3.12. Whipping of a catheter and its effects on the vascular wall.

vantage of side holes on a curved portion of the catheter is the entrance of a guide wire through one of the side holes into a vessel. In addition, if a single selective vessel is perfused, opacification of other unwanted branches may occur. These catheters are not recommended for venous hormone sampling because of contamination by blood entering through the side holes.

End Hole Catheters

End hole catheters are meant for selective opacification of a branch and its distal arborization. They are also used for *venous sampling*. Failure to aspirate blood from one of these catheters stems from a clot in the tip, impaction under a plaque, or suction of the wall of the vessel up against the orifice of the catheter. The *disadvantages* of this type of catheter are an increased chance of recoiling during an injection, improper perfusion of right angled branches, or intimal damage due to increased whipping. During whipping there may be accidental engagement of a small branch, thereby delivering the entire amount of contrast into a small vessel (Fig. 3-13). *"Angiographic coning"* is another disadvantage of selective opacification of one small vessel and its arborization.

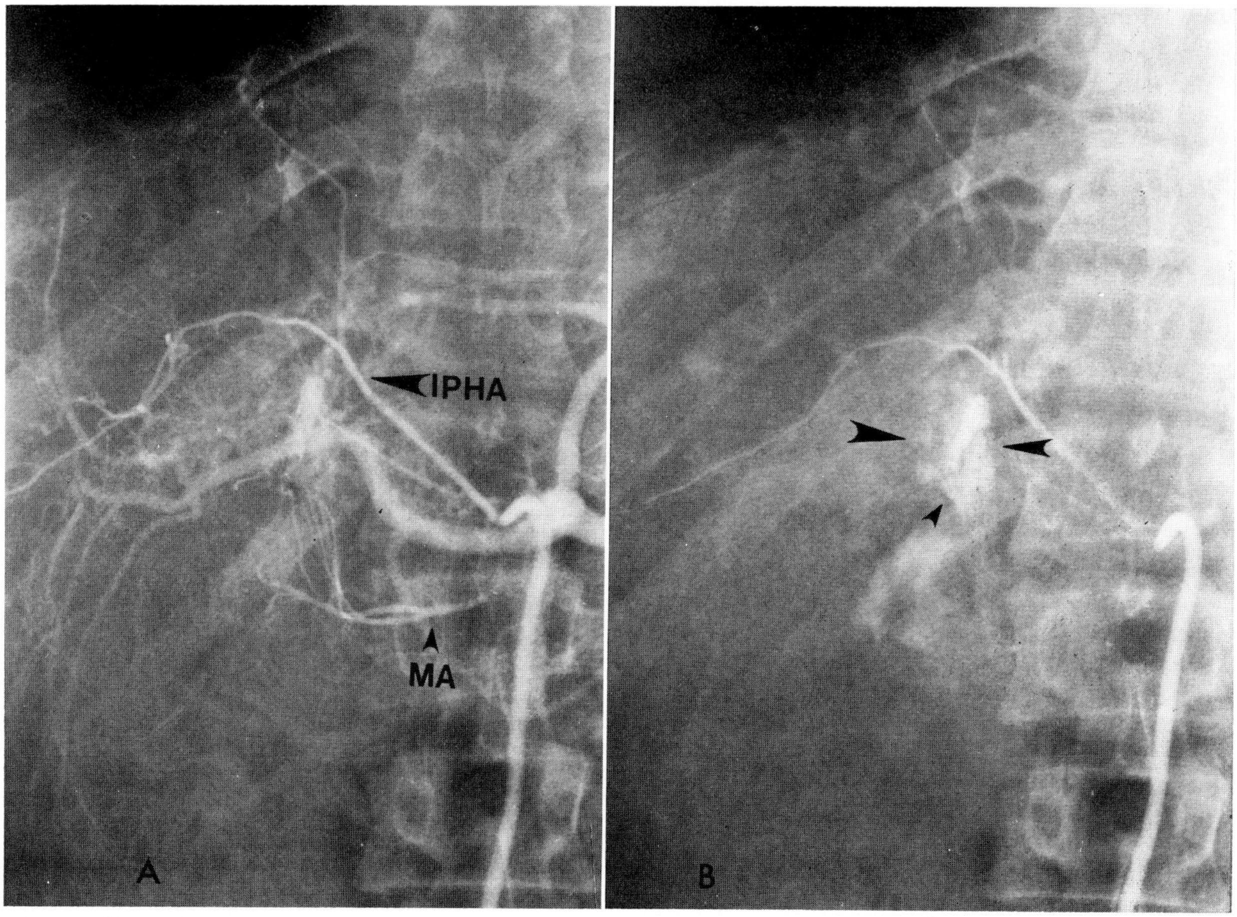

Figure 3.13. Celiac Arteriogram. *Arterial phase:* There is excellent opacification of the inferior phrenic artery (I.P.H.A.), with perfusion of the adrenal gland and filling of the middle adrenal arteries (M.A.). *Venous phase:* There is stain of the adrenal gland (Arrow). *Comment:* The catheter was originally placed in the celiac axis but recoiled into the inferior phrenic artery during injection. The increased perfusion of the inferior phrenic artery revealed the circulatory complex of the adrenal in one injection.

By not perfusing adjacent vasculature, the true blood supply to a lesion or its parasitic circulation may not be visualized.

Blunt Tipped Catheters with Side Holes

These are meant for injection into the cardiac chambers. They have less tendency to whip or recoil or to cause jet stream injury. They provide good perfusion to the right angled branches of some main trunks, such as the thyrocervical artery, when injected into the subclavian artery, subselective renals, aortic bifurcation and distal branch opacification, and left gastric opacification from the celiac axis. There is no significant distal or proximal jet stream effect, depending on the route of catheterization to cause opacification of other branches. These catheters[35, 45] require special sheaths[48] for their percutaneous introduction (Fig. 15-3).

Pigtail Catheters

Pigtail catheters[49] are those whose tips are twisted into a loop with an end hole and have multiple holes applied in the sides of the straight distal portion. This design is intended to deliver a concentrated bolus in a horizontal manner toward the right angled branches of the aorta. When used, the loop is placed slightly proximal to the desired level, with the tip pointing to the opposite side of the arterial puncture site. The *advantage* of this catheter is semiselective opacification of horizontal

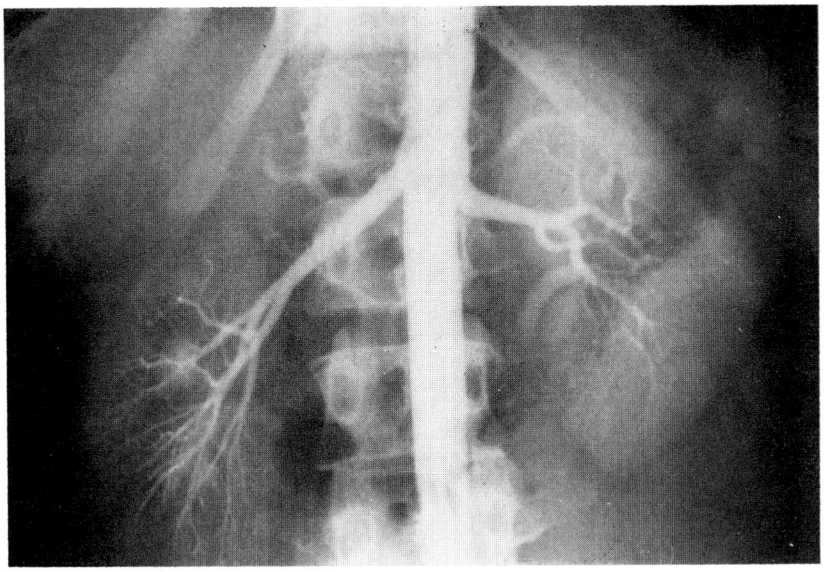

Figure 3.14. Abdominal Angiogram. The study was performed with a pigtail catheter. This opacifies the renal arteries and prevents filling of the other visceral branches. Thus, there is no interference with overlapping vessels.

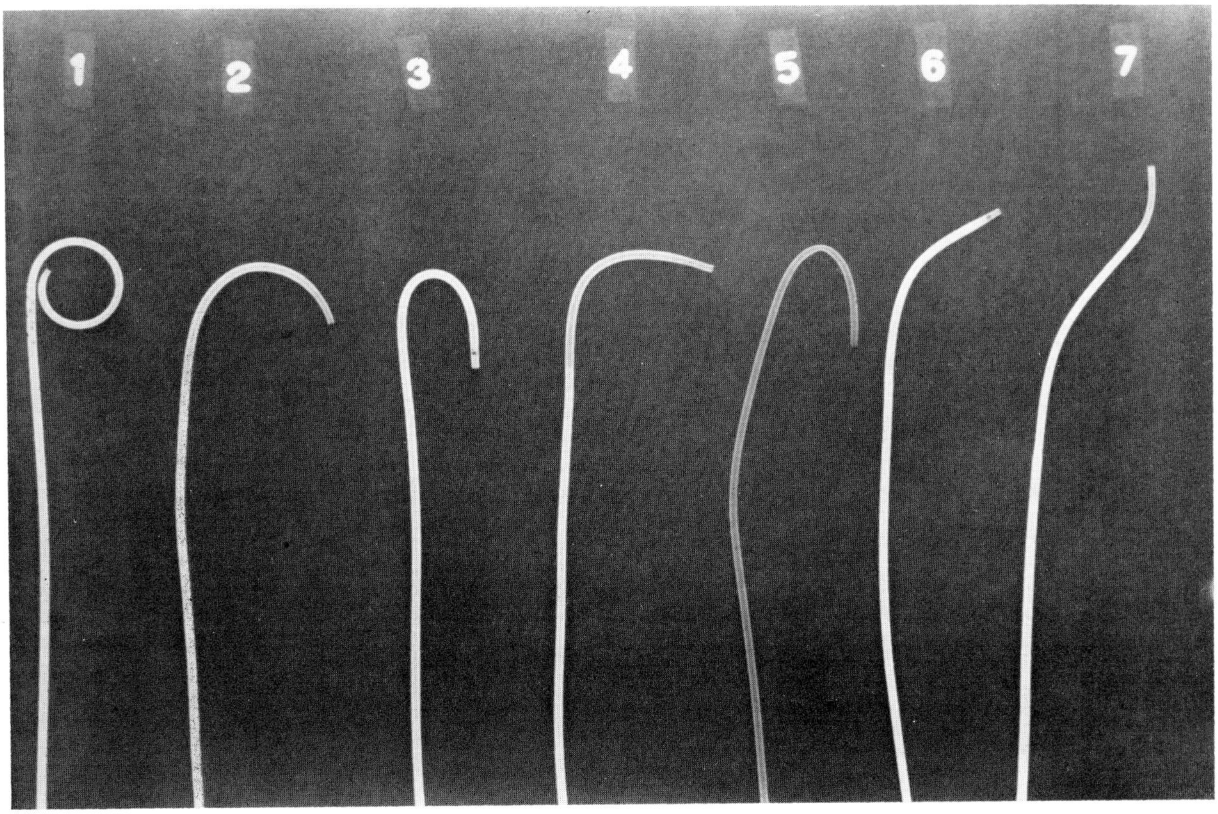

Figure 3.15. Basic Curves of the Catheter. 1. Pigtail, 2. Umbrella Handle, 3. "U" bend, 4. Horizontal, 5. Acute angle, 6. Obtuse, 7. Reverse.

branches and branches distal to the site of injection. There is negligible overlapping of other vessels. This avoids unnecessary perfusion of the branches proximal to the injection site. The injection rate and the total amount of contrast used is comparatively less (Fig. 3-14). The pigtail catheter is primarily used for opacification of both renal arteries simultaneously, for visualization of pelvic vessels and the abdominal aortic bifurcation, and for injections into the ascending aorta.

These catheters have *disadvantages* as well. Lesions proximal to the site of injection cannot be demonstrated; this also applies when there are aberrant origins to the renal arteries. Pigtail catheters tend to give poor performance in a dilated aorta. On occasion, arterial insertion may be difficult, particularly in obese individuals. This can be overcome by the routine use of a Teflon vessel dilator.[35] These catheters have an increased potential to form knots in narrow aortas. It is recommended that the catheter be removed only after being straightened with the guide wire. Sometimes the loop may uncoil with accidental perfusion of a small vessel with an excess amount of contrast. If the tip lodges in a lumbar or intercostal artery, neurologic deficits may occur.[50]

Curves

To seek an orifice of a branch which is at an angle in relationship to the long axis of a main vessel, the tip of the catheter should be turned in approximately the same direction. This is achieved by giving bends or curves to the distal most portion of the catheter. The length of the curved segment may vary. *However, if too long, intimal damage may occur, and if too short, the tip may be unable to reach the orifice of the vessel.* The type of curve created is based upon the anatomic mold of the main route (trunk), the existing natural exit (not a created one), and, of course, the route of entry (Fig. 3-15).

The curve for a particular artery will vary, depending on which major artery is used as the point of entrance. In other words, an "M" seen through the femoral approach can look like a "W" from the axillary route.

The selection of a *proper catheter curve* depends on (1) anatomical configuration and course of the vessel to be catheterized, (2) age and body build of the patient, (3) route of entry, and (4) any associated vascular abnormality. *The lack of identical anatomic course and origin of the vessels precludes a universal curve for the same vessel in different individuals and different vessels in the same patient.* Dependency on only one type of curve can result in suboptimal examinations, and of course, extreme frustration for the angiographer (Figs. 17-1, 17-2).

If the *curve* of the catheter *corresponds* to the anatomical course and angle of origin of the vessel, then the catheter easily moves with the flowing blood into the distal portion of the catheterized vessel (Fig. 3-16). On the contrary, if the catheter *curve does not correspond* with that of the vessel, then catheterization may be difficult, if not impossible (Figs. 3-17 and 3-18). In such situations, attempts to engage the tip into an orifice or further advancement of the catheter may damage the intima or dislodge an arteriosclerotic plaque. Even if it is engaged into the orifice, the initiation of injection will most often dislodge the unstable catheter tip.

The route of entry also influences the shape of the catheter, i.e. a curve meant for a cephalad celiac axis via the femoral route can also be used for a caudal superior mesenteric artery when approaching it via the axillary route. Therefore, the *catheter shape can be molded according to the anatomic arrangement of the vessels and the route of entry chosen.*

Gentle Curves Versus Acute Bends

The following descriptions are applicable when the route of entry is via the femoral artery. *A gentle curve with a smooth arc* closely resembles a semicircle. The diameter of this semicircle varies in relation to the width of the aorta at the point to be used or of the inferior vena cava. It is also used for further distal manipulation into a catheterized vessel. If the diameter of this curve is too small, the catheter will be unable to reach the orifice of a vessel. If the curve is too large, the catheter will

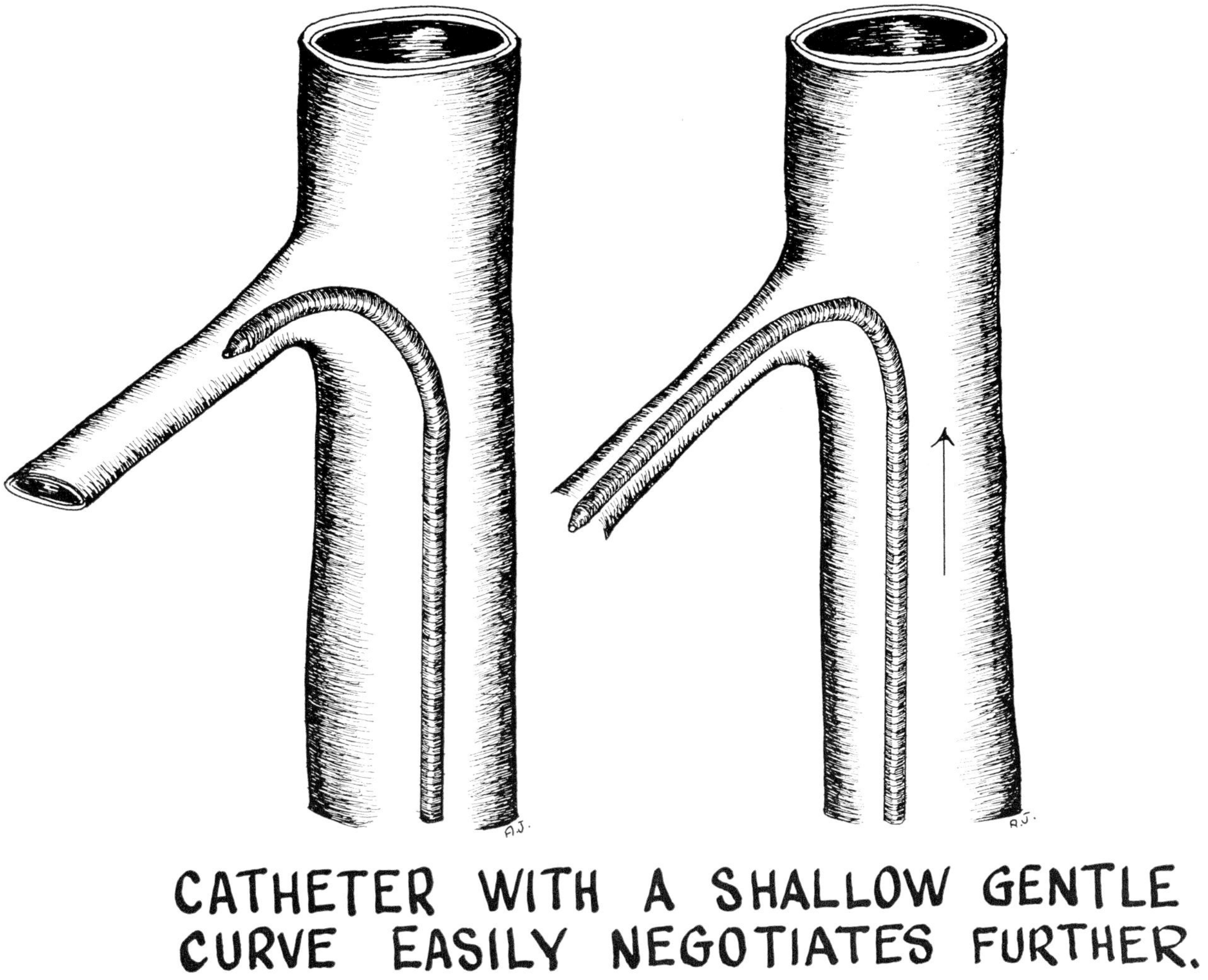

Figure 3.16

fold on itself or may dislodge arteriosclerotic plaques. When the anatomy is favorable to the use of this curved catheter, further manipulation into distal portions of a vessel is almost effortless. This results in good catheter stability; selective perfusion, which is very important during the perfusion of drugs; and an easy path for the superselective exchange of the guide wire. This type of catheter is *limited* when trying to engage the orifice of vessels oriented caudally or cranially from the main trunk. During ascent in the abdominal aorta, before reaching its final destination, this catheter has a tendency to peep into every orifice that it comes across. *Therefore, fluoroscopic monitoring during its use is mandatory* (Fig. 3-16).

Acute bends on the distal portion of a catheter reminds one of the letter "U." The width of the "U" and the length of the free limb depends on the width of the main vessel and the room available for catheter manipulation. The *advantage* to this catheter is that orifices which run in a caudal manner from the main trunk are very easy to catheterize. Furthermore, there is excellent stability of the catheter.

Its *limitations* are related to a greater tendency to fold and form knots if the "U" is too big. If too small, the orifice may not be engaged. It is very difficult to negotiate these catheters into the distal segment of the main vessel being catheterized (Fig. 3-20).

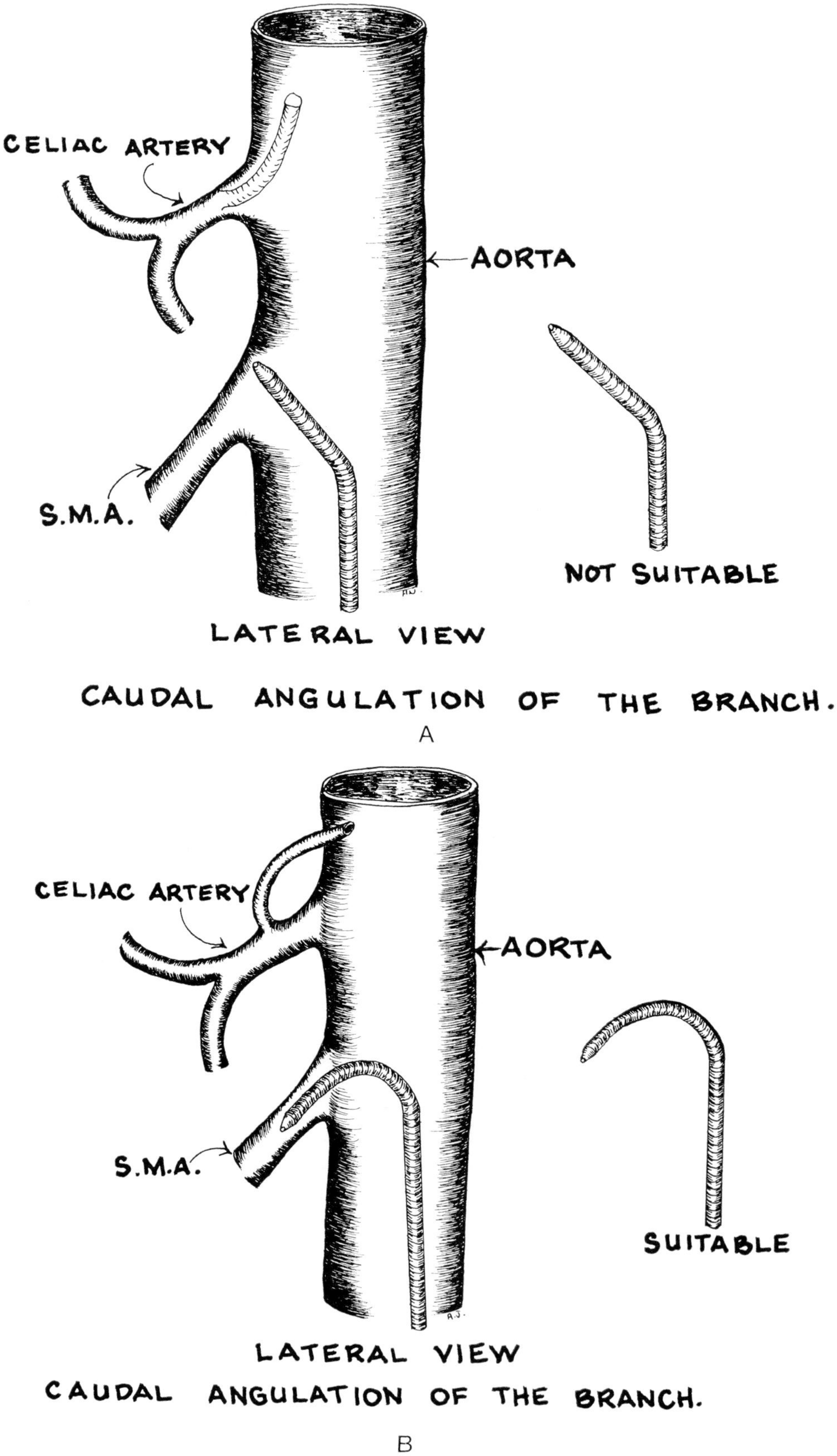

Figure 3.17. Catheter curve and arterial angulation.

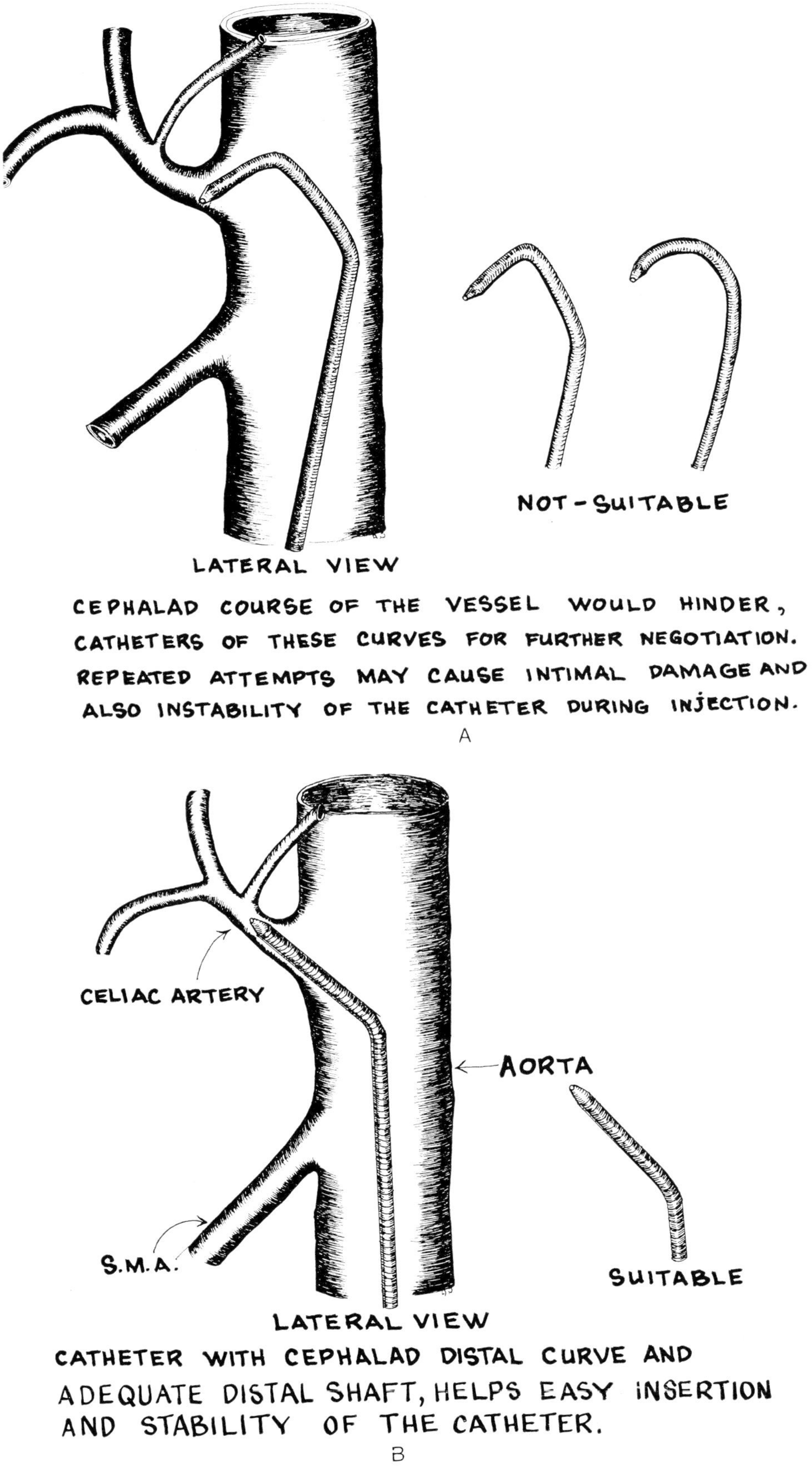

Figure 3.18. Catheter curve and arterial angulation.

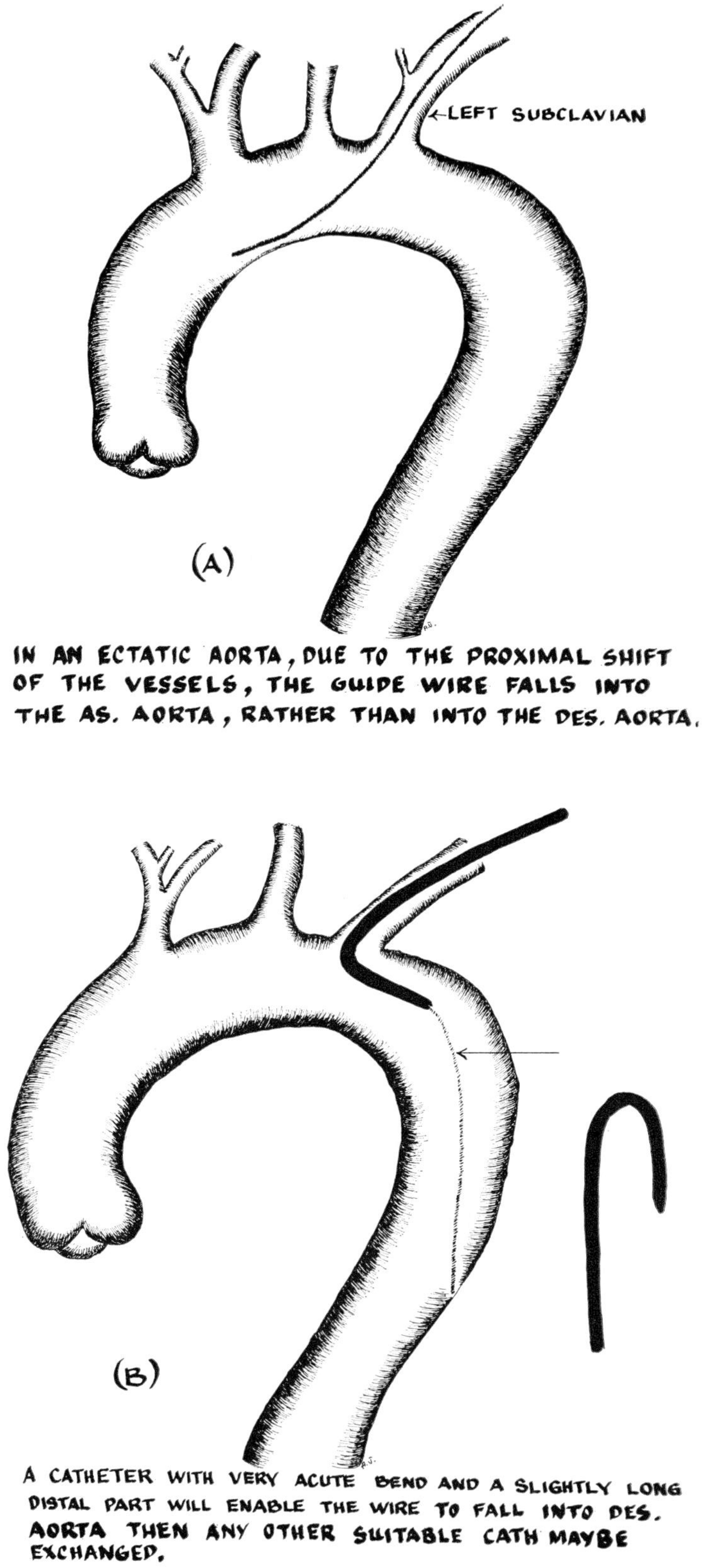

Figure 3.19. Catheterization of abdominal aorta via left axillary artery.

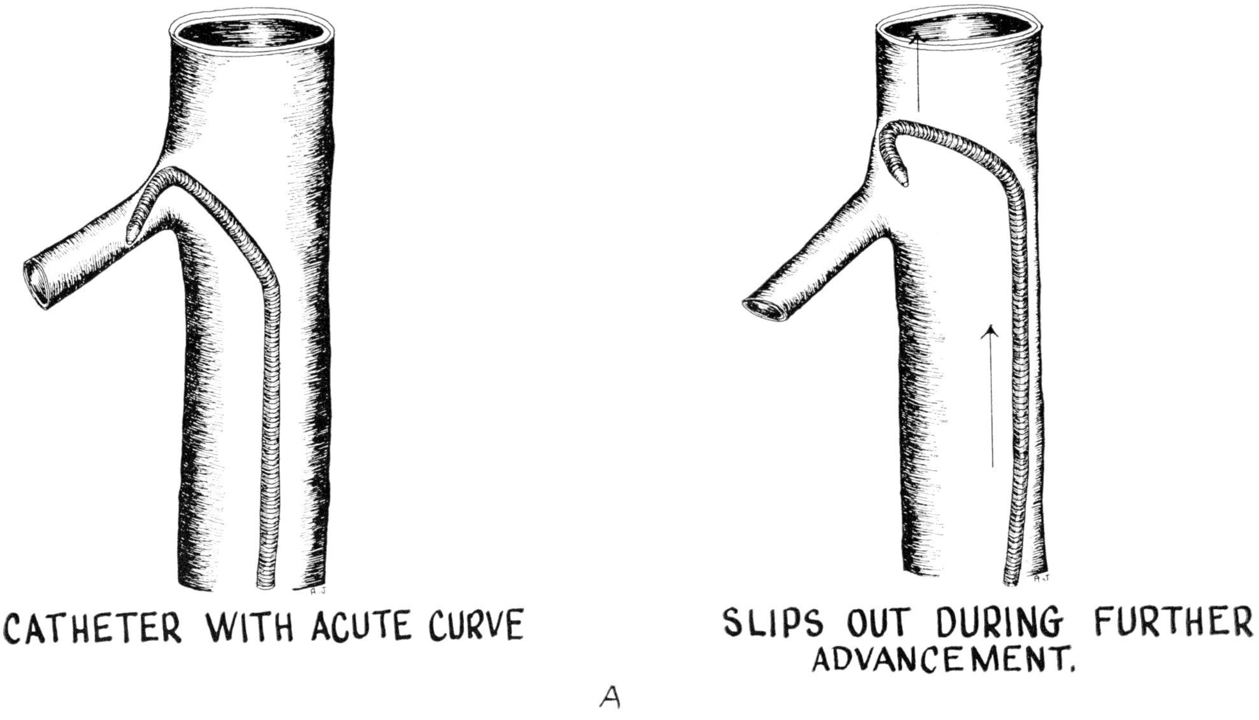

Catheters with Angled Bends

These catheters have the distal portion bent at an angle in relationship to the main shaft. This may be *acute* (less than 90°), *right angled* (90°) *or obtuse* (greater than 90° but less than 180°). The length of the distal segment beyond the bend is variable, depending on the width of the aorta. The degree of angulation has the same angulation as that of the vessels arising from the aorta (caudal, horizontal or cephalad). The acute angled catheters are *extremely good in seeking the orifices,* even in a tortuous aorta. An acute angled catheter is helpful in *changing the direction* of the guide wire (Fig. 3-19). However, because of the shoulder formed by the angulated bend it may be very *difficult, or even impossible,* to further advance the catheter distally into the catheterized vessel (Fig. 3-20). Its stability is unpredictable, occasionally recoiling during injection. The *right angled type* of catheter performs efficiently in vessels which have a horizontal orientation from the aorta. The *obtuse* angled catheters may vary anywhere from 120 to 160 degrees in

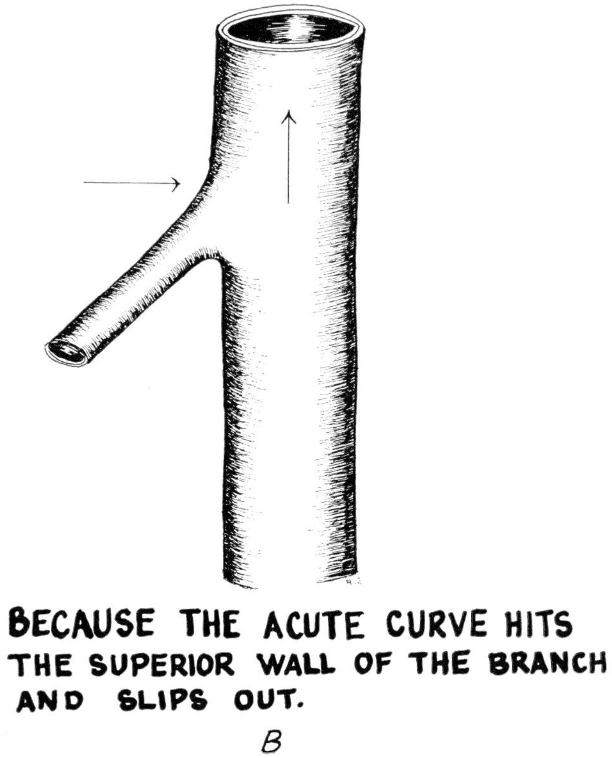

Figure 3.20

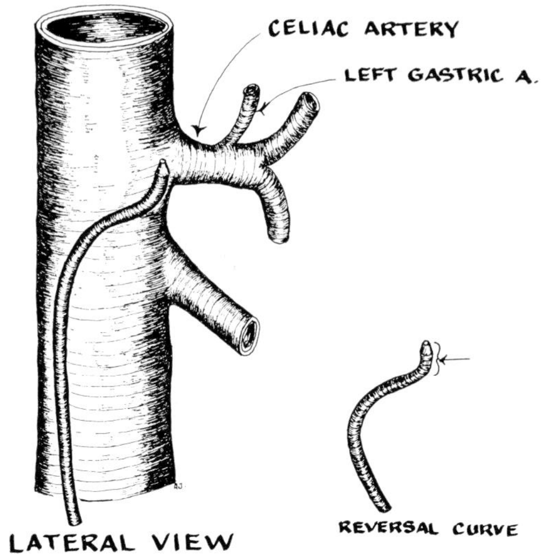

THE REVERSED PORTION OF THE SHAFT (ARROW) SLIDES ON THE ORIFICE, WITHOUT ENTERING THE ORIFICE. THE DIAMETER OF THE ORIFICE IS SMALLER THAN THE LENGTH OF THE REVERSED PART.

Figure 3.21

relationship to the main shaft. This position makes it easy to manipulate into cranially oriented branches and aortic arch vessels (Fig. 3-18).

Reversed Curve Catheters

Reversed curve catheters are those whose distal most tips are pointed in a cephalic direction in relationship to the proximal segment. This is an excellent shape *to catheterize cephalad directed branches from a primary branch* off the aorta or vena cava. (Examples: left gastric from the celiac; left adrenal from the left renal vein; left or middle hepatic arteries from the main hepatic.) Use of this catheter is *limited* by the fact that the tip is not an orifice seeking one in the lumen of the aorta or in the cava. Instead of falling into the orifice, it slides along the opening of the vessel except in unusual circumstances. If the main branch can be engaged by the tip, then catheterization of the right angle branch of that vessel is much easier (Figs. 3-21 and 3-22). There are numerous devices available to engage these type of curves into the parent vessel with subsequent facilitation of catheterization of smaller branches. Unfortunately, however, in the hands of beginners they do not perform as well *in vivo* as they do *in vitro*.[35, 37, 60–61] Eventually, however, when the angiographer gains experience and control of the catheter, he will invent his own ways of catheterizing small branches.

Selection of the Catheter

The tip of the catheter should be smooth and not frayed. The margins of the hole should also be smooth. The *tip* of the catheter should be *tapered* if needed, *fit the guide wire snugly*, and be *smaller than the branch vessel* to be catheterized. There should be no *kinks* in the catheter and it should be able to withstand the high pressure of injection. The catheter should have a wide internal diameter, reasonable torque control, and be at least 30 cm shorter than the selected guide wire. The curve should be appropriate; if not, it should be exchanged for one that is. *A curved catheter should not be used in a straight vessel; conversely, a straight catheter should never be used in a curved vessel.*

Only end hole catheters should be used to study the *aortic arch vessel* or *venous sampling* or for *superselective* angiography. *Only a side hole* catheter with no end holes should be used for injection into the *cardiac chamber*. End and multiple side hole catheters should be used to deliver large volumes of contrast.

The Care of the Catheter

It is preferable not to reuse a catheter, but soaring costs and increasing number of examinations demand reuse. Since polyethylene catheters are damaged if they are exposed to high temperatures, they must be either gas sterilized or cold sterilized. Teflon, mylar or dacron catheters may be autoclaved providing the temperature does not exceed 120 degrees Centigrade. Our technique for cold sterilization of catheters is:

1. After removing the catheter from the bloodstream, it is immediately flushed with cold water repeatedly.
2. The catheter is then soaked in hydrogen

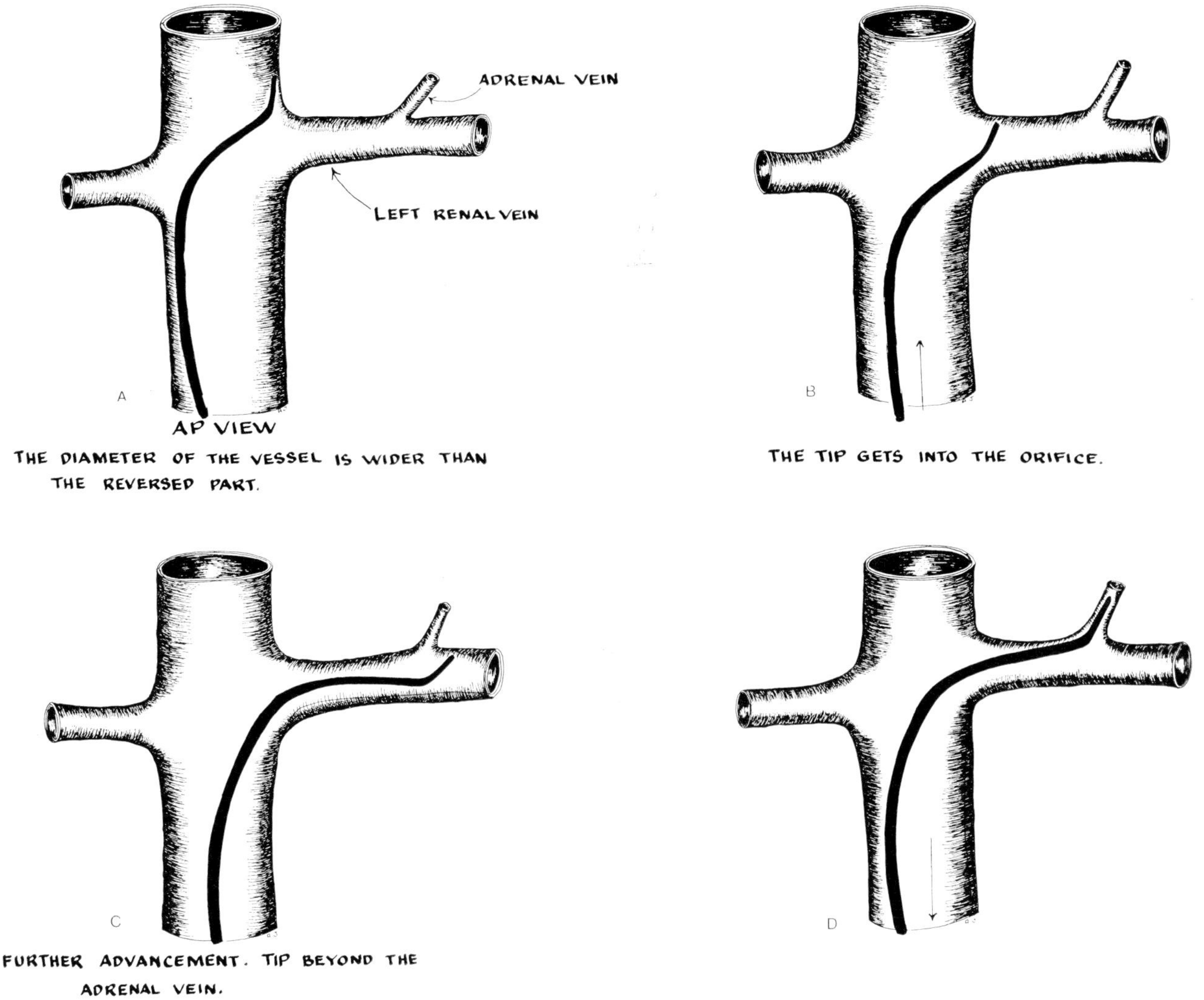

Figure 3.22. Uses of a reversed curve catheter.

peroxide solution for at least twelve hours.

3. It is again flushed frequently with cold water.
4. It is stored in cold sterilization solution for at least thirty minutes before each use.
5. Before being used, the catheter should be flushed with sterile cold water and the external surface wiped often with a sterile, wet sponge.

The cold sterilization solution may be obtained commercially[35] (Detergicide®), or can be prepared by the hospital pharmacy. The cold sterilization solution should be changed often and according to the manufacturer's or pharmacy's instructions. The same instructions apply to the use of vessel dilators.

After all, catheters are like batons: if gracefully handled with the waves of contrast and the vibrating vessels, one can record a unique vascular symphony.

THE INJECTOR

The mechanical features[54] of an acceptable injector should permit:

1. Instantaneous interruption of the injection to avoid accidental injection of a large bolus at high pressure.
2. The ability to make a test injection at the same delivery rate as the final injection.
3. Accurate and reproducible flow rates.

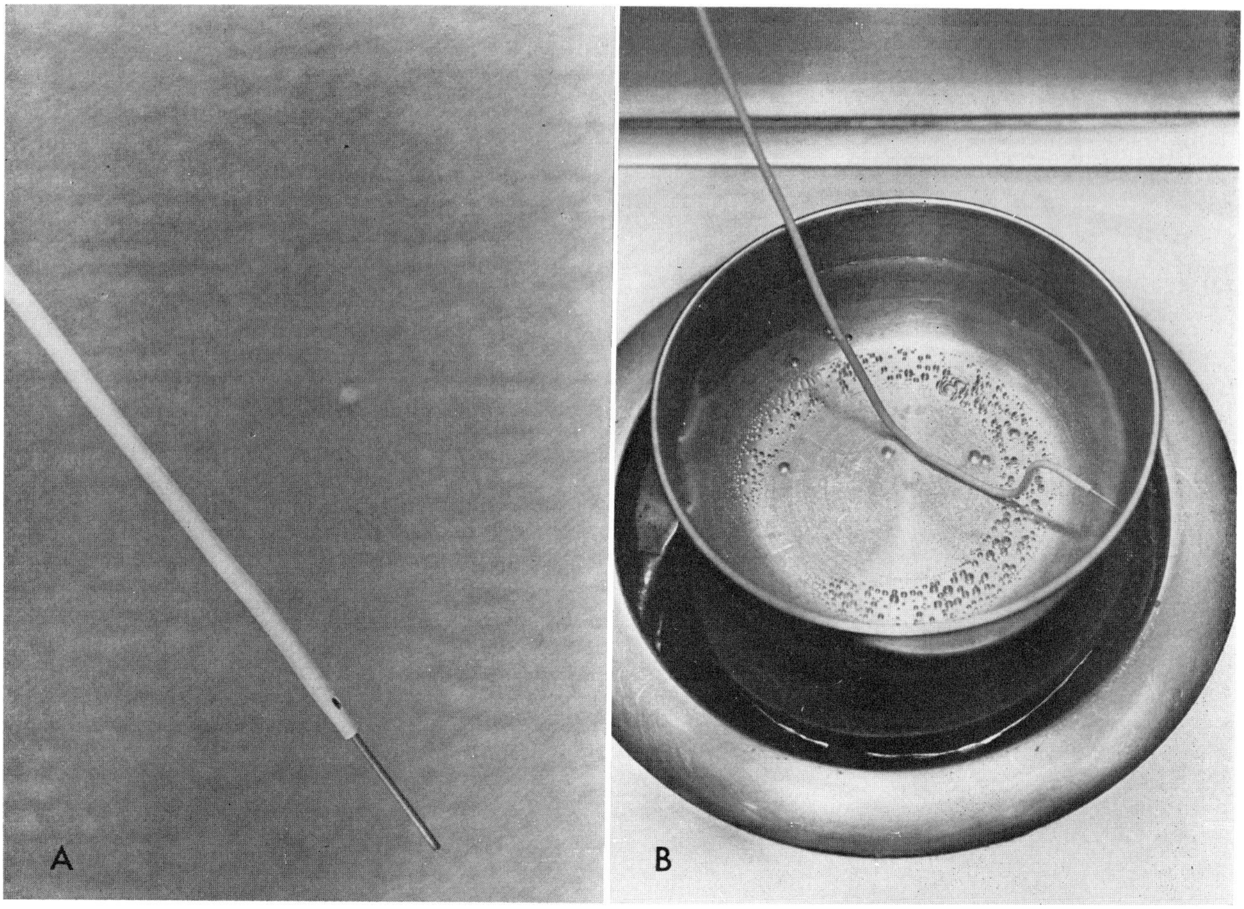

Figure 3.23. A straight catheter is bent into the desired curve with the help of the forming wire and immersed in boiling water for 2 minutes.

4. Avoidance of air embolism.
5. Prevention of electrical hazards which may cause ventricular fibrillations.

All injectors should have ground safety detectors; adequate grounding does not preclude the potential hazard of inducing electrical shock. Leakage may occur from various appliances in contact with the patient, and dangerous arrhythmias may occur. The inability to obtain a good EKG is a signal of poor grounding. *All equipment in contact with the patient should be at the same ground potential.*[54]

The principle of automatic flow rate control designed injectors[55] assures that with certain limitations, a desired flow rate will be delivered by the injector regardless of the catheter used. It should also insure that injection of force over 1000 psi—which can cause tissue damage by the injection jet, backlash of the catheter, or even rupture—cannot be exceeded. These built-in safety devices should assure that this pressure is not exceeded.[53] We have been using an automatic flow rate control injector[55] which operates on the principle of metered delivery rate, thus eliminating the use of time-consuming charts. The selection is easy; one dial controls the duration of injection, and a second, the delivery rate. Thus, within certain limits, a selected volume can be delivered in a selected time, irrespective of the design, length and diameter of the catheter or the viscosity of the contrast.[53]

There is still no substitute, however, for the individual angiographer's knowledge of the performance and limitations of his equipment in advance of its use in a patient.

FILM CHANGERS

We have used Schoënander cut film changers, Franklin roll film changers, and Elema roll film changers[56] in biplane configurations. The *advantage* of the *cut film* changer is its 14″ x 14″ exposure area. It is dependable and trouble free, with less jamming except in time of severe humidity change when the emulsion of the film expands. The primary *disadvantage* is the loss of sequential order when the films are mixed up. This has been avoided by marking each film with sequential numbers. Furthermore, in a teaching institution, films seem to disappear faster than the exposure rate. The *roll film* changers have the advantage of ease of handling and daylight loading. The individual films are in sequential order and there is less possibility of their disappearance. However, storage of these films is difficult unless individually cut, and the exposure area is smaller than on the cut film changer.

An *exposure rate* of more than four films per second is not necessary in general angiography. Most of the time the rapid sequence used will be two films per second. A total range of coverage of thirty seconds is useful.

Roentgen Techniques

To obtain films with good resolution, pleasing contrast, and visible detail, the shortest exposure time possible, highest M.A., and optimal K.V. should be used. The patient must be lying motionless with respiration suspended.

Magnification

Using a focal spot of 0.3 mm with the patient lying midway between the focal spot and the X-ray film, a 2× linear magnification may be obtained. This gives a fourfold increase in surface area.[57, 58] Using this technique, vessels up to 90 microns may be seen.[57]

Local Anesthetic

We have been using Lidocaine® 1% for local infiltration at the puncture site. One should always aspirate prior to injection to assure that direct intraluminal injection is not made. The angiographer should be aware of the *adverse effects*[59] of this local anesthetic which includes rare hypersensitivity and anaphylactic reaction, convulsions, or hypotensive cardiovascular collapse and even death.

CHAPTER 4
THE CONTRAST

An ideal contrast should have the least pharmacological activity and negligible histological and systemic toxicity. It should be physiologically acceptable without hemodynamic changes, completely excreted without any damage to the excretory organ. And, of course, it should give better opacification of the small vessels. Asking for too much? . . . not at all!! Sometimes we wish that physiological saline were radiopaque. An increase in the opacification of the small vessels can be achieved only by an increase in the concentration of iodine injected, rather than an increase in the injection rate.[62]

We have been using Reno-M-60® (meglumine diatrizoate—Squibb) for peripheral, cerebral, pulmonary and aortic arch studies; Renografin 60 (meglumine and sodium diatrizoate—Squibb) and Renografin 76 (meglumine and sodium diatrizoate—Squibb) for abdominal angiography. Meglumine has a protective action on coronary and cerebral vessels; it is used, therefore, in individuals with heart disease to avoid sodium overload. There is, however, an increased tendency of bronchospasm with the use of these salts. Subsequently, in asthmatic patients, one should use the sodium salts.[63]

ELIMINATION OF THE CONTRAST

Presently available contrast media are triiodobenzoic acid derivatives. They have a molecular composition precluding significant protein binding, and a molecular size allowing them to be freely filtered across the glomerular membrane. *They are excreted primarily by glomerular filtration.* If the glomerular filtration is decreased because of decreased blood flow or glomerular dysfunction, elimination of the contrast medium from the blood is impaired. Dehydration and salt depletion do not affect the elimination of contrast media from the blood, but they may reduce the glomerular filtration rate.

As tubular excretion and reabsorption of contrast are negligible, osmotically active, nonresorbed contrast produces salt and water diuresis, which is less marked in a dehydrated patient. Higher concentrations of contrast do occur regionally in underperfused kidneys. This may predispose to nephrotoxicity. The osmotic concentration will reach an end point, beyond which there is no further rise, but rather a fall in final urine concentration in spite of the high dose of contrast.[64]

Elimination

Normal half-time:	20 minutes
Patients with bilateral nephrectomy: half-time	30 hours
Normal biliary excretion:	1%
Patients with bilateral nephrectomy:	25%

There is also an enterohepatic circulation for the injected contrast. Diarrhea and dialysis in anuric patients can eliminate contrast quickly. At least 50 percent of the given dose can be removed by dialysis.[65] Renal excretory mechanisms and hepatic detoxification of contrast are

TABLE 4-I
PHYSICAL CHARACTERISTICS

Contrast	*Iodine content mgms/cc*	*Sodium content meq/cc*	*Viscosity Cps*	*Milli osmolarity/L*
Reno-M-60	282 mgms/cc	0.04 meq/cc	4.61 Cps at 25° C	1500 mosm
Renografin 60	288 mgms/cc	0.16 meq/cc	4.41 Cps at 25° C	1510 mosm
Renografin 76	370 mgms/cc	0.19 meq/cc	9.74 Cps at 25° C	1689 mosm

reduced in infants. There is a difference in the LD 50 between infants and adults.[66] Even with patients in *hepatic or renal failure,* there are no significant changes noted except for minimal changes in acid base balance and prolonged increase in the serum levels of contrast. Usually, there is no alteration in the clinical course.[67–70]

CONTRAST AND ANAPHYLAXIS

Acute anaphylactic reactions due to contrasts are unpredictable on the basis of history or pretesting techniques. There is a higher incidence of reaction in patients with histories of allergies. Asthmatics have a higher incidence of bronchospasm with methylglucamine salts than with the sodium salts. At pharmacologically active concentrations, methylglucamine salts are potent histamine liberators. Some of the anaphylactic reactions of contrast resemble the actions of histamine on tissues, such as its effect on smooth muscles (laryngospasm) and increased capillary permeability (angioneurotic edema). Allergic patients have a higher release of histamine as do patients who receive larger doses.

Subcutaneous or intradermal injections are useless predictors since different organs in the body have different amounts of releasable histamine. A conjunctival test is worthless, as mucosa does not liberate histamine. A 1 cc intravenous injection of contrast is below the threshold in many individuals for histamine release and bears no relationship to the amount of histamine released during a full dose. Furthermore, idiosyncratic patients may release massive amounts of histamine with only 1 cc of intravenously administered contrast and develop serious reactions to the test dose itself. In some cases there is even a potentiating effect for subsequent sequential repeated injections.[63, 181, 183–186]

CONTRAST AND THE BLOOD

The rapid infusion of a large bolus of hyperosmolar solutions of contrast (1500 mosm to 1700 mosm) causes *a sudden change in the internal environment* due to its *hypertonicity.* The increase in the milliosmolarity of the injected solution increases these adverse changes. *Red blood cells* begin to *crenate* at about 340 mosm; at 450 to 650 mosm arrest of spontaneous contraction of lymphatics and venules oc-

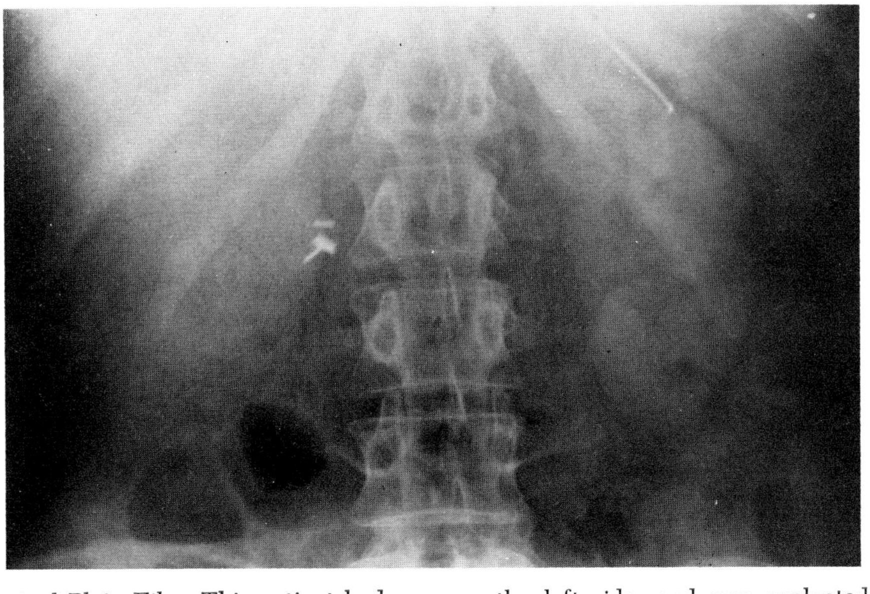

Figure 4.1. Abdominal Plain Film. This patient had an arteriogram 36 hours before. Notice the size of the right kidney and also dense opacifications of the renal parenchyma bilaterally. The patient had renal arterial embolus on the right side, severe renal artery stenosis on the left side, and was evaluated angiographically with a total of 50 cc of contrast material into the aorta. There was recirculation of the contrast material in the body. The patient's condition improved after dialysis.

curs. *Agglutination* of red blood cells, *rouleaux* formation, and *sludging* of red blood cells are the result of this injected hypertonic solution. This sets up a vicious cycle in which the red cells are trapped in vessels of 200 microns and less. This decreases tissue perfusion and further increases crenation and aggregation of red cells and platelets. In turn, this causes further damage to the endothelium which manifests itself in increased endothelial permeability thereby causing increased extravascular diffusion of contrast. *Capillary thrombosis and microembolism* climaxes the end of the cycle.[143–152]

A *large bolus* of contrast which has to travel first through systemic and then the pulmonary circulation, or the other way around, increases blood volume by shifting water from the intracellular and extravascular compartments. This sets up an adverse chain reaction; *increased cardiac load, increased end diastolic pressures in the cardiac chambers, increased pulmonary capillary venous pressure.* Finally, the excess fluid enters into the alveoli which results in frank *pulmonary edema.* Patients with *valvular heart disease and* other cardiac abnormalities are particularly *vulnerable* to this cycle. Solutions with an osmotic activity higher than 1500 mosm/L may produce *pulmonary hypertension, acute cor pulmonale,* and even *death.*[153]

The magnitude of the above changes depends on the volume of contrast injected, its concentration, rate of injection and injection site. *Therefore, larger volumes, higher concentrations, faster injection rates, and the injection closer to the heart all cause adverse hemodynamic changes.* These changes may be well compensated for in a physiologically well individual who is well hydrated and has good cardiac reserve. These changes appear to be greater with contrasts having sodium rather

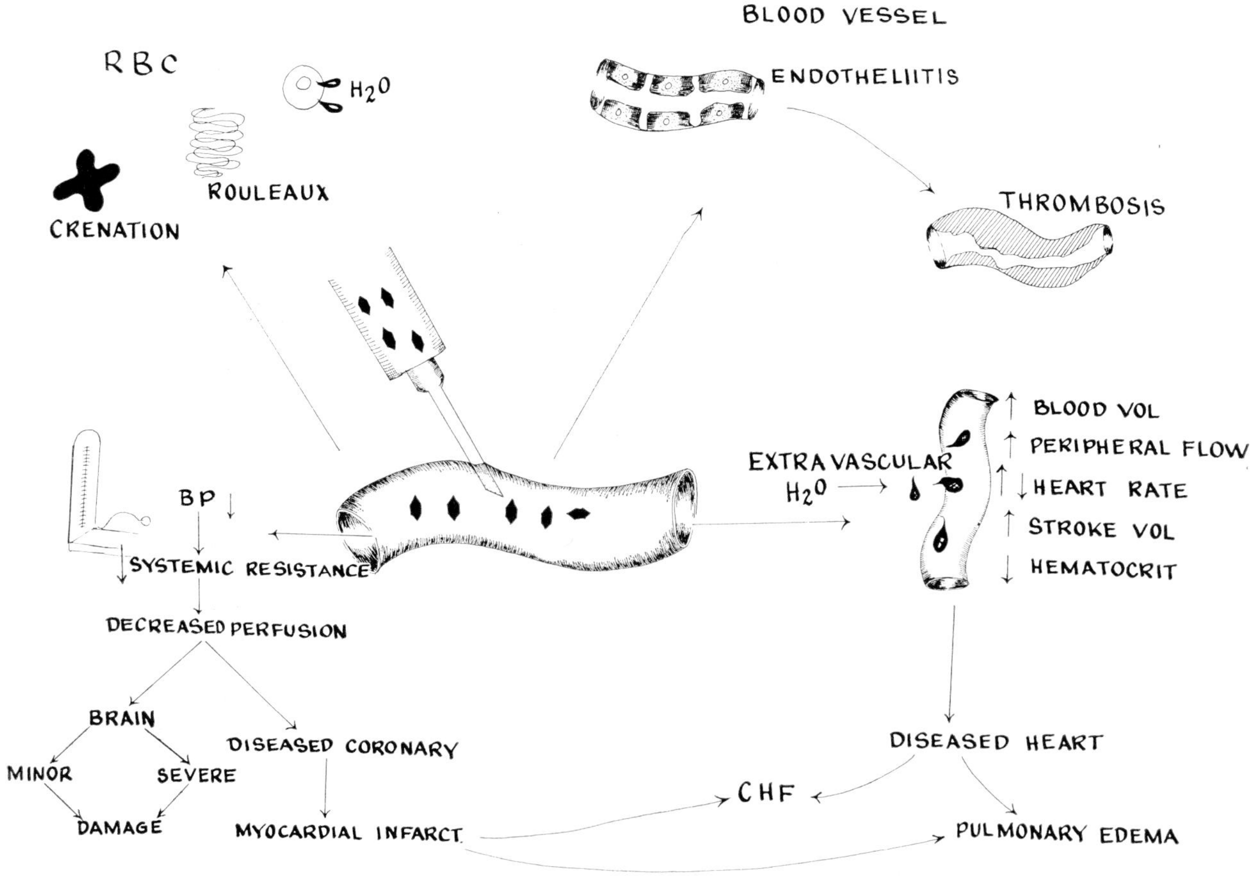

Figure 4.2. Hemodynamic alterations due to the contrast material.

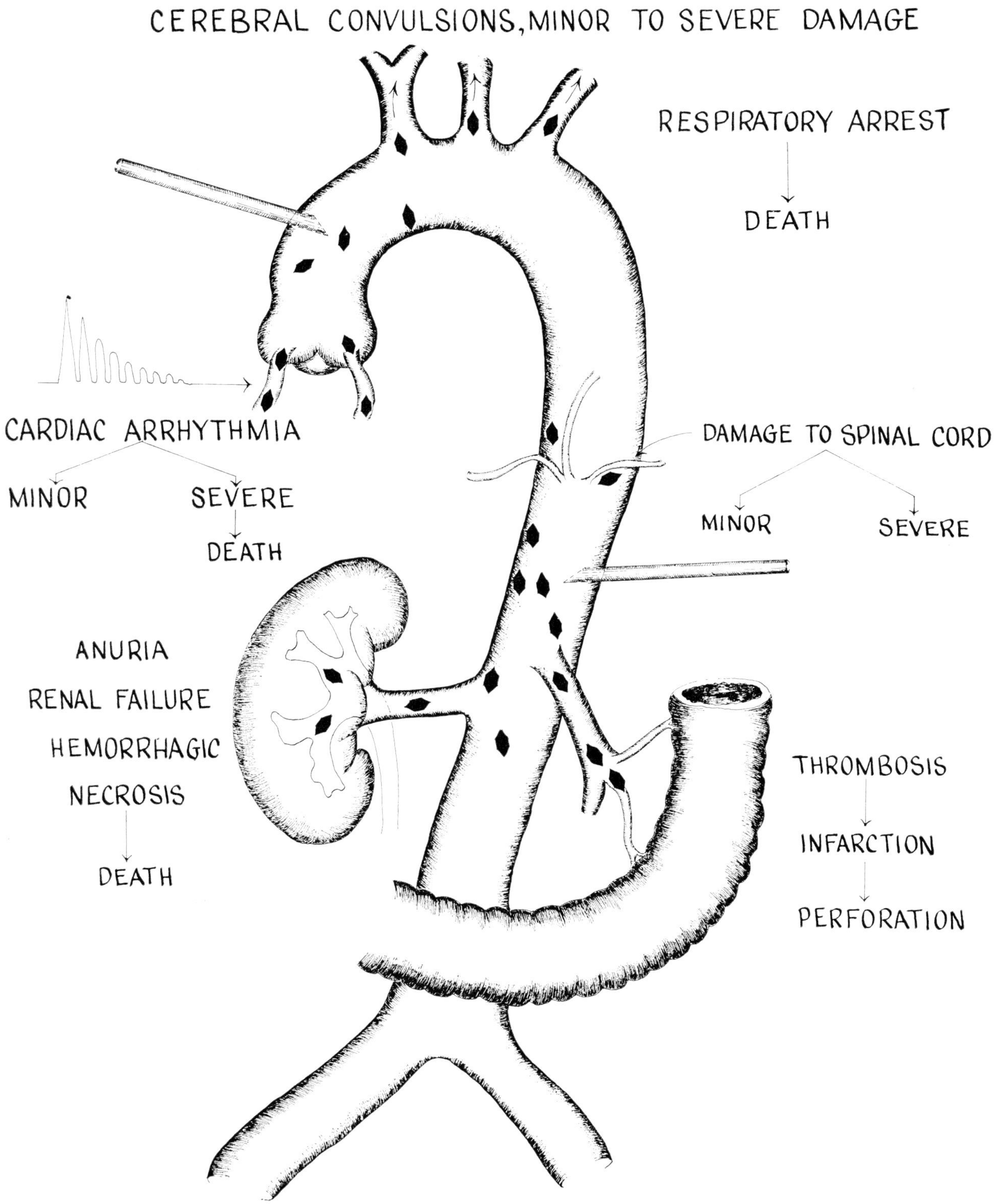

Figure 4.3. Complications due to the contrast material.

than methyl glucamine salts. The intensity of these reactions diminishes as one injects contrast further from the heart. The response then is only a local increase in blood flow because of decrease in local vascular resistance.[154–157]

CONTRAST MATERIAL AND REGIONAL HEMODYNAMICS

Renal Artery

Selective intraarterial injection of contrast elicits a *biphasic response* unique to the renal vasculature. Initially, there is transient *vasodilatation* followed by a long period of *vasoconstriction.* This type of biphasic response may be due to the *activation of renin.* In a hypertensive patient, renal arteriography may influence renal blood flow studies and renal vein renin determinations.[20]

Superior Mesenteric Artery

A *triphasic response* of the systemic blood pressure occurs, with an *initial rise* followed by a *decrease* in the mean blood pressure, followed by a *decrease* in the diastolic blood pressure. There is uniform increase in cardiac output and stroke volume. *Vasodilatation* increases superior mesenteric vascular blood flow, reaching a peak in ten to twenty-four seconds following injection. It is 10 to 60 percent above base line at five minutes and returns to normal within fifteen minutes.[162]

Cerebral

Only the external carotid vessels show evidence of dilatation. There is *no dilatation* of the *internal carotid* circulation.[154]

Brachial Artery

There is local vasodilatation.[163]

Femoral Artery

There is local vasodilatation.[164]

Coronary Arteries

There is an increase in the blood flow.[164]

Aorta

Ascending aortic injections reveal *greater change in systemic arterial blood pressure* than do abdominal aortic injections. This is the result of perfusion of the coronary arteries. The hypertensive patient is more susceptible to such and demonstrates a consistent and significant fall in blood pressure.[165–168]

CONTRAST INTERACTIONS

In a broad sense, the pharmacological effects of contrast media may reside chiefly in the projected role of protein and contrast combination. Protein binding may exert a buffer action on the toxic contrast; it also alters the critical protein structure and interferes with delicate enzyme-controlled metabolic pathways. The inhibition of acetylcholinesterase causes decreased resistance in the region where the contrast is injected.[158–160]

Contrast materials do not interfere with the electrophoretic pattern of sera, plasma or whole blood. This does not happen even in individuals with multiple myeloma, macroglobulinemia, liver disease or jaundice. The mobility may, however, be changed in patients with myeloma and macroglobulinemia.[169, 170]

Renal

No significant changes were seen during ordinary situations except for a slight increase in urinary excretion of enzyme.[171, 172] There were no appreciable changes in patients with hepatic or renal failure in relation to changes in acid base balance or prolonged levels of contrast in the serum.[67–70] As contrast is an osmotic diuretic, increased diuresis is not uncommon.[174] Transient proteinuria may occur after intravenous or intraarterial infusion of contrast.[173]

Superior Mesenteric Artery

There is slight elevation of the SGOT and alkaline phosphatase probably due to some hepatic perfusion. When given in usual doses, contrast causes only nonspecific histological changes of varying degrees.[175–177] Renografin® seems to be the better contrast available for visualizing bowel vasculature.[178]

Hepatic Artery

Renografin injected into the hepatic arteries or perfusing the portal venous circulation does not produce significant change in liver profile tests.[179, 180] Multiple *wedge hepatic injections* into the hepatic vein cause only transient increases in serum transaminase.[179] If extravasation occurs during wedge injections, resulting in perivenous hemorrhage, then fibrosis limited to the injected area occurs.[303]

CHAPTER 5

INDICATIONS AND CONTRADICTIONS

THE COMBINATION of an aggressive angiographer and a well-informed clinician increases the number of procedures performed. Potentially, such a combination may abuse the procedure when other, simpler methods can produce the same information. However, the inverse combination may actually be depriving the needy of the needed. The proper selection of patient, meticulous technique and a positive diagnostic yield convinces the clinician, rewards the angiographer, and expedites the application of further appropriate treatment to the ailing.

Indications:

1. To confirm or exclude the clinical suspicions.
2. To aid a surgical procedure.
3. To locate the clinically diagnosed lesion.
4. As a last resort.

TO CONFIRM OR EXCLUDE CLINICAL SUSPICIONS

As different diseases may have similar manifestations, angiography is indicated if other, more simple diagnostic studies are nonproductive.

A. Vascular diseases.

1. Hypertension: diseases of the renal vessels or aorta *as opposed* to essential hypertension.
2. Postprandial abdominal pain: abdominal angina due to vascular occlusion or angiitis *versus* other causes of abdominal pain.
3. Edema and albuminuria: thrombosis of the renal veins or inferior vena cava *as opposed* to other etiologies.
4. Sudden or gradual onset of ascites with or without lower extremity edema: Hepatic, portal or inferior vena caval occlusions.
5. Central nervous system: lesions of the great vessels of the aortic arch *as opposed* to intracranial lesions.
6. Vascular diseases: arteriovenous malformations, aneurysms, dissecting aneurysms, traumatic penetrating lesions in the vicinity of vessels, angiitis. Thoracic outlet syndromes *as opposed* to Raynaud's phenomena, etc.
7. Masses adjacent to the great vessels: aneurysms *as opposed* to extravascular mass lesions.

B. Evaluating mass lesions.

1. Renal masses: asymptomatic renal masses found on routine intravenous pyelograms, benign *versus* malignant.
2. To confirm the presence of a mass or masses: lymph nodes above the right renal pedicle (the inferior venacavogram) or in the mediastinum (azygous venogram).
3. Unexplained splenomegaly: space occupying lesions *versus* other causes.
4. Unexplained hepatomegaly: especially with defects on isotope scans.
5. Painless jaundice: obstruction by carcinoma or other mass *versus* other nonobstructive causes of jaundice.
6. Hypoglycemia: pancreatic endocrinal tumors, connective tissue tumors *versus* other causes (functional). Islet cell hyperplasia as a cause of hypoglycemia cannot be excluded angiographically.
7. Ulcerogenic tumors: endocrinal (pancreatic) tumors *versus* other causes.
8. Backache, loss of weight: pancreatic carcinoma or other retroperitoneal tumors *versus* other causes.
9. Placental malpositions: presence or absence of placenta previa. It is question-

able as to whether or not a procedure for this purpose is ever indicated.

TO AID IN SURGICAL PROCEDURES

In the *evaluation of masses*, angiography may reveal the nature of a mass, its anatomical extent (operable or inoperable), the feeding and draining vessels, the amount of vascularity, the variations in the vascular arrangement, the parasitic blood supply, the presence of metastasis, the site for biopsy of soft tissue tumors, and the status of the contralateral organs in paired organs such as the kidney, or carotid body tumors[23] occurring bilaterally in the neck.

Knowing the *arrangement of the vessels* is important during such surgical procedures as hepatectomy or renal transplants. The extent of vascular abnormalities in *aneurysms* or *dissecting hematomas* should be determined. A relatively avascular surgical zone may be created by infusing vasopressin into the superior mesenteric artery during *portocaval shunt operations*.[24]

Angiography is used to evaluate the extent of *vascular* and *parenchymal injuries* resulting from blunt or penetrating trauma. In *acute gastrointestinal hemorrhage*, angiography is used to locate the bleeding point and hopefully determine its cause, to exclude other sites of bleeding in a patient with known cause of bleeding, or to locate postsurgical bleeding. The *patency of vessels* can be determined prior to shunt procedures such as portal to systemic venous circulation. The patency of the portal, superior mesenteric, and splenic veins may be determined in addition to selecting eligible candidates for the procedure.

The status of the *vena caval system* before plication procedures or before ligation procedures (is the hepatic portion of the inferior vena cava absent?[21]) may be visualized. Angiography may also be used to evaluate postplication results for repeated thromboembolic disease.

TO LOCATE THE CLINICALLY ESTABLISHED LESION

When the presence of a lesion is strongly suspected by clinical and laboratory methods, then the primary responsibility of angiography is to locate the lesion and its numbers by using the most informative and least morbid procedure. This is especially valuable in evaluating *endocrinal disorders*.

Venous Samplings

Although arteriography cannot localize microscopic tumors, venous samplings can.[25] This same possibility applies to localized hyperplasias of endocrinal organs. In addition to the evaluation of endocrinally active adrenocortical lesions, venous sampling may be helpful in the assessment of hypertension caused by adrenal medullary hyperplasias.[22] Venous sampling is also very helpful in evaluating infarcted,[26] avascular,[27, 28] or extraadrenal[31] pheochromocytomas. Renal vein sampling is used to determine renin levels.[29, 30] Thoracic venous samplings are obtained for establishing thyrocalcitonin levels in lung tumors.[25] Parathyroid venous sampling is used to evaluate parathyroid lesions.[15, 16] Ovarian venous samplings may have certain potential in evaluating ovarian endocrinal tumors.

Arterial Evaluation in Endocrinal Lesions

This procedure is particularly useful in evaluating *pheochromocytomas*. Malignant endocrinal or nonendocrinal lesions of the *adrenal* may be evaluated to determine the extent of involvement of adjacent structures. *Parathyroid* angiography may localize a small lesion. *Pancreatic* endocrinal tumors as a cause for hypoglycemia may be found, although hyperplasias may not be demonstrated at all. Ulcerogenic disorders (Zollinger-Ellison Syndrome) may be evaluated to establish the biological behavior of these tumors (malignant versus benign) depending on the presence of liver metastasis. Renal *renin secreting tumors*[32] may be evaluated. Angiitis and telangiectasia may be diagnosed by angiography, and certainly the involvement of the visceral arteries can be determined.

Venous Studies

Venography demonstrates the morphological abnormalities related to deviation, distortion or stretching of the intrinsic venous system of an organ. The functional significance of any of these morphologic abnormalities may be confirmed by venous assay. In our series we encountered several *nonendocrinal lesions* causing hormonal abnormalities. Hypercalcemia was noted in two cases of hypernephroma and one case of benign mesenchymoma. Increased corticosteroids were found in one carcinoid tumor of the lung and one oatcell carcinoma of the lung. Hypoglycemia was seen with one retroperitoneal fibrosarcoma.

AS THE LAST RESORT

When all the other diagnostic facilities have failed to demonstrate a lesion, then, in some instances, angiography may be undertaken as a *last diagnostic technique*. Chronic gastrointestinal bleeding can be evaluated by angiography to search for the following obscure lesions: vascular ectasias, Meckel's diverticulum, aneurysms of the splanchnic vessels, arteriovenous malformations, hemangiomas, hemobilia, leiomyoma, or portal vein thrombosis. Small malignancies of the kidney may be established as the cause of painless hematuria. And finally, obscure abdominal complaints, possibly related to abdominal angina, malrotation with volvulus, or internal hernias of the bowel may be evaluated by angiography.

CONTRAINDICATIONS

A previous *allergic* response to contrast may be a relative contraindication, but any previous occurrence of recognizable anaphylactic reaction is an absolute contraindication. *Pregnancy*, especially in the first trimester, is an absolute contraindication; but after the second trimester the life-saving benefit from the study should be weighed against the unpredictable effects of radiation on the fetus. And finally, if the diagnosis has already been established by other methods, then angiography is obviously contraindicated.

CHAPTER 6

ZONAL SOMATIC RESPONSE

CONTRAST MEDIA, due to its hypertonicity, vasodilatory effect or transient ischemic effects (because of replacement of the blood), may elicit transient zonal responses. These may be reflected *somatically* as intense heat, pain or even *reflex* reactions. The stasis of contrast due to sluggish circulation or occluded vessels increases the duration and intensity of these responses. Although they produce discomfort or even interference during roentgen exposures, these responses can be *diagnostic clues* during either catheter placement or catheter recoiling, add *pathologic significance* to an anatomic lesion, or act as a *provocative test.*

CATHETER PLACEMENT

Knowing the somatic response of a patient to test injections of contrast can aid in catheter placement. Injections into the *intercostal* and *lumbar* artery create the sensation of intense burning or pain localized to that dermal segment. A cough reflex may be elicited when the *bronchial artery* is catheterized. Injection into the *inferior phrenic artery* causes pain and burning in the anterior lower intercostal, mammary, ipsilateral shoulder, and suprarenal areas. Inferior and middle *adrenal artery* injections produce intense heat and burning localized to suprarenal area. If the pain persists, extravasation of contrast may have occurred. The response to *internal iliac artery* injection includes pain in the gluteal area and occasionally a sense of defecation.

Peripheral artery injection results in severe burning and pain in the region perfused by those vessels. The intensity increases if there is stasis of contrast flow. *Visceral artery injection* (celiac, superior mesenteric, inferior mesenteric arteries) gives warmth in the abdomen and occasionally epigastric discomfort. The sensation of warmth may be due to vasodilatation and/or increased blood flow. Occasionally the discomfort may be due to the stretching of the celiac plexus. If the inferior phrenic arteries arise from the celiac axis, then that zonal somatic discomfort is also felt.

Renal artery injection causes warmth in the flank posteriorly. If there is a reflux of contrast into the aorta, then segmental discomfort may occur due to perfusion of lumbar arteries. If the inferior adrenal artery is also perfused, then there may be additional discomfort in that region. Occasionally, if the inferior phrenic or gonadal arteries arise from the renal artery, then the reference of pain or discomfort is to those specific areas. Awareness of the variation in the normal anatomic arrangement of blood vessels will spare the angiographer from unnecessary tension or suspense during the procedure.

When great vessels, such as the aortic arch or abdominal aorta, are injected, all the areas that are perfused have the sensation of heat and/or discomfort.

Venous injection into any peripheral vein will induce nausea, vomiting and a feeling of generalized warmth. When the retroperitoneal veins, such as the adrenal, are catheterized, the heat may persist for a long time. If excruciating pain develops when the adrenal vein is injected then perivenous extravasation has occurred. When the peripheral veins are injected, there is intense burning and pain if stasis occurs. As can be expected, anxious and nervous individuals tend to exaggerate the intensity of these responses.

CATHETER RECOIL

If an unstable selective catheter recoils during an injection, this can be detected by questioning the patient regarding the localization of the discomfort. Thus the angiographer may quickly determine whether the study was successful or not. For example, if a catheter recoils out of the celiac axis, the patient will complain of discomfort in the lumbar areas and lower extremities.

PATHOLOGIC SIGNIFICANCE OF AN ANATOMIC LESION

Faithful reproduction of the clinical symptoms by contrast perfusion of the major feeding artery of a circulatory unit may aid in evaluating the pathological importance of the demonstrated anatomic lesion (Fig. 25-17). Reproducing the tearing pain of dissecting hematoma of the aorta during accidental injection into the false lumen further correlates the clinical and radiographic presentation of this lesion.

PROVOCATIVE

The sudden transient rise in the blood pressure of patients with *pheochromocytoma,* especially when the feeding arteries are perfused with contrast, may aid not only in detecting the location of the lesion, but also in the number and their sites.[18] Injected contrast or just the placement of the catheter tip into the thymic vein may trigger a myasthenic crisis in patients with *myasthenia gravis.*[19] In these cases appropriate medication should be available to counteract the effects of the angiography. The release of *angiotensin* during renal arterial injection of contrast[20] advises the angiographer to study the renal arteries and also to collect blood from the renal veins for renin assay on two separate occasions.

CHAPTER 7
DRUGS AND THE VESSEL

THE CHOICE of pharmacologic agent for enhancing visualization in angiography depends upon the indication for the diagnostic study, the initial observation from the control study, and the specific vascular bed studied. Tumor visualization may be enhanced by using vasoconstrictors, while inflammatory lesions or small tumors may be seen more clearly using vasodilator drugs. However, conflicting results are not unusual.[71]

Vasoconstrictors: epinephrine, vasopressin, angiotensin.

Vasodilators: tolazoline hydrochloride, glucagon, papaverine, acetylcholine, histamine.

VASOCONSTRICTORS

Epinephrine

This drug is a powerful vasoconstrictor of renal arteries and even veins.[59] It decreases the renal blood flow from 1500 cc per minute to 900 cc per minute.[72] By constricting the renal arteries, the arterial phase is prolonged, with a diminished or no nephrogram. There is increased venous tone. By increasing intrarenal resistance there is reflux of contrast into the aorta and the right angled branches of the renal artery, such as the inferior adrenal and capsular arteries. When epinephrine is injected, there is slight transient elevation in blood pressure, increase in heart rate, and mild excitement and anger.[73–75] *Following epinephrine injection, the effect of contrast material can be very nephrotoxic if it is injected ten minutes after infusion of epinephrine, rather than in the usual twenty to thirty seconds.*[76] Epinephrine is used for (1) renal phlebography, (2) detecting neovascularity, (3) enhancing splenic detail, and (4) evaluating the functional significance of an anatomical lesion.

Postepinephrine Renal Phlebography

The selective intra-arterial injection of epinephrine causes reduction of renal blood flow and increases the venous tone, thereby reducing the renal venous pool. This results in increased perfusion of the tributaries when contrast is injected into the renal vein[74, 77] (Fig. 7-1).

Identifying Neovasculature

Epinephrine may be used to detect neovasculature, *but may not be able to differentiate between benign and malignant neovasculature.* The responsiveness of a vessel to the vasoconstricting effects of epinephrine requires the presence of contractile elements in its wall. Unlike normal vessels, *malignant tumor vessels* behave differently to humoral agents,[80–82] as they lack contractile (muscular) elements in their walls.[85, 94] *Benign processes* like hamartomas with abnormal components in their vascular architecture and also different proportions of the normal constituents, are noted for their vascular dysplasias found in the tumor mass. The vascular structure may consist of angiomatous lacunae,[96, 97] sinusoids or vessels with thin musculature, or vessels with no musculature but excessive hyalinization.[95] Therefore, it is only logical to expect variable responses to epinephrine from these tumors, depending on the type of dysplastic vessels they possess.[83, 84] The vascular structure of neurofibromas resembles, more or less, that of hamartomas with excessive collagenization or hyalinization of their walls in certain areas. They also contain vessels with excessive musculature in other areas. Again, the term *dysplastic vessels* is appropriate. It is obvious that variable responses to epinephrine are not unusual.

Vascular responses of *inflammatory granula-*

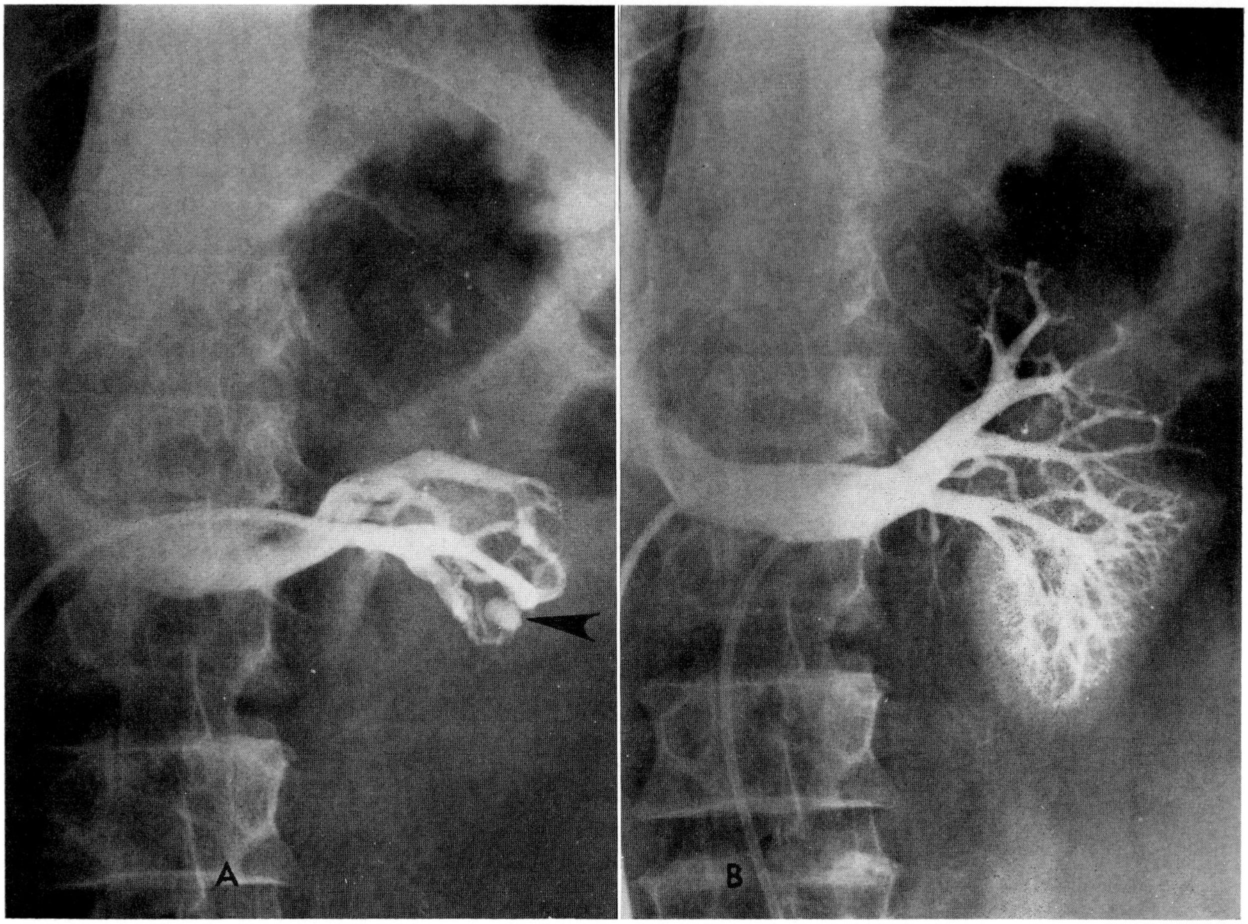

Figure 7.1. Renal Phlebography. (A) Without epinephrine. (B) With epinephrine. *Comment:* The good opacification of the small branches is obvious.

tion tissue when epinephrine is injected can resemble that of a malignant tumor vessel response. This is not unusual, as the granulation tissue has sinusoids in the early stage (ten to fifteen days) before differentiation into regular thick-walled capillaries occurs.[79]

Even malignant tumors may have variable responses[87, 98] depending on the nature of the vascular stroma of the tumor. This is true if the *stroma* has been *appropriated* from the parent organ and retains its ability to respond to vasoconstrictors, unlike its counterpart, *"the newly generated vessels,"* which lacks contractile elements.[85] In addition to these, vessels, if encased or infiltrated by malignant tumors or benign desmoplastic processes or atherosclerosis with degeneration of its wall, may be devoid of contractile elements. There may be a parasitic blood supply or siphonage from a preexisting collateral or dual blood supply, all of which may modify the vascular response to epinephrine. In addition, different individuals may have a different threshold for epinephrine response. If the parent branch supplying the tumor is

---

Figure 7.2. Renal Arteriogram. (A) Early arterial phase: There is deviation and stretching of intrarenal branches in the upper and lower poles of the same kidney. (B) Avascular filling defects of different sizes can be seen. (C) Postepinephrine renal arteriogram on same side. There is severe constriction of the intrarenal arterial branches, delayed intrarenal arterial circulation, and reflux of contrast into the aorta. (D) Poor nephrogram—stasis of contrast in the intrarenal branches occurs. *Diagnosis:* Multiple cysts. Effect of epinephrine on the intrarenal circulation is noted.

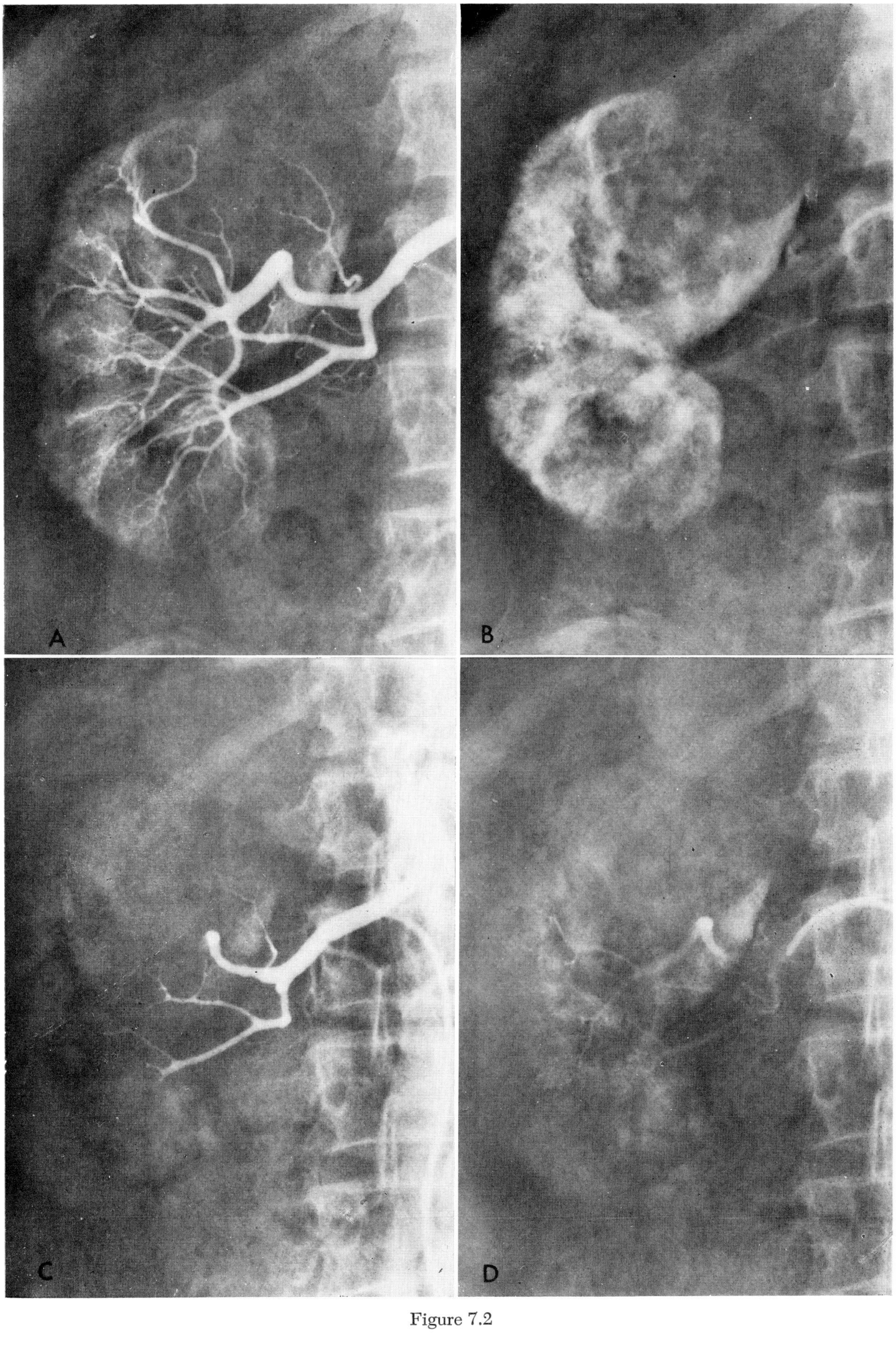

Figure 7.2

constricted markedly by epinephrine, there is no way for contrast to reach the peripheral abnormal vessels. Therefore, *conflicting angiographic and pathologic results are not unusual,* as the angiographer bases his diagnosis solely on the fibrovascular stroma of a lesion, while his colleague, the pathologist, looks to abnormal cellular parenchymal architecture to make his decision. The practical *value of epinephrine studies exists when the control angiogram is normal, and the postepinephrine angiogram is abnormal.*[86]

Lack of vasoconstrictive responses may occur in the following benign processes: angiomyolipoma;[83, 84] lipoma;[88] renal cyst;[89] inflammation;[91, 92] neurofibroma, multicystic kidney;[98] and hemangioma.[112] Vasoconstrictive responses from malignant tumor vessels may occur with soft tissue tumors[87] (fibrosarcoma) and probably with Wilm's tumor.[98]

Enhancing Detail in the Splenic Parenchyma

By contracting the splenic capsule and decreasing the size of the spleen, details are enhanced following the injection of epinephrine.[59] When injected into the splenic artery or the celiac axis following injury to the spleen, the details due to trauma are enhanced. There is no effect on lacerated vessels or change in the rate of blood leakage and pooling of contrast

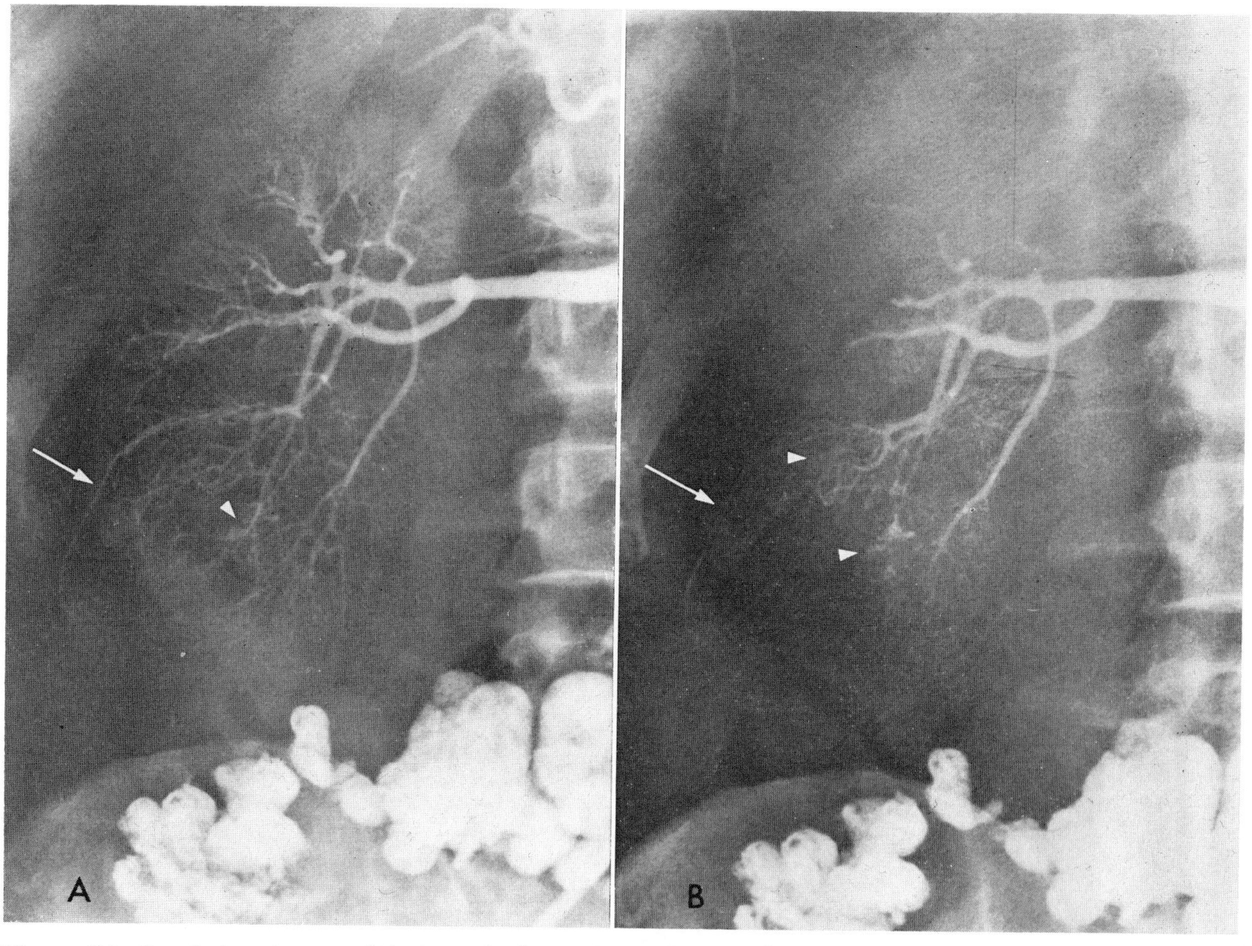

Figure 7.3. Renal Arteriogram. (A) Arterial phase: A very prominent perforating capsular vessel courses beyond the renal contour. (Arrow) Small subtle abnormal vessels with irregular caliber are in the lower portion of the kidney. (Arrow Head) (B) Postepinephrine renal arteriogram shows the perforating capsular vessel to better advantage (Arrow) with abnormal collections of islands of contrast material. (Head) Incidentally, note the constriction of the renal branches. *Diagnosis:* Renal tumor with abnormal vasculature, which is nonresponsive to vasoconstrictors because of lack of contractile elements. *Pathology:* Hypernephroma.

material.[99] There is increased opacification of the splenic vein after infusion of epinephrine into the celiac axis.[100]

Functional Significance of Anatomical Lesions

Epinephrine can be used to demonstrate the direction of blood flow in renal artery stenosis in an attempt to evaluate the hemodynamic significance of the stenosis.[78] When injected into the hepatic artery, moderate doses of epinephrine increase hepatic blood flow by dilating the mesenteric blood vessels and increasing the portal pressure and flow.[59] There can also be a direct effect on collateral vessels.

Vasopressin

This powerful vasoconstrictor of arterioles has no effect on veins. Unlike epinephrine, whose action is mediated through the autonomic nervous system,[59] vasopressin does have *a direct action on small vessels.* It is an antidiuretic and its other adverse effect is on coronary circulation.[59]

The small bowel blood vessels are very responsive to vasopressin. It decreases the superior mesenteric arterial flow and thereby decreases portal venous flow and portal venous pressure. There is at least a 50 percent decrease in portal hypertension in portal hypertensives, and a 20 percent decrease of portal pressure in normal patients. There is no change in cardiac output. When vasopressin is infused for treatment of gastrointestinal bleeding, the blood gases do not

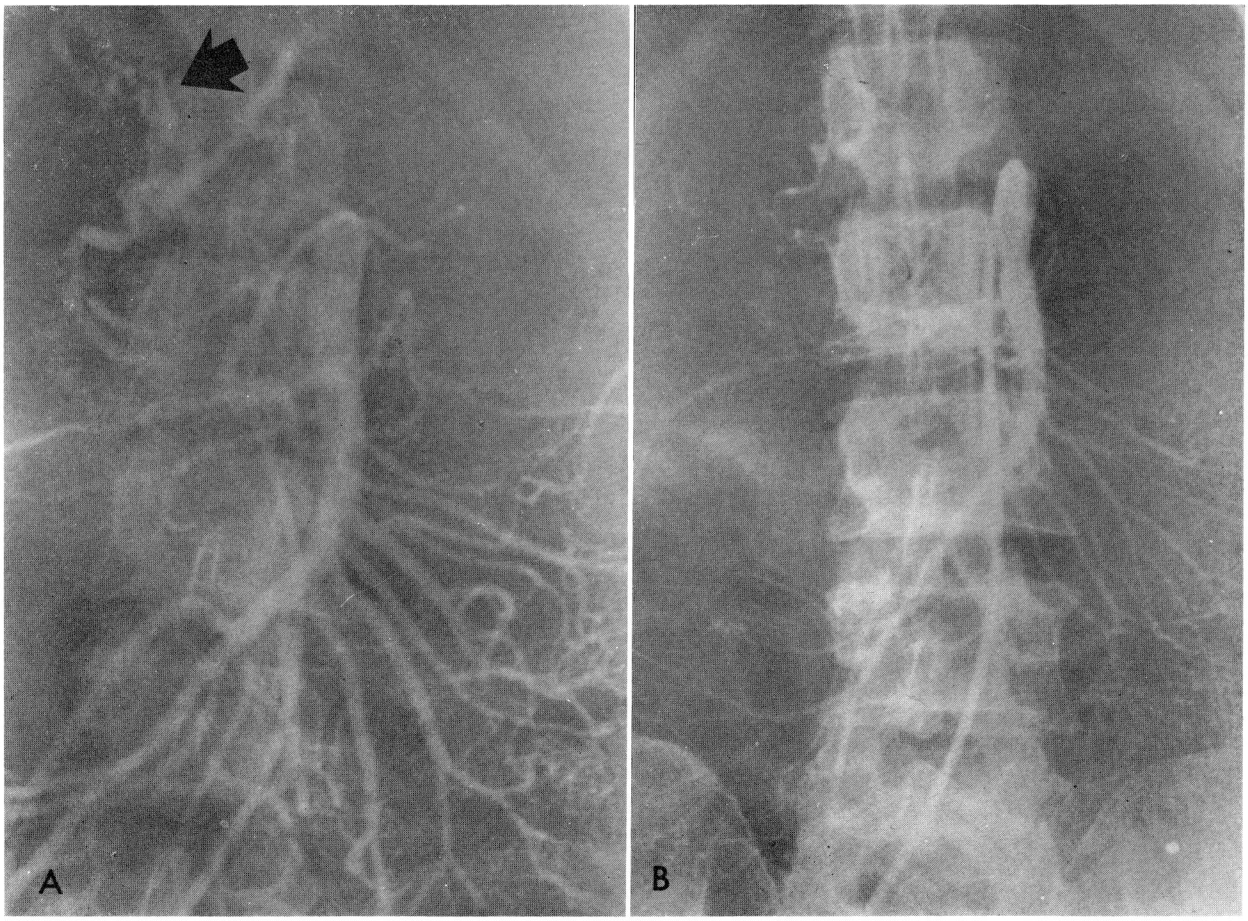

Figure 7.4. Superior Mesenteric Arteriogram. (A) Arterial phase: There is reflux into the hepatic artery (Arrow), via the gastroduodenal artery. (B) Vasopressin infusion into the superior mesenteric artery; notice the sudden dramatic change in the caliber of the main trunk as well as its branches. *Comment:* Vasoconstriction due to vasopressin infusion.

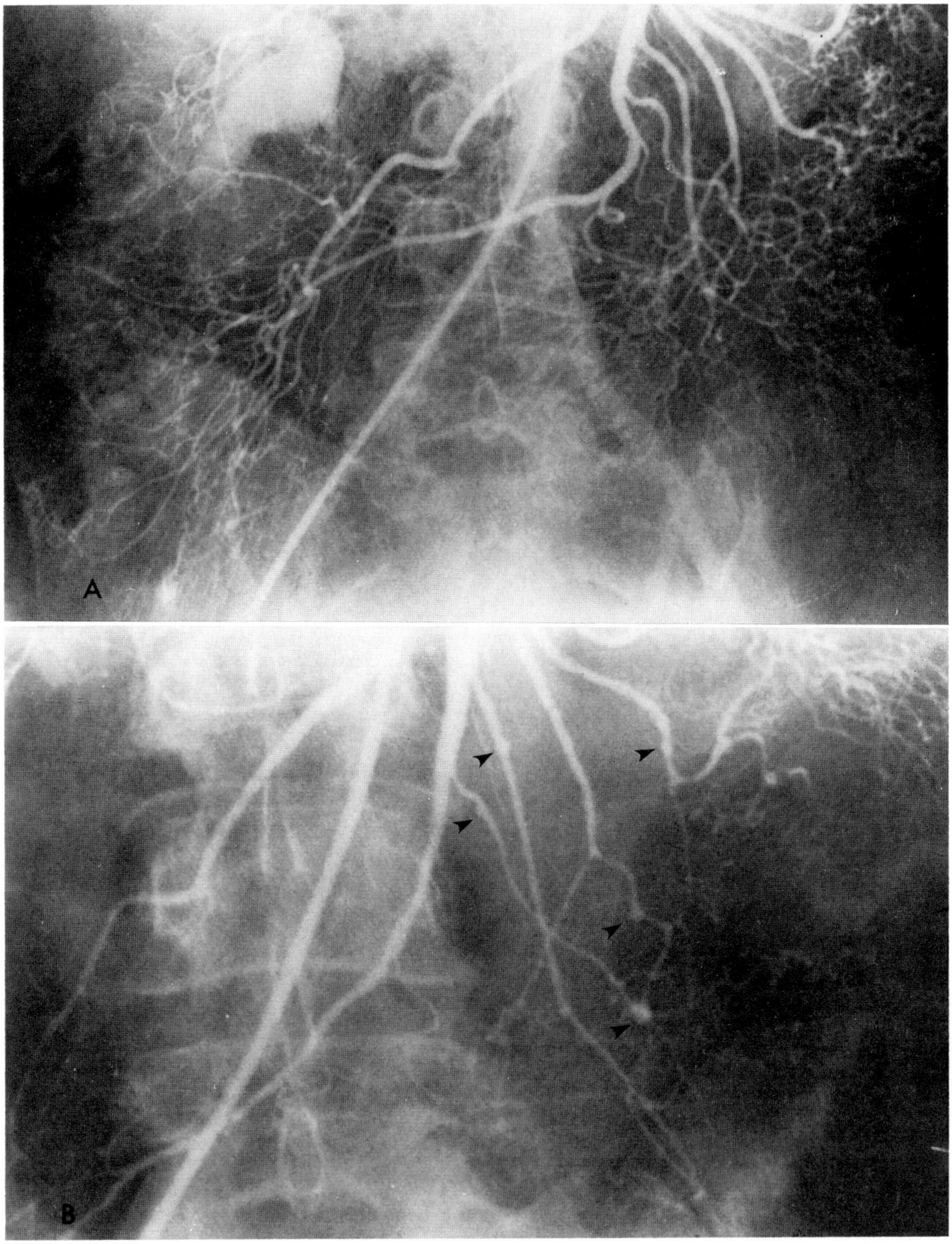

Figure 7.5. Superior Mesenteric Arteriogram. (A) Arterial phase: No apparent abnormalities are seen. (B) Postvasopressin infusion: Notice the marked vasoconstriction of those vessels with contractile elements, yet there is no ability to contract in certain areas probably because of atherosclerosis. Possibly more aneurysms of small branches can be detected by this method. (Courtesy of Dr. Pavitra Singh, Aurora, Illinois.)

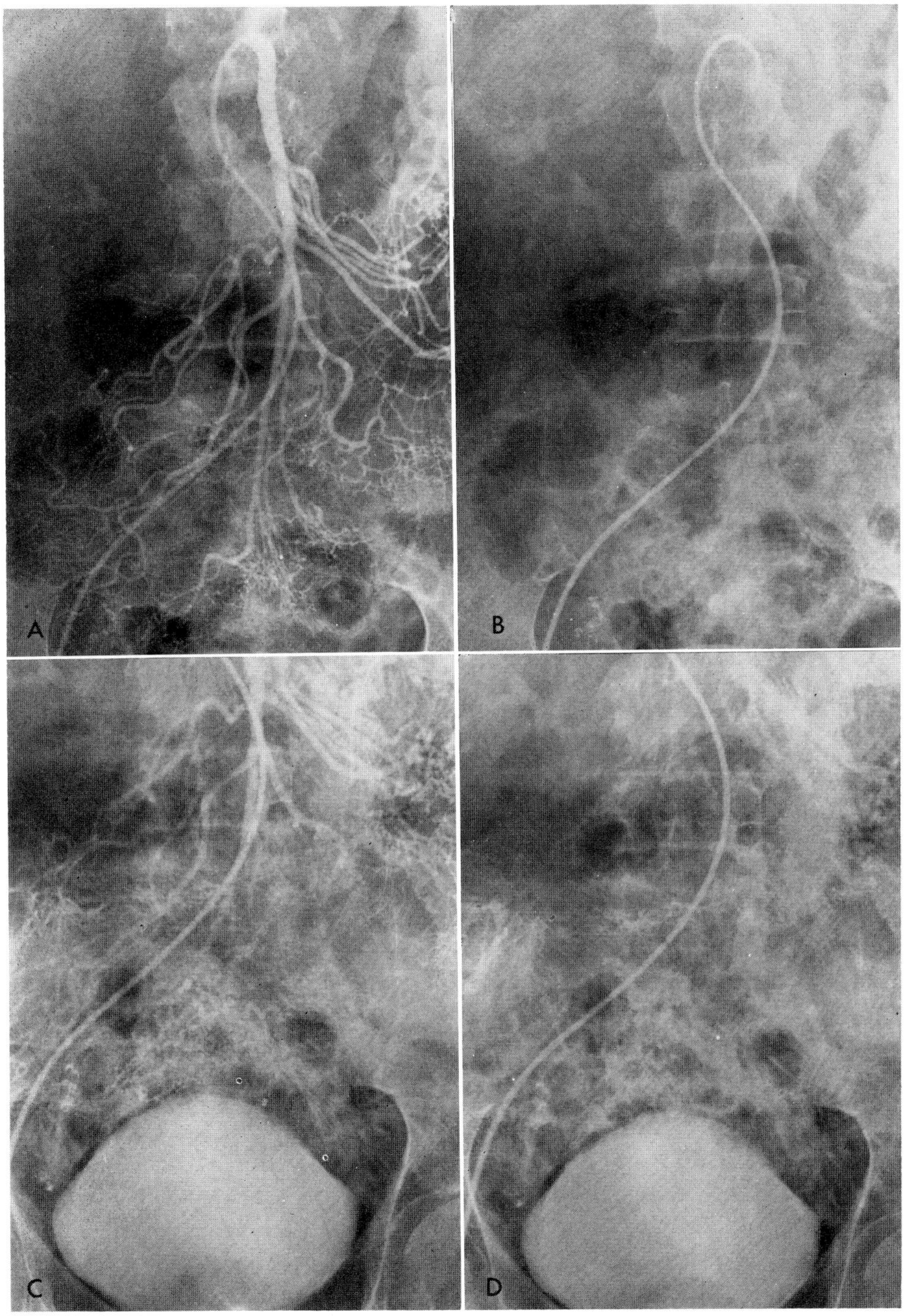

Figure 7.6. Superior Mesenteric Arteriogram. (A) Superior mesenteric arteriogram: Note the caliber of the main trunk and the branches. (B) Venous phase: There is faint opacification of the mucosa and veins. (C) After prescoline infusion into the superior mesenteric artery: Notice the blurring of the major and minor branches with increased early staining of the mucosa. (D) Late phase: Increased staining of the mucosa of the bowel with early good venous opacification is revealed. *Comment:* Vessel dilatation and excessive contrast perfusion is due to prescoline.

change in the portal or superior mesenteric venous bed (Ref. Ch. 25). The gastroduodenal, left gastric, splenic and superior mesenteric arteries are constricted. Despite continuous infusion, however, the hepatic arteries are dilated.[102–105]

In hypersplenism, a fifteen-minute perfusion of vasopressin at the rate of 0.2 units per minute can help preoperative evaluation to determine if there is an endogenous or exogenous increase of platelets.[106] The effect on the kidney is the same as that of epinephrine.[107] Vessels denuded of muscle, necrotically digested vessels (pancreatitis), or inflammatory vessels may not respond.[108] Lack of response is also noted in atherosclerotic vessels and vessels with periarterial fibrosis (Fig. 7-5).

The *adverse effects* of vasopressin include an antidiuretic effect,[59] tissue ischemia[109] with doses greater than 0.4 units per minute, and thrombosis of small mesenteric veins. Anuria may also occur. Therefore, intermittent infusion and monitoring of the serum lactic acid levels are necessary to protect the bowel from ischemic necrosis.[110] Frequent cardiac monitoring for elderly patients is also advisable.

Angiotensin

This powerful vasoconstrictor of arterioles, like vasopressin, has no effect on veins. This hormone is formed in the blood in response to renin, a substance formed in the juxtaglomerular cells of the kidney.[52] It acts directly on the precapillary region[59] and enhances perfusion

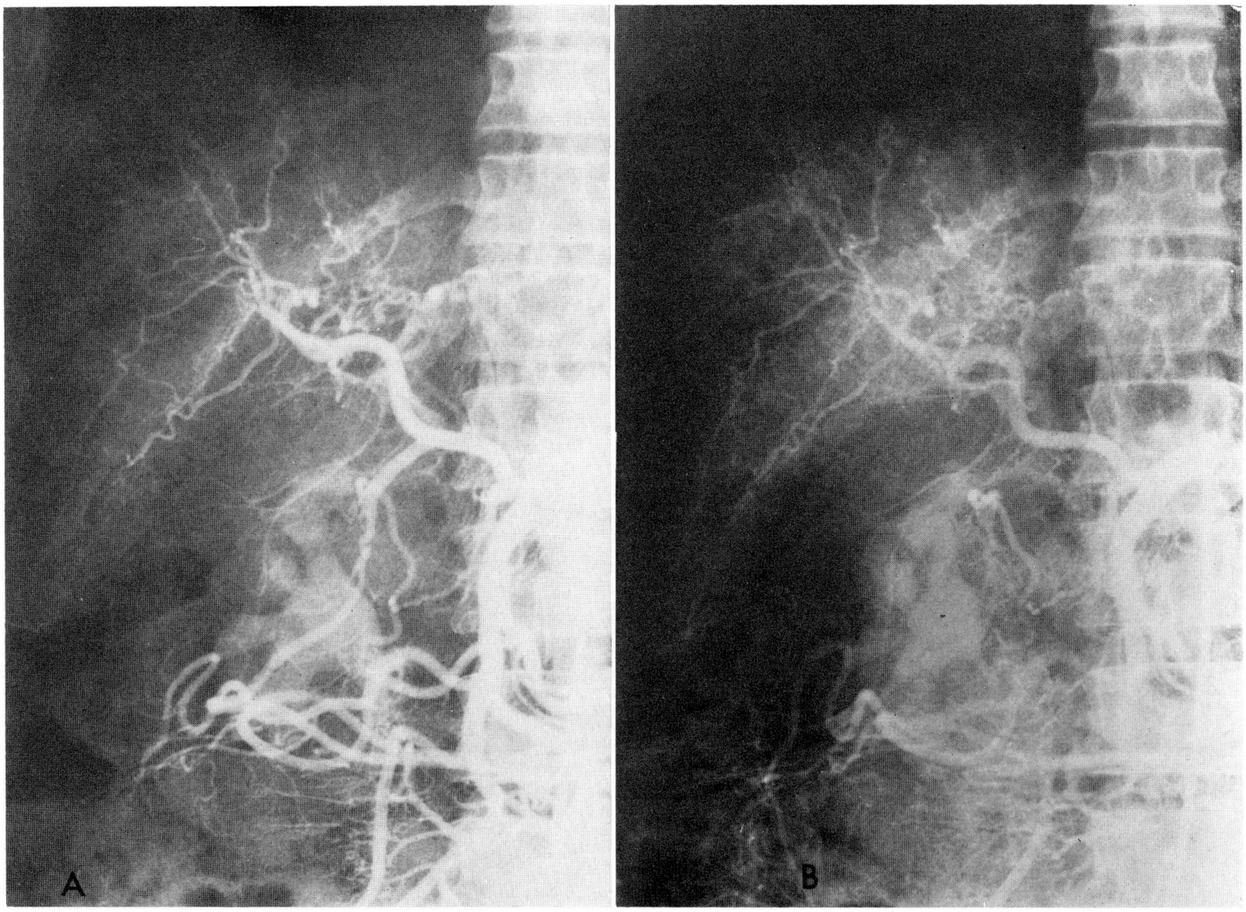

Figure 7.7. Superior Mesenteric Arteriogram. (A) The right hepatic artery originates from the superior mesenteric artery. The gallbladder is distended due to obstruction. The patient was known to have carcinoma of the head of the pancreas. (B) After perfusion of prescoline into the superior mesenteric artery, there is increased early staining of the liver parenchyma. There is blurring however, of small branches. The gallbladder wall is better opacified. *Comment:* The above effects are due to vasodilatation.

of small vessels by contrast material. It is a powerful vasoconstrictor of the splanchnic and renal vascular beds.[59]

Tumor vessels are better shown after selective intraarterial injection of angiotensin. In some cases described, tumor vessels were shown only after angiotensin was injected. Like any other vasoconstrictor, it prolongs the arterial phase, decreases parenchymal staining, and decreases or completely eliminates visualization of the veins.[112, 113] When angiotensin is infused, there is good opacification of inflammatory vessels and good demonstration of hemangiomas.[112]

VASODILATORS

Tolazoline Hydrochloride (Prescoline®)

This vasodilator has a direct effect on the vascular smooth muscle. It causes cardiac and gastric stimulation, producing tachycardia, *arrhythmias, and may precipitate myocardial infarction.*[59] The dose used, however, in clinical angiography is below the level required to produce any adverse cardiac or gastrointestinal manifestations in individuals with normal cardiovascular function. Because of its vasodilatory effect, it can enhance better opacification of the superior mesenteric and portal veins, portocaval shunts, and collateral veins by contrast injected into the superior mesenteric artery[114] (Figs 7-6, 7-7 and 7-8).

Tolazoline hydrochloride can be used in peripheral arteries to enhance the visualization of collaterals and to decrease the circulation time.[115] It can also be used to demonstrate the presence of arteriovenous fistulas, malignant tumors, venous malformation,[116] and small aneurysms due to angiitis.[117]

It is a helpful drug for young individuals with a tendency to develop vascular spasm at the puncture site. To prevent spasm the artery may be perfused immediately after puncture and catheter insertion, and a second time just before the catheter is withdrawn.

Papaverine

This smooth muscle relaxant has the *potential to cause cardiac arrhythmias.*[59] Side effects, however, are comparatively less with papaverine

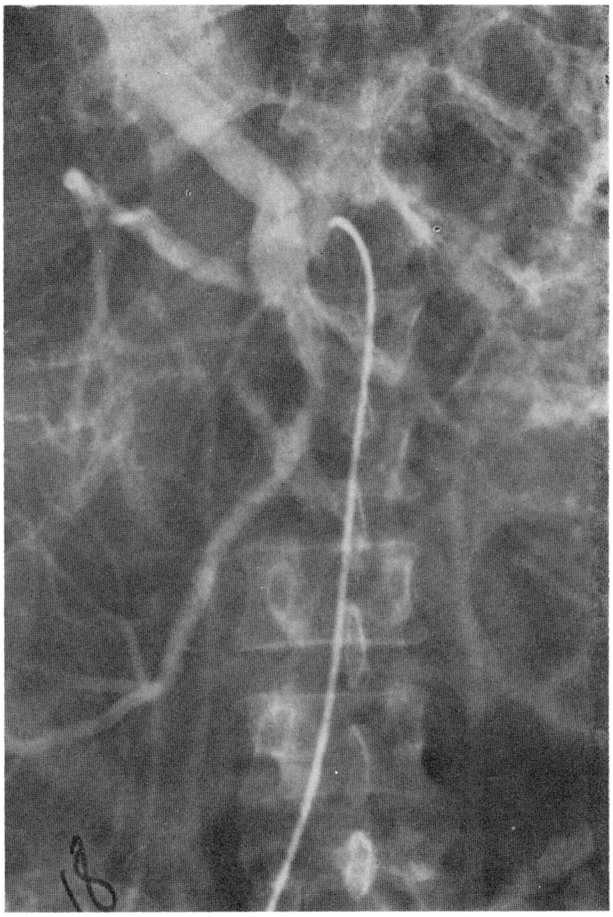

Figure 7.8. Postprescoline Superior Mesenteric Venography. The superior mesenteric vein and its branches are well opacified.

than with tolazoline. Hence the visualization of the portal venous system can be obtained after the superior mesenteric artery is infused with papaverine and the contrast is immediately injected.[118]

In *reversible mesenteric arterial vasoconstriction* due to low flow syndromes (cardiogenic shock, arrhythmias, congestive heart failure, prolonged hemorrhagic hypotension) infarction of the bowel may be overcome by selective infusion of papaverine into the superior mesenteric artery. A test infusion of 45 mgm of papaverine diluted with 50 cc of normal saline is infused over fifteen minutes into the superior mesenteric artery at the rate of 3 mgm per minute. At the conclusion of the infusion another 30 mgm of papaverine with 30 cc of saline is injected as a bolus into the artery. A repeat superior mesenteric angiogram is conduct-

TABLE 7-I
PHARMACOANGIOGRAPHY

Study	*Drugs and Dose*	*Site of Injection*	*Contrast*	*Filming*
Superior mesenteric phlebography	Prescoline 30 to 40 mgm in 5 cc of saline	Superior mesenteric artery over 4 to 6 seconds	20 seconds after infusion of the drug, 60 to 70 cc of contrast is injected over 8 to 10 seconds into the superior mesenteric artery	1 film every other second for 30 seconds
Renal phlebography	Epinephrine 0.2 micrograms per kg up to 70 kg (15 micrograms is maximum for 70 kg and above)	Corresponding renal artery over 4 to 6 seconds	20 seconds after infusion of the drug, 24 to 30 cc of contrast is injected over 2 seconds into the same renal vein	1 film every second for 8 to 10 seconds
Renal arteriography	Epinephrine 0.2 micrograms per kg up to 70 kg (15 micrograms is maximum for 70 kg and above)	Renal artery over 4 to 6 seconds	20 seconds after infusion of the drug, 10 cc of contrast is injected over 4 to 5 seconds into the same renal artery	2 films/second for 5 seconds and 1 film/second for 10-15 seconds
Peripheral arteriography	Prescoline 25 to 40 mgm in 5 cc of saline	Desired peripheral artery	15 seconds after infusion of the drug, standard injection of contrast for that artery	2 films/second for 3-4 seconds and 1 film/second for 6 seconds

ed. If there is improvement showing relief of vasoconstriction, then 45 mgm of papaverine per hour is infused into the artery for sixteen to twenty hours.[132] If no signs of improvement after the test infusion of papaverine are found, then surgery is contemplated.[132]

Papaverine is not effective in reversing mesenteric vasoconstriction when the stimulus initiating the vasoconstriction, low cardiac output, persists. In such situations, early recognition of the vasoconstriction and a combination of circulatory assistance and papaverine infusion into the superior mesenteric artery may be beneficial.[132]

Acetylcholine

Acetylcholine increases the blood flow to the renal cortex and decreases the flow to the medulla. This is due to vasodilatation and decrease in vascular resistance. The effect returns to normal in ten to twenty minutes. The older the patient, the lesser the response.[125–127, 131] This drug is useful in demonstrating the irreversibility of vascular changes due to malignant nephrosclerosis, chronic pyelonephritis and the rejection phenomena in renal transplantation.[128, 129] There is an exaggerated vasodilatation due to increased resting vasomotor tone in essential hypertension. The dose of acetylcholine used in clinical angiography is many times lower than the dose which can cause side effects. But in patients lacking serum cholinesterase, adverse effects can be seen. This can be screened clinically by a simple test.[130] Acetylcholine has also been used to evaluate the functional significance of renal artery stenosis and the direction of blood flow in the collateral vessels.[78]

Secretin

This drug causes increased oxygen consumption and increases blood flow to the pancreas which improves visualization of the pancreatic parenchyma and pancreatic veins. It is contraindicated in pancreatitis.[133, 134]

Histamine

As a potent vasodilator, histamine increases the blood flow to the stomach, especially to the fundus. Normally, the increased flow is to the gastric antrum.[135] A nice mucosal blush to the stomach may be demonstrated with the assistance of intramuscular histamine.[136, 137]

Adrenocorticotropic Hormone (ACTH)

This drug triples the blood flow through the adrenal gland within ten minutes after injection.[142]

Glucagon

This vasodilator increases renal,[121] hepatic[120] and superior mesenteric arterial blood flow.[119, 124] Selective injection into the renal artery may cause dilatation for up to two hours afterward.[121] It can be used for further enhancement of the splanchnic venous circulation. Nausea and vomiting are the side effects. It is *contraindicated in diabetics* because of its hypoglycemic effect. It is also contraindicated in patients with *pheochromocytoma* because of its stimulating effect.[123]

MISCELLANEOUS

Diet

Angiography done immediately after the ingestion of a high caloric diet (a milk shake or ice cream) increases opacification of the upper gastrointestinal tract mucosa. There is rapid arteriovenous shunting and comparative increase in flow to the active area of absorption,[138, 139] enhancing visualization of small areas of abnormality.

Digoxin

Digoxin causes splanchnic vasoconstriction with its adverse effects on the bowel.[140, 141]

Ergot

This drug causes vasoconstriction, endothelial damage, vascular stasis, thrombosis and even gangrene. Patients with occlusive vascular disease are more susceptible to the side effects of this group of drugs.[59]

CHAPTER 8

COMPLICATIONS

MURPHY'S LAW (an axiom of scientists and engineers): "If anything can go wrong, it will at the worst possible time" (Figs. 8-1 to 8-7).

When the blood vessels, blood and organs are exposed to foreign materials such as needles, guide wires, catheters and contrast, they can only respond with a spectrum of undesirable end results. These results may be at the unrecognized histological level or at the obvious clinical level. *Every catheterization procedure is associated with some degree of injury regardless of the duration of the examination, the attention paid to meticulous technique, or the use of sophisticated instruments.* Fortunately, many of these injuries are cleverly compensated for by nature's capacity to heal. When the extent of injury exceeds nature's reparative abilities, mor-

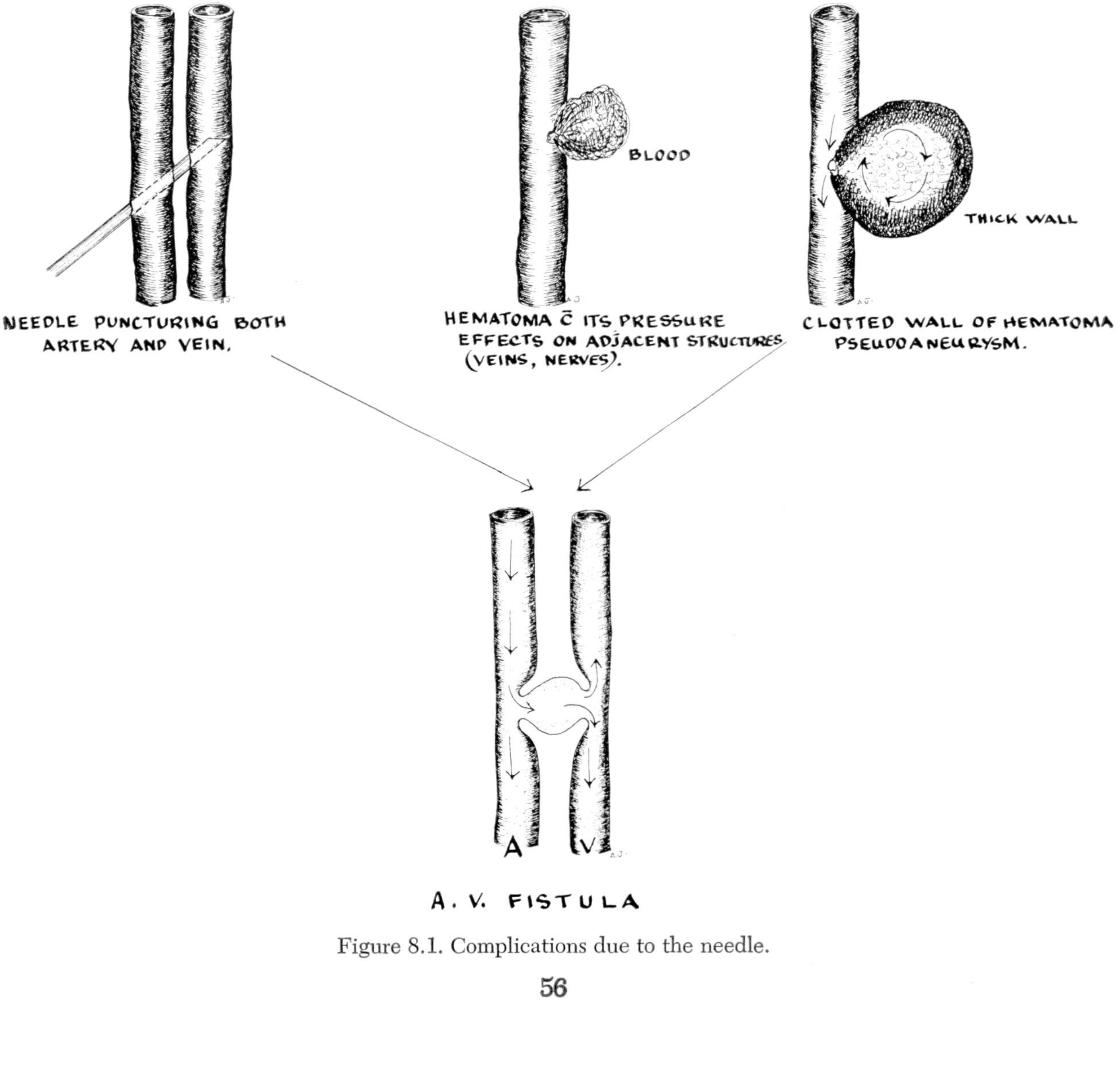

Figure 8.1. Complications due to the needle.

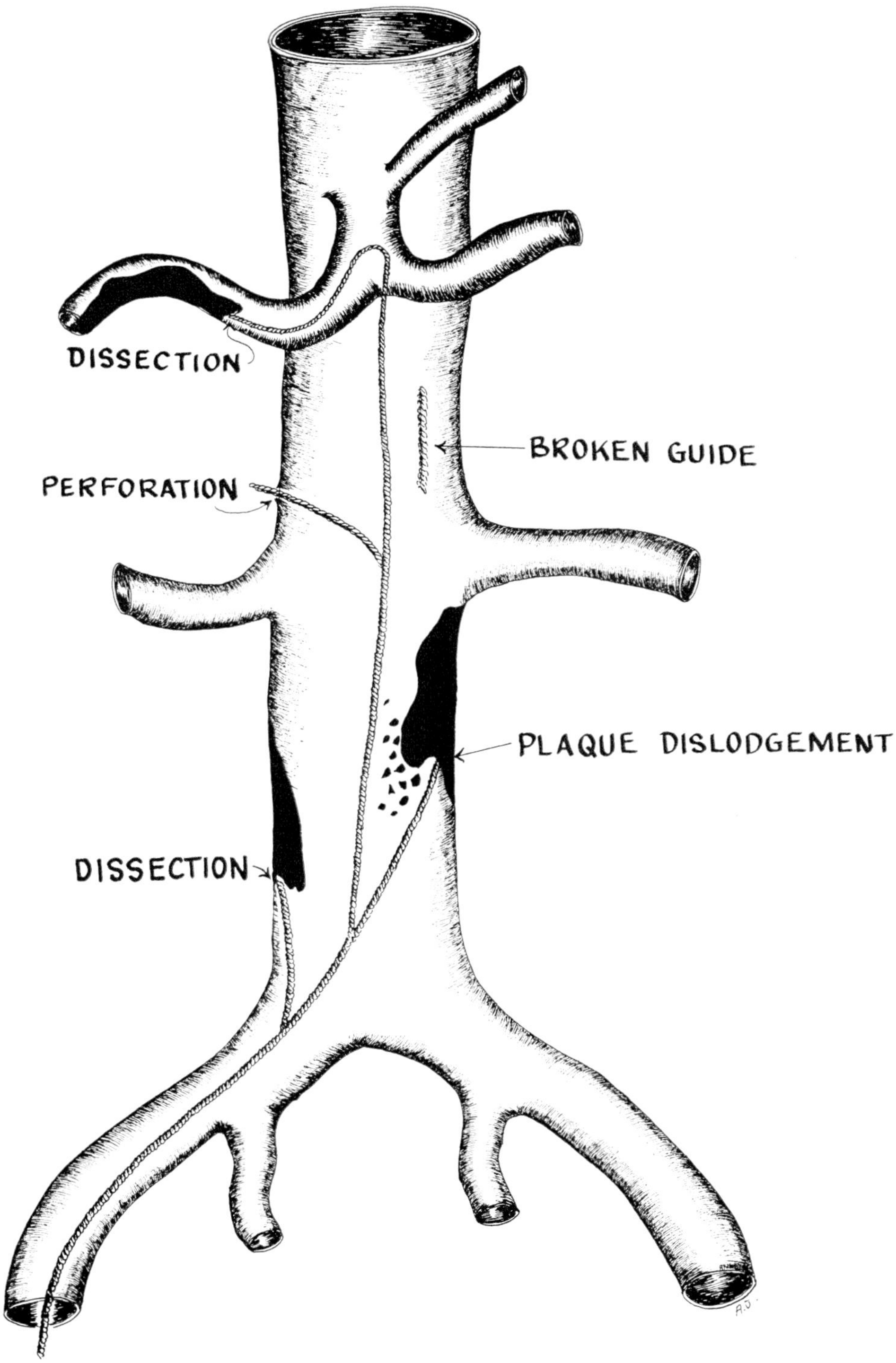

Figure 8.2. Complications due to the guide wire.

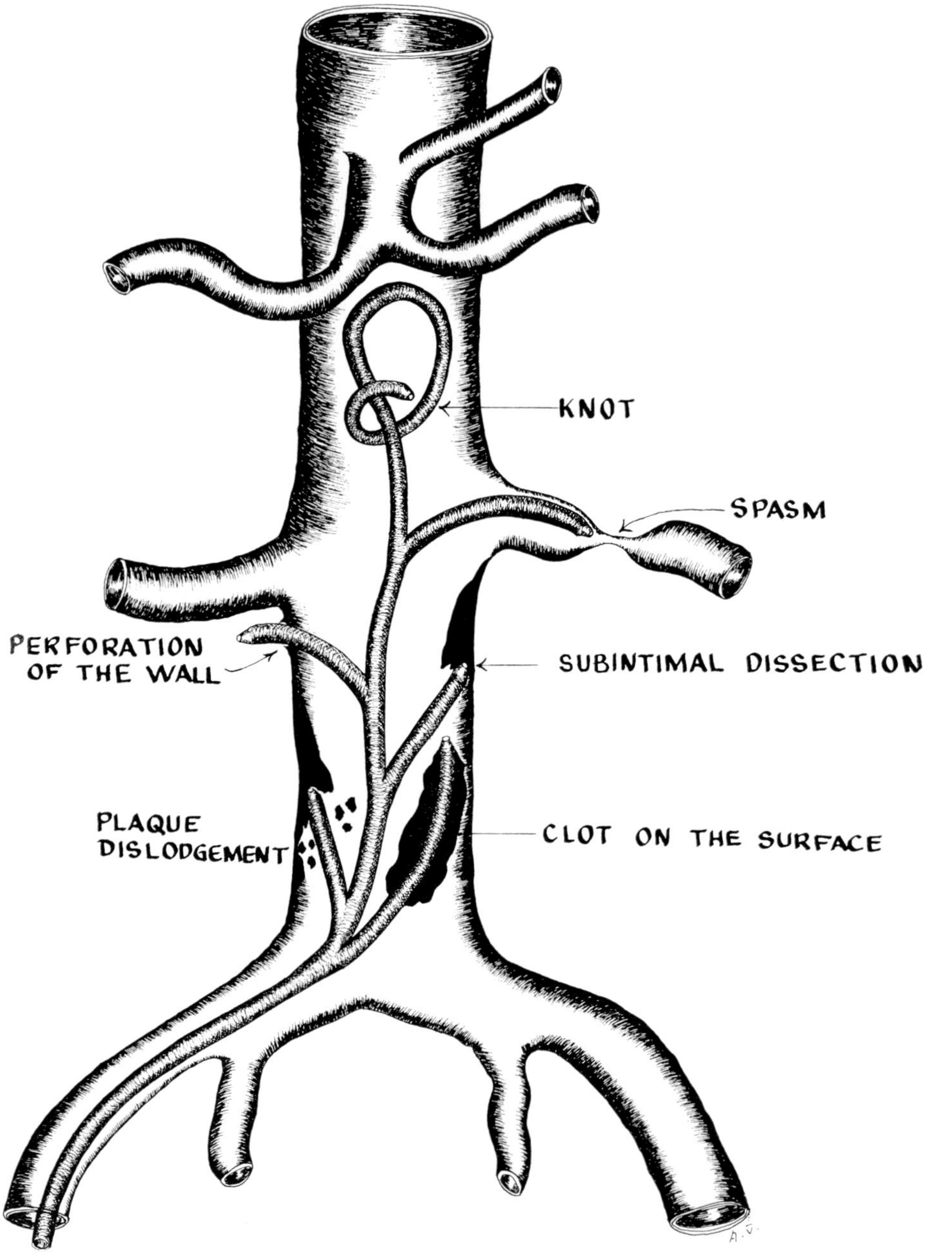

Figure 8.3. Note some complications of an intravascular catheter.

bidity ensues. Were it not for nature's reserves, there would be fewer angiograms done today.

Unfortunately, individuals predisposed to complications such as atherosclerotic vascular disorders, valvular cardiac diseases, and hypercoagulable disorders have already exhausted nature's reserves. They are, therefore, more vulnerable to complications when exposed to the stress of angiography. One simple complication may set the stage for a vicious play which may have a tragic ending.

On the other hand, if the desire is to perform angiography without any injury to the structures involved, then it must be done without the assistance of the presently available tools and contrast. *Learning to work within the safety parameters of nature's reserve definitely decreases morbidity and mortality.*

CONTRAST AND DEATH

Though newer contrasts are available, mortality has not decreased. Most deaths occur within five to ten minutes and are usually due to cardiac arrest. Autopsy usually shows that contrast deaths are nonspecific, apart from demonstration of coronary artery disease of variable degree, or fluid-filled blebs in the tracheobronchial tree due to angioneurotic edema.[63] The use of intravenous epinephrine to circumvent an oncoming reaction may cause ventricular fibrillation. In patients taking digitalis, death may be due to sensitization of the heart by a sodium overload, with subsequent fibrillation and death. The rate and severity of reactions increases with age.

SPINAL COMPLICATIONS

Spinal cord injury following angiography is due to injection of *highly concentrated or excessive amounts of contrast* into the vessels from which *spinal radiculomedullary arteries* arise. These small vessels arise from the vertebral, costocervical, thyrocervical, intercostal, lumbar, ilio-lumbar-arteries and sacral branches of the internal iliac artery.[188] The end result may be tetraplegia, hemiparesis, transient blindness, paraplegia, etc.[189, 192, 193] The accidental injection of a large bolus of contrast into spinal cord feeders, multiple injections into the aorta, the tip of an uncoiled catheter sticking in a small vessel, or excessive manipulation of the guide wire may cause transient or permanent damage.[195–199] Further complications have been reported with dislodgement of a mural thrombus or atheromatous plaque.[190, 194] In addition, cotton fiber embolization from an open bowl of saline used to flush the catheter, or cotton sponge,[191] may also contribute to unwanted, disastrous results.

If spinal complications occur, immediate consultation with a neurologist or neurosurgeon is advised. Reportedly, immediate lumbar puncture and replacement of equal volumes of spinal fluid with 10 cc of isotonic saline may improve the situation.[188]

RENAL COMPLICATIONS

A kidney which has been *overzealously dehydrated* and is *clinically in oliguria* may respond to contrast injection with the *precipitation of Tom Horsfall proteins* (constituents of tubular casts), causing blockage of the renal tubules.[200] In patients with *polycythemia,* hemolysis and hemoglobinuria due to increased hematocrit and decreased plasma volume, with an associated insult from dehydration, may cause *renal shutdown.* Adequate hydration prior to, during and after a study associated with urine-made alkaline may serve to decrease the complications[201] in polycythemic individuals.

Acute renal failure either due to aortography[202] or cholesterol emboli due to catheter manipulation[203] need special mention. Although rare, nephrogenic diabetes insipidus and azotemia may also result after angiography.[204] It must always be remembered that the renal artery is not exempt from becoming a victim of a clot at the tip of the catheter.[205]

ADRENAL COMPLICATIONS

Frequent complications may not be unusual with catheterization of delicate vascular structures like the adrenal veins. This may occur due to *wedging* of the catheter into the vein or *excessive pressure* during contrast injection. Infarctions may occur either due to extravasation or thrombosis. There may be high incidence of these complications in patients with aldosterone secreting adenomas. Adrenal insufficiency can be the end result of these complications.[259–261] One should be alert to *hypertensive crises* during venography for pheochromocytomas.[27]

CATHETERS AND CLOTS

The interaction of *platelets by adherence* either to the injured arterial wall or to the catheter surface initiates the most important stimulus in the creation of a chain of events resulting in the formation of a *dangerous thrombus.*[206] Platelet adhesiveness increases by 10 percent after catheterization. The longer the length of a catheter, the greater the development of adhesiveness.[207, 208] Clots on the sur-

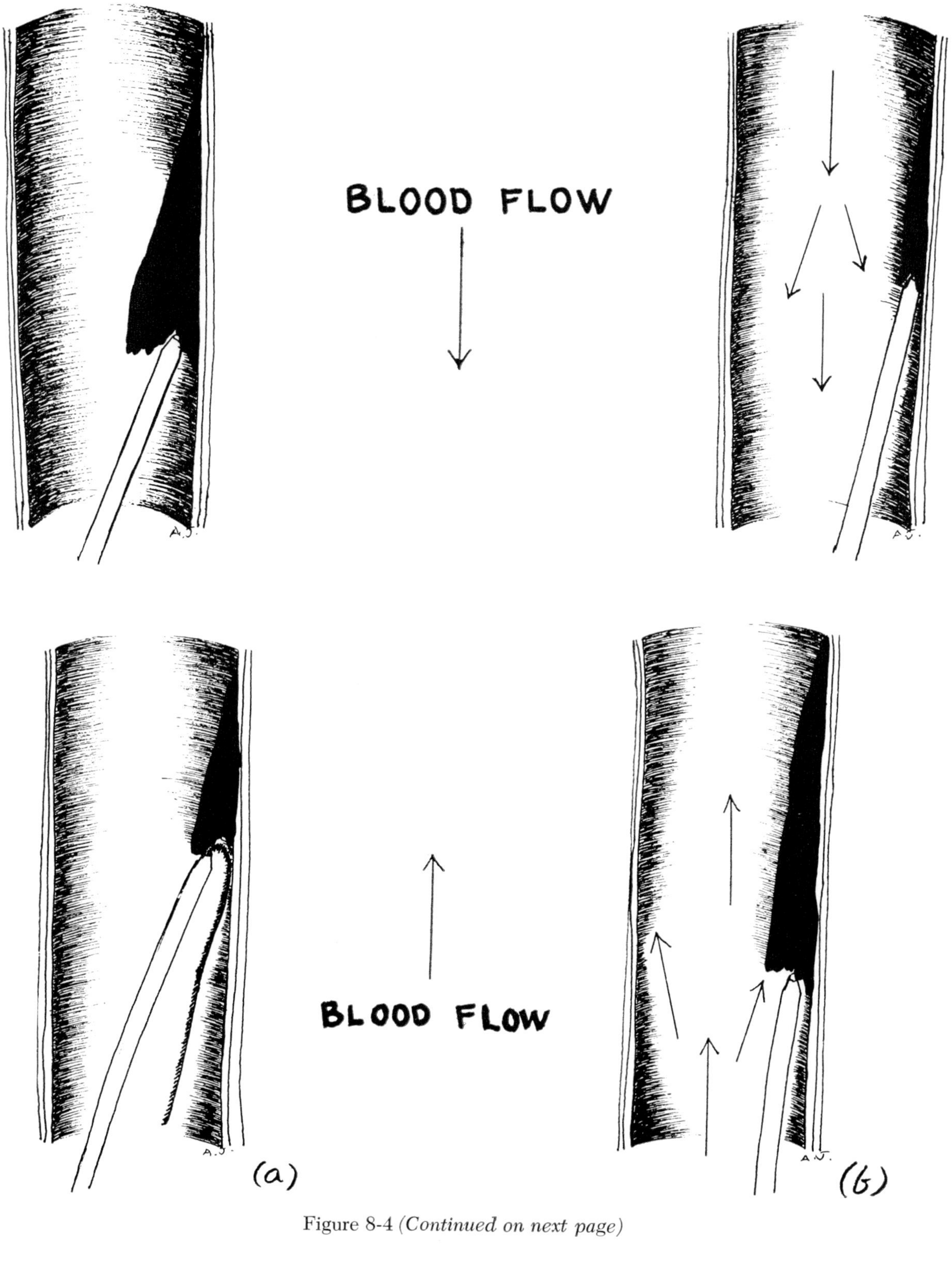

Figure 8-4 *(Continued on next page)*

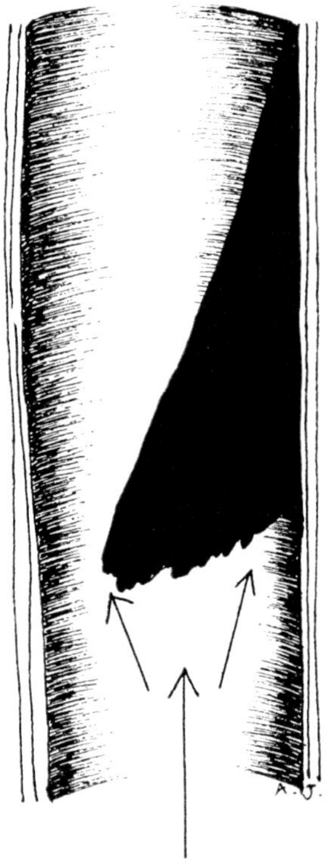

Figure 8.4. Effects of iatrogenic dissections of the wall of the artery in relation to the direction of contrast injection.

(C)

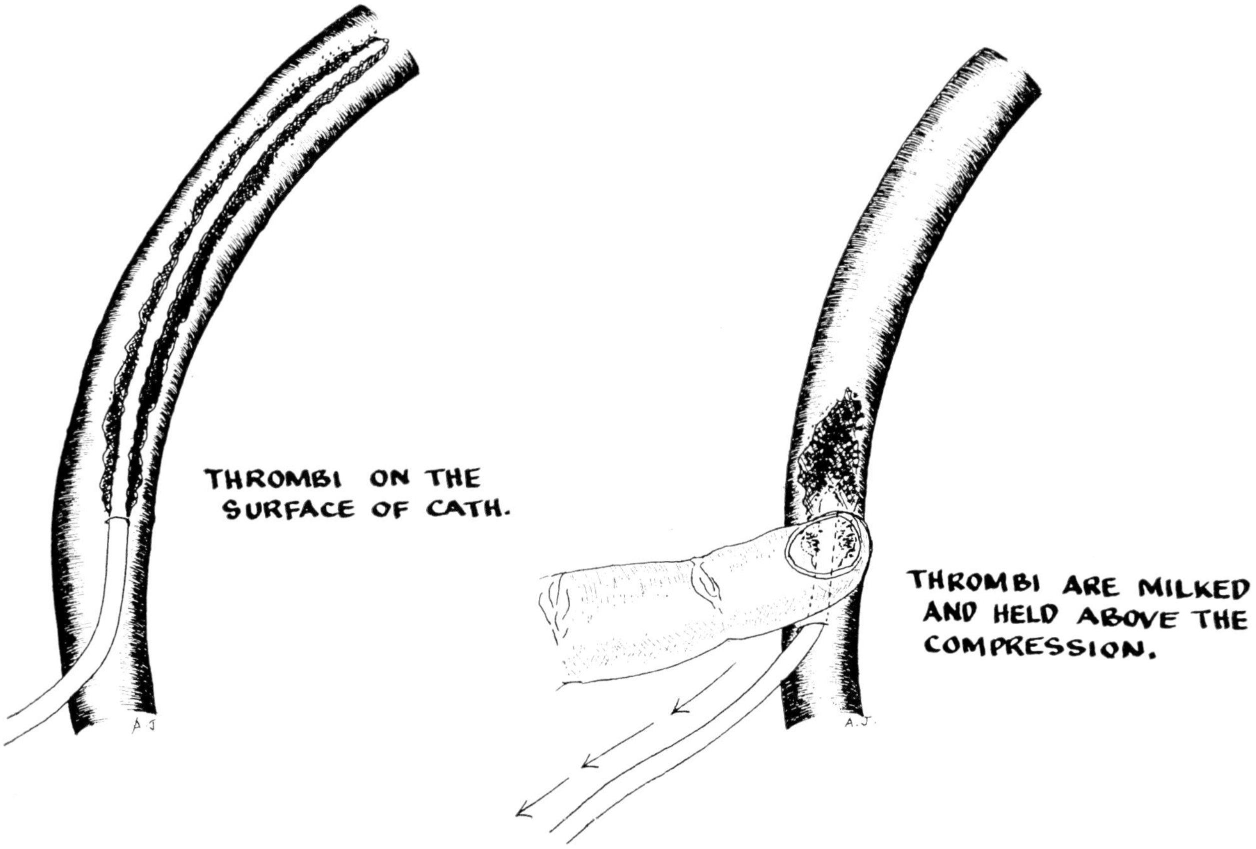

Figure 8.5 Note clot formation on the catheter surface and its distal embolization.

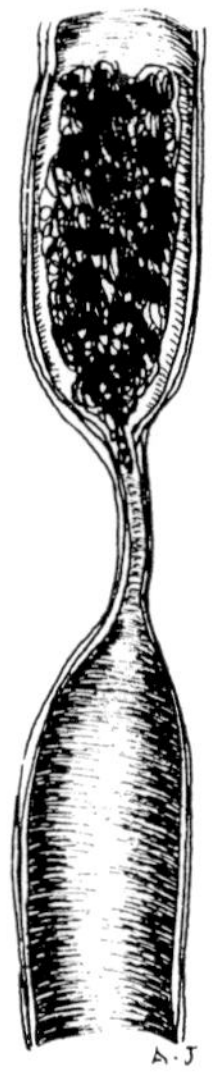

SPASM OF THE ARTERY c̄ STASIS OF BLOOD PROXIMALY LEADING TO SECONDARY CLOT FORMATION c̄ TOTAL OCCLUSION OR FRAGMENTATION OF CLOT AND DISTAL DISSEMINATION.

Figure 8.6

face of the catheter are noted as early as fifteen minutes after insertion. If left inside the blood vessel for a day, 100 percent of catheters will develop deposition of thrombi.[209]

Increased viscosity of blood due to diabetes,[210] premenstrual periods, menopause, posthysterectomy,[211] polycythemia,[212] rapid dehydration and restoration of compensation in patients with cardiac decompensation,[213, 214] diarrhea and vomiting, hastens the process of thrombogenesis. *Increased coagulability* after myocardial infarction,[215] pregnancy,[216] and the use of oral contraceptives[217] helps the blood to solidify earlier. *Increased platelet adhesiveness* in postoperative states, or myocardial infarcts,[218] is no less a competitor in hastening the process of thrombus formation.

The formation of *fibrin sleeves* is not uncommon, originating from areas of intimal injury, the puncture hole and at the tip of the catheter which is in contact with the intima.[44,219] When the catheter is withdrawn, these thrombotic deposits are wiped off inside the artery as a last parting gesture of catheterization.[221] Clots which are bigger than 2.5 mm at the puncture site may have objective evidence of decreased circulation peripheral to the puncture site.

Bilateral simultaneous catheterizations, though impressive, *should not be encouraged* as there is extensive friable clot formation in the space between the crossing of the catheters and the bifurcation of the aorta. This is due to turbulence, decreased blood flow and twice as many foreign surfaces.[223]

The higher incidence of thromboembolic phenomena in patients suffering from *homocystinuria* warns one to avoid vascular trauma in these individuals. There is also a higher incidence of *neonatal arterial thrombosis* and occlusion of aortic branches due to umbilical arterial catheterizations in neonates. One should thus be warned to leave the catheter tip as distal as possible in the aorta.[225]

VENOUS COMPLICATIONS

The effects of prolonged contact of contrast in the presence of venous stasis produces more extensive and severe inflammatory change in the veins, with eventual development of thrombus.[226] Although rare, gangrene formation following peripheral phlebography in patients with venous thrombosis may occur.[227]

CAPILLARY CHANGES

Increased capillary permeability may present itself as *petechiae* in the areas of perfusion distal to the catheter tip. Injections into the ascending aorta may manifest themselves with diffused petechiae, while injections in the abdominal aorta may result in petechiae formation in the lower part of the body.[228]

SALINE, DEXTRAN AND BLOOD

Morphologic changes in red blood cells that occur with contrast can be reversed by immediately washing erythrocytes with physiological saline.[229] Low molecular weight dextran has the ability to maintain a normal apparent red blood cell viscosity, decreased platelet aggregation, and decreased platelet adhesiveness. Thus a normal blood flow may be maintained by decreas-

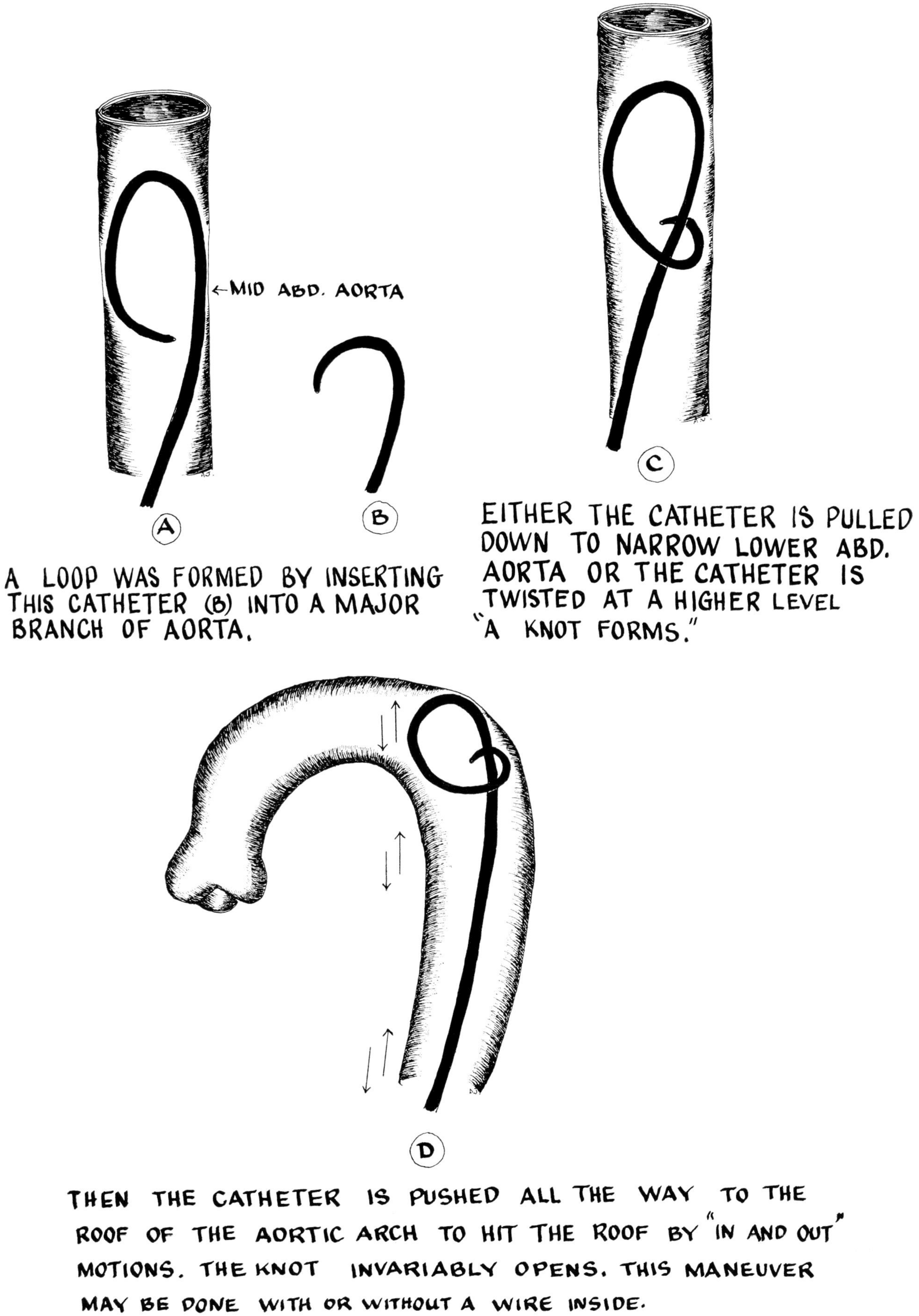

Figure 8.7. Note the knot formation of a catheter and its untying.

ing the viscosity.[230-233] *Dextran is contraindicated* in patients with pulmonary edema, localized septic processes, debilitation, and also in patients with long bleeding times, as they may develop pseudoaneurysms. Perivascular infiltration of dextran may cause edema.[207, 235] Because of osmotic nephrosis, renal failure may also develop.[236]

AIR EMBOLISM

This may occur because of malfitting plastic connectors[237] or accidental injection from an empty syringe or the creation of low pressure at the tip of the catheter, causing cavitation.[238] *The signs and symptoms*[239] *of venous air embolization* includes cyanosis, unconsciousness, apnea, dyspnea, convulsions, dilatation of the pupils, chest pains or restlessness. *Cardiac massage should not be attempted until all the froth has been aspirated.* In healthy people, 100 cc of air injected through the venous route is enough to cause death. A fraction of that amount is enough to cause death via the arterial route. The *coronary arteries, left ventricle* and *middle cerebral arteries* are the *critical areas.*[239] When air is injected into the artery, marbling of the skin or pallor of a portion of the tongue may occur.

THE VESSEL AND INJECTION PRESSURE

Excessive injection pressure with an end hole catheter may cause a forceful forward jet from the catheter resulting in *angiographic jet collapse and rupture of the aorta* involving all the layers. This is especially true in the newborn. In the *newborn,* not more than 6 cc per second, or not more than 275 psi effective pressure should be applied to the aorta. Even with low injection pressures of 220 psi effective pressure, the pliable walls may be pulled inward causing collapse. This happens more often in venous injections.[240] Markedly negative pressures exerted by the forward jet effect may be transmitted to the vessel, resulting in collapse. Disruption of the intima and media may occur. The maximal positive pressure occurs if the catheter is in direct contact with the vessel in a right angle position. In such a situation transmission of the pressure in the syringe may disrupt both intima and media. Again, this is more common in young individuals.[251]

Pressure induced extension of the catheter in a longitudinally curved spacious vessel like the aorta causes the orifice of the catheter to rest firmly against the aortic wall. This results in varying degrees of injury to the wall, ranging from microscopic subintimal hematoma to frank dissection. This adverse effect is hastened by the presence of diseased vessels or hypertension. This complication can be reduced by employing low injection pressures or by using a catheter with a curved configuration similar to the aorta, which results in less whipping.

Catheters in straight vessels, like the descending or ascending thoracic aorta, have less tendency to whip and damage the intima.[241]

THE HEART AND ELECTRICITY

Ventricular fibrillation, especially following selective angiocardiography, may be caused by malfunctioning of the electrically powered injector or the EKG machine due to inadequate grounding of these accessory apparatus. Experimental ventricular fibrillation can be caused by 35 microamperes, and 0.06 volts of electricity.[242-244]

NEEDLES, CATHETERS, HOLES

The vessel wall, which is traumatized by the needle and the catheter, responds in return by *spasm* if there are adequate contractile elements present (not uncommon in young people). The secondary *effects of spasm* include *stasis* of blood flow, *thrombosis and distal embolization.* Conversely, the *hole* made by the catheter may remain open with a formation of a sizeable *hematoma,* or even a *pseudoaneurysm.* This is more common in hypertensive patients and those with calcified peripheral vessels. *Continued bleeding into the neurovascular sheath* during axillary artery puncture may cause median and ulnar nerve injury, the damage being permanent if not recognized early. This can be detected by the onset of diminished sensation, numbness, or weakness soon after the effect of anesthesia wears off (after one hour).[252, 253]

TABLE 8-I

COMPLICATIONS IN OUR SERIES

Site	*Nature*	*Predisposing Factors*	*Study*	*No.*	*Outcome*	*Comment*
Arterial	Aortic dissection	Failure to inject test dose. Catheter tip impacted subintimally.	Aortogram	2	Asymptomatic	? Ignorance
	Celiac dissection	Excessive manipulation of the catheter.	Celiac angio	1	Asymptomatic	Too much fooling around
	Splenic A. dissection	Same	Splenic angio	1	Infarct of the spleen	Same as above
Renal	Post angio renal shutdown	Rt. Renal embolus Lt. Renal A. stenotic	Flush aortogram (contrast 50 cc)	1	Dialysis	Wish saline was radiopaque
		Severe atherosclerosis	Renal angio	1	Dialysis	Cholesterol emboli
		Multivalvular heart disease	Celiac and mesenteric angio 110 cc contrast	1	Dialysis	. . . . . .
Cardiac	Ventricular fibrillation	Bad cardiacs	Aortic arch	2	Medical management	Inevitable?
		Accidental injection into coronary artery graft	Aortic arch 50 cc over 2 sec	1	Medical management	Test dose was not injected. Inexcusable
	Pulmonary edema	Fragile heart	Abd aorta and renal artery	1	Medical management	We had no choice
Neurologic	Transient cerebral symptoms	Old patients	Aortic arch	3	Recovered	
Catheter	Knots	Too wide a curve	Selective studies	3	Untied by manipulation	Initially a nightmare

TABLE 8-II

COMPLICATIONS IN OUR SERIES

Site	*Nature*	*Predisposing Factors*	*Age*	*Number*	*Outcome*	*Comment*
Puncture site	Arterial thrombosis (Femoral Artery)	Females	10 yrs. to 40 yrs.	11	Surgical removal	. . . Young Females . . .
	Arterial spasm (Femoral Artery)	Females and males	6 yrs. to 35 yrs.	5 Females 1 Male	Medical management	. . . Unlucky . . . Male
	Uncontrolled bleeding (Groin)	Accidental high dose of Heparin	Young	2	Medical management	A medical student, another the wife of an attorney
		Severe hypertensive	Young	1	Symptomatic treatment	. . . No comments
		Inefficient post angio care	Different age groups	4	Symptomatic management	. . . Negligence . . .
	Severe testicular pain	High puncture	Young	1	? Spermatic cord injury	. . . He is probably O.K.
	Periarterial extravasation	Improper placement of the needle	Different age groups	5	Symptomatic management	
	Perivenous extravasation	? Improper placement of Teflon sleeve	Different age groups	3	Symptomatic management	. . . It . . . Happened

If there are clots larger than 2.5 mm shown by pull-out angiography at the puncture site, the patient may have objective evidence of decreased distal circulation.[254] *Oscillographic evaluation is more reliable* than clinical methods in recognizing the presence and levels of occlusion.[255] Growth discrepancy of the catheterized leg in young individuals is not an unusual end result.[256] Some advocate the removal of the postcatheterization clot by applying the pressure on the artery distal to the puncture site. The catheter is then withdrawn while applying suction. If no bleeding occurs through the puncture site, milking and massaging the artery above this point is done to extrude the clot.[257] Iatrogenic clots, if recognized, may be removed by using suction on the catheter (Fr. 8 catheter).[258]

Patching the "Holey" Vessel

The hole made after the needle puncture and catheter insertion is repaired by: (1) formation and consolidation of a fibrin plug; (2) endothelialization of the fibrin plug; (3) organization of the plug from the adventitia in approximately ten days; and (4) maturation of the scar in approximately thirty days. As early as *eighteen hours* after angiography there is evidence of *endothelialization* which smooths the irregularities of the vessel wall.[249] *Multiple catheterizations* at the same site of entry can cause intimal hyperplasia, collagen deposition, fibroblastic proliferation, and organization of thrombus with recanalization. The presence of these lesions does not correlate with the number of catheterizations. Partial occlusions with slow flow, intraarterial localized excrescences, or

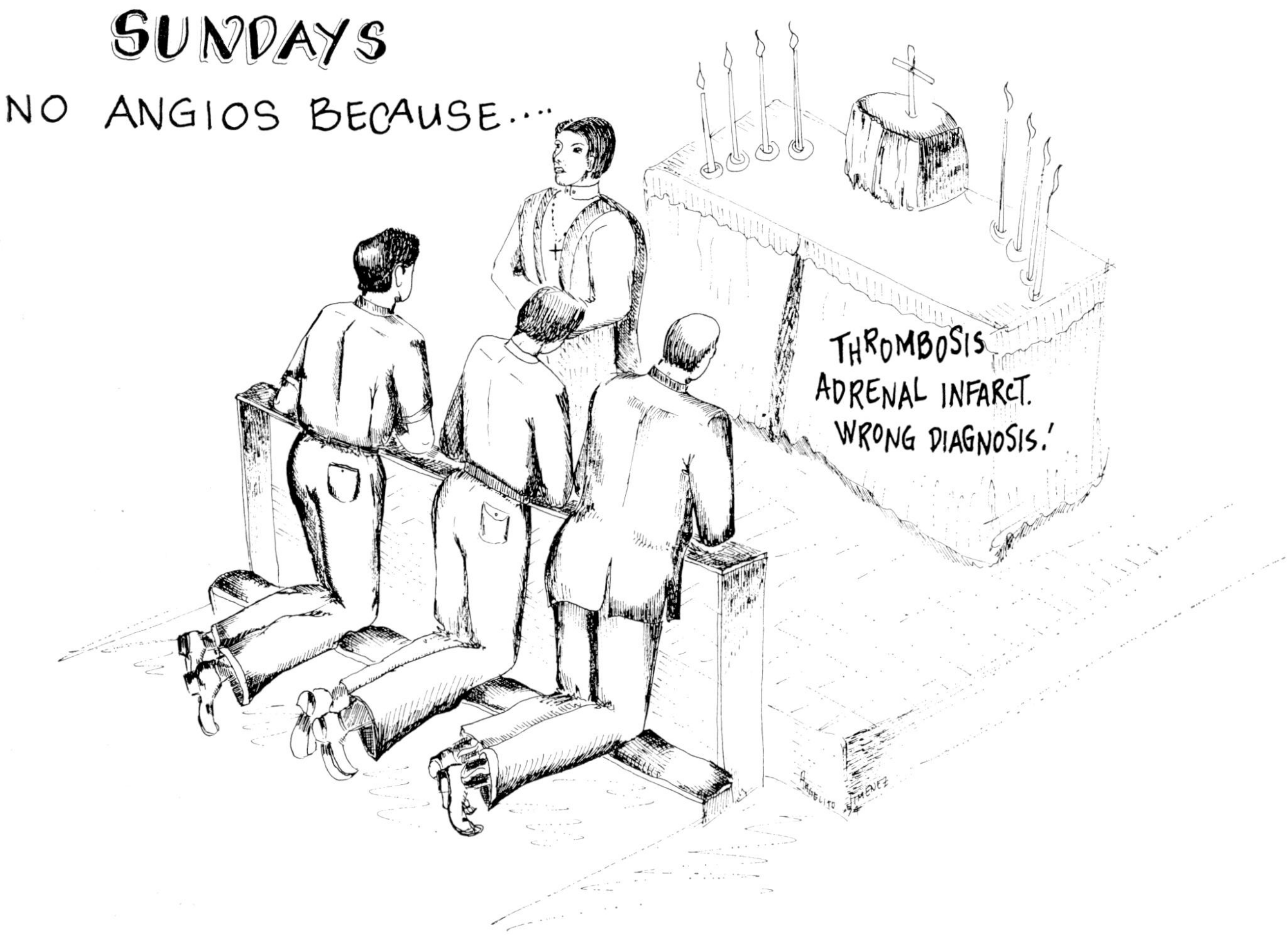

Figure 8.8

small dissections may be significant in persons with already compromised circulation and limited collaterals.[250]

COMPLICATIONS—WHOSE FAULT?

All complications occurring within forty-eight hours following vascular opacification are considered as secondary to the procedure. An overall survey revealed a total complication rate of 1.02 percent, mostly renal or neurological. Fatal complications occurred in 0.28 percent of the cases and nonfatal complications in 0.74 percent.[245–247] In actuality, *some of the postangiographic complications were the result of the underlying primary disease for which the angiography was performed.* There was a striking similarity in the incidence and character of untoward reactions occurring within forty-eight hours prior to angiography and those occurring in the forty-eight hours following the procedure. In other words, myocardial infarctions, thrombophlebitis, atrial fibrillation, etc. occurred as frequently before as after angiography.[248]

CHAPTER 9

TREATMENT OF COMPLICATIONS

EMERGENCY MEDICATIONS

CONSULTATION with an anesthesiologist and a cardiologist is mandatory before setting up an emergency cart with all the necessary aids to combat anaphylaxis, cardiac arrest, convulsions, etc. *This emergency cart should be available at all times in the special procedure room.* Biweekly inventory and immediate replenishment of the used medications following an emergency will avoid tragic embarrassments at subsequent time of need. All medications should be clearly labeled and arranged in order to facilitate administration at the time of emergency. If there is standardization of emergency carts throughout the hospital, then the cart in the angiographic suite should conform with those used elsewhere.

It goes without saying that blood pressure apparatus, stethoscope, EKG monitor and defibrillator are essential. Plenty of needles and syringes, intubation equipment, padded tongue blades, intravenous fluids and connecting tubing, suction apparatus, and oxygen cylinder should be within reach of hands in the angiography room. Emergency medications on the cart should include aminophylline, atropine sulfate, epinephrine (1:1000), sodium bicarbonate, calcium chloride, Benadryl®, barbiturates, steroids, isoproterenol, levophed, pronestyl, and digoxin.

TREATMENT

The uncommon and infrequent occurrence of severe complications tends to make the radiologist complacent and ill-prepared to cope with an emergency that will one day come.[161, 263] The cardiac arrest team is called immediately and at the same time *cardiac compression* is started at the rate of sixty per minute in adults and sixty to ninety per minute in infants and children. The *airway* should be restored and every third or fourth cardiac compression, ventilation should be instituted. If the heartbeat is not restored in three minutes, *intracardiac epinephrine* (0.2 cc of 1:1000) should be administered. For allergic reactions epinephrine (0.3 to 0.5 cc of 1:1000) should be administered. Benadryl may be given for allergic reactions at the dosage of 25 to 50 mgm intravenously. The dose of prednisolone phosphate is 100 mgm intravenously. Asthmatic patients are given aminophylline 500 mgm intravenously.

If one practices at a hospital with other specialists available, consultation with them regarding the management of complications is mandatory. In addition, when patients with diseases that have a higher complication rate have angiography, it is advisable to have a consultant available in the department during a procedure. It is reassuring to both radiologist and patient to have a cardiologist available when doing an arch study in someone with known arteriosclerotic coronary artery disease or pheochromocytoma.

Spinal Complications

Treatment involves immediate lumbar puncture with removal of cerebrospinal fluid, 10 cc at a time, replacing it with the same amount of isotonic saline.[188]

Arterial Spasm

Heparinization and injection of papaverine hydrochloride is beneficial. However, papaverine is contraindicated in patients with cardiac disease. Venospasm is treated by the local application of hot, moist packs, and if no prompt return, heparinization is begun.

Hematomas

Local application of hot packs and bed rest is beneficial. If they are sizeable, causing pressure effects on adjacent nerves, then surgical drainage of the hematoma should be considered.

Convulsions

Intravenous barbiturates are administered until the convulsions cease.

CHAPTER 10

VASCULAR STRUCTURES, FLOW, VELOCITY AND PRESSURES

THE STRUCTURE OF VESSELS

Arteries

Large conducting arteries such as the aorta, innominate, subclavian, beginning of the common carotid, and origin of the pulmonary arteries are rich in elastic tissues. Arteries of *medium size* are rich in muscular tissue. *Distributing arteries* such as the renals, superior and inferior mesenterics, radial, ulnar, popliteal and deep femoral arteries have a large amount of muscular tissue in the media and more nervous tissue in the adventitia. The different layers of the vessels which are very distinct in large vessels are indistinguishable in the arterioles. The smaller arteries are 2 mm or less in size; arterioles occur within the organ. Any artery which is less than 100 microns in diameter is considered an arteriole. As the smooth muscle increases, there is a relative decrease in the amount of elastic tissue; and at the level of arterioles, there is no elastic tissue at all[111] (Fig. 10-1).

It is interesting to note the higher incidence of *nonatherosclerotic diseases* involving the *medium and small distributing arteries.* These diseases include angiitis; thromboangiitis; hyperplastic diseases of intima, media, and adventitia, with the exception being aortitis. *Atherosclerotic diseases* tend to spare medium and small vessels, demonstrating an affinity for the *large, elastic, conducting arteries.*

Veins

These are thin-walled vessels with poorly developed media and uneven distribution of a thin adventitia[111] (Fig. 10-1). The cross-sectional area of the large cavae are at least four times greater than the aorta.[52] When an artery or vein bifurcates, the sum of the cross-sectional area of its branches exceeds that of the parent vessel.[182] The walls of large arteries and the large veins are thick and tough. Their bursting pressures range in the thousands of millimeters of mercury.[187]

FLOW, VELOCITY AND PRESSURE

In an artery, the layer of blood immediately adjacent to the wall of the vessel moves at a very slow rate. As one moves toward the lumen of the vessel, subsequent layers of blood flow at progressively faster velocities. When the velocity exceeds a critical level, turbulence of flow occurs.[187] Distal to the aortic and pulmonary valves the flow is very turbulent, and laminar flow occurs only in the center of the descending aorta.[220] *Bloodflow*[52] varies from vessel to vessel. In the liver the flow rate is 1450 cc per minute, contributed to by the mesenteric and gastric circulation (850 cc per minute), splenic and pancreatic flow (250 cc per minute), and the hepatic artery (360 cc per minute). The flow[234] in the left gastric artery is 5 cc per second (300 cc per minute); in the hepatic artery it is 6 cc per second (360 cc per minute), and to the kidney 10 cc per second (600 cc per minute).

Venous Flow

In the superior and inferior vena cava, venous flow is phasic and pulsatile, varying with different phases of circulation and different times in the cardiac cycle. Flow in the inferior vena cava is two to three times faster than in the superior. Tachycardia and bradycardia influence flow in the superior vena cava, but not in the inferior. During inspiration, velocity increases and flow decreases.[300, 354, 407]

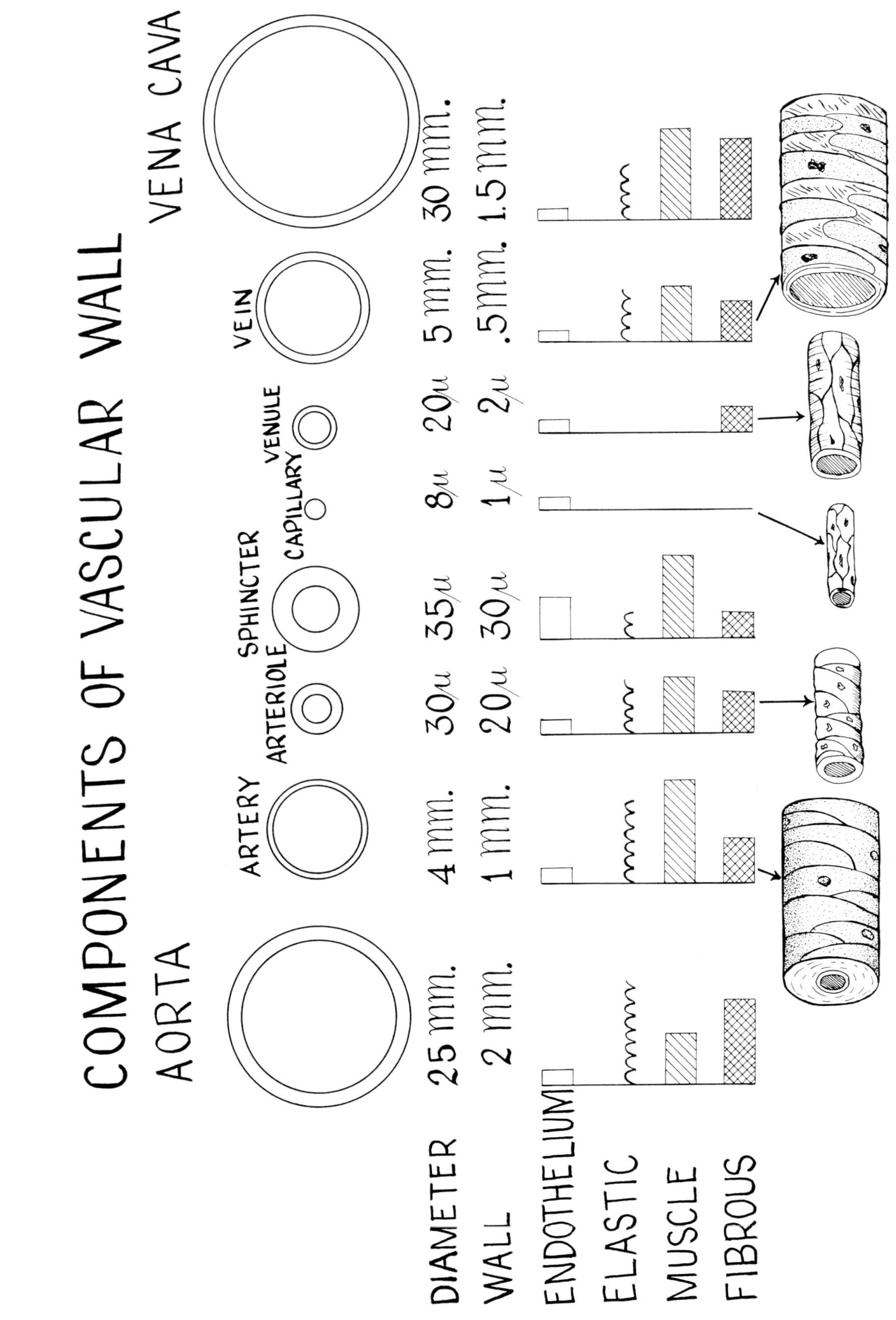

Figure 10.1. (Courtesy of Dr. Robert F. Rushmer, Professor of Physiology and Biophysics, University of Washington Medical School and W. B. Saunders and Company from *Cardiovascular Dynamics*, second edition, 1961.)

Vertebral Veins

The flow in the vertebral veins is influenced by the position of the body. In the upright position cerebral circulation drains through the vertebral veins, while in a head down position the vertebral veins drain the distal part of the body. In other words, as the body becomes erect the upper part of the vertebral plexus opens and the lower part closes. The reverse happens when the head is down. In decubitus position, both ends are closed.[403]

Vertebral Artery

Blood flow in the vertebral artery decreases when the face is turned away from the side being measured. Even temporary occlusion of the subclavian, proximal to the origin of the vertebral artery, causes increased blood flow in the vertebral artery.[270]

Hepatic Veins

Normally there is reflux into the hepatic veins from the inferior vena cava during expiration. This does not occur in people with hepatic cirrhosis.[407]

Valsalva Maneuver and the Vessel

At the beginning of the valsalva maneuver the blood in the lungs and heart is squeezed out of the thorax, causing a transient increase in the systemic blood pressure. This is immediately followed by decreased venous return to the heart causing the systolic pressure to fall, reaching a plateau in seven to eight seconds. By now the systolic blood pressure has diminished by 50 percent and the diastolic pressure by 30 percent. The cardiac output diminishes by 48 percent. *This is an opportune time to inject contrast after eight seconds of sustained straining.* This injected contrast is driven into the smaller peripheral vessels due to the rebound phenomena that follows the sustained straining.[413, 424] *Syncope* can occur after valsalva due to decrease in the cerebral blood flow and associated hyperventilation. The fall in cerebral blood flow is obviously related to fall in the systolic pressure.[493] At the same time *coronary artery perfusion will also be decreased.*

The caval flow decreases markedly with even a segmental collapse due to the fluid from a high pressure chamber flowing into a low pressure chamber.[494] During an increase in intra-abdominal pressure above 40 cm of water, pelvic venous flow is directed by ascending lumbar veins, vertebral veins, and the azygos veins.[495] Contrast in the peripheral (upper extremity) veins may stop at the first rib simulating obstruction, and the pressure in the antecubital vein may rise to 500 to 700 mm of water. The normal is 40 to 80 mm of water.[496]

Velocity[52]

Under basal condition the flow rate in the aorta is 33 cm per second—mean velocity, and almost nothing during diastole. The flow in other arteries is 25 cm per second, in capillaries 0.5 mm per second, and in the veins 8 cm per second.

Normal Venous Pressures

In the portal system[11, 52] portal vein pressure is 10 mm Hg, splenic pulp pressure 3 to 13 mm Hg, free hepatic vein pressure (FHVP) 1 to 5 mm Hg, and wedge hepatic vein pressure (WHVP) 3 to 11 mm Hg.

WHVP—FHVP equals corrected sinusoidal pressure. *The normal corrected hepatic sinusoidal pressure is approximately 5 mm Hg.*

Pressure in the inferior vena cava[52] is close to 0 mm Hg.

The Kidney

Blood flow to the kidney is approximately 10 cc per second per kidney.[111] The average renal vein capacity is 24 cc, and the average renal artery capacity is 6.2 cc.[498] The normal pressure difference from aorta to renal artery is 13 mm Hg.[497] The dual nature of the intrarenal circulation with its cortical and medullary component results in early rapid perfusion of the cortex and slowed perfusion of the medulla.[264] Functional intrarenal distribution of the blood is characterized by reduction or even complete cessation of flow to the outer two thirds of the cortex with maintenance of normal, or even increased, medullary circulation.[265] Contrast media entering the renal arterial system passes through an excretory site before reaching the venous system.[266] The *nephrogram* may be due to glomerular filtration[267] or contrast in the tubular cells, ducts and veins.[268] The width of the cortex of the kidney is measured from the arcuate veins to the renal margin. The normal cortical width is usually about 45 to 55 percent of the calyceo-marginal distance. This ratio is maintained in many renal diseases except in *sickle cell anemia* where the medulla hypertrophies and the cortex thins.[269]

PART II
TECHNIQUES

CHAPTER 11
ARRANGEMENT OF THE VESSELS

Normal Arrangement Is in Reality One of the Variations[350]

Lumbar Arteries

THESE PAIRED VESSELS arise from the aorta on its posterior surface at the level of the intervertebral disc spaces. They course over the lateral surface of the vertebral bodies and then behind the psoas and quadratus lumborum muscles, giving rise to an *anterior short ramus* and a *longer posterior ramus.* The orifice may be 2.5 to 3.5 mm in diameter. Usually there is one ostium per lumbar artery. Comparatively larger arteries at the level of L. 1 and L. 2 are not unusual. Branches are given to the spinal cord, peritoneum, retroperitoneum and associated muscles[306, 307] (Fig. 11-1 and 11-2).

Inferior Phrenic Arteries

The right and left inferior phrenic arteries arise in order of frequency from either the celiac axis, the aorta, or from the renal arteries. They divide into anterior and posterior rami, supplying the diaphragm inferior vena cava, retroperitoneum, esophagus, renal capsule and pericardium. The posterior branch gives ten to sixty small ramifications to the adrenal gland (Figs. 11-3 and 11-4).[370–373]

CELIAC AXIS

Pancreatic Vessels

There are multiple vessels supplying the head, body and tail of the pancreas.[308–310] Typically, two arise from the gastroduodenal artery;

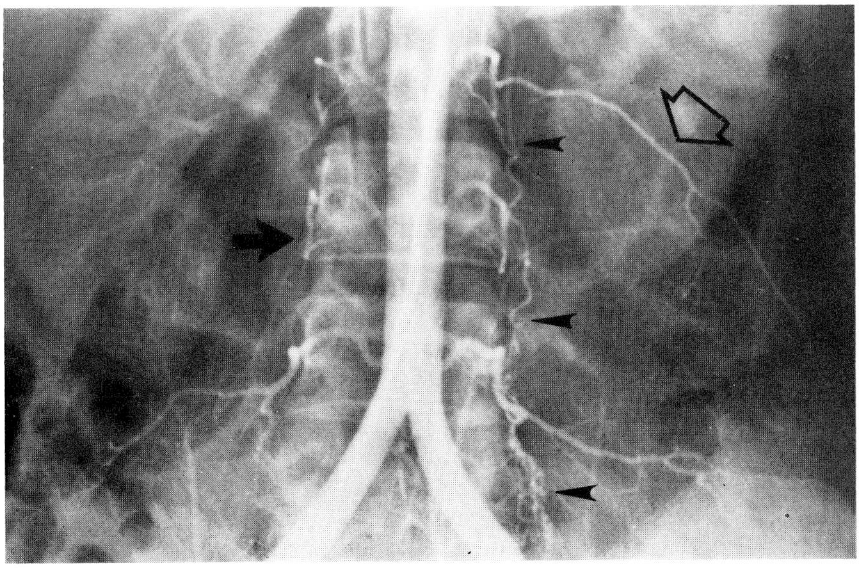

Figure 11.1. Abdominal Aortogram. The lumbar arteries arise from the posterior wall of the aorta and cross the vertebral pedicle. They give off an anterior ramus (Arrow) and a posterior ramus (Blank Arrow). The gonadal artery is also opacified (Arrow Head).

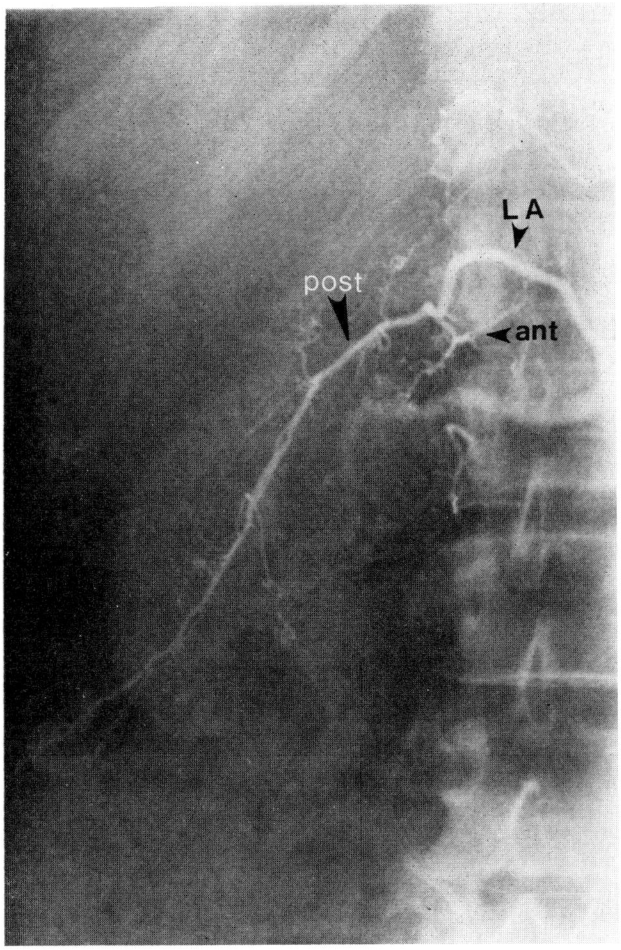

Figure 11.2. Selective Lumbar Arteriogram. Anterior branches (Anterior). Posterior branch (Posterior). *Comment:* Normal lumbar arteriogram.

two from the superior mesenteric artery; one from the splenic, hepatic, or celiac arteries; and multiple small branches from the splenic artery. Except for the vessels arising from the anterior arcade, the other vessels lie predominantly on the posterior surface of the pancreas. The two branches arising from the gastroduodenal artery are the *anterior and posterior superior pancreatico-duodenal arteries.* These anastomose with the corresponding branches from the superior mesenteric artery, via the inferior pancreatico-duodenal arteries. This artery may arise as a single stem and then bifurcate into the anterior and posterior inferior pancreatico-duodenal arteries. This pancreatico-duodenal arcade supplies the head and neck of the pancreas (Fig. 11-6).

The dorsal pancreatic artery supplies the uncinate process and the neck of the pancreas. It may arise from the celiac axis, hepatic artery, or splenic artery. The diameter is usually 1.5 mm, but may vary (Fig. 11-5).

The transverse pancreatic artery is formed by contributions from the dorsal pancreatic, superior mesenteric and pancreatico-duodenal arteries. It courses along the long axis of the pancreas within the pancreatic parenchyma (Fig. 11-5).

The *pancreatica magna* arises from the splenic artery and supplies the tail of the pancreas (Fig. 11-7).

The *short pancreatic branches* from the splenic artery supply the tail of the pancreas (Fig. 11-7).

The dorsal surface of the neck of the pancreas is the site of the confluence of the portal venous circulation. The splenic vein is very intimately related to the superior border of the pancreas. At its origin the middle colic artery has a very important relationship just below the pancreas.

Gastroduodenal Artery

This is one of the main branches of the right hepatic artery and supplies the pancreas via the pancreatico-duodenal arteries.[318] It then continues along the greater curvature of the stomach as the right gastroepiploic artery to anastomose with a corresponding left gastroepiploic artery, which in turn is a branch of the splenic artery. Branches of the gastroepiploic arteries supply the greater curvature aspect of the stomach and epiploic vessels which course into the greater omentum. One of the very important first branches of the gastroduodenal artery is the retroduodenal artery (Fig. 11-6).

Cystic Artery

The cystic artery[322] usually arises from the right hepatic artery. It divides into deep branches to the gall bladder bed and superficial branches to the peritoneal surface. The deep and superficial branches may have separate origins. The cystic artery occasionally arises from the middle or left hepatic or gastroduodenal artery (Figs. 11-35 and 11-36).

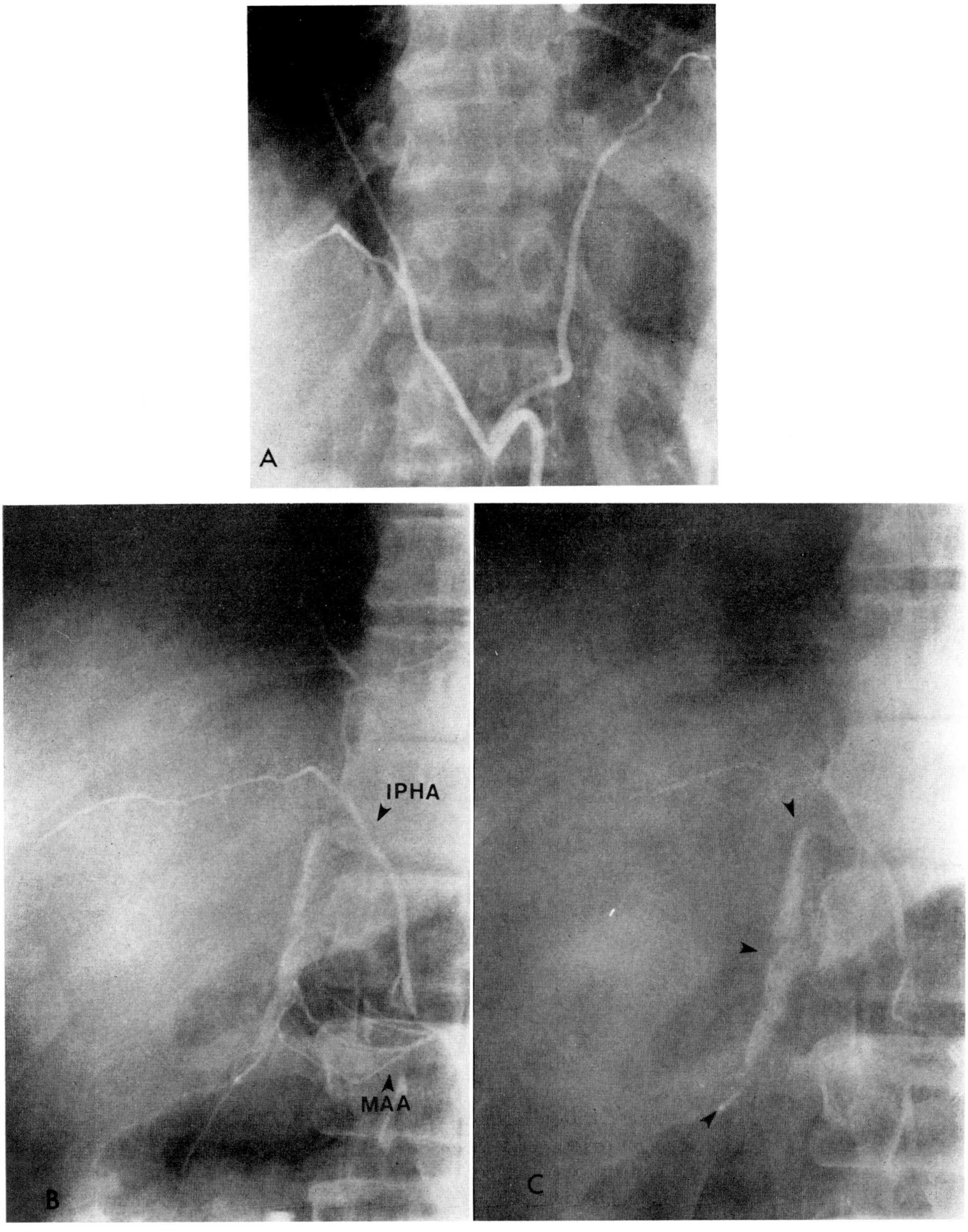

Figure 11.3. Inferior Phrenic Arteriogram. (A) Both the inferior phrenic arteries arise from a common stem in a normal patient. (B) Inferior phrenic artery (I.P.H.A.), middle adrenal arteries (M.A.A.). (C) Stain of the normal adrenal gland. *Comment:* Normal inferior phrenic arteries.

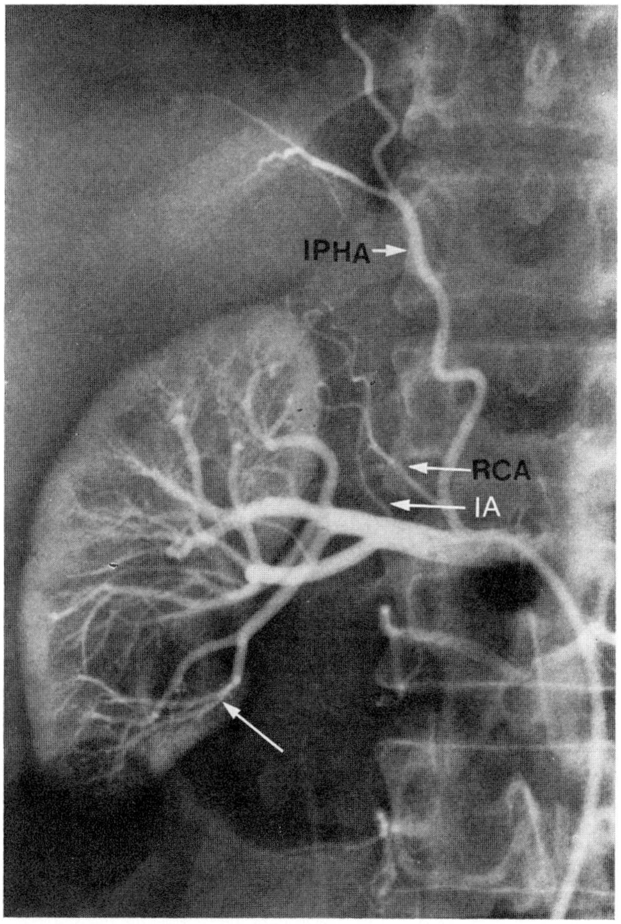

Figure 11.4. Renal Arteriogram. There is opacification of the inferior phrenic artery on the right side (I.P.H.A.), the inferior adrenal artery (I.A.) and the capsular artery (R.C.A.). *Comment:* Note inferior phrenic and renal capsular arising from a common stem. An incidental cyst is also noted in the lower portion of the right kidney (Arrow).

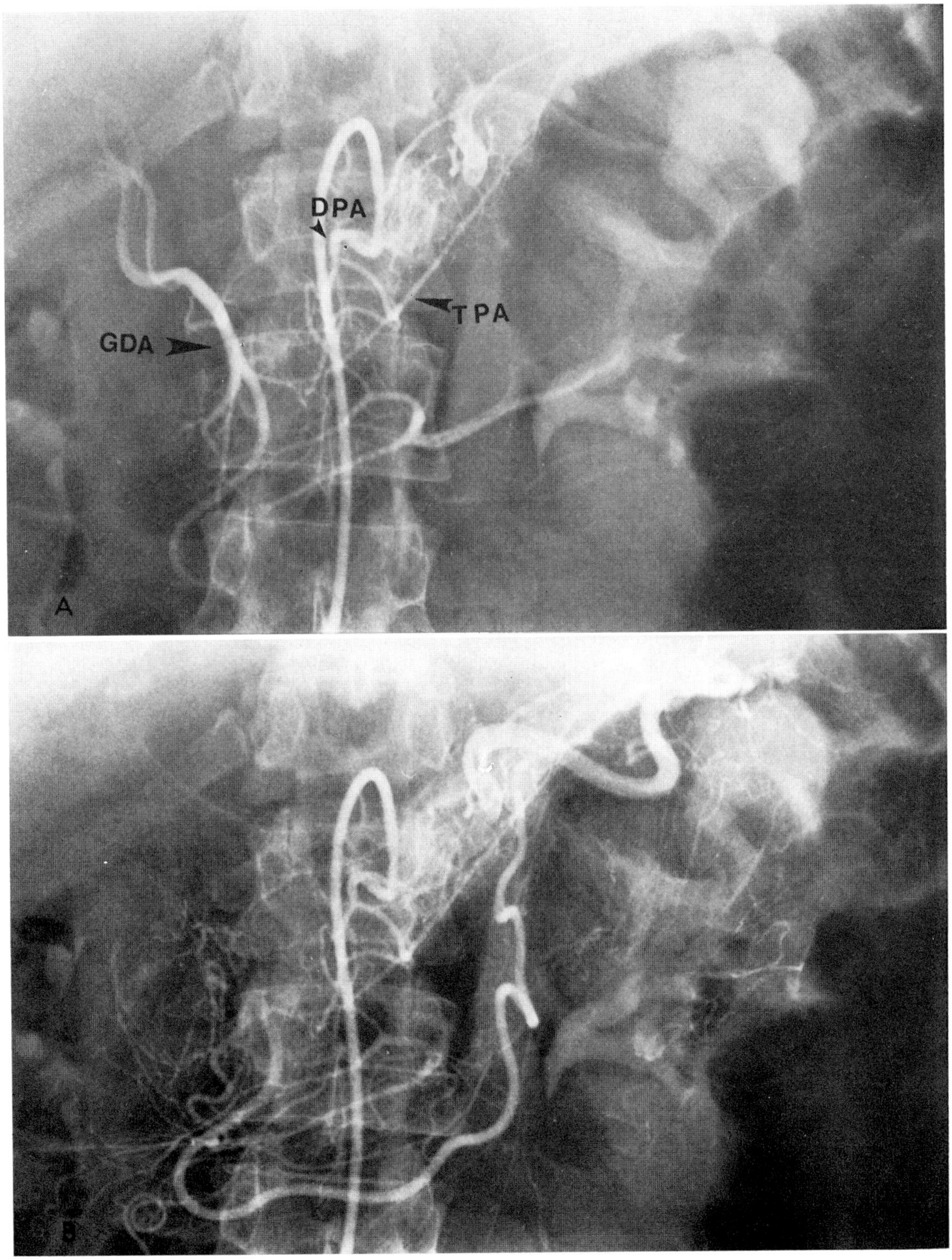

Figure 11.5. Dorsal Pancreatic Arteriogram. (A) Transverse pancreatic artery (T.P.A.), dorsal pancreatic artery (D.P.A.), gastroduodenal artery (G.D.A.). (B) Pancreaticoduodenal branches. *Comment:* Normal.

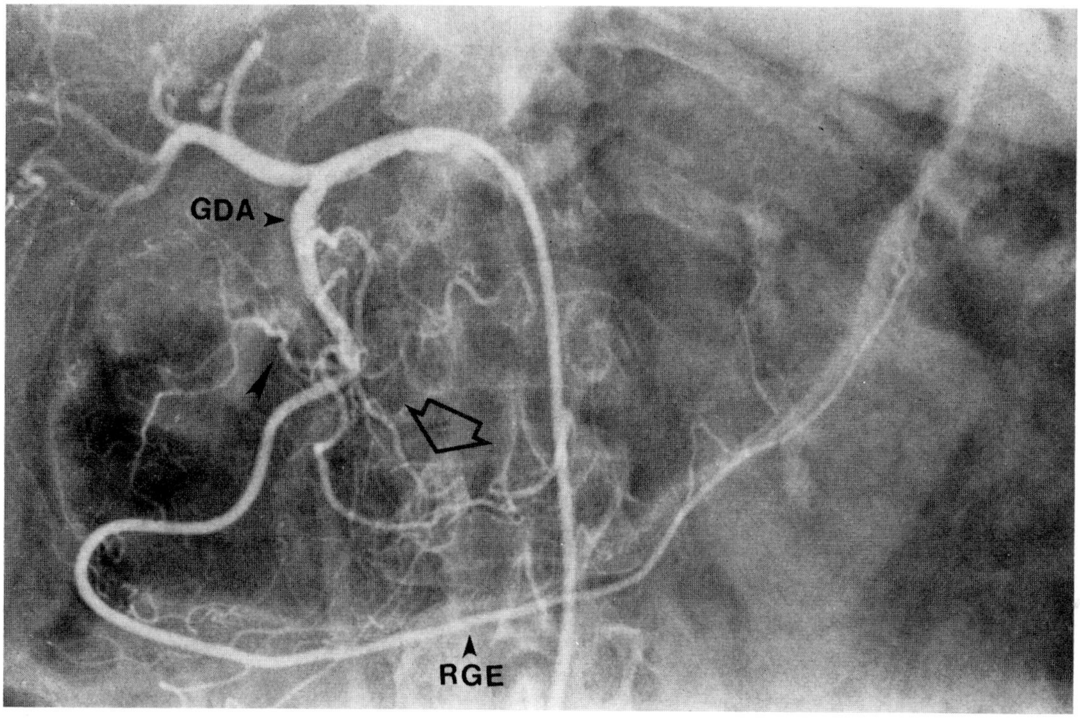

Figure 11.6. Gastroduodenal Arteriogram (G.D.A.). Duodenal branches (Arrow Head), pancreatic branches (Arrow), right gastroepiploic artery (R.G.E.).

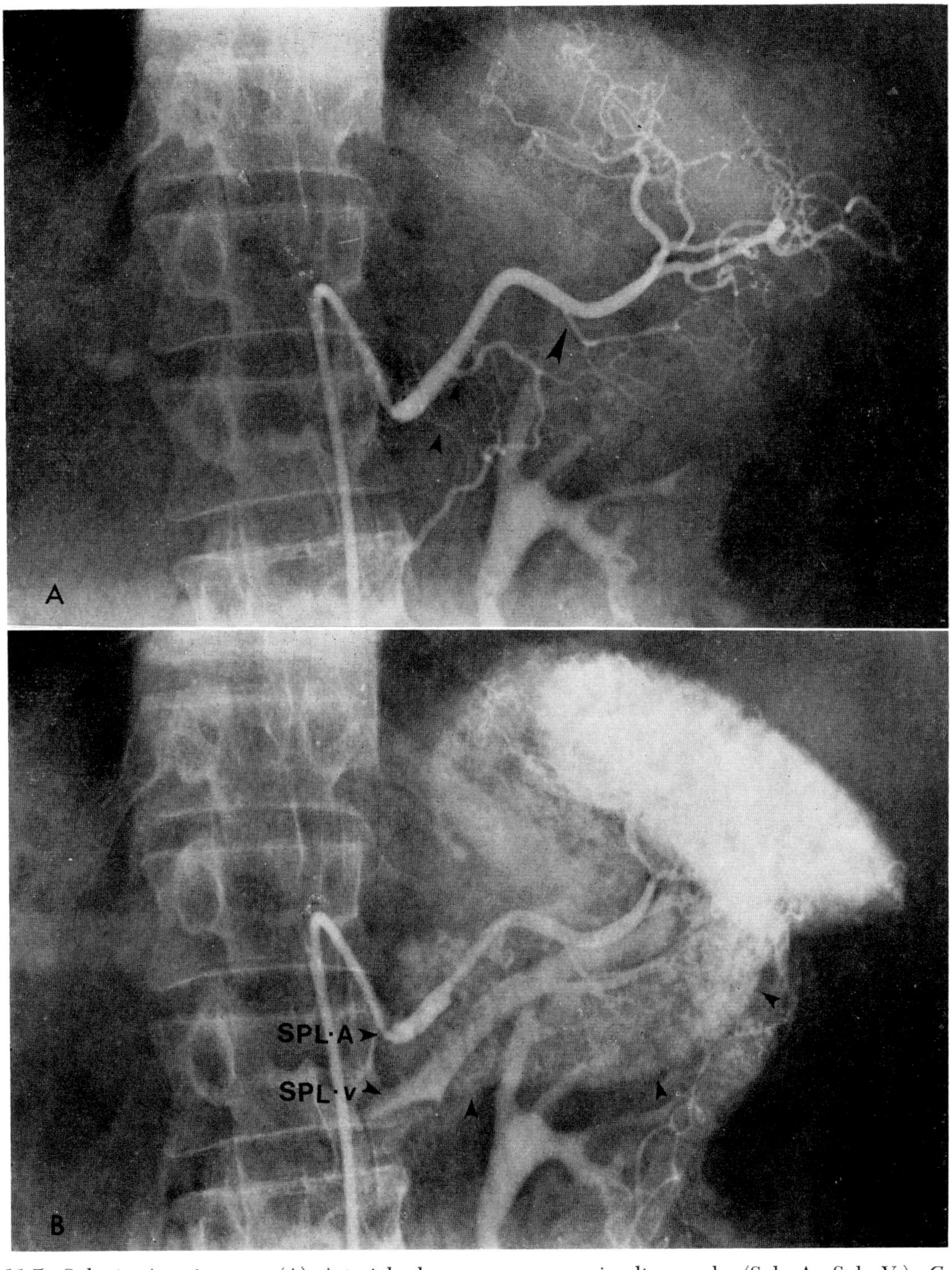

Figure 11.7. Splenic Arteriogram. (A) Arterial phase: Multiple pancreatic branches to the body and tail are seen to arise from the splenic artery. (B) Venous phase: After eight seconds the pancreatic body and tail have a stain (Arrow). Both the splenic artery and vein are seen simultaneously (Spl. A. Spl. V.). *Comment:* Simultaneous opacification of artery and vein are due to prolonged injection of contrast. This may occur anywhere else also during a prolonged arterial injection.

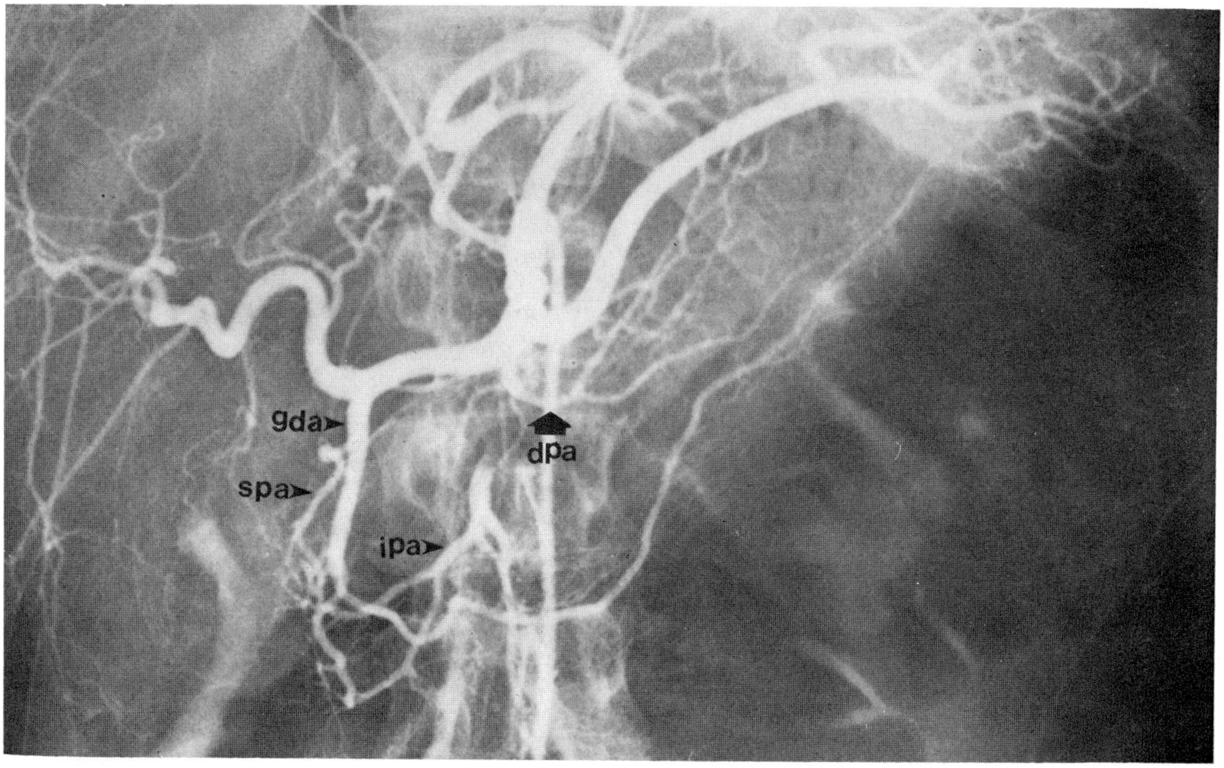

Figure 11.8. Celiac Arteriogram. Gastroduodenal artery (G.D.A.), superior pancreaticoduodenal artery (S.P.A.), inferior pancreaticoduodenal artery (I.P.A.), dorsal pancreatic artery (D.P.A.). *Comment:* Note anatomy of the pancreatic vasculature.

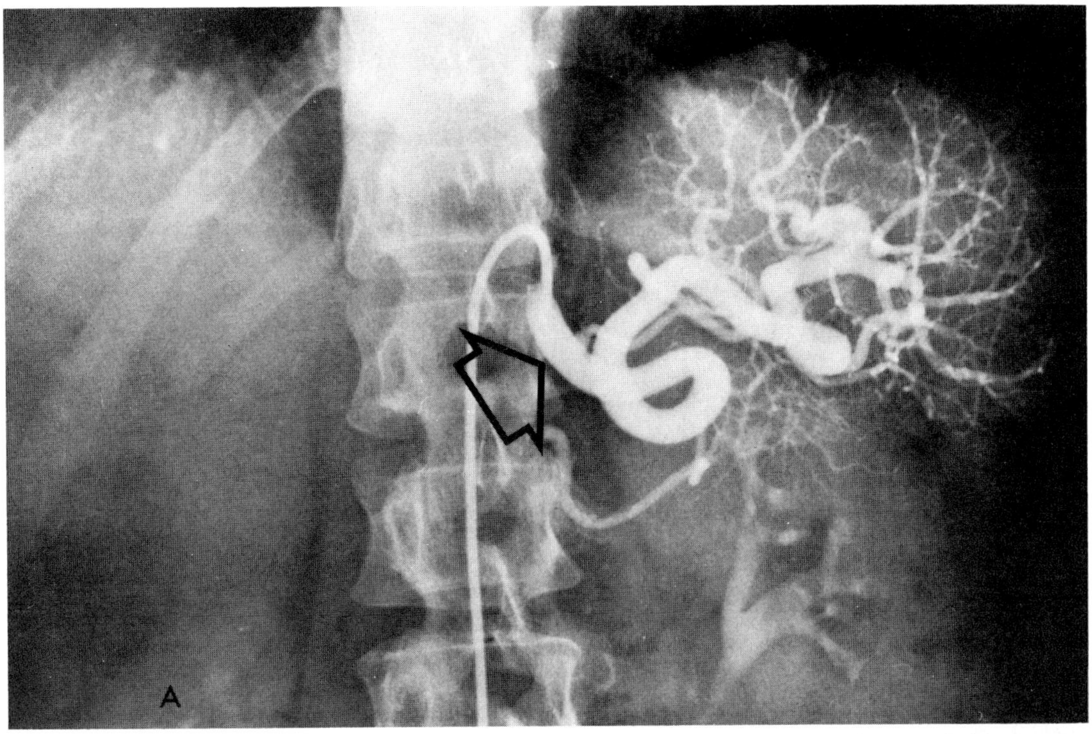

Figure 11.9. Splenic Arteriogram. (A) Arterial phase, (B) Venous phase: Demonstrates diffuse homogeneous opacification of the spleen. Normal staining of the fundus of the stomach (Arrow Heads) and the splenic vein (Blank Arrow) in a normal but recently married young female. Please note the accessory spleen (Arrow) which is very diagnostic of a recent marriage!

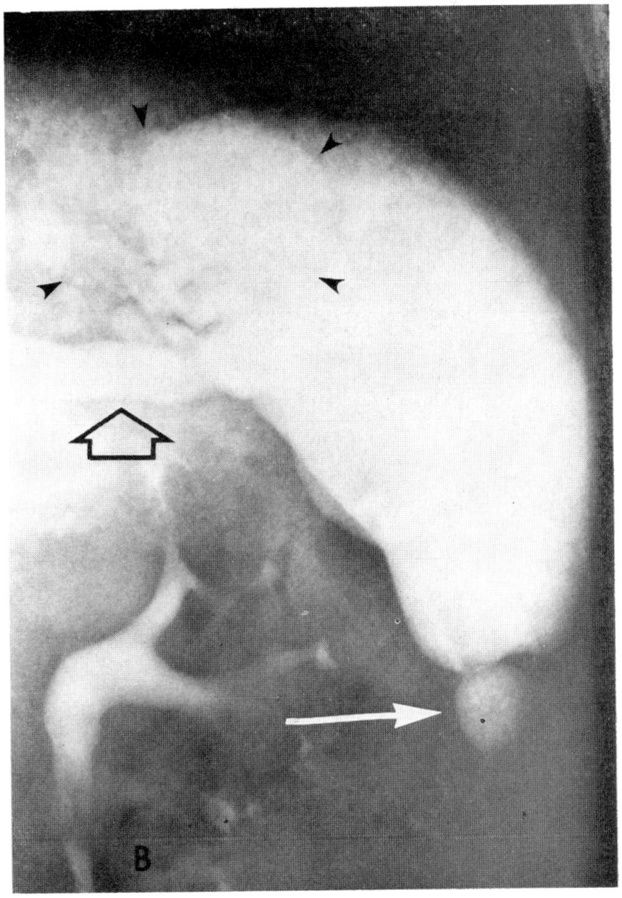

Splenic Artery

This artery[311, 312] usually originates from the celiac artery, but occasionally can have variable origin from the left gastric, left hepatic, superior mesenteric, or other arteries. Rarely there are two splenic arteries. The splenic artery may be arbitrarily divided into different segments in relationship to the pancreas. This would include the suprapancreatic, pancreatic, prepancreatic and prehilar segments. The *suprapancreatic segment* is the first two to three centimeters of the splenic artery. The *pancreatic segment* may be above, behind or even beside the pancreas. This segment is the most tortuous segment of the artery and as it gives pancreatic branches, never stays away from the pancreas. This segment also gives rise to the arteria pancreatica magna. The *prepancreatic segment,* coursing anterior to the

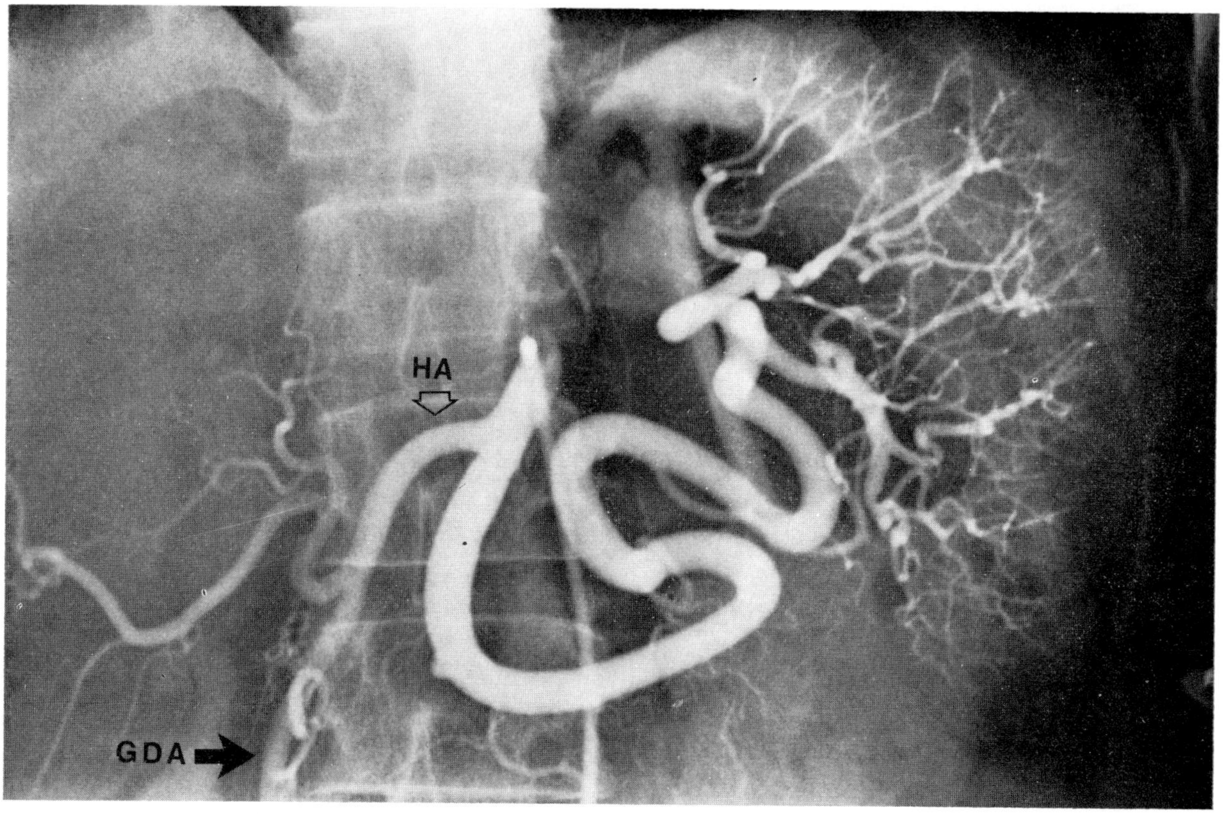

Figure 11.10. Celiac Arteriogram. This is a normal but tortuous splenic artery. In addition, please note the gastroduodenal artery (G.D.A.) and hepatic artery (H.A.). *Comment:* Note dominant splenic artery.

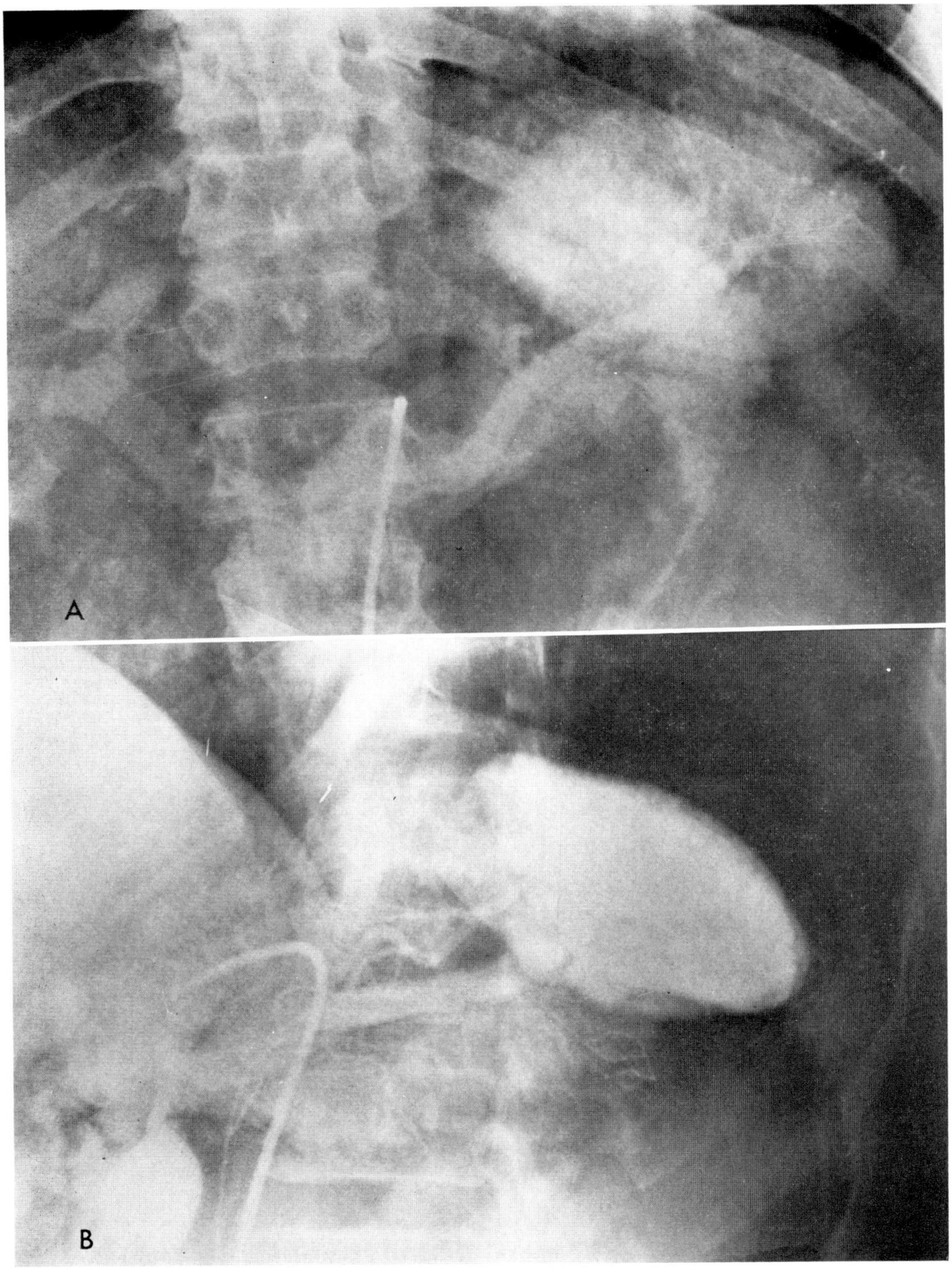

Figure 11.11. Splenic Arteriogram. (A) Venous phase: A.P. projection. This demonstrates a normal splenic parenchymal stain. (B) Venous phase: Right posterior oblique projection. *Comment:* This is a normal spleen. The oblique projection helps to separate overlapping, confusing shadows of the gastric fundus.

Figure 11.12. Celiac Angiogram—venous phase. The right posterior oblique projection reveals the splenic borders well. The bullet is anterior to the spleen.

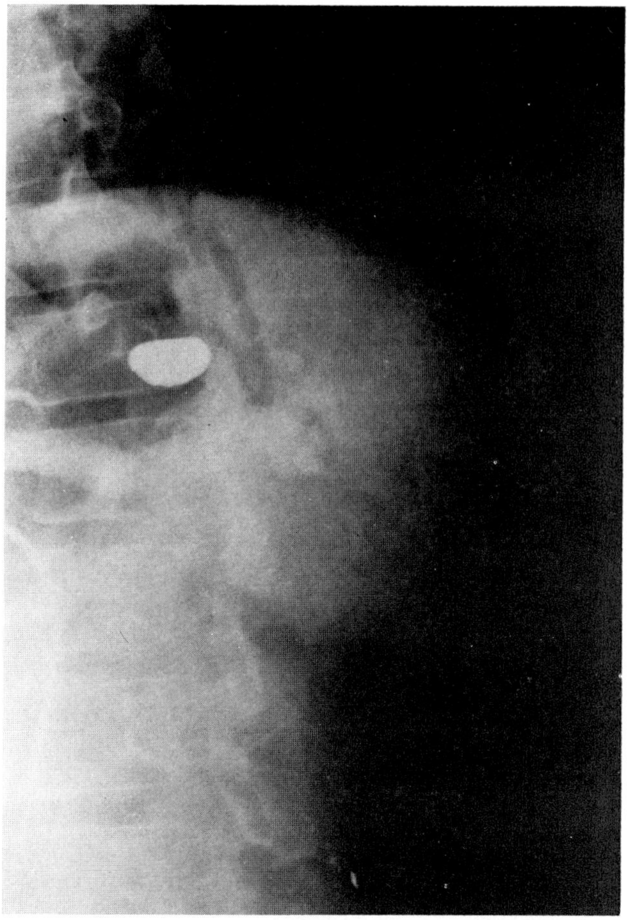

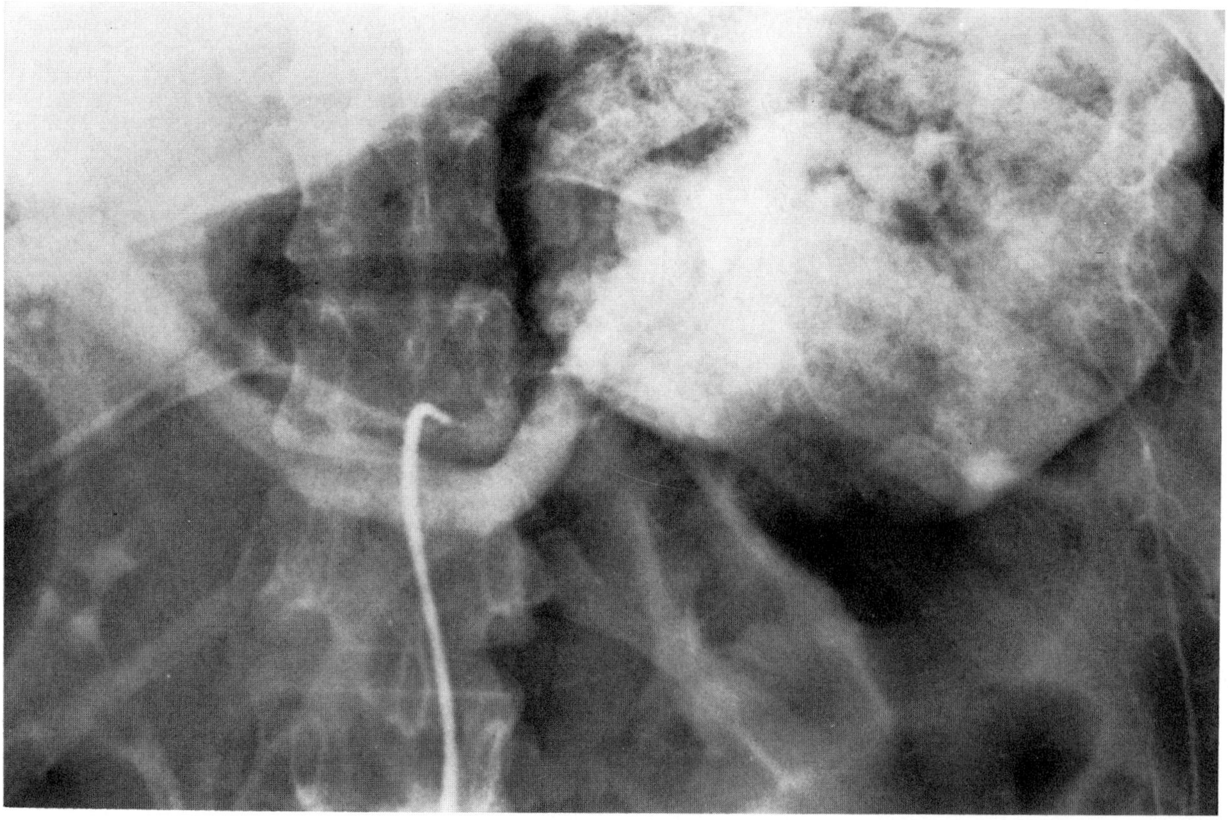

Figure 11.13. Celiac Arteriogram—Venous Phase. The hilum of the spleen faces anteriorly giving an enface projection.

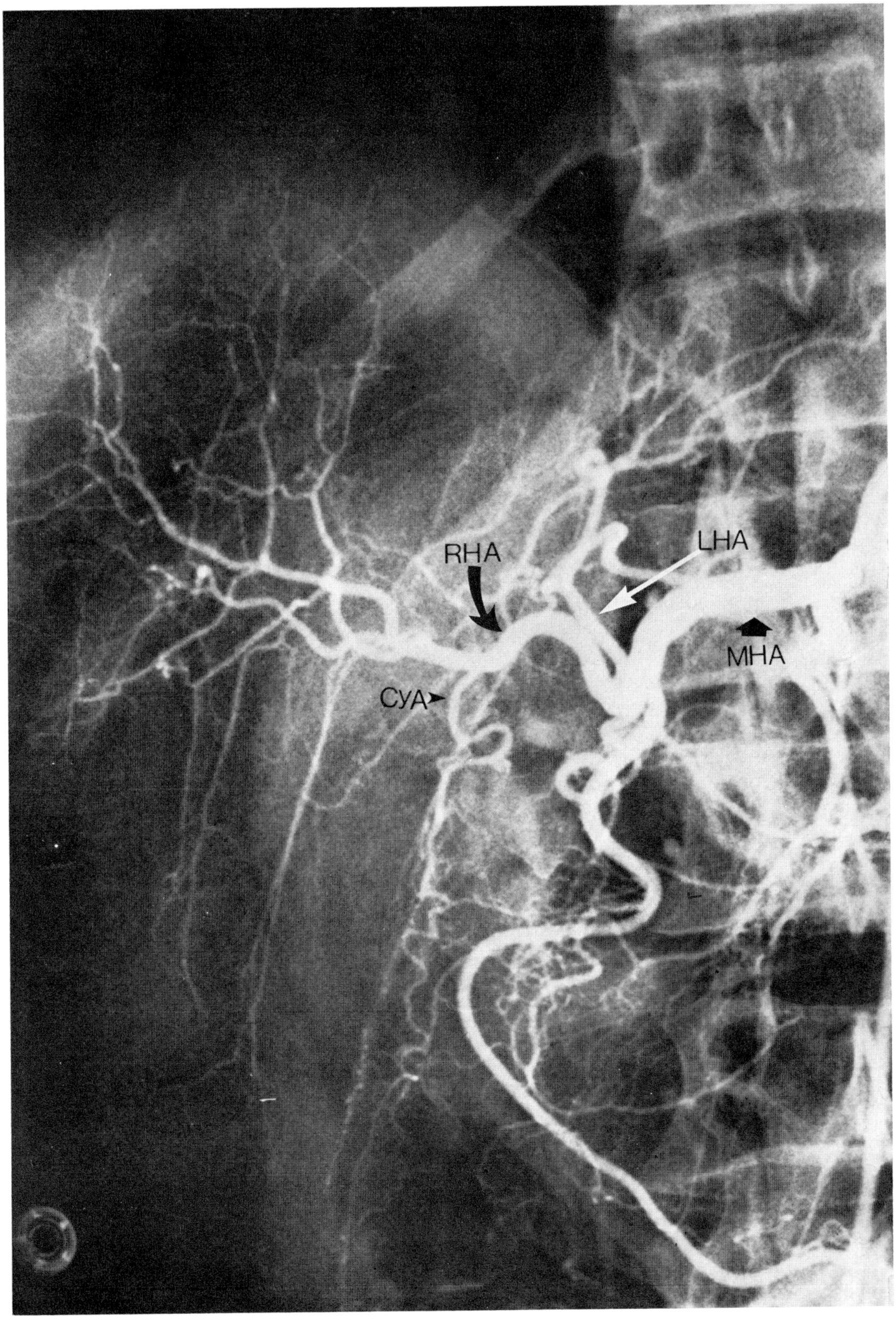

Figure 11.14. Hepatic Arteriogram. Good opacification of main hepatic (M.H.A.), right hepatic artery (R.H.A.), left hepatic artery (L.H.A.), cystic artery (Cy. A.). *Comment:* Normal.

pancreas, gives rise to the left gastroepiploic artery. The prehilar segment is the terminal segment lying between the tail of the pancreas and the hilum of the spleen. The splenic artery may divide into its hilar branches either from the distal segment (magistral type—30%) or from the proximal segment (distributed type).

The size of the spleen does not decide the number of intrasplenic branches. Notched spleens have more branches than smooth spleens. Supernumerary branches from the splenic artery are not unusual. These would include the left hepatic, left gastric, accessory left hepatic, middle colic, right gastric, and dorsal pancreatic arteries. The spleen is covered by the peritoneal sac except at the hilus. It is not fixed by any peritoneal folds. The splenic capsule has smooth muscle within, but comparatively less in humans than in animals[313] (Figs. 11-9 to 11-13).

The Left Gastroepiploic Artery

The left gastroepiploic artery[311] originates from the splenic artery either proximal to its termination or from its inferior terminal branch. It courses along the greater curvature of the stomach in the anterior layer of the greater omentum. It may be adjacent to or far removed from the gastric border. This artery terminates by anastomosing with the corresponding artery from the right side via numerous branches rather than as a single vessel. It supplies branches to the fundus of the stomach and tail of the pancreas, and epiploic vessels to the omental plexus (Fig. 11-16).

Hepatic Arteries

If there is a conventional arrangement of the blood vessels arising from the celiac axis, then the common hepatic artery[318] gives rise to the right, middle and left hepatic arteries (Fig. 11-14). The hepatic arteries may also be derived from the superior mesenteric artery or the left gastric arteries either partially or totally. The intrahepatic supply is segmental with more variations in the left hepatic segmental supply.[320, 321] The middle hepatic may arise from either the left or right hepatic artery; it supplies the caudate lobe. There are no accessory hepatic arteries, as each one is an end artery with a selective distribution to a definite area of the liver. They cannot be sacrificed without necrosis of that portion of the liver.[322]

When a hepatic artery arises from a vessel other than the celiac, it is aberrant. There are two types of aberrant vessels, an "accessory" artery and a "replaced" artery. An *accessory* artery is the term used when there is also a normal right and left hepatic artery arising directly from the celiac axis. It is a *replaced* artery when the normal right hepatic from the celiac is absent and arises instead from the superior mesenteric or left gastric arteries. "Accessory" is an additive; "replaced" is a substitute. An aberrant right hepatic artery usually arises from

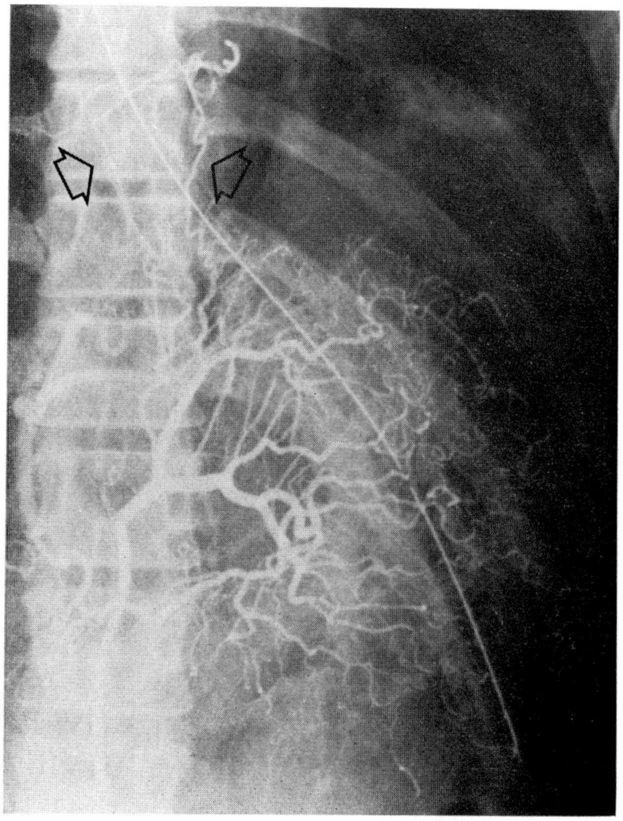

Figure 11.15. Normal Left Gastric Arteriogram. Notice also the esophageal branches (arrows).

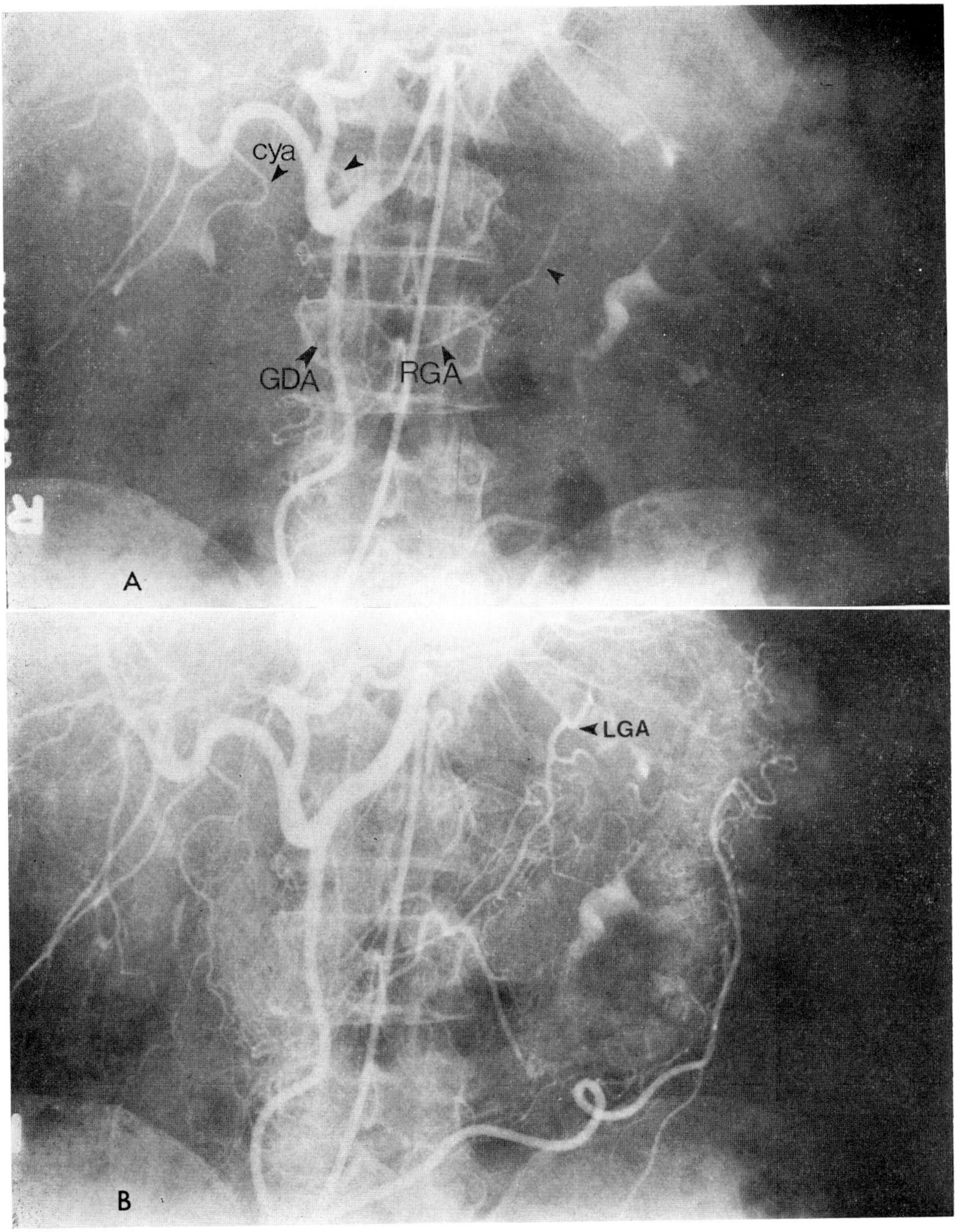

Figure 11.16. Hepatic Arteriogram. (A) There is good opacification of right gastric artery (R.G.A.), cystic artery (Cy. A.), gastroduodenal artery (G.D.A.). (B) The same right gastric artery perfuses the left gastric artery (L.G.A.). Further opacification of the branches of the cystic artery is noted. *Comment:* Normal. Also seen is the opacification of the left gastroepiploic artery along the greater curvature of the stomach.

the superior mesenteric artery, and an aberrant left hepatic artery usually arises from the left gastric artery.[318]

The liver has an anterior and posterior segment in the right lobe and a medial and lateral segment in the left lobe.[323]

Left Gastric Artery

The left gastric artery,[337] which is the smallest of the three branches of the celiac axis, has an average diameter of 4 mm. It courses first upward and then to the left toward the cardiac end of the stomach. Then the artery passes between the layers of the lesser omentum to follow the lesser curvature of the stomach, eventually anastomosing with the corresponding artery from the right side. This artery supplies the distal end of the esophagus and the proximal portion of the stomach. It is not unusual for it to give origin to an aberrant left hepatic artery (Fig. 11-15).

Right Gastric Artery

A very infrequently seen branch during angiography, the right gastric artery is usually a branch of the common hepatic artery. Sometimes it arises from the left hepatic, or even the gastroduodenal artery. It anastomoses with the corresponding left gastric artery[318] (Fig. 11-16).

Celiac Artery

This median unpaired trunk arises from the anterior border of the aorta between T. 12 and L. 1. In relation to the diaphragm, it may be above the arcuate ligament or at the same level. This is due to a low ligament rather than a high origin. This is more common in endomorphic or mesomorphic individuals, or in females.[317] The celiac artery has a mean diameter of 7 mm and passes horizontally above the upper margin of the pancreas to divide into three branches.[337] In the most common, conventional arrange-

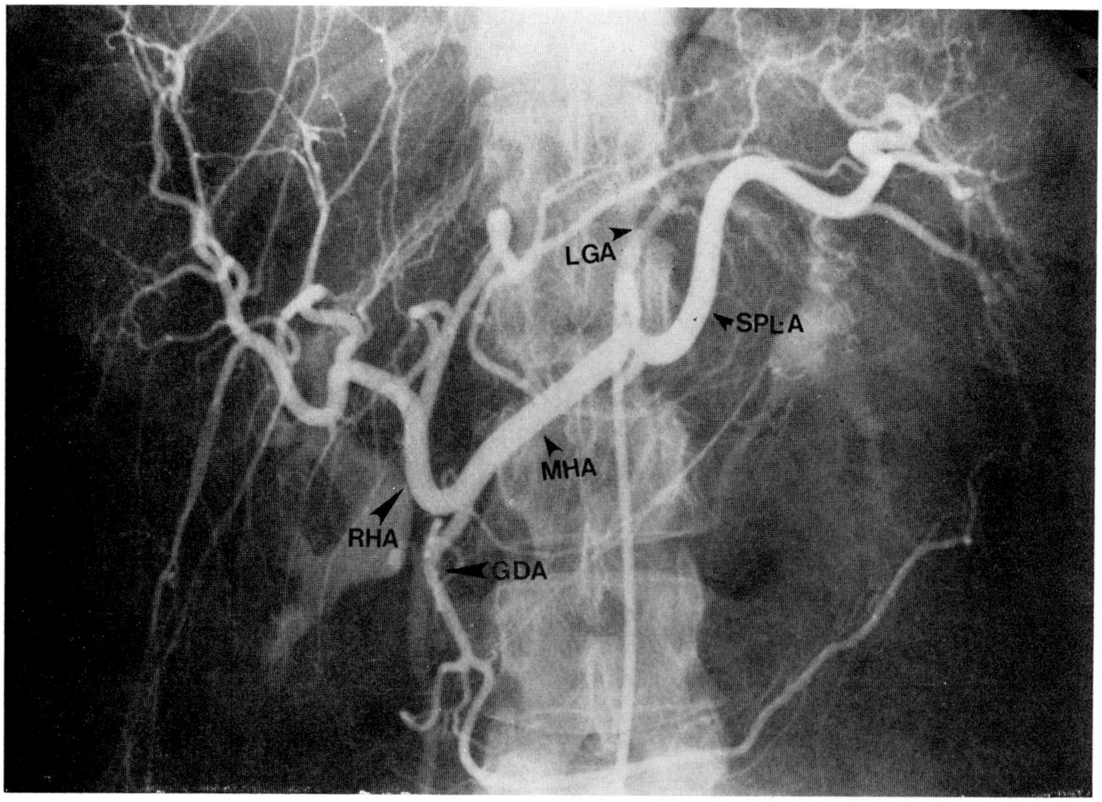

Figure 11.17. Celiac Arteriogram. Main hepatic artery (M.H.A.), gastroduodenal artery (G.D.A.), right hepatic artery (R.H.A.), left gastric artery (L.G.A.), and splenic artery (Spl. A.). *Comment:* Note conventional arrangement of the vessels.

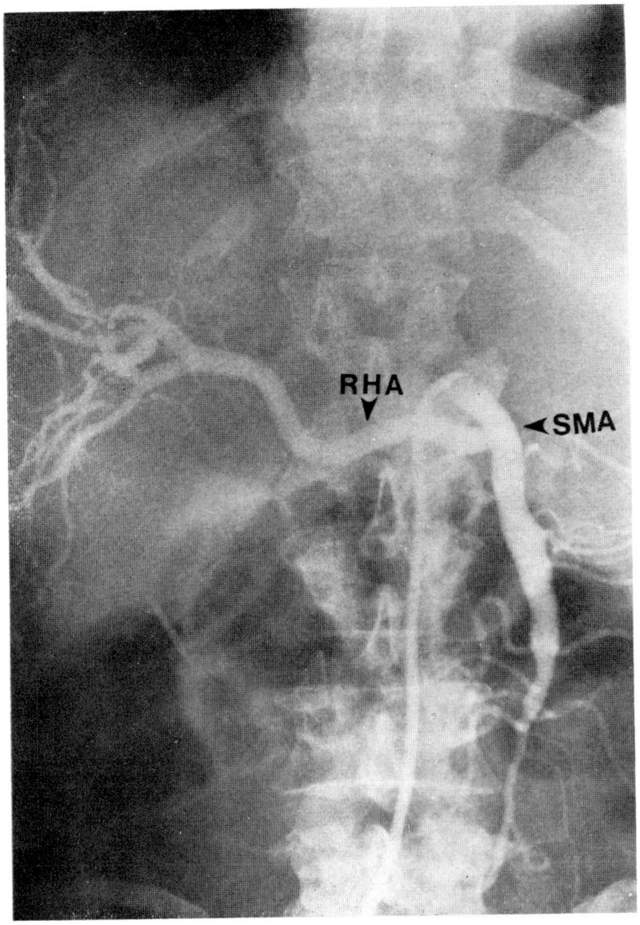

Figure 11.18. Superior Mesenteric Arteriogram. The superior mesenteric artery and the replaced right hepatic artery opacify simultaneously.

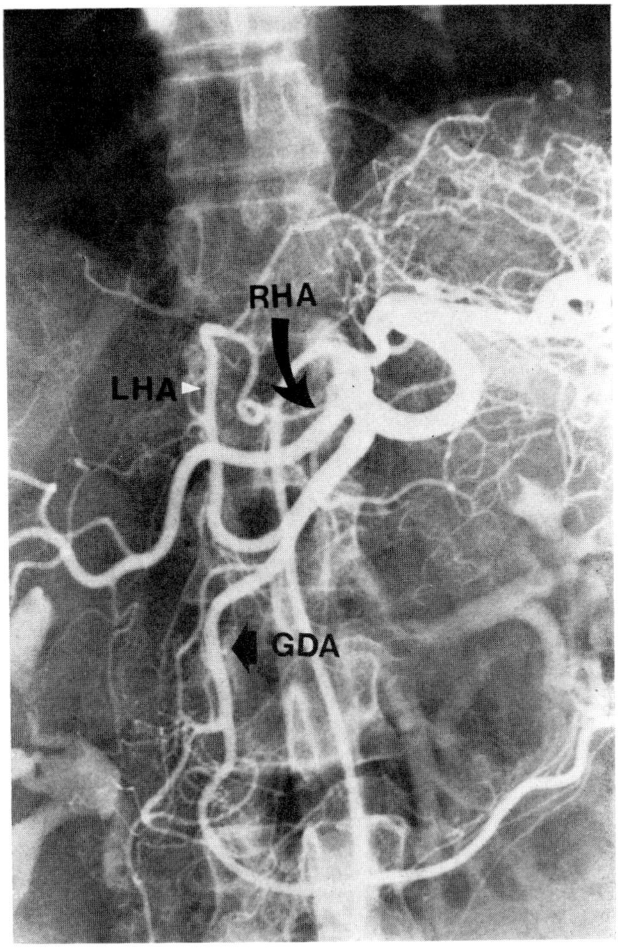

Figure 11.19. Celiac Arteriogram. The right hepatic artery arises directly from the celiac axis (R.H.A.). There is a common origin of the left hepatic and gastroduodenal (L.H.A.) (G.D.A.) arteries.

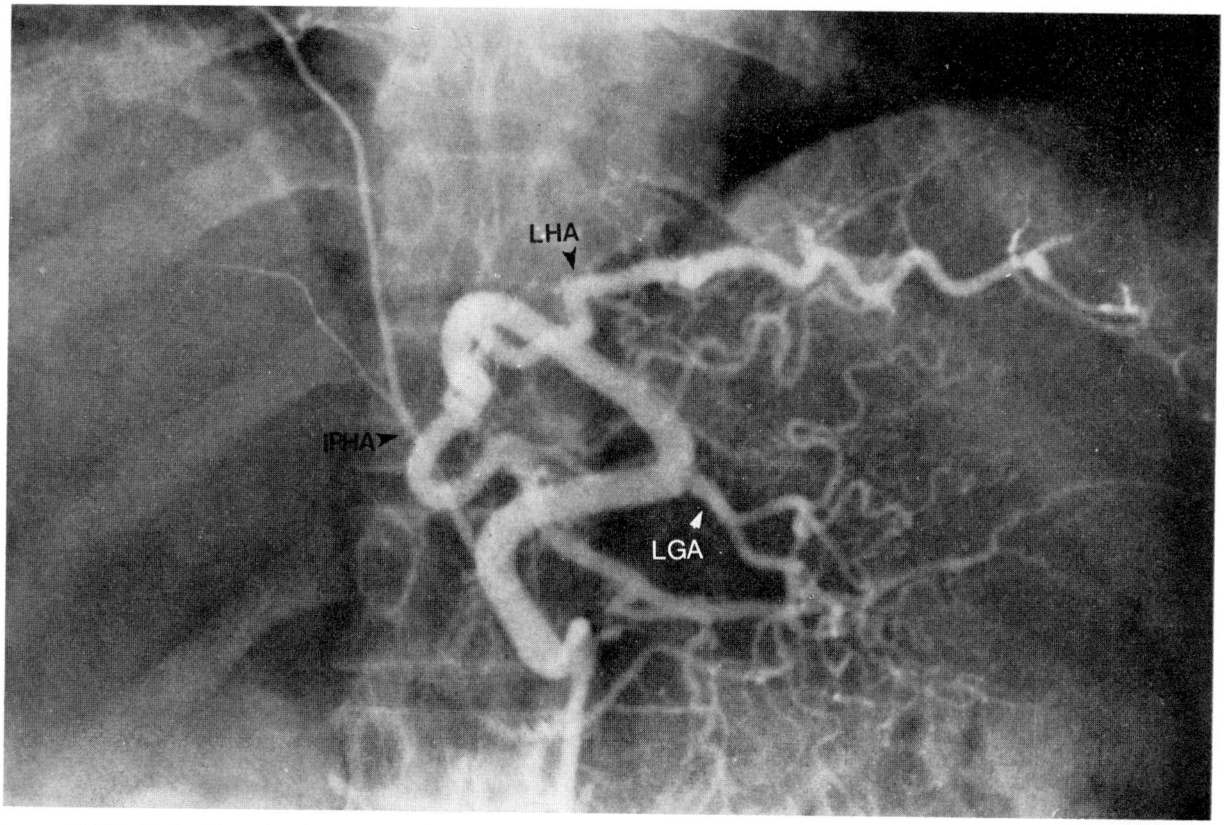

Figure 11.20. Left Hepatic Arteriogram. Left hepatic artery (L.H.A.), left gastric artery (L.G.A.), right inferior phrenic artery (I.P.H.A.). *Comment:* There is variation in a normal arrangement here, with the left hepatic and the left gastric arteries arising together.

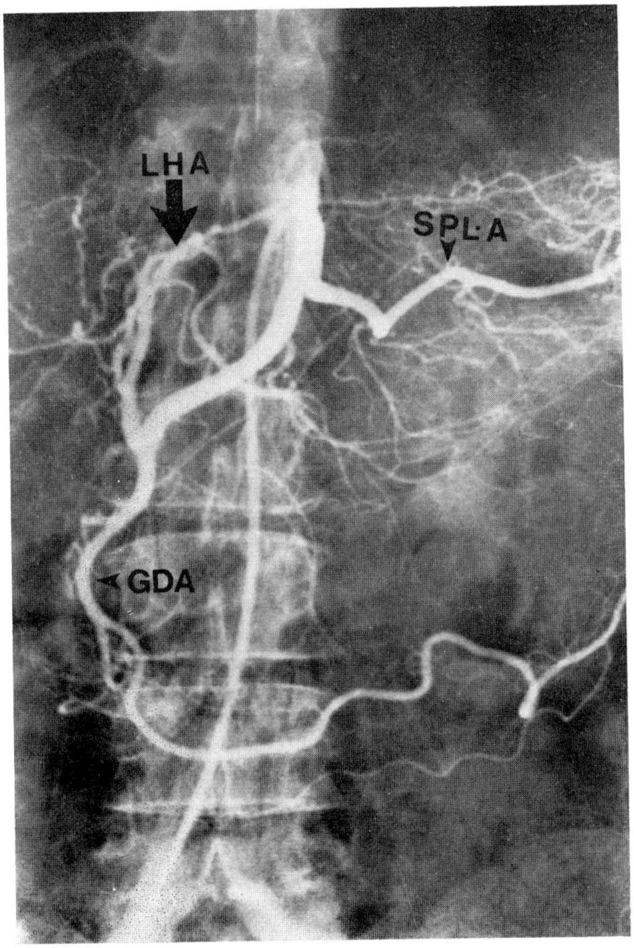

Figure 11.21. Celiac Arteriogram. Variations in normal anatomic arrangements. There is a common origin of the splenic (Spl. A.), left hepatic (L.H.A.), and gastroduodenal (G.D.A.) arteries. The right hepatic originated from the superior mesenteric artery.

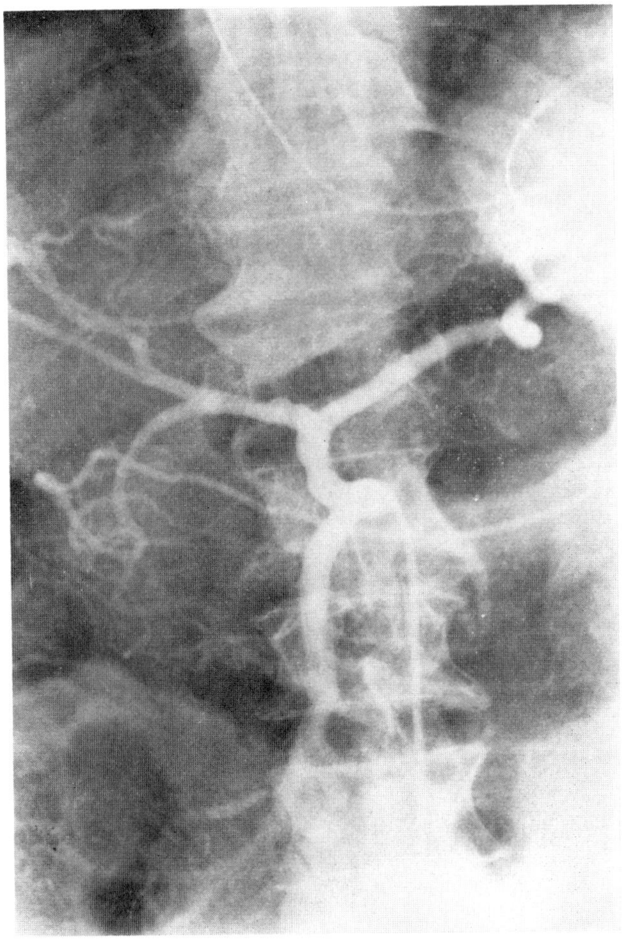

Figure 11.22. Celiac Arteriogram. There is simultaneous opacification of the celiac and superior mesenteric arteries which originate from a common trunk. The left gastric artery arose directly from the aorta. *Comment:* Common celiacomesenteric axis with independent origin of the left gastric artery.

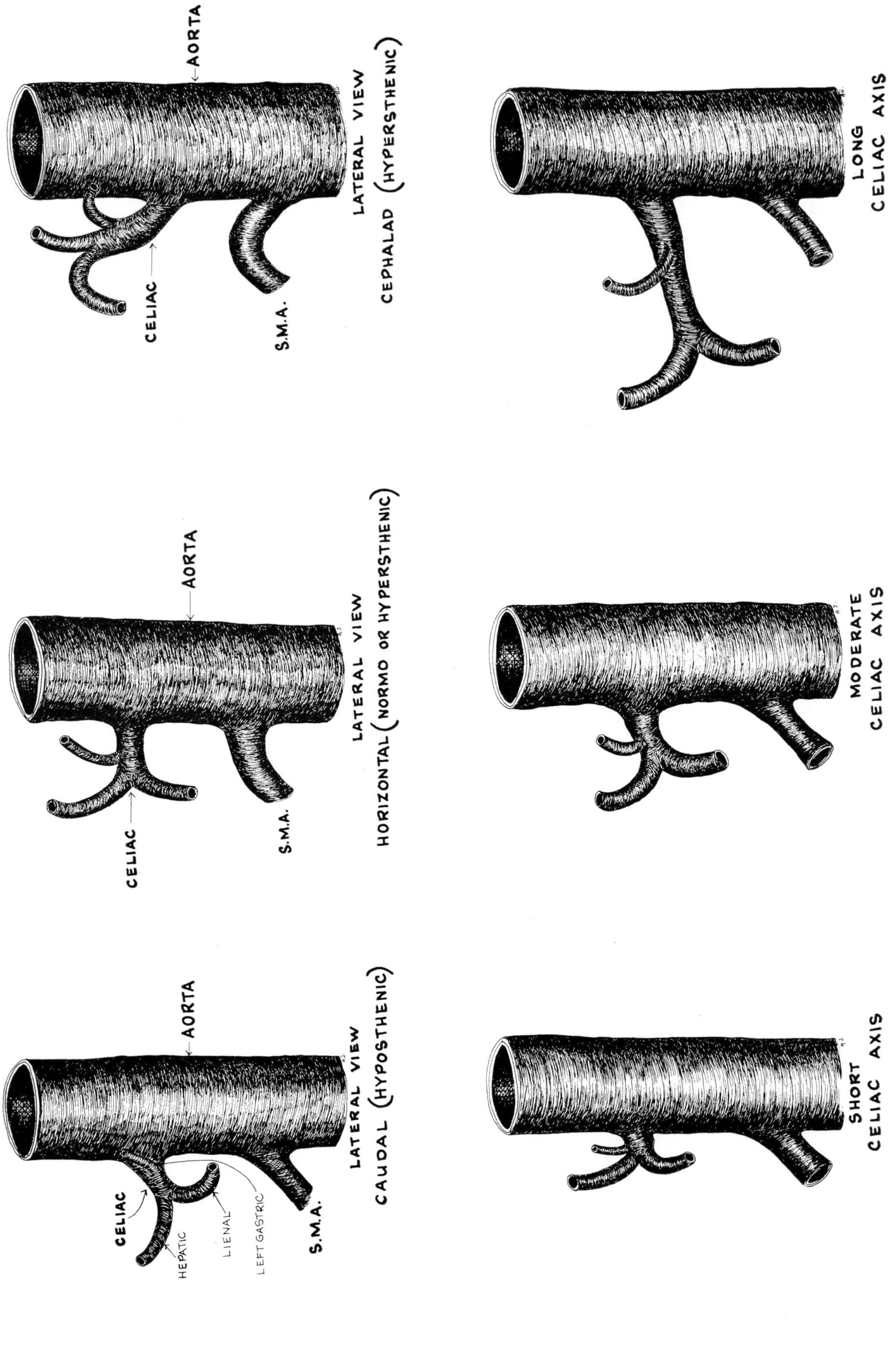

Figure 11.23. Variations in the directions and lengths of the celiac and superior mesenteric arteries as seen from a lateral direction.

ment, this artery divides into the main hepatic splenic and left gastric artery, and actually occurs in about 55 percent of the population (Fig. 11-17). Replaced origins of the hepatic or various combination of origins of the remaining arteries are not at all unusual.[318] These variations in the origins are explained on the basis of abnormal atrophy of the segmental, ventral arteries of the aorta which occur while joining the omphalomesenteric artery[319] (Figs. 11-18 to 11-29).

MESENTERIC VESSELS

Superior Mesenteric Artery

The second median unpaired branch of the abdominal aorta arising after the celiac is the superior mesenteric artery.[326, 337] It arises from the anterior surface of the abdominal aorta 1 to 20 mm caudal to the origin of the celiac axis. The origin ranges from the level of T. 12 to L. 2 vertebral body.[324] It is *crossed by the neck of the pancreas at its origin,* while the vessel itself courses in front of the uncinate process of the pancreas. The average diameter is 7.7 mm. The course of the first portion depends on the amount of adipose tissue present in the abdomen.[325]

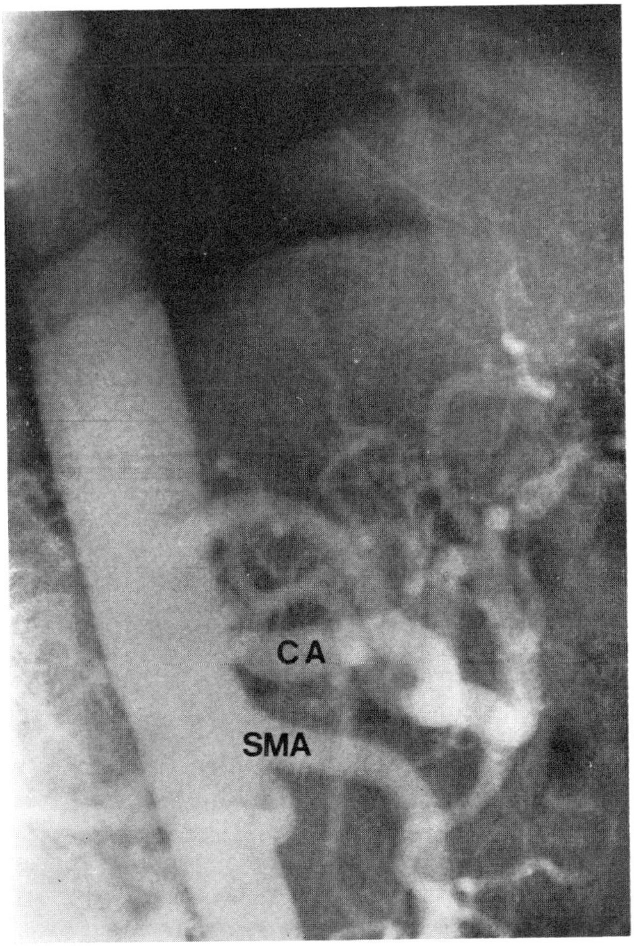

Figure 11.24. Cross-table Abdominal Aortogram. The celiac and superior mesenteric arteries have a horizontal course in this eusthenic patient.

The *branches* of the superior mesenteric artery are the inferior pancreatico-duodenals, intestinal branches (12-20), middle colic, right colic, and the ileo-colic arteries. Inconsistently occurring branches such as the dorsal pancreatic and right hepatic arteries, splenic artery are not at all uncommon. The inferior pancreatico-duodenal arteries anastomose with the corresponding superior pancreatico-duodenal arteries from the gastroduodenal artery. From the ultimate loops formed by the intestinal branches are the relatively straight branches, "vasa recta." The middle colic artery arises proximally from the superior mesenteric arterial trunk just distal to the origin of the inferior pancreatico-duodenal artery. This artery courses toward the transverse colon and divides into two branches, the right and left, which anastomose with the right colic and left colic arteries respectively.

The right colic artery courses toward the ascending colon and divides into ascending and descending branches. The former anastomoses with the middle colic artery and the latter with the ileo-colic artery. The ileo-colic artery reach-reaches the cecum and divides into numerous branches supplying the terminal ileum, cecum and appendix (Figs. 11-37 to 11-40).

Inferior Mesenteric Artery

The third, and last, unpaired branch[337] of the abdominal aorta arises between the vertebral levels of L. 2 and L. 4.[324] It originates from the anterior surface of the aorta, more often towards the left, and gives rise to the left colic, sigmoid and superior rectal arteries. The

(Text continues on page 110)

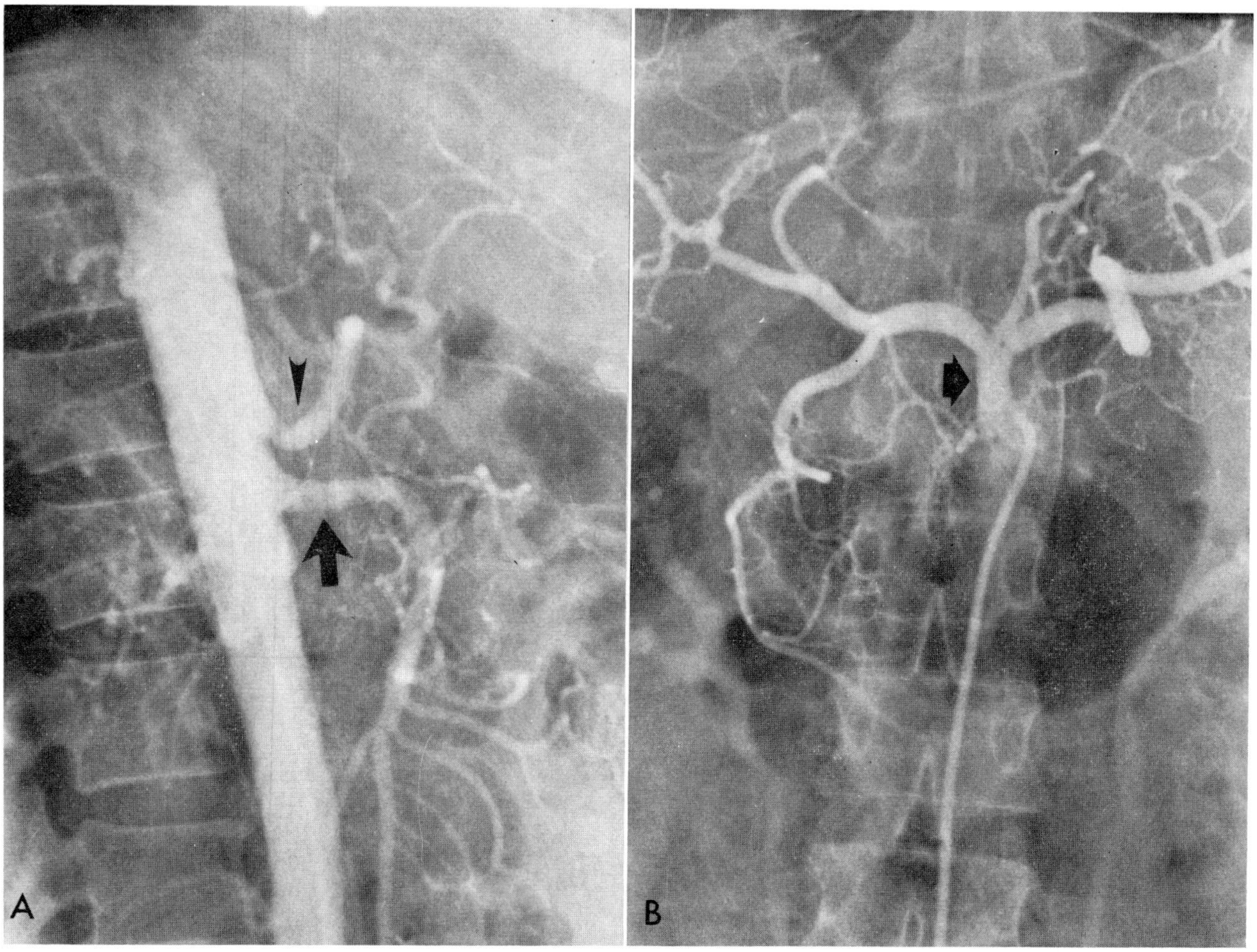

Figure 11.25. (A) Lateral aortogram: The celiac axis (arrow head) points in a cephalic direction. The superior mesenteric artery is horizontal (arrow). (B) The celiac axis points in a cephalic direction.

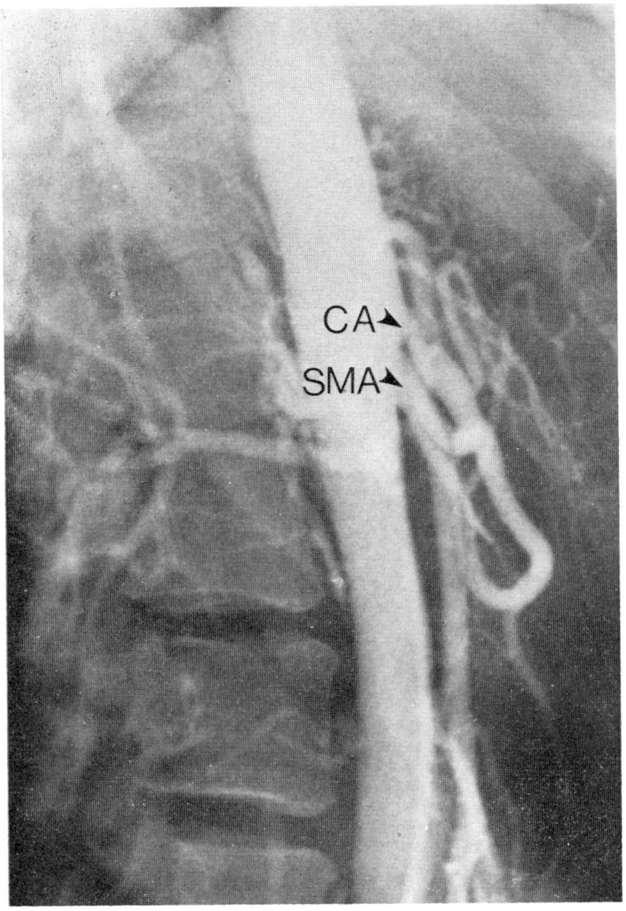

Figure 11.26. Cross-table Abdominal Aortogram. The celiac (C.A.) and superior mesenteric (S.M.A.) arteries have a caudal direction in a hyposthenic patient.

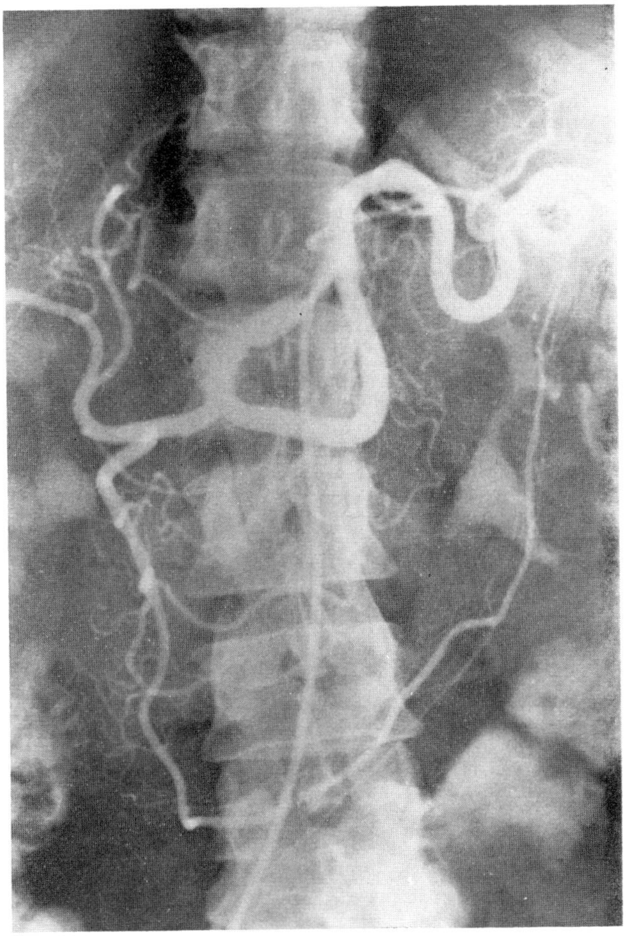

Figure 11.27. Celiac Arteriogram. Notice the long stem of the celiac axis and a tortuous elongated splenic artery.

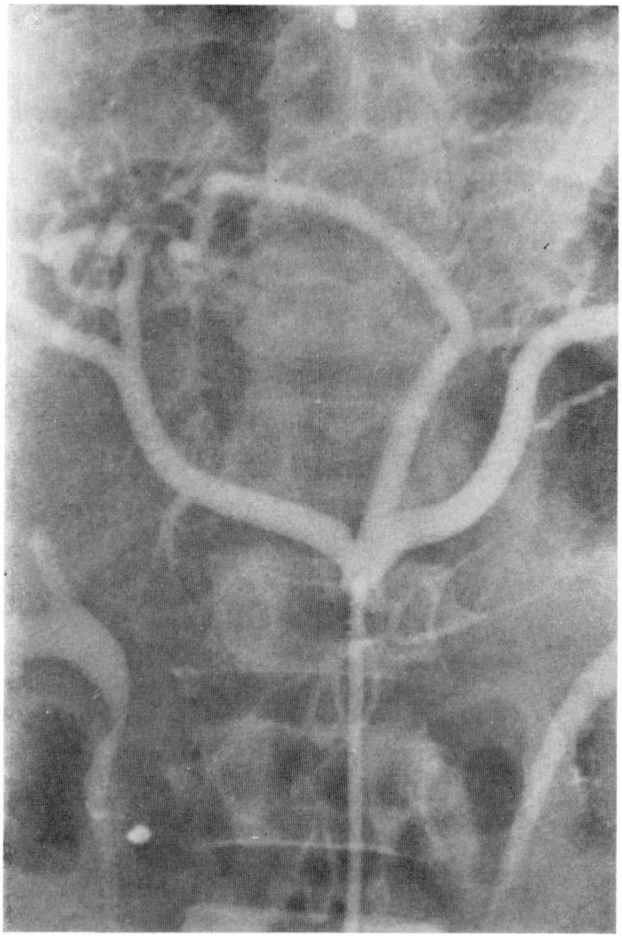

Figure 11.28. Celiac Angiogram. Note short celiac axis with a cephalic course.

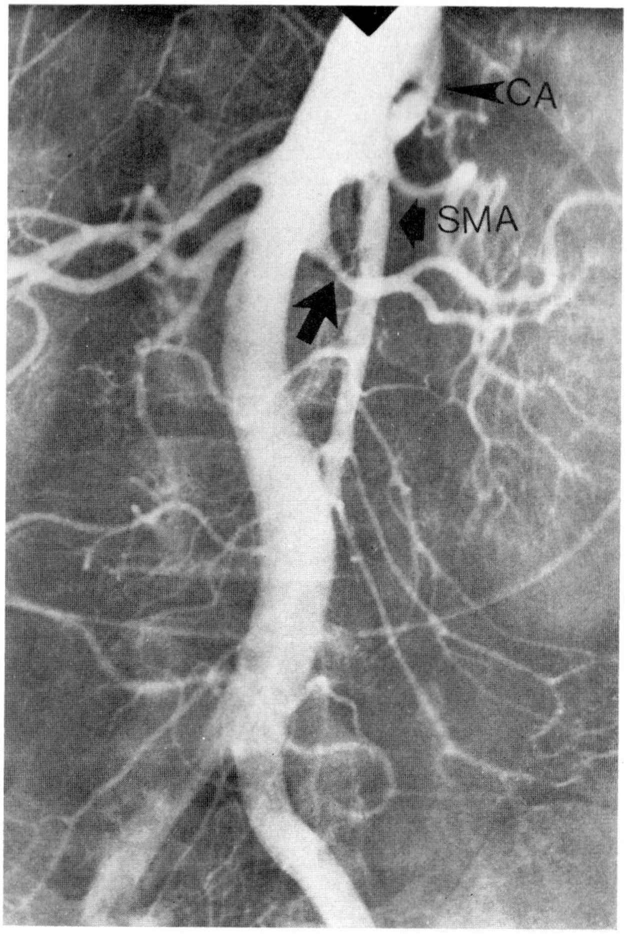

Figure 11.29. Flush Abdominal Aortogram. The aorta is tortuous and the orifices of the celiac axis (C.A.) and superior mesenteric artery (S.M.A.) have almost a lateral position. Incidentally seen is atherosclerotic narrowing of the left renal artery (Arrow). *Comment:* This hint should be helpful while searching for these arteries during a procedure.

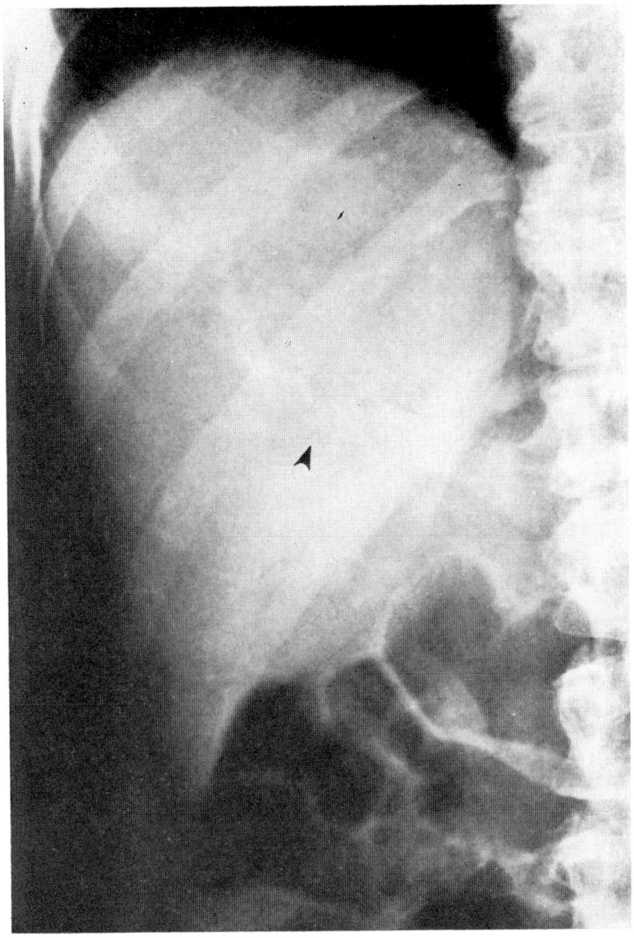

Figure 11.30. Celiac Arteriogram—venous phase. There is homogeneous stain of the right lobe of the liver and visualization of portal vein radicles (Arrow). *Comment:* Normal.

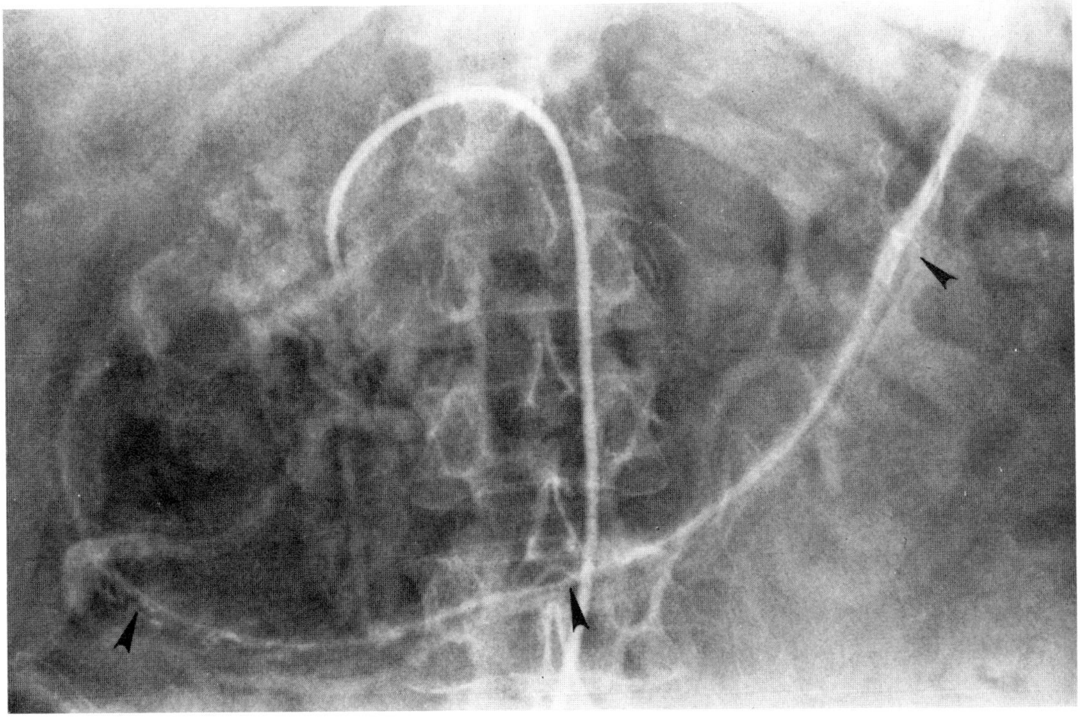

Figure 11.31. Gastroduodenal Arteriogram—venous phase. Shows uniform staining of the normal gastric mucosa.

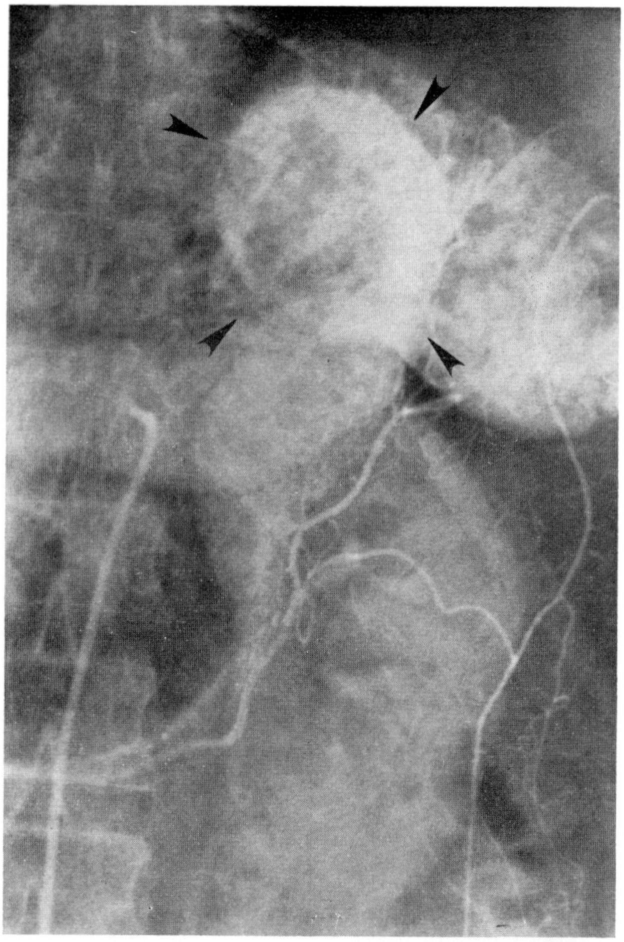

Figure 11.32. Celiac Arteriogram. During the late phase of the study there is discrete staining in the left upper quadrant. *Comment:* Note staining of the fundus of a normal stomach.

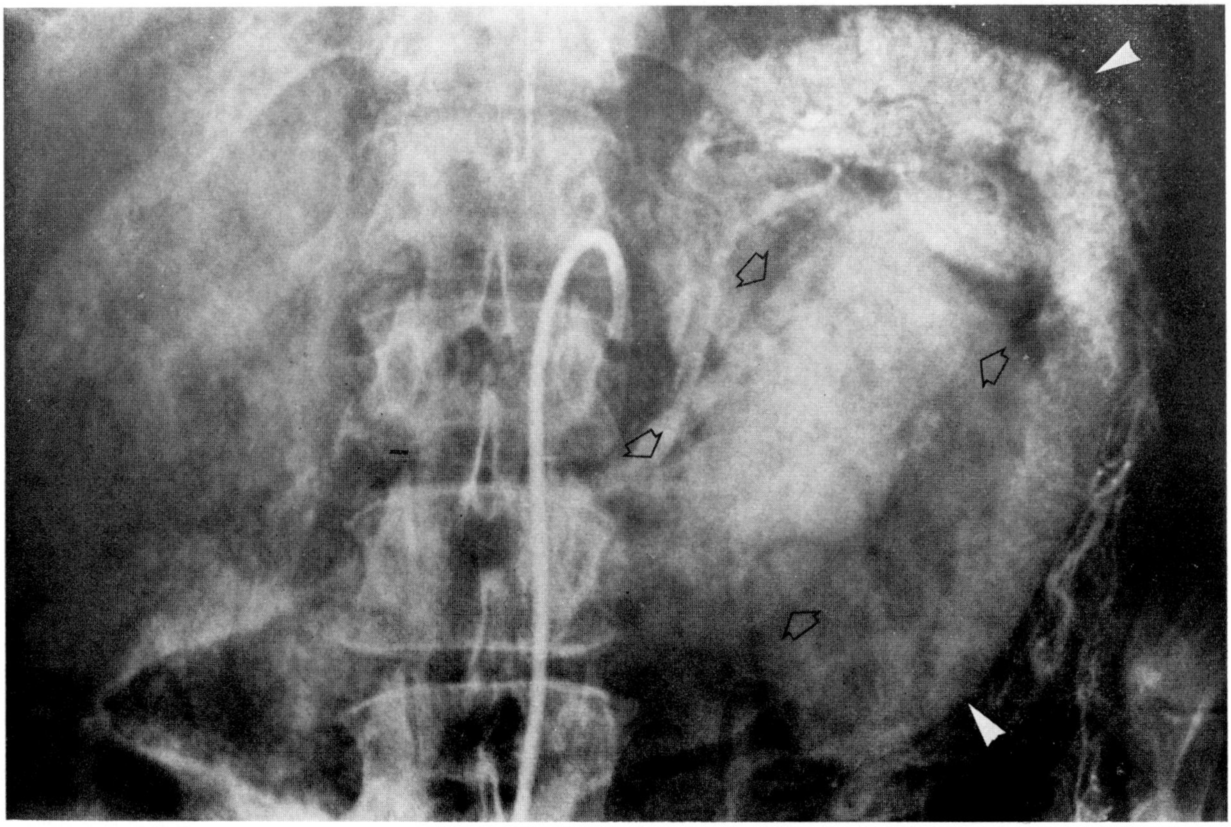

Figure 11.33. Celiac Arteriogram—late phase. There is parenchymal stain of the pancreas (Blank Arrow) and wall of the stomach (Arrow Head). *Comment:* Note normal staining.

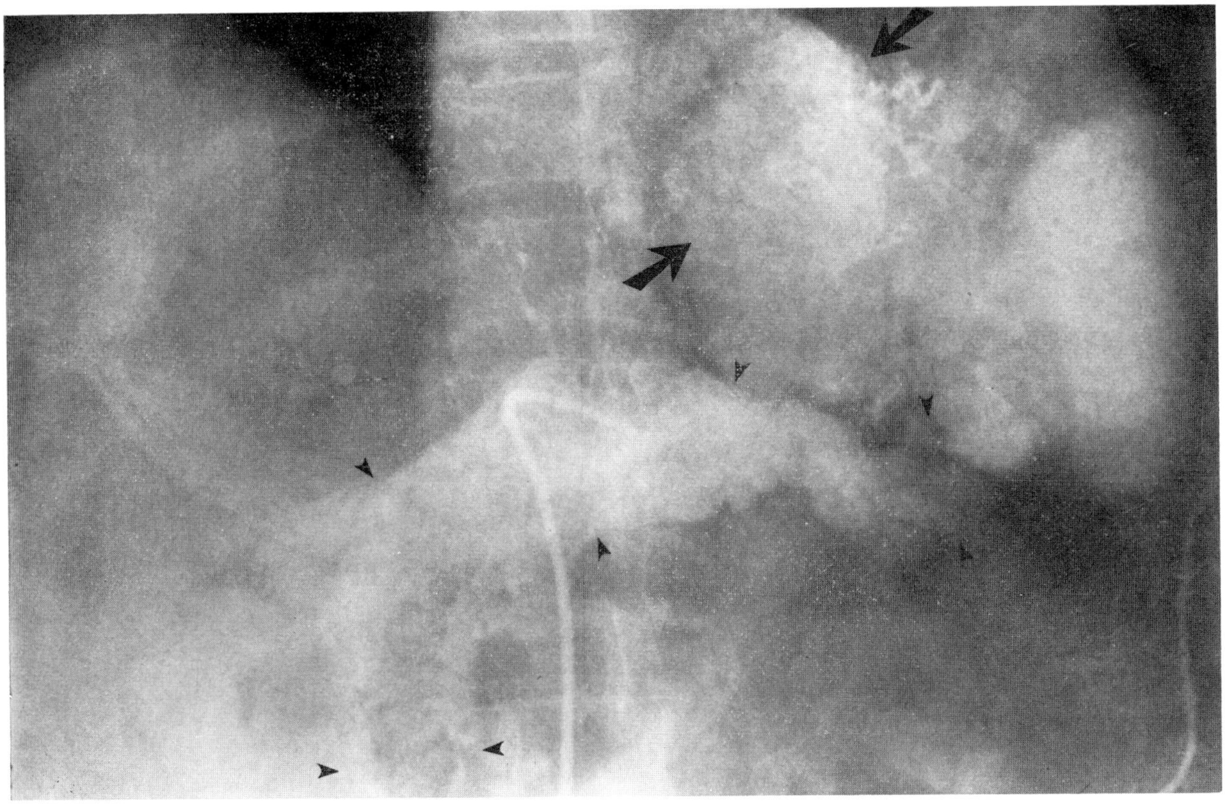

Figure 11.34. Splenic Arteriogram. Venous phase: There is good staining of the normal pancreas (Arrow Heads), fundus of the stomach (Arrows), and the spleen. *Comment:* Note normal staining of the pancreas and fundus of the stomach.

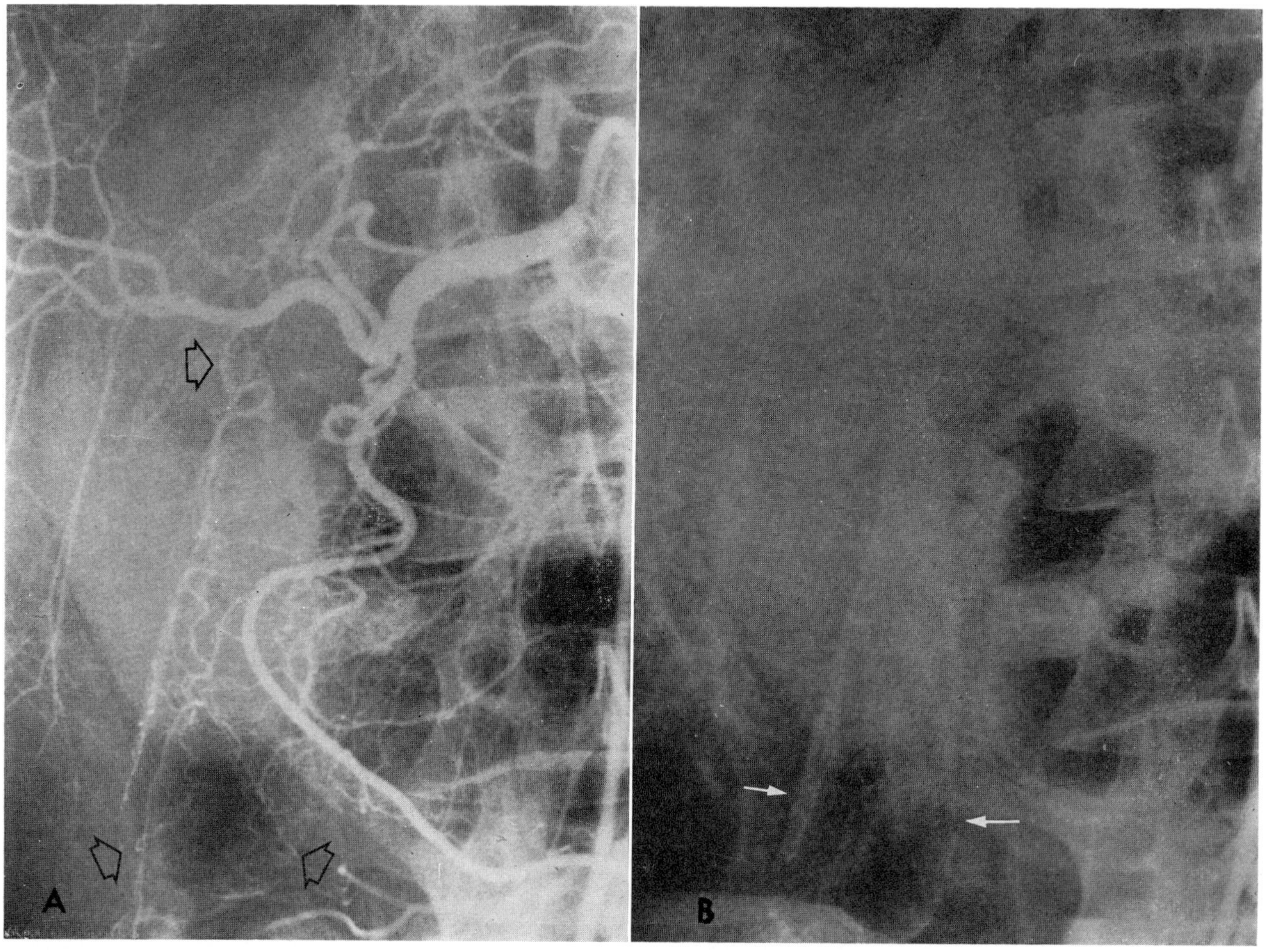

Figure 11.35. Hepatic Arteriogram. (A) Please note the cystic artery arising from the right hepatic artery. (B) Venous phase reveals the well-stained wall of the gallbladder. *Comment:* Normal.

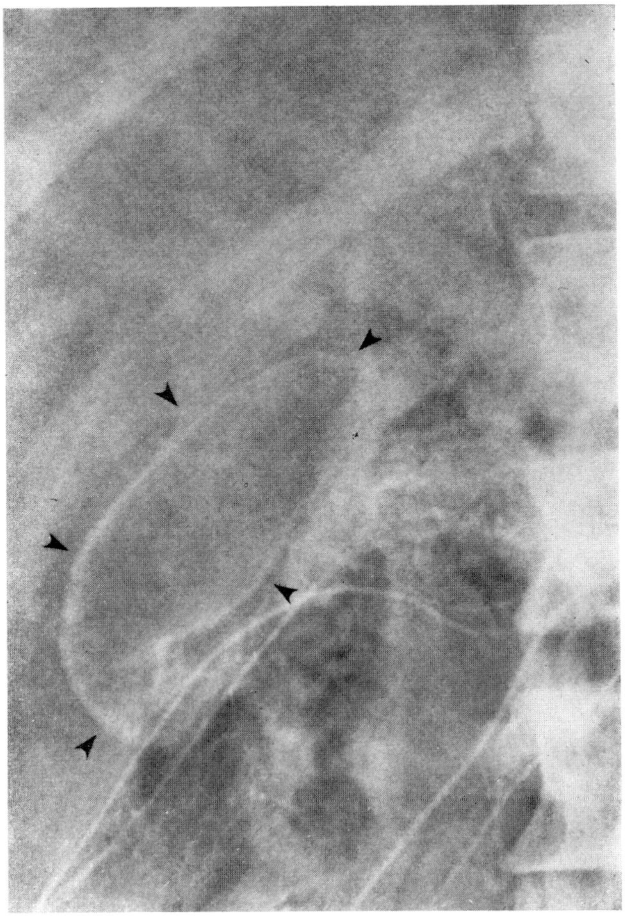

Figure 11.36. Celiac Arteriogram. During the late phase there is staining of the wall of a normal gall-bladder.

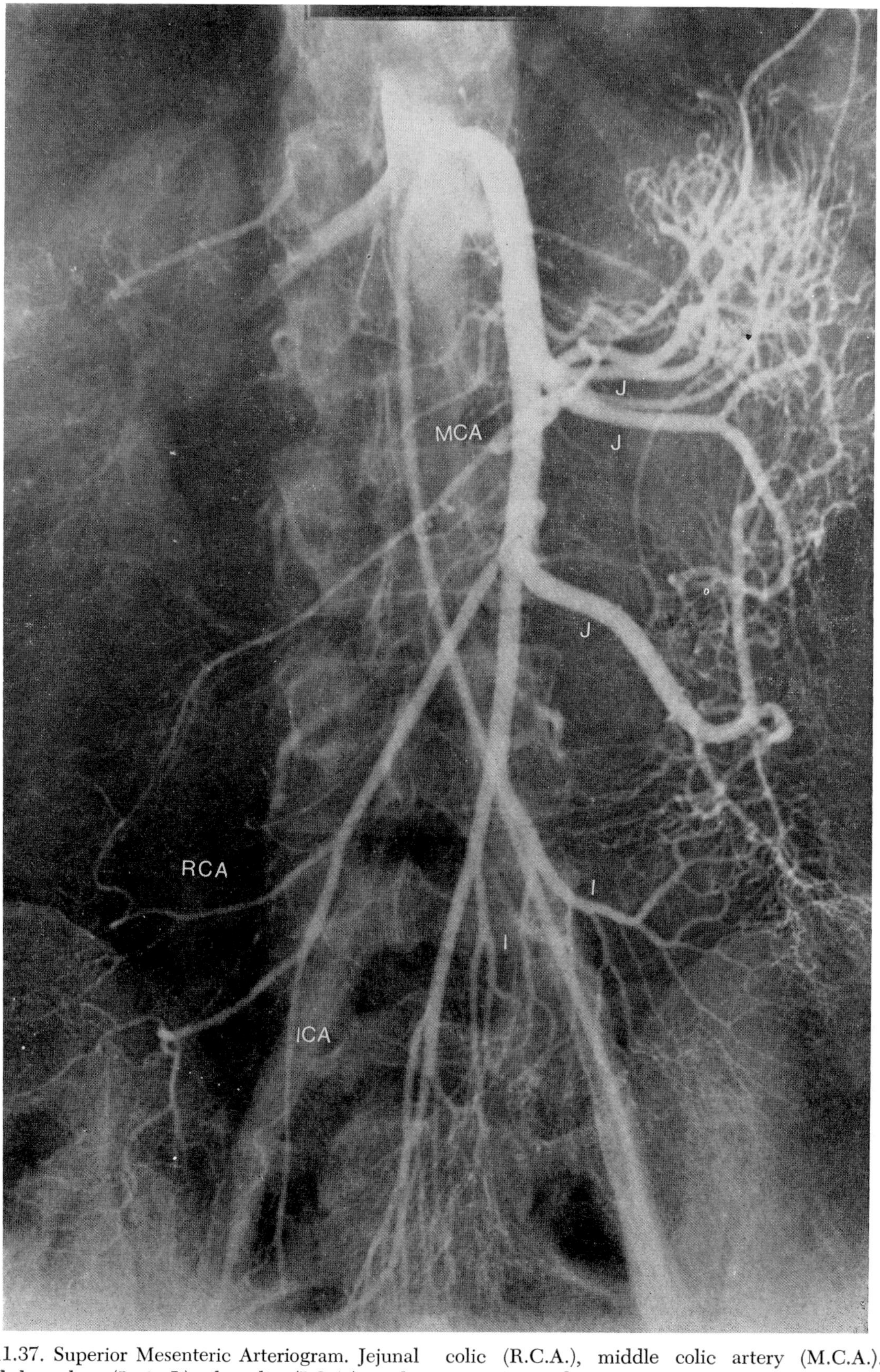

Figure 11.37. Superior Mesenteric Arteriogram. Jejunal and ileal branches (J. & I.), ileocolic (I.C.A.), right colic (R.C.A.), middle colic artery (M.C.A.). *Comment:* Normal.

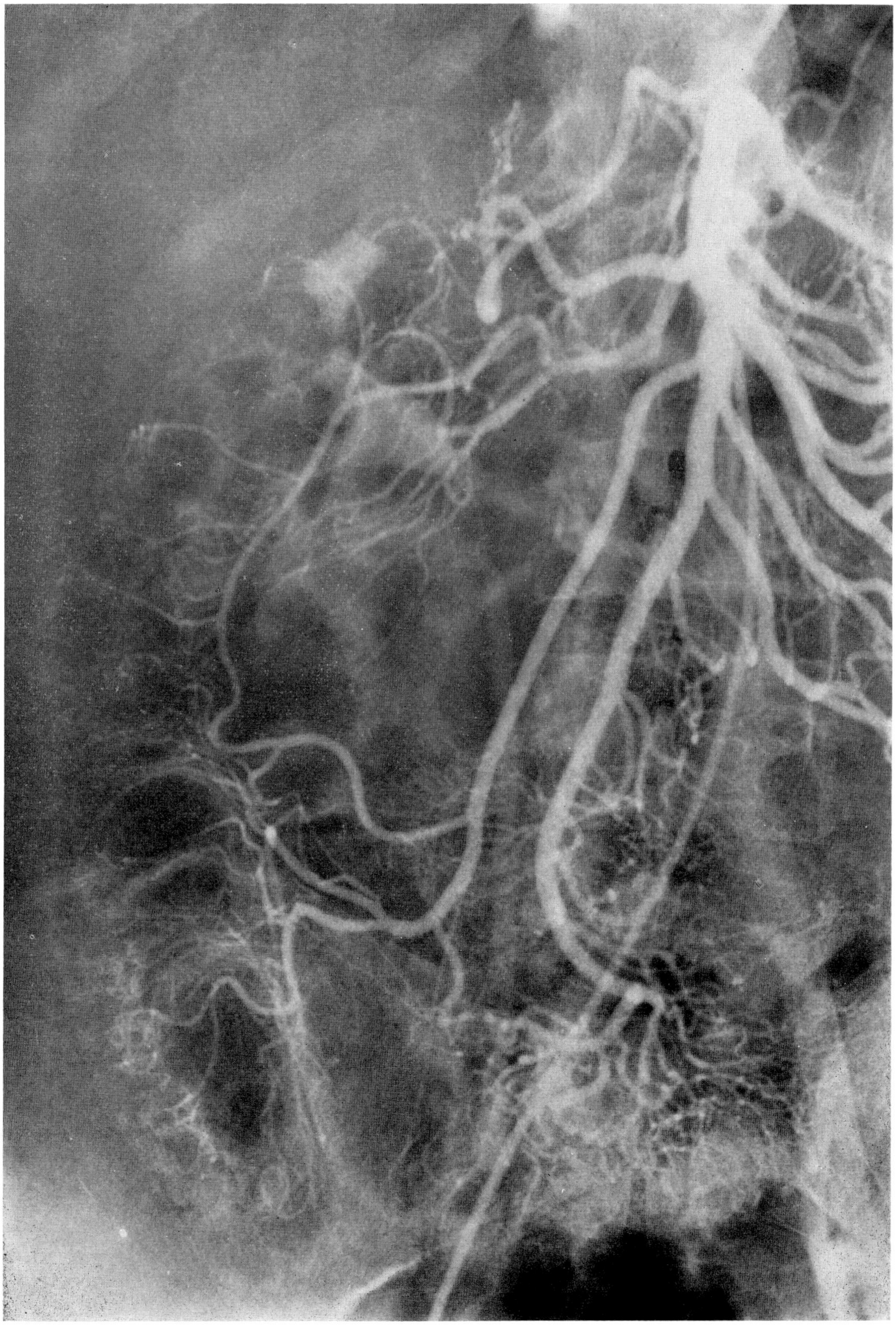

Figure 11.38 A *(Continued on next page)*

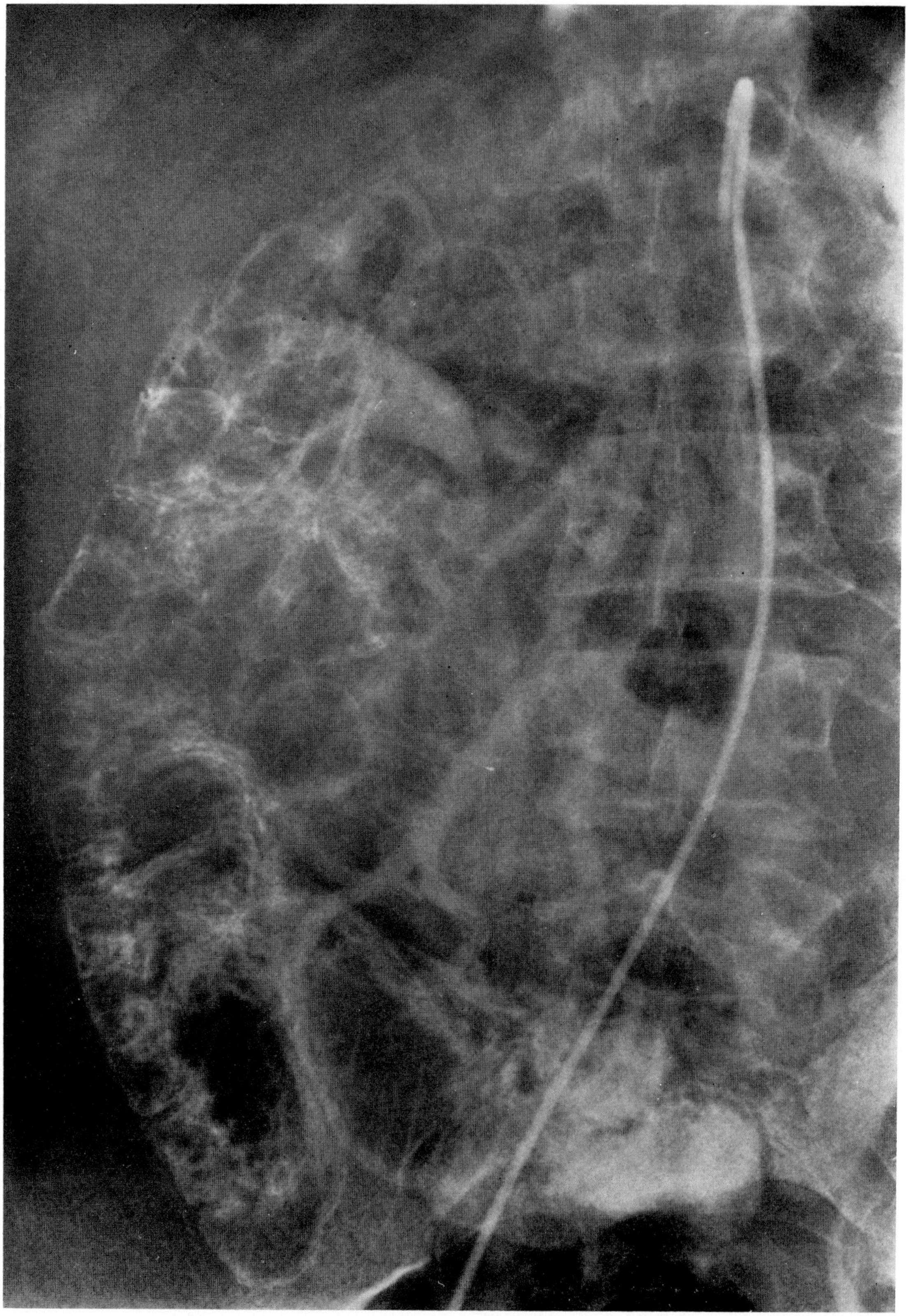

Figure 11.38. Superior Mesenteric Arteriogram. (A) Demonstrates ileocolic and right colic arteries. (B) Normal staining of the cecum and ascending colon. *Comment:* Normal.

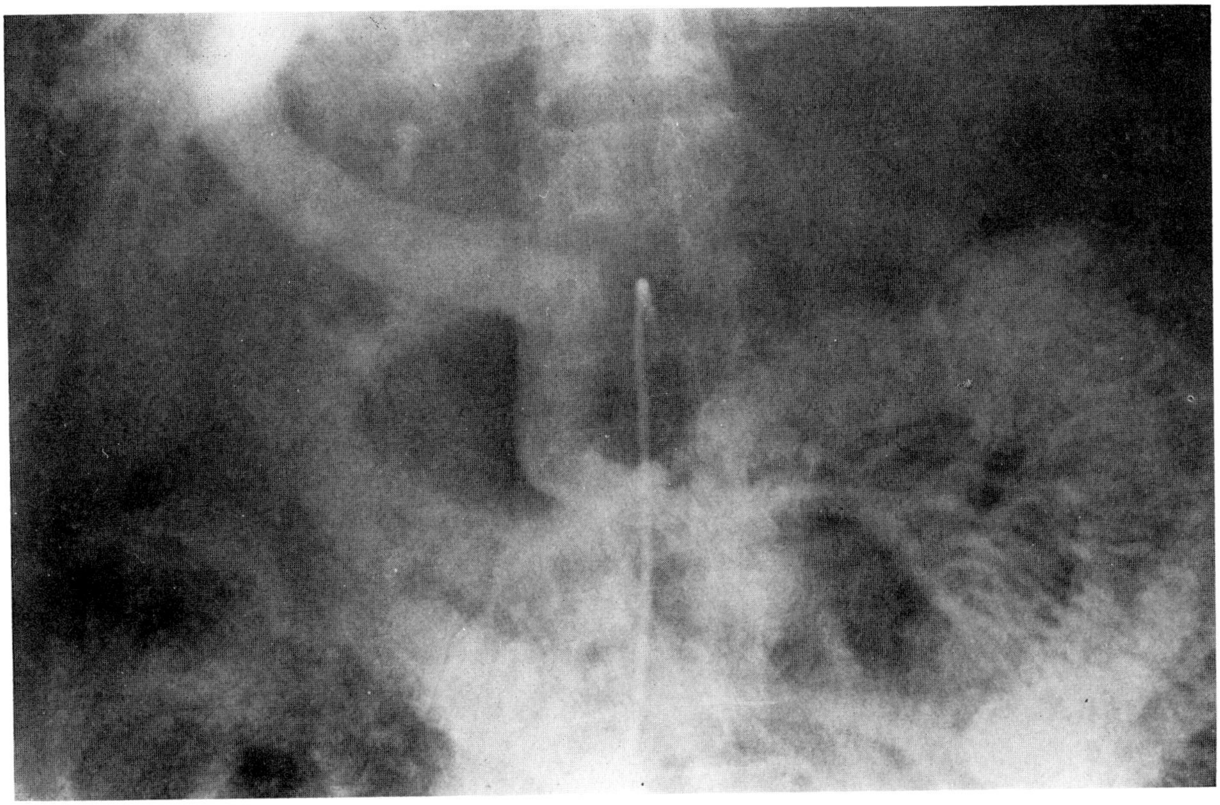

Figure 11.39. Superior Mesenteric Arteriogram. Venous phase: There is good staining of the walls of the small bowel and good opacification of the branches of the superior mesenteric vein. *Comment:* Note staining of the normal bowel wall.

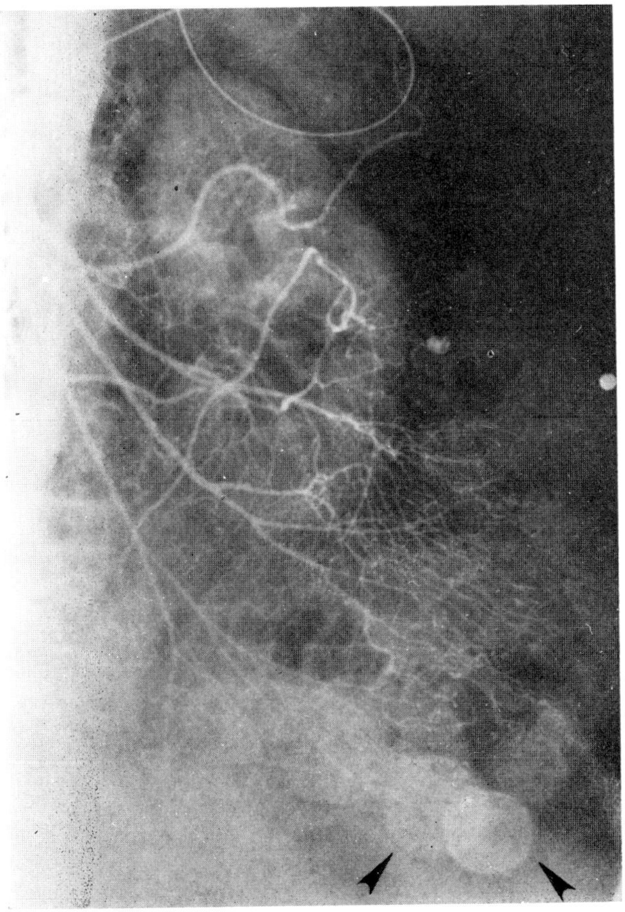

Figure 11.40. Superior Mesenteric Arteriogram. *Comment:* Note end on bowel with discrete staining of the mucosa.

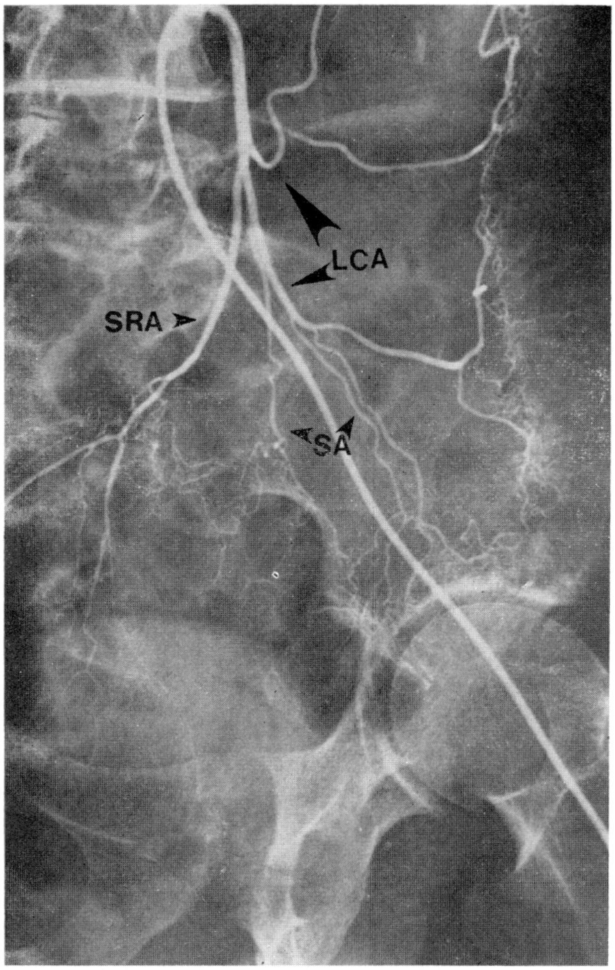

Figure 11.41. Inferior Mesenteric Arteriogram. (A) Arterial phase: left colic artery (L.C.A.), sigmoidal arteries (S.A.), superior rectal artery (S.R.A.). *Comment:* Normal inferior mesenteric arteriogram.

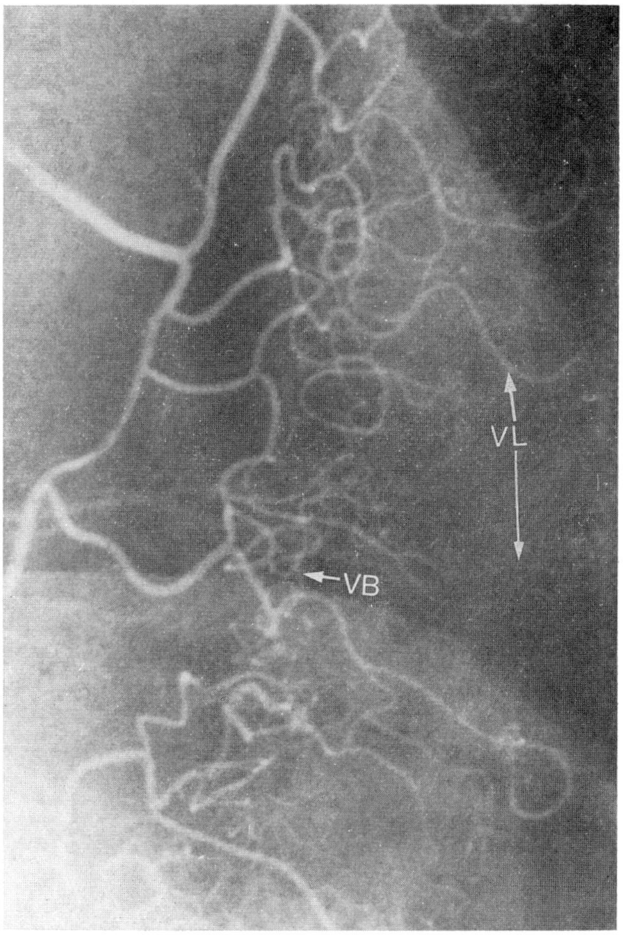

Figure 11.42. Inferior Mesenteric Angiogram. Note normal vasa longa (Arrow) and vasa brevia (Arrow Head).

left colic artery anastomoses with the middle colic artery to supply the descending colon. The sigmoid arteries supplying this portion of the colon are one to four in number. The superior rectal artery, the continuation of the inferior mesenteric artery, descends toward the rectum to anastomose with the middle rectal arteries, which are branches of the internal iliac artery. The middle rectal arteries, in turn, anastomose with the inferior rectal arteries from the internal pudendal arteries (Figs. 11-41 and 11-42).

COLLATERAL PATHWAYS

Marginal Artery

This is a paracolic vessel of anastomoses between the adjacent branches of the ileo-colic, right colic, middle colic, left colic, and sigmoidal arteries.[337] Usually it is a single, uninterrupted vessel. When it is interrupted,[342, 343] it is usually between the ileo-colic and right colic arteries, or between the middle colic and left colic arteries (Fig. 11-43).

Arc of Riolan

This is a short loop from the superior mesen-

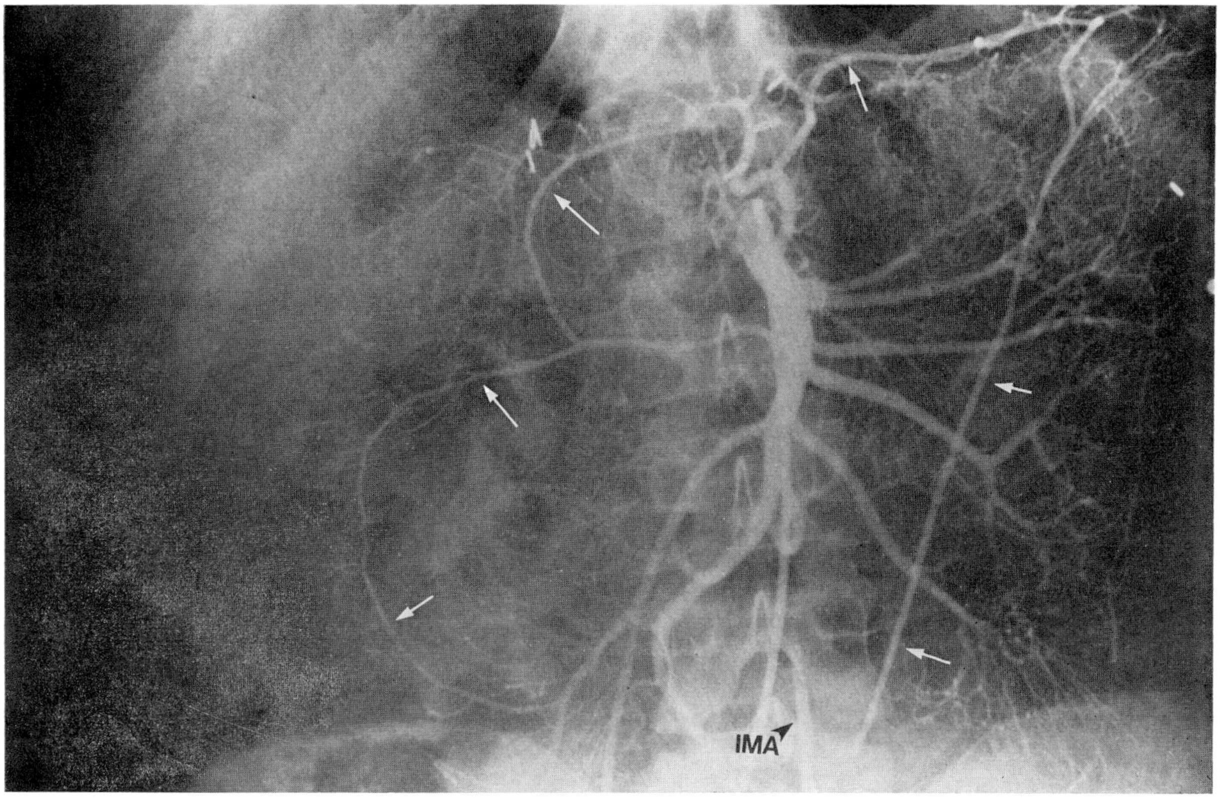

Figure 11.43. Superior Mesenteric Arteriogram. Note the continuous marginal arcade from the right ileocolic artery to the right colic artery, to the middle colic artery and then to the left colic artery towards the inferior mesenteric artery (I.M.A.). *Comment:* Note continuous marginal arcade from the ileocolic artery all the way to the inferior mesenteric artery.

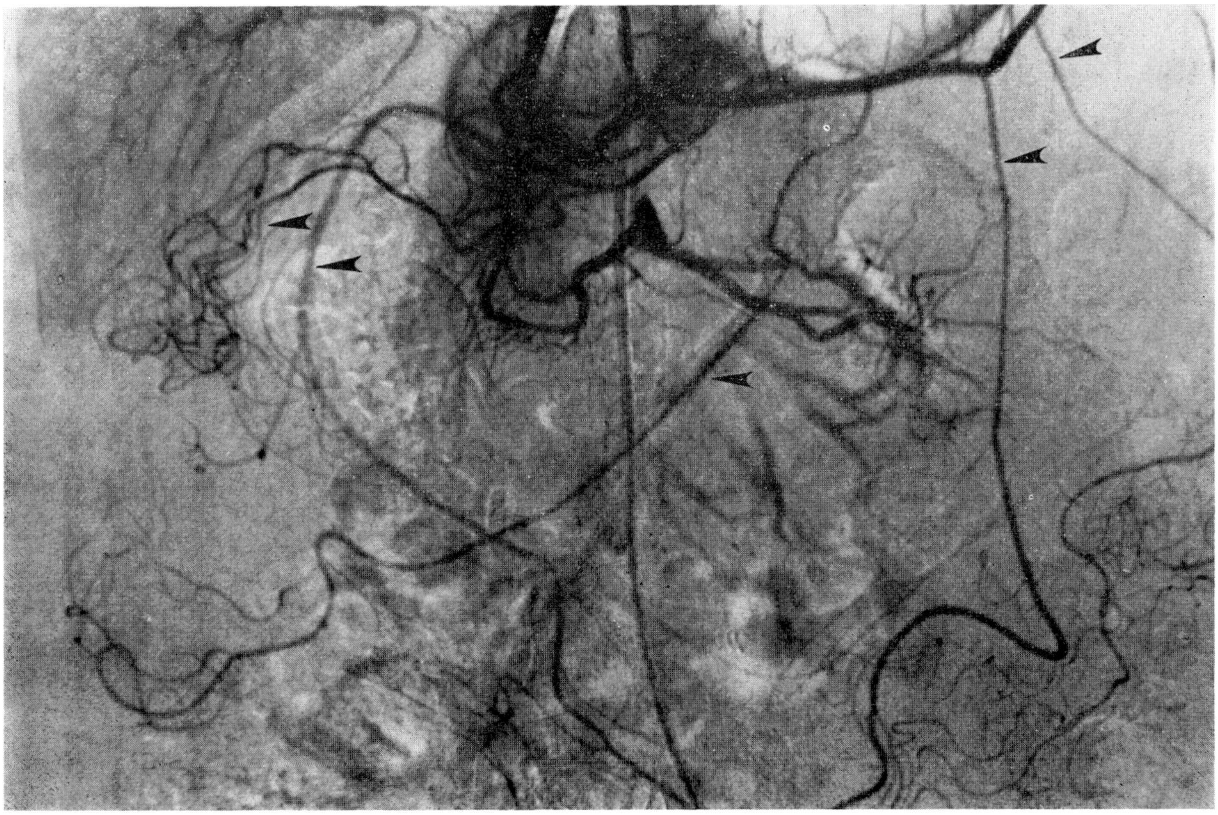

Figure 11.44. Omental Arcade. There are prominent omental epiploic vessels arising from the gastroduodenal artery (Arrow). This patient had marked ascites. *Comment:* Hypertrophied omental vasculature is not uncommon in individuals with ascites.

teric artery or its branches to the inferior mesenteric artery or its branches.[338]

Plexus of Turner

This retroperitoneal plexus affords communication between the visceral and parietal branches of the aorta. It is formed from parietal twigs originating from the intestinal branches and anastomosing with the adipose capsular vessels arising from the renal and adrenal arteries. This plexus has excellent potential for bidirectional flow.[370]

Splanchnic Circulation

In a broad sense, the splanchnic vasculature is actually a single vascular unit with intercommunications at the junctional zones, reinforced at both ends by the systemic vasculature. Proximally it is reinforced by the inferior phrenic through its esophageal branches and distally by the internal iliac via its rectal branches. In very drastic circumstances it can lean back on the "Turner's plexus" for an additional supply.

Omental Blood Supply

This blood supply[365] forms the pathways of Hyrtl and Barkow. Hyrtl's pathway is formed by the right and left gastroepiploic arteries as they anastomose along the greater curvature of the stomach. They give rise to omental branches named the right epiploic and left epiploic arteries. These vessels descend in the greater

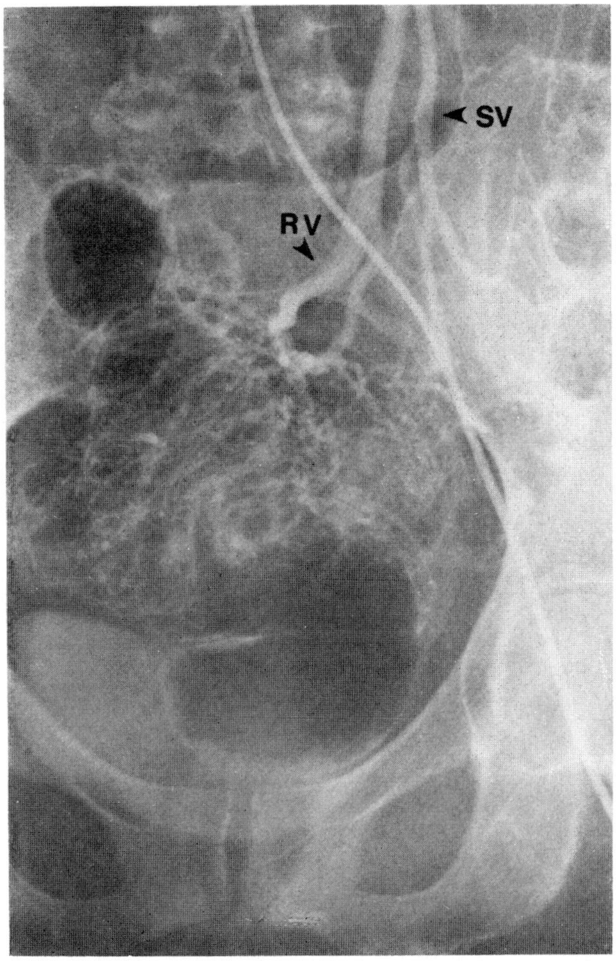

Figure 11.45. Venous phase—inferior mesenteric arteriogram. Good filling of the rectal (R.V.) and sigmoidal veins (S.V.). *Comment:* Normal venous phase.

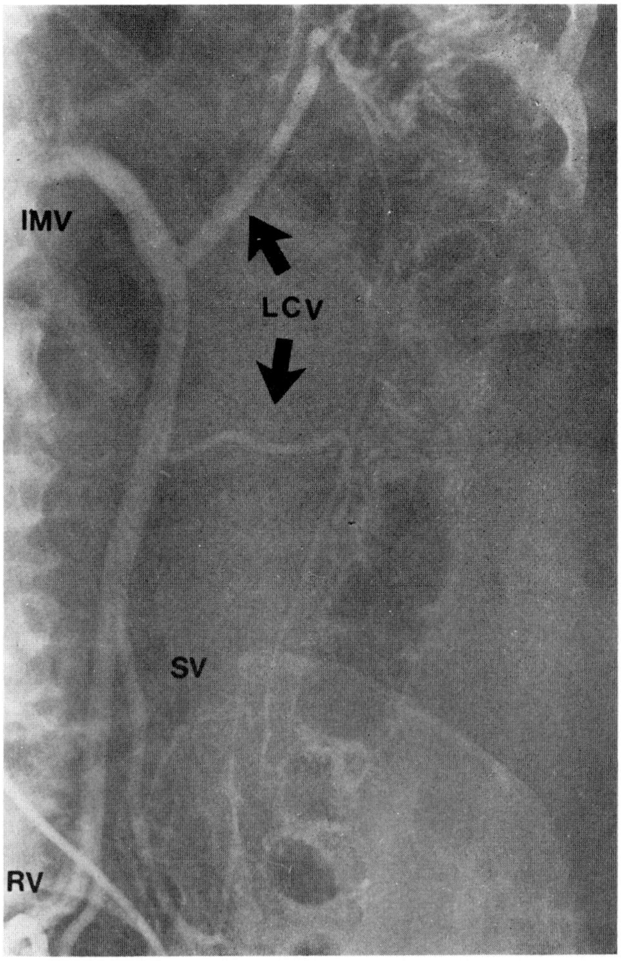

Figure 11.46. Inferior Mesenteric Arteriogram—venous phase. Rectal veins (R.V.), sigmoidal veins (S.V.), left colic vein (L.C.V.). *Comment:* Normal inferior mesenteric venous phase.

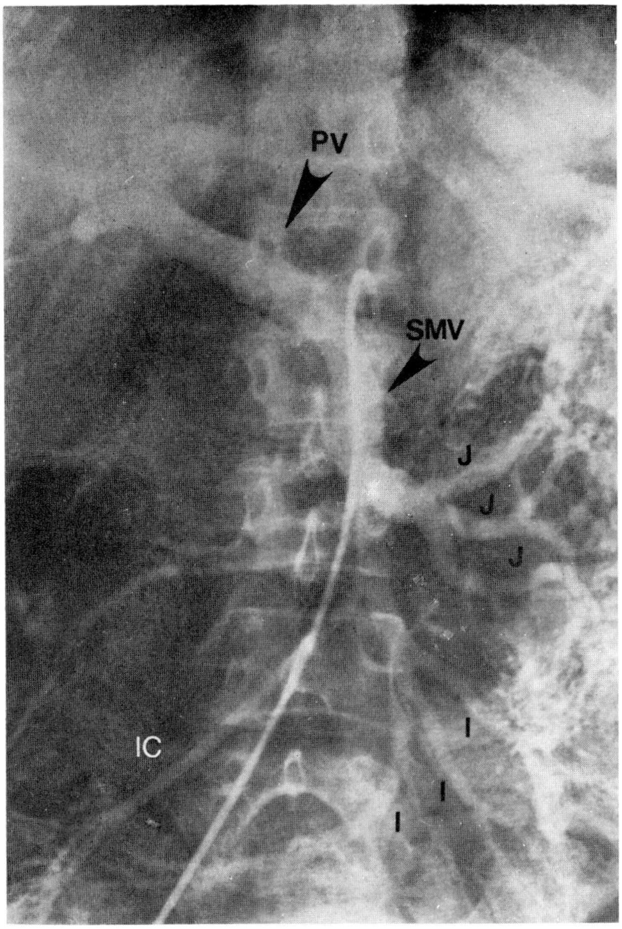

Figure 11.47. Postprescoline Superior Mesenteric Venogram. Jejunal and ileal veins (J & I), ileocolic vein (I.C.), superior mesenteric vein (S.M.V.), portal vein (P.V.). *Comment:* Normal superior mesenteric venogram.

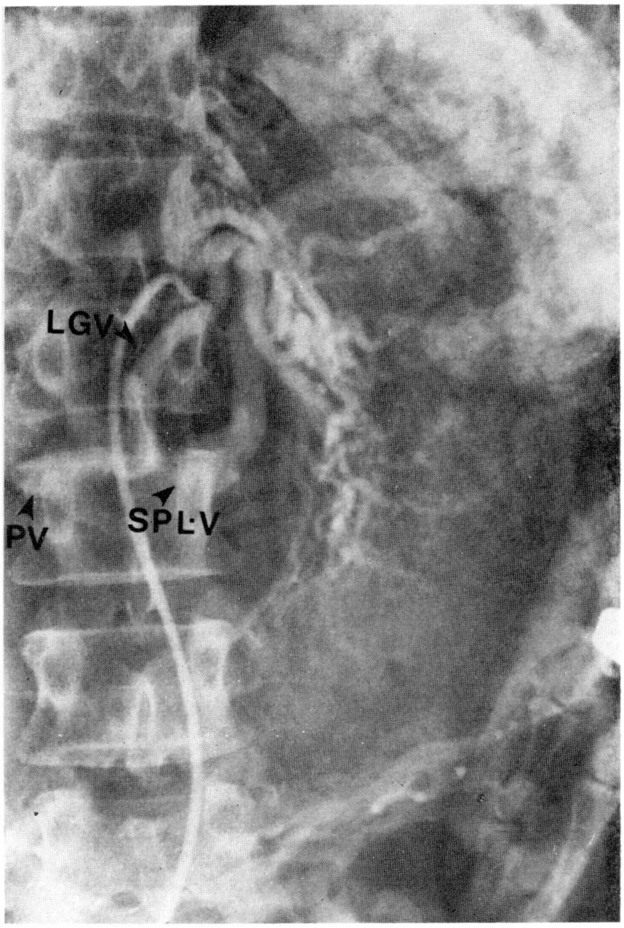

Figure 11.48. Celiac Arteriogram. Venous phase: Splenic vein (Spl. V.), left gastric vein (L.G.V.), portal vein (P.V.). *Comment:* Normal.

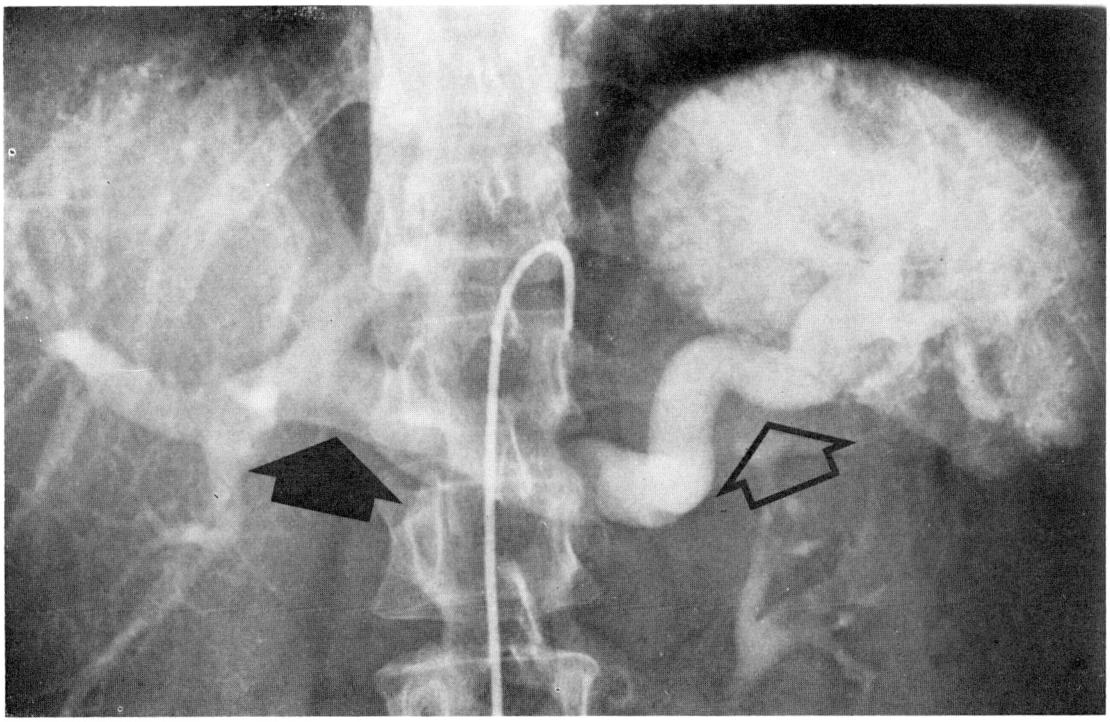

Figure 11.49. Splenic Arteriogram. Venous phase: Splenic vein (Blank Arrow), portal vein (Arrow). *Comment:* Normal.

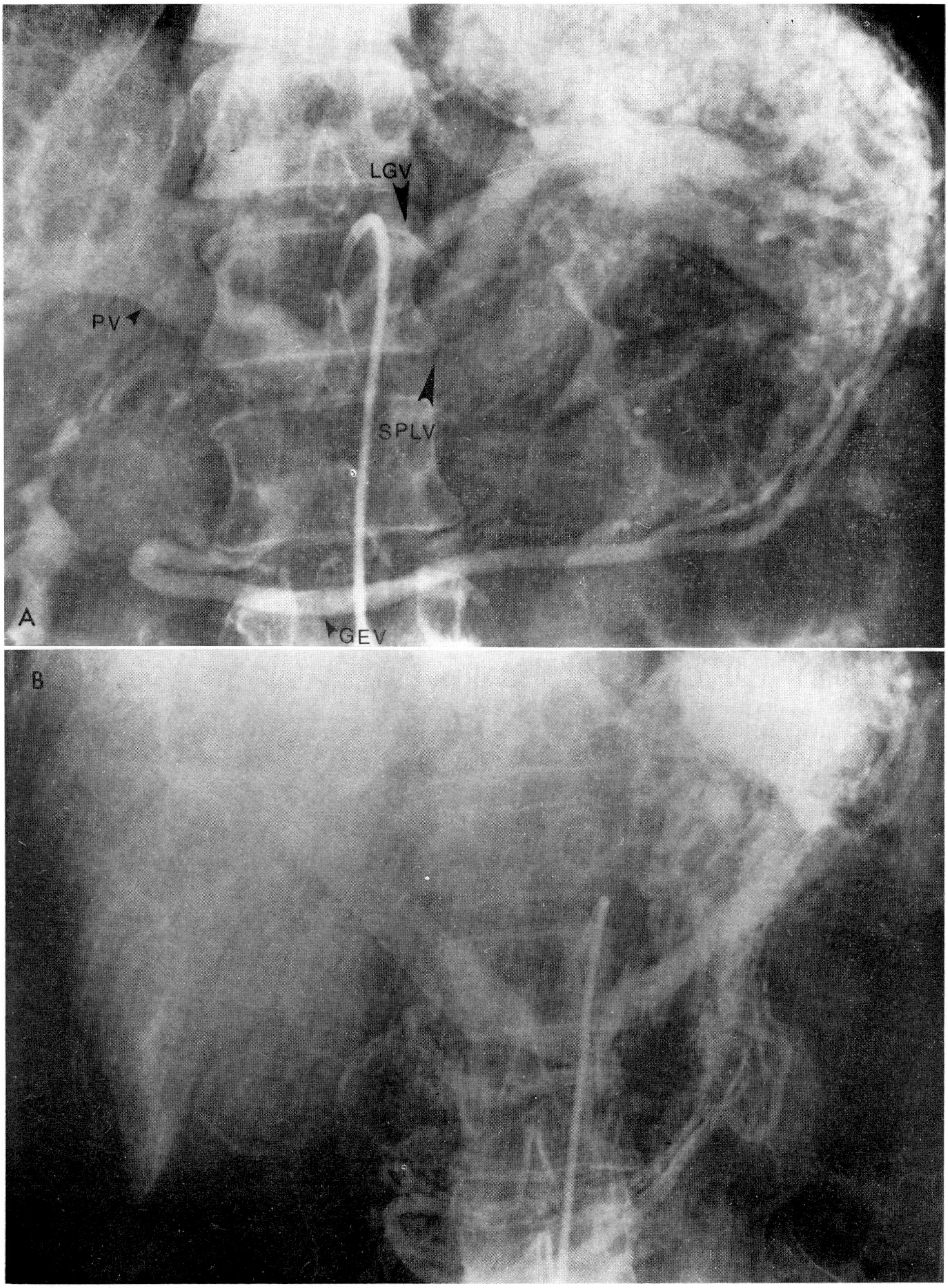

Figure 11.50. Celiac Arteriogram—normal venous phase. (A) Splenic vein (Spl. V.), left gastric vein (L.G.V.), gastroepiploic vein (G.E.V.), portal vein (P.V.). (B) Second patient. *Comment:* Note normal splenoportal veins.

omentum for 2 to 4 cm below the greater curvature of the stomach and then form an arc connecting on the right with the gastroduodenal artery, and on the left with the vessels at the gastroesophogeal junction and the fundus of the stomach (Fig. 11-44).

Barkow's pathway is a retro-omental vascular arcade formed by the right and left epiploic arteries 2 to 4 cm below the level of the transverse colon.

PORTAL VENOUS SYSTEM

The portal venous system is comprised of the superior mesenteric, inferior mesenteric, splenic and portal veins, and their tributaries. The main trunk, formed by the confluence of the splenic and superior mesenteric veins, enters the liver. This valveless venous system is unique in that the collecting veins of the system drain blood which has already passed through a capillary plexus in the splanchnic viscera, again to break up into capillaries within the liver, before the enteric blood reaches the right atrium.

Inferior Mesenteric Vein

This[363, 396] is formed by the superior hemorroidal, sigmoid, and left colic veins and terminates into the splenic or superior mesenteric vein behind the body of the pancreas. Very

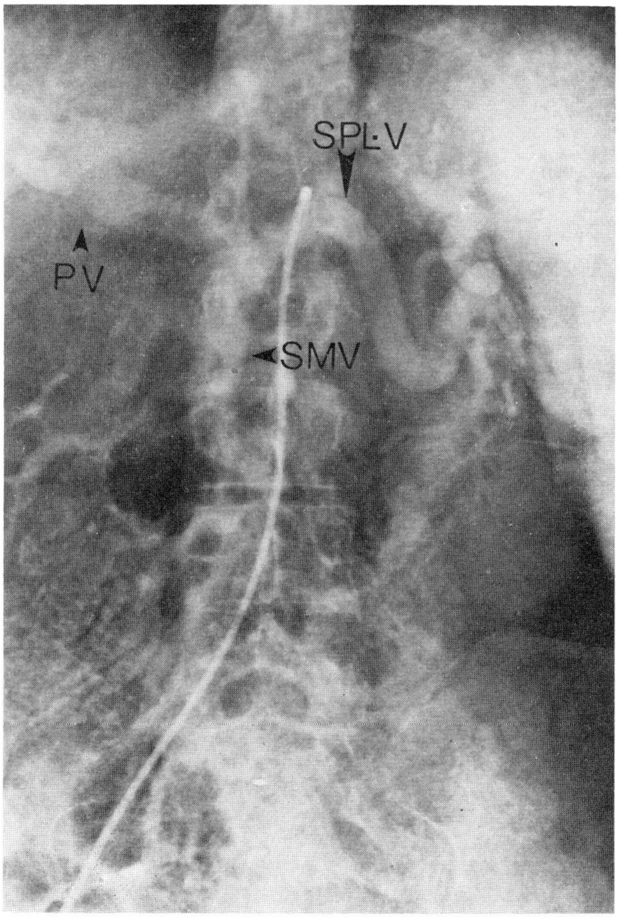

Figure 11.51. Superior Mesenteric Arteriogram—venous phase. The splenic (Spl. V.), superior mesenteric (S.M.V.), and portal veins (P.V.) are seen in a patient who had occlusion of the celiac axis and collateral circulation to the celiac axis via the pancreatic vessels. *Comment:* Note the enlarged spleen.

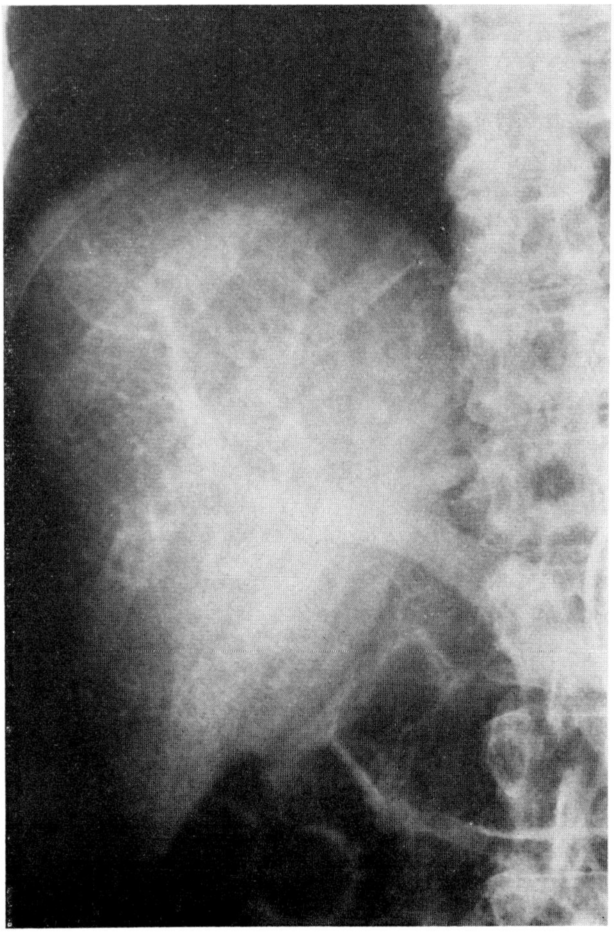

Figure 11.52. Celiac Arteriogram—venous phase demonstrates the portal vein and its intrahepatic ramifications. *Comment:* Normal.

rarely the inferior mesenteric vein may be blessed with two trunks (Figs. 11-45 and 11-46).

Superior Mesenteric Vein

Angiographically, this is a very resourceful vein for demonstrating a variety of anatomical lesions pertaining to different pathological entities.[363, 396] It is formed by the colic, ileal and jejunal branches from the bowel, and by the inferior pancreatico-duodenal veins and the right gastroepiploic veins from the pancreatic arcade and greater curvature of the stomach. The superior mesenteric vein merges with the splenic vein behind the pancreas to form the portal vein (Fig. 11-47).

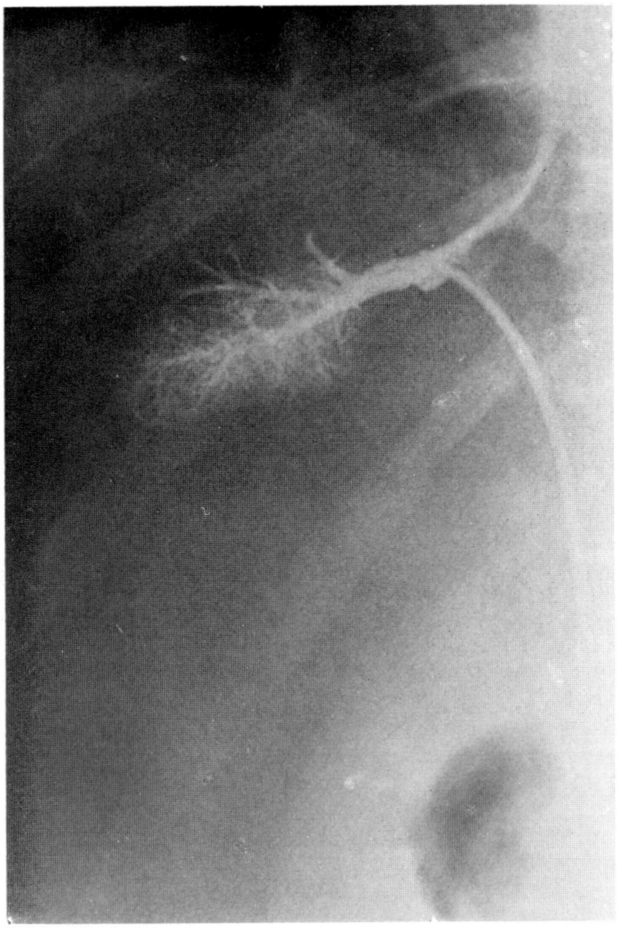

Figure 11.53. Wedge Hepatic Venogram. There is good opacification of the normal hepatic venules and homogeneous perfusion of the normal hepatic sinusoids.

Splenic Vein

The splenic vein,[363, 396] an inferior accompaniment to the splenic artery, courses across the posterior aspect of the body and tail of the pancreas. Posterior to the neck of the pancreas, it unites with the superior mesenteric vein at an angle of approximately 90 degrees to form the portal vein. The tributaries of the splenic vein are the short gastric veins from the fundus of the stomach, the left gastroepiploic vein from the greater curvature of the stomach, the coro-

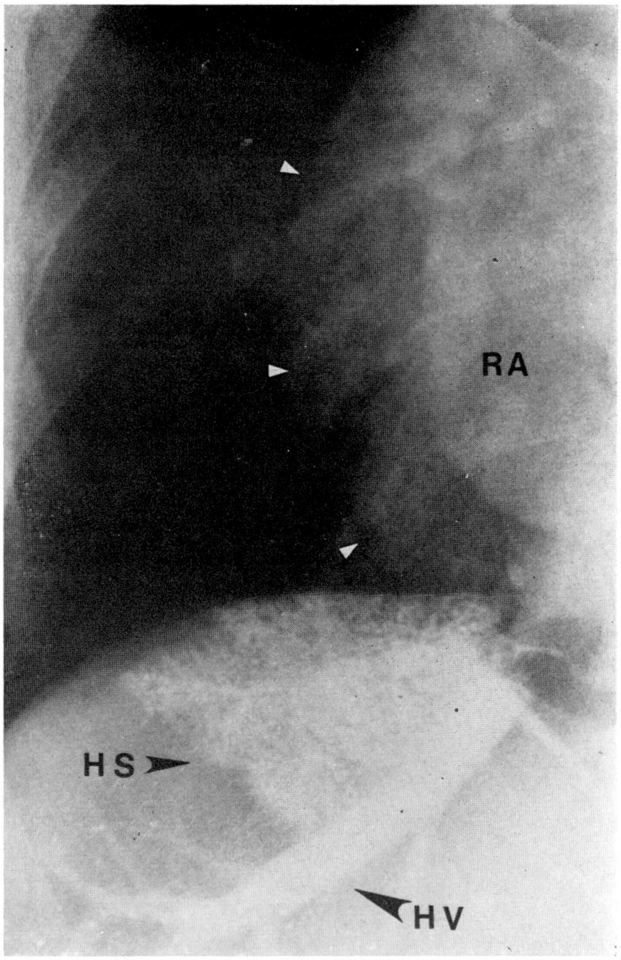

Figure 11.54. Hepatic Venogram. A granular collection of contrast material is seen in the hepatic sinusoids (H.S.) with good opacification of the hepatic veins (H.V.) and increased distance between the contrast material in the right atrium and the cardiac contour. *Diagnosis:* Opacification of the normal hepatic sinusoid and pericardial effusion.

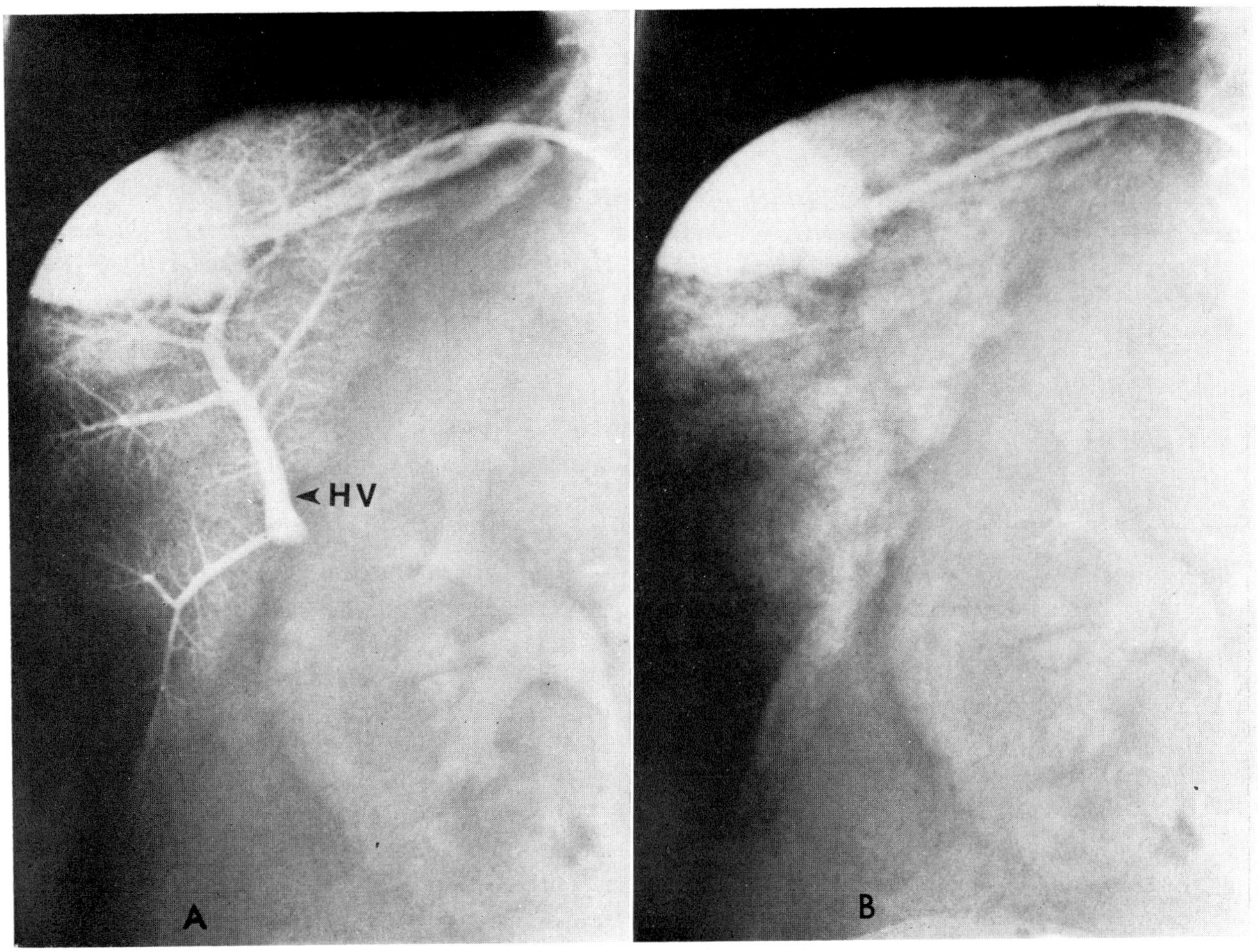

Figure 11.55. Hepatic Venogram. (A) The hepatic veins are well opacified with intense staining of a segment of the liver. (B) Excellent wash out of contrast from the hepatic veins with persistent staining of a segment of the liver. This is a normal hepatic venogram. The perivenous extravasation of contrast is due to excessive injection pressure.

nary (left gastric) vein from the lesser curve of the stomach, the pancreatic veins from the body and tail of the pancreas, and, of course, the inferior mesenteric vein (Figs. 11-48 and 11-49).

The Left Gastric Vein

This is a very popular vein because of its communication with the submucosal esophogeal plexus via the gastric fundal veins. It curls back on itself along the lesser curvature to terminate at the splenic vein, or at the junction of splenic and superior mesenteric veins (Fig. 11-48).

Portal Vein

This vein[363, 396, 397] represents the confluence of the great splanchnic venous drainage. It is formed *behind the neck of the pancreas* and in front of the inferior vena cava by the junction of the splenic and superior mesenteric veins. On its way to the liver, it receives the last contributions from the superior pancreaticoduodenal vein, cystic vein, perhaps the coronary vein, right gastric vein, and paraumbilical veins. The combination of a double capillary bed, a comparatively higher venous pressure with the opportunity for bidirectional flow during times of crises because of lack of valves and its communication with the hepatic arterioles in the hepatic sinusoids, creates a great venous bed (Figs. 11-50, 11-51 and 11-52).

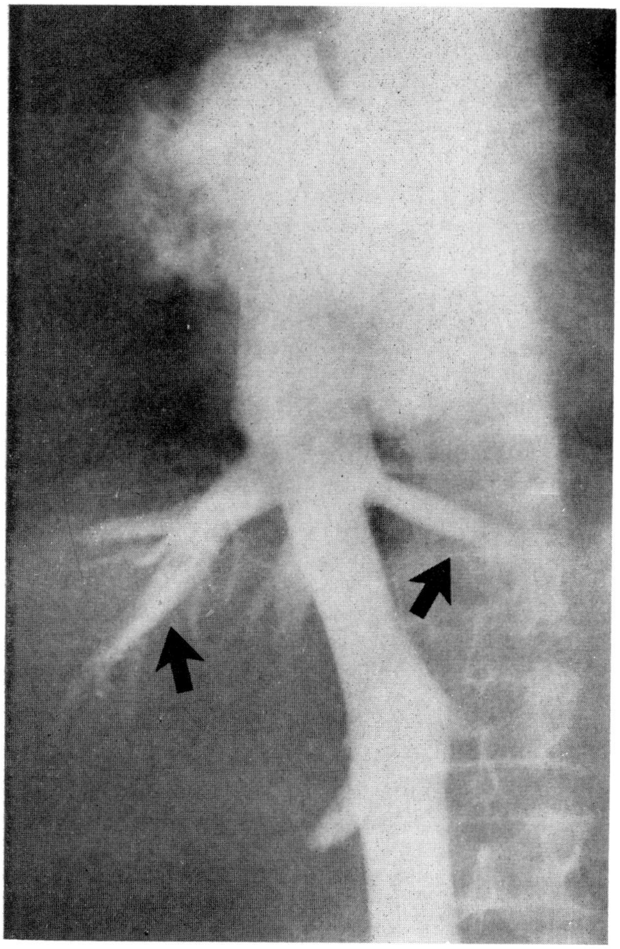

Figure 11.56. Inferior Venacavagram. Please note the reflux of contrast into the normal hepatic veins.

Hepatic Vein

These veins[395] drain into the inferior vena cava within an approximate span of 7 cm of the cranial portion of the cava. The average number of hepatic veins is about eleven, and sometimes may even number up to twenty-five in order to keep an angiographer busy (Figs. 11-53 to 11-57)!

RENAL VESSELS

Renal Arteries

The renal arteries[330, 331] originate from the lateral surface of the aorta, usually at the level of L. 1. They supply the five different segments of the kidney by dividing into an anterior (ventral) and a posterior (dorsal) branch. The *dorsal* branch is usually the first branch and descends vertically and parallel to the posterior hilar lip of the kidney to supply the posterior segment.[332] The *ventral* branch supplies the remaining four segments; the apical, upper, middle and lower segments. The ultimate terminations of the renal vasculature are end arteries in the strictest sense[328] (Figs. 11-58 and 11-59). Unfortunately, this type of conventional anatomy is not stereotypical. Varying courses of the renal arteries and their branches through the renal hilus are a common, rather than an uncommon, occurrence. The aberrant arteries actually are normal segmental arteries with precocious origins, whose blood flow in no way constitutes an extra supply. Two or more renal arteries in normal kidneys represent persistent mesonephric arteries which do not enter the hila, but enter the parenchyma directly. *Aberrant arteries* may arise from the aorta, or from the internal spermatic, suprarenal, middle sacral, internal iliac artery, or other arteries (Figs. 11-60, 11-63, 11-65 and 11-66).

The arterial supply to an *ectopic or fused kidney* may come from persistent lower mesonephric arteries (Figs. 11-68 and 11-69). The arterial supply to a *horseshoe kidney* is usually multiple, arising from the aorta and/or the common iliac arteries.[329]

The right renal orifice, and less frequently the left, may arise close to the ventral midline of the aorta.[333] Although rare occurrences, unusual vascular supplies to the kidney include vessels from the medial sacral vessels,[334] the right renal artery arising from the left renal artery,[335] and even less frequently, there may be arterial connection between the lower poles of the two kidneys.[336]

Perirenal Arterial Circles

These may be formed by the adipose capsular arteries, renal, mesenteric, spermatic, lumbar, inferior phrenic, and the aorta.[370]

Renal Veins

The *right renal vein* joins the inferior vena cava around the level of the L. 1 vertebral

(Text continues on page 143)

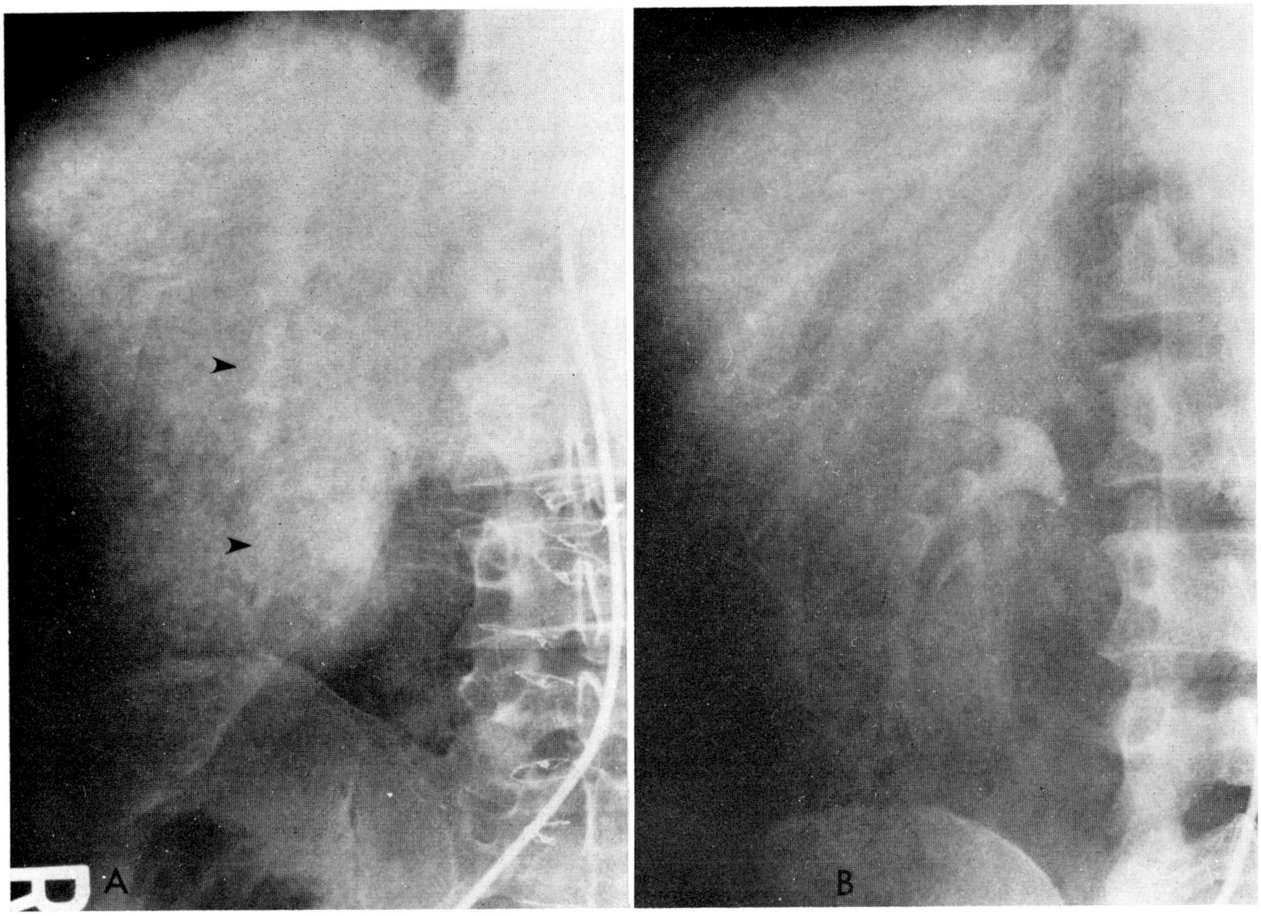

Figure 11.57. Hepatic Arteriogram. A and B are two different patients. The late phase reveals opacification of the normal hepatic veins. *Comment:* Hepatic vein visualization after selective hepatic arteriogram is rarely seen, probably because the contrast is diluted by the nonopacified portal venous blood.

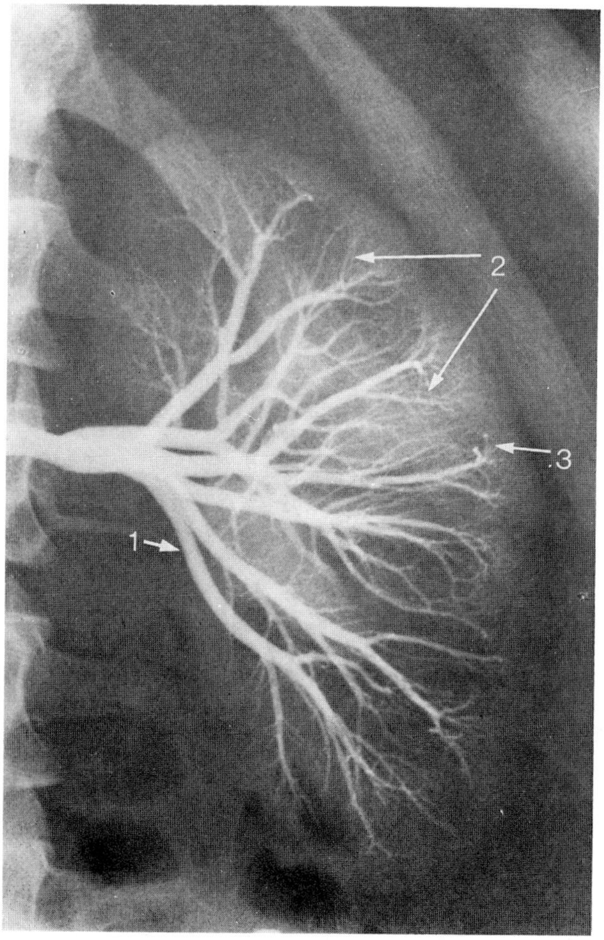

Figure 11.58. Renal Arteriogram. 1. Hilar branches, 2. Interlobar branches, 3. Arcuate arteries. *Comment:* Note normal renal arterial anatomy.

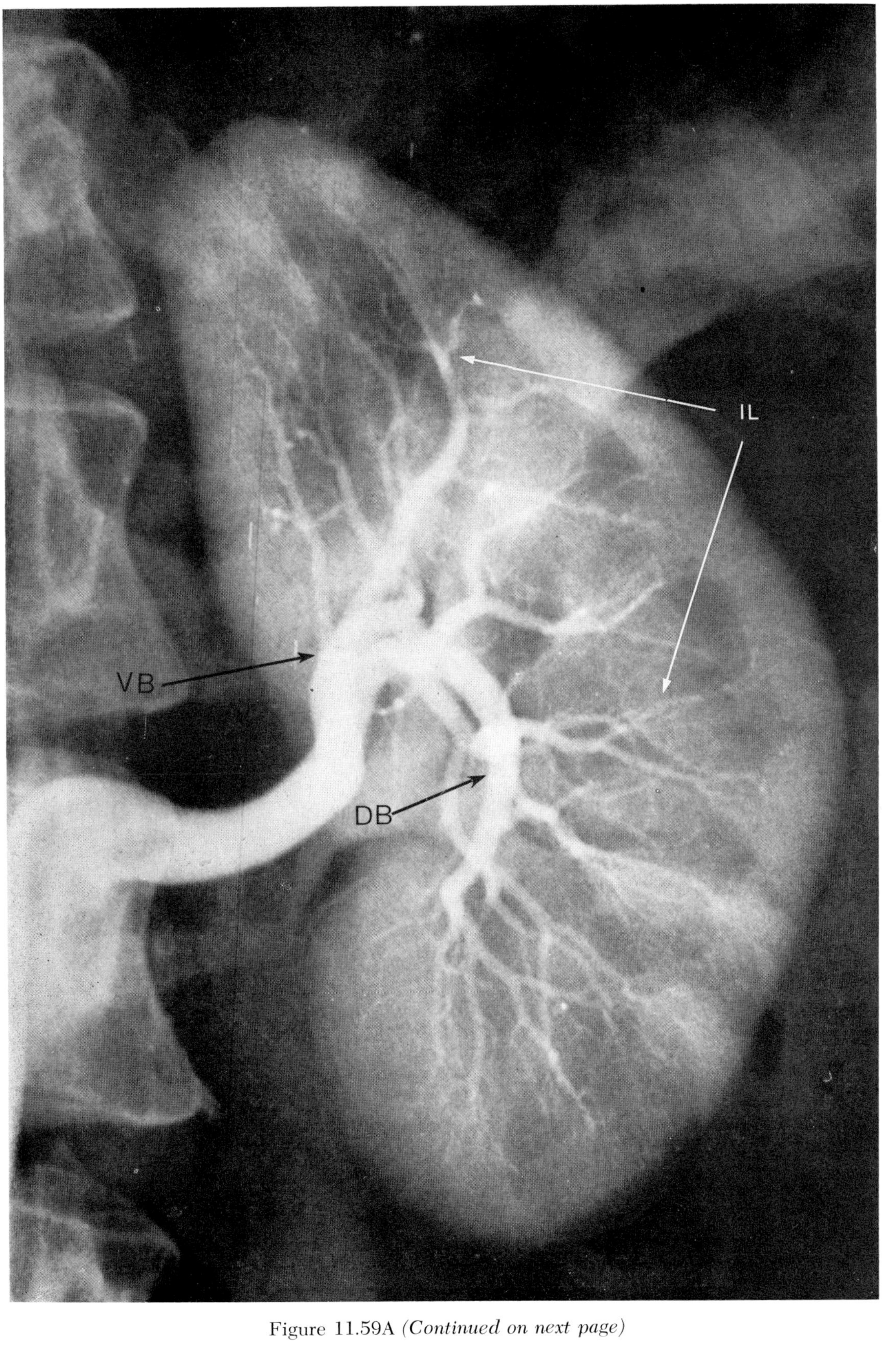

Figure 11.59A *(Continued on next page)*

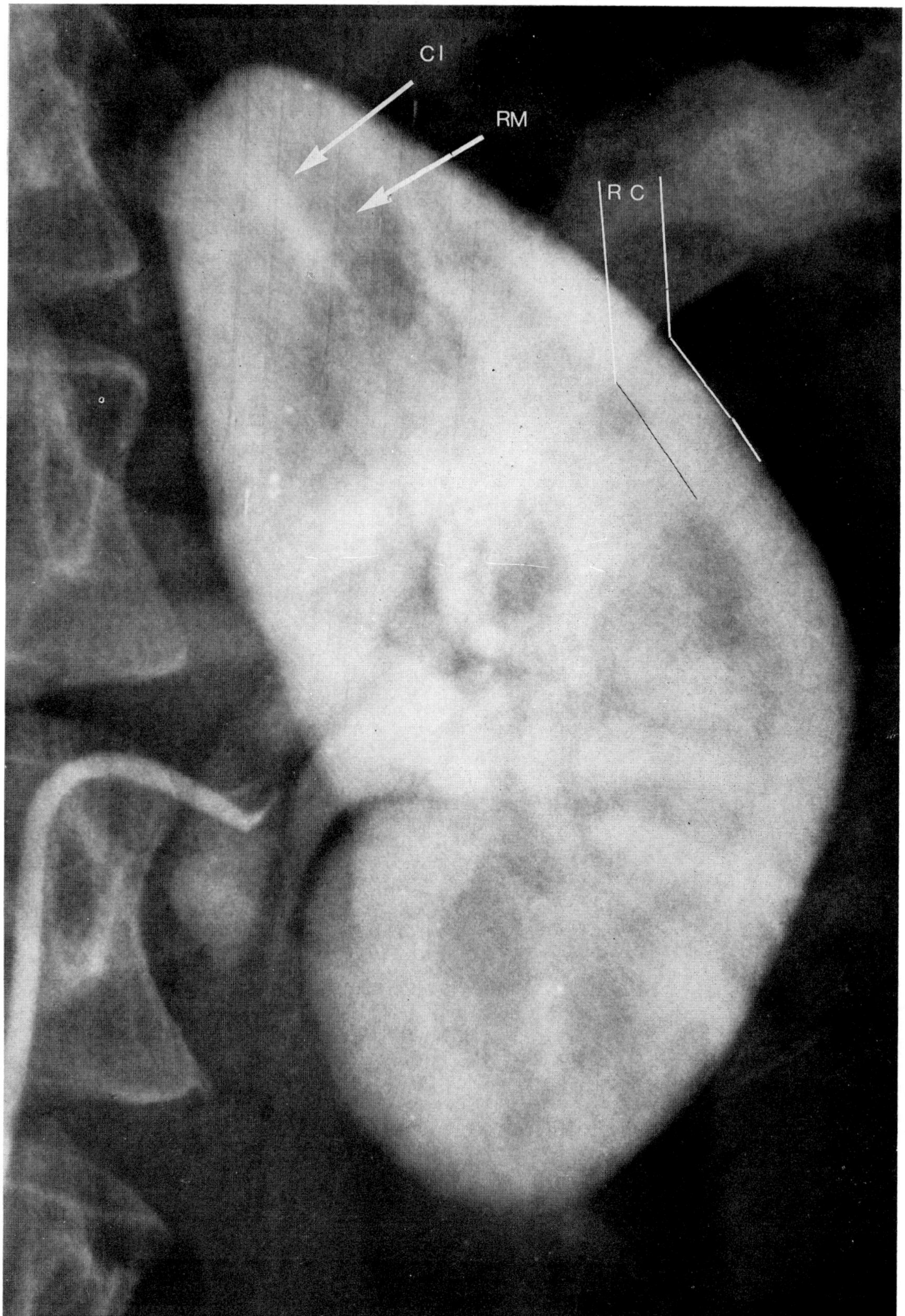

Figure 11.59. Renal Arteriogram. (A) Arterial phase: Ventral branch (V.B.), dorsal branch (D.B.), interlobar branches (I.L.). (B) Parenchymal phase: Renal cortex (R.C.), renal medulla (R.M.), cortical invagination into the medulla (C.I.). *Comment:* Note normal renal arteriogram.

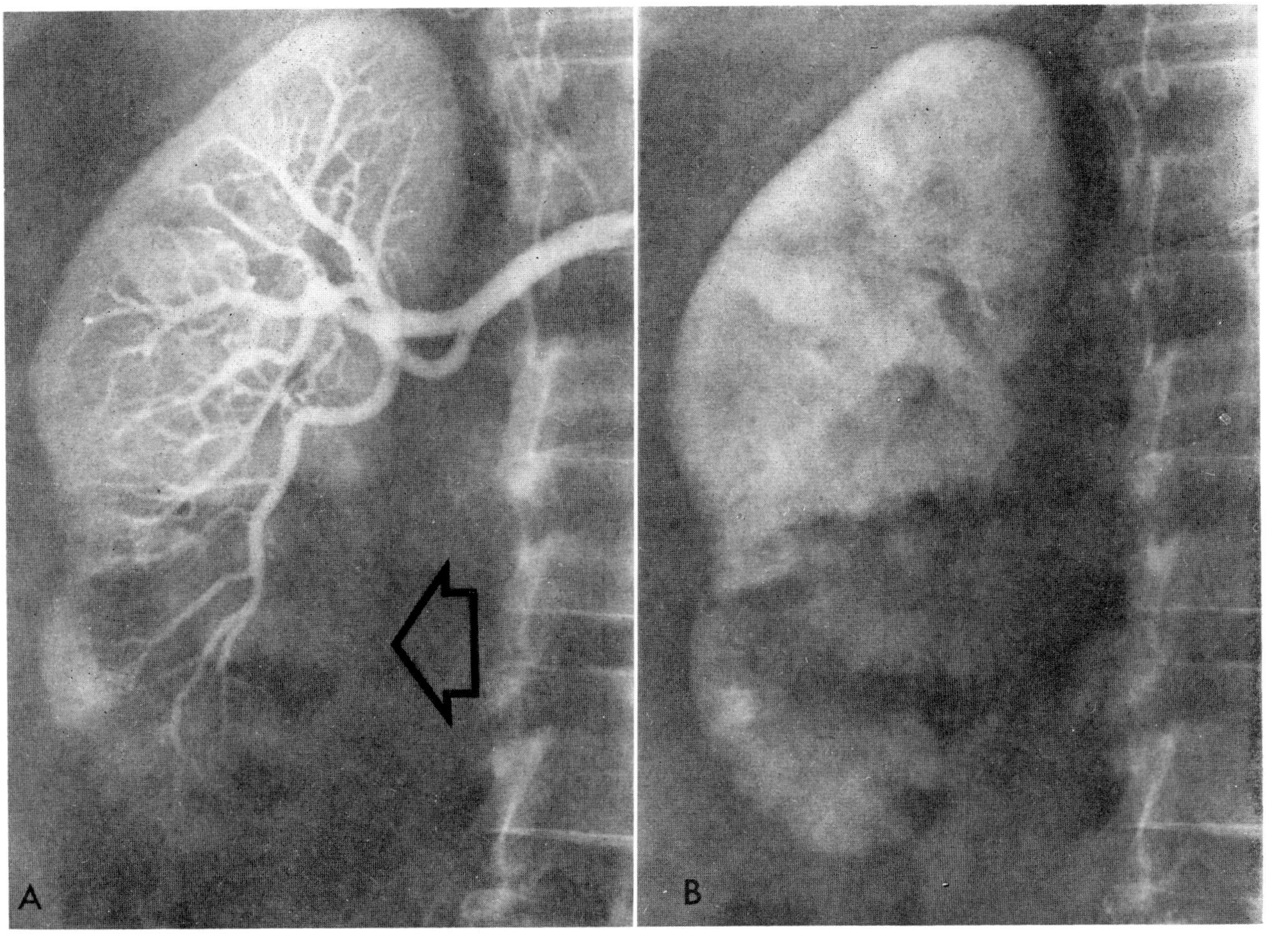

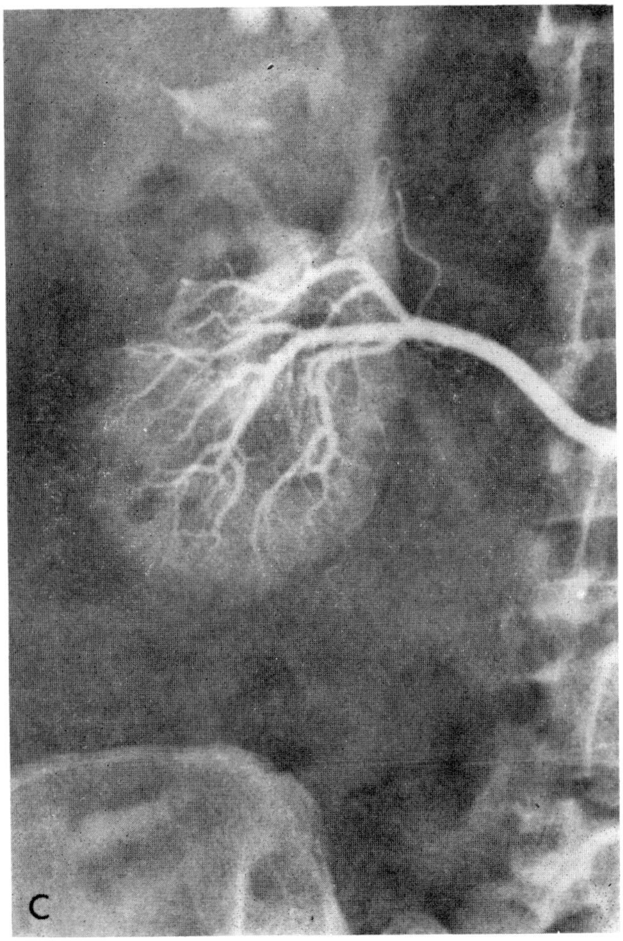

Figure 11.60. Renal Arteriogram. (A) Arterial phase: The intrarenal branches to the lower medial portion of the kidney (Arrow) are sparse. (B) Renal parenchymal phase: Irregular geographic filling defects are in the lower half of the kidney. (C) Catheterization of the aberrant renal artery on the same side. *Comment:* Note aberrant renal artery.

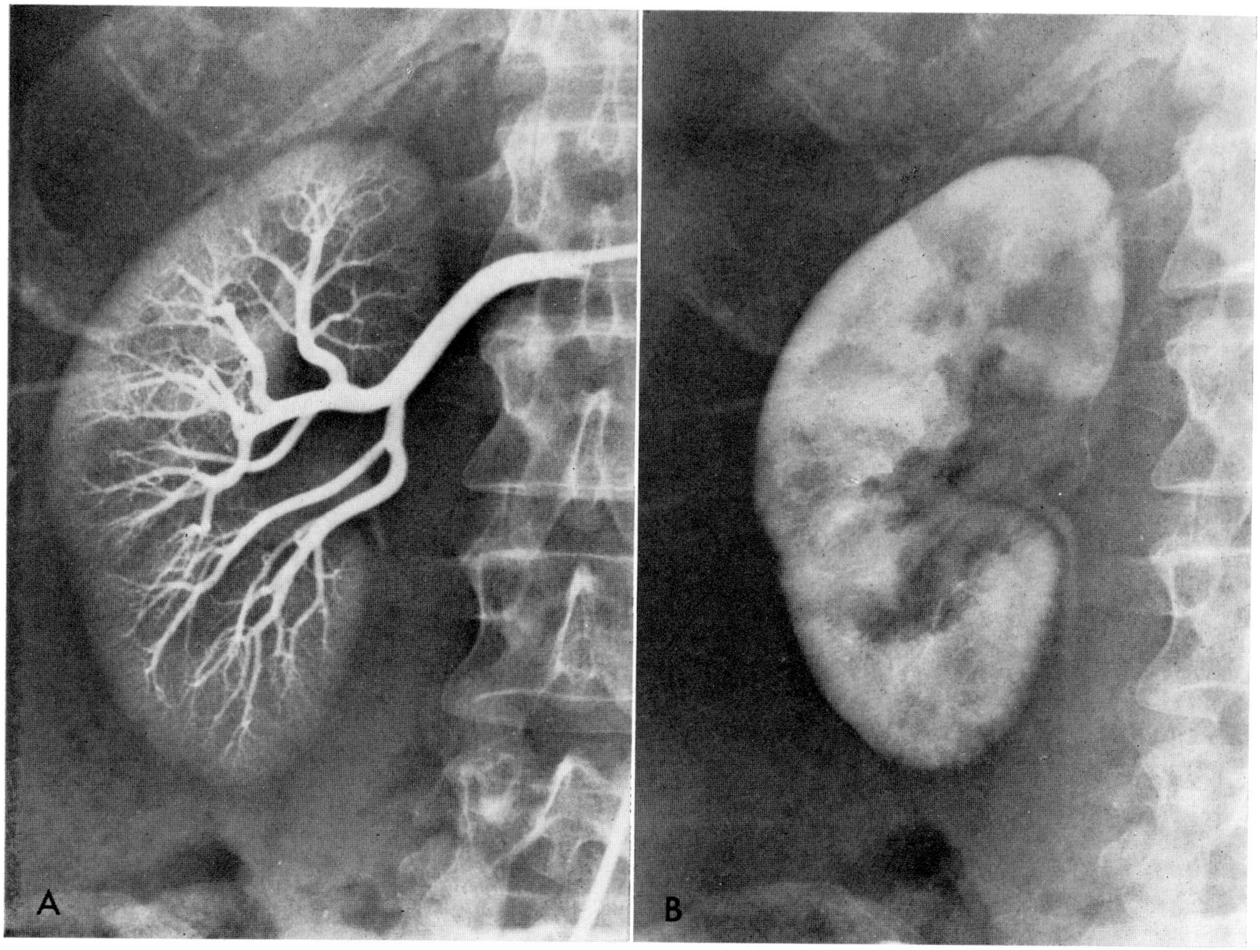

Figure 11.61 A and B *(Continued on the next page)*

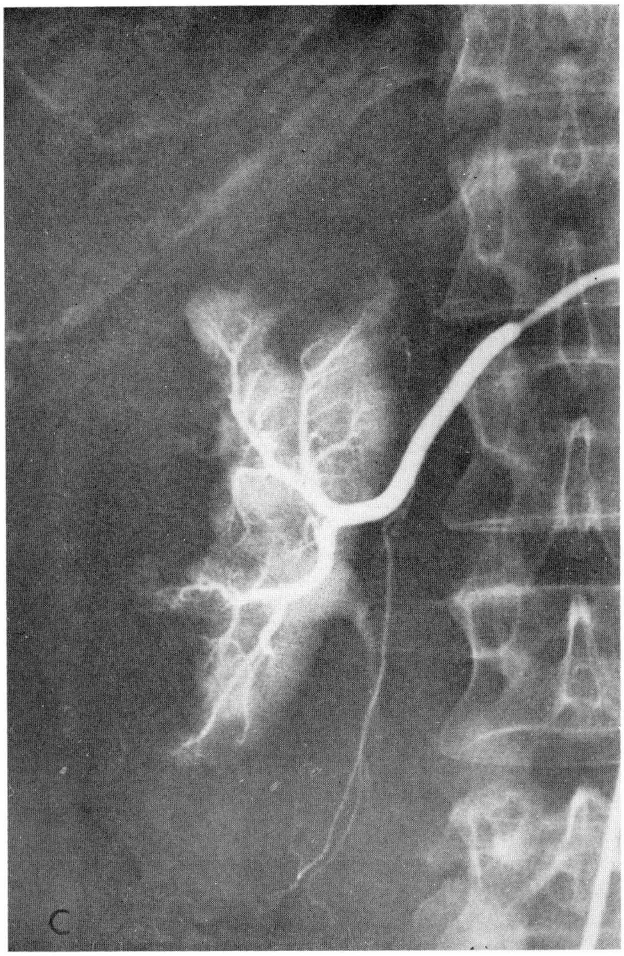

Figure 11.61. Renal Arteriogram. (A) Arterial phase: Any abnormality? (B) Parenchymal phase: Note a geographic filling defect. (C) Same patient after catheterization of the dorsal renal artery. Notice the perfusion of the previously seen geographic filling defect from the dorsal renal artery. *Comment:* Early division of the dorsal and ventral branches.

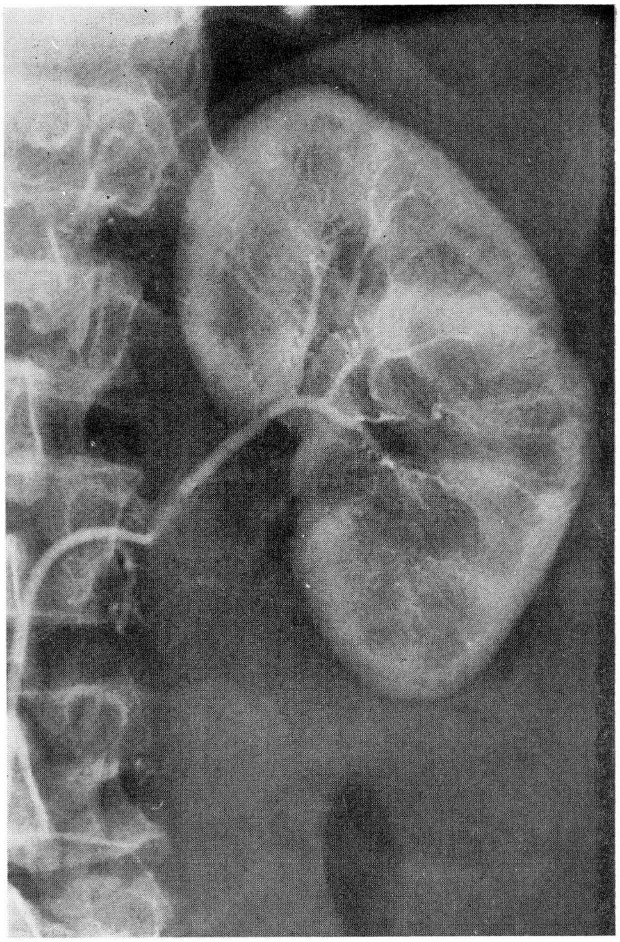

Figure 11.62. Renal Arteriogram—midphase. Good opacification of the dorsal branch of the renal artery due to stasis is revealed.

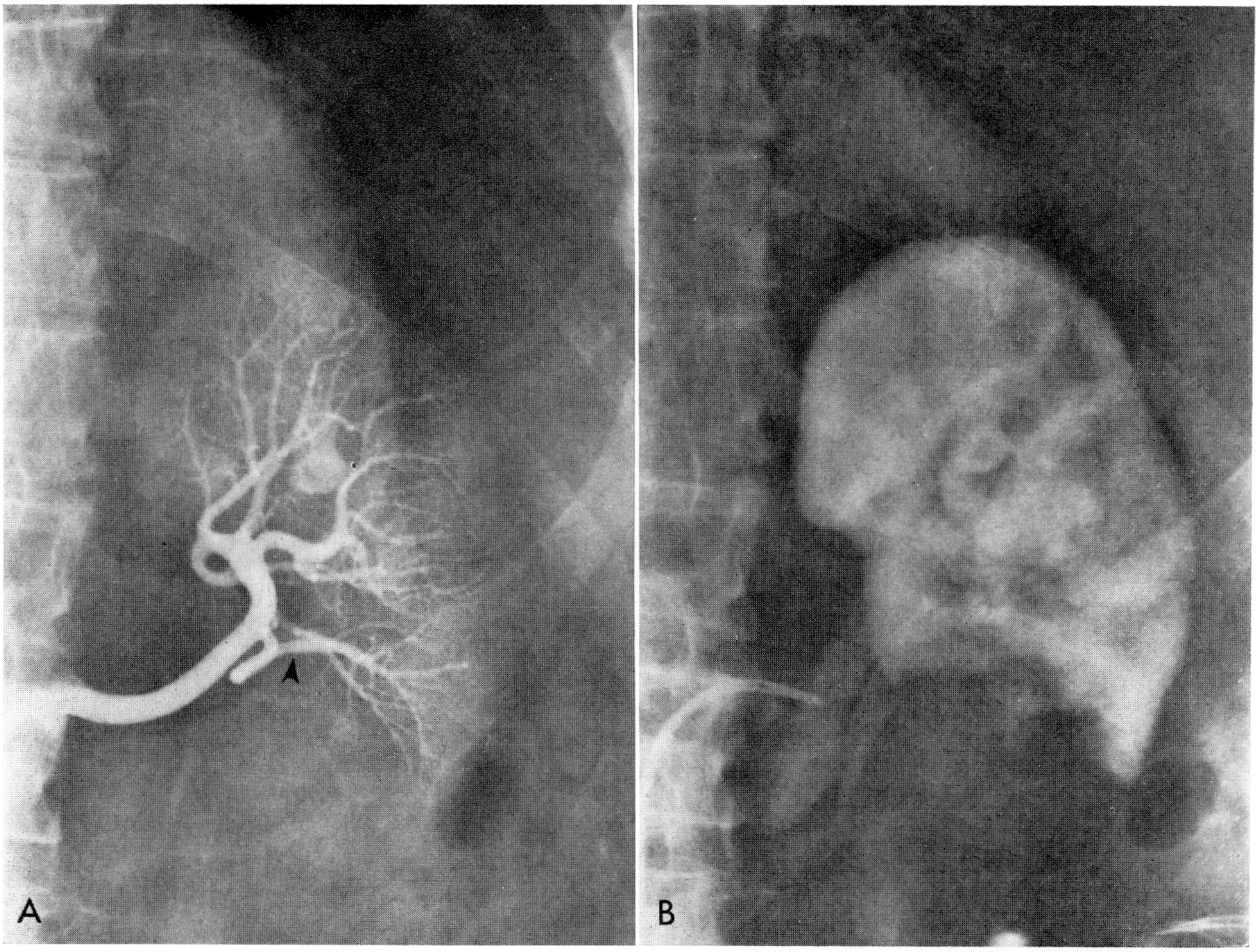

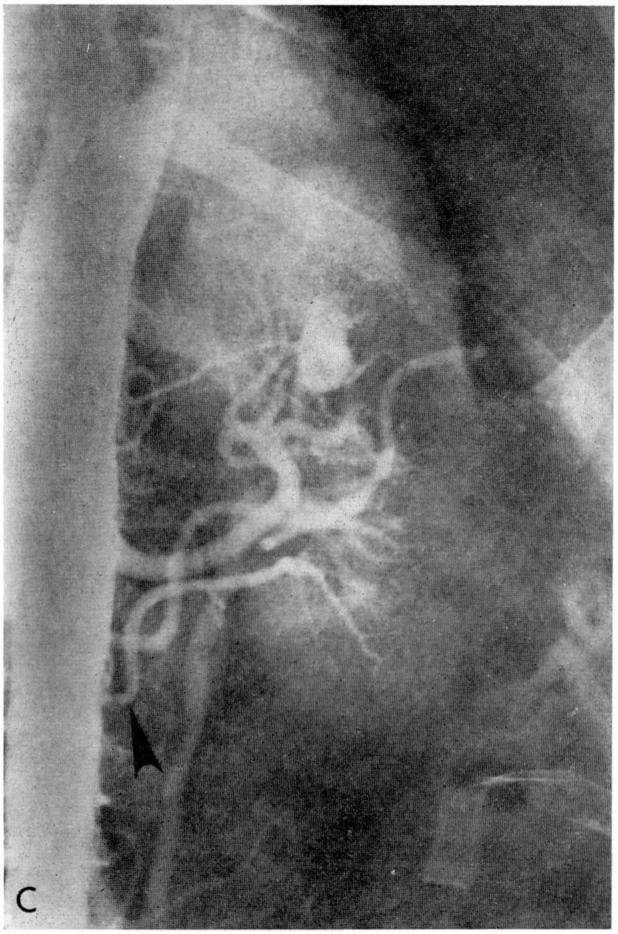

Figure 11.63. Renal Arteriogram. (A) Arterial phase: There is deviation and stretching of the lower intrarenal branch. (B) Parenchymal phase: A well-defined filling defect is seen in the same lower pole with a sharp interface with the renal parenchyma. This patient has had left flank trauma. (C) A flush aortogram reveals an aberrant renal supply to the lower pole.

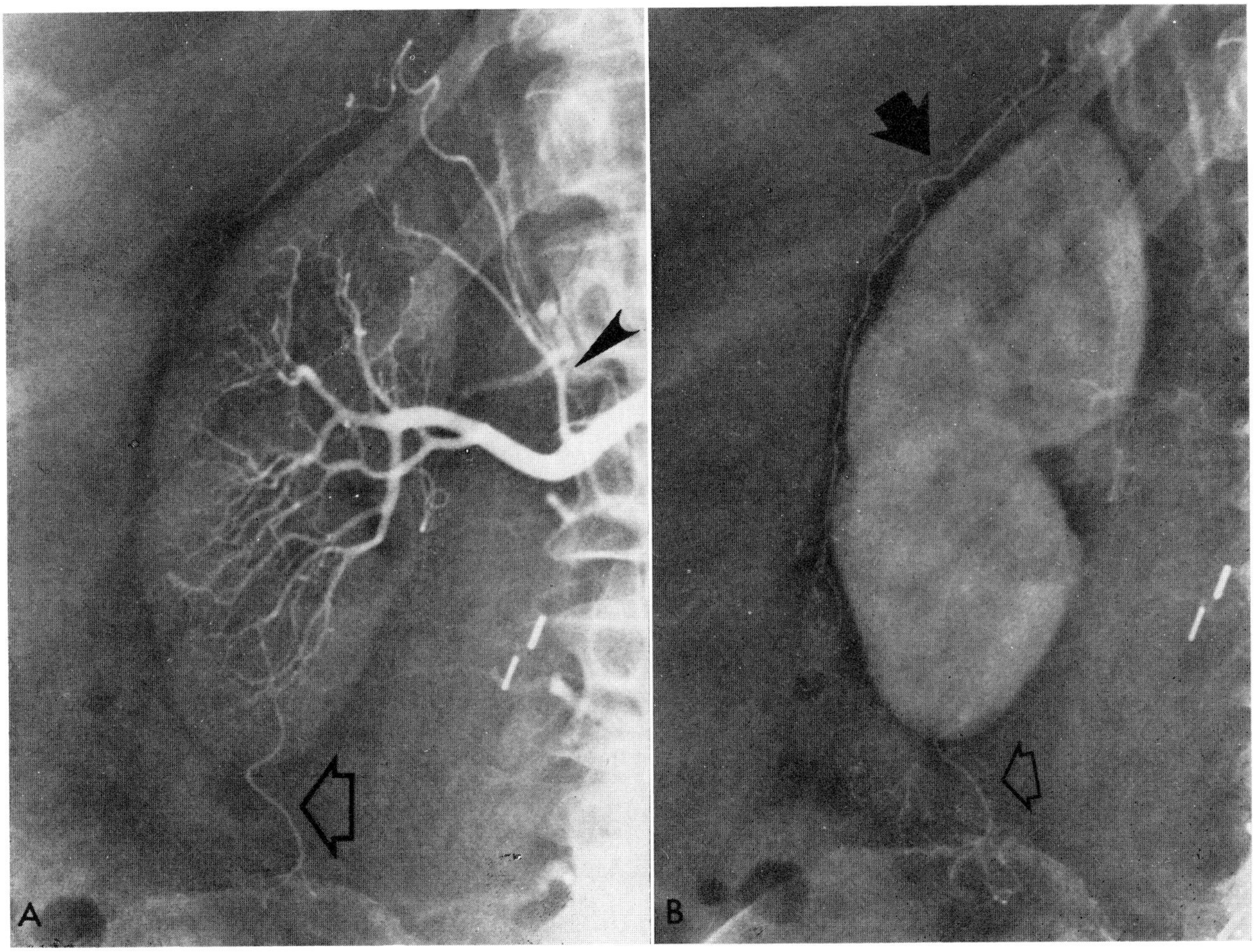

Figure 11.64. Renal Arteriogram. (A) Arterial phase: A prominent adrenal capsular branch is seen. The same adrenal capsular branch also gives an aberrant artery to the upper pole of the kidney. Note prominent perforating capsular artery. (B) Late arterial phase: Note good opacification of the renal capsular branch (Arrow) as well as perforating capsular branch. *Comment:* It is not uncommon to have a common stem for renal capsular as well as the inferior adrenal artery. At the same time, small areas of vascular supply to the kidney from this branch is also not unusual.

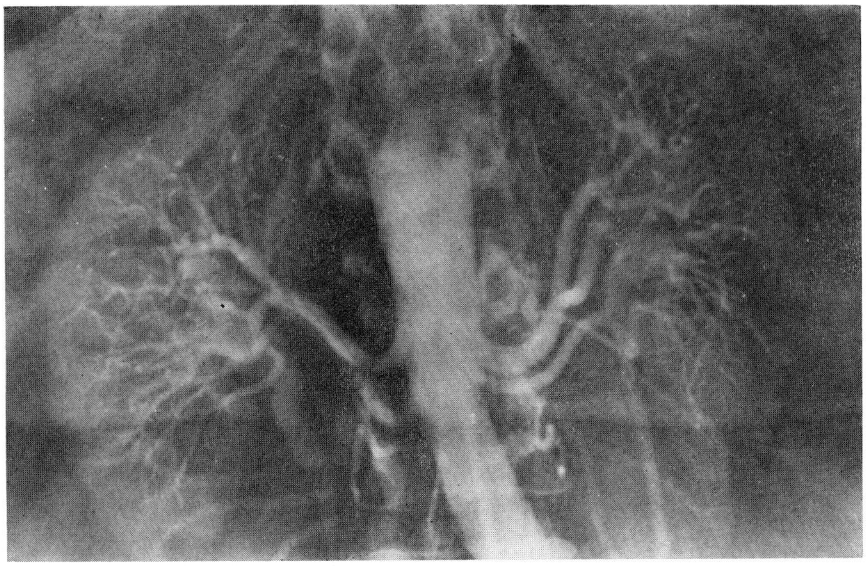

Figure 11.65. Flush Aortogram. Notice the two renal arteries located bilaterally.

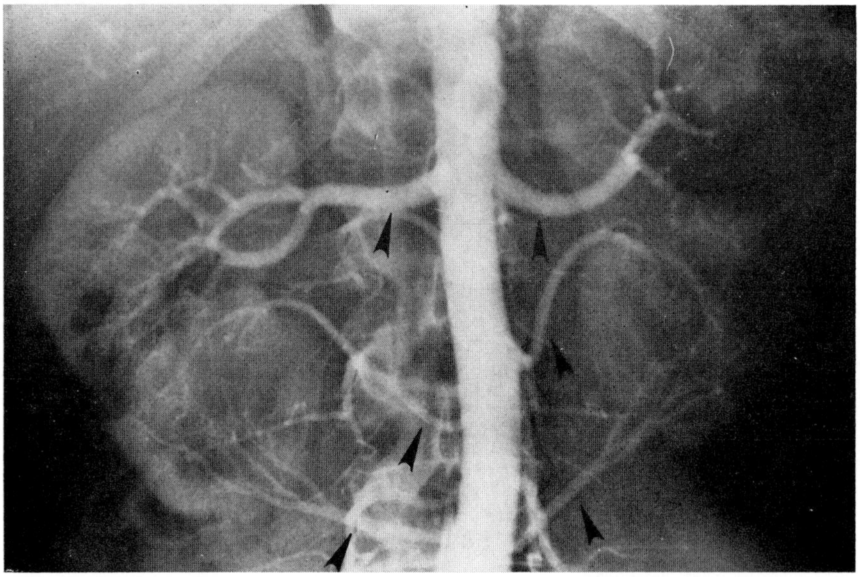

Figure 11.66. Flush Aortogram. Notice the multiple renal arteries.

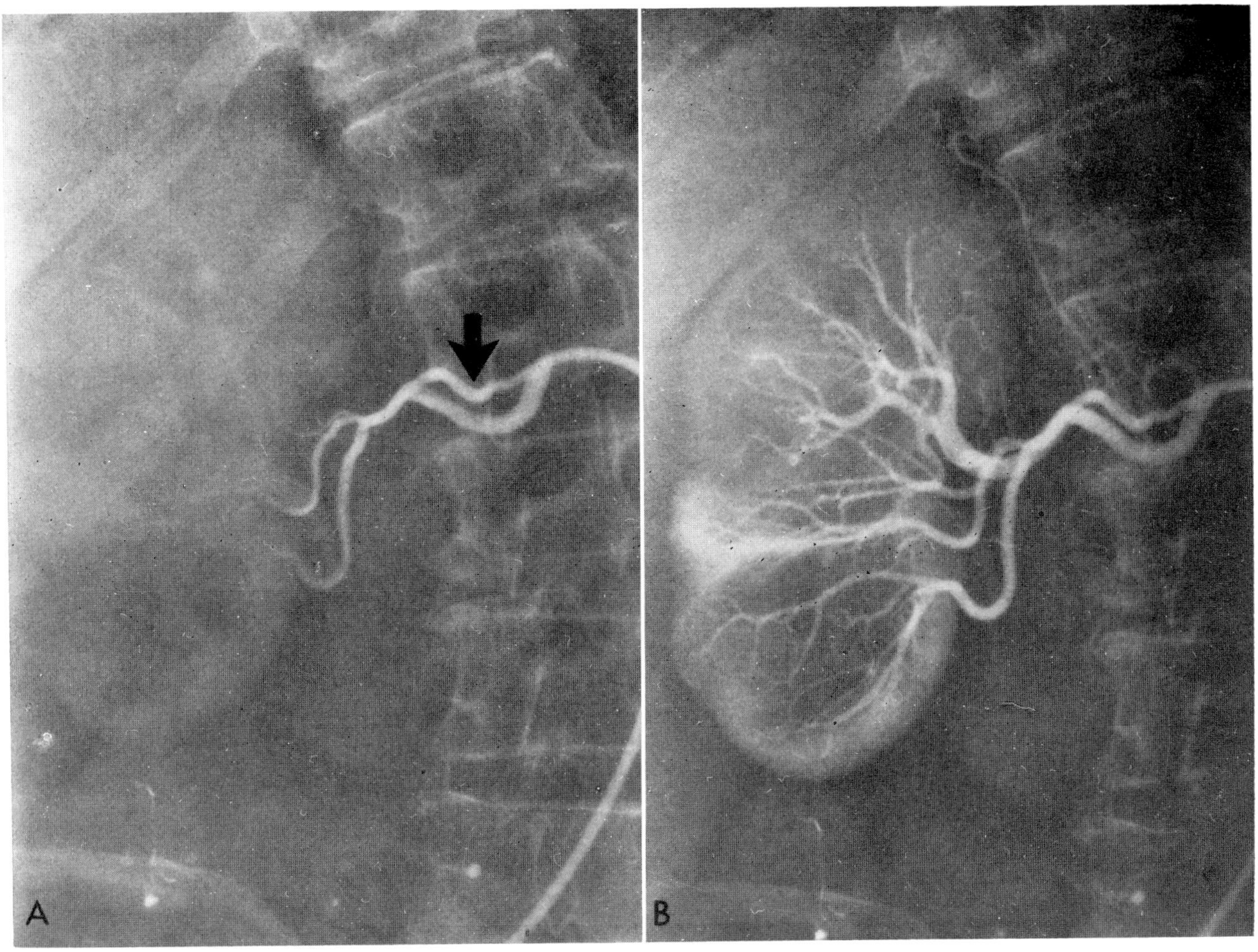

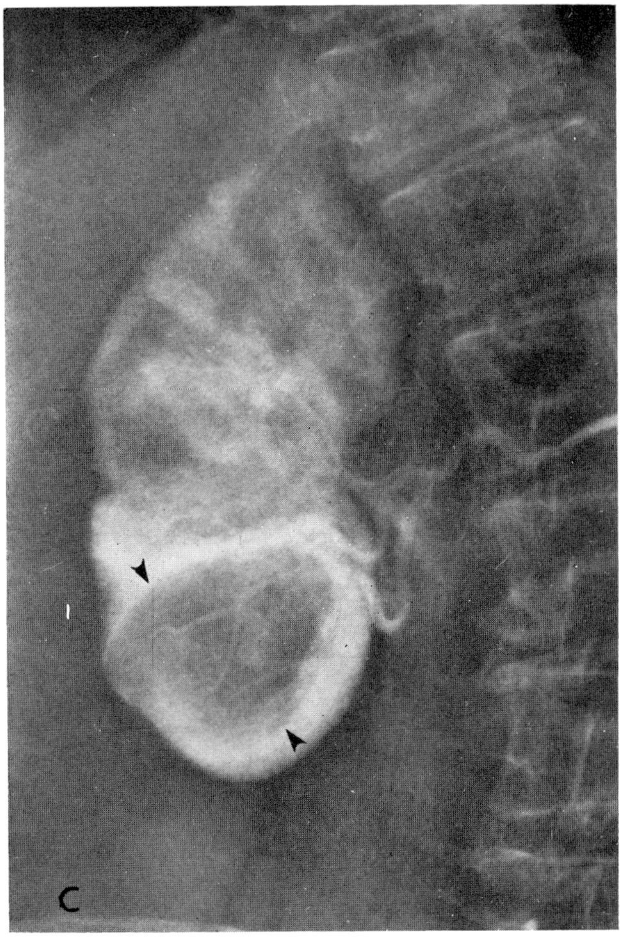

Figure 11.67. Renal Arteriogram. (A) Early arterial phase: Notice the early bifurcation of the renal artery. (B) Midarterial phase: The catheter tip engages in a small branch of the early bifurcation supplying an avascular mass in the lower pole. (C) An avascular filling defect is in the lower pole of the kidney with a sharp interface with the renal parenchyma. *Diagnosis:* Simple renal cyst. *Comment:* Early bifurcation of the renal artery is a technical problem during catheterization.

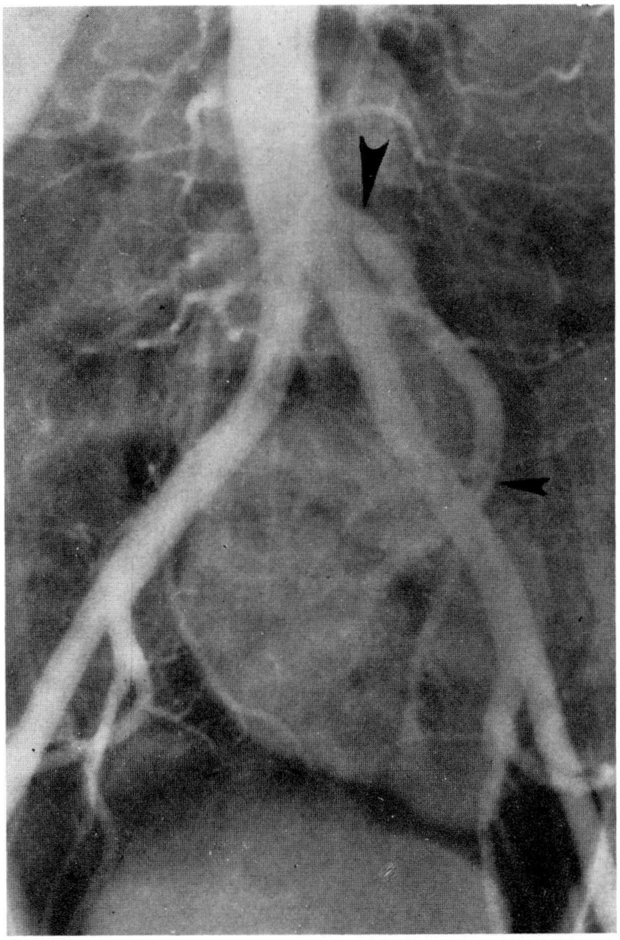

Figure 11.68. Flush Aortogram. A strange vessel arises from the distal abdominal aorta (Arrow) supplying the kidney in the pelvis. *Comment:* Ectopic pelvic kidney supplied by the lower abdominal aorta.

Figure 11.69. (A) An aortogram reveals multiple strange vessels arising from the aorta, right common iliac and left internal iliac arteries (Arrow). (B,C,D) Selective catheterizations of these vessels reveals perfusion of pelvic kidneys.

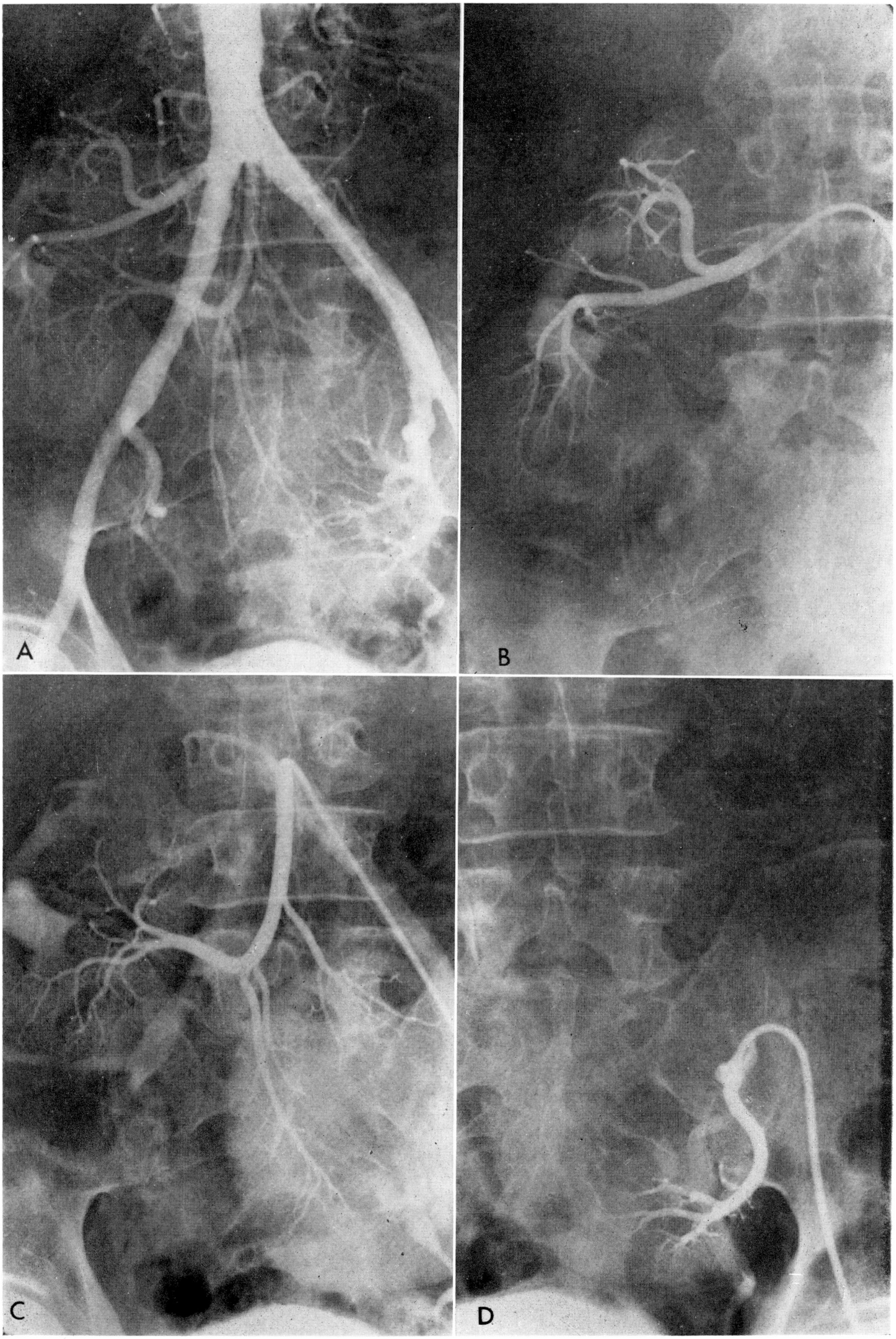

Figure 11.69

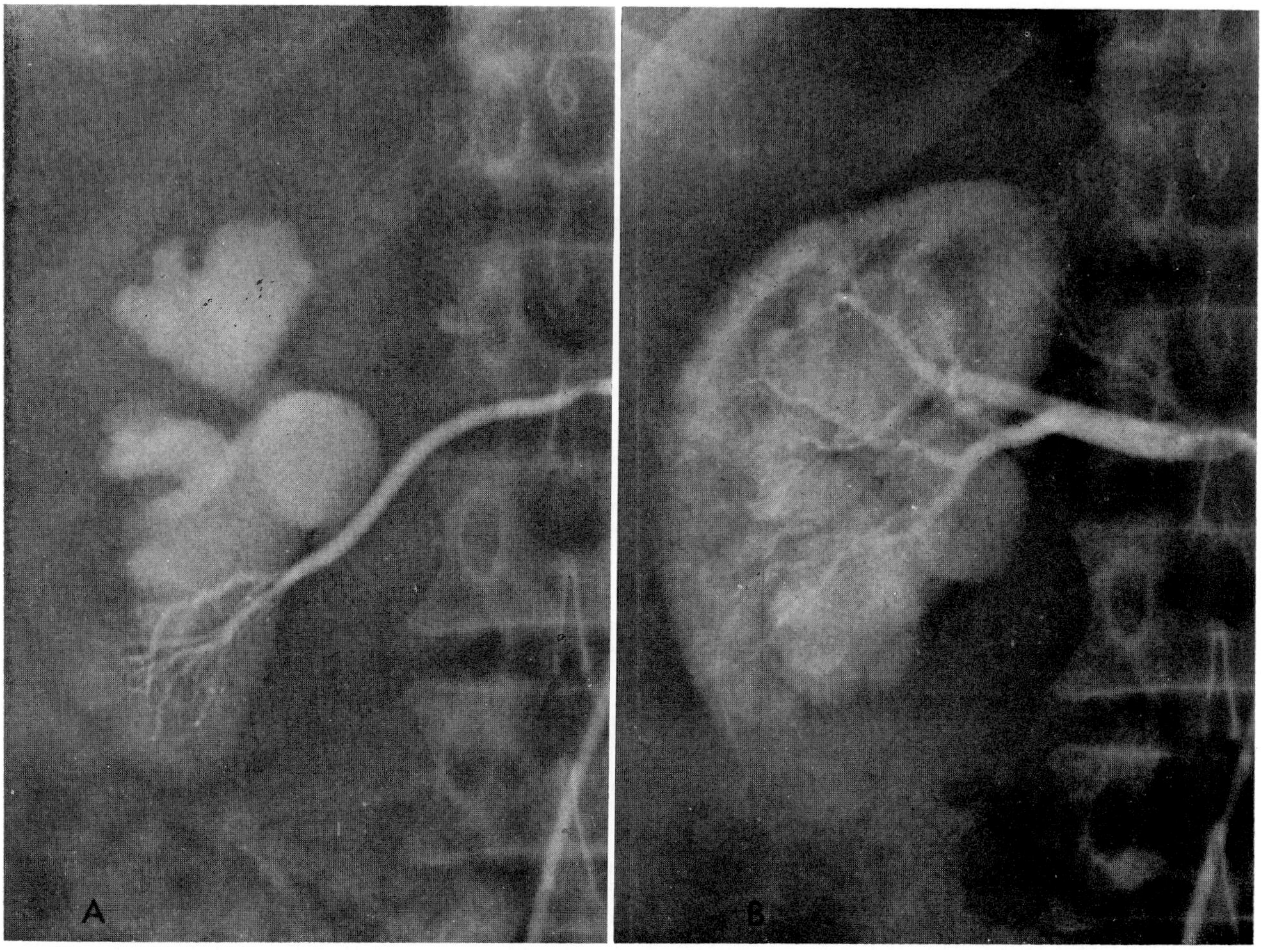

Figure 11.70. Renal Arteriogram. (A) The catheter is in an aberrant renal artery which is coursing across the ureteropelvic junction. Notice the proximal hydronephrosis. (B) A renal arteriogram of the main renal artery supplying the rest of the renal parenchyma. *Diagnosis:* Aberrant renal artery with secondary extrinsic pressure on the ureteropelvic junction causing proximal hydronephrosis.

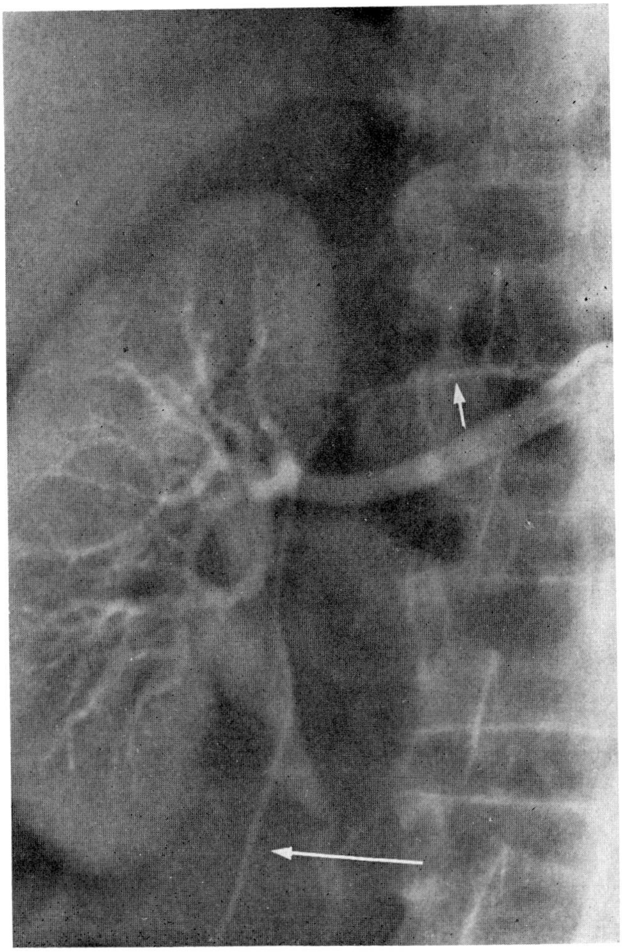

Figure 11.71. Renal Arteriogram. A prominent branch arises from the proximal artery and courses in the retroperitoneal area (Arrow). A patient who complained of right testicular pain and warmth during the injection of the contrast material. *Comment:* Origin of the testicular artery from renal artery.

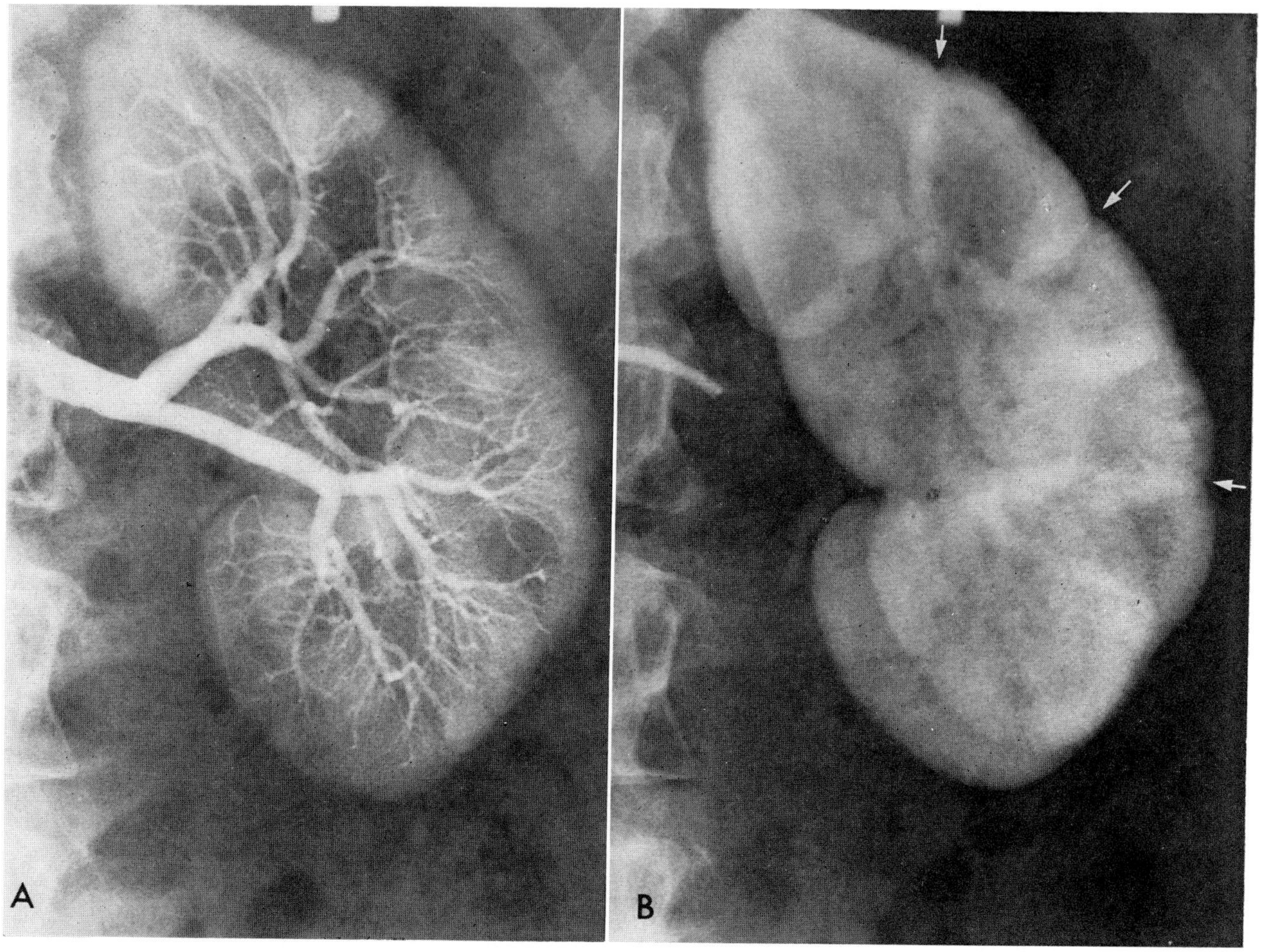

Figure 11.72. Renal Arteriogram. (A) Arterial phase: No apparent abnormalities are seen. (B) Multiple indentations of the renal contour are seen at the level of cortical invaginations into the medulla. *Comment:* Fetal lobulation. Unlike pyelonephritic scars, the indentation of fetal lobulations are at the levels of the cortical invaginations.

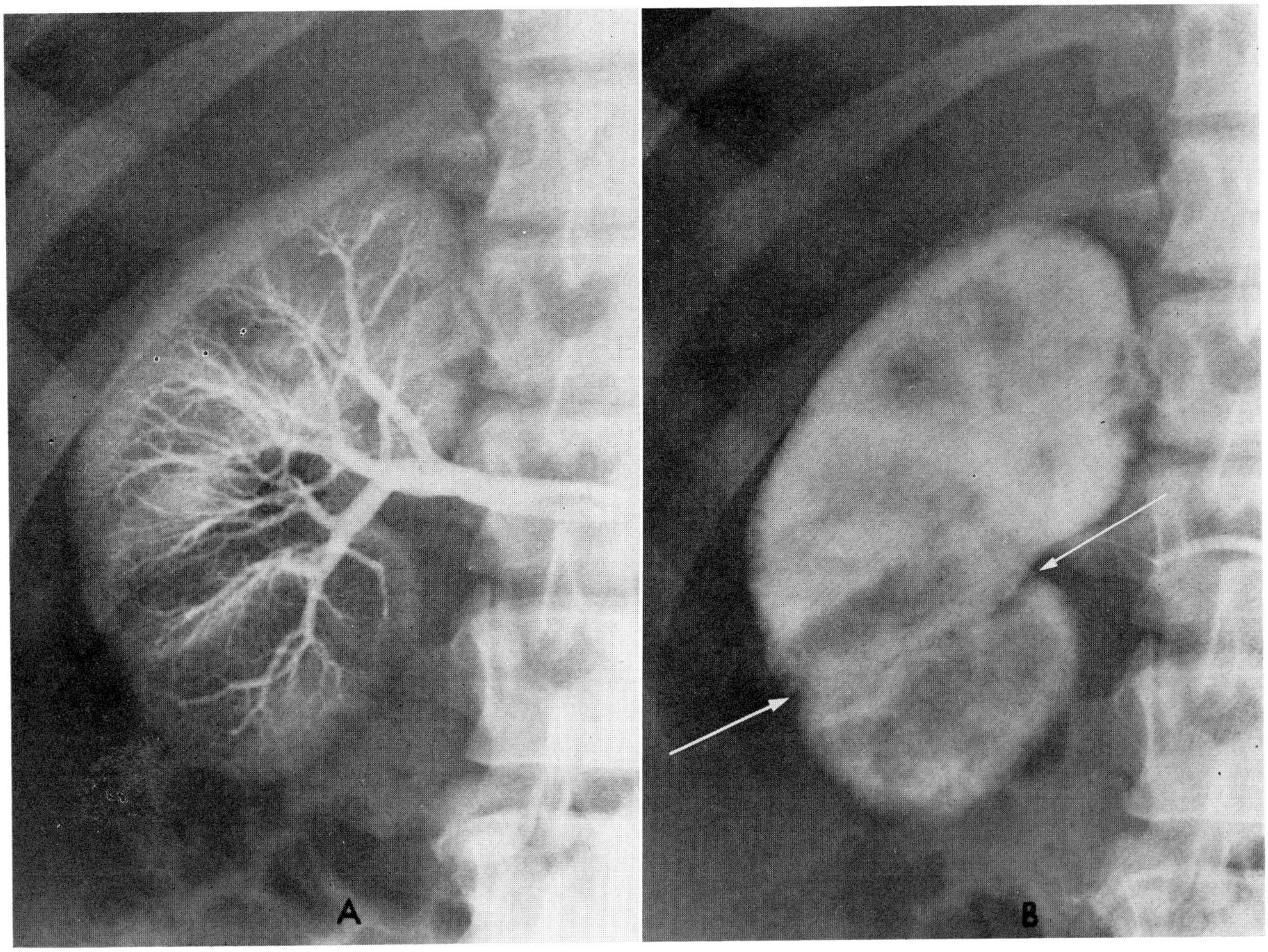

Figure 11.73. Renal Arteriogram. (A) Arterial phase: No apparent abnormalities are seen. (B) Parenchymal phase: A depression is seen on the renal cortical border (Arrow) with a translucent line in the same axis (Arrow) and an overlapping renal hilus. *Comment:* Renal lobule uniting with the rest of the kidney.

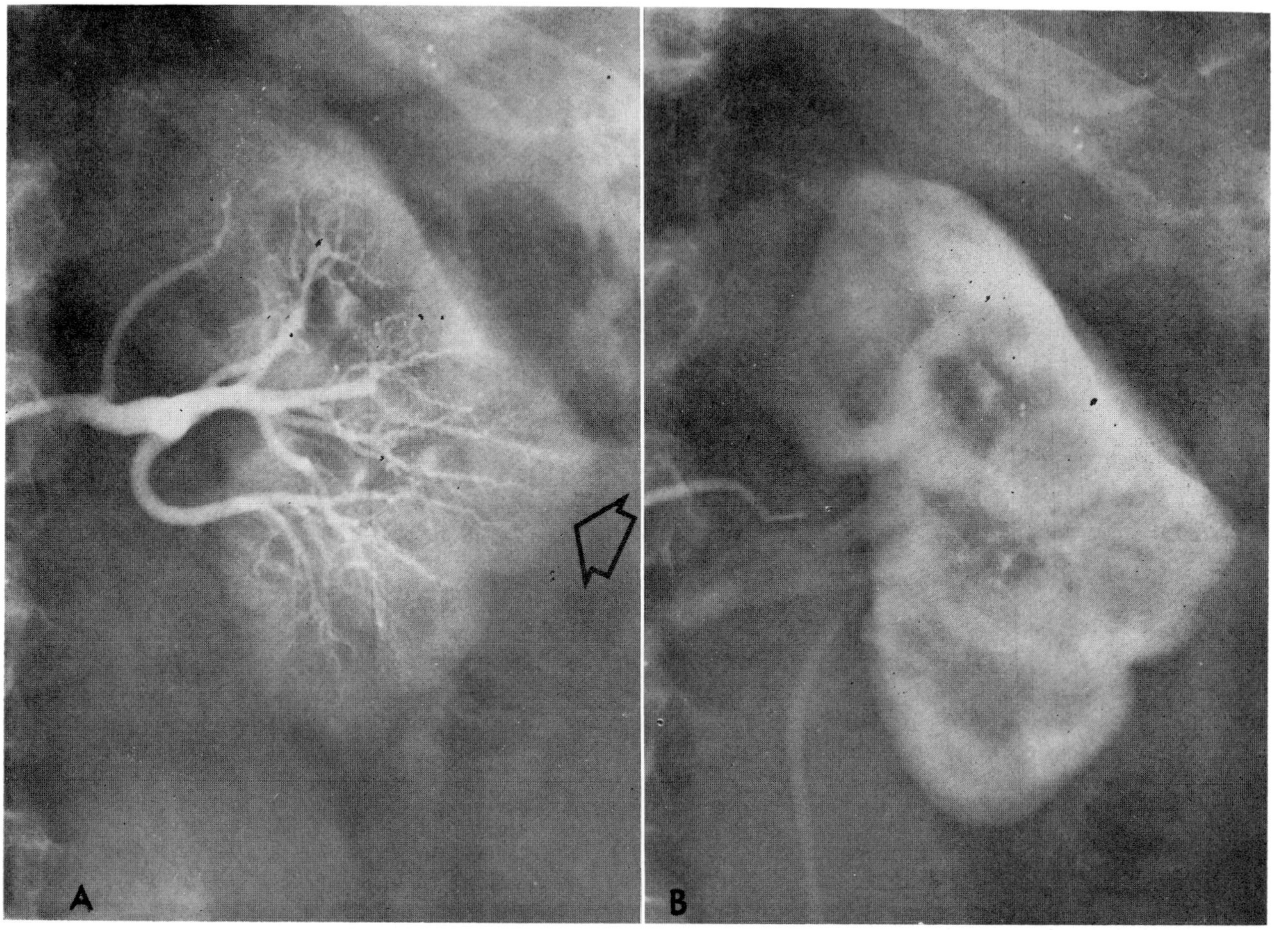

Figure 11.74. Renal Arteriogram. (A) The renal parenchyma is prominent with normal perfusion. (B) Nephrographic phase: Normal staining of the cortex and the medulla with a notch.

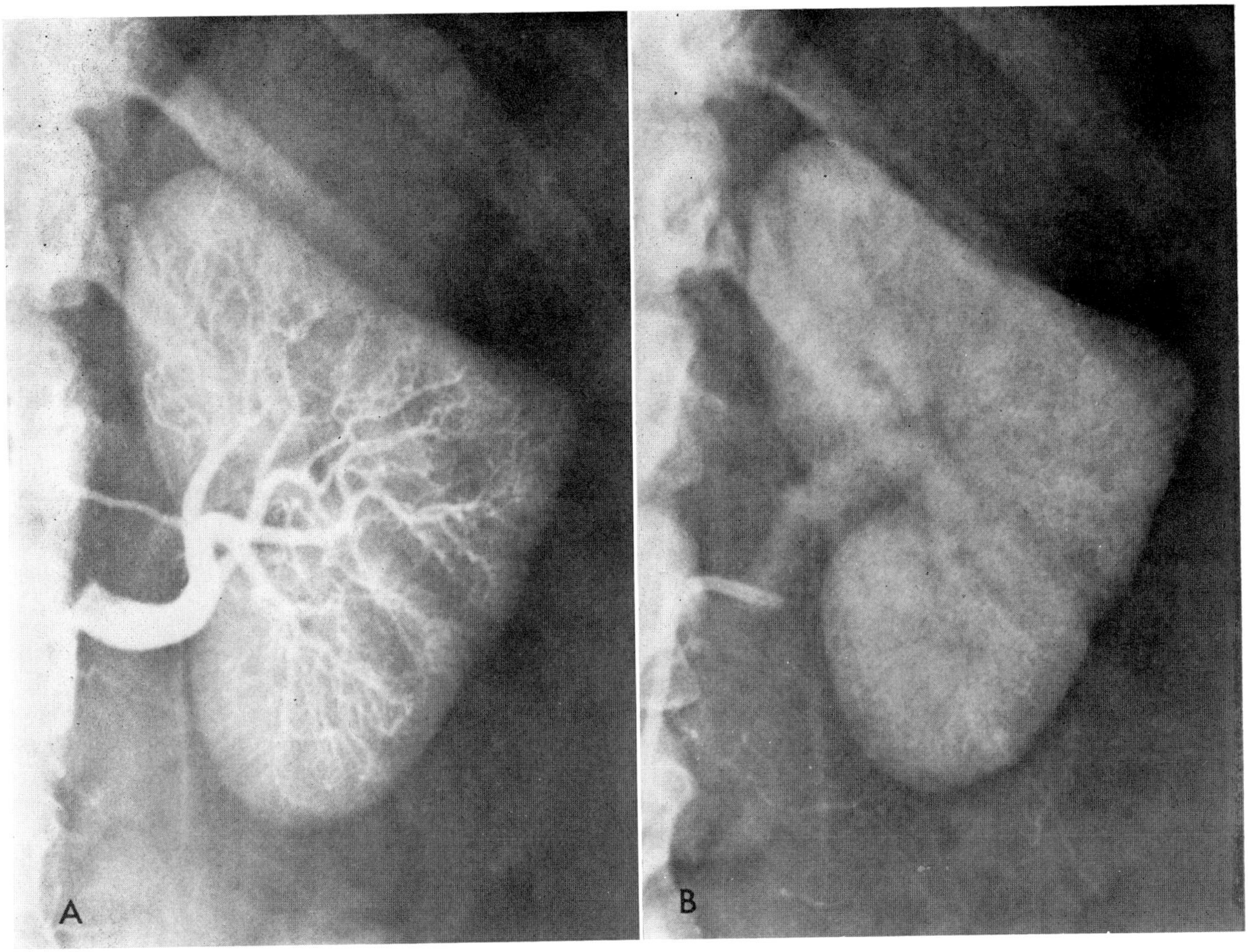

Figure 11.75. Renal Arteriogram. (A) Early arterial phase: An unusual bulge of the lateral border of the left kidney with normal vasculature is seen. (B) Parenchymal phase: There is no abnormal staining or filling defect. *Comment:* Dromedary hump.

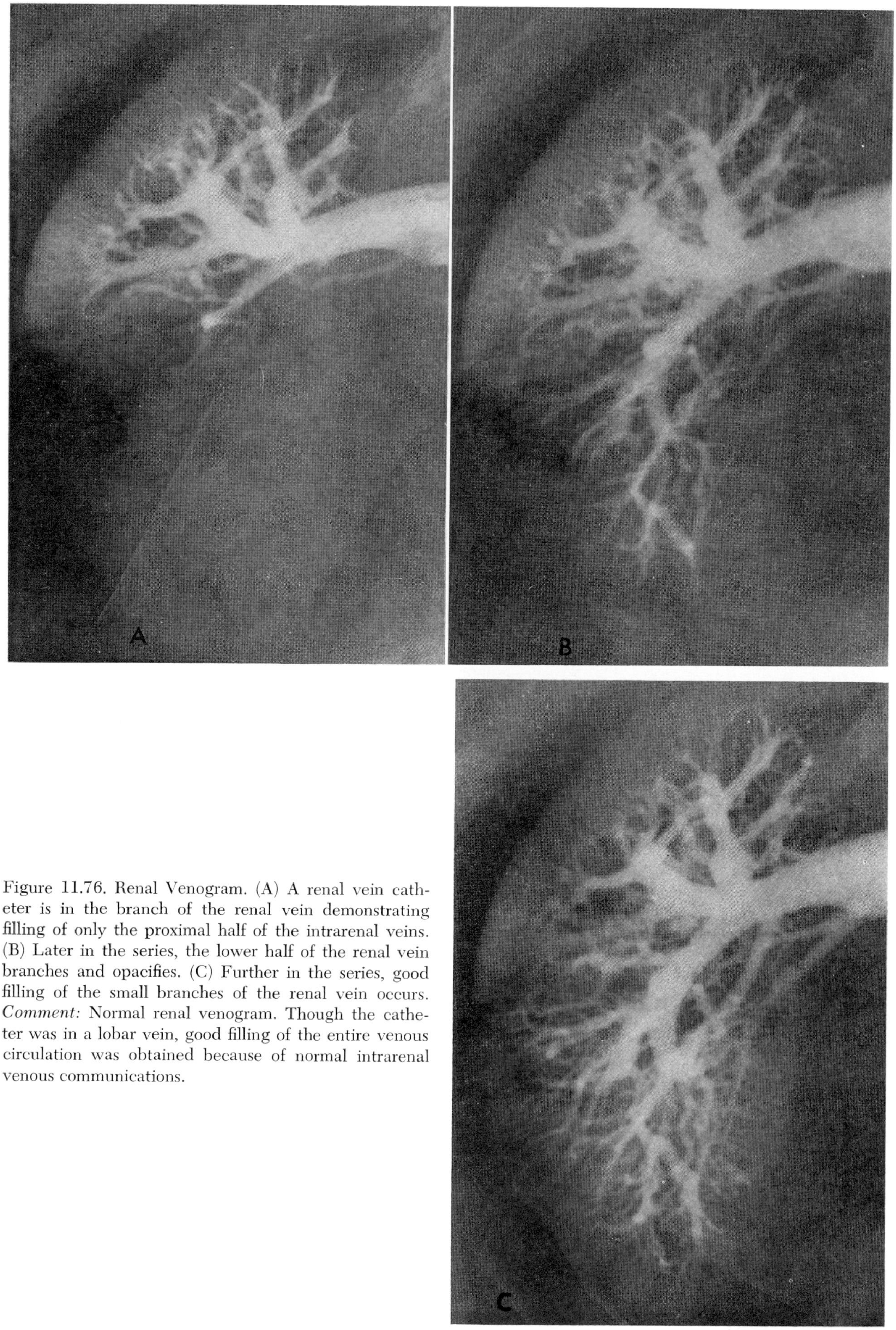

Figure 11.76. Renal Venogram. (A) A renal vein catheter is in the branch of the renal vein demonstrating filling of only the proximal half of the intrarenal veins. (B) Later in the series, the lower half of the renal vein branches and opacifies. (C) Further in the series, good filling of the small branches of the renal vein occurs. *Comment:* Normal renal venogram. Though the catheter was in a lobar vein, good filling of the entire venous circulation was obtained because of normal intrarenal venous communications.

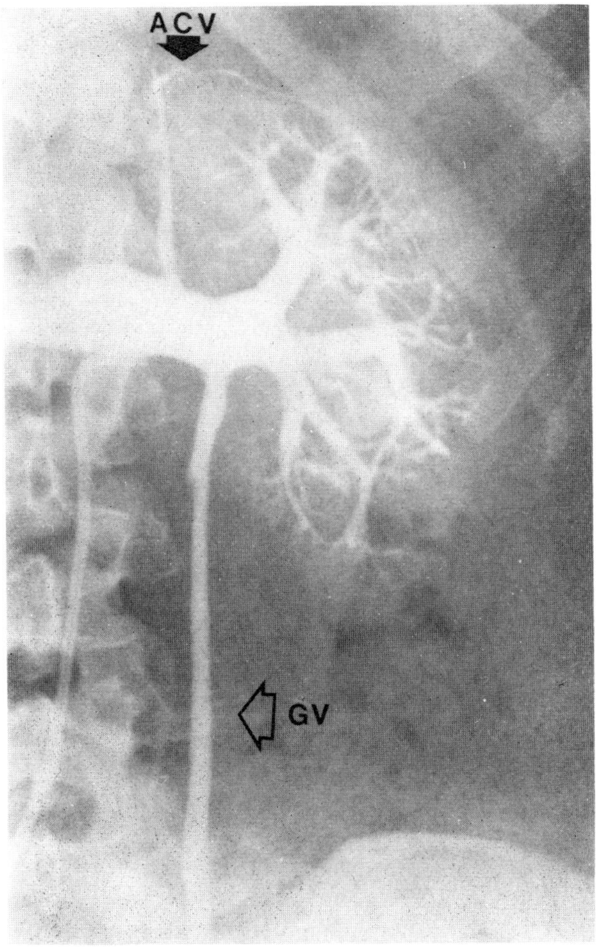

Figure 11.77. Postepinephrine Renal Phlebography. There is good opacification of the intrarenal venous ramifications and good filling of an incompetent gonadal vein in a female (G.V.) and incidental opacification of the adrenocapsular vein (A.C.V.).

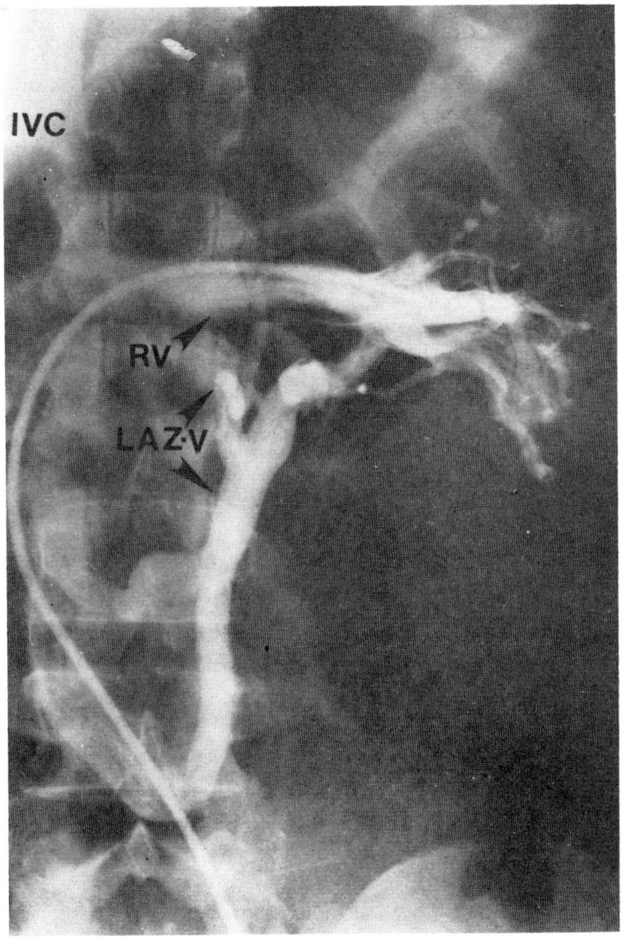

Figure 11.78. Left Renal Venogram. Left renal vein (R.V.), lumbar azygous vein (LAZ.V.), communication with inferior vena cava (I.V.C.). *Comment:* A renal lumbar azygous communication is not unusual.

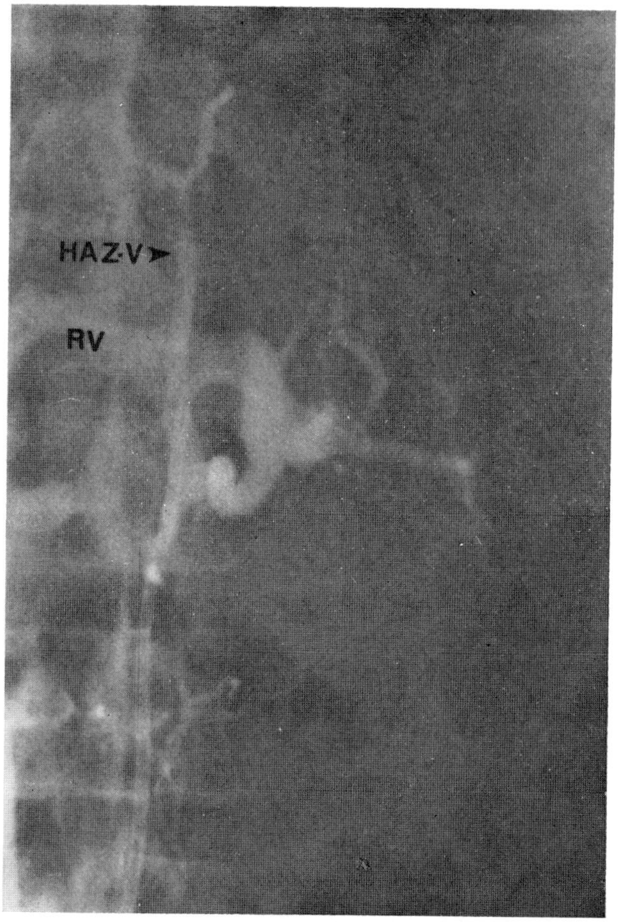

Figure 11.79. Left Renal Venogram. Notice the catheter in the left renal vein (R.V.). Note simultaneous filling of the lumbar veins. Opacification of the beginning of the hemiazygous vein. (HAZ.V.) is seen. *Comment:* Normal renolumbar azygous communication.

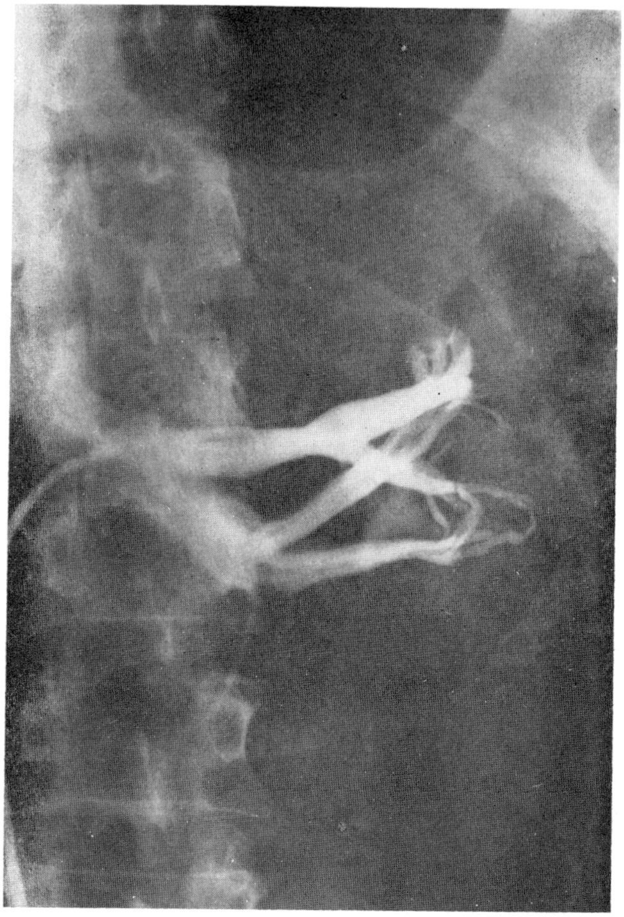

Figure 11.80. Renal Venogram. Notice the distal reunion of the hilar branches with a very short main trunk of the left renal vein. *Comment:* This is a variant.

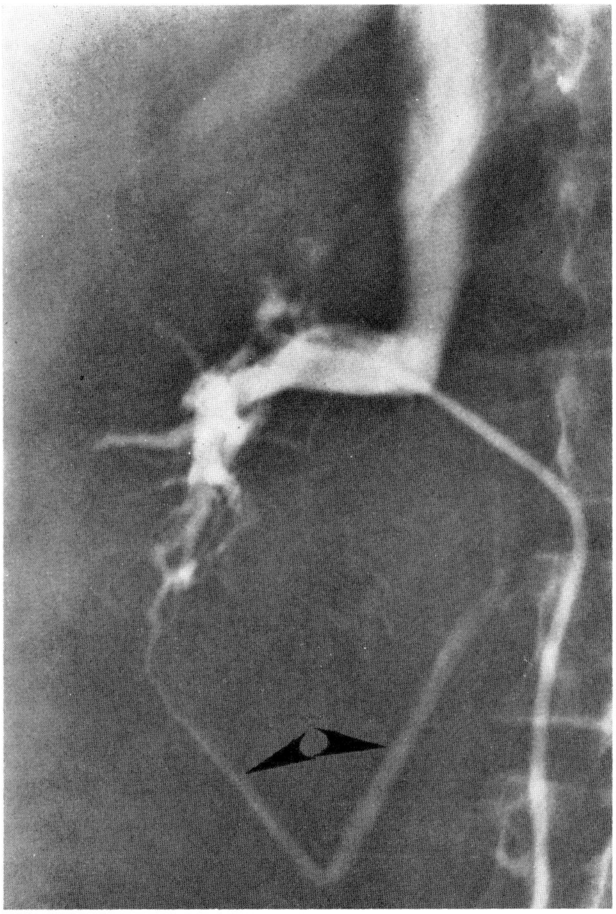

Figure 11.81. Right Renal Venogram. The catheter is in the right renal vein. Another perforating capsular vein drains from the intrarenal branches into the inferior vena cava. *Comment:* Example of a good collateral route. This may contaminate the inferior vena caval sampling for venous assays of renin.

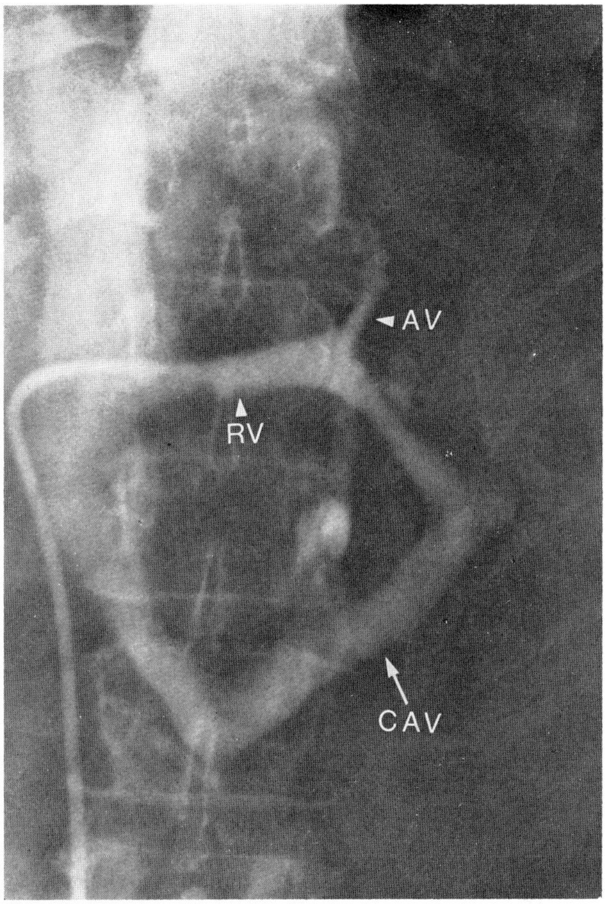

Figure 11.82. Left Renal Venogram. A catheter is inserted in the left renal vein. Another dilated vein arises from the renal hilus and joins the inferior vena cava. Notice the adrenal vein joining the proximal limb of this venous ring. *Comment:* Circumaortic renal vein (C.A.V.).

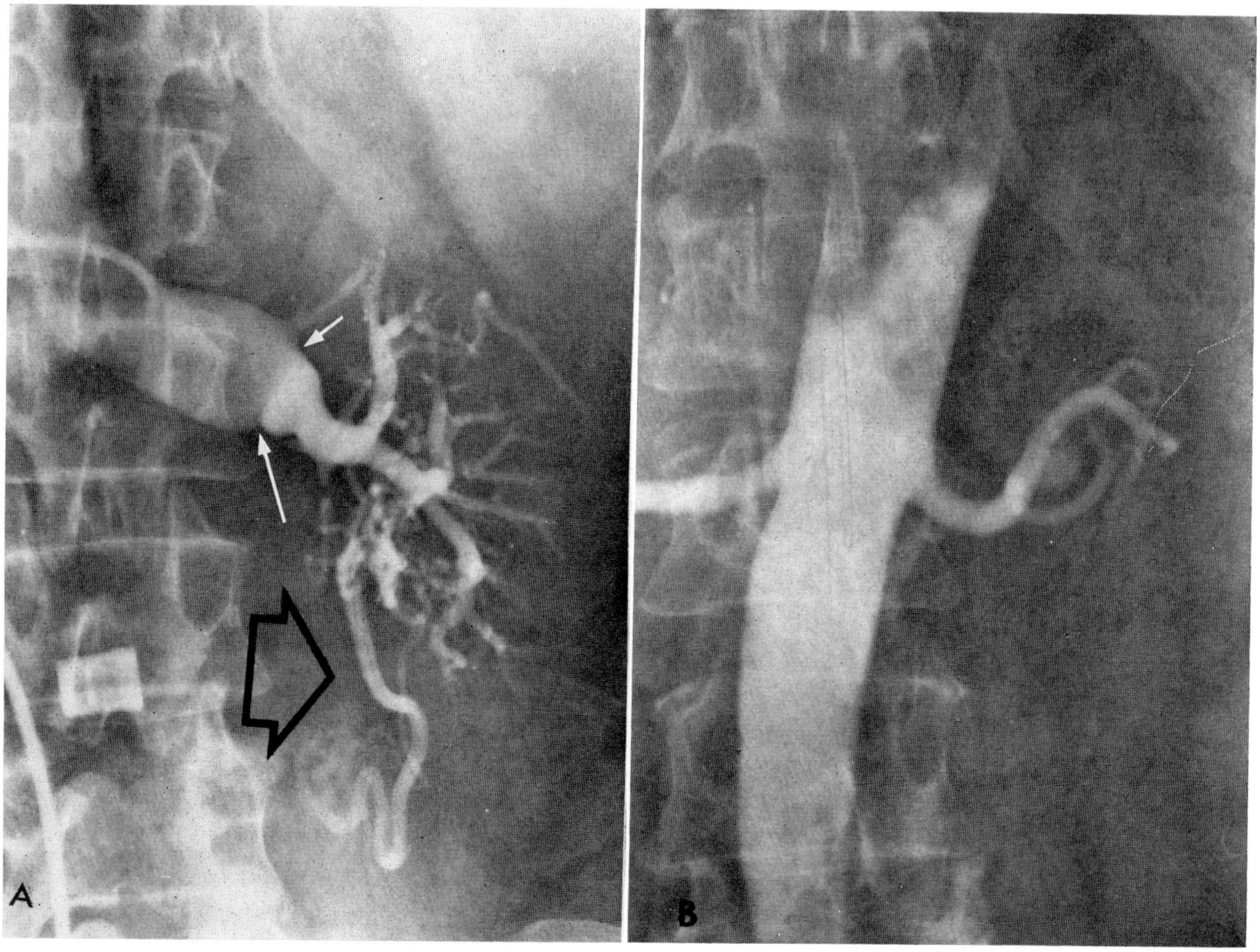

Figure 11.83. Left Renal Venogram. (A) Left renal venogram: Multiple dilated tortuous veins in the left renal pelvic area and left retroperitoneal area (Large Arrow). Notice the splaying of the left renal vein and the pad affect (White Arrow). (B) Aortogram: The corresponding course of aorta and the tortuous left renal artery at this area of splaying and pad affect is revealed. *Diagnosis:* Tortuous aorta with secondary pressure on the left renal vein with associated varices in the renal pelvic and retroperitoneal areas. A retro-aortic left renal vein was confirmed by autopsy at a later date.

body. On occasion it may receive the right gonadal vein. The *left renal* vein is longer than the right, situated at the core of an impressive set of venous plexuses and veins. In relation to the left renal vein, the inferior phrenics and adrenal veins are above; the gonadal, capsular and ascending lumbar veins and the lumbar communication with the hemiazygos and vertebral plexus are below. This complexity of the left renal vein is due to the embryologic proximity of the various structures resulting in venous intercommunication. The terminal portion of the left renal vein is wider than its segment of origin[390] (Figs. 11-76 and 11-81). Tributaries of the left renal vein are the suprarenal vein, left inferior phrenic vein, and left gonadal vein.[331, 387, 388]

There are several well-known normal variations in the anatomy of the renal veins. The *circumaortic renal vein* occurs on the left. Such a left renal vein is bifid, forming a pre- and postaortic venous ring. The cranial limb of this ring is wider and anterior to the aorta, receiving the adrenal, inferior phrenic and gonadal veins. The small caudal limb of this venous ring courses posterior to the aorta receiving lumbar and azygos veins (Fig. 11-82). The *retroaortic left renal vein*[389] is a single vein which, instead of having a normal course ventral to the aorta, courses posterior to the aorta to terminate in

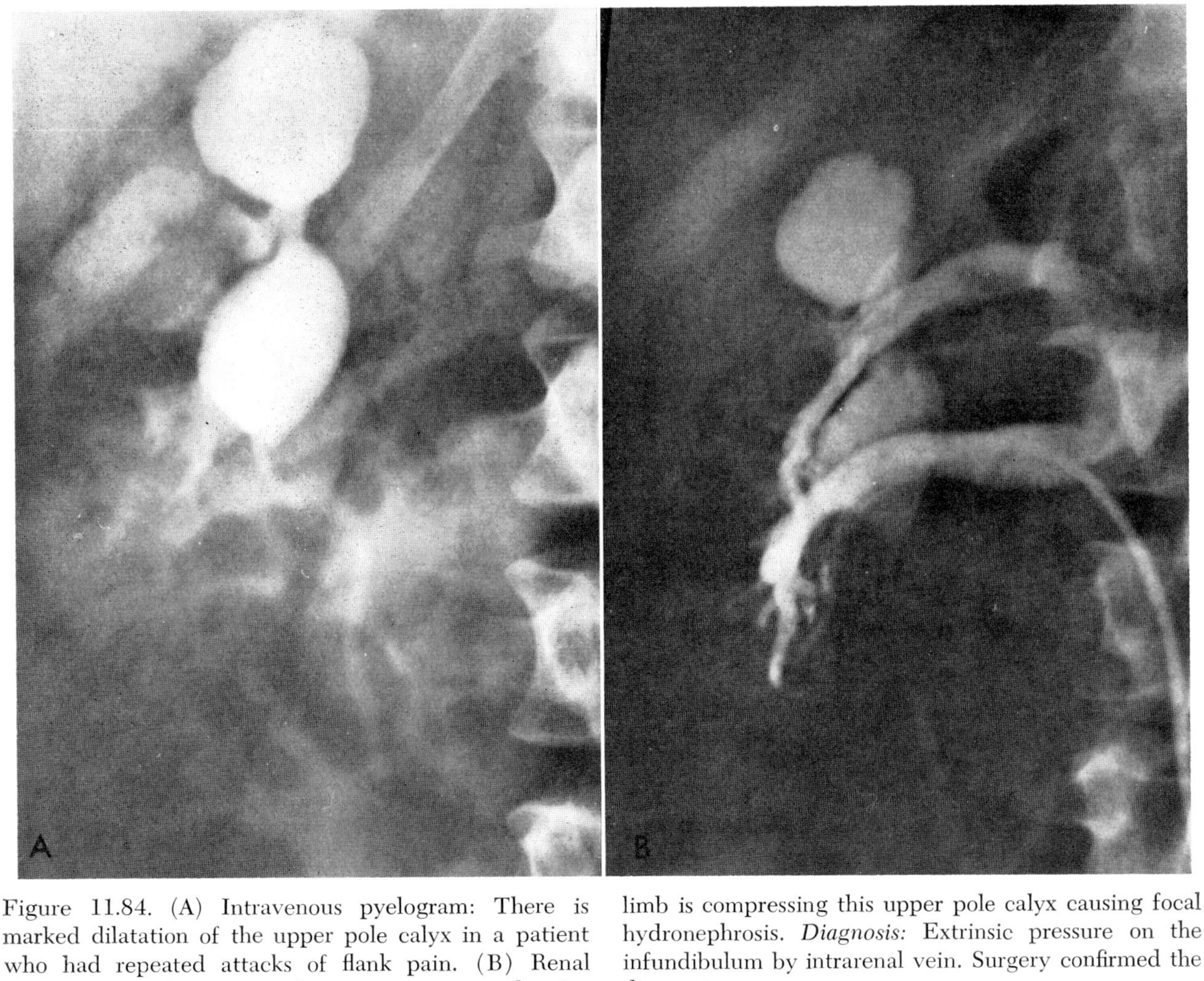

Figure 11.84. (A) Intravenous pyelogram: There is marked dilatation of the upper pole calyx in a patient who had repeated attacks of flank pain. (B) Renal venogram on the same side: Two major renal veins course towards the inferior vena cava. The proximal limb is compressing this upper pole calyx causing focal hydronephrosis. *Diagnosis:* Extrinsic pressure on the infundibulum by intrarenal vein. Surgery confirmed the diagnosis.

the inferior vena cava (Fig. 11-83).

A circumrenal venous network is mainly formed by the capsular veins in the perirenal fat. There they anastomose with the subcapsular veins of the kidney; parietal veins of the body wall; and gonadal, ureteric, phrenic and adrenal veins. These capsular veins may also communicate with the superior and inferior mesenteric veins along the posterior abdominal wall.[337]

ADRENAL VESSELS

Adrenal Arterial Supply

The adrenal gland is bounded superiorly by the inferior phrenic artery, medially by the aorta, inferiorly by the renal artery, and laterally by the renal margin. As three out of the four boundaries are vessels, one may expect an arterial supply from each one (Figs. 11-85 and 11-86).[370, 374–377] The superior adrenal artery arises from the inferior phrenic (ten to sixty branches), the middle adrenal artery arises from the aorta, and the inferior adrenal from the renal artery. The middle adrenal artery may also arise from the lumbars, superior mesenteric artery, or even the celiac artery. On rare occasions the inferior adrenal may arise from the aorta, gonadal artery, or even from the inferior phrenic arteries. The superior adrenals are the best supply, the middle adrenals are the poorest.

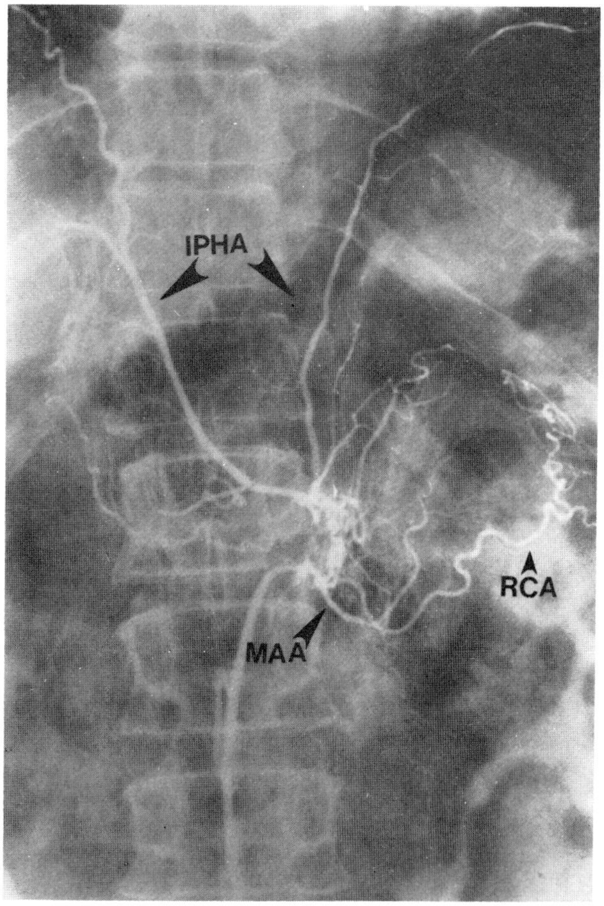

Figure 11.85. Middle Adrenal Arteriogram. (A) Middle adrenal artery (M.A.A.), renal capsular artery from the middle adrenal artery (R.C.A.), retrograde filling of the inferior phrenic artery (I.P.H.A.), branches to the right adrenal from the right inferior phrenic (I.P.H.A.). *Comment:* Normal. (Courtesy of Dr. T. Grant, Toledo, Ohio.)

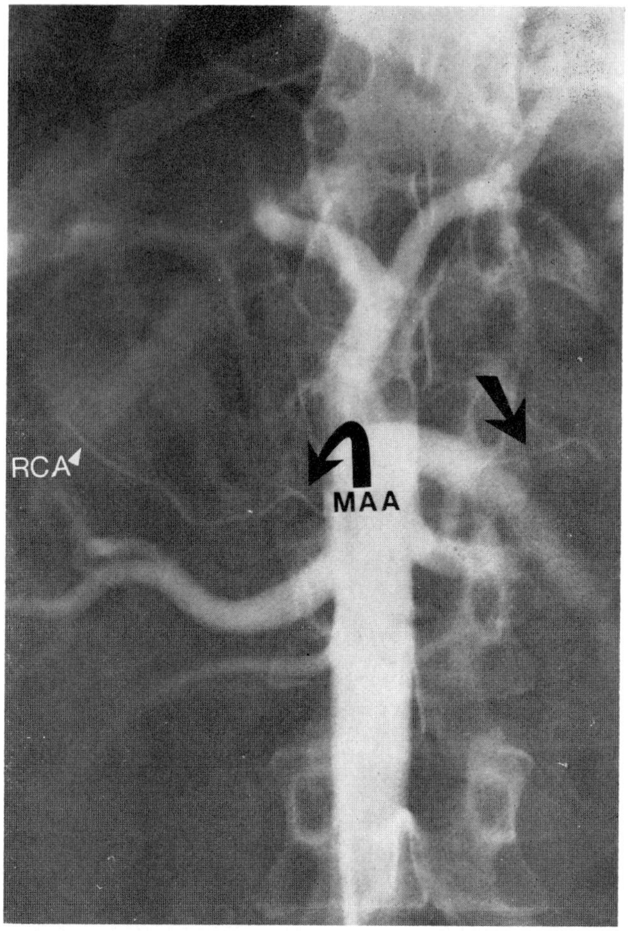

Figure 11.86. Flush Aortogram. There is good opacification of the middle adrenal arteries (M.A.A.) and the renal capsular artery from the right middle adrenal artery. *Comment:* It is very unusual to opacify normal middle adrenal arteries.

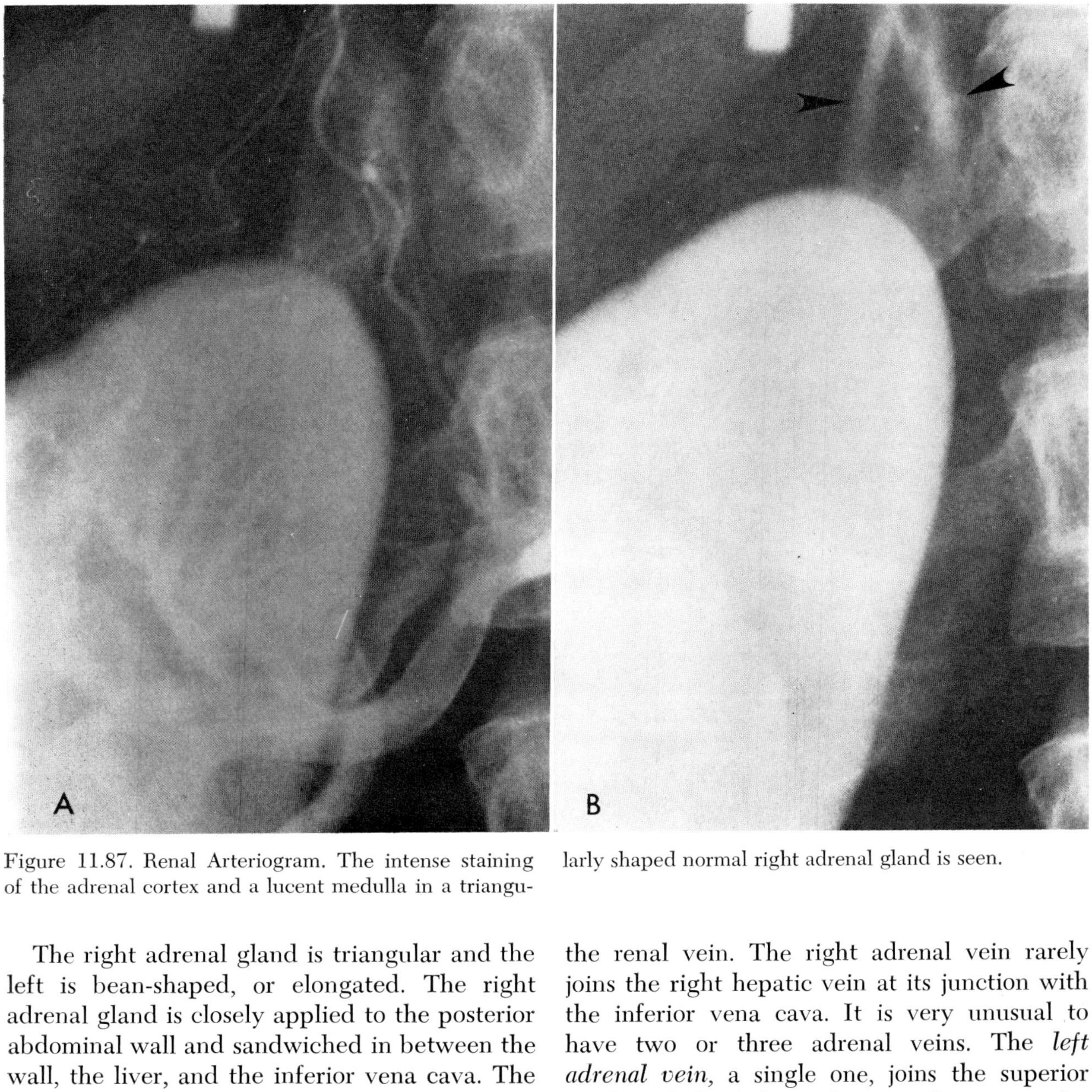

Figure 11.87. Renal Arteriogram. The intense staining of the adrenal cortex and a lucent medulla in a triangularly shaped normal right adrenal gland is seen.

The right adrenal gland is triangular and the left is bean-shaped, or elongated. The right adrenal gland is closely applied to the posterior abdominal wall and sandwiched in between the wall, the liver, and the inferior vena cava. The left adrenal gland is tucked between the pancreas and the posterior abdominal wall.

Adrenal Veins

The *singularity* of the adrenal vein stands in contrast to the multiplicity of its arterial supply.[331, 378–380] The vein is usually between 1 to 4 mm in diameter. *The right adrenal vein* is a very consistent single vein, joining the inferior vena cava posteromedially around the level of the T. 12 vertebral body and above the level of the renal vein. The right adrenal vein rarely joins the right hepatic vein at its junction with the inferior vena cava. It is very unusual to have two or three adrenal veins. The *left adrenal vein,* a single one, joins the superior border of the left renal vein adjacent to the left vertebral border. It may also unite with the inferior phrenic vein. Extra glandular connections with the capsular, lumbar and splenic veins are not uncommon. Multiple venous anamolies may complicate catheterization.[383]

At the *adrenal cortex* there exists a portal type of circulation with juxtamedullary sinuses. The intraparenchymal portion of the central vein has a unique thick- and thin-walled structure. At certain areas the wall lacks longitudinal

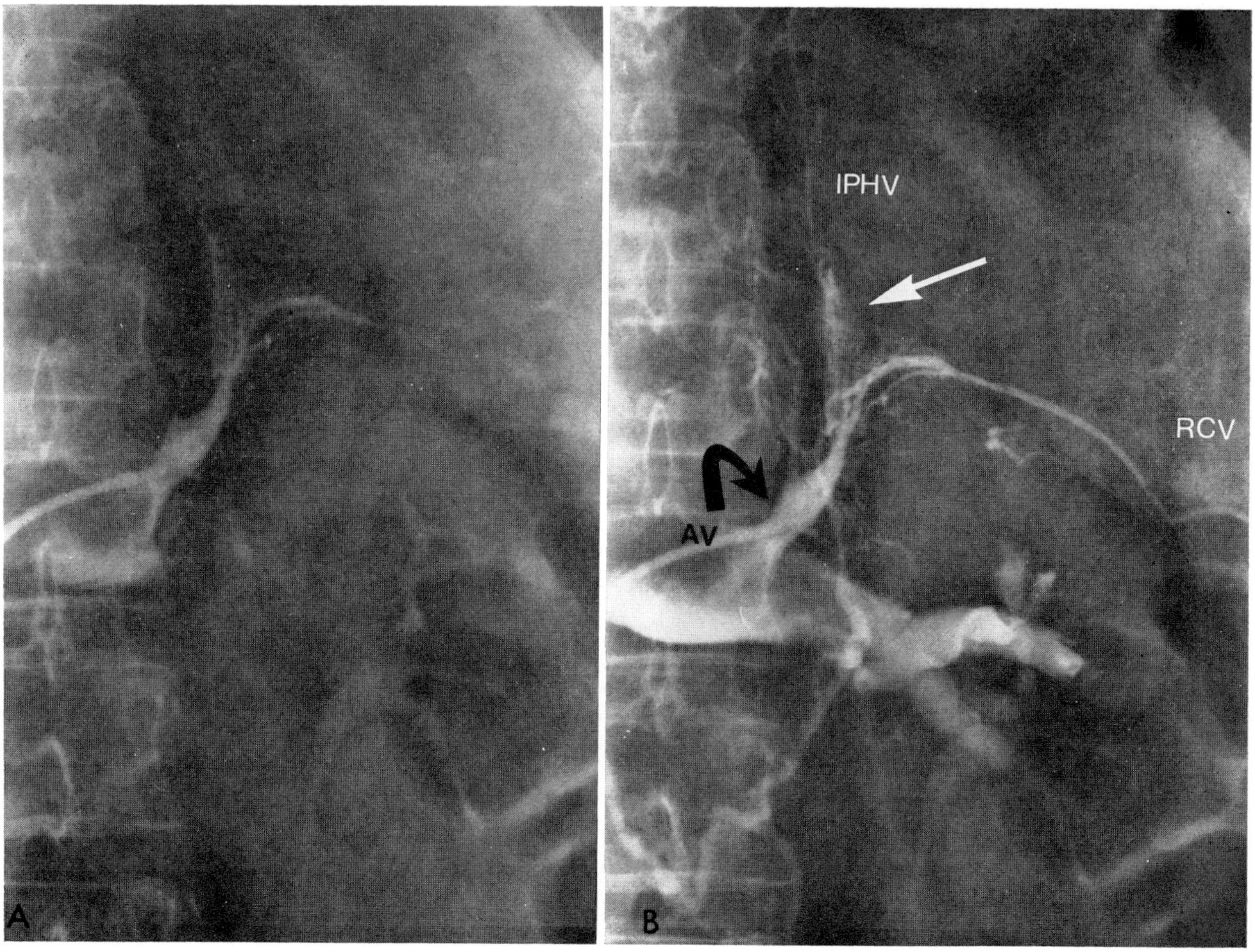

Figure 11.88. Left Adrenal Venogram. (A) Note left adrenal vein (A.V.). Intraadrenal branches (Arrow) in turn fills the renal capsular vein (R.C.V.). (B) Later: Further filling of the renal capsular vein (R.C.V.) and reflux into the inferior phrenic vein (I.P.H.V.) noted. *Comment:* Normal adrenal venogram and its normal communication with the renal capsular and the inferior phrenic veins.

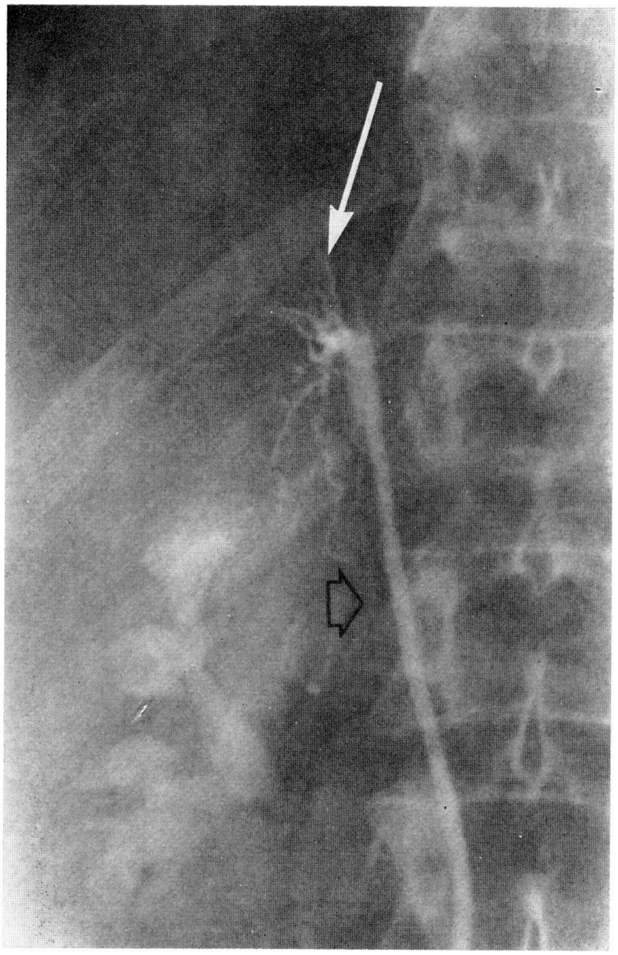

Figure 11.89. Right Adrenal Venogram. Adrenal veins (White Arrow), retroperitoneal and capsular veins (Arrow). *Comment:* Normal right adrenal venogram.

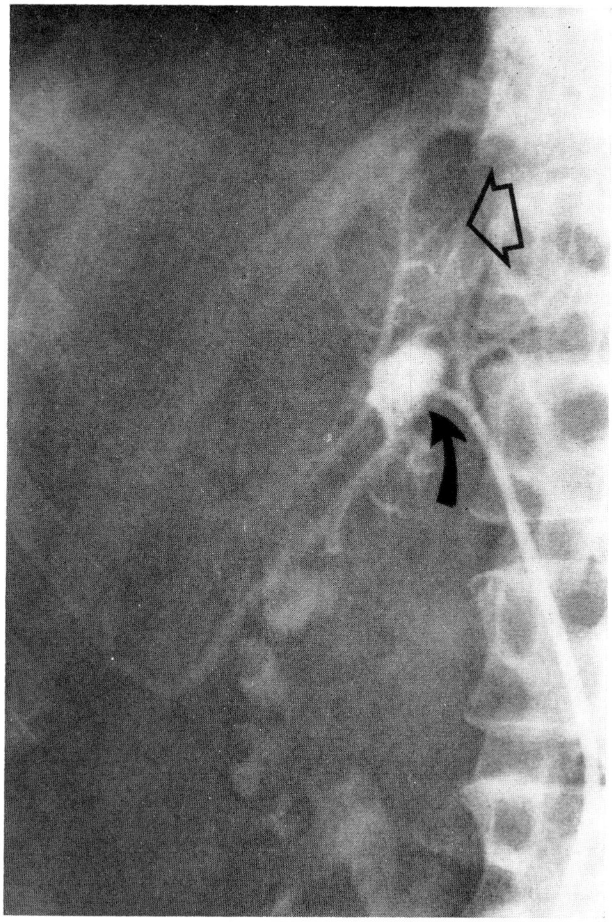

Figure 11.90. Hepatic Venogram. Amorphous collection of contrast material (Arrow) and a hepatic vein with herringbone pattern (Blank Arrow) are seen. *Comment:* An unsuccessful attempt to catheterize the right adrenal vein. The catheter fell into the hepatic with extravasation and opacification of the small hepatic veins.

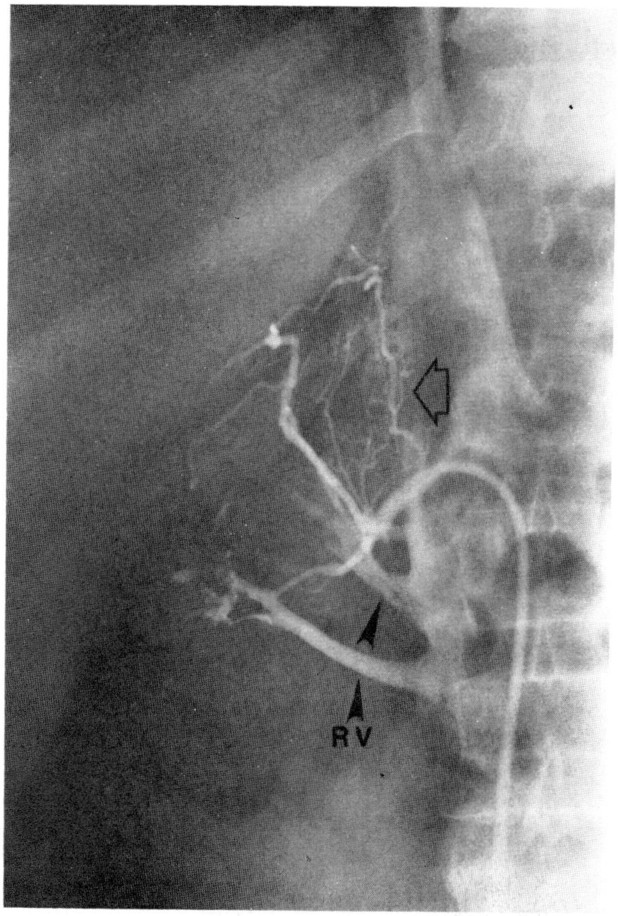

Figure 11.91. Right Retroperitoneal Venogram. Opacification of a retroperitoneal vein (Arrow) with reflux into the renal veins (R.V.) is seen in a patient on whom an adrenal venogram was attempted.

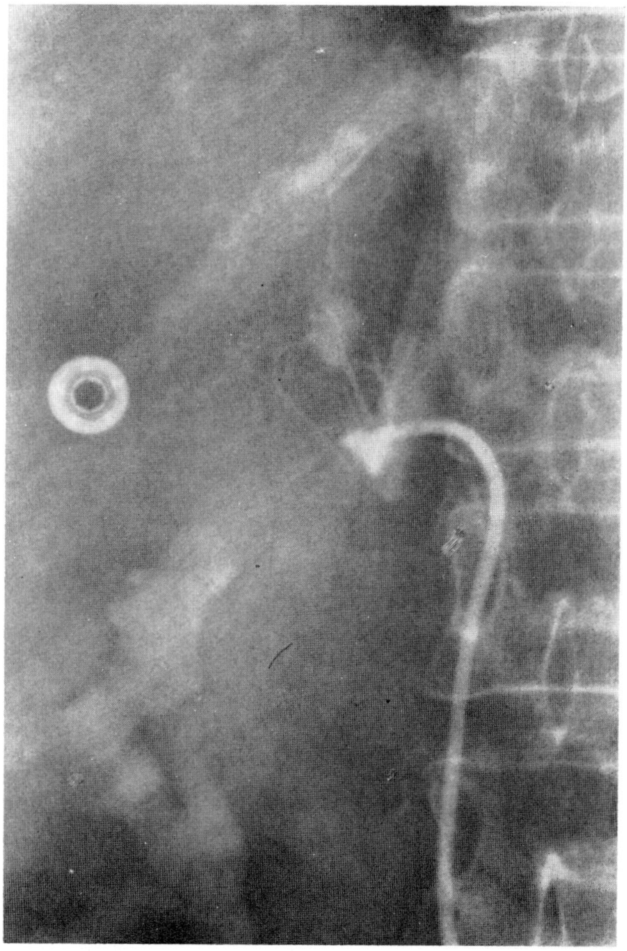

Figure 11.92. Adrenal Venogram. The catheter tip is inserted in the retroperitoneal vein with minimal extravasation of the contrast material. *Comment:* This illustrates an unsuccessful attempt to catheterize the right adrenal vein and accidental entry of the catheter into a small retroperitoneal vein.

muscle and is lined only by endothelium. This predisposes the vein to frequent ruptures[142, 327, 381, 382] (Figs. 11-88 and 11-89).

GONADAL VESSELS

The Gonadal Arteries

They usually arise from the aorta between the levels of the superior mesenteric and renal arteries on the anterolateral surface. It is not unusual to have their origin from the renal, adrenal or inferior phrenic arteries. On rare occasions there may be two arteries on each side[314, 370] (Fig. 11-93).

Gonadal Veins

The right gonadal vein terminates in the lateral or anterolateral surface of the inferior vena cava within the 5 cm segment below the right renal vein.[384, 385] There may be two gonadal veins on the right side. The left gonadal vein usually drains into the left renal vein. There are frequent retroperitoneal anastomoses between the gonadal and retroperiotneal veins. The presence of valves in these veins may be a frequent occurrence (Fig. 11-94).

PARATHYROID VESSELS

Parathyroid Arteries

The main arterial supply is through the inferior thyroid artery.[355, 356] The *inferior thyroid* is the larger, but less constant artery, and

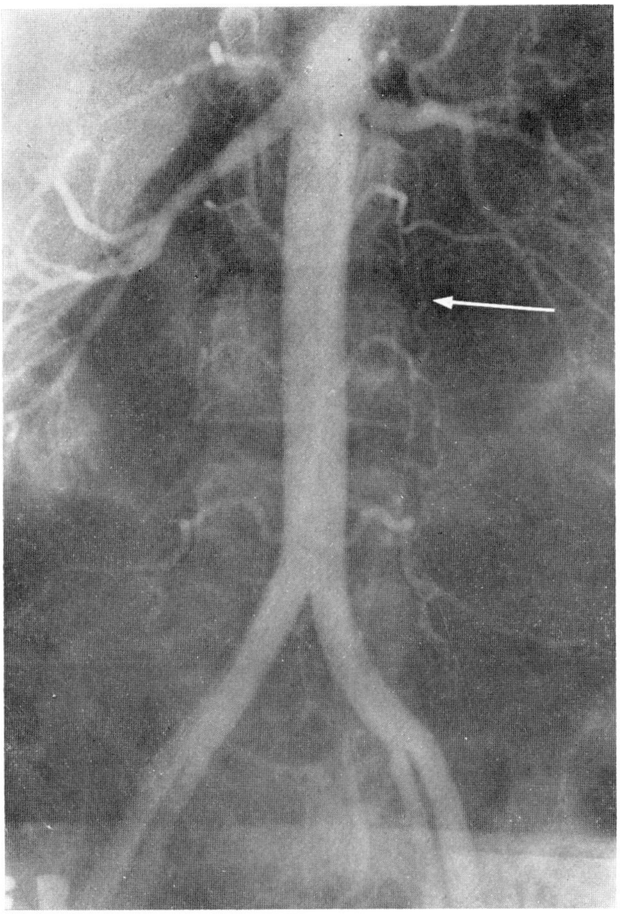

Figure 11.93. Flush Aortogram. There is good filling of the left ovarian artery. *Comment:* Normal flush aortogram.

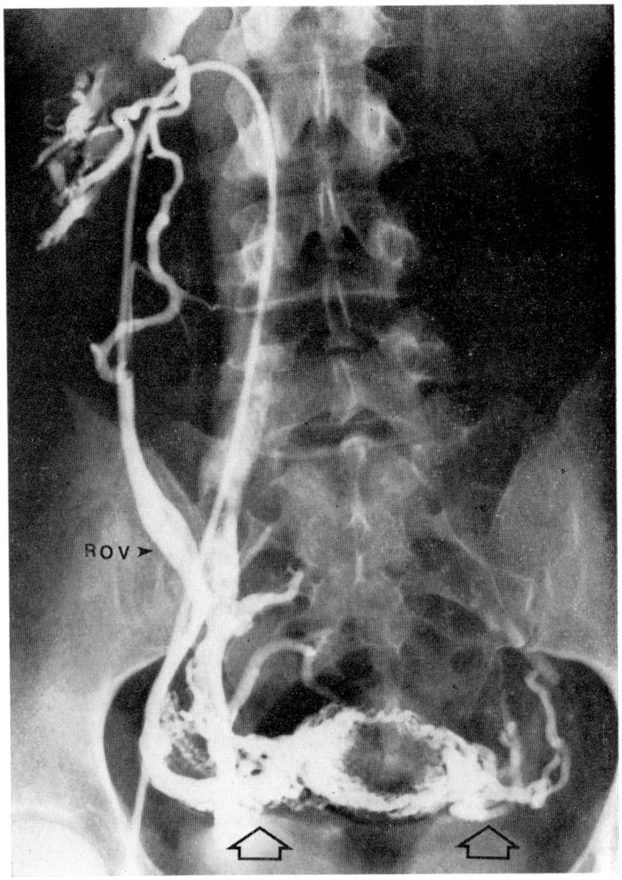

Figure 11.94. Gonadal Venogram. The catheter is in the right ovarian vein (R.O.V.). Notice the ovarian pedicular veins (Arrows). Also notice the good filling of the myometrial veins. *Comment:* Normal gonadal venogram.

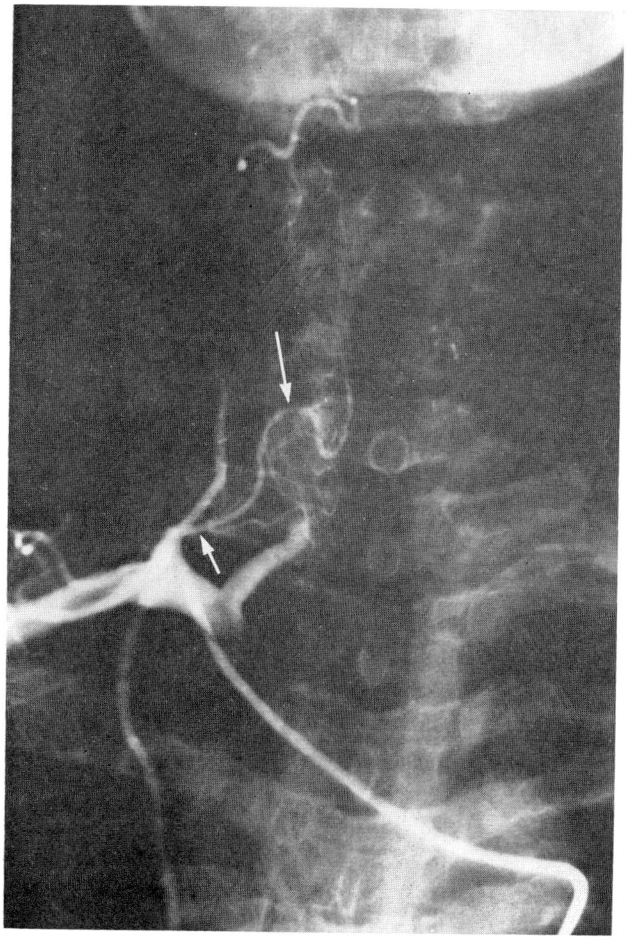

Figure 11.95. Right Thyrocervical Arteriogram. Notice a normal S-loop of the inferior thyroid artery and also filling of the cervical branches.

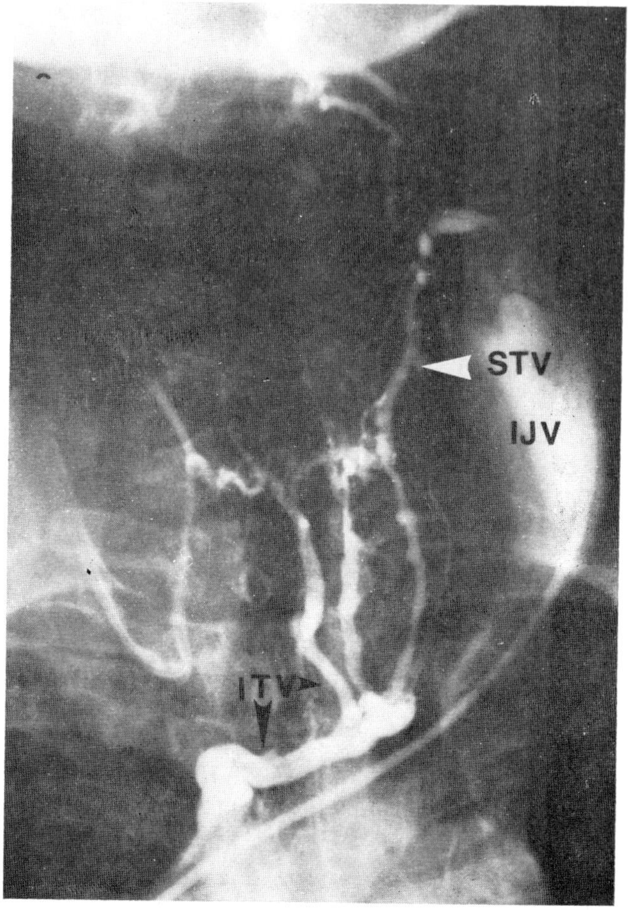

Figure 11.96. Left Superior Thyroid Vein Injection. Left superior thyroid vein (S.T.V.), inferior thyroid vein (I.T.V.), left internal jugular vein (I.J.V.). *Comment:* This is a normal superior thyroid venogram with reflux into the inferior thyroid veins as well as to the right superior thyroid vein.

may be absent or duplicated. It may arise directly from the subclavian artery when the thyrocervical artery is absent. The inferior thyroid rarely arises from the vertebral, common carotid, innominate, or distal subclavian artery. In almost every instance a separate branch arises from the inferior thyroid artery to the inferior parathyroid gland. The superior parathyroid gland may be fed by the inferior thyroid artery, or by an anastomoses between the inferior thyroid artery and the superior thyroid artery. The *superior thyroid artery* is small and primitive, but constant[355, 356] (Fig. 11-95).

Parathyroid Veins

They[386] consist of a venous plexus about the parathyroid gland with diffuse anastomosing vessels without valves. The superior and middle thyroid veins drain into the ipsilateral internal jugular vein. The inferior thyroid veins drain into the corresponding innominate vein, either separately or through a common stem. They may have valves just prior to the termination into the innominate veins[337] (Fig. 11-96).

VASCULATURE OF TUBULAR STRUCTURES

Esophageal Arterial Supply

Compared to the ureters, the esophagus is probably the next most inaccessible viscus for the angiographer.[337] This is not because it is avascular, but rather because the esophagus, like the ureter, obtains its vascular supply in a segmental manner from multiple sources along its journey. The arterial supply comes from the inferior thyroid arteries, thoracic aorta, bronchial arteries, inferior phrenic arteries, and the left gastric artery. The venous plexus drains into the left gastric vein caudally and into the azygos and thyroid veins cranially, thus establishing a portosystemic communication.[339–341]

Ureteric Arterial Supply

The ureter receives its blood supply from many sources.[316] The *proximal* segment is supplied from the renal hilar branches. The *middle* segment has a poor vascular supply, mainly from the aorta and common iliac arteries. The *inferior* segment, which has increased vascularity as it approaches the bladder, is supplied from the common and internal iliac arteries and the superior and inferior gluteal arteries.

Spinal Cord Arterial Supply

The arterial supply to the spinal cord comes from the vertebral arteries, the deep cervical branch of the costo cervical artery, the ascending cervical branch from the thyrocervical artery, the intercostal, lumbars, ilio lumbars, and sacral branches of the internal iliac arteries.[188] The *arteria radicularis magna* arises from the intercostal or lumbar arteries in the majority of the population. This occurs from the level of the eighth thoracic to the first lumbar vertebral bodies.[366, 367]

THORACIC AORTA

The *ascending aorta* begins at the cranial end of the left ventricle at the semilunar valves, gives rise to the coronary arteries, and continues as the arch of the aorta.[337] The arch curves gently and superiorly and continues as the descending thoracic aorta. At its origin it is approximately 3 cm in diameter, and after giving off its main branches becomes approximately 2 to 3 cm in diameter. The branches of the aortic arch are in order: the innominate artery, the left common carotid artery, and the left subclavian artery. On occasion a *thyroidea ima* branch may rise from the arch between the in-

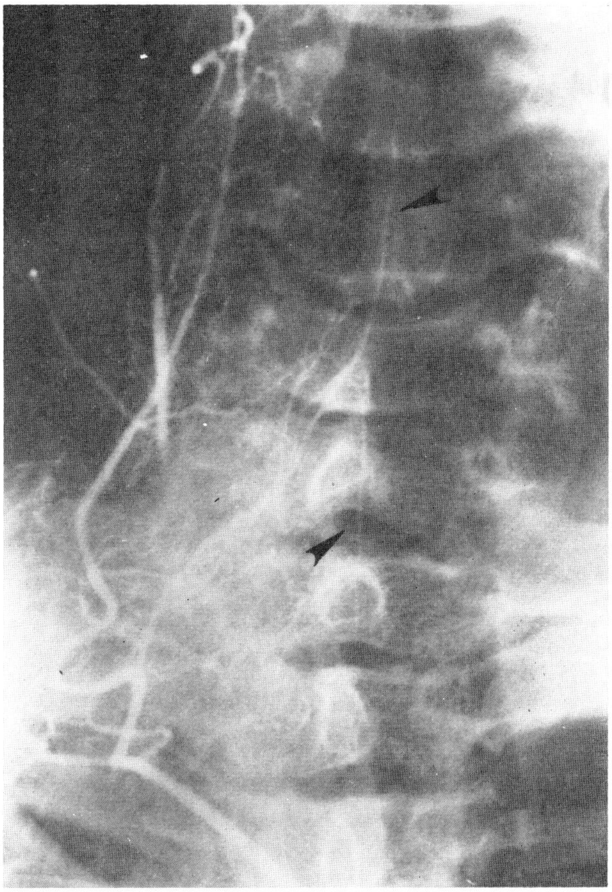

Figure 11.97. Accidental injection into the cervical branch of the subclavian artery which reveals the artery to the spinal cord.

nominate and left common carotid arteries (Fig. 11-98). Variations in the origins of the great vessels from the arch of the aorta are not unusual[347, 348] (Figs. 11-99 to 11-102).

The *descending thoracic aorta* extends from the termination of the aortic arch to T. 12 vertebral level where it becomes the abdominal aorta. The branches of the descending thoracic aorta are both visceral and parietal. The *visceral* branches include the bronchial, esophogeal, pericardial and mediastinal arteries, while the *parietal* branches include the posterior intercostals, the subcostals, and the superior phrenic arteries.

Common Carotid Arteries

The right common carotid artery arises as a branch of the innominate, and the left has an independent origin from the aortic arch.

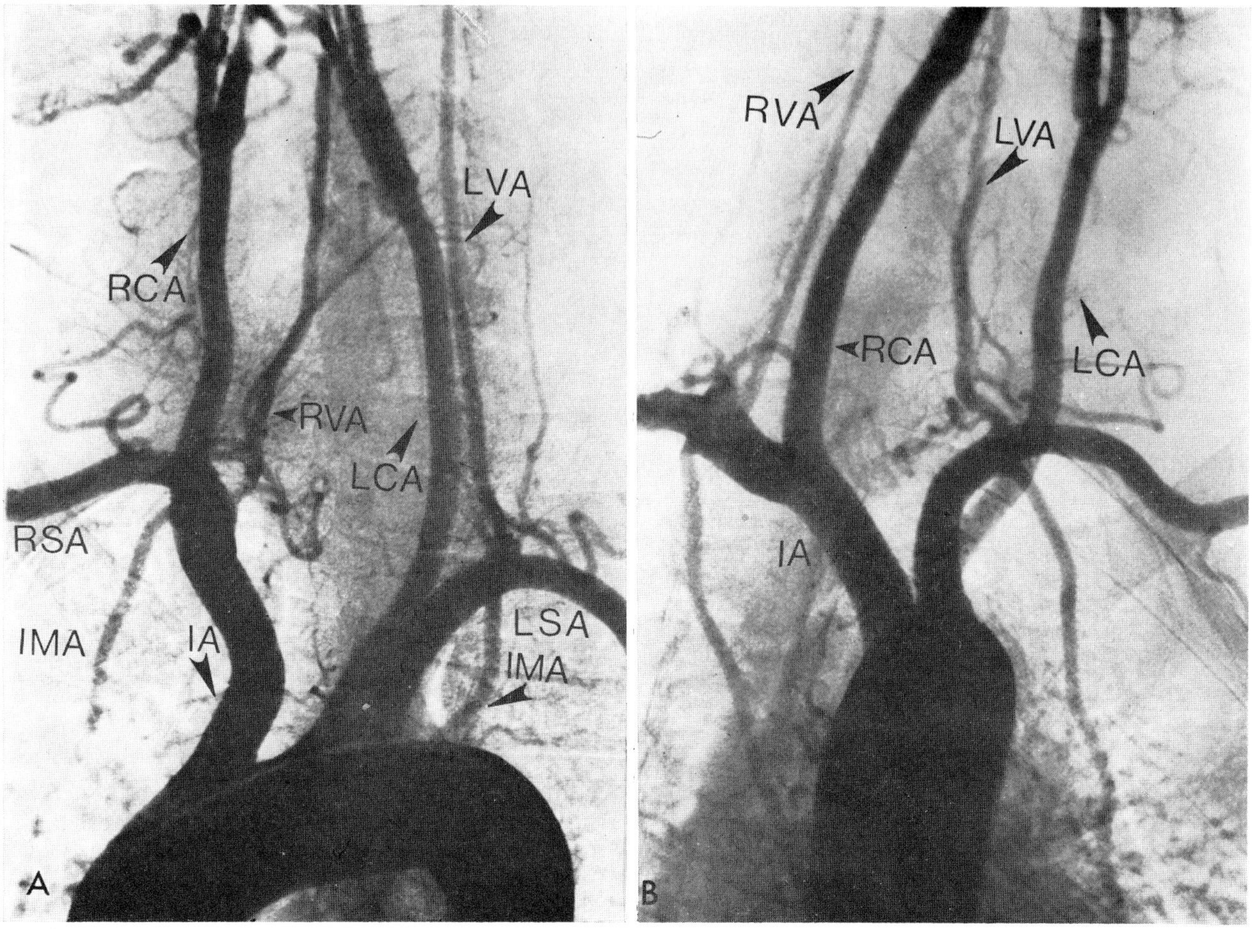

Figure 11.98. Aortic Arch Angiogram. (A) Left anterior oblique projection: Innominate (I.A.), right common carotid (R.C.A.), right subclavian (R.S.A.), right vertebral (R.V.A.), left common carotid (L.C.A.), left vertebral (L.V.A.), left subclavian (L.S.A.), right internal mammary (I.M.A.), left internal mammary (I.M.A.). (B) Right anterior oblique projection. *Comment:* Normal.

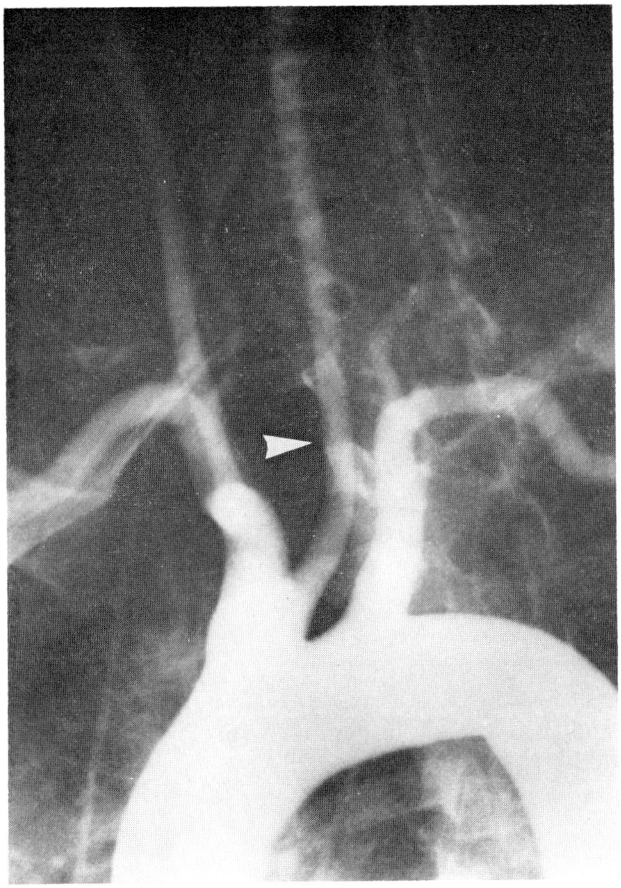

Figure 11.99. Aortic Arch Arteriogram. The left common carotid artery is arising from the innominate artery. *Comment:* This is a variant.

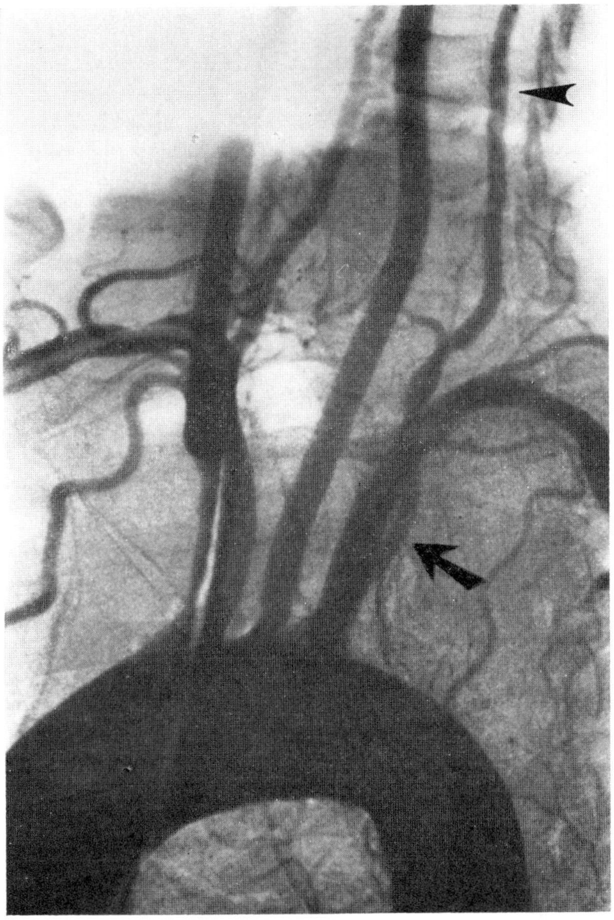

Figure 11.100. Aortic Arch Angiogram—left anterior oblique projection: The left vertebral artery arises directly from the aortic arch (Arrow). *Comment:* This is a rare variant.

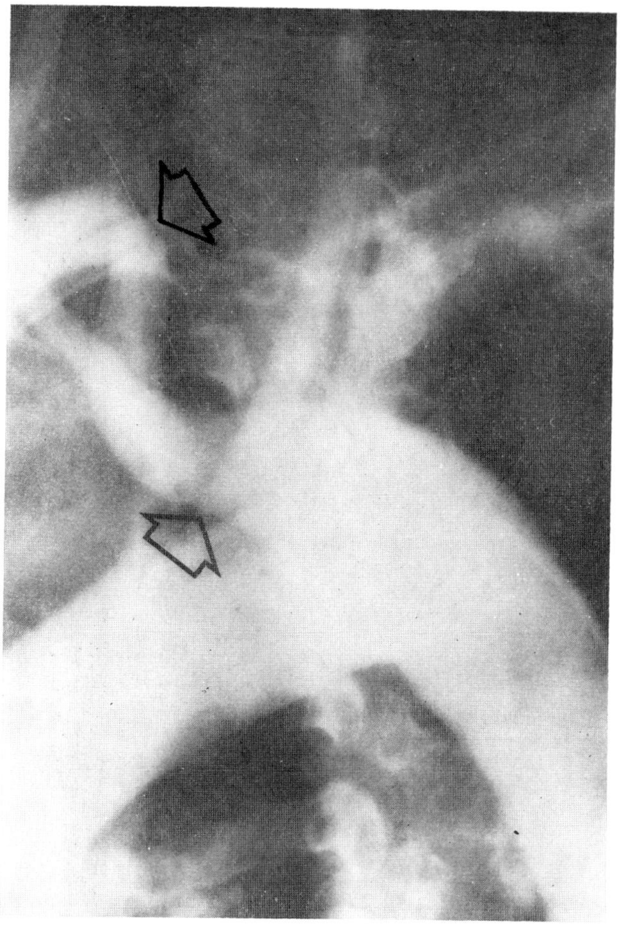

Figure 11.101. Aortic Arch Angiogram. The right subclavian artery has a direct distal origin from the aortic arch. *Diagnosis:* Aberrant right subclavian artery.

Neither has any branch within its cervical portion, and both bifurcate into internal and external carotid branches. The external carotid branches supply the neck, face and mouth. The internal carotid arteries, without any branches in the neck, continue on to supply the intracranial circulation.

UPPER EXTREMITY VESSELS

Arteries of the Upper Extremity[337]

The *subclavian arteries* arise from the innominate on the right and as the last branch of the aortic arch on the left. From its origin to its termination at the lateral border of the first rib, this artery is divided into three segments, the middle one being overlapped by the anterior scalene muscle. The branches include the vertebral, thyrocervical, internal thoracic and costocervical arteries. The vertebral arteries are the most consistent branches. The *vertebral* is also the largest branch of the subclavian, lying between the longus colli and the anterior scalene muscles before entering the vertebral foramina. In addition to supplying the brain, it also supplies the spinal cord and the muscles of the neck. Variation in its origin is not uncommon (Fig. 11-103).

The *thyrocervical* artery arises from the antero-superior border of the subclavian artery, usually opposite the internal thoracic artery. It divides into the inferior thyroid, transverse cervical, and supra scapular arteries. The thyrocervicals may be variable, or even absent. Instead of the thyrocervical, only the inferior thyroid artery may be present.[355]

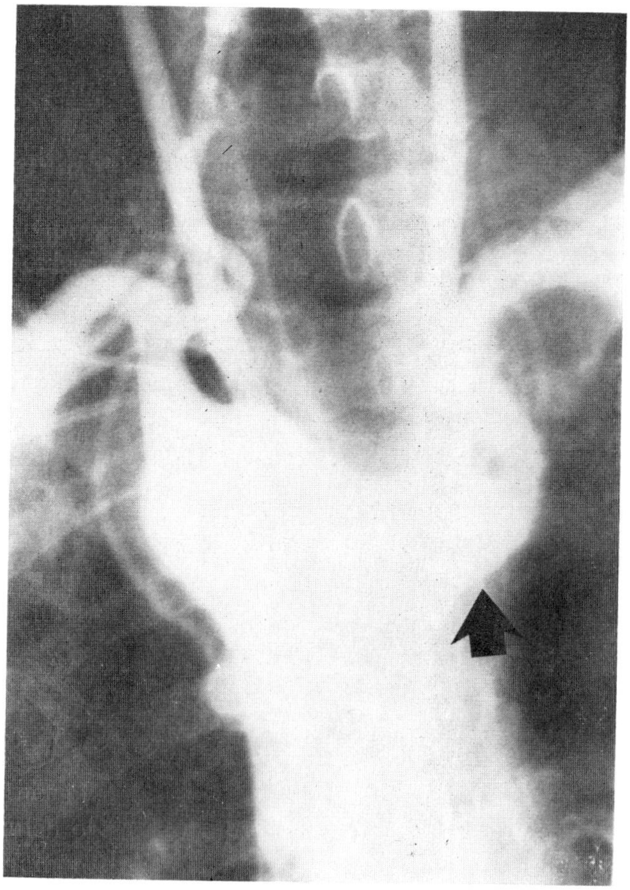

Figure 11.102. Thoracic Aortogram. Notice right-sided aortic arch with an infundibular origin of the left subclavian artery (Arrow).

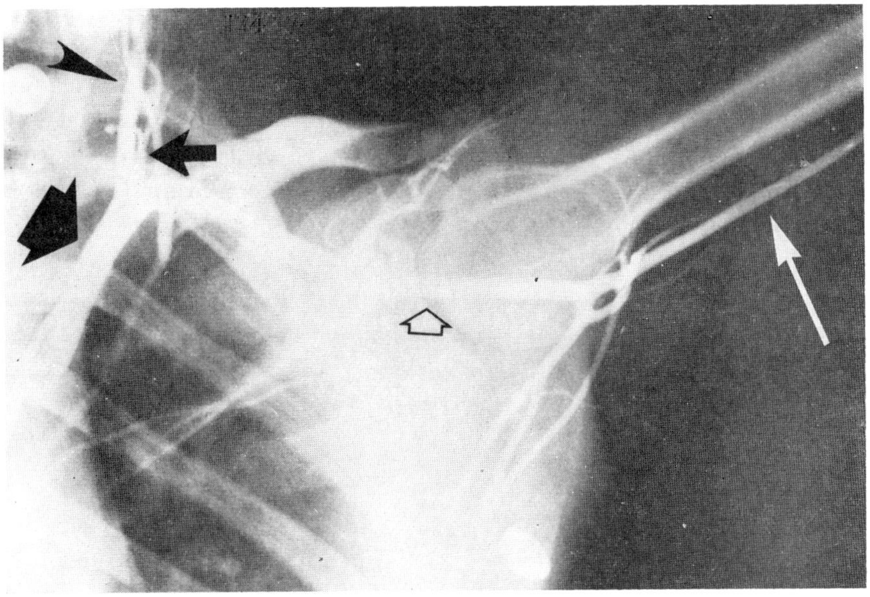

Figure 11.103. Subclavian Arteriogram—normal anatomy. Subclavian artery (Large Arrow), vertebral artery (Arrow Head), thyrocervical artery (Small Arrow), axillary artery (Blank Arrow) and brachial artery (White Arrow).

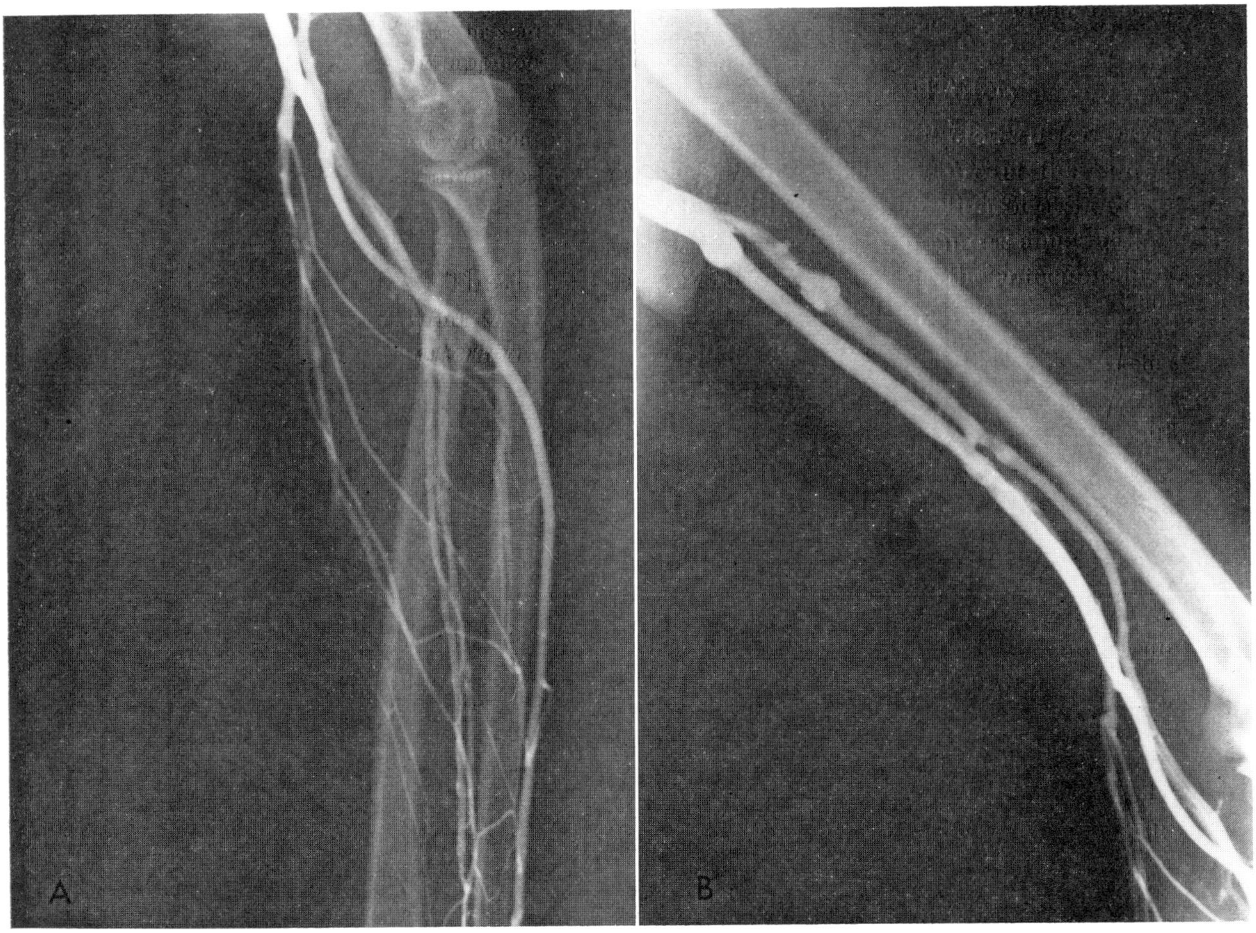

Figure 11.104. Upper Extremity Venogram. There is good filling of the superficial and deep veins of the forearm as well as the deep veins of the upper arm. *Comment:* Normal upper extremity venogram.

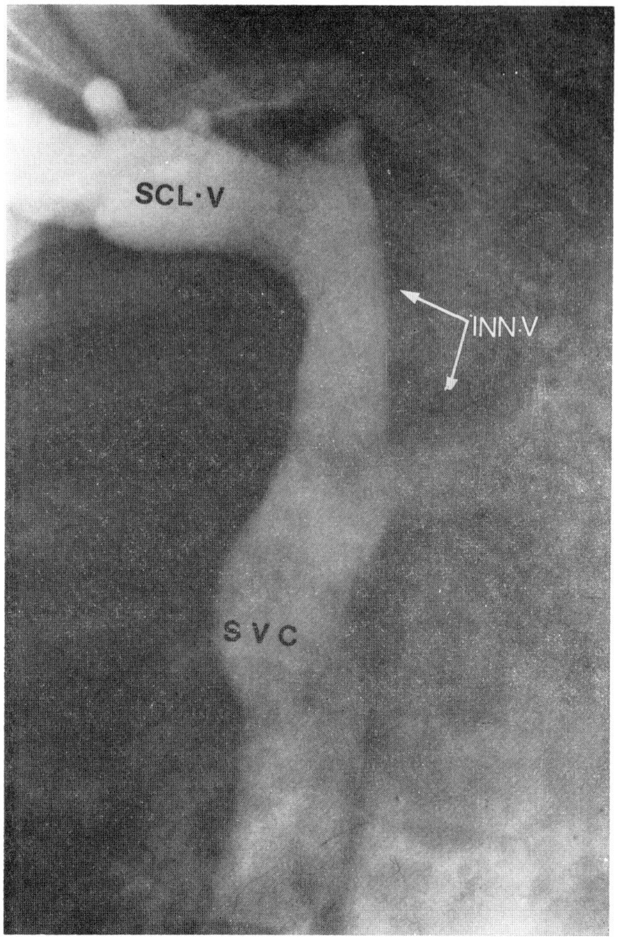

Figure 11.105. Superior Vena Cavogram. Subclavian vein (SCL.V.), innominate veins (INN.V.), superior vena cava (S.V.C.). *Comment:* Normal.

The *axillary artery* is a continuation of the subclavian distal to the lateral border of the first rib. It terminates as the brachial artery beyond the distal border of the teres major muscle. The cords of the brachial plexus are around the axillary artery, and together they are enveloped by the axillary sheath. The *brachial artery* is the continuation of the axillary artery at the lower border of the teres major muscle to the apex of the antecubital fossa. At this point it divides into the radial and ulnar arteries. In its proximal course it lies medial to the humerus and as it passes distally, it courses anterior to this bone.

Variation in the level of the bifurcations of the axillary artery or direct branching of the axillary into the radial and ulnar artery without a brachial artery is a rare event.[357, 358] Bilateral or unilateral variations of the brachial arteries with a high bifurcation or unusual courses are not infrequent either.[359] The absence of the radial artery, although unusual, does occur.[360] Incomplete palmar arches may occur in 20 percent of the population, making these individuals more susceptible to minor trauma with resultant digital ischemia.[361]

Veins of the Upper Extremity

The radial and ulnar veins formed by the palmar arches course proximal through the forearm, uniting at the bend of the elbow to form the brachial vein. The brachial vein courses toward the axilla to terminate as the axillary vein. At the same time, it receives the basilic vein. The axillary vein then receives other tributaries and the cephalic vein and continues as the subclavian vein at the lateral border of the first rib. The subclavian vein is the continuation of the axillary vein and receives the internal jugular vein to form the innominate vein. This, along with its contralateral colleague, forms the superior vena cava (Figs. 11-104, 11-105).

ABDOMINAL AORTA

The abdominal portion of the descending aorta[337] begins at the lower border of T. 12 and extends to its bifurcation, which can occur anywhere from L. 3 to L. 5 vertebral body.[324] At its origin the abdominal aorta is 2 cm in diameter, after giving its major branches; and below the level of the renal arteries it is about 16 mm in diameter. The *branches* of the abdominal aorta usually arise in the following descending order: right and left inferior phrenic arteries, celiac axis, right and left middle adrenals, superior mesenteric artery, right and left gonadal arteries, right and left renal arteries, inferior mesenteric artery, median sacral artery, right and left common iliac arteries, and four to five pairs of lumbar arteries in segmental manner. The common iliac arteries divide into the internal iliac arteries to the pelvis, and the external iliac arteries to the legs (Fig. 11-106).

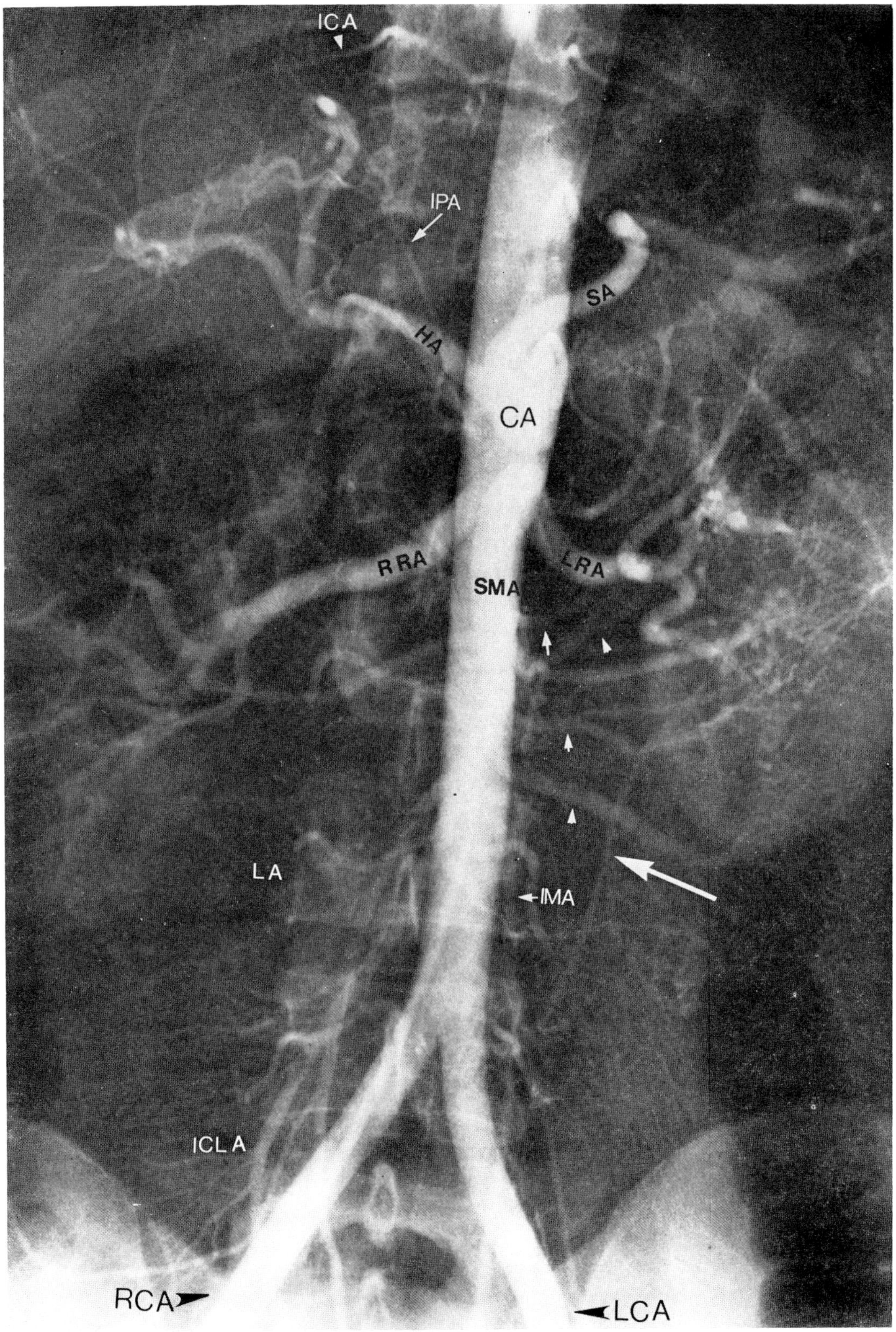

Figure 11.106. Flush Abdominal Aortogram. Intercostal artery (I.C.A.), right inferior phrenic artery (I.P.A.), celiac axis (C.A.), splenic artery (S.A.), hepatic artery (H.A.), superior mesenteric artery (S.M.A.), renal artery (L.R.A., R.R.A.), inferior mesenteric artery (I.M.A.), common iliac artery (R.C.A., L.C.A.), jejunal branches (Arrow Heads), left colic artery (Arrow), ileocolic artery (I.CL.A.), and lumbar artery (L.A.).

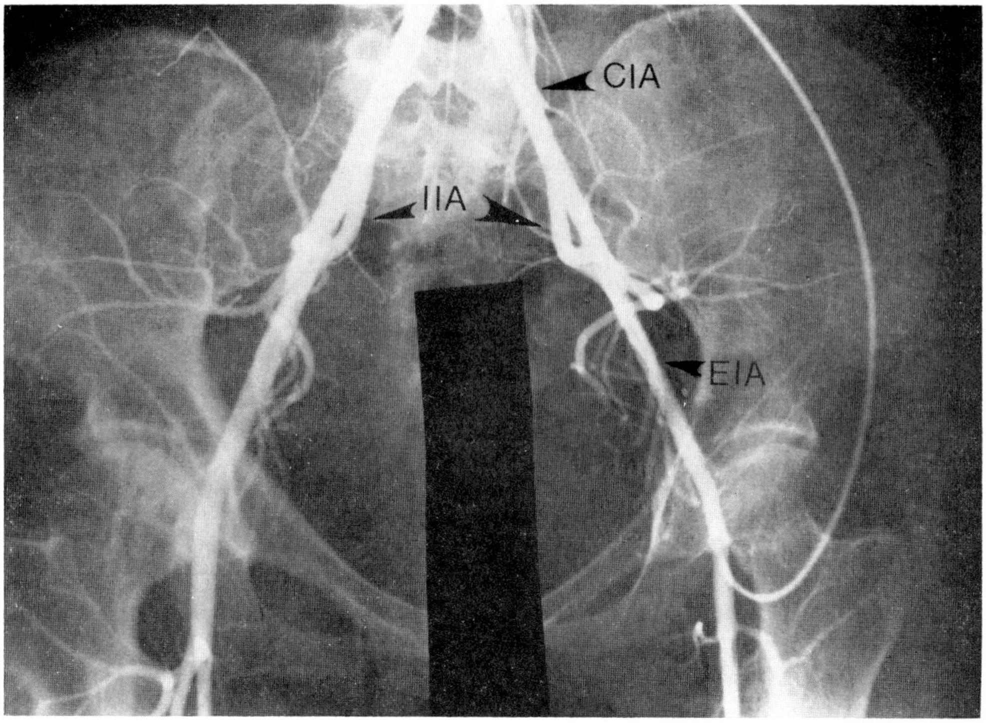

Figure 11.107. Pelvic Arteriogram. Common iliac artery (C.I.A.), internal iliac artery (I.I.A.) and external iliac artery (E.I.A.). *Comment:* Normal.

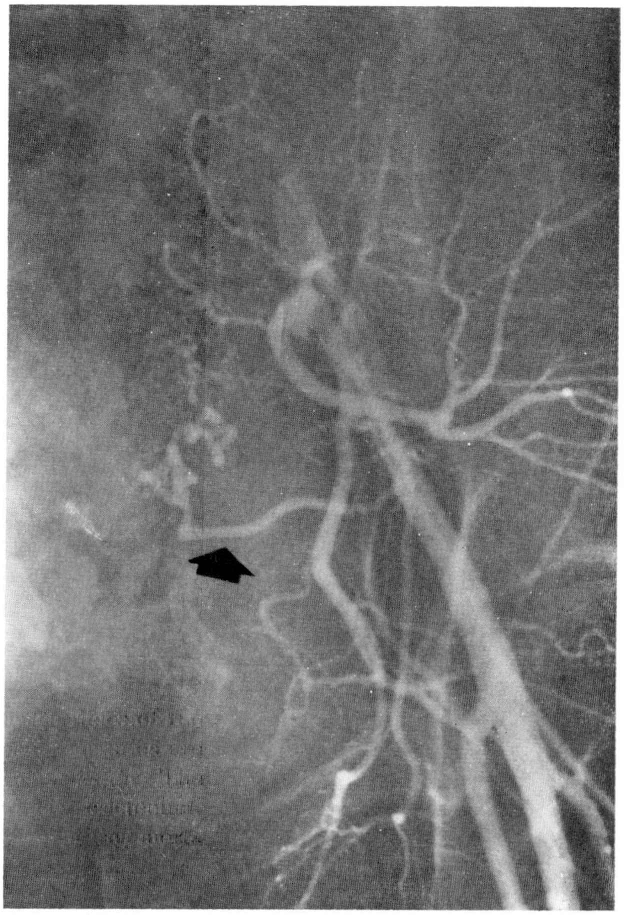

Figure 11.108. Left Internal Iliac Arteriogram. A slightly prominent left uterine artery is seen in its parametrial course (Arrow), giving good filling of the intramural branches of the uterus. The increased densities in the pelvis are due to a recent barium enema. *Comment:* Normal left uterine artery.

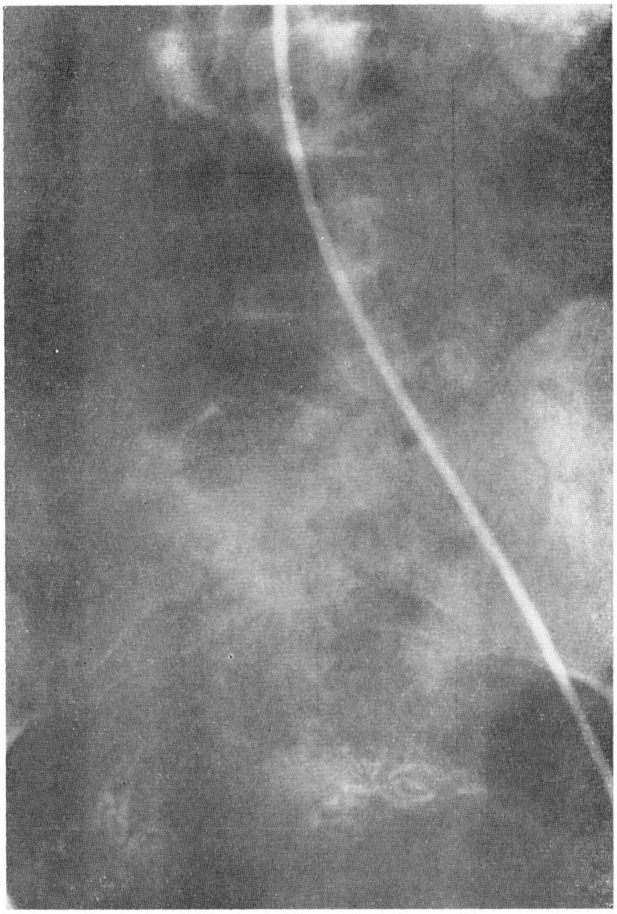

Figure 11.109. Flush Aortogram—late phase. There is demonstration of myometrial branches with their normal corkscrew appearance.

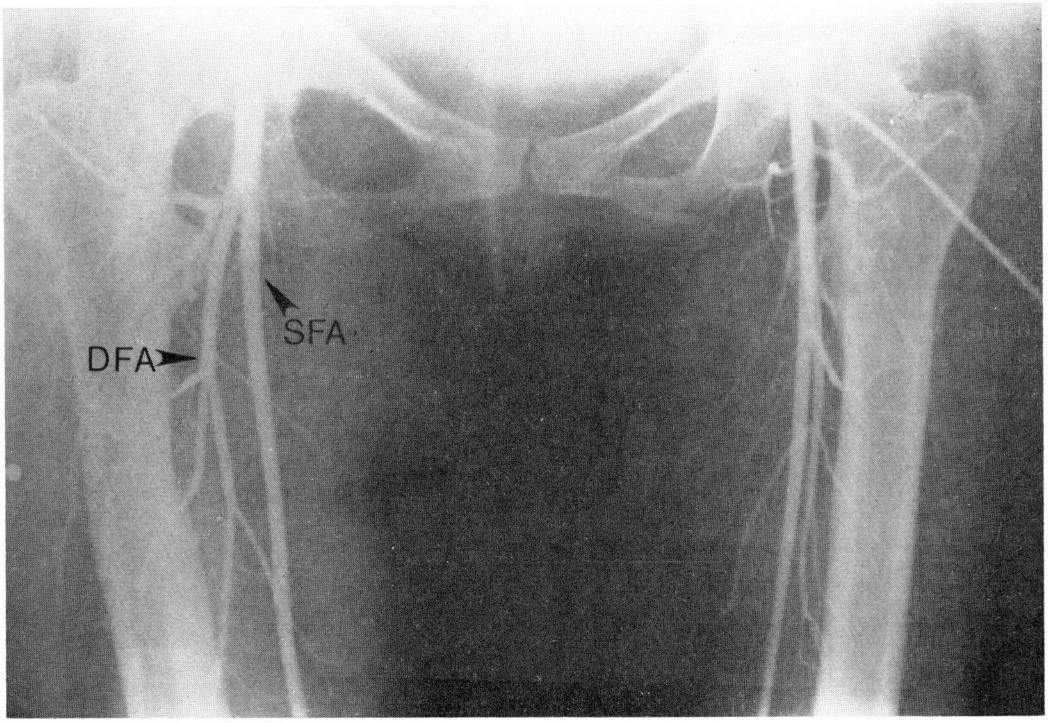

Figure 11.110. Femoral Arteriogram. Superficial femoral artery (S.F.A.), profunda femoris artery (P.F.A.).

Comment: This happens to be another normal situation.

Common Iliac Arteries

These are the major arteries to the lower extremities and pelvis, dividing into the internal iliac artery and the external iliac artery. The internal iliac artery supplies the pelvic structures and the buttocks; the external iliac continues as the common femoral artery. The internal iliac artery has an acute angle of origin and possesses a variable pattern in its branching into ventral (visceral) and dorsal (parietal) branches. The visceral branches include the inferior vesical, umbilical, middle rectal, and uterine arteries. The parietal branches are the obturator, internal pudendal, iliolumbar, lateral sacral, superior and inferior gluteal arteries. Variation in the parietal branches[352] and even absence of the iliac arteries[353] are not rare occurrences.

Uterine Artery

This arises from the anterior (visceral) branch of the internal iliac artery, courses caudally and medially through the pelvic connective tissue to reach the uterus at the isthmus of the cervix.[337] It then turns cranially along the lateral wall of the uterus (Fig. 11-108). Its tortuosity increases as it reaches the uterus, terminating as convoluted intramural branches to the uterus (Fig. 11-109). One of the uterine arteries may be narrow or absent, and the contralateral may be wide. Both may be narrow or absent, and when this occurs, the ovarian vessels may supply the uterus. These vessels are straight in a nulliparous woman and tortuous in a multiparous woman.[368, 369]

LOWER EXTREMITY VESSELS

The Femoral Artery

The femoral artery[337] is a continuation of the external iliac artery, extending from the caudal border of the inguinal ligament, passing through the adductor hiatus, and then entering the popliteal space to become the popliteal artery. In addition to other superficial branches, it also gives off the deep femoral artery (profunda femoris) anywhere from 2 to 4 cm below the inguinal ligament (Fig. 11-110).

Popliteal Artery

The popliteal[337] is a continuation of the femoral artery through the popliteal fossa. This artery terminates by dividing into anterior and posterior tibial arteries. The posterior tibial gives off the peroneal artery. High bifurcation of the popliteal artery, or absence of its major branches such as the posterior or anterior tibial, are not uncommon.[349, 351] These abnormalities are more often unilateral than bilateral. In general, asymmetrical patterns from right to left in the same individual are not an uncommon finding[350] (Fig. 11-111).

Lower Extremity Veins

The lower extremity venous[337] system can be divided into superficial and deep branches. The superficial veins communicating frequently

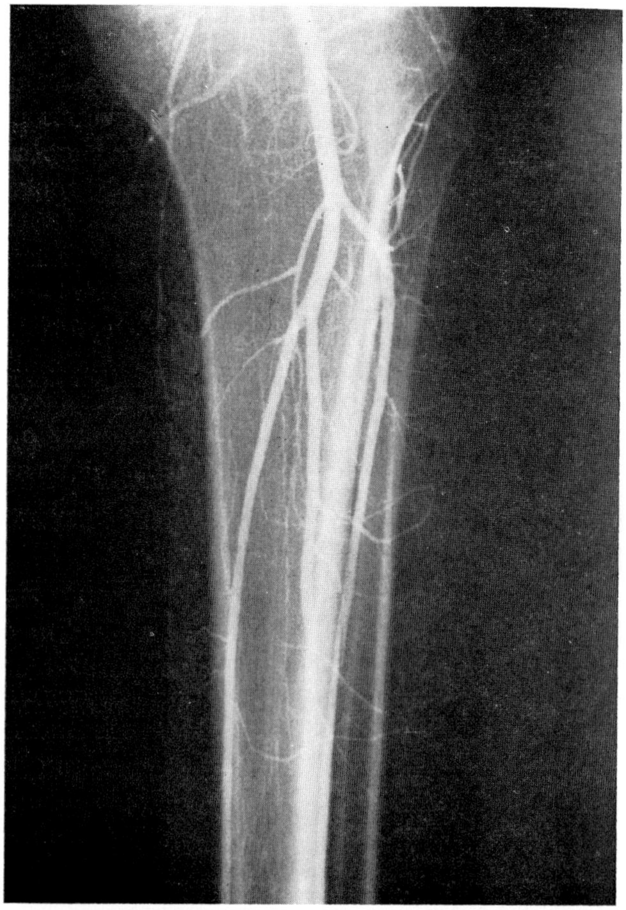

Figure 11.111. Femoral Arteriogram. Demonstrates the popliteal artery and its trifurcation. *Comment:* Normal.

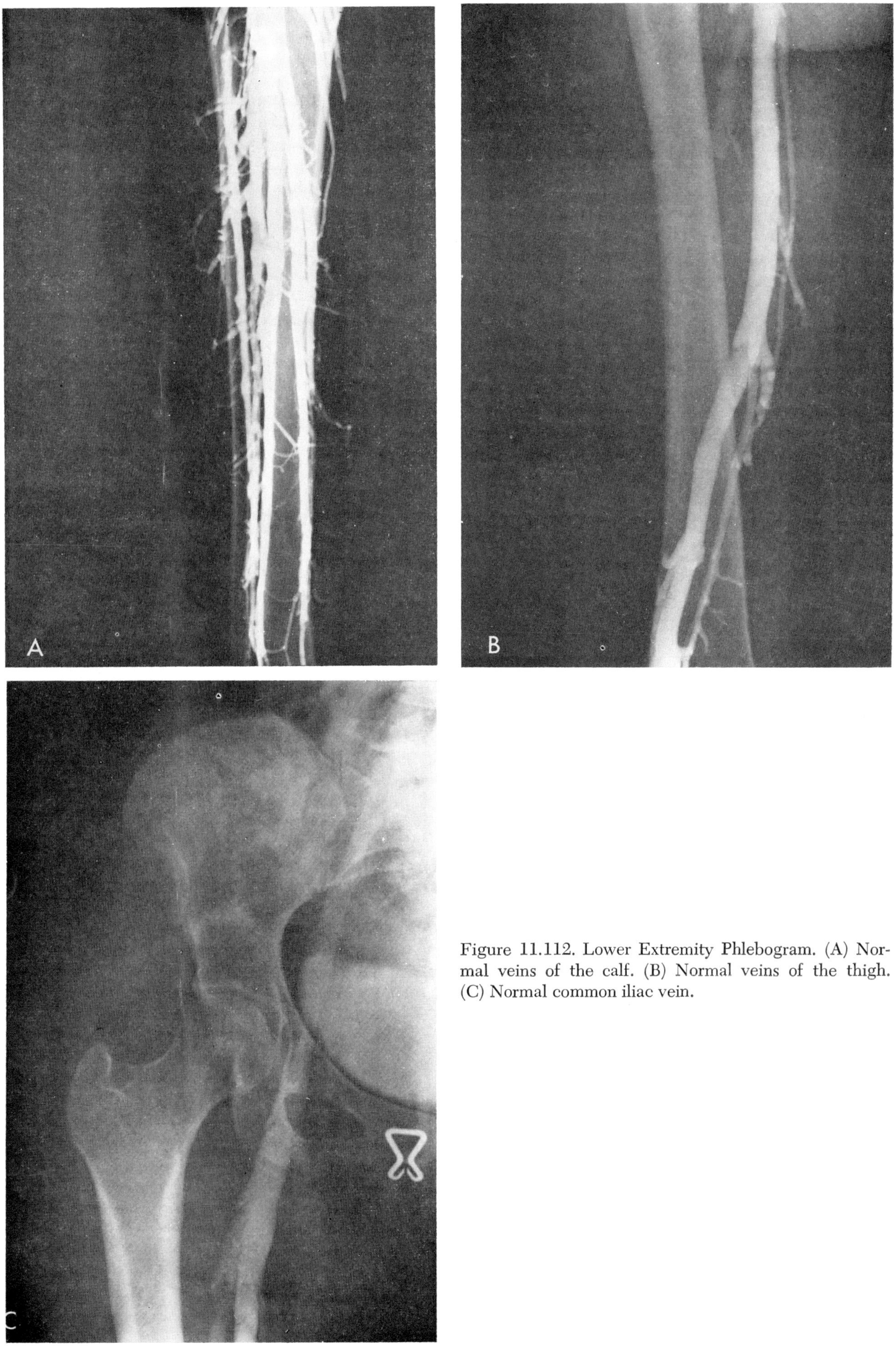

Figure 11.112. Lower Extremity Phlebogram. (A) Normal veins of the calf. (B) Normal veins of the thigh. (C) Normal common iliac vein.

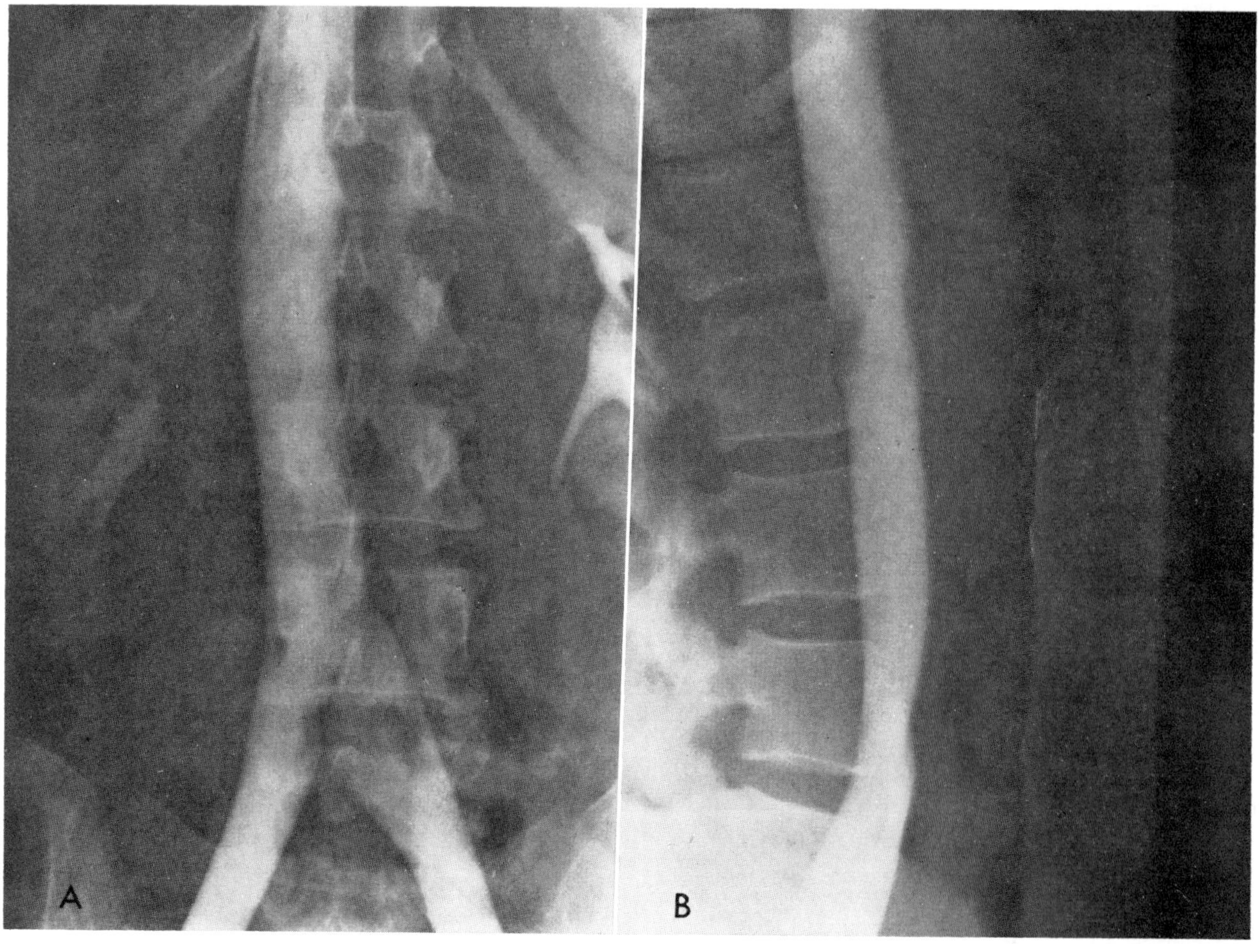

Figure 11.113. Inferior Vena Cavagram. (A) A.P. projection. (B) Lateral projection. *Comment:* Normal inferior vena cavagram.

with the deep veins via perforating vessels are collected chiefly into two main trunks. These are the greater saphenous vein anteriomedially and the lesser saphenous vein posterolaterally. The former joins the femoral vein in the groin, the latter joins the popliteal vein. The deep veins separate from the superficial in the foot, and course with the corresponding arteries to terminate in the popliteal vein. This continues as the femoral vein to the level of the inguinal ligament. It then continues cranially as the external iliac vein, and when it is joined by the internal iliac vein, becomes the common iliac vein. The two common iliac veins unite to form the inferior vena cava (Fig. 11-112).

Of interest in the distal two thirds of the leg is one paired vein to correspond with each main artery. When an artery is absent, it is associated with absence of the corresponding vein. Thus, variations are not uncommon, nor is it uncommon to have an accessory saphenous vein. The femoral vein is usually medial to the artery at the femoral triangle, but on occasion may be anterior or even posterior to the artery.

Perforating Veins

Incompetent perforating veins of the legs have a constant distribution despite the differences in body lengths.[409] The levels do not vary more than 0.5 cm, and the majority are on the medial side of the leg. They may, however, be found at any level in the limb. They serve to connect the superficial and deep venous system in the leg. Their numbers increase after deep venous thrombosis, and they may be the cause of skin ulcers.

CENTRAL VEINS

Pelvic Veins

The pelvic visceral veins[337] are valveless. The important ones are the ovarian pedicle, parauterine veins, and the uterine plexus which communicates with the vaginal plexus inferiorly and the ovarian veins superiorly. They are found between the layers of the broad ligament. The major venous drainage is through the internal iliac veins. The gonadal veins, though originating in the pelvis, terminate on the right in the inferior vena cava and on the left in the renal vein.

Inferior Vena Cava

The inferior vena cava is formed by the confluence of the common iliac veins at approximately the fifth lumbar vertebral body. It ascends toward the right atrium in a plane slightly ventral to the aorta and the lumbar vertebral bodies. When in contact with the liver, it lies in a deep fossa sometimes surrounded by liver parenchyma in a circumferential manner. At the same level the caudate lobe is to the left of the inferior vena cava. No doubt the cava here is comparatively well fixed on all sides and easily subjected to extrinsic pressure[394] (Figs. 11-113 to 11-115).

The Vertebral Veins

The vertebral veins[391, 392] are a set of valveless vessels carrying blood under low pressure subjected to constant arrest and reversal of the blood flow. They consist of epidural, perivertebral, thoraco abdominal wall, and head and

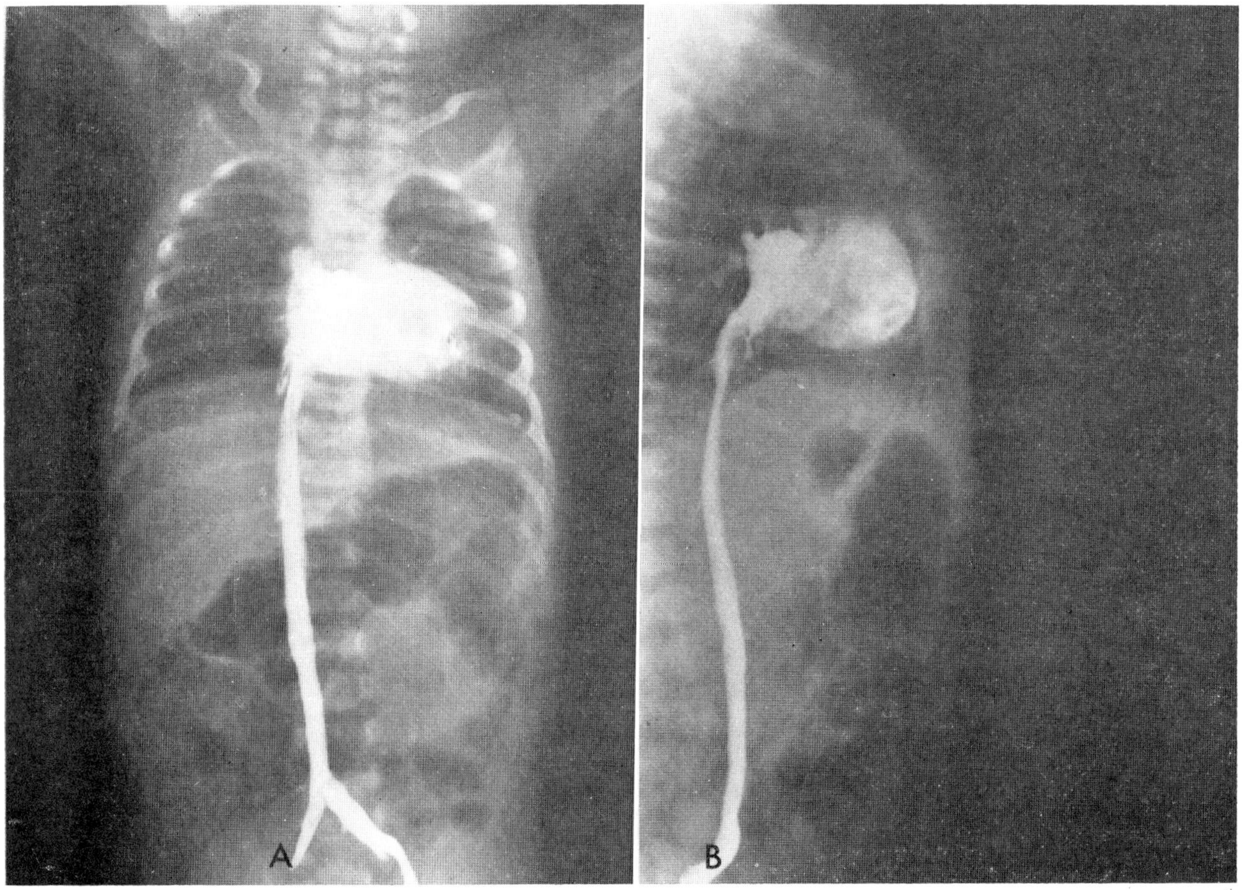

Figure 11.114. Inferior Vena Cavagram. (A) Normal inferior vena caval course. (B) Lateral view with a normal course of the inferior vena cava.

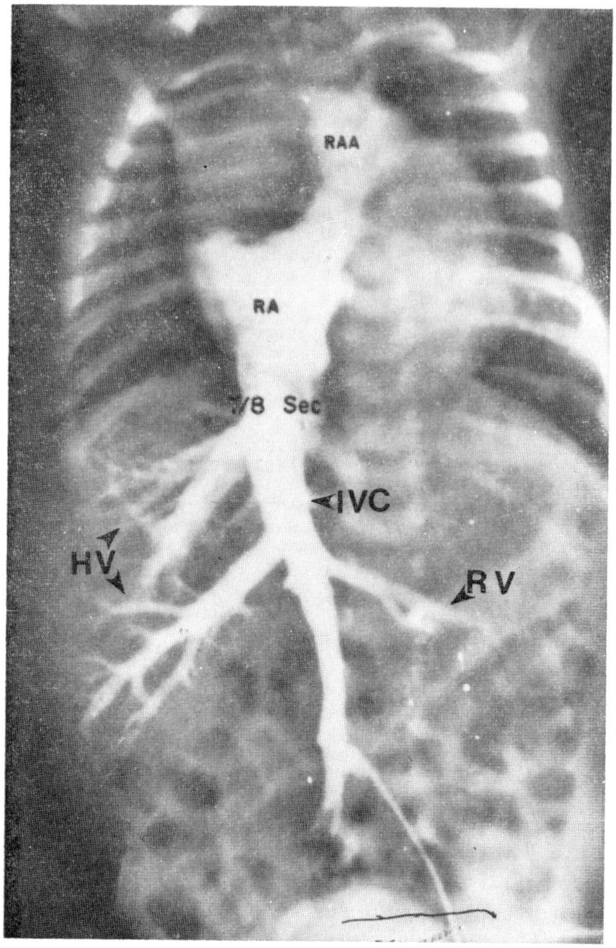

Figure 11.115. Inferior Vena Cavagram. Inferior vena cava (I.V.C.), left renal vein (R.V.) and hepatic vein (H.V.). *Comment:* Good reflux of contrast into the inferior vena caval branches in a patient with a hypoplastic right ventricle.

neck veins. This plexus parallels, connects and bypasses the caval, portal and pulmonary systems. It can provide in itself a pathway for disease between remote organs. It may act as a venous pool or bypass for other venous systems (Fig. 11-116). *Thus, the irrigation streams of life can also carry the ships of destruction.*

Azygos Veins

The azygos and ascending lumbar veins constitute a continuous channel for venous drainage of the posterior body wall.[337, 344, 345] The ascending lumbar veins receive the lumbar veins, while the azygos receives the posterior intercostal veins. Communication between the thoracic and abdominal portions of this system frequently occurs.

The azygos venous system of the thorax consists of longitudinal collecting trunks into which the vertebral plexus and the intercostal veins drain. The three primary channels comprising this system are the azygos, the right superior intercostal vein on the right, and the hemiazygos and the accessory hemiazygos on the left. The azygos vein on the right side empties into the superior vena cava posteriorly approximately at the level of the right tracheobronchial angle. The hemiazygos terminates in the azygos vein around the level of the ninth thoracic vertebral body. Variations in the arrangement of this system are not unusual[346] (Figs. 11-117 and 11-118).

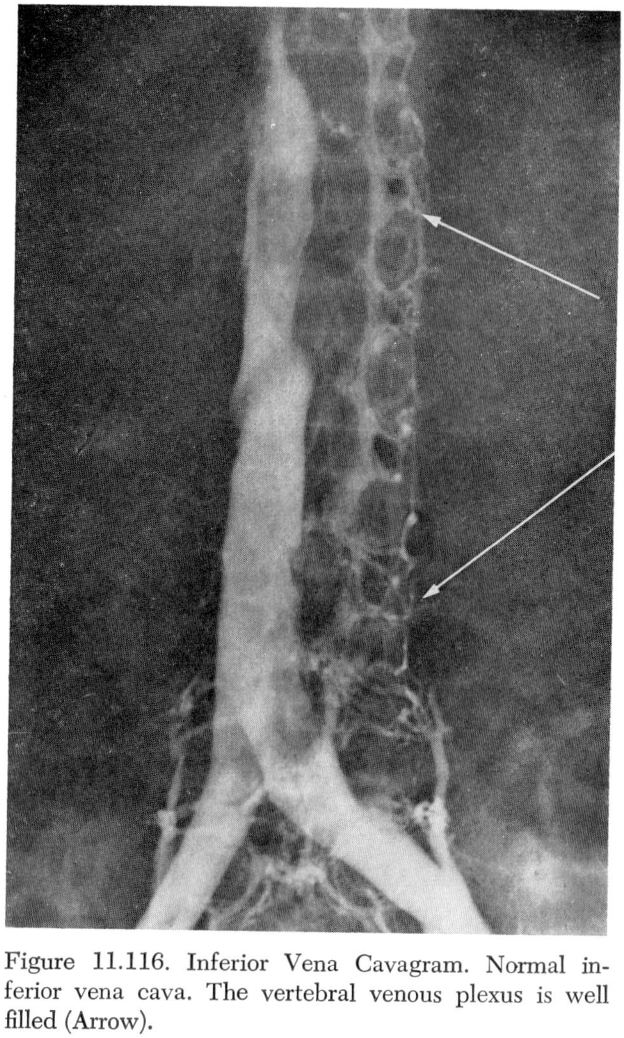

Figure 11.116. Inferior Vena Cavagram. Normal inferior vena cava. The vertebral venous plexus is well filled (Arrow).

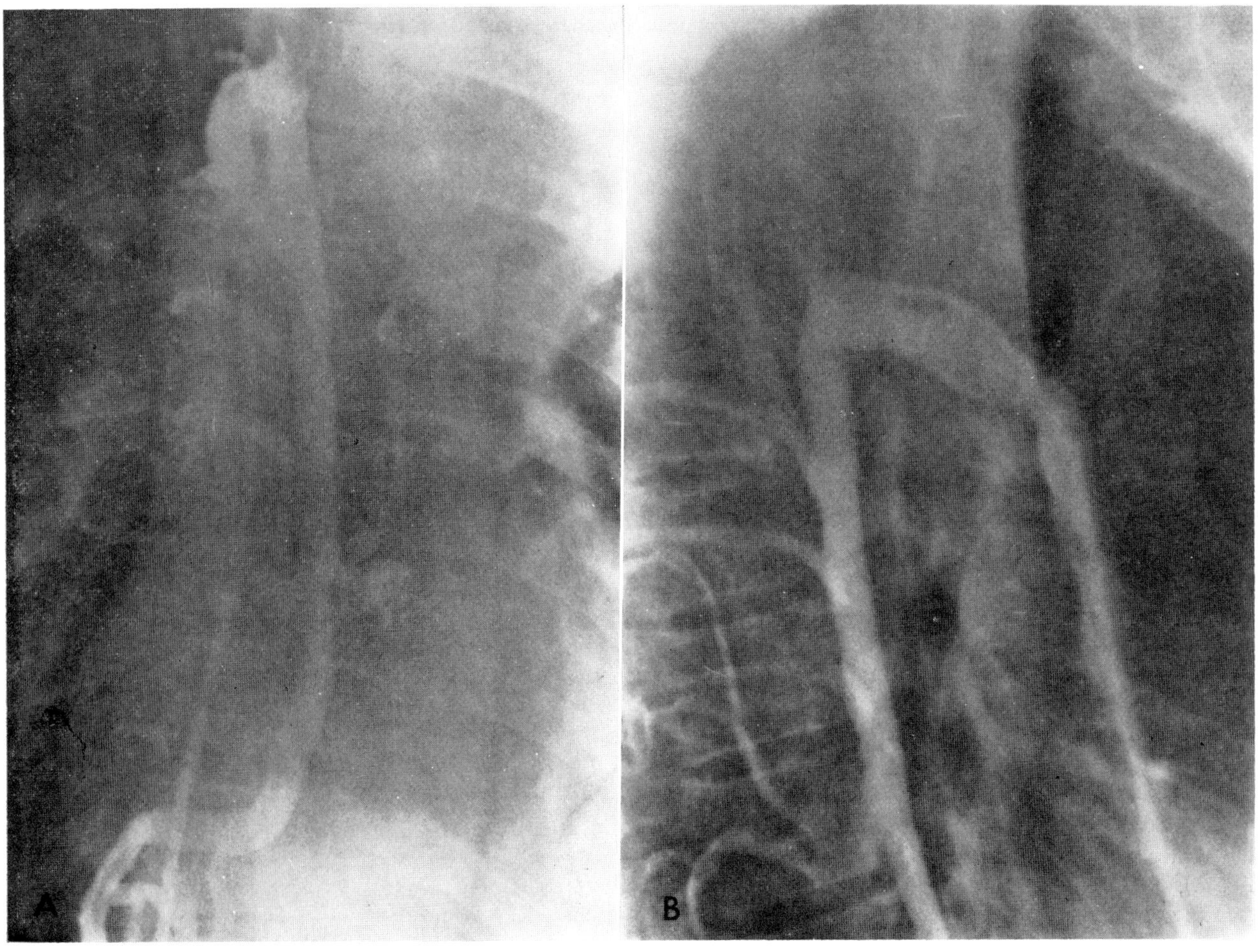

Figure 11.117. Azygous Venogram. (A) A.P. projection. (B) Lateral projection. *Comment:* Normal azygous vein.

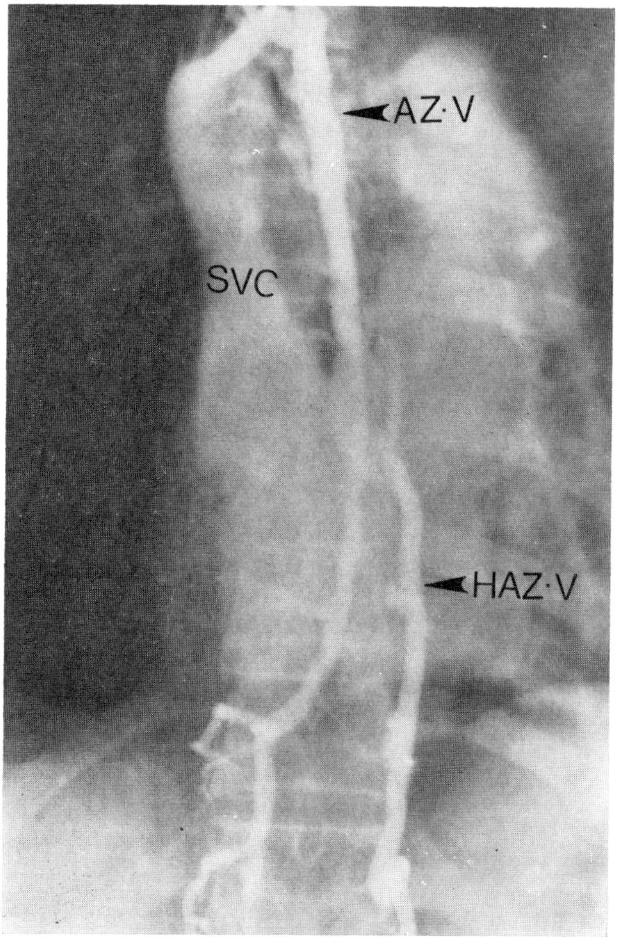

Figure 11.118. Ascending Lumbar Vein—Catheterization. Superior vena cava (S.V.C.), right azygous (AZ.V.), hemiazygous (HAZ.V.). *Comment:* Normal anatomy of the azygous venous system.

Venous Valves

These valves develop from intimal cushions lined by endothelium molding progressively into the semilunar valve form and growing constantly throughout their lives.[400, 401] Most valves are bicuspid. There are great variations in the number of valves present in the venous system.[402] Valves are usually found in areas where long columns of venous blood are flowing against gravity and in the tributary veins before they terminate in main channels. They are absent in very small and in very large veins. They have a passive function, collapsing against the wall during normal blood flow and opening during reversal of flow.[337] Adequate external compression, or Valsalva maneuver, demonstrates the valves to greater advantage. Some of the significant valves[402] are in the popliteal vein distal to the adductor opening, common femoral vein at the inguinal ligament, external iliac vein distal to the junction of the internal iliac vein, inferior vena cava occasionally as it terminates with the right atrium (eustachian valve), internal jugular vein[406] just above the confluence with the subclavian vein, azygos vein,[405] middle or posterior one third of the arch of the azygos, gonadal vein[403] on the left side, one at the pelvic brim level, and another before it enters the renal vein. The right gonadal vein also may have multiple valves. The left renal vein[404] occasionally (4% of the population) has a valve 1.5 cm medial to the gonadal vein junction, while the right renal vein more frequently (28% of the population) has a valve at the junction of the right renal vein and inferior vena cava.

The valveless veins include the portal, vertebral, pelvic, parathyroid plexus, superior vena cava, pampiniform plexus, and the hepatic veins. Complete thrombosis of a vein with or without recanalization produces a valveless vein.[408]

MICROANATOMY

Sinusoids

A *sinusoid*[327] is a large, variable size channel consisting of vessels with only an endothelial or endotheloid layer. These sinusoids are fitted closely against the cells of the organ from which they develop, their walls following the shape of the parenchyma of that part. They have free and wide communication with other sinusoids. A typical sinusoid has no connective tissue, or if any at all, a very little which is acquired and develops late. Sinusoids offer the main channel of circulation in the liver, heart, adrenal, parathyroid, aortic bodies and coccygeal bodies. A *capillary* differs from a sinusoid by possessing a wall of its own with definite caliber and shape. Capillaries are formed

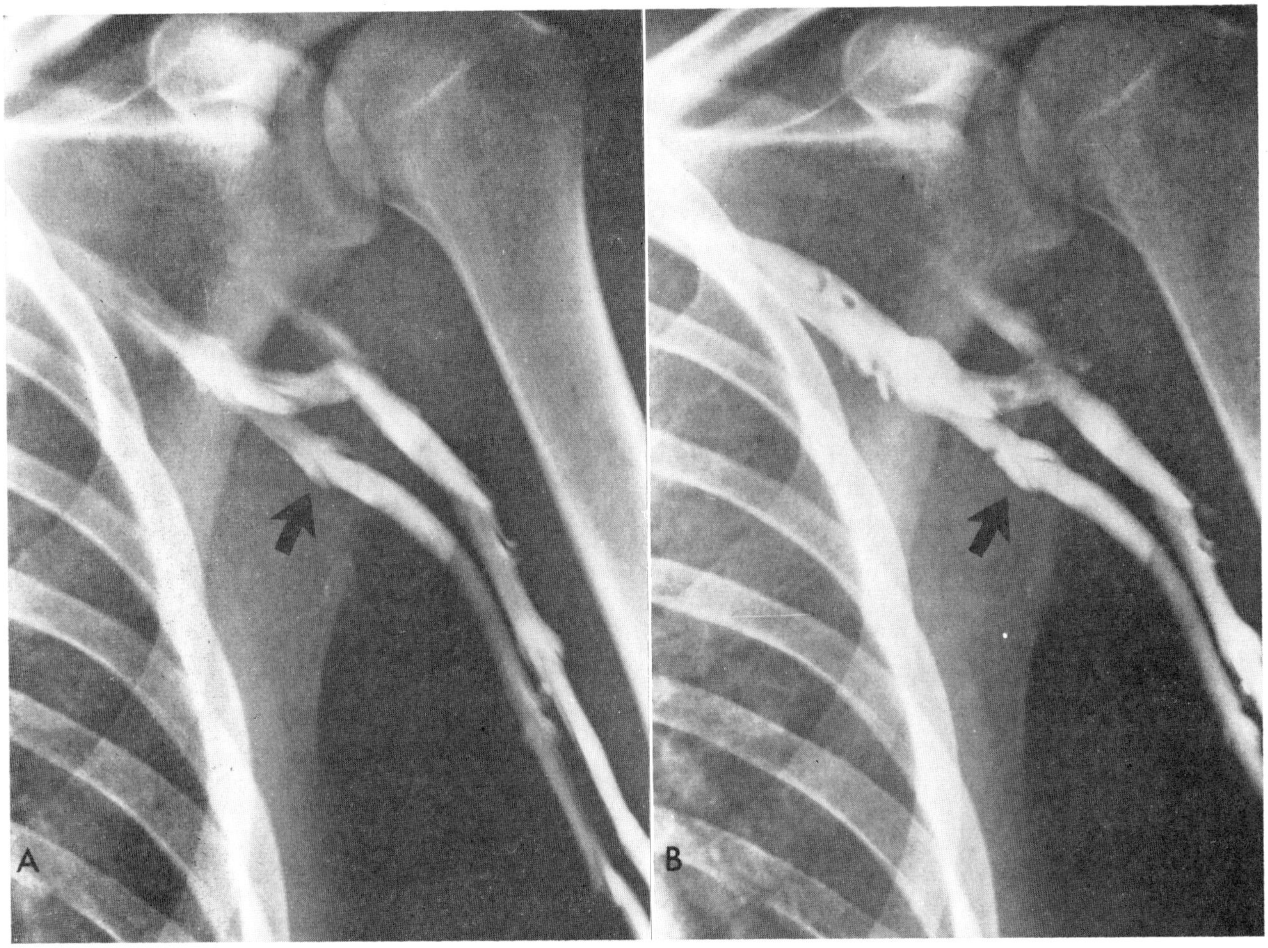

Figure 11.119. Upper Extremity Venogram A & B. (A) Normal deep veins: Notice the closed valves. (B) In the same patient, notice the open valves. *Comment:* Competent valves.

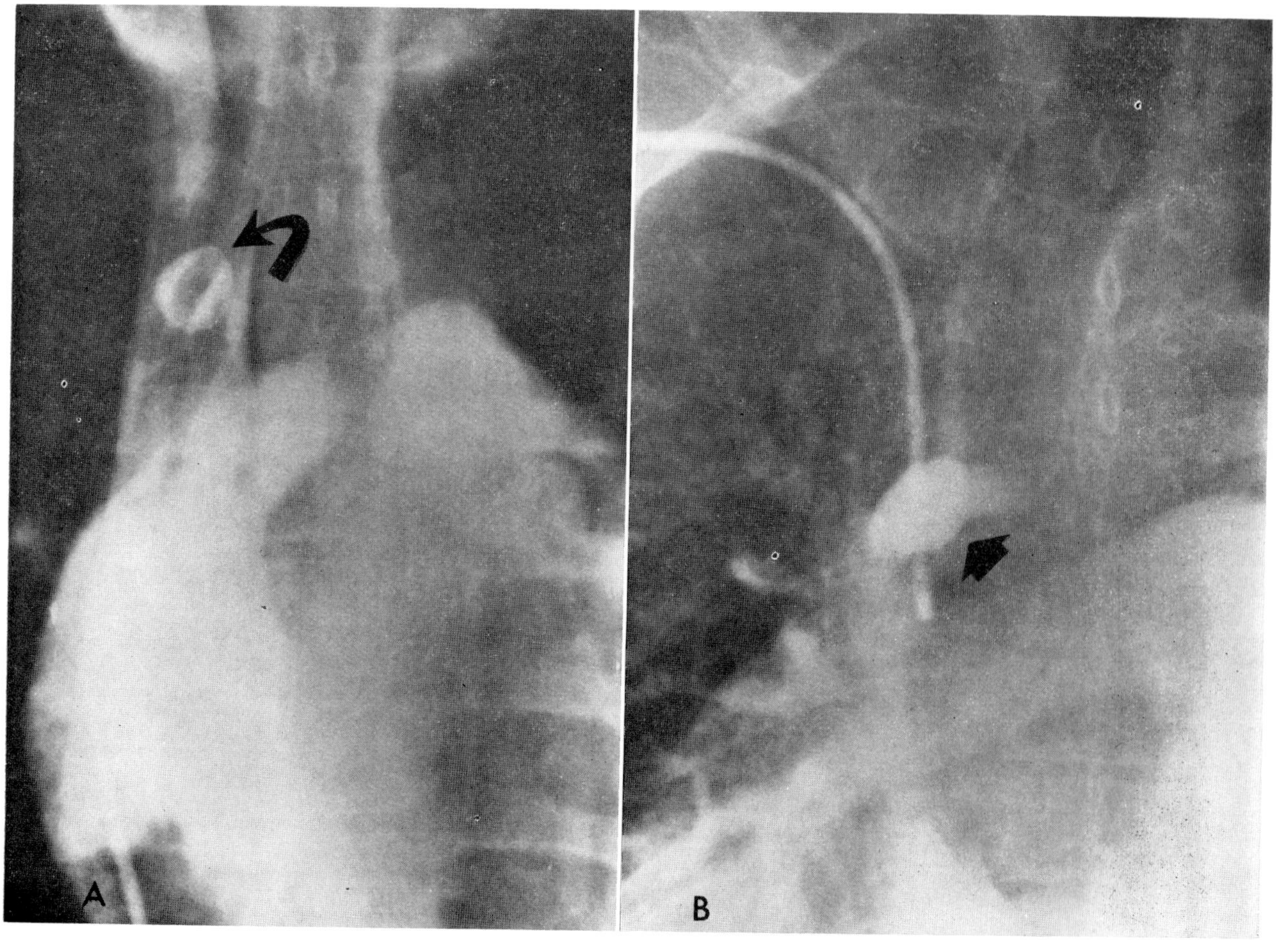

Figure 11.120. Intravenous Angiocardiogram. (A) A circumscribed collection of contrast material with a central band-like translucency is seen at the right tracheobronchial angle. *Comment:* Collection of contrast material in the valve pockets of the azygous vein. (B) Basilic vein catheterization demonstrates a dense collection of contrast at the right tracheobronchial angle. *Comment:* Collection of contrast in the normal azygous vein.

by a chain of vasoformative cells which become hollowed out and connect with other vessels at both ends. A sinusoid is not a product of new histiogenesis, but arises from the growth of the endothelial wall of a preexisting blood vessel or from the intercrescence of the growing endothelium of the organ. The physiological inferiority of the sinusoidal circulation has led to its modification and partial obliteration in the higher vertebrates.[327]

Myocardial sinusoids[410] exist in the intramural circulation of the heart. These embryonic sinusoids may persist and dilate even to the extent of diverticular communication with the coronary tree due to increased pressure in a hypertrophied small right ventricle,[411, 412] which may occur in disease entities like pulmonary atresia.

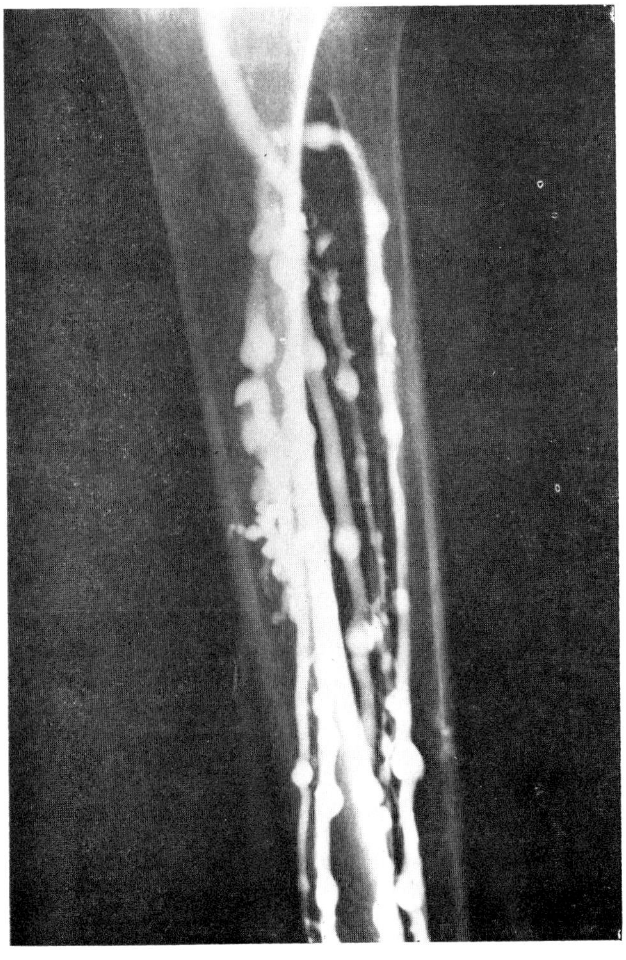

Figure 11.121. Lower Extremity Phlebogram. Numerous valves are in the calf veins.

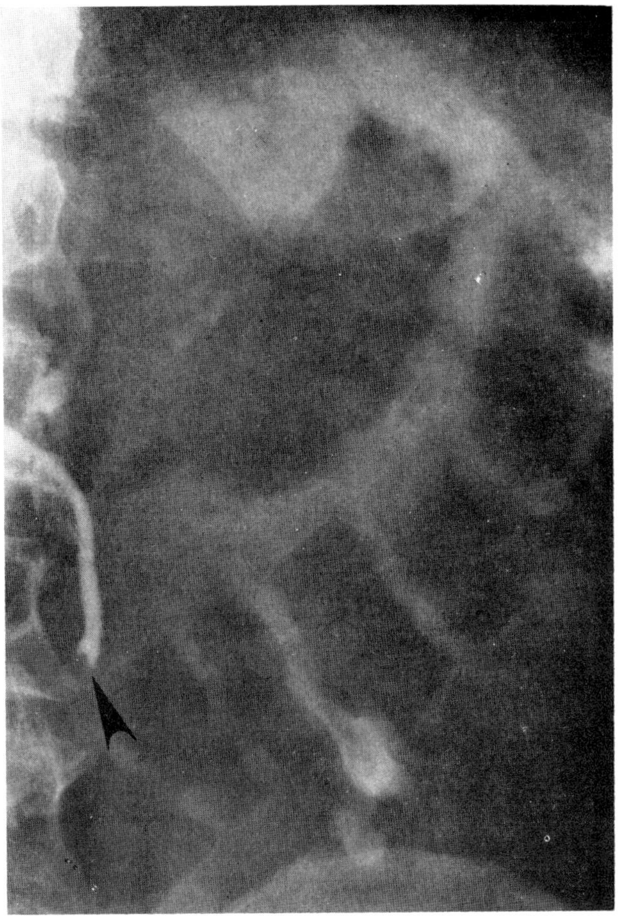

Figure 11.122. Left Gonadal Venogram. Note the abrupt termination of the contrast. *Comment:* A competent valve in the gonadal vein proximal to its termination. The presence of competent valves in the gonadal vein may be time consuming during catheterization when trying to insert a catheter distal to the valve.

Hepatic sinusoids[302, 361–364] may be purely arterial or venous or both. The outflow tract from these sinusoids is the central vein of the liver. These sinusoids are separated from one another by two cords of hepatic parenchymal cells lined by Kupffer cells. High pressure hepatic arterial and portal vein streams meet at the level of the hepatic sinusoids. The small arterioles may join the portal vein directly to maintain normal portal venous pressure. In normal individuals and in cirrhotic patients, no

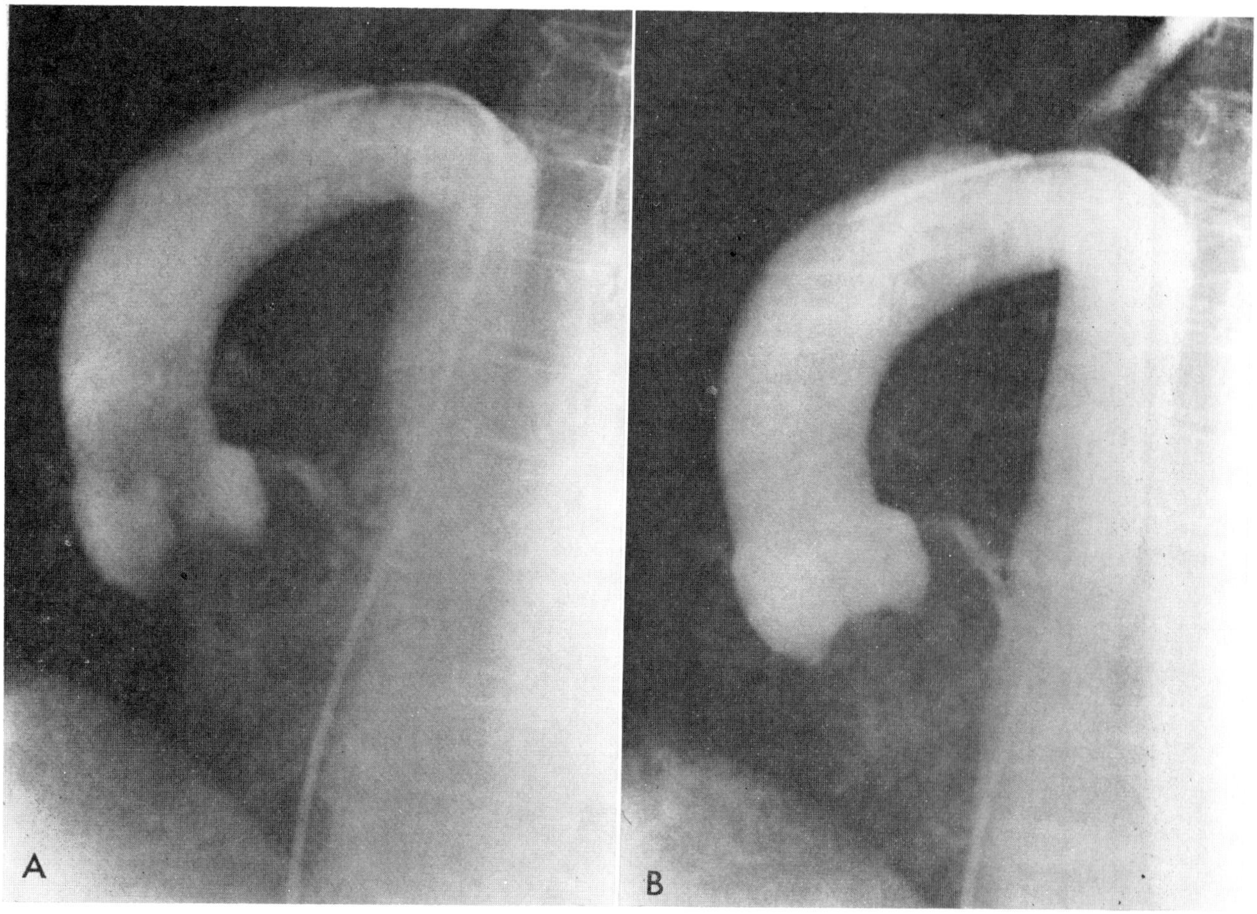

Figure 11.123. Aortogram. (A) Opening of aortic valve during cardiac systole. (B) Closure of the valve during cardiac diastole.

connections exist between the hepatic artery and the hepatic vein. No direct anastomoses are seen between the hepatic vein and portal venous radicles except through the sinusoids (Fig. 11-54).

Blood Circulation in Lymph Nodes

Studies of the microcirculation reveal marked dominance of the venous elements. The lymphatic circulation and the venous circulation communicate in the sinusoids.[315]

CHAPTER 12
ROUTES OF ENTRY

THE MAIN ROUTES of entry into the *arterial system* in adults are the *femoral or axillary arteries.* Brachial artery catheterization is contraindicated because of the high incidence of arterial thrombosis. In infants the umbilical artery is the route of choice.[225, 271, 285] For entry into the *venous system* either the *femoral, jugular or antecubital veins* can be used. Again in children, or on rare occasions in adults, the umbilical vein can be used.[287]

ARTERIES

Femoral Artery

This is the *route of choice* in almost all instances, unless the regional anatomy precludes its use. Entry through this site is contraindicated when there are masses overlying the artery, local infection, stenotic or occlusive vascular disease, or trauma. The presence of previous scars is not a contraindication but may make catheter insertion and subsequent manipulation difficult, if not impossible. With a properly curved catheter and cooperative anatomy almost all the primary and secondary arterial branches of the aorta may be catheterized from this route.

The right femoral artery is the more popular one, but the left acts as a good "standby" if the contralateral side develops spasm or happens to be tortuous. The left femoral route makes catheterization of the inferior mesenteric, left internal iliac, and left renal arteries less tedious, especially in older individuals. *Simultaneous catheterization of both femoral arteries should be discouraged.* The composite information obtained from such studies is no more informative than the diagnostic yield obtained from successive individual catheterization (celiac, mesenteric and internal iliac arteries). To avoid trouble a previously catheterized site should be shunned, if possible.

Axillary Artery

Selection of the axillary artery as the route of entry in preference to other available routes should be strongly discouraged. Associated

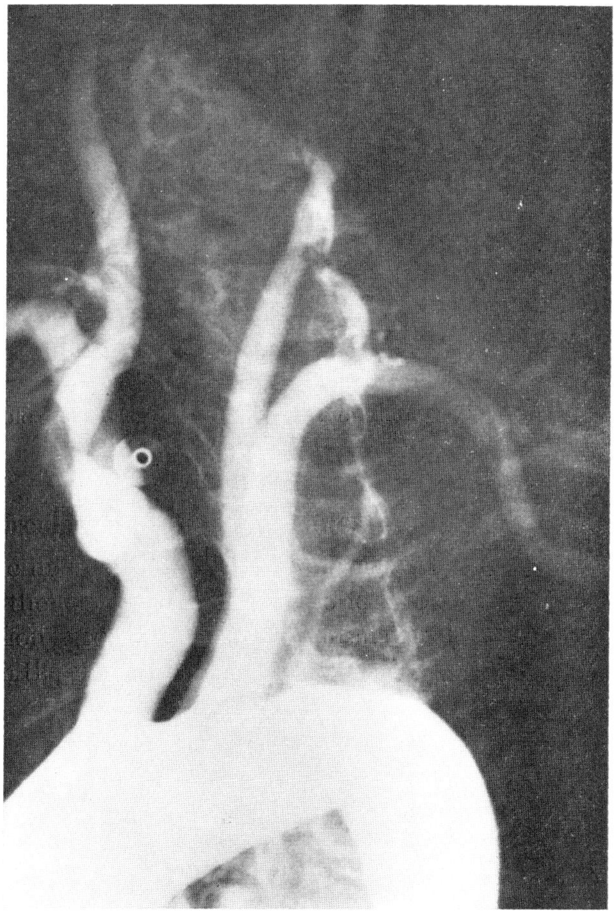

Figure 12.1. Aortic Arch Angiogram. The orifices of the left common carotid and the left subclavian arteries are shifted toward the ascending aorta. *Comment:* The change in position of the arterial origins causes technical difficulties in catheterizing the descending aorta from the left axillary approach.

crowding of vital structures like the brachial plexus about the artery in the "axillary cave" makes them vulnerable to the damaging effect of a hematoma or the dislodgement of a plaque or mural thrombus into the cerebral circulation en route to the aorta. *Thus, the risks are higher using this artery.* The axillary route is preferred only when the femoral sites of entry are unavailable due to severe atherosclerosis, occlusion or trauma and when selective catheterization of the arteries via the axillary artery is vital to solving the clinical problem. To demonstrate peripheral arterial occlusive disease, a translumbar aortogram in good hands is probably safer than the axillary artery approach.

The left axillary route is convenient for reaching the descending aorta, as the left subclavian orifice maintains a straight-line relationship with the descending aorta. Though the left subclavian orifice shifts anteriorly in an ectatic aorta, it is still the closest orifice for reaching the descending aorta (Fig. 12-1). *The right axillary artery* is the preferred route to opacify the ascending aorta when the femoral route fails. The innominate orifice maintains an almost straight-line relationship to the long axis of the ascending aorta. But this is not the situation in an ectatic aorta or in a buckled innominate artery. This may make it impossible to reach the ascending aorta from this route.

VEINS

Femoral Veins

Almost all the veins can be catheterized through this route provided that the femoral veins are not thrombosed and the regional anatomy is normal.

Jugular Veins

This vein is used as a route of entry only when the femoral veins are thrombosed, or during simultaneous catheterization of jugular and femoral veins to show proximal and distal extent of an occlusive process in the inferior vena cava. It is also used for the proper function of the presently available instruments for transjugular cholangiogram. The right jugular vein is preferred for transjugular cholangiograms because of better catheter control and less interference with the right atrial wall.

Antecubital Veins

Due to the presence of valves in these veins, at this route of entry a catheter with side holes only is used with the assistance of a sheath, short guide wire, and a dilator (Fig. 15-3). These sites are also the quickest and easiest for the opacification of the cardiac chambers to evaluate pericardial processes and for gross visualization of the pulmonary arterial tree.[272, 273] This opacification can very easily be achieved with the assistance of Teflon sleeve needles also.

CHAPTER 13
THE PUNCTURE SITE

THE ACTUAL puncture site for the route of entry should meet the following criteria:

1. The vessel should be easily accessible for percutaneous puncture with no vital structure anterior or posterior to it.
2. The vessel should not intermingle with important associated structures such as nerve roots or plexuses.
3. The vessel should be provided with a nonyielding posterior support (such as a bone) to insure effective compression of the vessel and proper closure of the hole in the wall.
4. There should be reasonably good potential collateral vessels proximal and distal to the puncture site in the event of local thrombosis.
5. The point of puncture should not be too close to a major branch whose patency may be very vital to the survival of the extremity in the present or future.
6. The puncture site should be free of infection, masses, scars or palpable thrills.
7. The site should be easily accessible for surgical exploration in the event of thrombosis.

FEMORAL ARTERY AND VEIN

The actual puncture site (Figs. 13-1 and 13-2) for the femoral artery is aimed at the level of the *midinguinal point* through a skin incision made approximately 3 cm below the midinguinal point. In this location the femoral artery courses through the above point and the vessel is easily palpable, fixable, and compressible against the head of the femur. No major branch (i.e. profunda femoris) is injured, and there are no vital structures either anterior or posterior to the artery. *The midinguinal point is located by palpating the anterior superior iliac spine and the pubic tubercle.* Dependency on the groin crease for the anatomic landmarks may result in unsuccessful puncture or damage to the deep femoral artery. The groin crease descends in relation to the inguinal fold and does not correspond anatomically to the level of the inguinal ligament, especially in obese individuals and/or in the elderly. *Aiming at a level proximal to the midinguinal point may result in a hole which is inaccessible for manual compression.* Subsequently, sizeable hematomas may develop (Fig. 13-3).

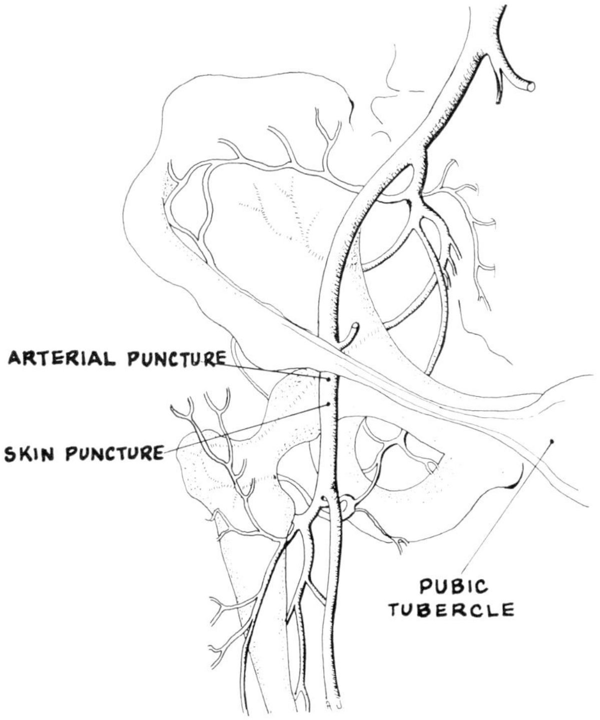

Figure 13.1. Femoral artery puncture site.

For the femoral vein, the *puncture is aimed at a point 1 cm medial to the midinguinal point.* The needle is advanced toward this point while

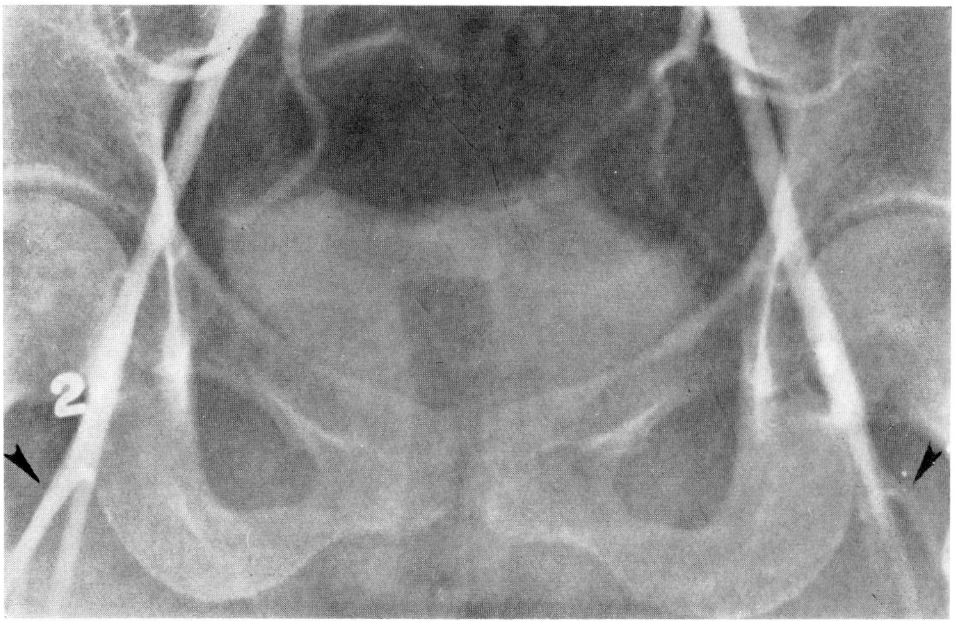

Figure 13.2. Pelvic Arteriogram. The radiopaque numbers are on the skin incisions. Arterial puncture should be approximately 1 centimeter proximal to this point. The origin of the deep femoral artery (Arrow Head) is usually below the head of the femur.

deviating the femoral artery laterally with the fingertips of the other hand (Fig. 13-5).

Axillary Artery

The patient should be lying in a supine position with his palm under his head. Then the *arterial puncture is aimed at a point just inferior to the axillary pectoral fold.* In this position the artery is not overlapped by too many nerves; it is easily fixed, palpable and compressible with provisions for good collaterals should thrombosis occur.

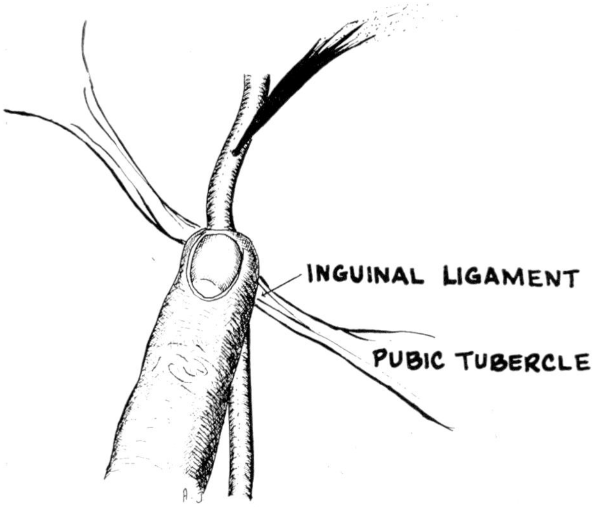

Figure 13.3. Effects of puncturing femoral artery proximal to the midinguinal point.

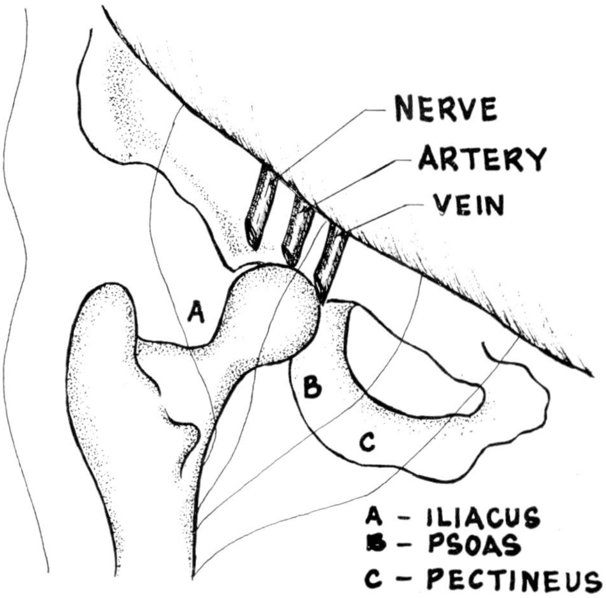

Figure 13.4. Femoral artery in the groin and its important neighbors.

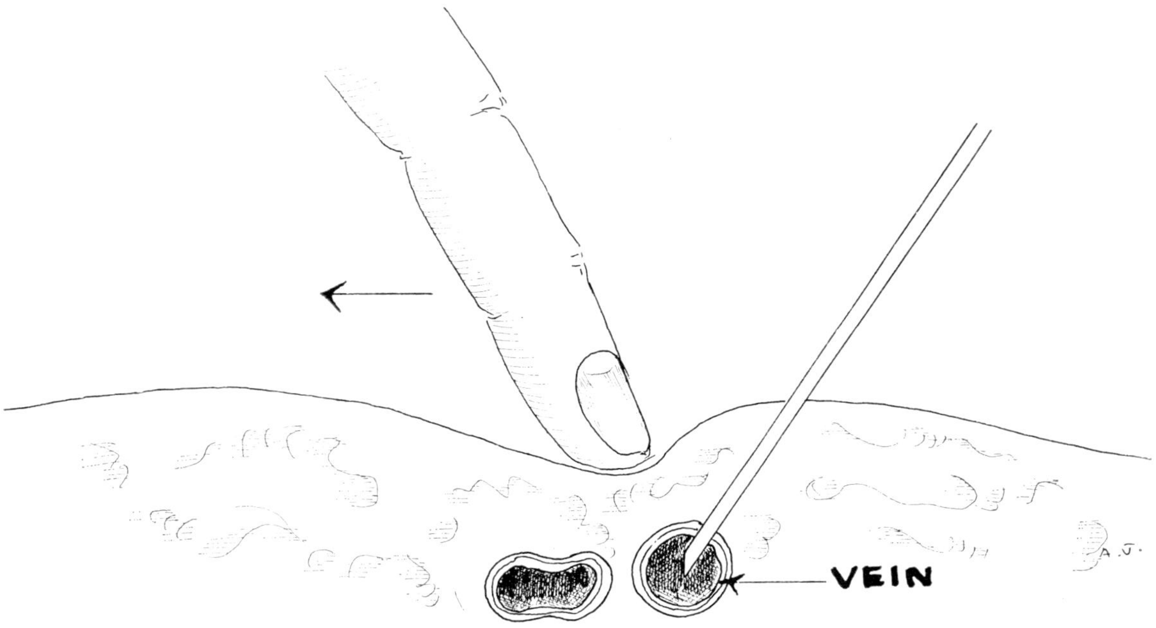

Figure 13.5. Puncture of the femoral vein.

Brachial Artery

This artery should not be used for catheterization procedures. Puncture at this site is intended only for the insertion of a short, Teflon sleeve. The arterial puncture is aimed at a point about 2.5 to 3.0 cm above the antecubital crease.

Jugular Vein

The puncture of the vein is aimed at a *point 5 cm below the angle of the mandible with the neck of the patient extended.* While advancing the needle, the carotid artery is deviated medially by the fingers of the other hand.

CHAPTER 14

THE TRAY

The standard, sterile angiographic tray should always contain the following equipment: guide wires, Seldinger needles, catheters, and Teflon sleeves. Other equipment may be added depending on the type of study being performed.

Needles

One 23 or 25 gauge needle for skin anesthesia. One 19 gauge 2″ needle for deep infiltration of anesthesia.

Stopcocks

One stopcock which can withstand high delivery rates.[35]

Syringes

Two 25 cc syringes for flushing the catheter. Two 10 cc syringes—one containing local anesthetic and one for injecting contrast material.

Routine habits should be developed to guard against drawing contrast into the same syringe as that being used to flush the catheter with saline. *Some means of identifying the syringe being used for anesthesia to differentiate it from the syringe being used for contrast should be devised* by each angiographer. For example, the needle used to infiltrate the anesthesia should be left on the syringe in order to positively identify its content.

Containers

Two containers about 8″ in diameter should be available. Each should hold approximately 500 cc of normal saline with 1000 units of heparin.

One is only used to flush the catheter, the other for cleaning needles, catheters, wires, etc. *The container with the saline to flush the catheter should not be used for any other purpose.* This should be covered by a sterile lid to keep out debris which may fall into it. If a closed system of irrigation[274] is used, then the basin to hold the flushing solution is unnecessary.

Three small containers should be available, one for local anesthetic, one for the antiseptic scrub solution, and one for contrast material. Again, care should be taken to insure that positive identification of the container holding anesthetic or contrast can be made. It is preferable to dilute the contrast for test injection by adding an equal volume of normal saline.

Linen

Six sterile towels and enough sterile drapes to cover the patient adequately. Disposable, sterile, prepackaged angiographic trays can be obtained at a nominal cost.[36] Sterile sheets, fenestrated for each femoral area and containing adhesive about the fenestrations to affix the drape to the patient are also available.

CHAPTER 15
STANDARD TECHNIQUE

FEMORAL ROUTE

After thorough cleansing with soap and water, the groin area is painted with antiseptic solution. The patient is properly draped with sterile towels and drapes. After *feeling the expansile pulsation* of the common femoral artery at the midinguinal point, ½ cc of local *anesthetic* is injected *intradermally* through a 23 or 25 gauge needle to raise a skin bleb about 2.5 to 3.0 cm below the midinguinal point. This should be in the same vertical axis as the vessel. Then with a regular 19 gauge needle, *deeper infiltration of anesthetic* is carried out. With each increase in the depth of infiltration, aspiration is attempted to insure that the injection is not made into an artery or vein.

A vertical *skin incision* (0.5 cm) is then made on the bleb to facilitate the catheter insertion and manipulation. External rotation of the lower extremity with slight abduction aids in good fixation of the artery. Then the *artery is well fixed* either by locking it in between the index and middle fingers or by stretching along its longitudinal axis. The latter is especially useful in thin individuals (Figs. 16-1, 16-2).

The *needle* is then advanced through the skin incision toward the midinguinal point at an angle of 45 degrees. It is inserted 1 cm deeper than the approximately estimated depth of the arterial location in order to *puncture both the anterior and posterior walls of the vessel* (transfixation). Then keeping the blunt cannula in place, the remaining stylet portion of the needle is removed. The cannula is then slowly withdrawn. If the needle has punctured the vessel, a sudden *pulsatile stream of bright red blood* with a forceful jet gushes from the cannula, indicating that its opening is in the lumen of the vessel. If a venous puncture is being done, there should be a steady trickle of dark red blood. The needle is then depressed horizontally and introduced slightly further into the vessel. The selected *guide wire* is then introduced through the cannula into the vessel with the *floppy leading segment entering first* for a distance of approximately 40 to 50 cm under fluoroscopic control. The cannula is withdrawn over the guide wire leaving the guide wire in the vessel. The guide wire should then be grasped between the thumb and second finger of the left hand while the third through fifth fingers of the left hand exert pressure on the artery proximal to the existing site of the guide wire to control bleeding. The guide wire is then wiped with a sterile gauze in the right hand of the angiographer, or it can be wiped by an assistant. By securing the guide wire between the first and second fingers of the left hand, accidental withdrawal while wiping it is avoided. The assistant then inserts the *dilator* over the guide wire and brings it up to the skin incision so that the angiographer can insert it through the vessel with a firm, but gentle, rotary, stabbing motion. This widens the puncture hole. The dilator can then be withdrawn, again grasping the guide wire in the same manner and wiping it off. Pressure must be kept proximal to the puncture site as the flow of blood through this enlarged arterial opening is great. The assistant then inserts the *selected catheter* on the guide wire, bringing it to the skin incision, and the angiographer inserts it into the aorta to a level slightly proximal to the desired point of selective catheterization.

Once the catheter has reached the level of the aortic bifurcation, it may be advisable to withdraw the guide wire partially, keeping it only 7 to 10 cm beyond the tip of the catheter

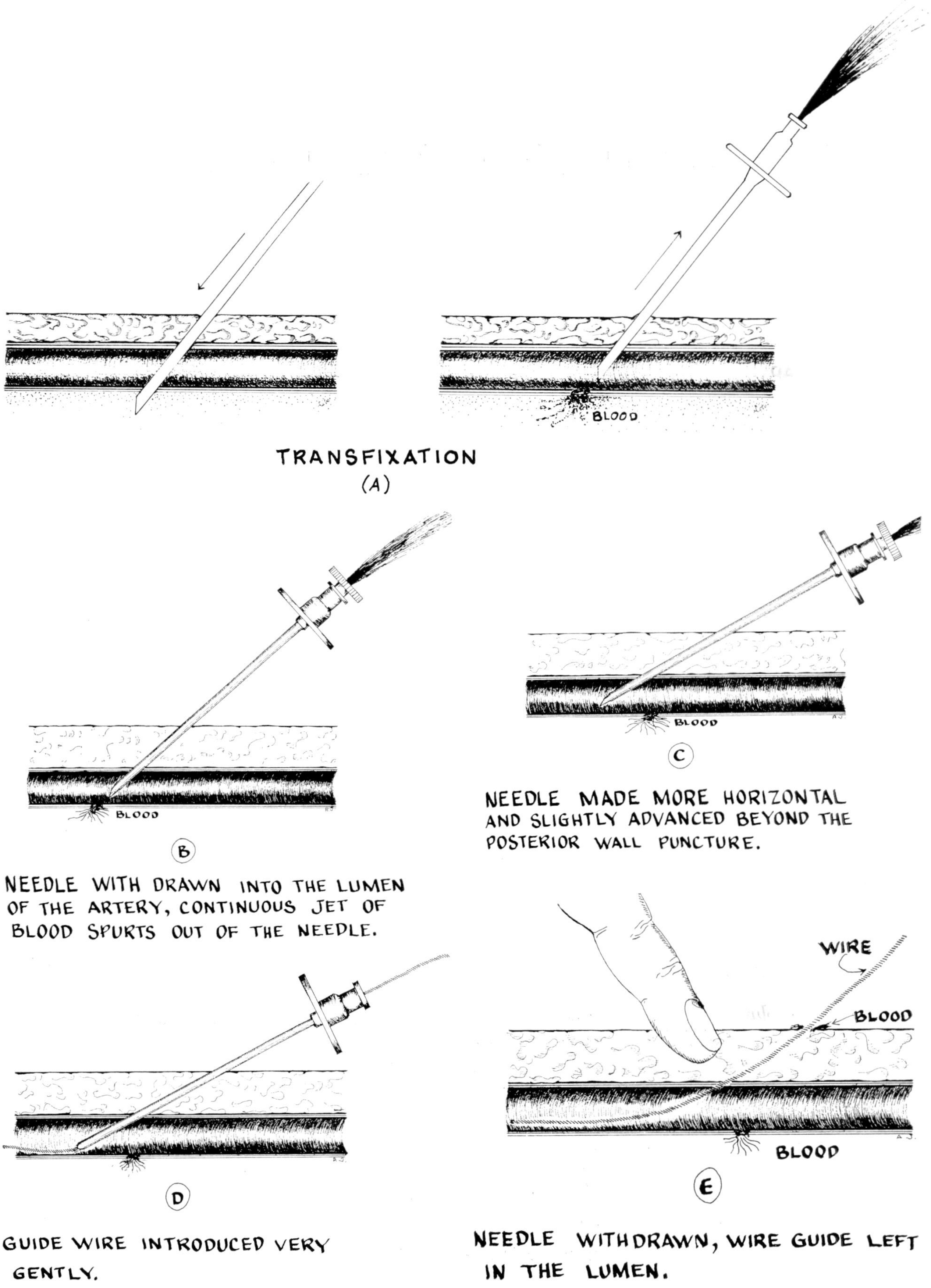

Figure 15.1 Standard Seldinger Technique.

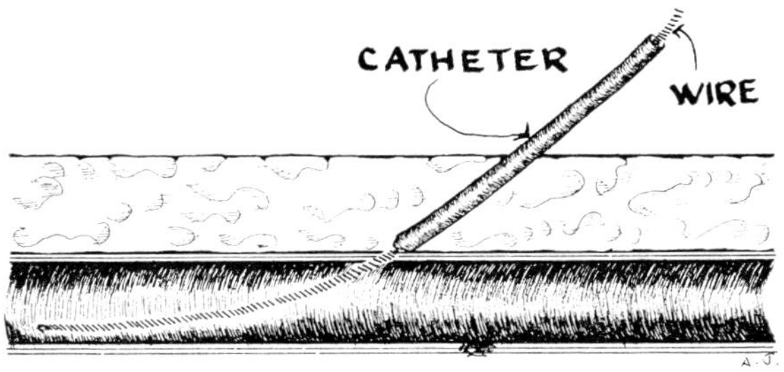

(F)

CATHETER ADVANCED ON THE WIRE.

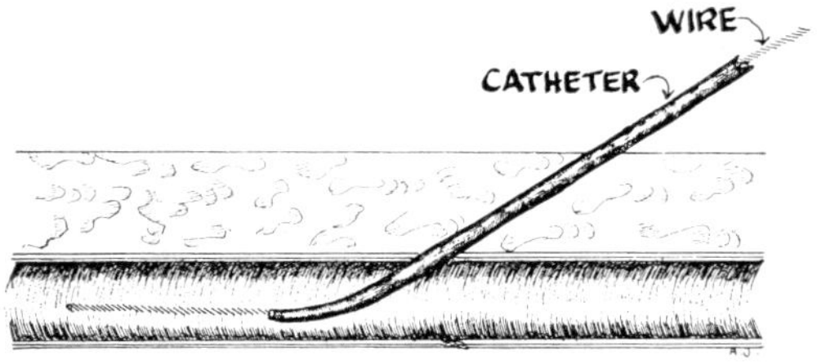

(G)

WITH GENTLE STABBING MOTION, CATHETER PERFORATES THE ANTERIOR WALL OF THE ARTERY AND FURTHER ADVANCEMENT OF THE CATHETER IS MADE.

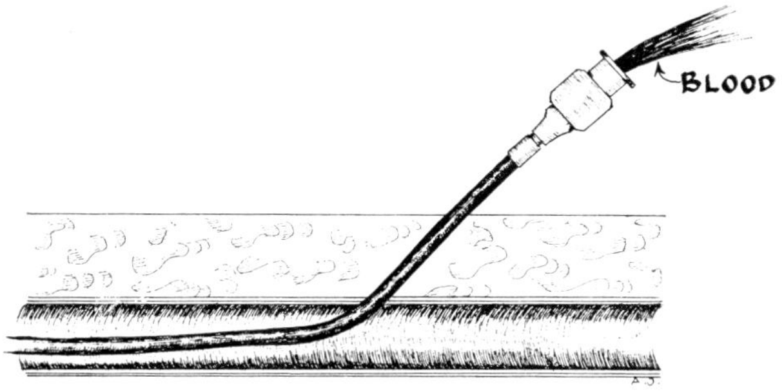

(H)

CATHETER IS ADVANCED ON THE WIRE, AND THEN THE WIRE IS REMOVED.

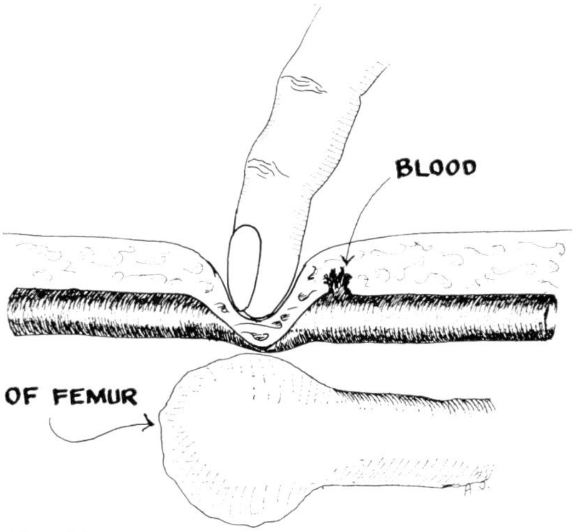

COMPRESSION OF THE ARTERY AFTER REMOVAL OF THE CATHETER.

(I)

Figure 15.1 *(Continued)*. Standard Seldinger Technique.

so that the tip of the wire will not damage the orifice of aortic arch vessels. As soon as the tip of the catheter reaches the desired level, the guide wire is immediately withdrawn and the *catheter is aspirated to check for good return of blood and then immediately irrigated with the flushing solution of normal saline and heparin.*

In order to keep a column of saline and not blood in the catheter lumen, *the locking and unlocking of the stopcock should be done while the flushing solution is being injected.*

If the study is a flush aortogram, a *test injection of contrast* is made to locate the exact position of the tip of the catheter and to insure that it is not impacted in the wall of the aorta. If a selective study is being performed, the tip of the catheter is withdrawn, pointing toward the direction of the orifice; and after the catheter enters the orifice, a test injection of contrast is made under fluoroscopic control to localize definitively the vessel being catheterized.

If it is necessary to change a catheter, the guide wire is reinserted so that approximately 40 to 50 cm extends beyond the tip of the catheter, the catheter is withdrawn, and the same maneuver described above is gone through (Fig. 15-2).

Exchange of a clotted catheter, or a catheter with only side holes and a blunt end, is done with the help of Desilet Hoffman sheath (Fig. 15-3).

Important Precautions after Catheterization

1. The catheter should be flushed every fifteen to twenty seconds with 1 to 2 cc of the flushing solution.
2. The arterial pulse immediately distal to the puncture site should be checked every ten to fifteen minutes.

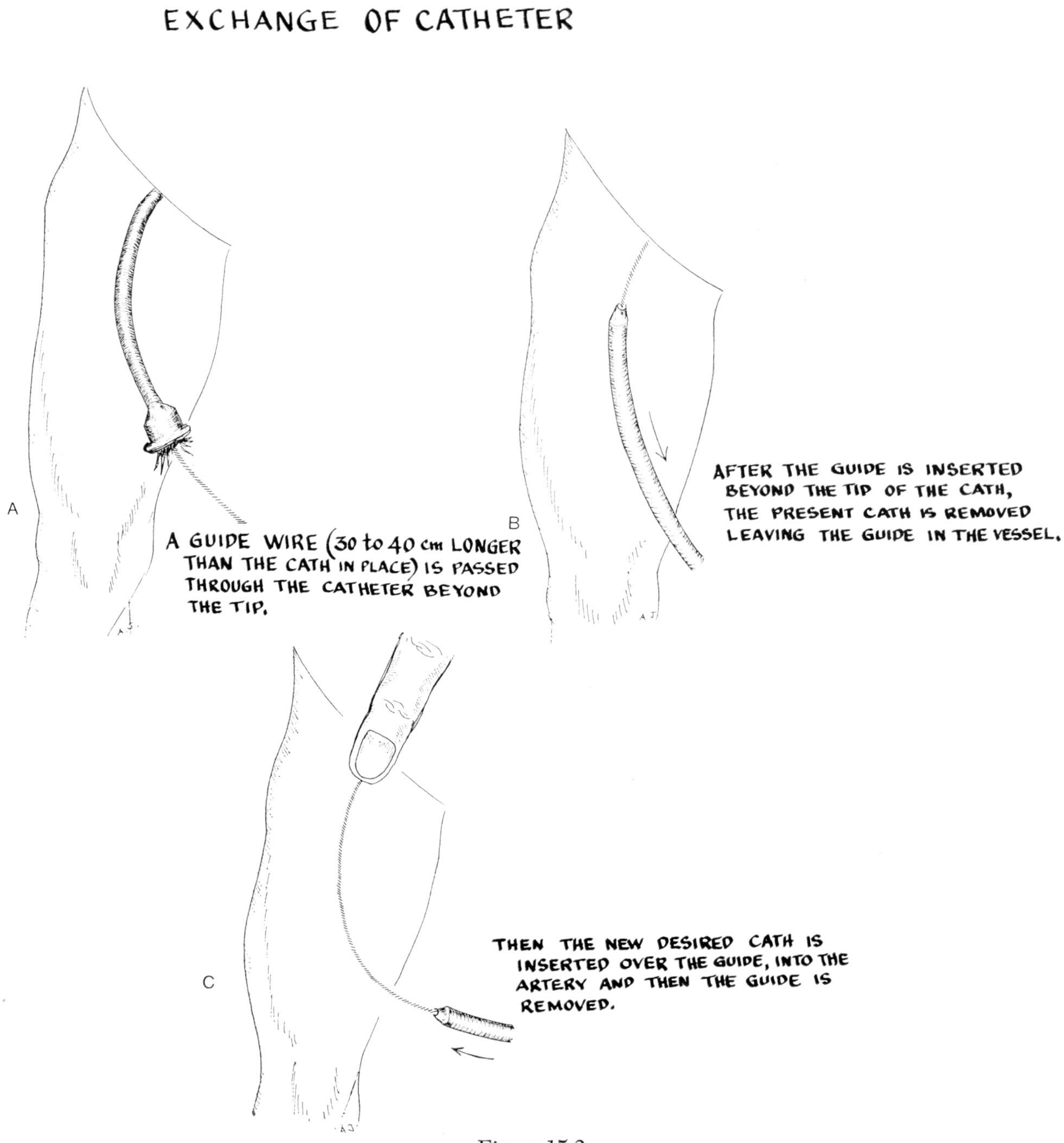

Figure 15.2

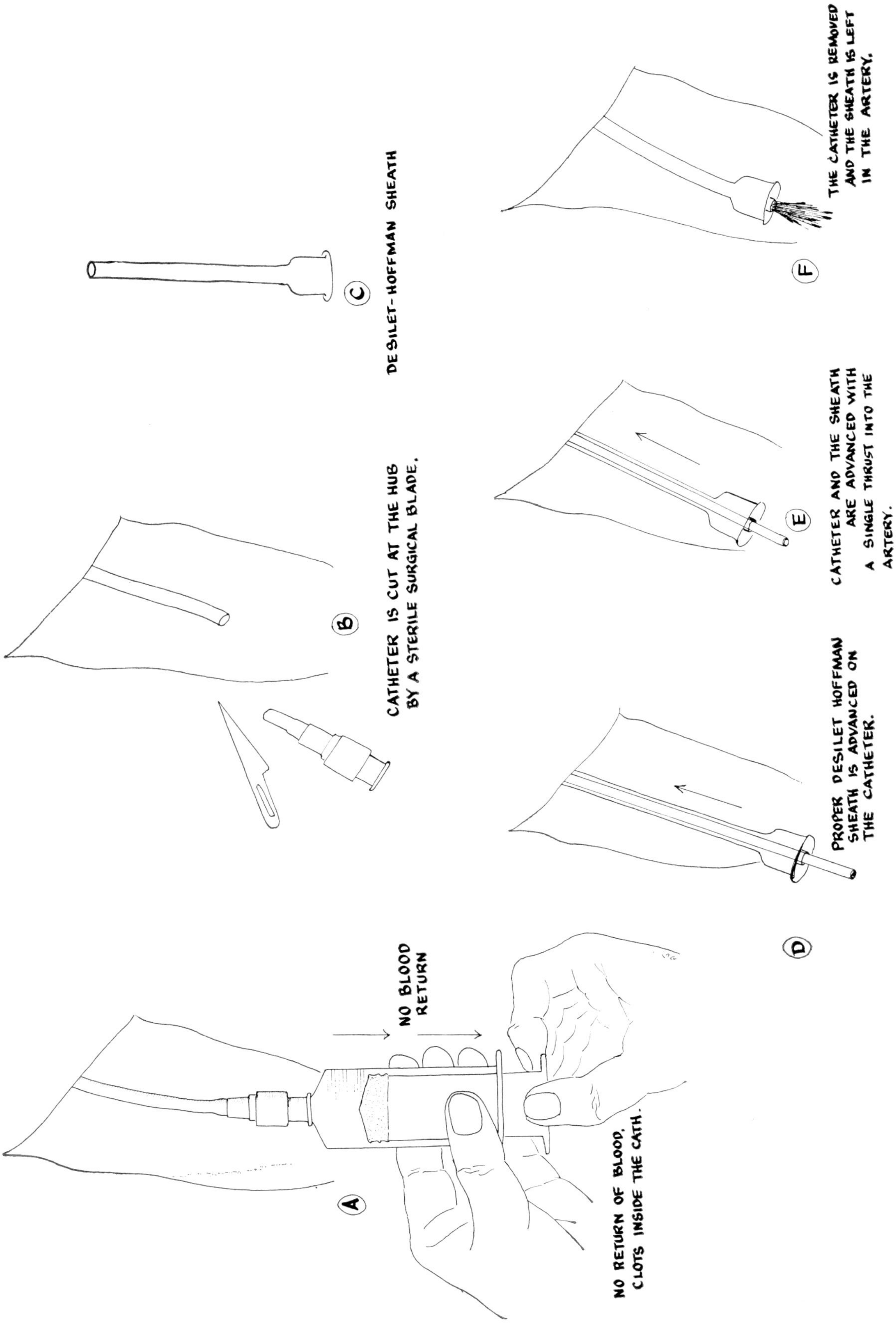

Figure 15.3. Exchange of a clotted catheter with the help of a Desilet-Hoffman sheath.

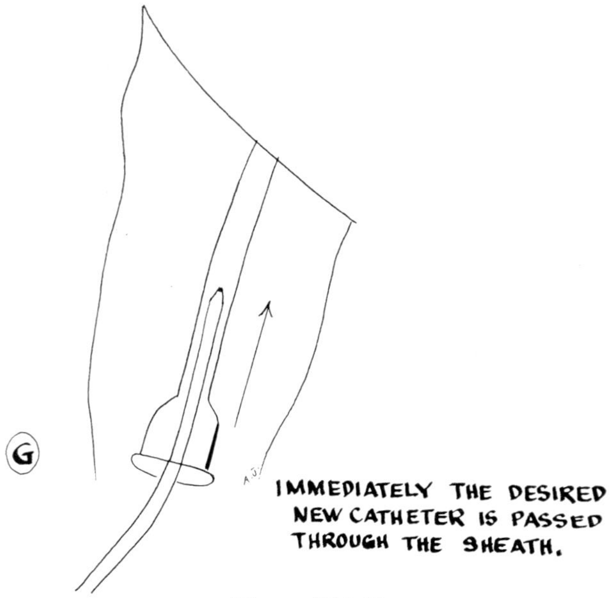

Figure 15.3 G

3. Diluted contrast should be loaded into its syringe, ready for test injection before catheterization of any branch.
4. Excessive manipulation of the catheter near atherosclerotic plaques should be avoided.
5. Catheterization of the great vessels of the arch of the aorta is contraindicated if there is evidence of atheromatous plaques near the orifices.
6. Accidental entry into an undesired vessel requires immediate withdrawal of the catheter from that orifice.
7. Test injections to localize the exact position of the catheter tip should involve only 1 to 2 cc of the diluted contrast. This will determine the caliber, washout time, and delicate nature of the vessel. This will also determine the appropriate amount of contrast to be used for the definitive study (Fig. 15-4).
8. If the vessel catheterized is of a smaller caliber than the catheter being used, it is exchanged for one with a narrower tip, and the study is completed without undue delay. The catheter should be withdrawn into the parent vessel after the films are exposed. In such a situation, continuous perfusion of that vessel with saline may reduce the chance of local ischemia.
9. If the vessel is too small to be catheterized, then a flush study is done, leaving the tip of the catheter at the level of the origin of that branch.
10. Every advancement of the catheter should be immediately followed by a small test injection, monitored fluoroscopically, to determine the position of the catheter tip. This is especially important during selective catheterization.
11. If the anatomy of a vessel is unclear, or if there are variations in the vessel arrangement, a pilot injection of contrast is made, exposing a few films. The amount of contrast used for the test injection and the magnitude of the force exerted during injection depends on the caliber of the vessel and its delicate nature. Thus the amount and force of injection varies markedly from the celiac axis compared to the adrenal vein.
12. The patient's complaints or undue somatic responses should be immediately investigated, as they may be the initial vital clues of an impending complication.
13. The stability of the catheter in the branch vessel should be checked by a forceful hand injection of normal saline before the final injector-made injection. Again, the amount of contrast used and the force exerted correspond to the caliber and delicate nature of the vessel.
14. Prior to the injection of the final bolus of contrast, a "selective bath" with normal saline to that segment of the vasculature will facilitate the receipt of the hypertonic contrast material. The amount of saline used for the "selective bath" is at least two to three times that of the amount of contrast being used for injection.
15. Connections between the catheter and the injector are well secured to avoid air and contrast leaks during injection.

16. Immediately following the exposure of the last film of the series, another selective bath with saline is given to that regional vasculature, and then the catheter tip is withdrawn from that branch orifice if it happens to be extremely small, or a vital one.
17. While the films are being developed or the decision being made concerning the next study, intermittent irrigation with 1 to 2 cc of saline is carried out every forty-five to sixty seconds. The alternative is to use a continuous perfusion arrangement during this time interval.

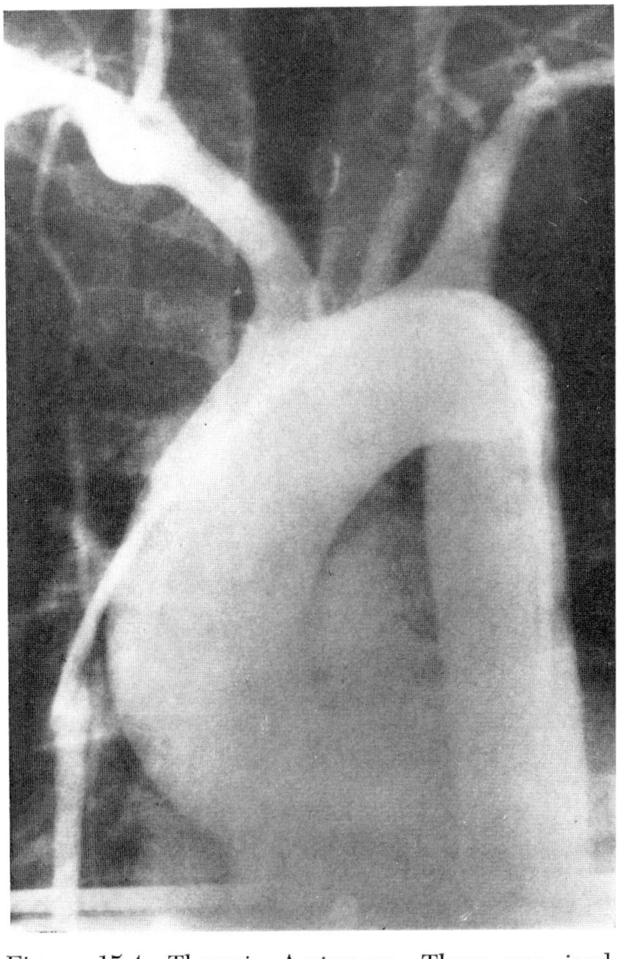

Figure 15.4. Thoracic Aortogram. There was inadvertant injection of contrast into the coronary artery bypass. The patient developed ventricular fibrillation with eventual recovery. Position of the catheter tip should always be checked with contrast under fluoroscopy, to avoid spasm of the radiologist's coronary arteries!

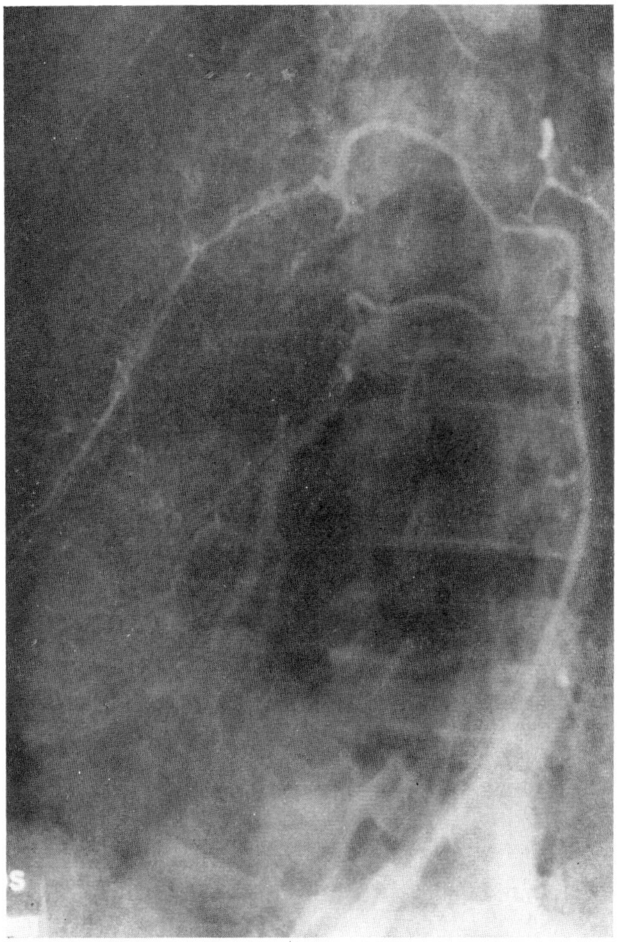

Figure 15.5. Flush Aortogram. There is accidental excessive perfusion of the lumbar artery. Originally this study was intended to be a flush aortogram, but this curved catheter whipped and became engaged to the lumbar artery. Fortunately, this patient did not develop any neurological complications.

18. A curved catheter should not be used for injections into a straight vessel (the descending aorta), nor should a straight catheter be used for injection into a curved vessel (the arch of the aorta) (Figs. 15-5, 3-11).
19. After a study using catheters with a looped configuration or deep curves is over, the catheter should be withdrawn under fluoroscopic control to avoid knot formation. An even better idea is to straighten the catheter with a guide wire prior to withdrawal to decrease further the possibility of knot formation, especially at the infrarenal aortic level.

CHAPTER 16
THE WHYS AND THE HOWS

PROBLEMS, PREVENTIVE MEASURES AND SOME SOLUTIONS

In most instances, a satisfactory study is obtained without undue technical problems or complications during the procedure. Unfortunately, this is not always the situation. Patients of different ages, with different body habitus and associated variations in the vascular arrangement, aging processes, and distortion of the normal anatomy by pathological processes pose problems during different steps of the catheterization procedure. Therefore, it is the angiographer's duty to be aware of these "whys" and to know some of the "hows" to prevent or to correct problems as they develop, or to terminate the procedure if problems exceed angiographic limitations.

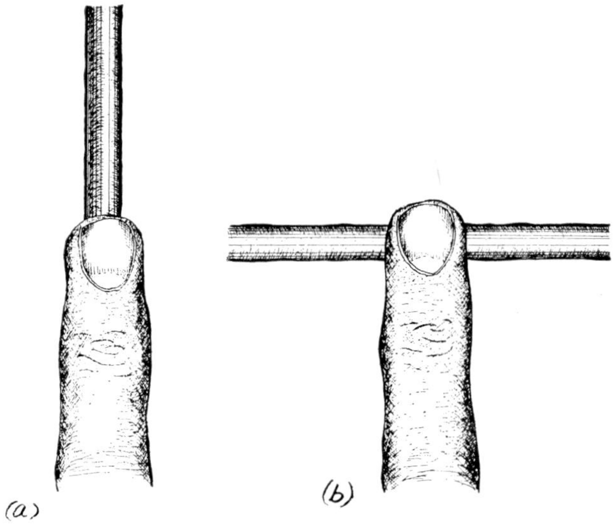

Figure 16.1. Palpation of the Puncturing Artery. (A) Along the longitudinal axis, (B) Along the transverse axis.

Unsuccessful Puncture of the Vessel

The Wrong Puncture Site

To determine the exact location of the artery before a skin bleb is raised with the local anesthetic, the *expansile direct pulsation* of the artery is felt by compressing the artery against the underlying bone. This is perhaps the key step in the puncture of the artery. Without it, repeated attempts elsewhere will result in frustrations and loss of self-confidence. This is extremely important in the small caliber vessels of pediatric age patients.

Improper Fixation of the Vessel

This is probably the most common cause of failure to puncture a normal artery facing the beginner. Both normal and obese individuals have sufficient surrounding tissue to support the vessel, thereby not allowing it to escape the puncturing tip of the needle. With these patients efficient digital pressure deep down to the bone along either side of the artery is essential to stabilize the artery (Fig. 16-2). On the other hand, in thin people and those with sclerotic arteries, the vessel has a tendency to escape the puncture by rolling from one side to another despite moderate fixation. This is akin to attempting to stab an apple in a bucket of water. Therefore, in these individuals the vessel is efficiently immobilized by stretching and applying pressure along the long axis of the artery (Fig. 16-2).

Needle Aimed in the Wrong Direction

The end result is accidental puncture of the adjacent vein medially or injury to the nerve bundles laterally. While aiming the needle, the *longitudinal axis of the needle* should correspond to the *longitudinal axis of the vessel.*

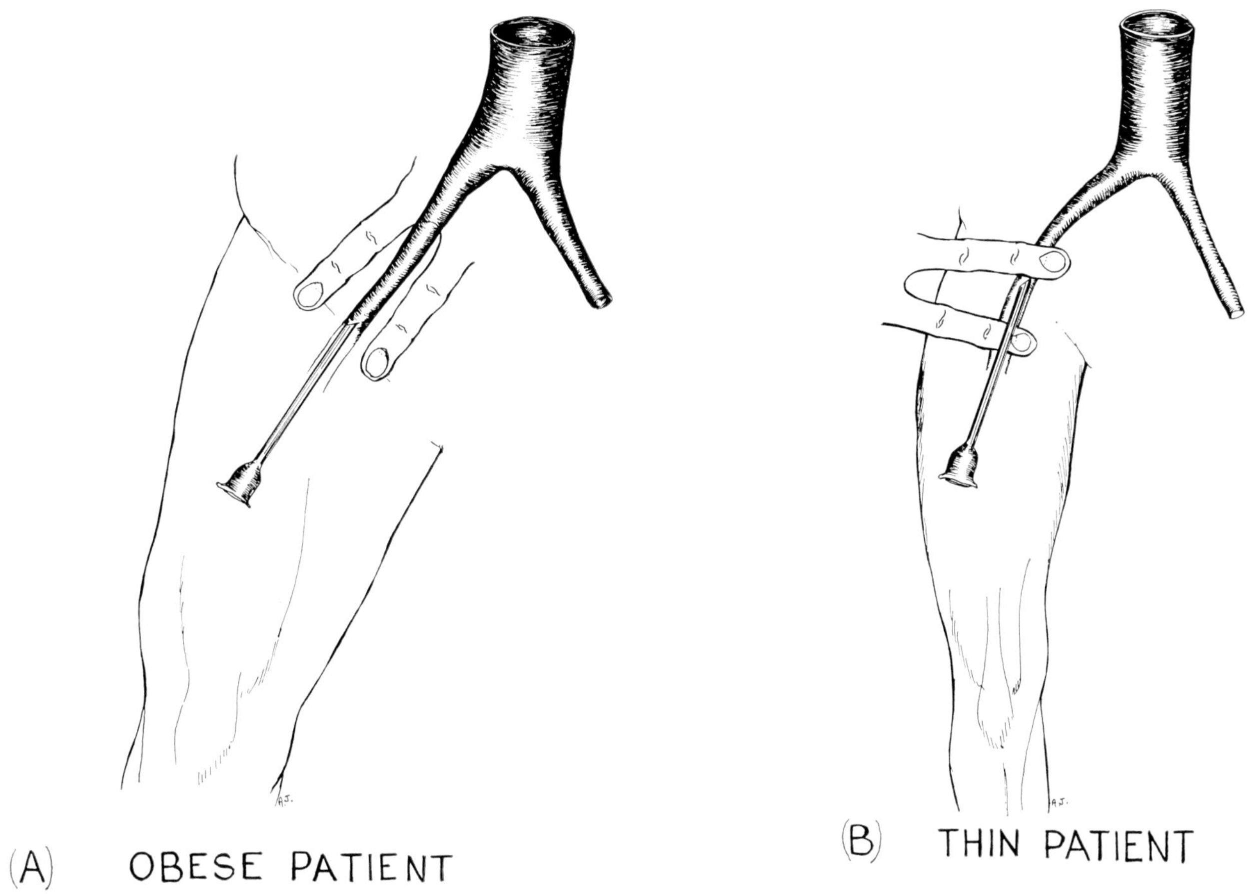

Figure 16.2. Fixing the femoral artery.

This is especially true in arteries of small diameter.

Improper Angle of Puncture

Even with proper arterial immobilization and accurate needle direction, the vessel may not be reached by the needle tip if the angle of puncture is less than optimal. The needle then slides superficial to the vessel wall rather than entering it. If the angle is greater than an optimal one, the artery then rolls away and escapes being punctured (Figs. 16-3 and 16-4).

Arterial Spasm

Every effort should be made to fix the artery properly in younger individuals and to puncture it during the first attempt. If not, every successive attempt initiates more arterial spasm, and even if the puncture is successful, post-catheterization complications such as spasm, stasis and thrombosis are more likely.

Stenotic or Occluded Arteries with Diffuse Pulsation Due to Collaterals

If there is a *thrill* felt or a *bruit* heard, especially with low amplitude diffuse pulsation, one

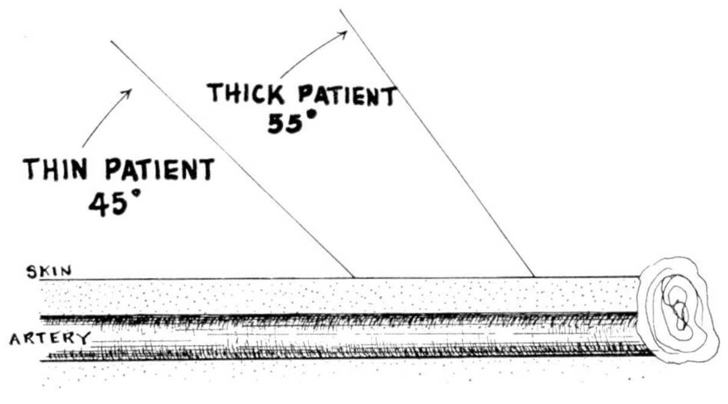

Figure 16.3. Angles of puncture.

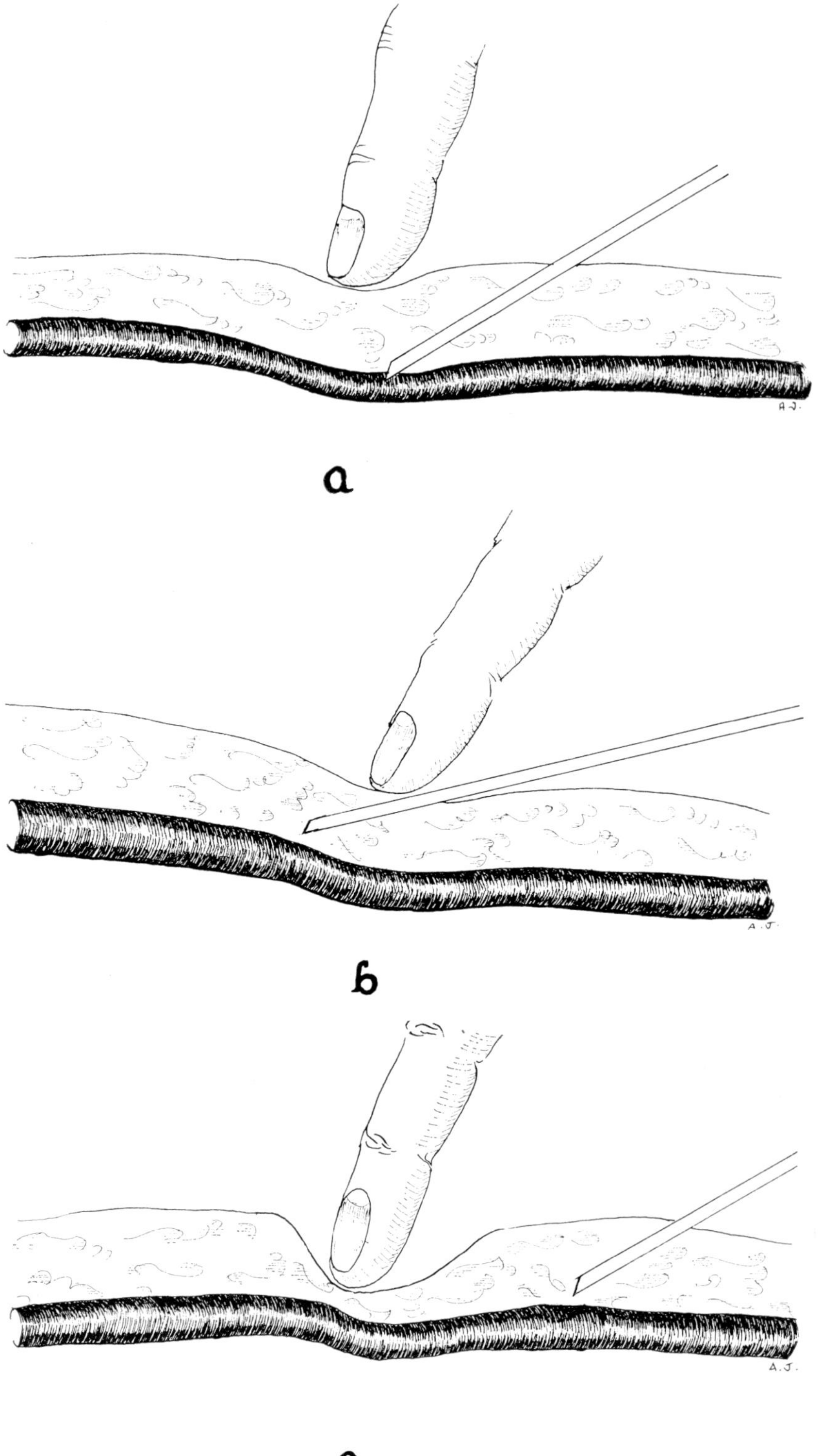

Figure 16.4. Puncturing the vessel at the proper level of fixation. (A) Proper, (B and C) improper. May result in unsuccessful punctures.

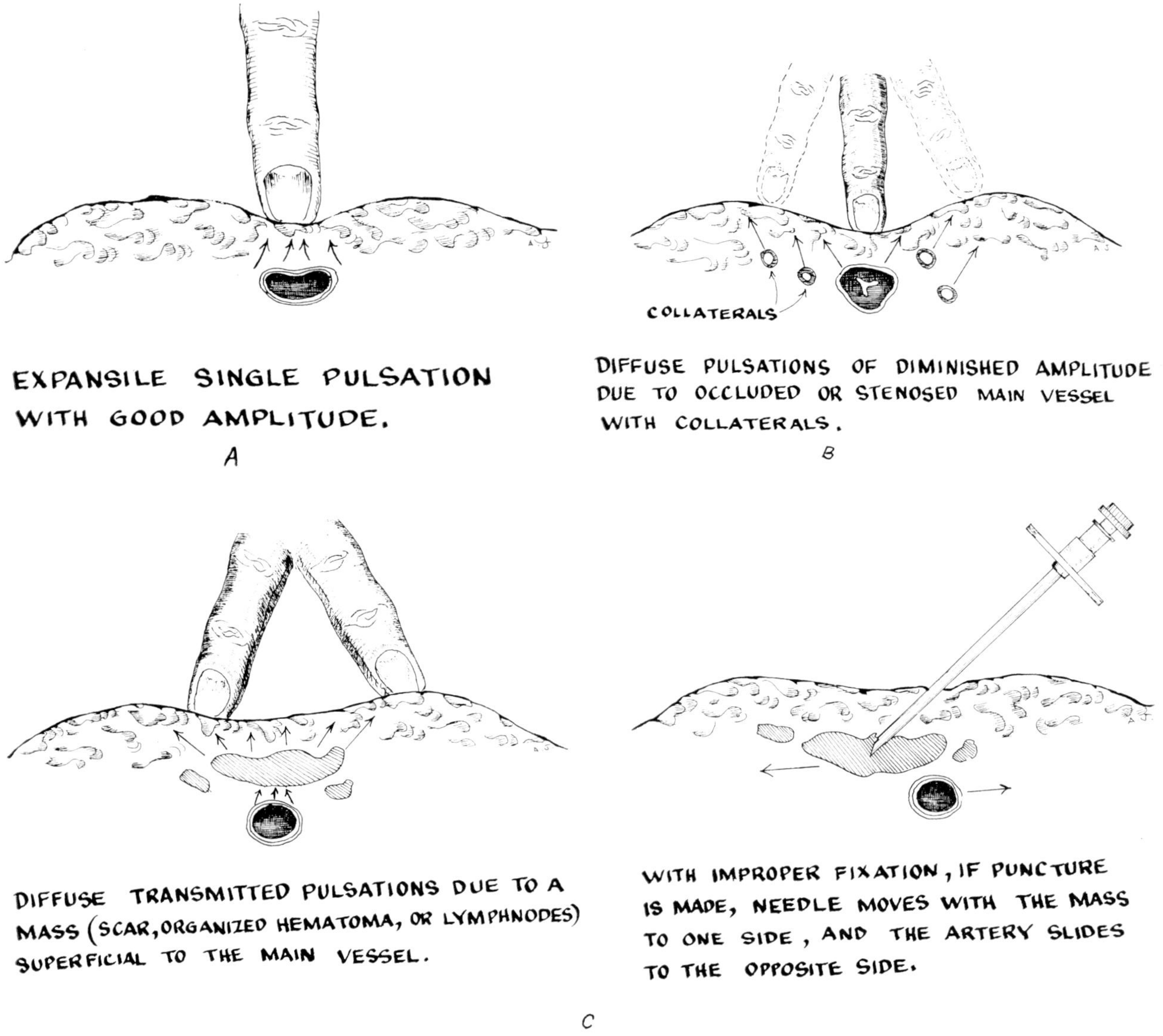

Figure 16.5. (B & C) May result in unsuccessful punctures.

should cleverly avoid that puncture site by choosing another (Fig. 16-5).

Scar Tissue or Masses Superficial to the Vessel

These lesions not only deceive the examiner by diffusely transmitting the arterial pulsations, but they also carry the needle tip to one side while the vessel slides to another (Fig. 16-5). The presence of masses at the puncture site is a contraindication to using that site; scar tissue is not. The difficulty due to scar tissue can be overcome by using a Teflon sleeve needle and locking the artery and scar mass together between the two fingers, pressing deep to the bone.

We learned it the hard way: no artery . . . no study.

Successful Puncture, but the Blood Return Is Either Intermittent or Trickling

It is presumed that in this case the patient is not in shock, nor has a sizeable intraabdominal mass compressing the vessels. In these indi-

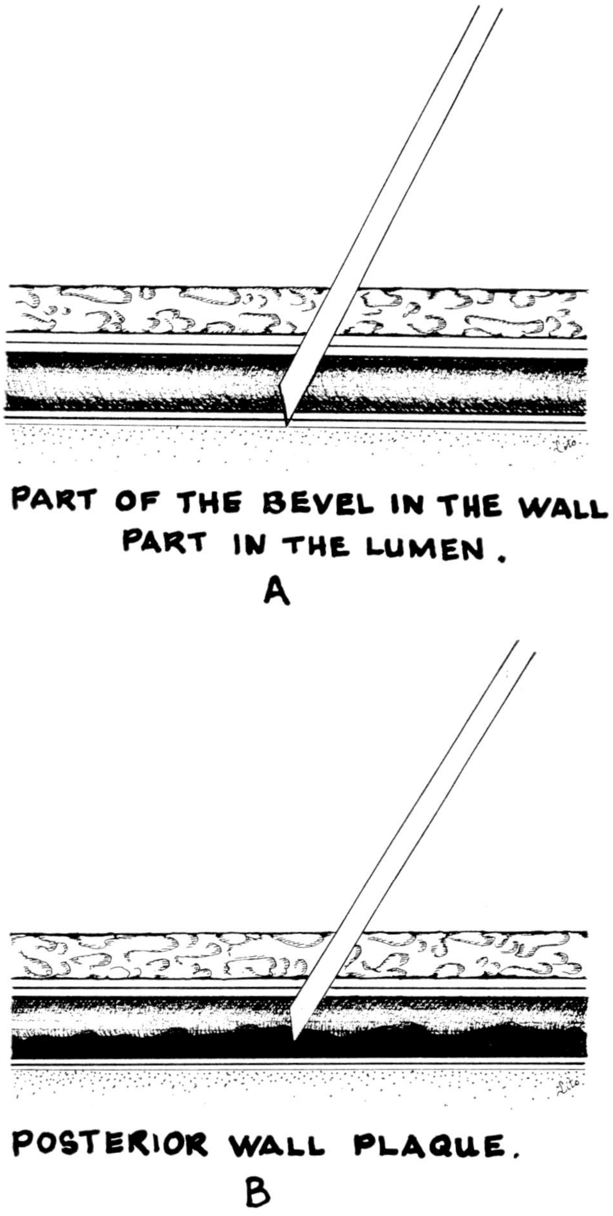

Figure 16.6

viduals a forceful, continuous jet of blood may not be obtained in spite of the needle being completely within the lumen of the artery.

Needle Bevel in the Wall

This problem is unlikely if, after transfixation of the artery, one removes all the parts of the Seldinger needle except the cannula. The problem can also be prevented by using a needle with a Teflon sleeve (Fig. 16-6).

The Needle in a Branch or Collateral Vessel

It is undesirable to damage a potential collateral vessel which may be needed for the existence of the extremity either at the present or in the future. This usually occurs when the *puncture site is lower* than the acceptable position, especially femoral artery puncture. Thus the *midinguinal point should be determined by the anatomic bony landmarks,* not by using the groin crease as the reference point.

Good Return of Blood, but the Guide Wire Cannot Enter the Lumen

A Long Beveled Needle

When a needle with a long bevel is used to puncture the artery, part of the bevel may stay in the wall and part may be in the lumen of the artery. If the angiographer then attempts to pass a guide wire, it will enter *subintimally* rather than enter the lumen. This can be avoided by using a needle with a short bevel, a cannula, or a Teflon sleeve needle (Fig. 16-6).

Perpendicular Angulation of the Needle

The needle in this case is directing the tip of the guide wire toward the posterior wall hole of the vessel, thereby preventing guide from sliding on the intimal surface. This can be prevented by proper initial angulation or, upon witnessing the return of blood, by slanting the cannula horizontally and introducing it slightly farther into the vessel.

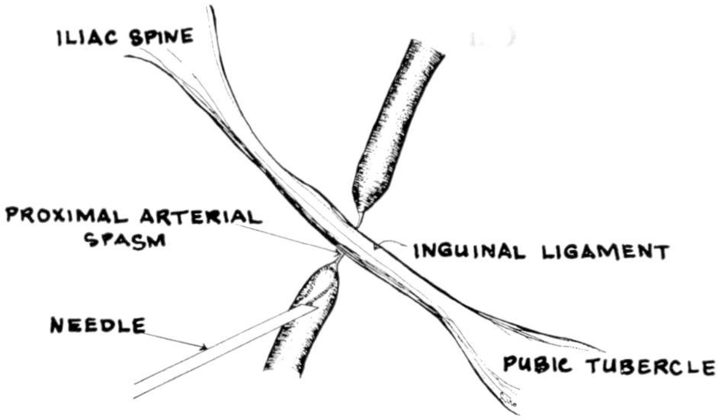

Figure 16.7. Spasm of the vessel proximal to the puncture site offering resistance for the introduction of the guide wire.

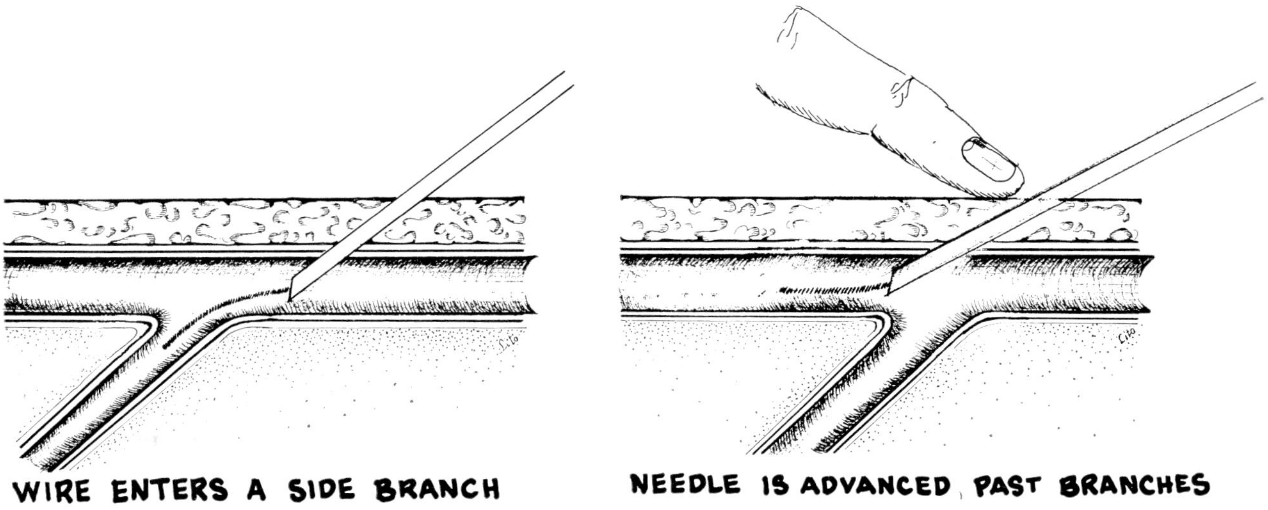

Figure 16.8

Narrowing of the Immediate Proximal Segment

If this is suspected, it can be demonstrated by injecting a small dose of contrast and exposing a film or two. If the stenosis is severe, another puncture site should be selected (Fig. 16-7).

Tip of the Guide Wire Met by Plaques. Bifurcation or the Arterial Wall

The cannula is oriented to one side and the wire is advanced gently. If the wire does not bounce off the arterial wall, then a very *small "J" wire* is used to bypass this point (Figs. 3-4 to 3-9). In fact, in older patients a "J" wire is routinely used to avoid inserting the tip of the guide wire under a plaque.

The Guide Wire Is Introduced to a Certain Level but Cannot Be Negotiated Further

Accidental Entry into a Side Branch

This happens either during femoral artery puncture with the guide wire entering the deep circumflex iliac branch, or during axillary arterial puncture with the guide wire entering the scapular branches or the vertebral artery (Figs. 16-8 and 16-9). This situation can be avoided by using *a "J" wire* having a width wider than the diameter of the orifice of the branch artery to be bypassed.

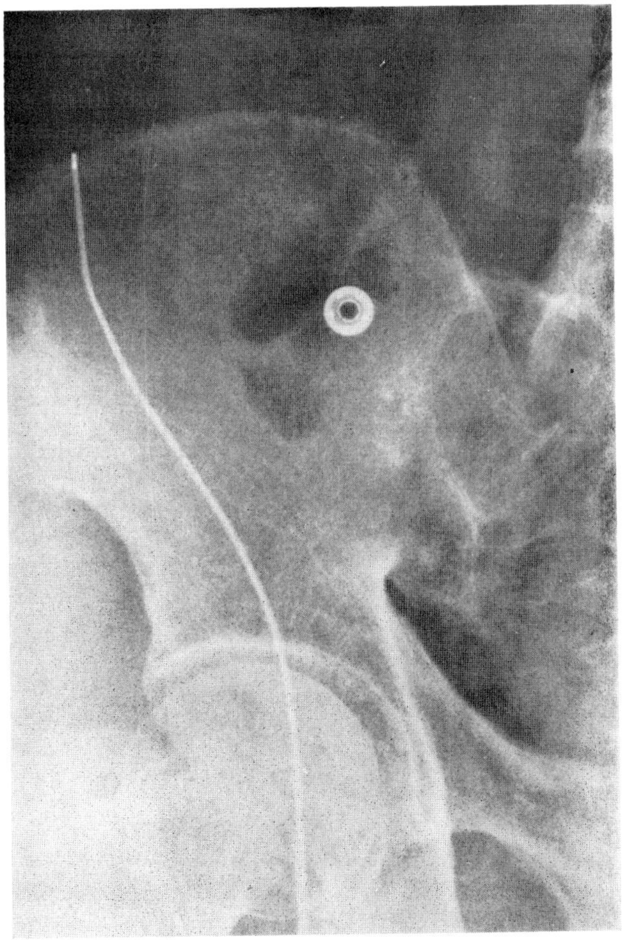

Figure 16.9. Femoral Artery Puncture. The course of the guide wire was noticed at the same time the patient began to complain of a catching pain in this area. *Comment:* The guide wire was unintentionally passed into the superficial circumflex iliac artery.

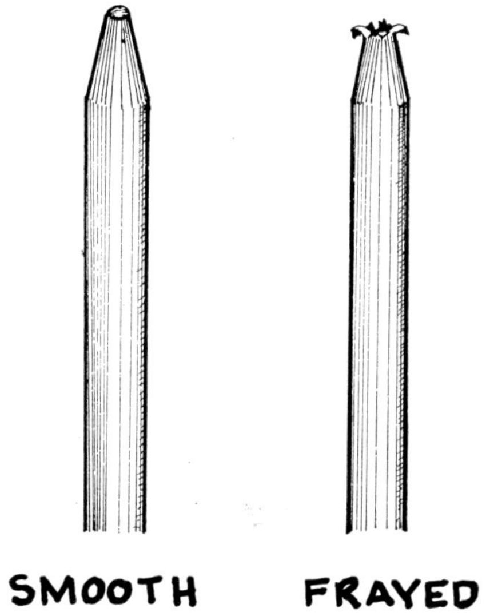

Figure 16.10

Kinks, Tortuosities and Plaques

Invariably these obstacles can be bypassed with the assistance of a suitable "J" wire, or a long, floppy guide wire. Occasional failures require selection of another puncture site or another route of entry, depending on the importance of the study.

The Wire Is in the Vessel, but the Catheter Cannot be Inserted Through the Vessel Wall

Tip of the Catheter Frayed

It is very difficult to insert a catheter with a frayed tip through the wall even after a dilator has been used. Repeated attempts to insert a damaged catheter will result in injury to the wall of the vessel. Even if it does enter, the ragged tip will lacerate the intima. For smooth entry either the tip must be amputated and retapered, or the catheter replaced with a new one (Fig. 16-10).

Mismatching Guide Wire

An ill-fitting guide wire results in the formation of kinks at the juncture of the catheter tip and the vessel wall. This is most frequent in obese individuals. In individuals with scar tissue, the catheter curls superficial to the scar. This can be prevented by using an appropriate guide wire which fits the tip of the catheter snugly.

Obese Patients

Subcutaneous *kinking* of the guide wire and curling of the catheter occurs frequently in obese individuals. This is particularly true if the *catheter is soft,* if the *tip is frayed,* or if the *guide wire does not fit the catheter* well. Occasionally, even with proper materials, the catheter may not enter the vessel. Then a Desilet Hoffman sheath and its accessories may be used to make a tunnel in the soft tissues (Fig. 16-11).

Scars Superficial to the Vessel

The same methods as described for obese individuals can be used (Fig. 16-12).

The Wire Meets Resistance Internally While Inserting the Catheter

A very important concept to remember, is that

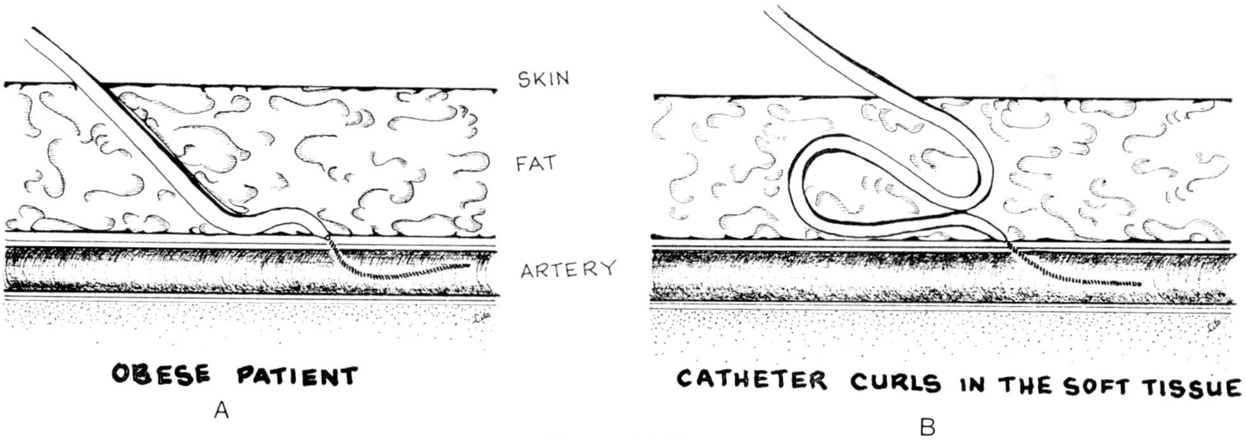

Figure 16.11

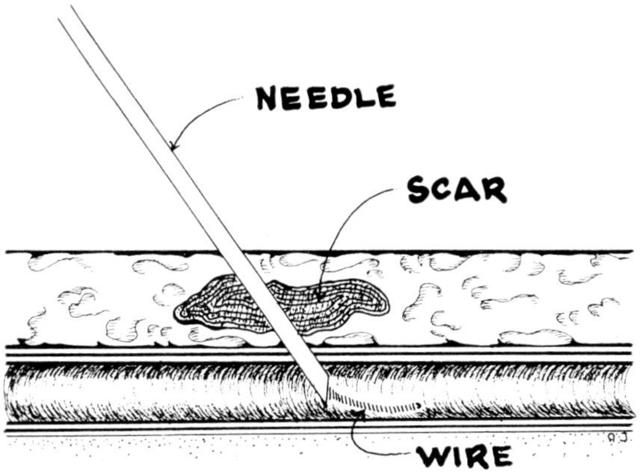

A

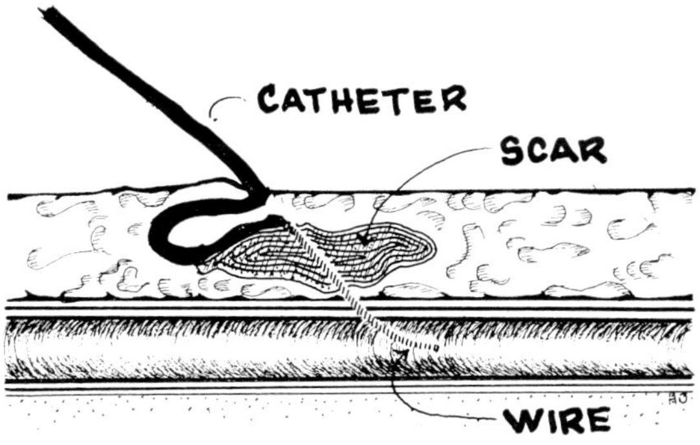

B

Figure 16.12

the catheter and the guide wire move together as a single unit during catheter insertion. The catheter does not just slide over the guide wire by itself. During catheter insertion, if the tip of the guide wire encounters a point of resistance inside the vessel, catheter entry may be prevented. This can be avoided by withdrawing the guide wire a short distance away from the focus of resistance to facilitate the smooth entry of the catheter into the lumen. This prevents the exiting of the guide wire through the arterial wall (Fig. 16-13).

Catheter Is Advanced Over a Kink

A catheter cannot be advanced over a kink in the guide wire or over the floppy segment.

Right Angled Puncture

Refer to the preceding discussion on kinks (Fig. 16-14).

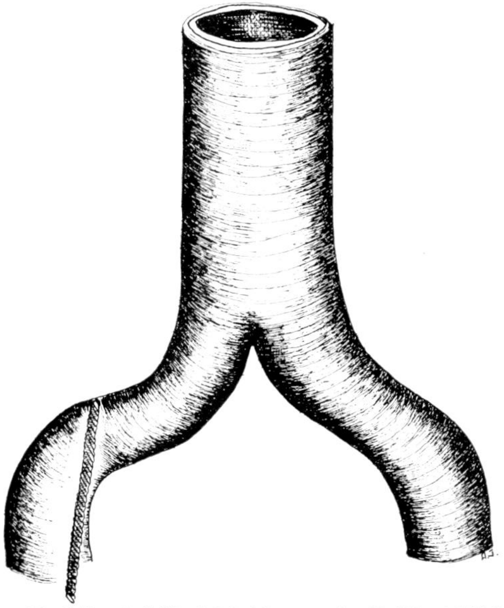

A

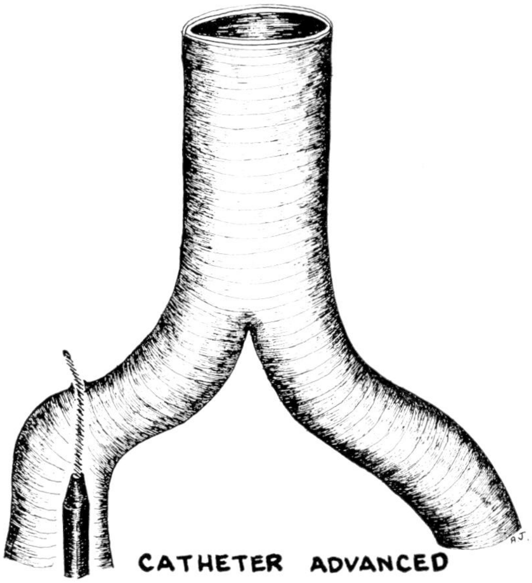

B

Figure 16.13

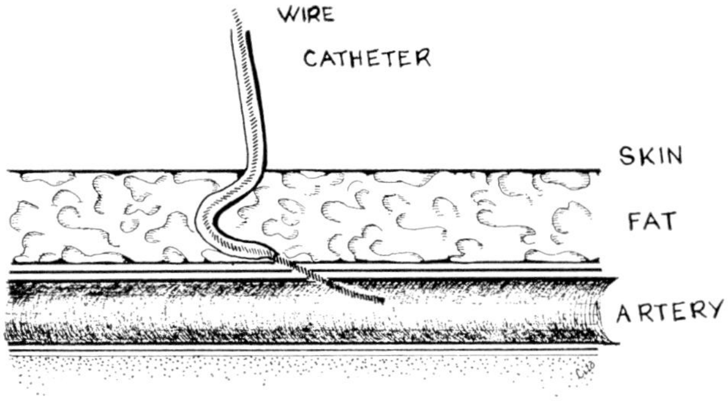

Figure 16.14

The Catheter Is in the Vessel Up to a Certain Level, but Cannot Be Rotated

Poor Catheter Torque

The torque of a catheter can be improved by using a comparatively more rigid catheter material which will still retain the given shape of the catheter. This is easily achieved by using catheters with metallic braid in the shaft.[37]

Tortuosity of the Conduit Vessel

If a catheter with good torque also fails despite repeated meticulous attempts, then a flush aortogram is done. The quality of the films and the available information should suffice (Figs. 16-15 to 16-18).

Excessive Scar Tissue at the Puncture Site

Occasionally the amount of scar tissue at the puncture site causes such excessive friction on the sides of the catheter that it cannot be successfully manipulated.

The Orifice of a Branch Cannot Be Reached

The Tip Is Not Pointing Toward the Orifice

If the tip is pointing elsewhere, even though it is at the same level as the orifice, it is impossible for the tip to fall into the opening. This frequently happens while searching for the celiac or mesenteric orifices. After a test injection, the immediate realization is that the catheter tip is pointing posteriorly and engaging a lumbar artery will enable one to rotate the catheter 180 degrees and aim the tip anteriorly. If in doubt, the tip is engaged into a renal artery orifice, then a counterclockwise rotation from the left renal, or a clockwise rotation from the right renal, while dislodging it from the renal artery will aim the tip anteriorly.

The Curved Segment of the Catheter Is Not Long Enough

This can be corrected by giving appropriate length to the curved segment as soon as one realizes the problem (Fig. 16-19). If the curved segment is longer than necessary, then buckling of the catheter or frequent dislodgment of plaques occurs (Fig. 16-20).

Atherosclerotic Plaques About the Orifice of a Branch Artery

This will make the tip of the catheter bounce from one plaque to another (Fig. 16-21), preventing the tip from falling into the orifice. Too many attempts will dislodge plaques, causing distal or local embolization. If this problem arises, a flush aortogram is acceptable as a last resort.

Change in the Direction of the Orifice

This happens when a tortuous aorta shifts the anterior orifices laterally and the lateral orifice posterolaterally. Some of the orifices (renal artery) may not always arise from their conventional location. If the aorta or inferior vena cava have been deviated by a sizeable mass, then the orifices of the branches may also change direction (Fig. 11-29) (Fig. 29-23).

Variation in Arrangement

Though the levels of origin of vessels are supposed to be at certain conventional levels, they do not always obey this rule.

Replaced or Aberrant Origins

Variation in the origin of the hepatic arteries, developmental chaotic confusion at the celiaco-mesenteric area, or aberrant renal arteries can confuse the angiographer. Thus an awareness of these variations enables one to search not only along the circumference of the

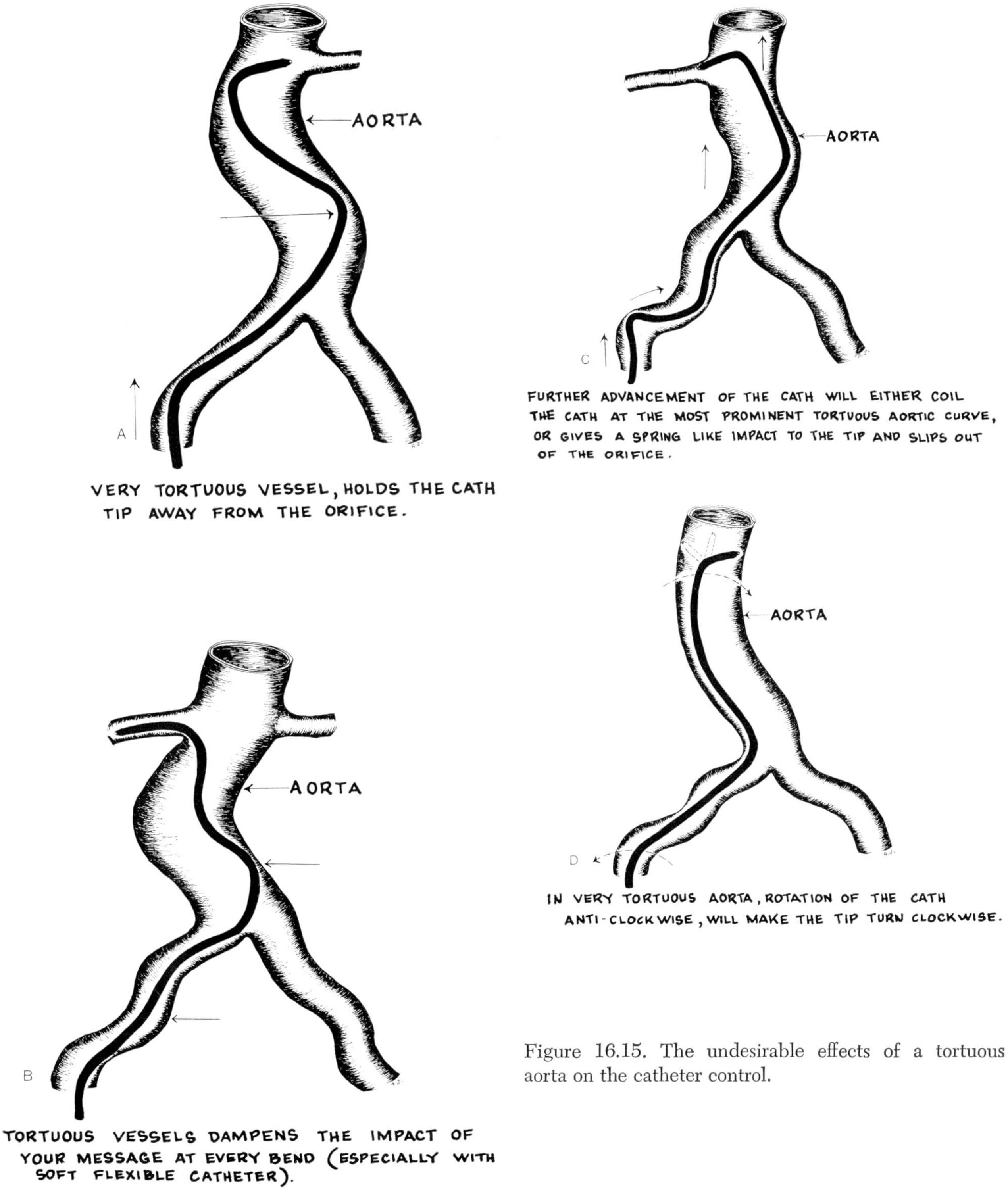

Figure 16.15. The undesirable effects of a tortuous aorta on the catheter control.

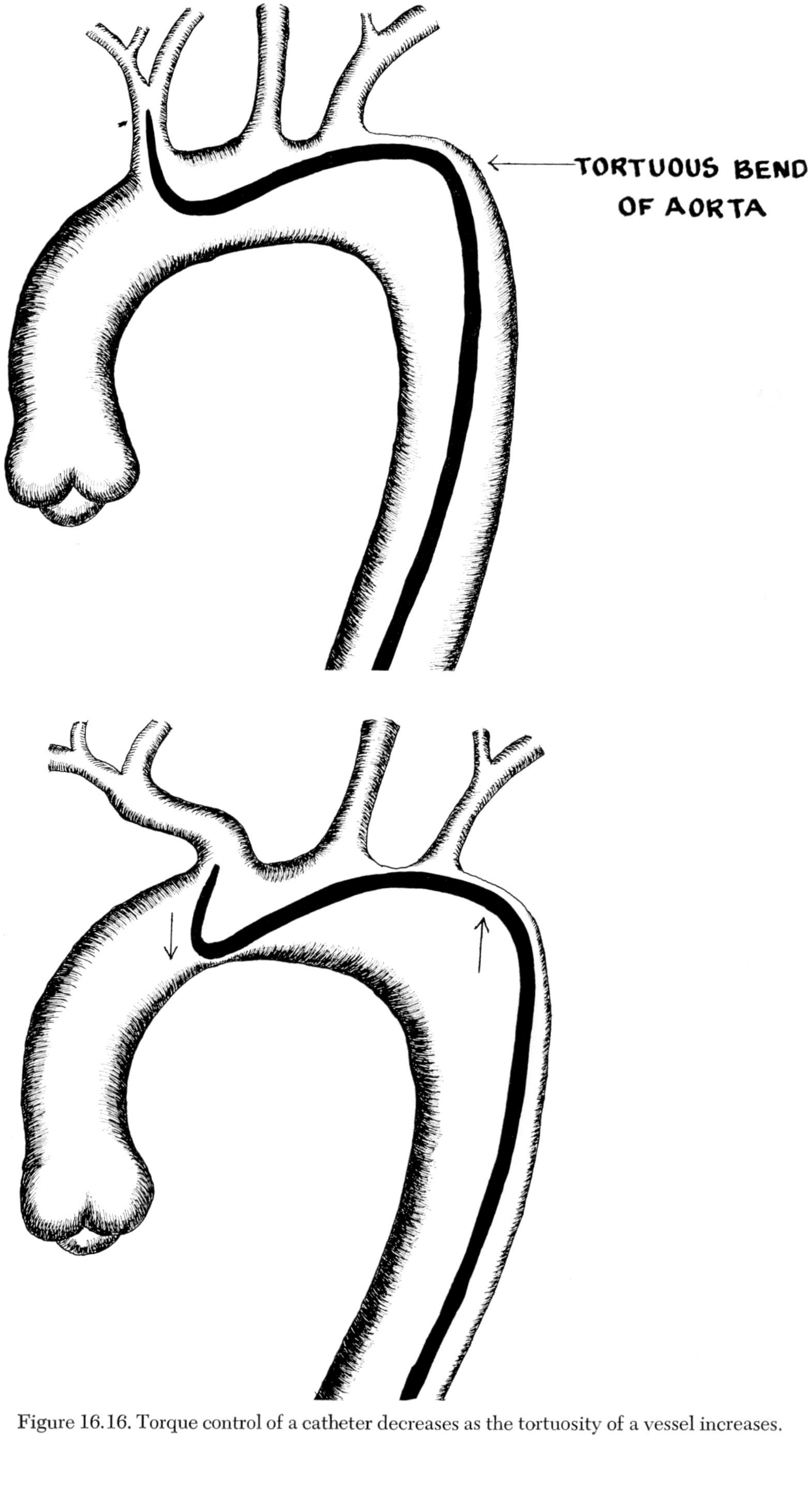

Figure 16.16. Torque control of a catheter decreases as the tortuosity of a vessel increases.

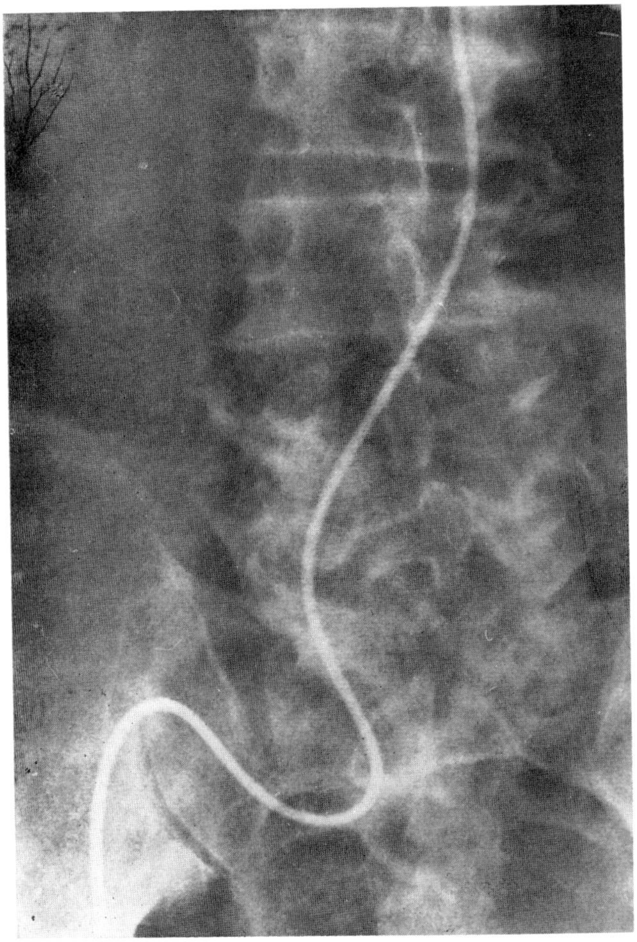

Figure 16.17. There is severe tortuosity of this arterial route. This condition diminishes the ability to conduct the message from the external portion of the catheter to its tip.

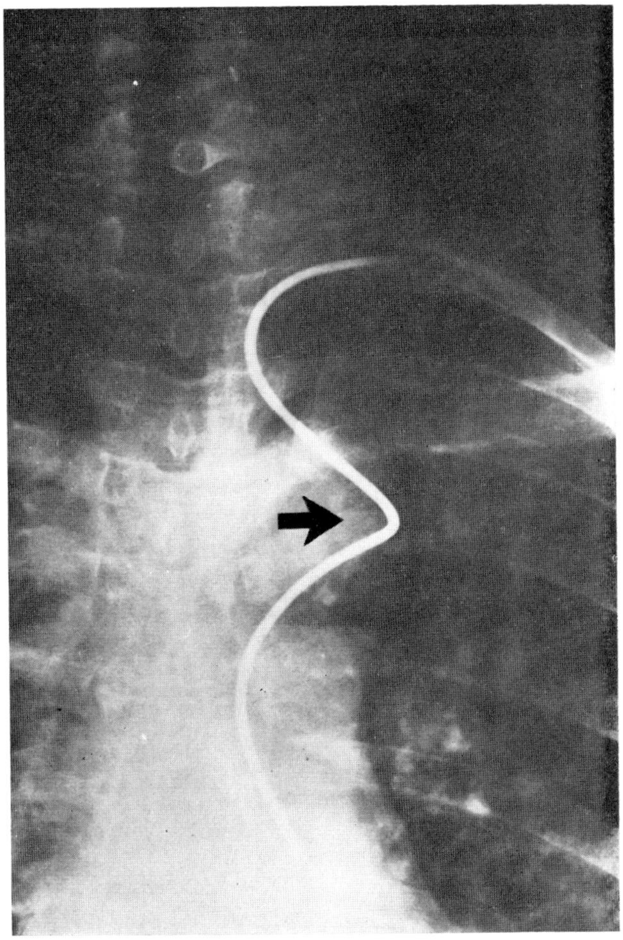

Figure 16.18. The catheter is in the left subclavian artery via the thoracic aorta. Note the tortuosity (Arrow) which hinders manipulation of the catheter.

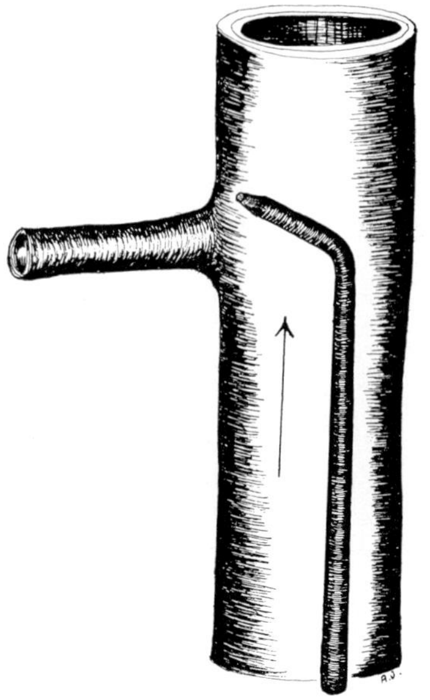

DIAMETER OF AORTA WIDE, OR, DISTAL SHAFT OF THE CATHETER SHORT. TIP CANNOT REACH THE BRANCH ORIFICE.

A

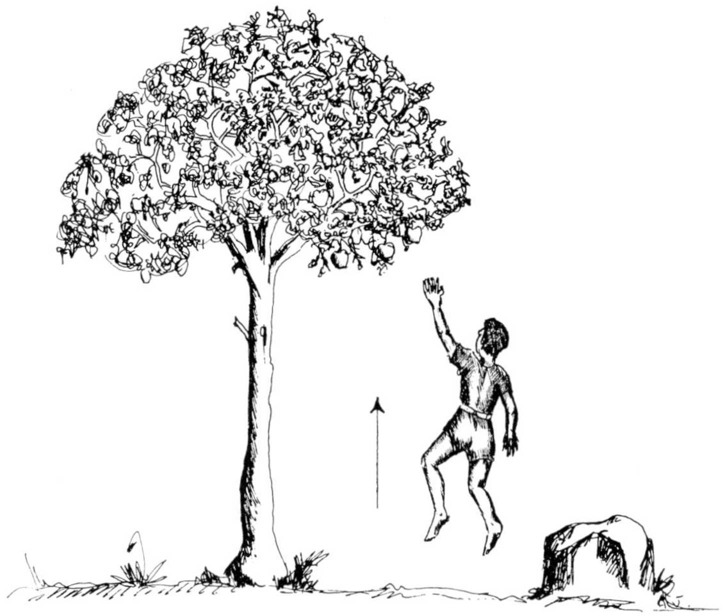

SMALL BOY JUMPING TO REACH THE APPLE.

B

Figure 16.19

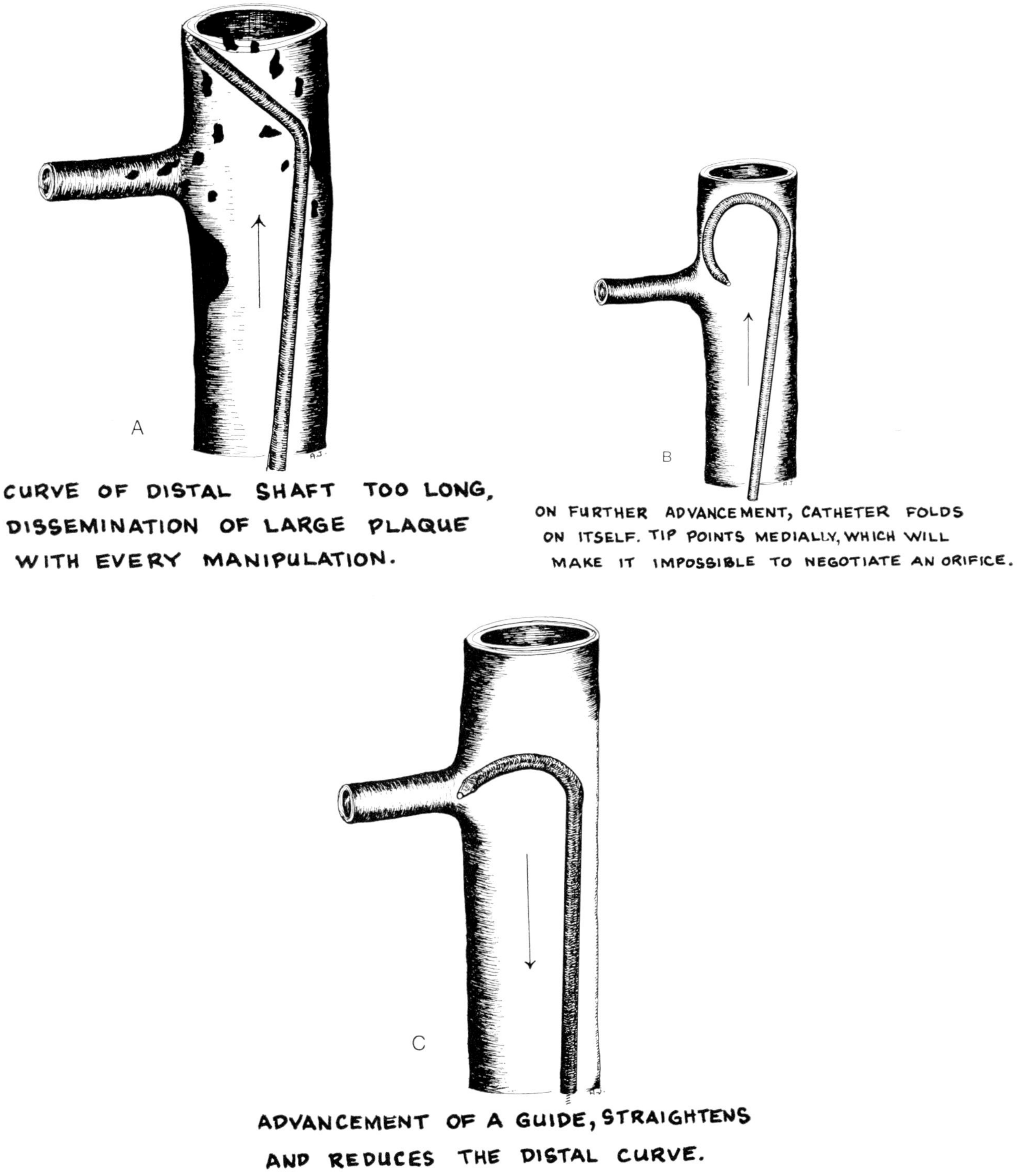
A
CURVE OF DISTAL SHAFT TOO LONG,
DISSEMINATION OF LARGE PLAQUE
WITH EVERY MANIPULATION.
B
ON FURTHER ADVANCEMENT, CATHETER FOLDS
ON ITSELF. TIP POINTS MEDIALLY, WHICH WILL
MAKE IT IMPOSSIBLE TO NEGOTIATE AN ORIFICE.
C
ADVANCEMENT OF A GUIDE, STRAIGHTENS
AND REDUCES THE DISTAL CURVE.

Figure 16.20

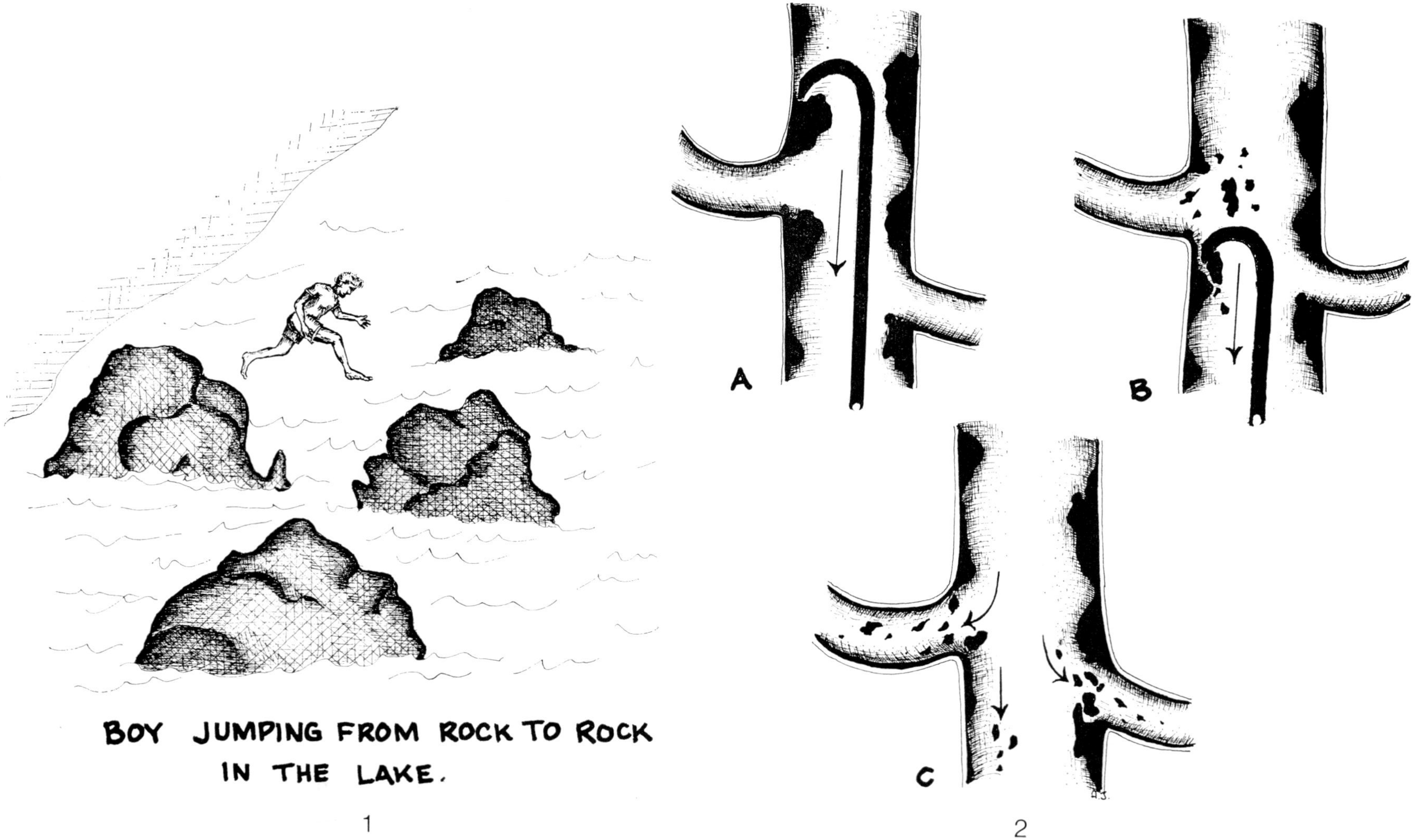

Figure 16.21. Atherosclerotic plaques and their effects on catheter tip control.

main vessels (or aorta inferior vena cava), but also at different heights along the circumference of these major trunks (Figs. 11-18 to 11-28).

Absent Orifices

The orifice of a branch may be either congenitally absent or occluded or stenotic because of acquired disease. An awareness of these pathologic processes enables one to obtain a flush aortogram for orientation purposes when appropriate. Recognition of such abnormalities will prevent the angiographer from occluding the vascular supply by engaging the catheter into a stenotic vessel if any.

Tortuous Conduit

If the iliac arteries and abdominal aorta are tortuous, it will prevent delivery of the given message along the long axis of the catheter and may even change the direction of branch orifices along the circumference of the aorta. Appropriate measures to improve the torque or proper direction of the tip are essential (Figs. 16-15 to 16-18).

The Orifice Is Reached but the Catheter Cannot Be Advanced Further

Inappropriate or Divergent Curves

It will be almost impossible to advance a catheter into a branch of a vessel if a caudally oriented catheter curve is used for a cranially oriented vessel curve or vice versa (Figs. 3-17 and 3-18). Immediate recognition of this situation demands exchanging the existing catheter for one with an appropriate shape.

Catheters with Shoulders or Angled Bends

These catheters (Fig. 3-20) invariably slip out of the orifice during attempts to further advance them into the catheterized vessel. This disadvantage can be overcome by using a catheter with a smooth, gentle curve similar to that of an umbrella handle (Fig. 3-15).

Stenotic Vessels

If a tip of a selected catheter cannot be placed proximal to the stenosis in a side branch artery during selective injection, then a flush aortogram is performed to delineate the stenotic area. This is done to ensure that a catheter does not plug a stenotic vessel of an organ whose blood supply is of the end artery type distribution. This will also avoid the catheter tip bypassing the stenosis.

Abrupt Change in the Course of a Vessel Distal to Its Origin

Gentle attempts with a floppy wire or a small "J" may be tried during different phases of respiration to further advance the catheter. Sometimes, even with all the available facilities, it may be impossible to negotiate the catheter beyond the kink. In fact, vessels with such a course are a limitation for superselective studies. In such situations, either the injection rate is modified or a simple selective injection is carried out. One must accept philosophically this limitation.

Tortuous Main Conduit

As before in this situation, measures to improve the torque of the catheter may aid in further negotiation into branch vessels.

Recoil—the Catheter Is in the Branch; When the Final Bolus Was Injected, the Catheter Recoiled Out of the Orifice or There Was Significant Reflux of the Contrast into the Aortic Lumen

Stability

The stability of a selective catheter during injection cannot be assured just because the tip of the catheter has reached the orifice. A well-stabilized selective catheter effectively withstands reasonable injection rates without recoiling, unlike one which is proximally placed in the vessel. Not only may the catheter recoil, but in the process it may engage itself into another orifice perfusing the entire volume of contrast into that vessel. This occurs more frequently when the catheter has only an end hole (Fig. 16-22). Stability, of course, can be tested prior to injecting the final bolus by a forceful hand injection of saline into the catheter and by fluo-

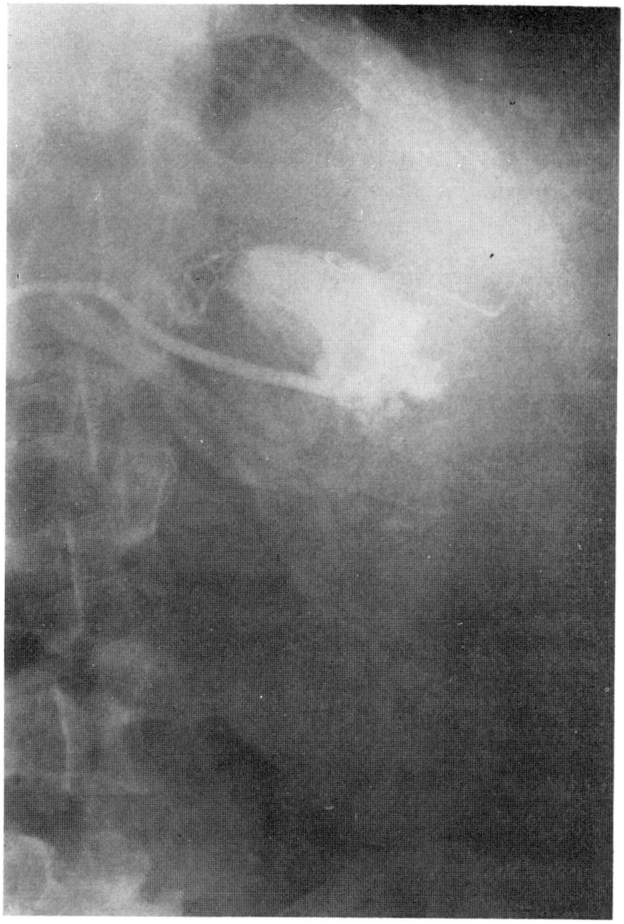

Figure 16.22. Left Renal Arteriogram. The catheter perfuses a small branch of the renal artery because of early bifurcation. *Comment:* Originally the catheter was placed in the main renal artery, but during injection the catheter whipped into the small branch with subsequent excessive perfusion. Luckily, there were no obvious after effects.

roscopic monitoring. In order to stabilize the catheter well, it may have to be advanced deeper into the branch artery. This in itself may raise some problems. In the celiac axis, for example, if the catheter is advanced too far for stability, the most important proximal branch, the left gastric, may not be opacified with contrast. In the renal arteries, early bifurcation of the main artery may again fail to perfuse a certain part of the kidney. And in a short celiac trunk, the catheter may enter only the splenic or only the hepatic artery; thus, the other organs are not visualized. If the main trunk of the vessel is sufficiently long, two holes on the superior wall of the catheter, each 1 cm apart and 1 cm from the tip of the catheter, will perfuse right angled branches and at the same time stabilize the tip of the catheter. In cases of very early bifurcation or short main trunks, individual selective opacification of branches may be advisable. If the vessel is small and of end artery type, a flush aortogram is acceptable.

Tortuous Main Conduit

Appropriate measures to improve catheter torque are attempted.

Undue or Excessive Injection Rates

This may cause reflux of the contrast into the aortic lumen despite a stable catheter. This occurs in elderly patients with low output failure or in patients with aortic valvular insufficiency. Reflux into the aorta can also occur if there is regional increase in vascular resistance due to prior infusion of vasoconstricting drugs.

Blood Oozing Around the Catheter Near the Puncture Site

Catheter Problems

Either too many catheters of the same size were exchanged, or a catheter of wider diameter was replaced by one with a small diameter. Oozing may also develop if there has been excessive manipulation of one catheter.

Low Prothrombin Reserve

A properly planned study with an established protocol avoids this interference during catheterization. In patients with low prothrombin levels such oozing occurs more frequently. Pressure applied for a few minutes between catheter manipulation may help stop the bleeding. The study in these patients should be completed without any undue delay. If the oozing is excessive, then the study may have to be terminated. Certain prophylactic measures taken before the technical part of the procedure will help retain the catheter for longer times in those patients (i.e. gastrointestinal bleeding) who are receiving intra-arterial therapeutic drugs.

No Pulses Distally in the Middle of the Procedure

This may be due to an excessively large catheter being used, or an extremely sensitive vessel which develops spasm or other predisposing factors. Perivascular infiltration and intravascular perfusion of accepted vasodilating drugs may be tried. The study should be completed without undue delay, and a pull-out angiogram is performed to show the level of obstruction in the route of entry or at the puncture site.

Arterial Catheter Removed, and No Bleeding From the Puncture Site

This may be due to spasm which will hopefully respond to vasodilators, or due to arterial thrombosis. An initial attempt to milk out the clot may be done as described in the section under "Treatment of Complications." If this is unsuccessful, then further surgical consultation should be obtained.

Excessive Bleeding from the Puncture Site After Removing the Arterial Catheter

This may be due to (1) accidental use of excessive heparin, (2) inefficient and insufficient pressure, (3) pressure applied at the wrong location, (4) an extremely obese individual, (5) a hypertensive patient, (6) coagulation disorders, and (7) a high puncture site (Fig. 13-3). Appropriate measure should be taken as soon as the nature of the problem is determined.

The Guide Wire Removed from an End Hole Catheter with No Return of Blood

Clot

If a clot occurs at the tip of the catheter, forceful suction may dislodge the clot which may then be aspirated into the syringe. If this is unsuccessful, then the catheter can be exchanged with the assistance of a mylar sheath (Fig. 15-3).

Tip Impacted Under a Plaque

Withdrawal of a short segment of the catheter should result in the return of blood.

Suction Pressure

Suction pressure exerted upon the wall of a collapsible vein can be recognized by withdrawal of a short segment of the catheter. In some small veins like the parathyroid or thymic veins, it may be very difficult, if not impossible, to aspirate blood samples.

Veins—Puncture Problems

Accidental Venous Punctures Are More Common Than Intentional Ones

Because the vein is located by its anatomical landmarks rather than by direct palpation, accidental puncture is not uncommon, nor is failure to puncture the vein. It is a good practice to aspirate while withdrawing the transfixed needle since in some individuals, even though the needle is in the lumen of the vein, the pressure is not sufficient to cause blood to trickle out through the needle lumen. In individuals with increased pressure due to obstructing lesions, a forceful jet of blood may emanate from the needle hub. However, the *color differences* will indicate that the needle is in a vein rather than in an artery. Just as in arterial route studies, the guide wire may make accidental entry into side branches such as the ascending lumbar vein. This can be prevented by fluoroscopic monitoring of the guide tip or be overcome by using a proper "J" wire.

CHAPTER 17
STANDARD RECIPES*

THE RANGE OF LESIONS with their different etiologies, biological behaviors, modes of extension, influence by adjacent structures, and variation in feeding and draining vessels requires tailoring of the angiographic studies to the information needed. For example, a superior mesenteric arteriogram done for opacification of the portal vein is entirely different from one done to determine a point of gastrointestinal bleeding. The angiographic approach to evaluate renovascular hypertension differs from a study being done to assess renal malignancy. A preliminary diagnosis made with the assistance of other available information will shorten the duration of the procedure and determine the amount of contrast used, thereby decreasing morbidity.

I. ARTERIES

A. Flush Angiography

Abdominal Aortogram

Catheter
Shape
Straight: End and multiple side holes
Size
Adults: 7 Fr.
Children: Smaller (3, 4, or 5 Fr.)
Contrast
Adults
20-25 cc/sec. for 2 sec.
Children
3-6 years 6-10 cc/sec. for 2 sec.
6-16 years 10-15 cc/sec. for 2 sec.
Filming sequence
2 films/sec. for 3 sec.
1 film/sec. for 6 sec.

Comment: The tip is positioned at least 2 cm below the level of the orifices to be visualized. To obtain a *panoramic view of the intraabdominal vasculature* a flush abdominal aortogram is performed. Initially this looks like a road map, but further scrutiny will yield a great deal of valuable information which helps to focus on the area of interest. Unlike a selective study, *surprises during a flush aortogram are common.* The flush abdominal aortogram is indicated as a preliminary study to (1) renal vascular pathologies and mass lesions, (2) aortic pathology, (3) abdominal masses, (4) pheochromocytoma, (5) blunt abdominal trauma.

Aortic Arch Angiogram

Catheter
Shape
Curve with a 4 cm radius to conform to the curve of the aortic arch. End and multiple side holes.
Size
Adults: 7.5 Fr. or 7 Fr.
Children: Smaller
Contrast
Adults
30-35 cc/sec. for 2 sec.
Children
3-6 years 8-12 cc/sec. for 2 sec.
6-16 years 12-18 cc/sec. for 2 sec.
Filming sequence
2 films/sec. for 4 sec.
1 film/sec. for 3 sec.

Comment: The predilection for *atherosclerosis* to involve the *origins of the great vessels* from the aortic arch, or the *bifurcation of the carotids,* causing either transient ischemic attacks or major cerebral catastrophies, places the study of this vessel in the prerogative of the general angiographer. However, it is preferable that the patient be on continuous cardiac monitor-

* Standard recipe includes the curve of the catheter, amount of contrast and the rate of filming for that particular vessel in consideration.

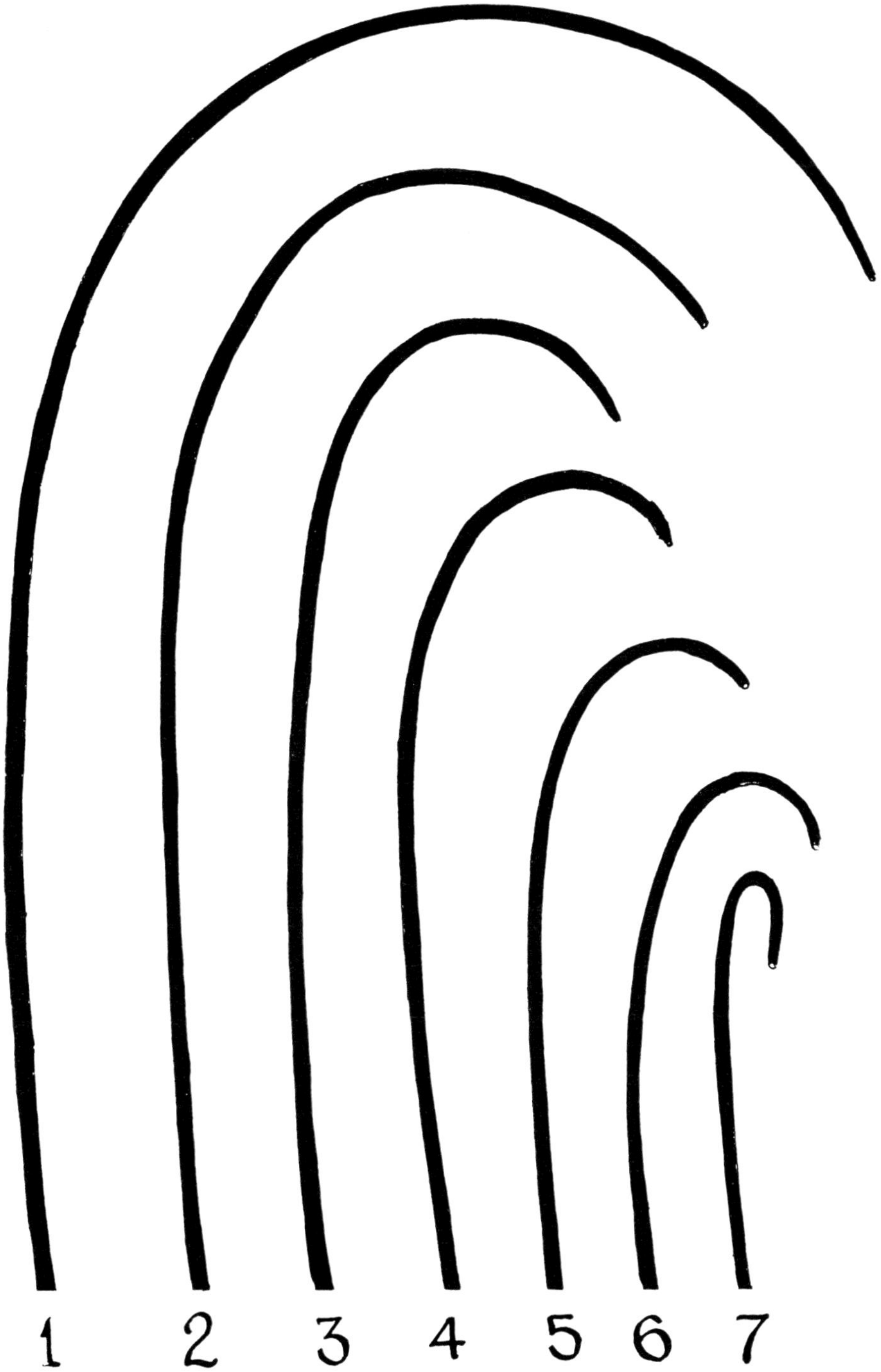

Figure 17.1. Some curves (via femoral route): 1. (a) Hepatic veins, (b) Left renal vein, (c) Wide ectatic aortic arch. 2. (a) Right and left renal veins, (b) Hepatic veins, (c) Azygous vein, (d) Aortic arch. 3. (a) Right renal vein, (b) Azygous vein, (c) For celiac superior mesenteric renals arising from a very wide aorta. 4. (a) Right renal vein, (b) Azygous vein, (c) Celiac, superior mesenteric, renals arising from a wide aorta, (d) Left renal vein (pediatric). 5. (a) Celiac, superior mesenteric and renals, (b) Inferior mesenteric artery arising from a wide aorta. 6. Celiac, superior mesenteric renals (young individuals). Standard inferior mesenteric artery catheter. 7. (a) Internal iliac artery catheter, (b) Caudal celiac, superior mesenteric in young individuals, (c) Abd. Aorta via left axillary route in ectatic aorta as a leader to the guide.

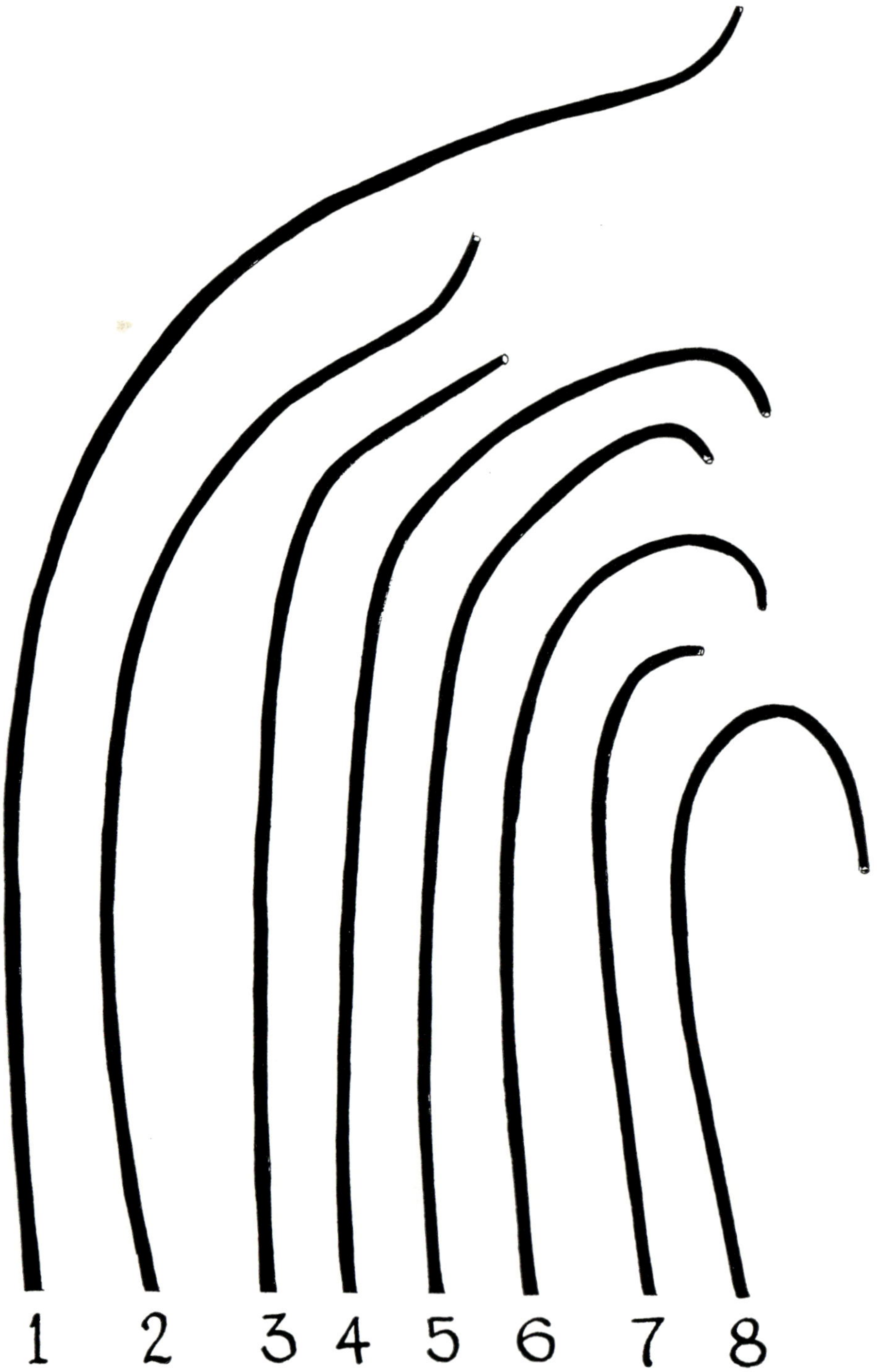

Figure 17.2. Some curves (via femoral route): 1. (a) Left adrenal vein, (b) Parathyroid vein (inferior). 2. Mostly superselective: (a) Left gastric artery (from celiac), (b) Left adrenal vein, (c) Vertebral arteries, (d) Left hepatic artery (from celiac), (e) Parathyroid vein (inferior). 3. (a) Cephalad celiac axis, (b) Cephalad superior mesenteric, (c) Carotids and vertebrals and subclavians, (d) Internal jugular veins, (e) ASc. Lumbar vein. 4. (a) Thymic vein, (b) Left gonadal vein, (c) Internal mammary vein. 5. (a) Right adrenal vein, (b) Thymic vein, (c) Left gonadal vein, (d) Lumbar artery. 6. (a) Dorsal pancreatic artery, (b) Left gonadal vein. 7. Superselective: (a) Gastroduodenal artery, (b) Hepatic arteries, (c) Selective lumbar artery, (d) Vertebral thyrocervical internal mammary arteries (via axillary). 8. (a) Caudal celiac, superior mesenteric arteries, (b) Left common iliac artery via right femoral artery or vice versa.

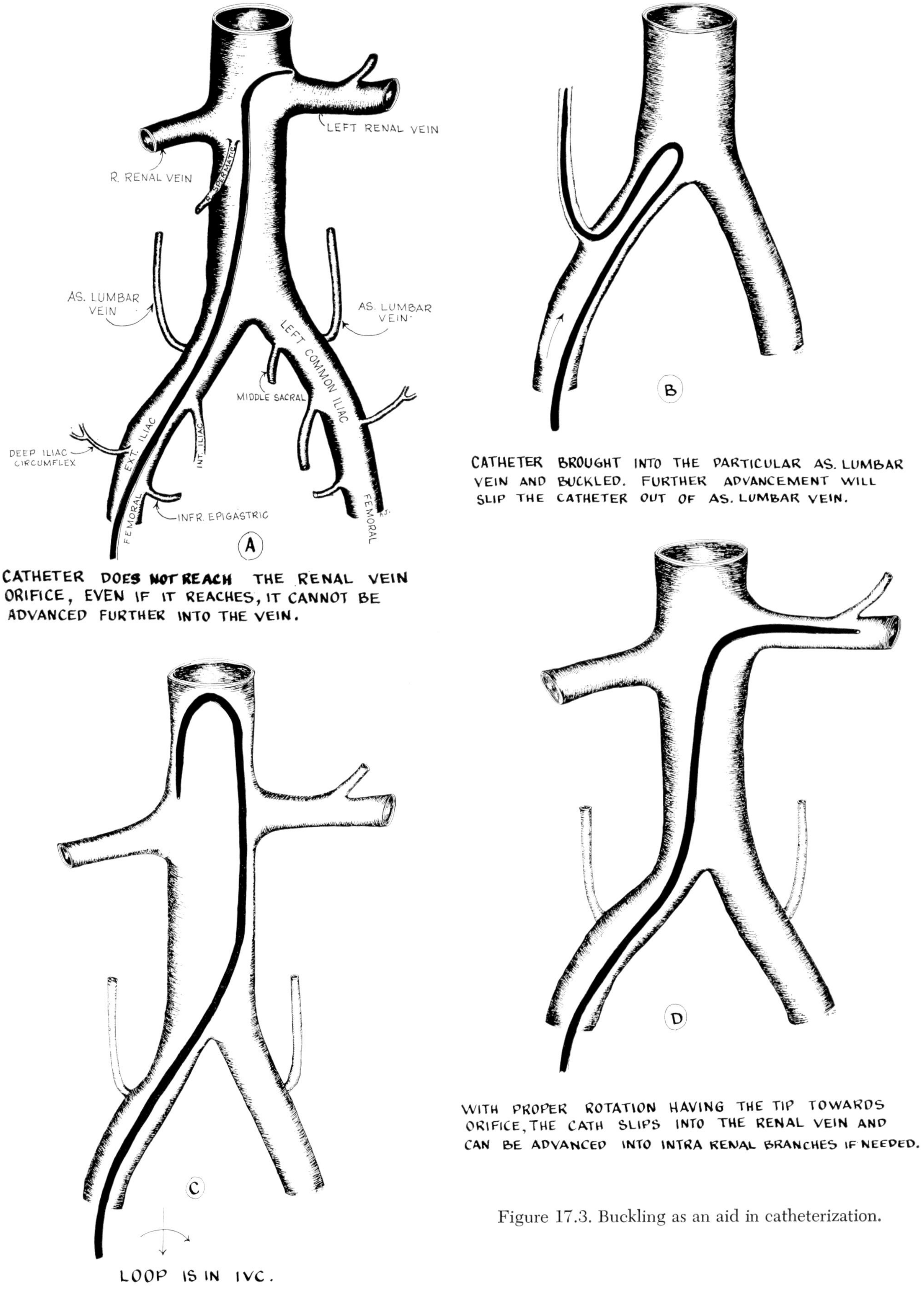

Figure 17.3. Buckling as an aid in catheterization.

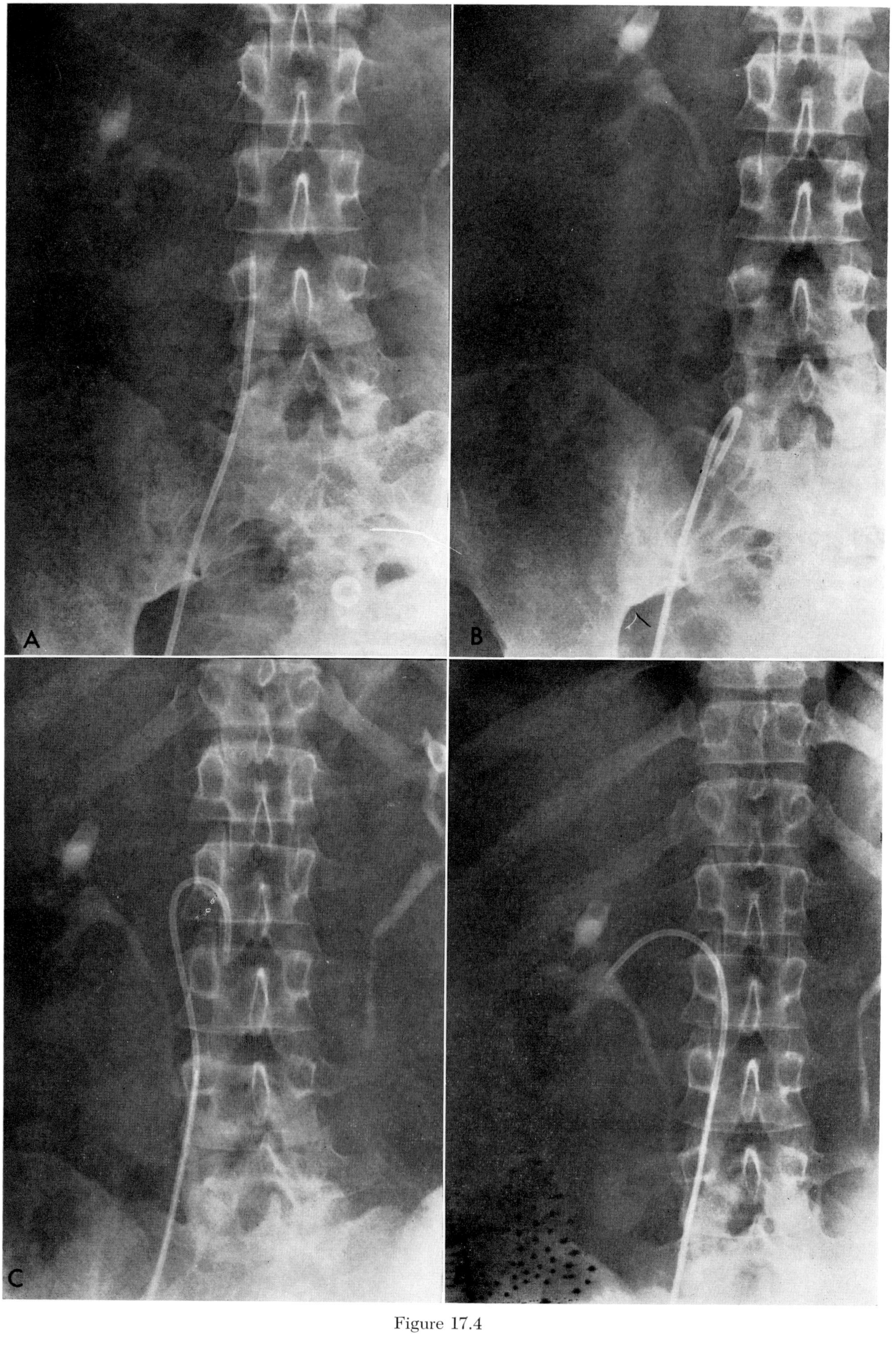

Figure 17.4

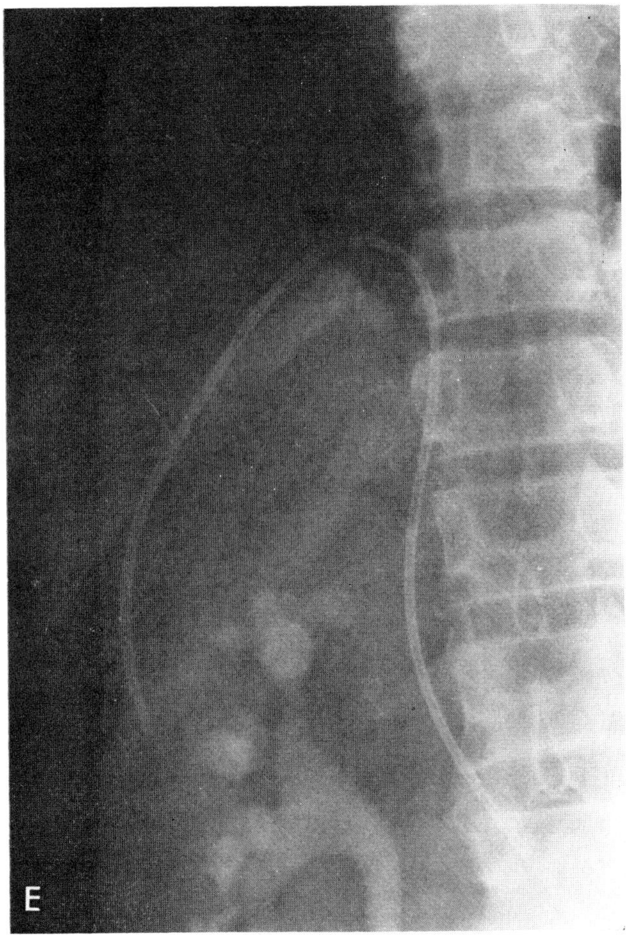

Figure 17.4. (A) An almost straight catheter in the inferior vena cava. (B) The catheter was withdrawn into the common iliac vein and engaged in the ascending lumbar vein to form a curve by buckling. (C) The buckled catheter ascends in the inferior vena cava. (D) The same catheter manipulated into the right renal vein. (E) The same catheter manipulated into the hepatic vein as far distally as one wishes. *Comment:* In some situations a very minimally curved catheter can be buckled to form a curve and then can be engaged into an orifice with easy distal manipulation of the tip into the distal portions of that vessel.

ing with intravenous catheter and fluids running. If the patient's cardiovascular status is fragile, and it usually is, a cardiologist should be in the immediate vicinity. Two or three studies may have to be done to show the origin and course of the great vessels from the aortic arch. The standard projection is in the *right posterior oblique* with the head turned to the same side. If however, visualization of the origins are not clear, then studies in the *anteroposterior, or even left posterior oblique,* positions may have to be performed.

Descending Thoracic Aortogram

Catheter
- Shape
  - Straight: end and multiple side holes.
- Size
  - Adults: 6.5 to 7 Fr.
  - Children: Smaller

Contrast
- Adults
  - 15 cc/sec. for 2 sec.
- Children
  - 3-6 years 6-10 cc/sec. for 2 sec.
  - 6-16 years 10-15 cc/sec. for 2 sec.

Filming sequence
- 2 films/sec. for 3 sec.
- 1 film/sec. for 5 sec.

Comment: This is occasionally needed in the field of general angiography to evaluate the presence of a possible pulmonary sequestration or spinal cord arteriovenous malformations.

Pediatric Angiography[286]

Route of entry
- 1-5 days—umbilical artery
- 5 days—percutaneous femoral approved.

Contrast
- ¾ cc per kg in the aorta.
- ½ cc per kg in the celiac or superior mesenteric artery.
- 0.1 cc per kg for renal.

Comment: The arterial technique has been described elsewhere.[285] Umbilical venography is probably the fastest way to diagnose right-sided intrathoracic herniation of the liver.[287]

Intravenous Angiogram

Catheter
- Shape and Size
  - Two 16 or 18 ga. needles with Teflon sleeves introduced into the antecubital veins. Each is connected via a plastic tube to a "Y" connector.

Contrast
- 20 cc/sec. for 3 to 4 sec.

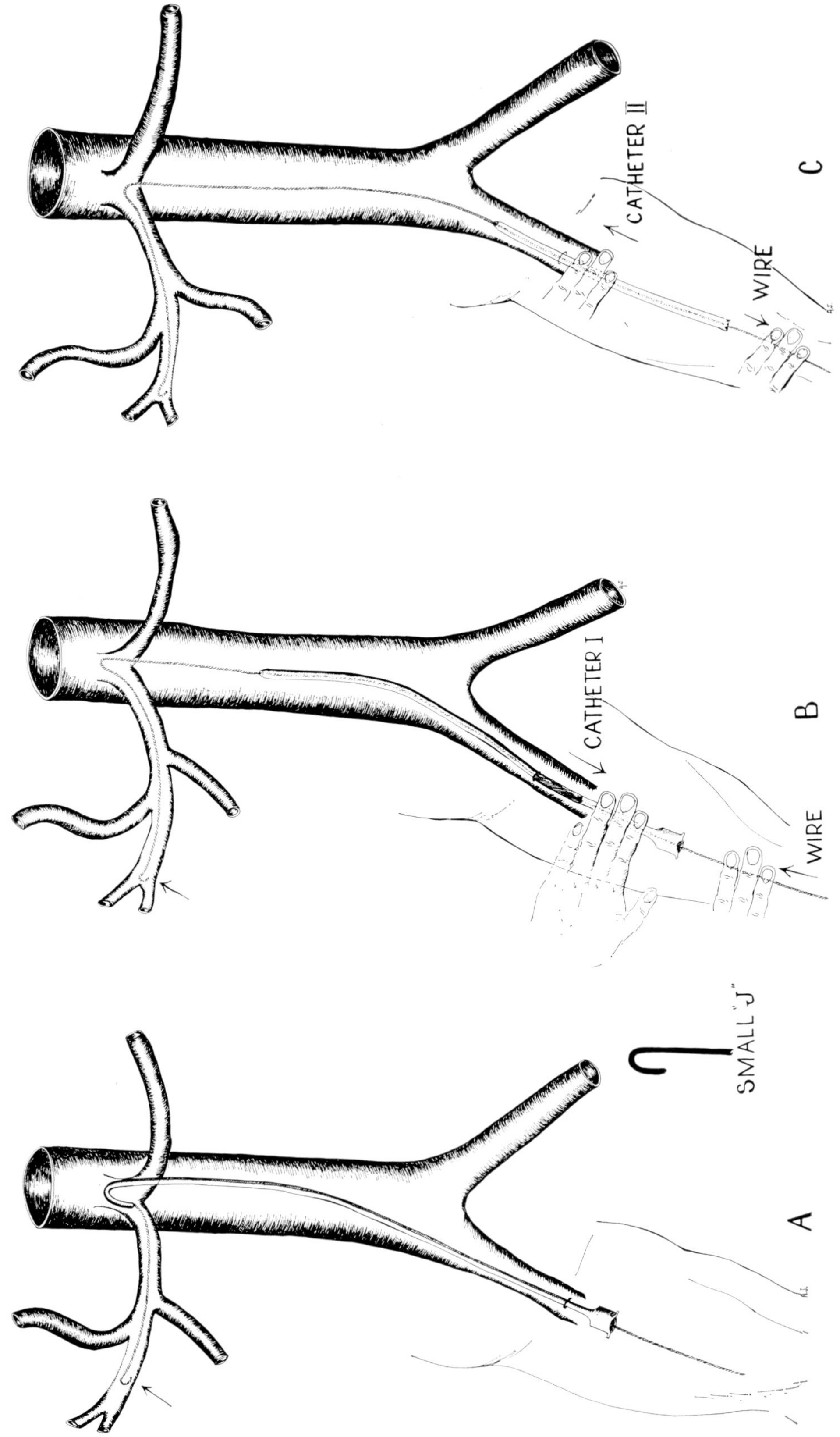

Figure 17.5 (*Continued on next page*).

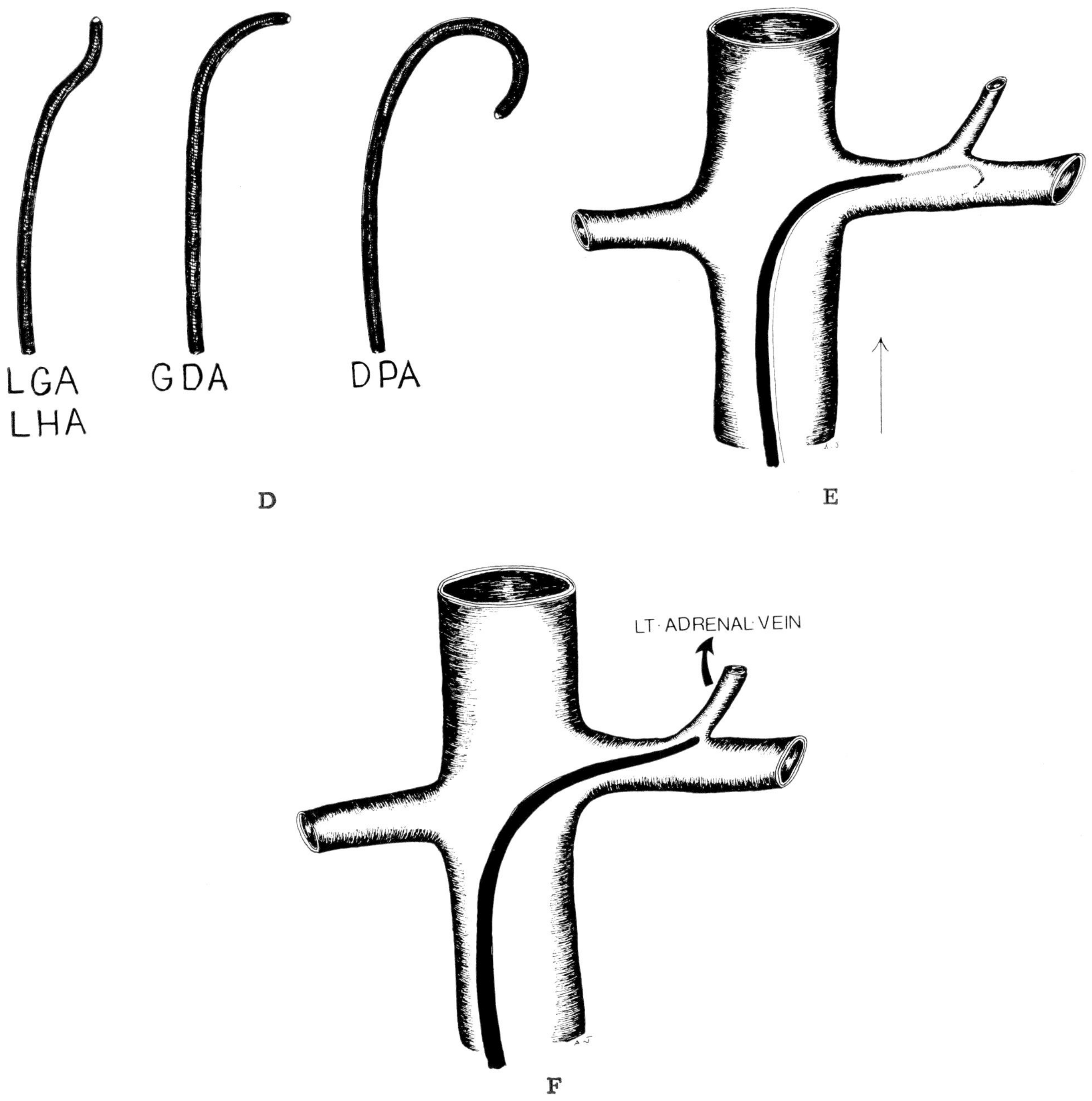

Figure 17.5. Superselective technique: Throughout the procedure, the tip of the wire is maintained as far distally in the parent branch (Arrow).

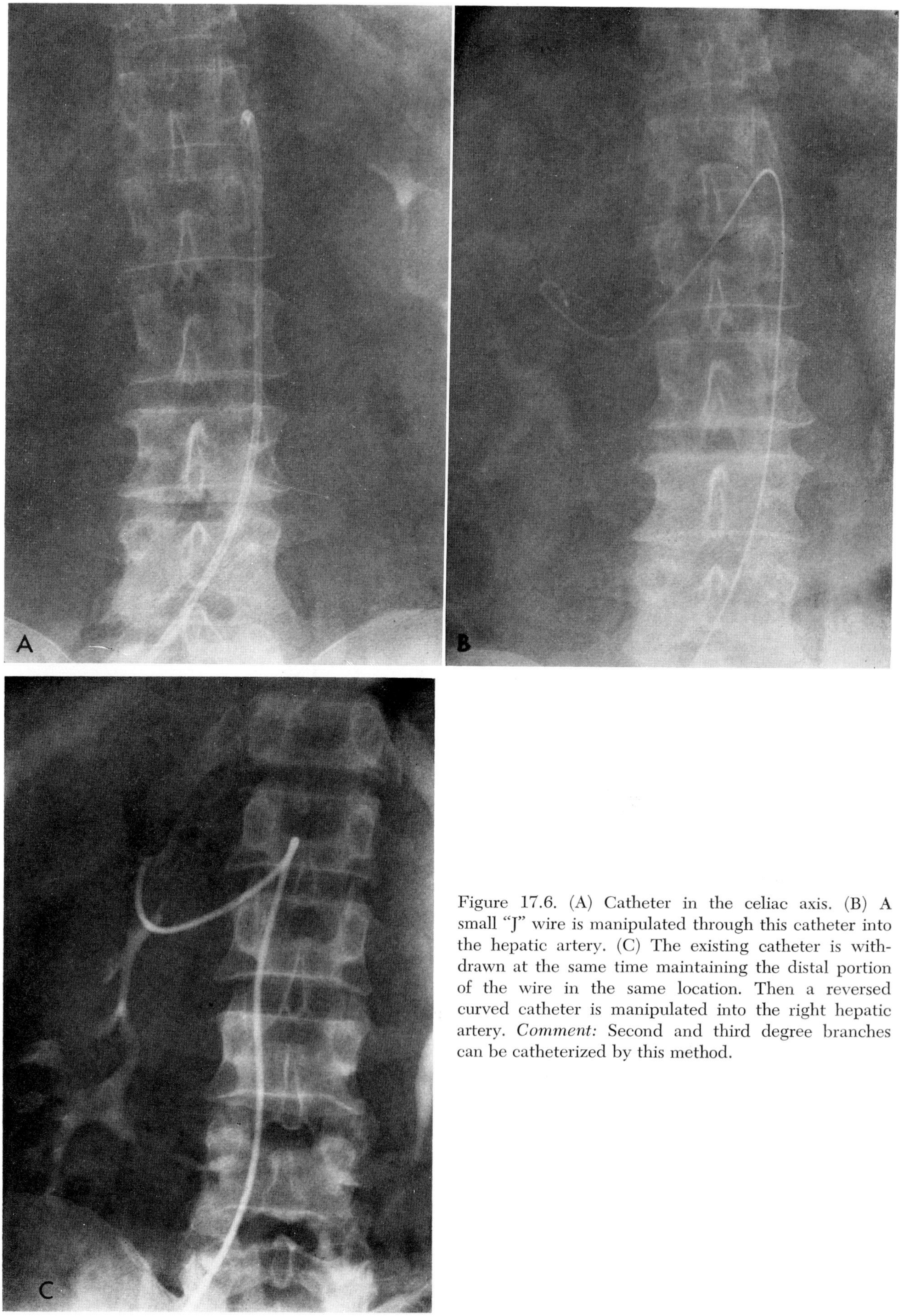

Figure 17.6. (A) Catheter in the celiac axis. (B) A small "J" wire is manipulated through this catheter into the hepatic artery. (C) The existing catheter is withdrawn at the same time maintaining the distal portion of the wire in the same location. Then a reversed curved catheter is manipulated into the right hepatic artery. *Comment:* Second and third degree branches can be catheterized by this method.

Filming sequence
(a) cardiac chambers and pulmonary arteries.
1 film/sec. for 20 sec.
(b) Superior vena cava.
1 film/sec. for 10 sec.
(c) Abdominal aorta and its branches.
1 film/sec. for 20 to 24 sec.

Comment: This is a fast, easy way to opacify the cardiac chambers for evaluation of *pericardial effusions,* to visualize the *superior vena cava,* or the *pulmonary arteries* (gross visualization), to demonstrate masses adjacent to the aorta, or as a last resort, to opacify the aorta and its branches.

B. Selective Angiography

Renal Arteriogram—Standard

Catheter
Shape
End and side hole, curved (Fig. 17-1 [4, 5, 6])
Size
Adults: 6 or 7 Fr.
Children: 3, 4 or 5 Fr.

Contrast
Adults
3 to 5 cc/sec. for 2 sec.
Children
3-6 years 1.5 to 3.0 cc/sec. for 2 sec.
6-16 years 2 to 4 cc/sec. for 2 sec.

Filming sequence
2 films/sec. for 3 sec.
1 film/sec. for 8 sec.

Comment: An initial flush abdominal aortogram is optional, but it may make the study easier if there are multiple renal arteries. If multiple arteries are present, then the total amount of contrast is proportionately divided amongst the number of arteries, depending on the area of distribution.

Lowering the injection rate using the same total amount of contrast and *prolonging* the filming will yield satisfactory films when there is increased intrarenal resistance. This may occur in *nephrosclerosis* or *hydronephrosis.* This same principle applies to all vascular beds when vasoconstricting medications have been selectively perfused into the artery. In the case of an *avascular mass,* an additional series of filming, if done in the *oblique projections,* may aid in mapping all of the borders of the avascular mass. To show the anastomotic area clearly in *renal transplants,* the patient is positioned in the lateral projection with the exposure done using an anterior posterior beam.

Celiac Arteriogram—Standard

Catheter
Shape
End and side holes (Fig. 17-1 [3, 4, 5, 6]).
Size
Adults: 6 or 7 Fr.
Children: A smaller French size is used.

Contrast
Adults
50 cc over 4 to 8 sec. The injection rate is decided by the caliber of the celiac axis and its branches.
Children
3-6 years, 12 to 20 cc over 3 to 4 sec.
6-16 years, 24 to 30 cc over 4 to 5 sec.

Filming sequence
2 films/sec. for 3 sec.
1 film/sec. for 3 sec.
1 film every third second for 18 seconds.

Hepatic Arteriogram—Standard

Catheter
Shape
End and side holes (Fig. 17-1 [3, 4, 5, 6]).
Size
Adults: 6 or 7 Fr.
Children: A smaller French size is used.

Contrast
Adults
30 to 40 cc over 5 to 6 sec.
Children
3-6 years, 8 to 16 cc over 2 to 3 sec.
6-16 years, 16 to 30 cc over 3 to 4 sec.

Filming sequence
2 films/sec. for 3 sec.
1 film/sec. for 3 sec.
1 film every third second for ten seconds.

Comment: If possible, the existing celiac catheter itself may be further manipulated distally into the hepatic artery. If not, another catheter is exchanged with the help of a "J" wire (Fig. 17-5 [7]).

The standard projection used is anterior posterior and will suffice in most instances, but for *segmental localization* of masses, either a right posterior oblique or even an additional lateral projection may have to be obtained. For better opacification of primary or secondary tumor masses, a low injection rate of contrast using a large amount is suggested.[283] In other words, 50 cc of contrast may be given over a ten-second period.

Splenic Arteriogram—Standard

Catheter
Shape
End and side holes (Fig. 17-1 [3, 4, 5, 6]).
Size
Adults: 6 or 7 Fr.
Children: A smaller French size is used.
Contrast
Adults
20 to 30 cc over 4 to 5 sec.
Children
3-6 years, 8 to 15 cc over 2 to 3 sec.
6-16 years, 12 to 20 cc over 3 to 4 sec.
Filming sequence
2 films/sec. for 3 sec.
1 film/sec. for 3 sec.
1 film every third second for 18 seconds.

Comments: If possible, the existing celiac axis catheter may be manipulated distally into the splenic artery, or another catheter may be inserted after exchanging over a "J" wire (Fig. 17-5 [7]). In cases of splenomegaly, 40 to 80 cc of contrast may be given over six to eight seconds, with the *amount of contrast used dependent upon the size of the spleen.* To prevent overlapping shadows from the fundus of the stomach, an additional study in the *left anterior oblique* may have to be obtained. This is especially true in traumatic abnormalities of the spleen. To *enhance visualization* of traumatic lesions of the spleen, a postepinephrine selective splenic arteriogram may be of benefit.[99]

Left Gastric Arteriogram—Standard

Catheter
Shape
End hole. Reversed curve (Fig. 17-2 [2], 17-5).
Size
Adult: Fr. 6
Contrast
Adult
12 to 16 cc over 3 to 4 sec.
Filming sequence
2 films/sec. for 3 sec.
1 film/sec. for 3 sec.
1 film every 2 sec. for 10 sec.

Comment: As the left gastric artery is an important blood vessel of the stomach, its selective catheterization is vital in many acute emergencies, either for the diagnosis of *esophogeal varices, Mallory-Weiss syndrome, hemorrhagic gastritis, or bleeding ulcers, or for therapy* by infusing vasoconstricting drugs. Since a reversed curve catheter cannot be engaged in a right-angled orifice of a branch of the aorta, the existing celiac axis catheter is exchanged with the help of a small width "J" wire for one with a reversed curve. Then the reversed tip of the left gastric catheter is engaged in the left gastric orifice. Deflector wires[37] can also be used to engage the reversed tip into the celiac axis. Occasionally, even with all the available facilities, it may be impossible to engage the reverse tip into the left gastric orifice. Then the appropriate celiac axis catheter with two holes on the superior wall of the curve, each hole 1 cm apart and 1 cm proximal to the tip of the catheter, will provide good opacification of the left gastric arborization. This may not, however, be satisfactory for the infusion of vasoconstricting drugs. One should be aware of the variations in the arrangement of the celiac axis and its branches; valuable time may be lost searching for a left gastric artery in the celiac axis, when it is actually arising from a separate origin.

To demonstrate *esophogeal varices*[284] and any active bleeding from them, a large bolus of contrast is injected (25 to 30 cc over five to six seconds) into the left gastric artery selectively.

Pancreatic Arteriogram—from the Gastroduodenal Artery for the Head of the Pancreas

Catheter
Shape
End and side holes (Fig. 17-1 [3, 4, 5, 6]).
Size
Adults: 6 or 7 Fr.
Contrast
12 to 15 cc over 3 to 4 sec.
Filming sequence
2 films/sec. for 4 sec.
1 film/sec. for 3 sec.
1 film every two seconds for six seconds.

Comment: The existing celiac axis catheter may be advanced into the gastroduodenal artery or exchanged to a simple curved 6 or 7 Fr. catheter (Fig. 17-2 [7], 17-5) meant for the gastroduodenal artery. This is exchanged with the help of a small width "J" wire (Fig. 17-5).

If magnification facilities are available, they are very helpful in demonstrating the vessels to greater satisfaction. Occasionally-filming in the right posterior oblique projection may be done to avoid superimposition of overlying bony structures. Variations in the normal arrangement of the gastroduodenal artery sometimes makes the procedure tedious.

Pancreatic Arteriogram—Dorsal Pancreatic Artery for the Body and Uncinate Process

Catheter
Shape
End and side holes (Fig. 17-1 [3, 4, 5, 6]).
Size
6 or 7 Fr.
Contrast
9 cc over 3 sec.
Filming sequence
2 films/sec. for 4 sec.
1 film/sec. for 6 sec.

Comment: If the existing celiac axis catheter happens to engage the orifice of the dorsal pancreatic vessel, then further exchange is unnecessary. If not, a proper 6 or 7 Fr. catheter (Figs. 17-2 [6], 17-5) is introduced in the same way as is done for the gastroduodenal artery. Preferably, the tip of this catheter is tapered over a .035 wire to facilitate engagement into the small orifice.

Awareness of the variation in the origin of the dorsal pancreatic artery avoids a futile search in only one location. If magnification facilities are available, visualization of the small branches to the pancreas is improved.

Pancreatic Arteriogram—Branches from the Splenic Artery for the Body and Tail of the Pancreas (Pancreatica Magna and Short Pancreatic Arteries)

Catheter
Shape
End and side holes (Fig. 17-1 [3, 4, 5, 6]).
Size
6 or 7 Fr.
Contrast
15 to 20 cc over 3 to 4 sec.
Filming sequence
2 films/sec. for 4 sec.
1 film/sec. for 3 sec.
1 film every two seconds for eight seconds.

Comment: Satisfactory opacification of the pancreatic branches from the splenic artery may be obtained by selectively infusing the splenic artery using catheter techniques described above.

Superior Mesenteric Arteriogram—Standard

Catheter
Shape
End and side holes (Fig. 17-1 [3, 4, 5, 6]).
Size
Adult: 6 or 7 Fr.
Children: Smaller French sizes.
Contrast
Adults
30 cc over 3 to 4 sec.

Children
3-6 years, 8 to 12 cc over 2 to 3 sec.
6-16 years, 15 to 20 cc over 3 to 4 sec.
Filming sequence
2 films/sec. for 3 sec.
1 film/sec. for 3 sec.
1 film every two seconds for twelve seconds.

Inferior Mesenteric Arteriogram—Standard

Catheter
Shape
See (Fig. 17-1 [5, 6]).
Size
6 Fr.
Contrast
16 to 20 cc over 4 to 5 sec.
Filming sequence
2 films/sec. for 3 sec.
1 film/sec. for 3 sec.
1 film every two seconds for ten seconds.
Comment: Catheterization is easier if the *route of entry* is via the left femoral artery.

C. Extremity Angiography

In reality each extremity vessel is a *single unit from the origin of its parent branch,* either from the bifurcation of the aorta or from the aortic arch, to its termination at the tip of the digit. Clinical manifestations distally may actually reflect either a very proximal lesion or two different lesions at two different levels, one masking the other due to severity or location. Thus, a cold hand may be due to either an embolus from the heart or to a mural thrombus from poststenotic dilatation of the subclavian artery caused by a thoracic outlet syndrome. Another common occurrence is an atherosclerotic lesion of the common iliac arteries with a second narrowed lesion at the femoral or popliteal level.

Lower Extremity Angiogram

Catheter
Shape
Pigtail.
Size
6 Fr.
Contrast
50 cc of diluted Renografin-60.
(25 cc of contrast plus 25 cc of normal saline) injected over five seconds
Filming sequence
(1) 1 film/sec. for 3 sec. at the pelvic area to include the distal abdominal aorta.
(2) Table moved cephalad to expose the proximal thigh. 1 film/sec. for 4 sec.
(3) Table moved again cephalad to cover the distal thigh and proximal leg. 1 film/sec. for 3 to 4 sec.
(4) Table moved cephalad again to visualize the calves, and if possible, the ankles. 1 film/sec. for 3 to 4 sec.
Comment: The catheter is inserted into the aorta approximately 7.5 cm above the bifurcation of the abdominal aorta. Each time the table is moved, the roentgenographic exposure factors are reduced for the lower extremities.

A standard *lower extremity arteriogram* is done through the femoral route provided there are no obvious diseases of the vessel. If the vessel is diseased, the *contralateral femoral* is selectively catheterized. If both femorals are compromised, a *translumbar aortogram* can be done. This is preferable to using the left axillary route. Catching the contrast material in the entire lower extremity after one injection is a matter of trial and error. This is influenced by the velocity of flow, the presence of occlusions and collaterals, and the skill of the angiographer. Most of the time one can visualize the entire vascular unit with two injections.

Lower Extremity Angiogram, Alternative Routes—Opposite Femoral Artery

If there is any hesitation about inserting the catheter into the femoral artery because of a doubtful pulse at the puncture site, then a Teflon sleeve needle #16 or 18 ga. may be inserted into the comparatively normal femoral artery, and a total of 48 to 60 cc of diluted Renografin-60 injected at the rate of 12 cc per second. This will give satisfactory opacification of the bifurcation of the aorta as well as the contralateral femoral artery. Again, serial filming down the length of the extremity is performed. Occasionally this method may not opacify the bifurcation of the aorta if the ipsilateral external iliac artery is very tortuous.

Left Axillary Approach

This alternative route should be used very reluctantly since the *risks are significantly higher* enroute to the aorta via an arteriosclerotic subclavian artery. The axillary artery is punctured as described in Chapter 12, and an acutely curved catheter is advanced to the aortic arch. A "J" wire is passed through the catheter into the descending thoracic aorta. The catheter then follows and is advanced to the level of the bifurcation. The same amount of diluted contrast material as described under the pigtail catheter is injected and the series filmed as described above (Fig. 3-19).

Comment: Exercising the extremity provokes reactive hyperemia causing a decrease in the transit time by increased flow and filling of the collaterals. The distal site of the occlusion is well delineated using this technique. It may not be very satisfactory for the hands and feet, as the blood may be diverted to the muscles.[289, 290] For demonstration of the atherosclerosis of the deep femoral artery, a lateral or oblique projection of the leg is indicated.[288, 291] Arteries situated in closed compartments (i.e. the anterior tibial compartment) with increased pressure due to edema or hemorrhage require a longer filming sequence to demonstrate the slow flow in the arteries.[1039]

Upper Extremity Angiograms

Subclavian Arteriogram Via the Femoral Route

Catheter
Shape
End and side holes (Fig. 17-2 [3]).
Size
7 Fr.
Contrast
Diluted. 12 cc given over 3 sec.
Filming sequence
1 film/sec. for 4 sec.

Comment: Both the axillary and brachial arteries may be opacified in the same way, but in atherosclerotic individuals the *potential complication* of dislodging a plaque into the cerebral circulation always exists.

Brachial Artery
Catheter
The preferred way to visualize the brachial artery is via a local puncture with a Teflon sleeve needle.
Contrast
Diluted. 10 cc over 2½ sec.
Filming sequence
2 films/sec. for 3 sec.
1 film/sec. for 4 to 6 sec.

Comment: If Prescoline®, 15 to 20 mgm, is injected into the artery prior to the injection of contrast, there will be better visualization and opacification of the distal vessels.

D. Small Vessel Angiograms

Inferior Phrenic and Adrenal Arteries

Catheter
Shape
End hole only (Fig. 17-1 [3, 4, 5]).
Size
7 Fr. with the tip tapered over a .035 inch wire.
Contrast
6 to 8 cc over 3 to 4 sec.
Filming sequence
2 films/sec. for 3 sec.
1 film every other second for 6 to 8 seconds.

Comment: Since the advent of adrenal venography,[414–418] catheterization of the inferior phrenic or adrenal arteries is not very essential. The inferior phrenic arteries usually arise from either the celiac axis or the aorta about the celiac axis. A thorough search in these areas aids in catheterization. Occasionally, the inferior phrenic originates from the renal artery.

It is very difficult to catheterize a normal size adrenal artery, particularly the middle adrenal artery. A normal middle adrenal artery rarely opacifies during a flush abdominal aortogram unless it is dilated. The inferior adrenal arteries are frequently opacified during renal arteriograms. To facilitate opacification of the inferior adrenal arteries, one to two holes on the superior wall of the curved segment of the catheter may be created. *Adrenal arteriograms may not detect small masses or hyperplasias, but are very useful in detecting adrenal carcinomas, sizeable adenomas and pheochromocytomas.*

Lumbar and Intercostal Arteriograms

Catheter
  Shape
    Refer to Figure 17-2 [5, 7].
  Size
    6 Fr. with a tip drawn over a .035 inch guide wire.
Contrast
  6 cc over 3 sec.
Filming sequence
  2 films/sec. for 4 sec.
  1 film every other second for eight seconds.
Comment: Unless there is a strong indication clinically, catheterization of these vessels *should not be intentionally overutilized.*

Internal Iliac Arteriogram

Catheter
  Shape
    Refer to Figure 17-1 [7]. End and side holes.
  Size
    7 Fr.
Contrast
  12 to 16 cc over 3 to 4 sec.
Filming sequence
  2 films/sec. for 3 sec.
  1 film/sec. for 8 to 10 sec.
Comment: Simultaneous catheterization of both internal iliacs should be done with caution. Only in very rare circumstances are these studies indicated, basically for the demonstration of gynecological pathology.

E. Veins

Inferior Vena Cavogram

The routes for catheterization include both femoral veins, the internal jugular vein, or the basilic vein.

The Femoral Vein Route

Catheter
  Each femoral vein is punctured at the groin with a Teflon sleeve needle.[36]
Contrast
  12 cc in each femoral vein/sec. for 2 sec. and injected through a "Y" connector.
Filming sequence
  1 film/sec. for eight seconds.
Comment: For evaluation of *paravertebral mass* lesions anteroposterior and/or a right posterior oblique or lateral projections should be obtained. For thromboembolic diseases only an anteroposterior projection is necessary. *Injection through both femoral veins* results in good mixing of the contrast and blood, avoids streamline flow or layering, and reveals unsuspected thromboembolic disease in the opposite common iliac vein. Very rarely a double inferior vena cava, if present, is also detected.

The Jugular Venous Route

This is used when the femoral veins are thrombosed or to demonstrate the proximal extent of an occlusion or tumoral thrombi in the inferior vena cava if the thrombus is completely occluding the cava. Either a straight catheter is used to inject into the inferior vena cava, or a catheter with side holes and no end holes is passed through a mylar sheath (Fig. 15-3) to inject into the right atrium.

Basilic or Antecubital Veins Venous Route

If for some reason the jugular vein cannot be reached, then a side hole blunt tipped catheter is used through a mylar sheath (Fig. 15-3) and placed to the desired level in the vena cava or right atrium.

Renal Veins

Catheter
  Shape
    End and side holes. Refer to Figure 17-1 [1, 2, 3, 4]).
  Size
    Adults: 7 or 8 Fr.
    Children: Smaller French size.

Contrast

Adults

24 to 30 cc over 2 to 3 sec.

Children

3-6 years, 6 to 8 cc over 1½ to 2 sec.

6-16 years, 8 to 18 cc over 1½ to 2½ sec.

Filming sequence

1 film/sec. for six to eight seconds.

Renal Phlebography with Pharmocologic Aids

A catheter is inserted via the femoral artery in the opposite groin into the desired renal artery, and epinephrine is injected intraarterially. This diminishes renal blood flow through the kidney and enhances venous visualization. The epinephrine is prepared by diluting one ampule of epinephrine (1:1000) containing 1 mgm of epinephrine in 250 cc of normal saline. This solution will yield 4 micrograms per cc of epinephrine. The *dose given into the arterial catheter is 0.2 mcgm per kilogram body weight up to 70 kilograms. For patients 70 kilograms or above, only 15 micrograms total dose of epinephrine is given.* The proper dose of epinephrine solution is injected into the corresponding renal artery over two to three seconds, and then the catheter is flushed with normal saline. *Fifteen seconds later,* the needed amount of *contrast is injected* into the corresponding renal vein.

Filming sequence

1 film/sec. for six to eight seconds.

Comment: If the catheter tip is in a *segmental vein,* the same amount of contrast is injected over a longer duration to perfuse the entire venous circulation of that kidney which occurs via intrarenal communications. The total amount of contrast used is in proportion to the volume of the kidney. The venous opacification may not be satisfactory if there is significant arterial venous shunting which may occur in malignancies such as hypernephroma. The presence of multiple renal arteries may pose a problem in obtaining total venous opacification in one composite roentgenogram.

Portal Venous System Via Splenic Artery Catheterization

Catheter

7 Fr. inserted into splenic artery.

Contrast

Adults

50 to 75 cc over 7 to 9 sec.

Children

3-6 years, 15 to 30 cc over three to five seconds.

6-16 years, 20 to 35 cc over four to six seconds.

Filming sequence

1 film every other second for thirty seconds.

Portal Venous System Via Superior Mesenteric Arterial Catheterization

Catheter

7 Fr. inserted into the superior mesenteric artery.

Contrast

Prescoline, 40 mgm diluted in 5 cc of saline is infused into the superior mesenteric artery over three to four seconds. The catheter is flushed with saline and twenty to thirty seconds later, 60 cc of contrast is injected into the superior mesenteric artery over a ten-second interval.

Filming sequence

1 film every other second for thirty seconds.

Hepatic Venogram

This potentially versatile study not only opacifies the hepatic vein, but lends itself to establish the abnormal physiology of the *hepatic sinusoidal circulation.* The pressure in this vascular bed reflects the altered hemodynamics and its effect on the entire splanchnic circulation. This route of trespassing has opened the avenue for opacification of the bile ducts.[14] In the same manner this route may sometime in the future open a path for creating portal systemic shunts. The route of entry is via the femoral vein or the right internal jugular vein. The femoral route is the more convenient and flexible for all of the studies, except for the bile ducts. The right internal jugular vein as a route is better for cholangiographic studies.[14]

Hepatic Venogram

Catheter
  Shape
    End and side holes (refer to Fig. 17-1 [1, 2, 3], 17-4).
  Size
    7 Fr.
Contrast
  15 cc over three seconds.
Filming sequence
  1 film/sec. for six seconds.

Comment: Using this method, only the trunk of the lobar vein catheterized is opacified.

Wedge Hepatic Venogram[296, 303, 304]

The femoral route is used.

Catheter
  Shape
    End hole only. (Fig. 17-1 [1, 2], 17-4).
  Size
    7 Fr. The tip is drawn over a .035 inch guide.
Contrast
  8 cc over four to six seconds.
Filming sequence
  1 film/sec. for eight seconds.
  1 film every two seconds for twelve seconds.

Comment: The catheter is advanced into the hepatic vein branches toward the small segments until the tip of the catheter gently impacts into the smallest tributary. Deeper negotiation may be achieved with the assistance of a floppy or deflector guide wire. Even a regular flexible guide wire with the flexible end as the leading segment, advanced only up to the tip of the catheter, may also be used. *Segmental withdrawal of the guide and simultaneous internal advancement of the catheter* may impact the tip into a tributary. At the same time, hepatic sinusoidal pressures[11, 298, 299] may be measured. This includes the wedge hepatic venous pressure (WHVP) and the free hepatic venous pressure (FHVP). *WHVP minus FHVP equals the corrected sinusoidal pressure* (CSP). Pressures may also be measured both in the right atrium as well as below the liver in the inferior vena cava.

WHVP − FHVP = CSP
Normal WHVP = 3 to 11 mm of Hg
Normal FHVP = 1 to 5 mm of Hg
Normal CSP = 5 mm of Hg
Mild portal hypertension: CSP = 6 to 14 mm of Hg.
Moderate portal hypertension: CSP = 15 to 30 mm of Hg.
Severe portal hypertension: CSP is greater than 30 mm of Hg.

The advantage[11, 298, 299, 301] of the *wedge hepatic venogram* is that it actually reflects the *sinusoidal pressure* and detects the presence and degree of *sinusoidal and postsinusoidal hypertension.* The wedge hepatic pressure is normal in presinusoidal type of portal obstructive disease.[302] It reveals the *patency of the portal vein* if it happens to be nonvisualized during arterial portography or percutaneous spleno-portography.[297, 304] It establishes the abnormal *direction of portal venous flow,* either hepatopetal or hepatofugal, thereby selecting eligible candidates for portal systemic shunts. Finally, *sinusoidal morphology* is well demonstrated.

Normally the wedge hepatic venous injection of contrast does not visualize the portal vein, but artefactual opacification may occur if undue force is exerted during injection. The flow, however, is antegrade in that portal vein with no evidence of stasis. *The WHVP is normal in presinusoidal type of portal obstructive disease.*[302] The *intrasplenic pulp pressure* measures the presinusoidal pressure (normal 3 to 13 mm Hg) which is elevated in presinusoidal and postsinusoidal types of obstructive diseases.[302] An absolute correlation may not be possible between the severity of the liver disease and the portal pressure, due to the variable efficiency of the collateral veins from one individual to another in decompressing the portal vein.[301] Inferior vena caval pressures obtained in the right atrium and in the inferior vena cava below the liver may show a significant gradient because of the constriction of the hepatic segment of the cava by a distorted regenerating liver.

Adrenal Venogram[417–419]

Catheter

Shape

End hole. The catheters for the right and left adrenal veins differ in their shape (Fig. 17-2 [1, 5], 17-5).

Size

7 Fr. with tips taped to .035 inch.

Contrast

4 cc over two seconds. One should decide the total amount of contrast after visualizing the size of the adrenal gland, as sizeable masses may require more than 4 cc of contrast.

Filming sequence

2 films/sec. for three seconds.

1 film/sec. for six to eight seconds. At times the oblique on the side of the adrenal may be necessary.

Comment: This is a very precise technique for localizing macroscopic endocrinal gland lesions. Arteriography, however, is still preferred for localizing and detecting vascular pheochromocytomas in intraadrenal as well as extraadrenal locations. Venography and venous sampling gain importance here if there is an infarcted or avascular pheochromacytoma or medullary hyperplasia. *Venography should not be undertaken without substantial clinical and laboratory evidence suggesting an adrenal lesion.*

The *right adrenal vein* is searched for in a meticulous manner at the lateral and posterior surface of the inferior vena cava above the renal vein at approximately the level between the twelfth thoracic and first lumbar vertebral bodies. Frequent test injections of small doses of contrast should be made. Accidental entry into the small retroperitoneal veins or hepatic veins is not unusual. Injection into the adrenal vein elicits a painful zonal somatic response which does not occur when the hepatic vein is perfused. When in doubt, a single film exposed after injection of contrast will reveal the true anatomy. The hepatic venous system has a herringbone-like pattern. When catheterizing the *left adrenal vein*, the same amount of contrast and filming techniques are employed (Fig. 3-22).

F. Extremity Venography

Like the arteries of the extremity, the *veins comprise a unit from their origin to their termination*, either from the inferior or superior vena cava.

Femoral Venogram

The most important aspects of venography are instantaneous, satisfactory opacification of the large venous pool to avoid the artefacts such as streamline flow and extrinsic pressure defects from muscles and fascia or the easy distal drainage through superficial system. The size of the subcutaneous needle used depends on the caliber and strength of the vein in the foot and its ability to withstand the pressure of injection. This may be tested by a forceful hand injection of saline. There should be at least four 14″ x 17″ films ready. *Two tourniquets* are very tightly applied, one above the ankle and one above the knee. Then 50 cc of contrast warmed to body temperature is injected as rapidly as possible. At the end of the injection of 40 cc, one film of the leg is exposed, and immediately after the entire injection is completed, a second film is exposed. The patient is immediately moved caudally to bring the thigh into the exposure area. *Both tourniquets are removed* as the third film is exposed. Finally, a fourth film may be exposed to try and visualize the pelvic area. It may sometimes be difficult to catch the contrast in the pelvic veins. Of course, every change of anatomical location requires a change in exposure technique. Delayed films may show thrombi, if any, in the veins.[292] At times venography may have to be obtained with flexion of the knee, as the plantaris muscle may cause extrinsic pressure on the vein, simulating an obstruction.[293] If the diagnosis is uncertain a repeat study is obtained in the lateral projection also.

Upper Extremity Venogram

This is performed using the techniques of lower extremity venography.

Azygos Venography

The unsung heroes of the venous system.

Catheter
Shape
End and side holes (Fig. 17-1 [2, 3, 4]).
Size
7 Fr. via the femoral vein.
Contrast
25 cc over five seconds.
Filming sequence
A/P and lateral projections
1 film/sec. for eight seconds.

Comment: Retaining its connection with the superior and inferior vena cava, *it lends its shoulder to support the superior, offers a hand to lift the inferior, and leans backwards to assist the portal circulation* during crises. This system is truly the *unsung hero* of the venous circulation. Yet studies of these veins are rarely indicated except in pulmonary malignancies or in the lymphoma group of diseases for evaluating the presence of *lymph node enlargement in the mediastinum.* The presence of azygos vein abnormalities in these situations may mean that a lesion is inoperable. The absence of findings, however, may not mean that the lesion is operable.

Both the azygos and hemiazygos system may be opacified simultaneously by introducing a catheter (Fig. 17-2 [3]) into each femoral vein, engaging the catheter tips into the ascending lumbar veins. Then 3 cc/sec. are injected into each for five seconds with serial filming of the chest area.

Gonadal Veins

Catheter
Shape
End and side holes. (Fig. 17-2 [6]).
The catheter is first inserted into the left renal vein and then advanced into the left gonadal vein.
Size
7 Fr.
Contrast
25 to 30 cc over five to six seconds.
Filming sequence
1 film/sec. for twelve to sixteen seconds.

Comment: Although radiologists are aware of the great potential of gonadal vein catheterization, most clinicians are not. For example, the diagnosis of tumors, venous sampling, or demonstration of pelvic varices and thromboembolic disease may be obtained.

The presence of valves in the proximal portion of the gonadal vein on the left may make catheterization time-consuming. If contrast is injected into the left gonadal vein there is invariably opacification of the right as well.

Jugular Veins

Catheter
Shape
End hole (Fig. 17-2 [3], 17-5).
Size
7 Fr.
Contrast
8 cc/sec. for two seconds.
Filming sequence
1 film/sec. for ten seconds (biplane) and preferably with a subtraction film.

Parathyroid Venography[386]

This is very useful for venous sampling and sometimes for detecting mass lesions of the parathyroid glands. Though time-consuming, it is highly rewarding. A catheter deflector system, or double catheter system[61] with a special "J" wire, has to be used for this study.

Thymic Venography

Catheter
Shape
End hole only (Fig. 17-2 [4, 5]).
Size
7 Fr. with tip drawn to .035 inches.

Contrast

12 cc over four seconds.

Filming sequence

1 film/sec. for eight seconds obtained in the A/P and lateral projections.

Comment: Though actual *histological interpretation is limited,* this study locates thymic masses if they are in the arborization of the thymic vein. Occasionally a venous sampling may be obtained from this vein to help localize a mediastinal parathyroid mass. The femoral vein is used with the catheter crossing the right atrial chamber and the tip is then manipulated toward the left innominate vein for the orifice of the thymic vein.

Internal Mammary Venography

The study is done in the same manner as the thymic venography. It may be helpful in evaluating lymph node masses when staging malignancies. It may be especially useful in staging breast malignancies.

CHAPTER 18

SPECIAL RECIPES—THE CORDON BLEU FOR ANGIOGRAPHERS

RENAL-HYPERVASCULAR MASSES (HYPERNEPHROMA)

When a *hypernephroma* is found, the following structures must be demonstrated to complete the study: (1) the tumor and its vascularity in its entirety, (2) the patency of that renal vein, (3) the status of the contralateral kidney, (4) demonstration of metastasis, if any. The study begins with a *flush abdominal aortogram* to demonstrate the number of renal arteries supplying that kidney, to obtain a preliminary idea about the vascularity of the mass, to see if there is any extraneous blood supply to the mass, and to evaluate for retroperitoneal satellite metastases. If, as determined by the flush aortogram, the lesion is hypervascular, then the straight catheter is exchanged for a curved renal catheter, and a *selective renal arteriogram* is done with 25 to 30 cc of contrast injected over five to six seconds. This *large bolus injection* is meant to opacify the tumor vasculature in its entirety, the renal vein and the inferior vena cava, and if possible to delineate any perinephric metastasis. The large bolus of contrast cannot do any more harm to the kidney than the cancer has already achieved. The film sequence for this study is two films per second for three seconds, and one film per second for ten to twelve seconds.

To rule out incidental, unsuspected lesions or to demonstrate any metastasis or a second primary, a *standard renal arteriogram of the contralateral side* is obtained. If magnification facilities are available, it is wise to use them when studying this kidney. Whether or not the angiographer evaluates the *liver for* evidence of hepatic *metastasis* depends in part on the philosophy of the surgeons practicing in that hospital and how they evaluate the rare favorable biological behavior of metastasis after the primary has been extirpated.

If involvement of the renal vein cannot be excluded by an antegrade injection of contrast into the arterial tree, then one is obliged to study the *inferior vena cava* and subsequently the renal vein to see if there is involvement of these structures by tumor thrombus. If the suprarenal portion of the inferior vena cava cannot be visualized, then that portion of the cava and *right atrium* should be opacified via injection *through the internal jugular or basilic veins.*

Special Situations

If a comparatively *hypovascular* or angiographically avascular mass is found after a flush aortogram or selective studies and a malignancy is still suspected, then the paired abdominal aortic branches such as the *lumbars, middle adrenals, and inferior phrenics* must be examined for abnormalities on the flush angiogram. If any of these vessels show any abnormality in their size or arborization, then that particular vessel must be selectively catheterized with the properly shaped tip; a standard angiogram, as previously described, should be done. It must be remembered that *so-called necrotic tumors have to beg, borrow or steal their nourishment from some vessels, somewhere or somehow.* A *renal venogram* showing occlusion or infiltration of the veins may aid in the diagnosis of an invasive, avascular mass lesion. *Epinephrine renal angiography* may be informative if there is a normal control angiogram and

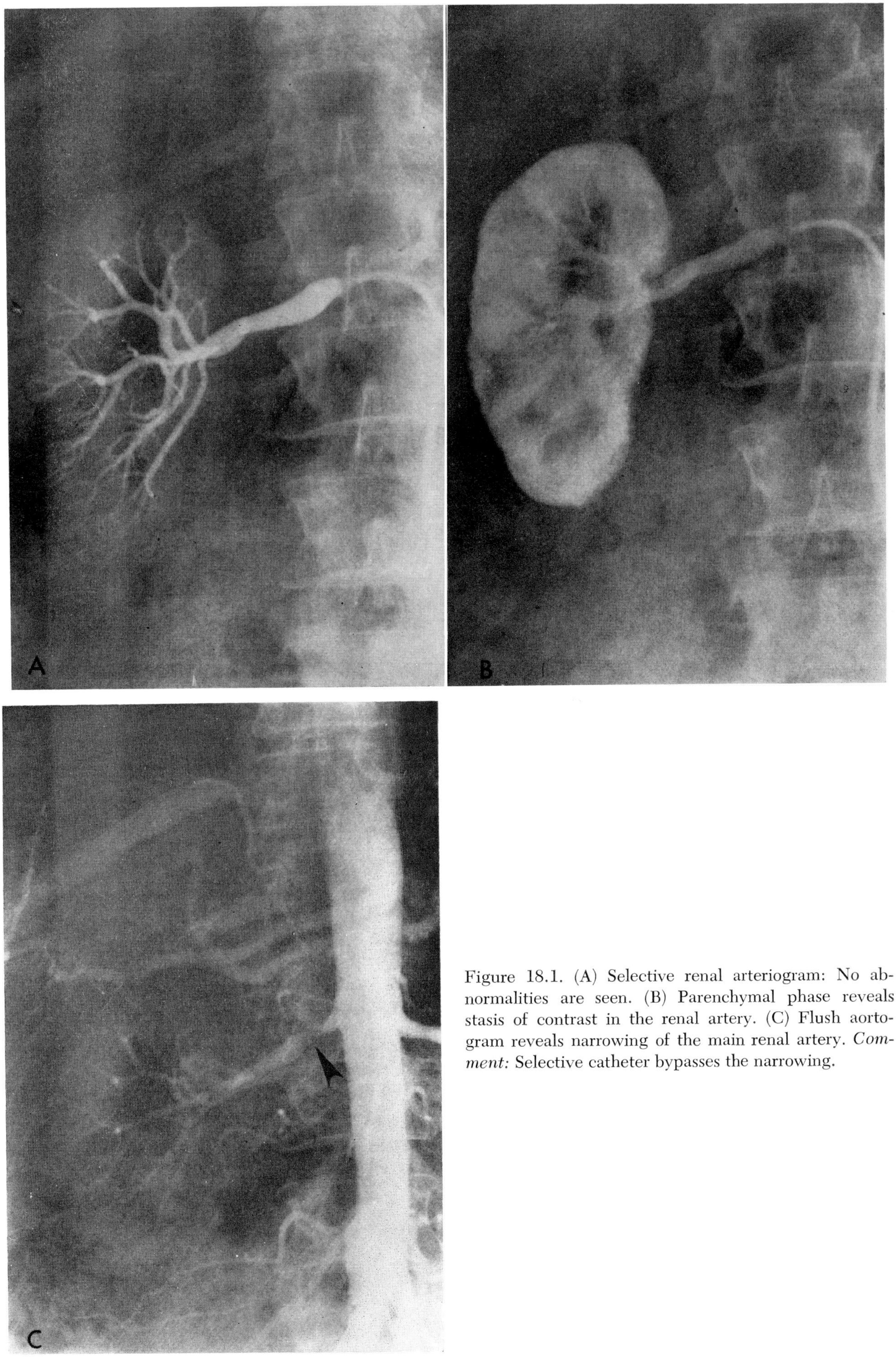

Figure 18.1. (A) Selective renal arteriogram: No abnormalities are seen. (B) Parenchymal phase reveals stasis of contrast in the renal artery. (C) Flush aortogram reveals narrowing of the main renal artery. *Comment:* Selective catheter bypasses the narrowing.

an abnormal postepinephrine angiogram. Twenty seconds after infusing that renal artery with epinephrine (0.2 micrograms per kg) a *standard* renal arteriogram is obtained with a slower injection rate and prolonged filming. Finally, if the nature of the mass lesion is still in doubt, a *percutaneous puncture* of the mass may be performed with aspiration of fluid and subsequent biochemical analysis.[305]

RENAL VASCULAR HYPERTENSION

This study is designed to demonstrate the *presence of anatomic lesions* in the renal vessels and the *functional significance* of these lesions, to evaluate *parenchymal* lesions and their significance in relationship to hypertension, and to determine any other unsuspected cause of hypertension.

Arterial Studies

A routine *flush abdominal aortogram* in deep inspiration[275] with a Fr. 6 or 7 pigtail catheter[38] is performed. This will demonstrate lesions at the origin of the renal arteries, visualize multiple renal arteries and their origins, define the perinephric area, delineate the status of the aorta for dissections, coarctations or aortitis and avoid the pitfall of spasm of the renal artery caused by selective catheter manipulation masquerading as an organic stenosis (Fig. 18-1). This also avoids the selective catheter tip bypassing a true stenotic lesion.

Projections

Apart from the standard *anterior/posterior projection, oblique* projections may have to be done to demonstrate variable origins of the renal arteries from the circumference of the aorta.[333] Because the renal arteries may arise either anterolateral or posterolateral from the margin of the aortic wall, the orifice may be hidden by the overlapping aortic wall on a flush angiogram. If the renal arteries arise anterolaterally, then that posterior oblique projection must be done, and if they arise posterolateral from the aortic wall, then that anterior oblique projection must be obtained. On occasion a prone aortogram may be needed to perfuse a renal artery which has an almost anterior origin from the circumference of the aorta (Fig. 18-2). After the abdominal angiogram, a *standard renal arteriogram* is performed for better demonstration of segmental vessels.

Venous Studies

Renal vein studies for assay of *renin* levels are done preferably at a separate sitting, or as the first part of the study to avoid the possibility of triggering the renin-angiotensin mechanism after intraarterial injection of contrast material.

Method: End hole renal vein catheter, Fr. 7 or 8 placed in the main branch of the renal vein beyond the origins of the tributary veins such as the gonadal or adrenals, especially on the left side. If more than one renal vein is found, the total amount of blood withdrawn is divided proportionately among the veins. Samples from the inferior vena cava are also obtained. Segmental renal vein samplings may be taken in cases of segmental arterial, or segmental parenchymal lesions.

Renal Vein Washout Time

This physiological test[276] demonstrates the rate of blood flow through the kidney and its relation to the presence of renal arterial narrowing involving the main artery or peripheral small vessels and the renal plasma flow. If there is significant renal arterial stenosis, the *normal one to three seconds* venous washout time is prolonged. *A prolonged washout time is also seen with profound arterionephrosclerosis without demonstrable main arterial lesions.* This is due to increased renin release from a kidney having nonstenotic, normal-looking vessels, with actual histological evidence of intrarenal arteriolar pathology.[277] This should further aid in determining the appropriate therapy.

This study is performed by injecting 15 cc of contrast into the renal vein in three quarters of a second. A cinevenogram is preferred. If not, two films per second for eight seconds are exposed.

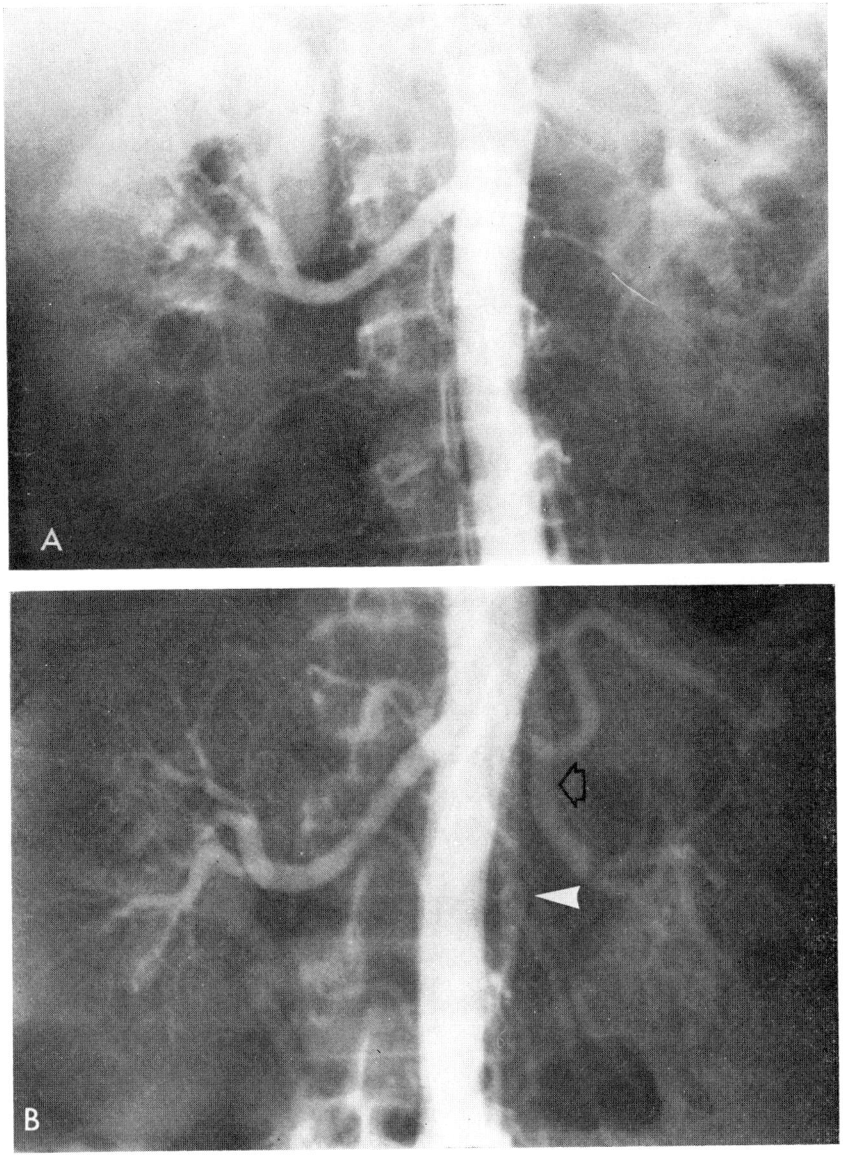

Figure 18.2. Abdominal Aortogram. (A) In the supine position the left renal artery and superior mesenteric artery do not visualize. (B) Prone Aortogram: Now there is filling of the left renal artery (Arrow) and superior mesenteric artery (Arrow Head) as they both have an anterior origin from the aorta in this patient. This young woman was being evaluated for hypertension. *Diagnosis:* Layering contrast due to gravity with nonvisualization of the left renal artery because of its anterior location. That is why it is seen only in the prone position.

Special Situations

Renal venography can be used to demonstrate *nonvisualized kidneys* arteriographically and pyelographically, with the intention of demonstrating the viability of nonfunctioning ischemic renal tissue.

Direct injection into the renal vein may show a renal vein stenosis as the cause of hypertension.[278] A cross-table lateral aortogram may be used to demonstrate occlusion or narrowing of the superior mesenteric artery origin and its relation to renal lesions and hypertension,[279–281] and also to show the celiac orifice to rule out splanchnic steal due to celiac occlusion and flow from the renal artery[282] via the inferior phrenic or capsular vessels.

Renal Vein Thrombosis

The involvement of the renal vein by thromboembolic disease is not only due to primary disease in the renal venous circulation, but may also be caused by disease extension from the inferior vena cava and its tributaries. The study is therefore incomplete unless the inferior vena cava and its conducting tributaries (common iliac veins) are opacified along with the renal vein.

Studies

A *standard inferior venacavogram* is performed, and if *the cava is free of thromboembolic disease, a renal vein catheter is advanced into the renal vein.* A total of 24 cc of contrast is injected over two seconds to opacify the venous circulation. If the opacification of the intrarenal veins is satisfactory, then the examination is terminated. If not, a renal arterial catheter is inserted from the opposite groin to obtain an *epinephrine renal phlebogram.* If the renal vein orifice cannot be located and is therefore totally obliterated, a *standard renal arteriogram* is obtained with an additional 4 to 6 cc of contrast injected, and the filming prolonged for an additional eight to ten seconds. This should demonstrate collateral perinephric venous drainage.

NONVISUALIZING KIDNEY

The causes of nonvisualizing kidneys include vascular insufficiency, hypoplasia or agenesis. The significance of a pyelographically nonvisualizing kidney increases if there is associated hypertension, hematuria or infection. Thus it is necessary to demonstrate both the cause of nonvisualization and the presence or absence of viable, ischemic, nonfunctioning renal tissue.

Studies

A routine *flush aortogram* to visualize the abdomen from the diaphragm to the symphysis pubis is performed. Failure to demonstrate renal vasculature, either from its conventional supply or collateral vessels, does not rule out the presence of renal tissue which may be fed by angiographically small inaccessible retroperitoneal vessels. Furthermore, lack of a conventional arterial supply may not deprive the kidney of its conventional venous drainage. Therefore, a *renal venogram* is obtained by direct injection into the renal vein. Absence of the renal vein also suggests absence of renal tissue. We learned about this entity after a young man, who had a pyelographically and arteriographically nonvisualizing kidney, happened to have a small but patent renal vein which drained that nubbin of renal tissue . . . *yesterday's mistake, tomorrow's curiosity.*

PANCREATIC MALIGNANCY

Besides the adrenal gland, the pancreas is probably the only organ which receives its blood supply from multiple sources. Let us forget about parathyroids for now. The pancreas, lying in front of the portal venous confluence, bordered by the great splanchnic vessels and their major branches with or without variations in their origins, is indeed *"nature's ecstasy; and the angiographer's agony."* This challenges the ability of the angiographer and the patience of the patient, and demands utmost sophistication of technical facilities. The confusion is increased by the similarity of abnormal angiographic patterns offered by a variety of disorders which mimic pancreatic carcinoma. This includes atherosclerosis, fibromuscular disease, pancreatitis, etc. Fortunately, the early clinical manifestations of lesions of the head of the pancreas and the late clinical presentation of lesions of the body and tail and its vascular invasiveness may make the situation easier for the angiographer, although not for the ailing. *A positive angiogram may ease the burden of diagnosis, while a negative study may haunt one until another explanation is found for the individual's complaint.*

Structures to Be Shown

1. The arterial supply of the area of the pancreas determined by the clinical find-

ings. Thus, with *obstructive jaundice,* the *head* must be demonstrated; with *backache and weight loss,* the *body and tail* must be demonstrated.

2. The venous confluence of the portal system must be demonstrated to delineate the *anatomic extent* of the lesions.
3. The *liver* must be visualized for primary or metastatic masses or to exclude cholangiocarcinoma, etc.
4. The size of the *gallbladder* must be determined.

Studies

1. A routine *celiac arteriogram* with a large volume of contrast (60 to 70 cc over six to seven seconds) is done to demonstrate the vascular road map and vessel variations and to visualize the splenic and portal veins, intrahepatic vasculature, and gallbladder. If the diagnosis and the anatomical extent of the lesion is established, the study may be discontinued. *If not. . . .*
2. A standard *gastroduodenal arteriogram* in the AP and/or RPO projection is obtained to show the vessels of the head of the pancreas.
3. A standard *splenic arteriogram* and, if possible, a *dorsal pancreatic arteriogram* is done to demonstrate the body and tail of the pancreas. Magnification facilities, if available, will aid in the establishment of the diagnosis.
4. A standard *superior mesenteric arteriogram* demonstrates its supply to the pancreas.
5. Finally, a *post-Prescoline superior mesenteric angiogram* will show the superior mesenteric vein and its confluence with the portal vein at the head of the pancreas.
6. Occasionally, a *selective inferior pancreatico-duodenal arteriogram* may have to be done if the celiac axis is occluded due to atherosclerosis, or infiltration by the malignancy.

Other Tumors of the Pancreas

Compared to the majority of pancreatic malignancies which are schirrous and invasive, the other pancreatic tumors are easily demonstrated by *standard celiac arteriography.* This is either due to bulk or abnormal vascularity as seen in cystadenomas, cystadenocarcinomas, anaplastic, medullary cancers of the pancreas, or due to discrete intense staining, which involves such endocrinal tumors as insulinomas or glucagonomas.

PORTAL HYPERTENSION

When evaluating patients with portal hypertension[11] one should try to establish the *location of the block,* either intra- or extrahepatic; *nature,* obstructive or nonobstructive; *type of venous flow,* hepato fugal or hepato petal; *patency of the portal,* superior mesenteric and splenic veins; presence or absence of esophageal varices; *status of the liver* in terms of hepatic vasculature for the magnitude of blood flow and for incidental mass lesions; and finally, *measurements of the sinuoidal pressures,* or postoperative evaluation of portal systemic shunts.

Studies

A *standard celiac arteriogram* or a hepatic arteriogram is done to evaluate the hepatic vasculature and/or hepatic masses. A *large bolus splenic arteriogram* is done for its venous phase to demonstrate the collateral circulation and patency of the splenic vein and the type of venous flow in relation to the liver. A *post-Prescoline superior mesenteric arteriogram* is done for its venous phase to demonstrate the patency of the superior mesenteric and portal veins and the direction of venous flow in relation to the liver. A *large bolus left gastric arteriogram* is optional for demonstrating the esophageal varices. A *wedge hepatic venogram* is done to demonstrate the type of venous flow in the portal vein and also to opacify a patent portal vein which may not have been opacified during arterial portography or during percutaneous splenoportography. *Hepatic venous pressure measurements* (free hepatic venous pressure and wedge hepatic venous pressure) are obtained to determine the corrected sinusoidal pressure necessary for the evaluation of the nature and severity of portal hypertension.

Postoperative studies are performed to evaluate the patency of surgical shunts via *post-Prescoline superior mesenteric arteriography.* In addition, an inferior vena cavogram, with or without selective catheterization of the shunt, may be done; and *pressure measurements* are made across the shunt to rule out any compromise of the newly created shunt.

JAUNDICE

If a patient is jaundiced, angiographic evaluation is used to demonstrate the nature of the lesion, *obstructive versus nonobstructive,* level of obstruction, if any; extent of the lesion in terms of operability; and etiology of the jaundice, if the histologic determination can be made. Prior knowledge of the available clinical and other roentgenographic information helps the angiographer to concentrate his attention to the area of suspicion.

The detection of the presence or absence of a *distended gallbladder* in a patient with jaundice can never be overemphasized, although it has some exceptions. The majority of the lesions which can cause the same clinical manifestations do occur around the head of the pancreas (ampulla of Vater, common bile duct or duodenum). The angiographic differentiation may be difficult, but at the present time it is mostly academic.

Studies

The same studies used to evaluate pancreatic malignancy are performed with particular attention paid to the head of the pancreas and the vicinity of the porta hepatis. Demonstration of the portal and superior mesenteric veins are vital to the diagnosis.

Standard Hepatic Arteriogram

This study is done to demonstrate *intrahepatic causes of jaundice* such as cholangiocarcinoma, hepatic masses, hemobilia, abnormalities of the choledochal apparatus such as cysts or diverticulum. It is also used to demonstrate the *size of the gallbladder.* The angiographic demonstration of a distended gallbladder when coupled with abnormal vascular changes in the vicinity of the pancreatic head lends moral support in establishing the presence and cause of obstructive jaundice distal to the formation of the common bile duct. But total dependency on the size of the gallbladder may lead one astray. The presence of *two odd lesions in the same individual* may result in diagnostic errors. For example, a normal pancreatic vasculature with previous hydrops of the gallbladder and recent nonobstructive jaundice, or a shrunken gallbladder due to previous inflammatory disease and a recent malignancy in the head of the pancreas obviously can present diagnostic difficulties. While confusion may be obviated, there is no diagnostic assistance to be gained when the gallbladder has been removed.

Cholangiogram

Either a percutaneous transhepatic or transjugular hepatic cholangiogram[14] represents the most definitive study for establishing the nature, location and cause of obstructive jaundice. The percutaneous technique has its associated risks; transjugular technique needs practice and may not be successful if the ducts are not dilated.

ABDOMINAL ANGINA

The only available *projection* to demonstrate the ostia and the proximal segments of the median unpaired visceral branches of the aorta (celiac superior mesenteric and inferior mesenteric arteries) is the *cross-table lateral abdominal aortogram* with a horizontal X-ray beam. The amount of contrast and the catheter are the same as those used for a standard flush abdominal aortogram. Depending on the patency of the origin of these vessels, further standard selective studies of the desired arteries may be obtained in the anterior/posterior projection. If the majority of the major splanchnic vessels are occluded, undue prolonged engagement of the catheter in the only feeding artery or *unnecessary excessive perfusion* of that vessel with contrast material may be *harmful.*

THORACIC OUTLET SYNDROME

Demonstration of the subclavian and axillary arteries is extremely important, not only with the arm in the *neutral position,* but also in the *desired stress position* as determined by a pre-angiographic clinical examination. A doubt rises in one's mind by lesions produced in such extreme physiological positions. Does an occlusion in a physiologic stress position definitely relate to symptoms? Perhaps it is like doing a toe-touch technique to demonstrate a hiatal hernia in many normal individuals.

Studies

First, an *aortic arch* in a right posterior oblique projection is obtained to exclude any other obstructing lesions. Then, after exchanging the aortic arch catheter for a selective one, a standard *selective subclavian arteriogram* is done. The subclavian arteriogram should be done both in the *neutral* position and in the *stress* position,[420] which clinically may cause dampening or absence of the radial pulse. The demonstrated vessels should include the subclavian and axillary arteries in their entirety.

Dissecting Aortic Aneurysm

The entire course of the variable extent of the dissection from its *origin* to its *termination* should be adequately shown to evaluate these patients. The *route of entry* is determined by the magnitude of the femoral and axillary pulses. As the *false lumen* of the dissection is usually on the *left* side, the left femoral or left axillary route is avoided if possible. A high-pressure retrograde injection into the false lumen may extend the dissection proximally and occlude the vessels of the aortic arch. The *right femoral route is* preferred with the intention of visualizing the entire aorta from one puncture site.

Studies

A standard aortic arch study is obtained in the right posterior oblique injection. The injection rate may have to be modified according to the diameter of the compressed true lumen and the velocity of flow in the false lumen.

Contrast. 50 cc to 75 cc of contrast material is delivered over three seconds, depending on the fluoroscopic observation made by test injection of contrast material.

Film sequence. Two films per second for four seconds, and one film per second for ten to twelve seconds. Provisions should be made to *include the proximal portion of the aortic arch vessels.* If the deflected intima is not shown in the right posterior oblique projection, then an anterior/posterior or left posterior oblique projection or even a lateral projection may have to be obtained at the same injection rate. Then the catheter is withdrawn to the level of the abdominal aorta and a standard abdominal aortogram is obtained with a lower injection rate if necessary.

The *abdominal aortic bifurcation* should be demonstrated if the distal extent of the dissection is not clear by this time. Occasionally it may be very difficult, or even impossible, to manipulate the catheter beyond the level of the diaphragm. This may be due either to the spiral nature of the dissection at this level or due to compression of the true lumen by a very distended false lumen. Aggressive manipulation at this juncture may result in the catheter's entering into the false lumen. *Intentional injection in the false lumen is not justified.* A test injection into the false lumen will reveal stasis, indicating to the angiographer exactly where the tip of the catheter is located. In this situation an abdominal aortogram is obtained with the existing catheter. Then a second puncture is made at the *right axillary route* for catheterization of the ascending aorta to opacify the ascending and the descending aorta. If manipulation of the catheter into the ascending aorta is difficult due to extension of the dissection into the innominate artery, then, as a last resort, *a standard intravenous aortogram* is obtained.

BLUNT ABDOMINAL TRAUMA

To evaluate this type of injury, a *flush abdominal aortogram* is performed for orientation. Then, depending upon the clinical and prior radiographic studies, the organ most likely to be injured is *selectively catheterized* and studied in detail. In individuals with left upper quadrant trauma, both the left kidney and spleen should be studied. In patients with right upper quadrant trauma, the right kidney and liver should be studied. These should be done on a routine basis to avoid overlooking an obscure traumatic lesion.

ABDOMINAL MASSES

If the anatomic origin of an abdominal mass is unclear, then a standard *flush abdominal aortogram* is obtained to evaluate for the presence of abnormal vessels or *hypertrophied vessels* coursing toward the mass. This helps to decide if further catheterization of these vessels for additional evaluation is necessary.

ACUTE GASTROINTESTINAL HEMORRHAGE

In cases of *hematemasis, celiac and superior mesenteric artery* catheterization is carried out with or without selective injection into the left gastric artery or gastroduodenal artery. In cases of *melena,* with or without bright red blood per rectum, *visceral branches* are catheterized in an *ascending order.* In other words, first the inferior mesenteric artery, then the superior mesenteric artery, and finally the celiac axis until the bleeding point is found. It is not unusual to find a bleeding duodenal ulcer without return from the nasogastric tube. Patients with cirrhosis may not only bleed from the varices, but may also bleed from the ulcers in the gastrointestinal tract.

ENDOCRINAL TUMORS

The main intention of angiography is to confirm the clinical suspicion of endocrinal tumor and find the anatomic location and number of lesions. *Venous assay* helps in evaluating the presence or absence of functioning endocrinal lesions confined to a specific anatomic location. Venous sampling to conduct an assay is very valuable in detecting *microscopic lesions* such as hyperplasia or tiny tumors which may not be discernable by venography or arteriography. The awareness of the presence of lesions in the nonendocrinal organs producing hormones will prevent embarrassing and tragic end results. For example, hypernephromas which produce hypercalcemia, sarcoidosis with hypercalcemia or Cushing's syndrome due to carcinoid or oat cell tumor of the lung.

PHEOCHROMOCYTOMA

The preangiographic use of *Dibenzyline*® (20 to 100 mg twice daily) until the individual is normotensive (usually three to seven days) and a *decrease in the concentration of the contrast* used have decreased the mortality during angiographic procedures.[295] The same precautions are used as for an aortic arch study. We usually have an *anesthesiologist* or internist *in the* immediate *vicinity* to assist us in case of a hypertensive crisis.

Studies

A flush abdominal aortogram to opacify the upper abdomen and pelvic structures is done first. If this does not reveal any abnormalities, then a *thoracic flush aortogram* is also obtained. If these studies adequately establish the diagnosis, the examination may be discontinued as selectively injecting contrast into the tumor may provoke a hypertensive crisis. If the arteriogram is negative, yet there is a high clinical index of suspicion, the angiographer should obtain *venous sampling* from the adrenal veins and an adrenal venogram to demonstrate avascular[27, 28] or partially infarcted[26] pheochromocytomas, or medullary hyperplasia.[22]

BUDD CHIARI SYNDROME

The number of etiologies for this syndrome are numerous, so it is the responsibility of the radiologist to demonstrate not only the presence of hepatic venous obstruction, but also the etiology.

Studies

An *inferior vena cavogram* to include the junction of the inferior vena cava and right atrium is performed first. If the vena cava is patent, then a *selective hepatic venogram* is performed. If the cava is obstructed at the hepatic segment, the presence of the anatomic lesion is established.

If the hepatic veins are thrombosed and cannot be catheterized, a *hepatic arteriogram* for indirect demonstration of the signs of hepatic venous occlusion and the presence or absence of hepatic masses, if any, is performed. Finally, an *intraparenchymal injection* of contrast into the liver may be done to demonstrate occlusion of the hepatic veins as well as the route of blood flow.[499, 500]

Comment

The causes of the Budd Chiari syndrome may be primary, such as hepatic venous occlusive disease, or secondary due to masses in the liver, or in the vicinity of the inferior vena cava, or tumor thrombi extending from adjacent organs via the inferior vena caval tributaries. Therefore, after establishing the presence of the anatomical lesion, further catheterization of other indicated vessels may be obtained to delineate the pathology further.

PART III
PATTERNS

CHAPTER 19
NORMAL PATTERNS

THE MAJOR ARTERY to an organ enters that organ through the hilus and then breaks up into smaller branches with a certain inherent pattern of arborization, constituting the intrinsic parenchymal vasculature. When contrast is injected intraarterially, it perfuses an organ via the major artery, passing through ultimate units of the arterial circulation to exit *via the veins through the same hilus.* The only exceptions to this pattern are the adrenal gland and pancreas.

In *cortico-medullary type of circulation* there is an increased blood flow to the cortex compared to the flow to the medulla (renal, adrenal). During stress there is an increase in flow to the adrenal cortex and a decrease to the renal cortex due to different physiological functions.

STAINING

Normal staining of parenchyma, mucosa, or the wall of tissue depends on the amount of contrast being perfused, which in turn depends on the amount of blood flowing through that circulatory bed. Regardless of the reason underlying the staining of normal tissue after contrast injection (capillaries, sinusoids, pulp, extracellular fluid[1481] or lymphatics), the stain disappears in a reasonable interval of time. This time variance depends on the volume and duration of injection, providing there is no "exit" problem. The homogeneity of the obtained stain depends on the integrity of the normal tissues present. Normal staining can be *enhanced* by the use of intraarterial vasodilators. Conversely, it can be *decreased,* or even eliminated, by using vasoconstrictors. The use of unreasonably large amounts of contrast to obtain a good stain may endanger the tissues involved. Staining of muscle tissue is not usually seen in spite of higher concentrations acquired during intravenous injection of contrast.[1481]

Composite staining of the entire organ is not always possible when there are multiple arterial supplies, unless a large amount of contrast is used with a high rate of injection. This is true for the pancreas and adrenal gland. This does not apply to organs with end artery types of circulations.

Since the staining of an organ or tissue depends on the perfusion of the entire circulatory complex, it is not seen after selective intravenous injections. The exception to this is the portal circulation with its double capillary bed. Stain of a normal structure may also be diminished or absent when there is precapillary arteriovenous shunting of sufficient magnitude and at various levels.

The intensity of venous opacification after arterial injection of contrast is a reflection of the intensity of the parenchymal stain. Different factors may prevent good opacification of the vein. For example, during a hepatic arteriogram, the contrast in the hepatic venous blood is diluted by the nonopacified portal venous blood; therefore hepatic veins are usually not visualized. In the renal circulation part of the injected contrast is excreted before it ever reaches the veins.[266]

CHAPTER 20

DISEASES OF THE VASCULAR WALL

A. Arteriosclerosis
   1. Atherosclerosis
   2. Medial calcific sclerosis
   3. Arteriosclerosis
B. Arteritis (Takayasu, or idiopathic)[624-627]
C. Necrotizing angiitis[608, 609]
   1. Polyarteritis nodosa
   2. Drug abuse and necrotizing angiitis[612]
   3. Lupus vasculitis[615]
   4. Hypersensitivity angiitis
   5. Wegner's granulomatosis
   6. Postsurgical[617]
   7. Idiopathic[616]
D. Fibromuscular dysplasia[628, 632, 633]
   1. Intimal fibroplasia
   2. Medial fibroplasia with aneurysm
   3. Medial fibromuscular hyperplasia
   4. Subadventitial fibroplasia
   5. Adventitial (periarterial fibrosis)[634] fibroplasia

Atherosclerosis

This is a disseminated, generalized disease involving the whole arterial tree with a *patchy* distribution.[111, 637, 638, 641-643] This may be segmental or diffuse. The lesions may occur as early as the fourth decade of life.

The predominating lesions of atherosclerosis are *raised plaques and fatty streaks.* The raised plaques occur at sites of turbulent flow such as the orifices of the branches from the abdominal aorta. The flat, fatty streaks occur where shearing strains are higher, such as the thoracic aorta. All lesions begin in the intima and as they progress and extend, affect the media. The threat of the disease lies in the secondary complication that can develop. *Hemorrhage* may occur into the atheroma causing ballooning; *ulcers* discharging their debris into the bloodstream cause embolization to vessels of variable caliber and secondary thrombosis.

In addition, *weakening of the media* due to injury of the fibromuscular elastic layer and weakening of the adventitia due to fibrosis cause secondary *dilatation* of the wall.

Although uncomplicated atheromas rarely cause total occlusion, *occlusion* ultimately occurs when they become ulcerated and superimposed by thrombosis. Thus, one must understand the unpredictable nature of the effects of atherosclerosis on the caliber of the vessel. It may be *unchanged, severely narrowed, totally occluded, or dilated.* The ultimate effect in any given instance depends on the balance between a number of factors, including the status of the blood pressure, medial damage, predisposing factors for formation of thrombus and its incorporation into the arterial wall, and the available external support to the vessels.

Sites of Involvement

The *conducting arteries* such as the aorta, iliac, femoral and popliteal arteries tend to be involved in either a *patchy* or *diffuse* manner. The *distributing vessels* such as the renals, celiac, mesenteric, or profunda femoris are usually involved *proximally* at their orifices. Certain areas of the vascular tree are more susceptible to the development of atheromatous plaques than others. *Factors* include:

1. *The nonyielding nature of the walls to the effect of pulsation.* An example is the posterior wall of the abdominal aorta whose pulsations are dampened by the spine, or the fixed nature of the superficial femoral artery at the adductor (Hunter's) canal.
2. *Repeated mechanical stress* in which fre-

quent bending or rotational movement may cause a change in the direction of blood flow resulting in turbulence. Examples include the origin of the common femoral artery at the hip, superficial femoral artery at the adductor canal, the popliteal artery at the knee joint, or the vertebral artery in the neck or before entering the bony canal.

3. *Changes in the direction of dynamic flow at either* right angled branches or arterial bifurcations. Examples include the proximal portion of the internal iliac artery and the distal portion of the superficial femoral artery as it changes direction from the adductor canal to the popliteal fossa.

Blood vessels which are considered a continuation of the parent vessels are relatively immune.[639] This includes the right common carotid artery as an extension of the innominate or the external iliac artery as a continuation of the common iliac. Some vessels show stenosis due to plaques predominately in their proximal segments. This includes the innominate, subclavian, vertebral, and left common carotid arteries. In others, such as the right common carotid artery, plaques predominate in the distal segment. The carotid sinuses are more affected than the cervical portion of the internal carotid arteries. The vertebral arteries show a decreased prevalence of severe disease, but an increased prevalence of stenosis. *By and large, distributing arteries are relatively free from disease in their distal portions and remain patent.* This may hold true long after the occlusion of the parent vessel. Examples include narrowing of the celiac and mesenteric arteries within 1.5 cm of their orifices,[640] and the orifices of the lumbar and intercostal arteries and of the profunda femoris.

Angiographically, there is little correlation between the clinical symptoms and the progression of the disease. There is uniform progression of the disease proximally, but rarely distally. Distal progression is more hazardous as it may involve the collateral vessels.[646] The occluded vessels neither recanalize nor widen.[646] It may not be a surprise to witness more lesions at autopsy than angiographically.[644, 645]

Medial Calcific Sclerosis

This occurs mostly in *muscular arteries of medium or smaller size* without encroachment upon the lumen of the vessel.[111] The femoral, radial, ulnar and tibial arteries are those most commonly involved.

Arteriosclerosis

This[111] involves the *small arteries* and *arterioles* with thickening of their intima and fibromuscular tissues.

ARTERITIS

This[624–627] includes aortitis, Takayasu's arteritis, and giant cell arteritis (superficial-temporal arteritis).[622, 623] The most frequent victims of this process are *young women*. Of unknown etiology, this group of diseases is characterized by *patchy* and *diffuse* involvement of the aorta and its branches, occurring anywhere from the aortic valve to the bifurcation of the abdominal aorta. Even the pulmonary arteries do not escape involvement.[621] Most of the symptoms are due to the involvement of the ostia of the branches and further extension. This disease is characterized by *panarteritis* with intimal proliferation, with or without thrombi and organization, which results in *stenosis* and *obstruction* with a characteristic *flame-shaped* thrombosis. There may be a *patchy destruction of the media* and even complete absence of the media in certain areas, causing *aneurysmal dilatation*. Irregular, wavy thickening of the adventitia reflects in a wavy roentgenographic shadow on the plain films of the chest.

Superimposed atheroma may cause more damage and change the roentgenographic appearance. Involvement of the superior and inferior vena cavae are not uncommon. Aortic insufficiency[620] or coarctation of the aorta[619] may add more insult to the already damaged great vessels. During the active stage of the disease, the erythrocyte sedimentation rate and "C" reactive protein may be elevated aiding in establishing the diagnosis.[618]

NECROTIZING ANGIITIS

This cluster of similar diseases have the same pathologic lesions afflicting the *muscular, medium small arteries, arterioles,* and *capillaries* of different areas.[111, 608–611] In some cases it is a reoccurring disease, in others it is self-limiting with predilections for certain organ systems. The basic pathology is a necrotizing angiitis. The spectrum may vary from pure angiitis to necrosis or granuloma formation.

Polyarteritis Nodosa

This *disseminated* vasculitis is characterized by focal, random and episodic necrotizing inflammation of the walls of medium and small size arteries. It mainly involves the *arterial bifurcations and branching areas.* There is progressive proximal and even distal extension of the lesions with associated involvement of the adjacent small veins as well. The pathologic lesions[111] depend on the stage of recognition. During the *acute stage,* inflammatory edema and exudate cause *narrowing* of the arterial lumen and *blurring* of their margins. These acute lesions may progress to *thrombosis* and *total occlusion. Fibrinoid necrosis* of the wall, either partial or circumferential, with destruction of the internal elastic lamina may cause the formation of *aneurysms.* In the *chronic form* it may progress to granulation tissue formation, collagenization, and even total obliteration. *Lesions of varying ages,* acute, chronic or healed, may be found in the same individual. There is a *predilection* for the involvement of vessels of the gastrointestinal tract, mesentery, liver, kidney, pancreas, lung or muscles. Almost any other vessel including the lumbar, intercostal and inferior phrenic arteries may be involved.[675, 676]

Drug Abuse Necrotizing Angiitis

Lesions resemble that of polyarteritis nodosa with more or less the same predilection and distribution of organ systems.[612–614] However, all *lesions are of the same age* since the disease is related to usage of a specific drug.

Lupus Vasculitis

There is diffuse irregularity of the small vessels of the superior mesenteric artery branches.[615]

Hypersensitivity Angiitis

This mainly involves the *intrinsic vasculature* of the heart and lung and progresses proximally with marked necrosis and thrombosis. Aneurysm formation is unusual.

Wegner's Granulomatosis

This necrotizing vasculitis has great affinity for the *small arteries and arterioles* of the kidneys, lungs, and upper respiratory tract.

Idiopathic

This is a disseminated focal arteritis of the *large and medium size vessels.* It occurs from the second to fourth decade. Multiple false aneurysms due to the focal arteritis are common.[616]

Postsurgical Angiitis

When the splanchnic vessels are exposed to high blood pressure, as occurs during surgical correction of a thoracic aortic coarctation, the small arteries and arterioles respond to the stress by way of necrotizing reaction and occlusion.[617]

FIBROMUSCULAR DYSPLASIA

This group of related, but nonatherosclerotic arterial lesions produce disruption and hyperplastic changes in the arterial wall.[628, 632, 633] The results are *narrowing, or narrowing and dilatation* of the involved vessel. Classification is according to the dominant layer of the arterial wall involved. Thus the *intima, media, or adventitia* may be the site of abnormality. *Women* are more frequently affected than men. It occurs predominantly in the distal two thirds of the renal artery and its branches. There is, however, a lower incidence of involvement of other arteries, such as the aorta,[629] external iliac, celiac, internal carotid,[630] and vertebral arteries.[631] Though most common in young people, newborns are not immune either.[636] The relationship of this disease to renovascular hypertension is fascinating when the renal arteries are involved.

The radiographic appearance of these disorders depends on the amount of *hyperplasia* causing *stenosis* or *thrombosis,* or the degree of *destruction* of the *internal elastic lamina* which causes *aneurysmal* dilatation. The added complication of *dissection* of the diseased arteries again is dependent upon the *integrity of the internal elastic lamina.* Therefore, any one of these appearances, or all, may be seen in the vasculature, depending on the type of involvement.[632, 633]

Intimal Hyperplasia

The age group involved ranges from eighteen months to forty-eight years. Fibrous intimal hyperplasia causes *smooth stenosis.* If the elastica is destroyed, then simple *aneurysms* or dissecting hematomas, causing irregular dilatation of the artery, may develop. Total occlusion of vessels can occur. This entity *cannot be differentiated* radiographically from the *fibromuscular type* of hyperplasia.

Medial Fibroplasia with Aneurysms

This occurs in people from thirty to sixty years of age. Thick ridges of collagen and muscle alternate with intervening areas of intimal and medial destruction, leaving only the adventitia to support the wall. Thus the appearance radiographically is of areas of *narrowing and dilatation,* giving a *string of beads* appearance to the vessel. The aneurysmal dilatations (beads) are wider than the diameter of the un-

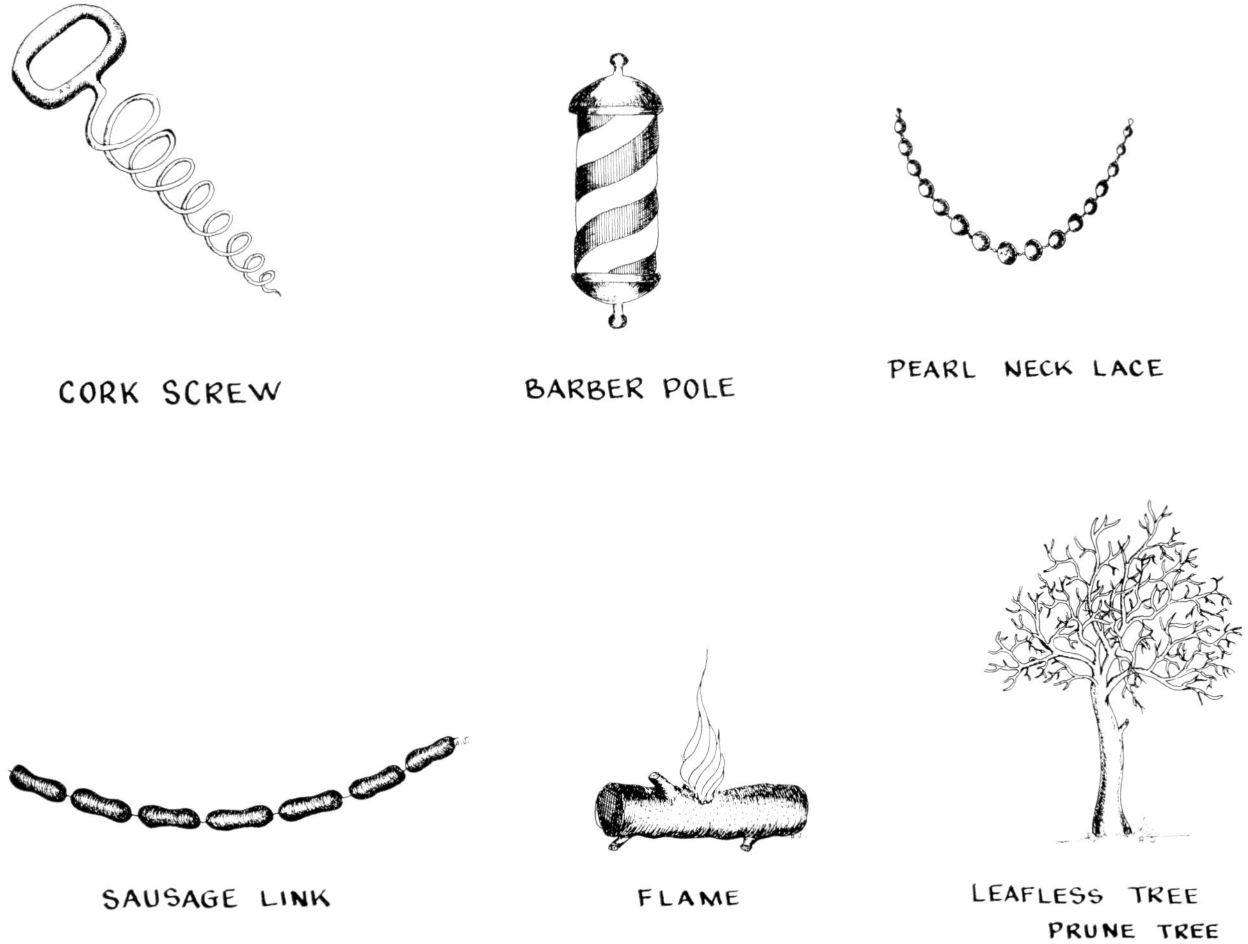

Figure 20.1. The patterns.

affected arteries unlike in subadventitial fibroplasia. Thrombosis and dissection do not occur, nor is it usual for the disease to progress after age forty. This is unlike its other related hyperplastic disorders.[635]

Medial Fibromuscular Hyperplasia

This occurs from childhood until about age forty-five. A rare lesion of this group can affect the proximal segment of the vessel (renal artery) also. Increased fibromuscular components causes *smooth stenosis.* If the internal elastica is destroyed, then *aneurysmal dilatation* may be seen. Dissection of the involved vessel can occur. From a radiographic point of view this entity *cannot be differentiated* from *intimal type* of fibroplasia.

Subadventitial Hyperplasia

This primarily involves young people. There is dense collagenous thickening of the outer media of the vessel of varying degrees and lengths, causing *stenosis.* However, thrombosis of the involved vessel is rare, and dissections are unlikely.

Adventitial (Periarterial Fibrosis) Hyperplasia

There is fibrous thickening of the adventitia and periarterial structures which causes *stenotic lesions* of the vessels.[634]

CHAPTER 21
DILATATION*

THE SPECTRUM of vascular lesions dealt with in the following chapters on dilatation, narrowing, narrowing and dilatation, and occlusion may be the end result of certain vascular disorders; or they may be a phase, however, in the life cycle of these disorders, either individually or collectively, occurring in various branches of the vascular tree at the same or different times.[650–652] Some, such as *atherosclerosis,* have a greater predilection for large and medium *conducting* arteries of an *elastic* nature. Others, such as *angiitis* or the *fibromuscular disorders,* tend to involve only the distributing arteries of medium and small caliber. These are the muscular arteries. Some diseases such as *aortitis* or *arteritis* may involve both types.

* Note: In this and following chapters, when the radiographic diagnosis concurred with the pathology, only one title, *Diagnosis,* has been used in the legends.

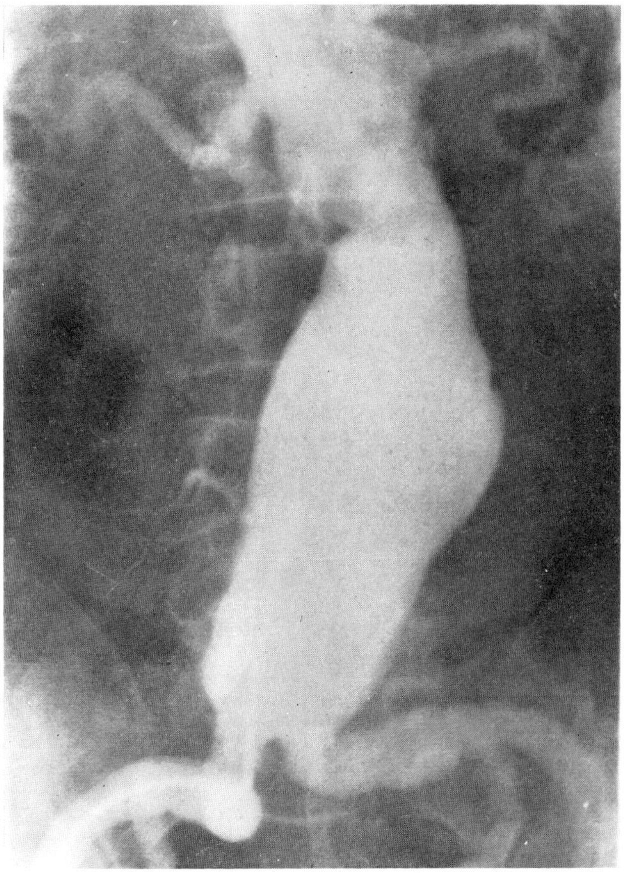

Figure 21.1. Abdominal Aortogram. Note the fusiform dilatation of the infrarenal abdominal aorta. *Diagnosis:* Arteriosclerotic aneurysm.

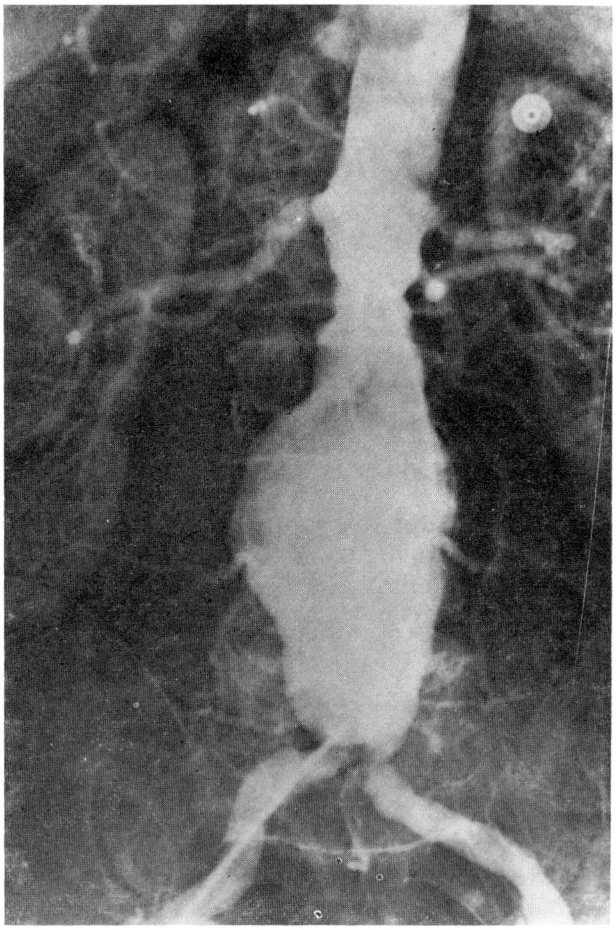

Figure 21.2. Abdominal Aortogram. There is fusiform dilatation of the infrarenal portion of the abdominal aorta. Contour defects are seen in the lumen. *Diagnosis:* Atherosclerotic abdominal aortic aneurysm.

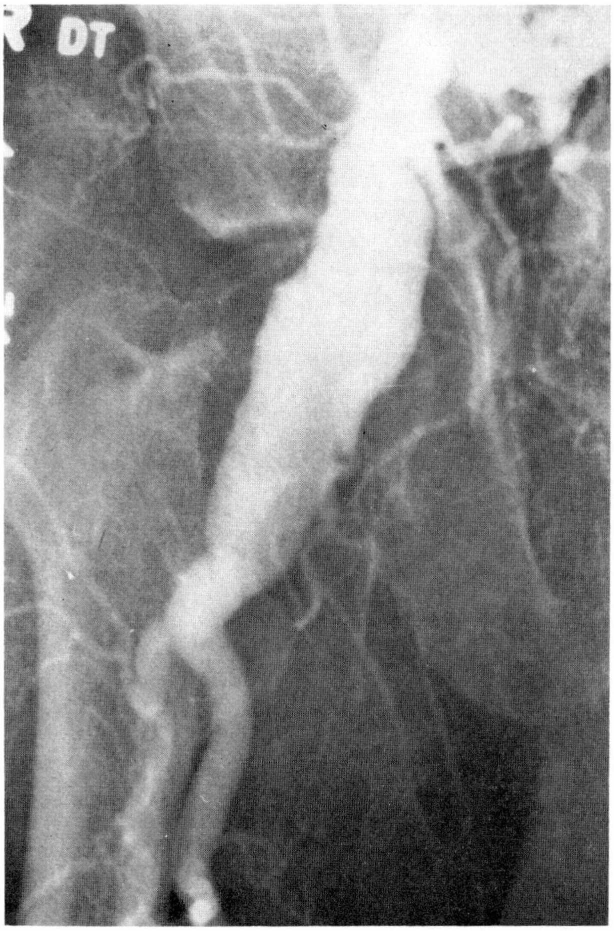

Figure 21.3. Femoral Arteriogram. There is fusiform dilatation of the common femoral artery without visualization of the superficial femoral artery. *Diagnosis:* Atherosclerotic aneurysm of the femoral artery with atherosclerotic occlusion of the superficial femoral artery.

PATHOLOGY

Dilatation of a vessel can be diffuse, segmental, fusiform or saccular. In old age, replacement of elastic tissue with fibrous tissue causes stretching and diffuse dilatation of the vessel. *Damage to the medial elastic layers* from spirochaetes, atherosclerosis, trauma, infection, necrotizing diseases, or collagen diseases leaves only the adventitia to support the arterial wall.[648, 649] Nature surrounds this area with fibrotic reaction and lines it with thrombus. Ischemic liquefaction of the laminated thrombus results in further weakening of the vessel wall with *subsequent enlargement and rupture.*

The initiating factor in the development of an aneurysm may be an area of proximal stenosis in the arterial lumen imposed by segmental atherosclerosis or fibrosis. Through this narrowed area a high velocity stream of blood flows into a normally distensible distal segment of the artery or into a weakened segment of the artery. A localized dilatation beyond the stenosis is thus produced. Lateral pressure relentlessly repeating with each systolic thrust produces structural fatigue and progressive dilatation, and even rupture.[647] Aneurysms may be single or multiple. A majority of aneurysms occur in a segment of an artery between two areas that are relatively fixed.[653] Common sites of aneurysms associated with the abdominal aortic ones may be in the thoracic aorta or the femoral or the popliteal arteries.[654] The high incidence of abdominal aortic aneurysms may be due to a relative decrease of the vasa vasorum in the abdominal aortic wall.[655] *Fusi-*

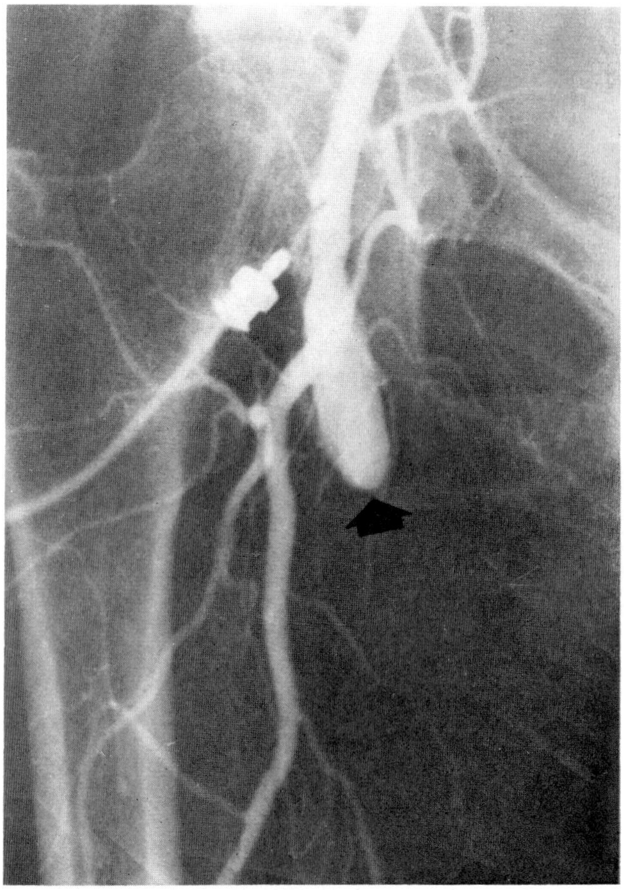

Figure 21.4. Femoral Arteriogram. Superficial femoral artery is dilated and totally occluded. *Surgical Diagnosis:* Thrombosed aneurysm.

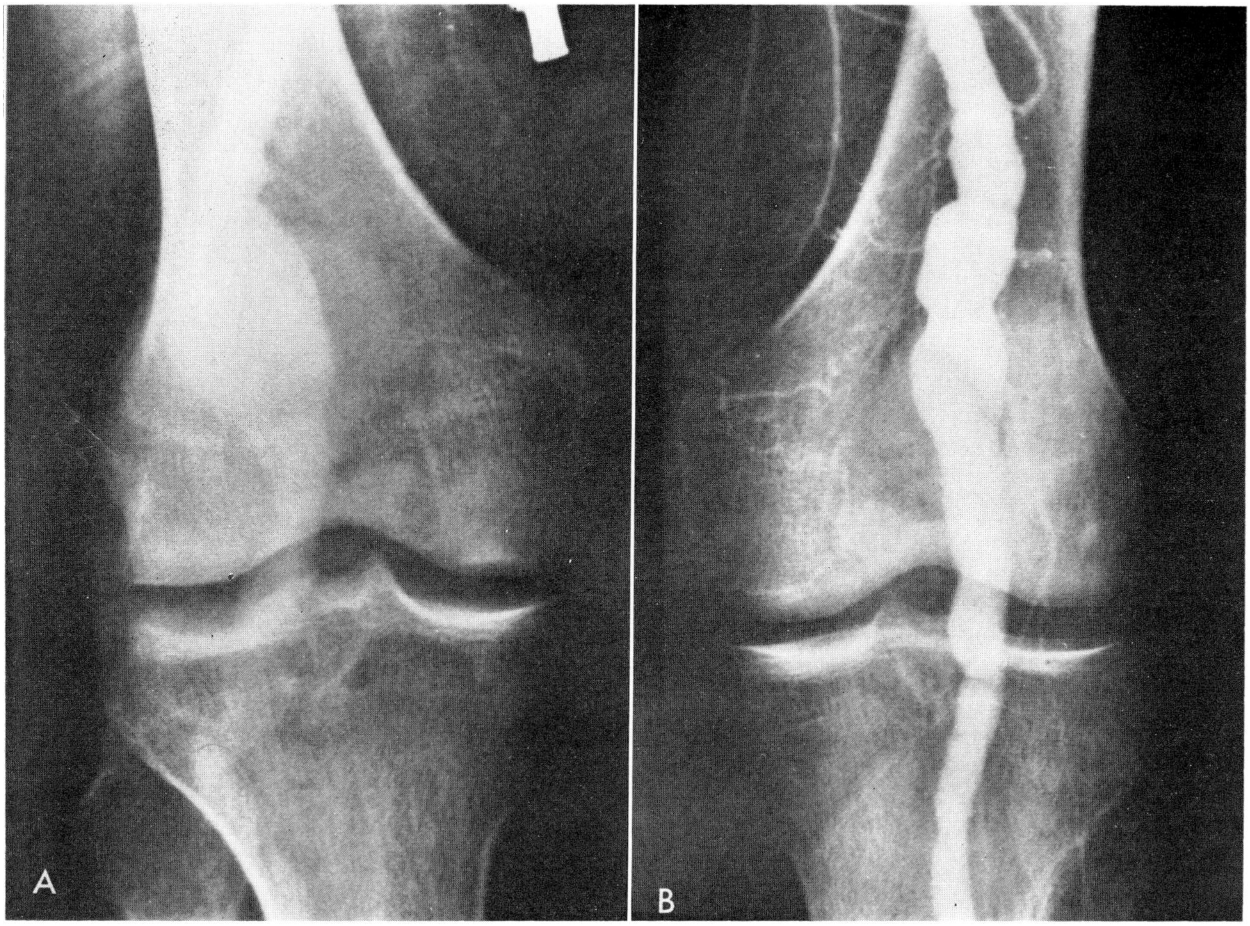

Figure 21.5. Bilateral Femoral Arteriogram. (A) Left side. (B) Right side. The distal femoral arteries are dilated and there is increased dilatation at the junction of the superficial femoral and popliteal arteries. *Diagnosis:* Aneurysmal dilatation superimposed on ectatic vessels.

form atherosclerotic abdominal aortic aneurysms usually occur below the level of the origin of the renal arteries. *Syphilitic aortic aneurysms,* usually saccular, are found primarily in the thoracic aorta and in the abdominal aorta above the level of the renal arteries.[642]

Effects of a Large Aneurysm

Unlike small aneurysms, large ones have a different whirl zone due to their size.[656, 657] They *may absorb all the blood supply,* causing transient ischemia to an important organ such as the kidney. On the other hand, they may *compress* the adjacent vessels and diminish distal circulation. Depending on their location, they may *rupture* into an adjacent vein creating an arteriovenous fistula, or into the gastrointestinal tract, biliary tree, pancreatic duct, peritoneal cavity, retroperitoneal space, or pleural cavity. The aneurysm may *completely thrombose* and curtail the circulation distal to that point. *Mural thrombi* in these aneurysms may dislodge and send off distal emboli causing symptoms while the aneurysm itself remains silent. There is a high incidence of rupture of larger aneurysms, particularly those greater than 5 cm in diameter.[658, 659] Also noteworthy is the high incidence of distal thromboembolic disease in smaller peripheral aneurysms.[660]

Radiographic Findings

In most cases there is obvious opacification of the fusiform or saccular aneurysms. *Stasis* of contrast in saccular aneurysms helps in bet-

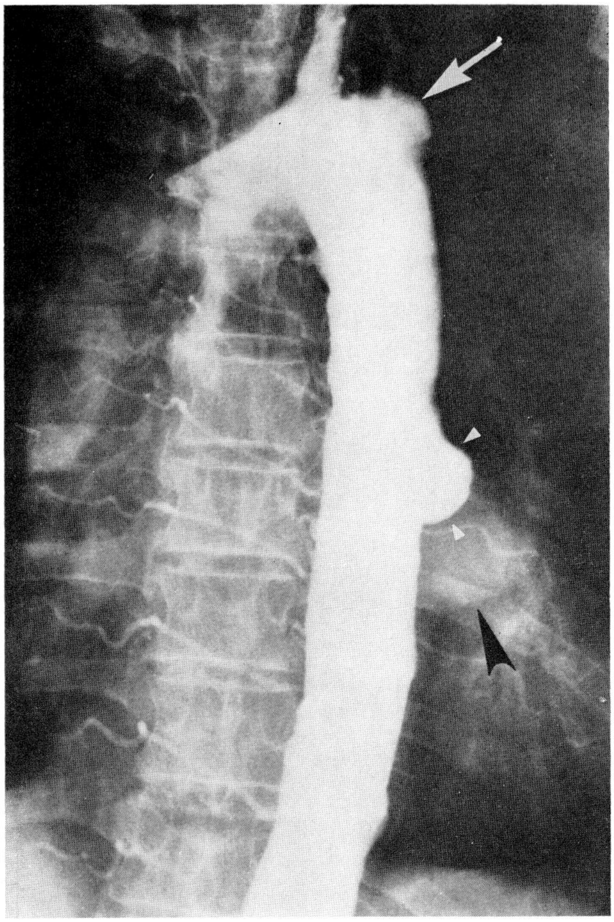

Figure 21.6. Thoracic Aortogram. There is a saccular collection of contrast along the left lateral border of the aorta (White Arrowhead), with a soft tissue density contiguous with it (Black Arrowhead). ***Diagnosis:*** Atherosclerotic aneurysm of the thoracic aorta with a thrombus along the wall. Note another aneurysm from the arch of the aorta (Arrow).

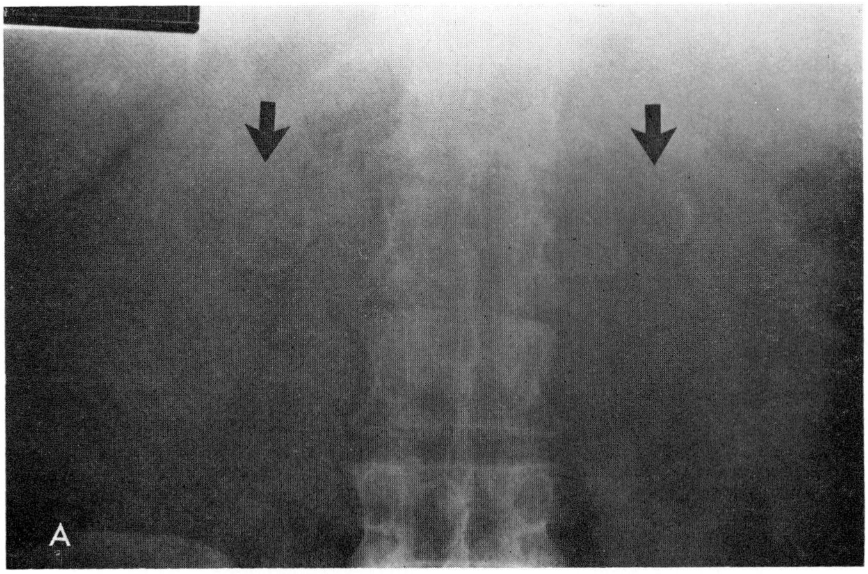

Figure 21.7 A *(Continued on next page)*

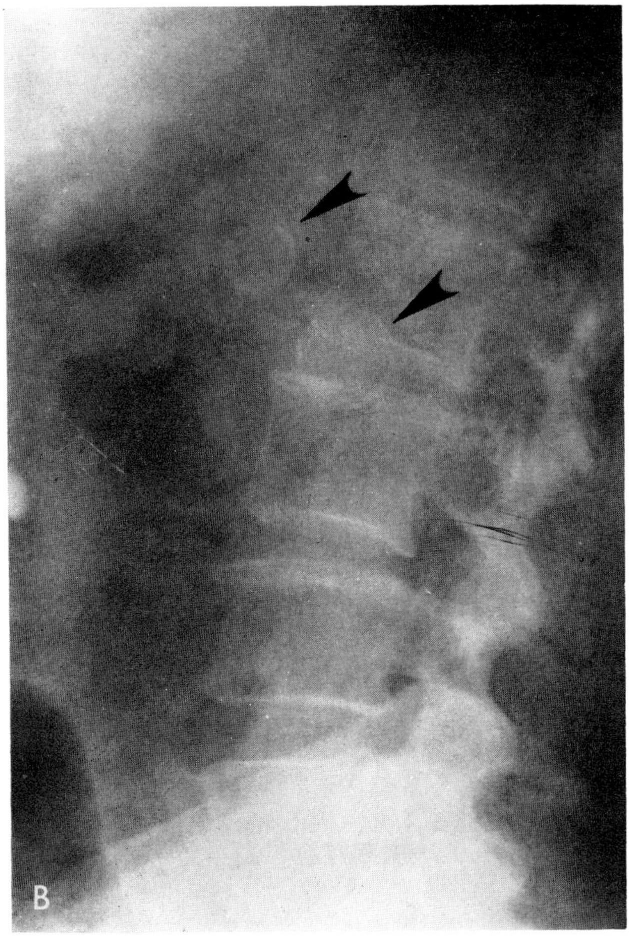

ter delineating these areas. If there are significant layers of thrombi in the aneurysms, the entire anatomical extent of the aneurysm may not be evident. Finally, if the aneurysm, either saccular or fusiform, is filled with sufficient layers of thrombi, the aneurysm may not opacify at all! Then indirect signs such as stretching and deviation of the adjacent vessels are sought. Simultaneously opacified channels of a dissecting hematoma may resemble a fusiform dilatation of the involved vessel; as an example, the aorta or renal artery.[550, 632] *Vessel kinks* may resemble an aneurysm which can be resolved by obtaining a different projection of that vessel. Lateral projections detect the presence and extent of aneurysms in the anterior and posterior walls of the aorta.

OTHER ETIOLOGIES

Traumatic Dilatation

Acute trauma or repeated chronic minimal trauma may cause *contusion* of an artery and results in weakening of a wall with progressive true dilatation.[532, 661] Examples of acute blunt injury resulting in aneurysms are those of the innominate artery[663] or of the palmar arch.[662] A crutch may produce repeated minimal trau-

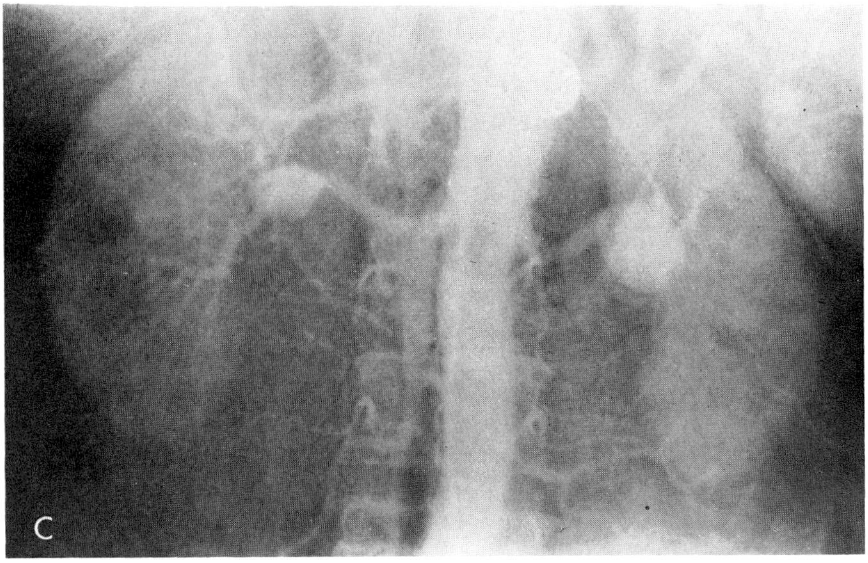

Figure 21.7. A & B reveals two ring-like calcifications in the renal hilar areas. (C) Flush aortogram: Two areas of saccular collection of contrast material are seen in the renal hilar areas. *Diagnosis:* Bilateral renal arterial aneurysms.

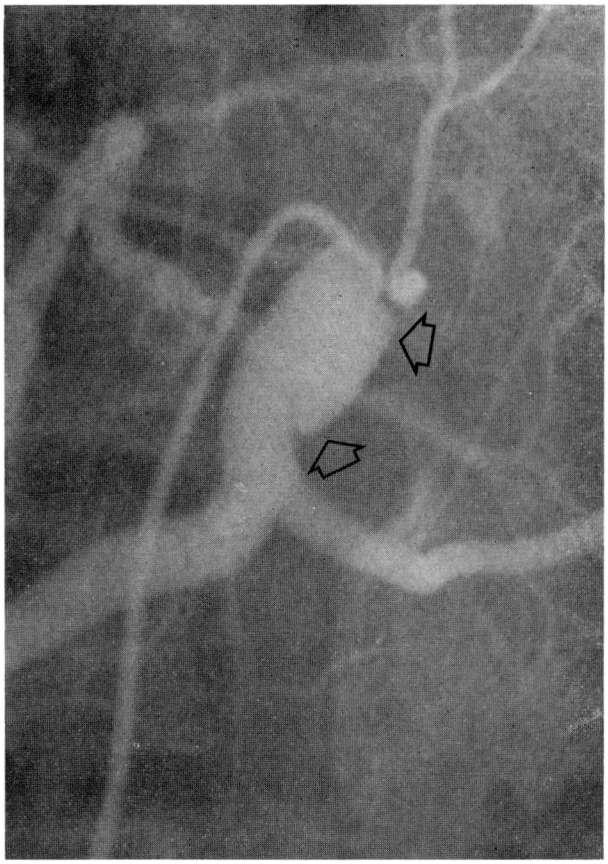

Figure 21.8. Celiac arteriogram reveals dilatation of the main stem in a middle aged man. *Diagnosis:* Aneurysm of the celiac artery. *Surgery:* Congenital aneurysm.

ma,[664, 665] giving rise to brachial and axillary artery aneurysms. Microaneurysms from nontraumatic percutaneous carotid punctures, occurring in both the walls, are of significant interest. This may be the site of mural thrombi with subsequent distal embolization[673] (Fig. 21-16).

Mycotic Aneurysms

Inflammatory destruction of the elastic walls of an artery result in dilatation.[554, 666, 667] Depending on the rapidity of infection and severity of destruction, fatal rupture may even occur. *Rapid growth is* very characteristic of a mycotic aneurysm.[664] Damaged intima due to atherosclerosis or thrombus in an aneurysm is fertile soil for implantation of the bacterial organisms. *In elderly individuals* atherosclerotic vessels of the extremities are frequent sites of enterobacterial or staphylococcal infection. *In younger individuals* the more common sites are vessels of the abdomen in which streptococci or diplococci may lodge and propagate. Direct extension from an adjacent inflammatory focus can also cause arterial wall destruction localized to a small segment. This may occur in tuberculous lymphadenitis involving the abdominal aorta,[668] or pulmonary tuberculosis involving the subclavian artery.[669] Other sites of involvement due to infection are at a coarctation of the aorta,[670] pulmonary arteries,[671] or hepatic arteries[672] (Figs. 26-26, 26-27).

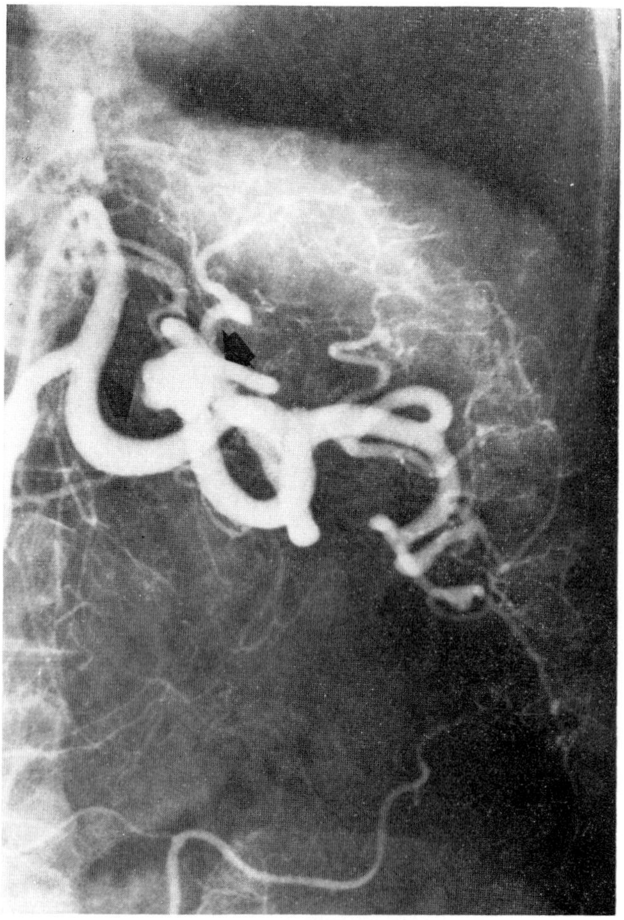

Figure 21.9. Celiac Arteriogram. There is localized dilatation of the splenic artery (Arrow). The patient was seventy years old. *Diagnosis:* Atherosclerotic aneurysm.

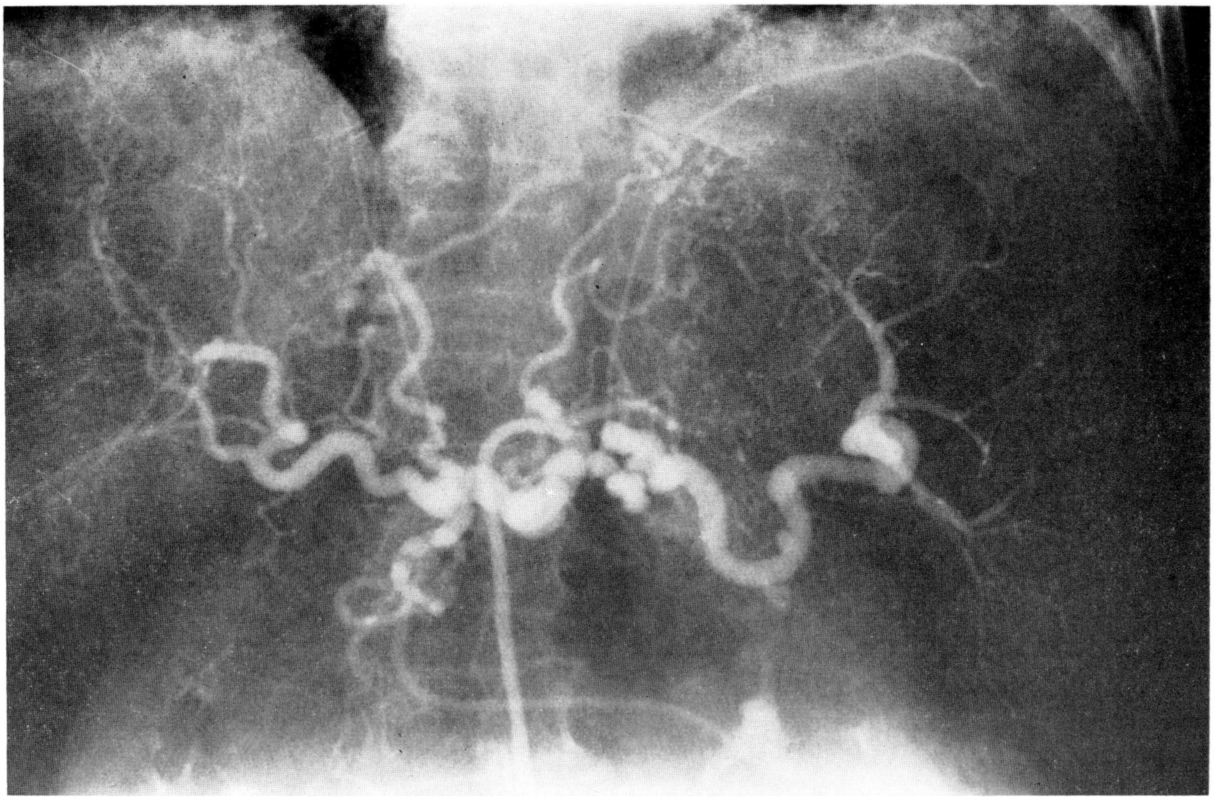

Figure 21.10. Celiac Arteriogram. There are multiple saccular dilatations of the splenic artery. The patient was seventy years old. *Diagnosis:* Atherosclerotic aneurysms.

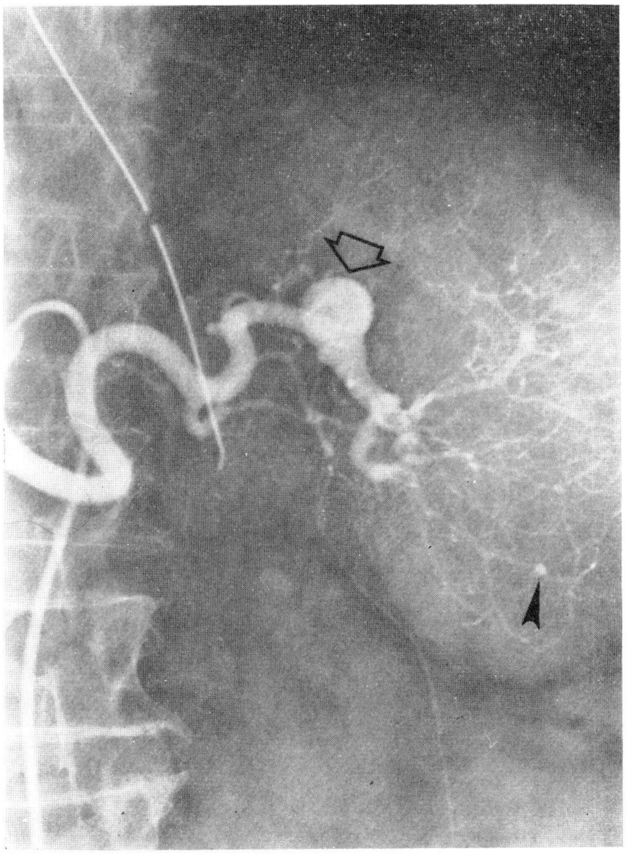

Figure 21.11. Splenic Arteriogram. Saccular dilatations of the terminal portion of the splenic artery (Arrow) and of parenchymal branches (Arrow Head). The patient had mild portal hypertension. *Diagnosis:* Aneurysms of the main splenic artery and intraparenchymal branch in an enlarged spleen.

Figure 21.12. Superior Mesenteric Arteriogram. There are circumscribed dilatations of the jejunal branches. *Diagnosis:* Aneurysms from the jejunal branches; not an uncommon cause of intraperitoneal bleeding.

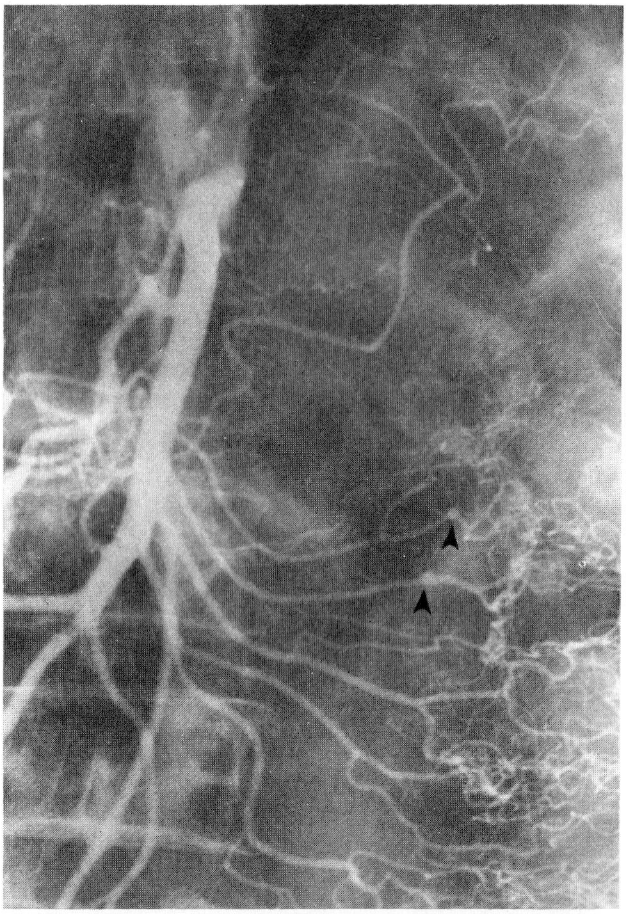

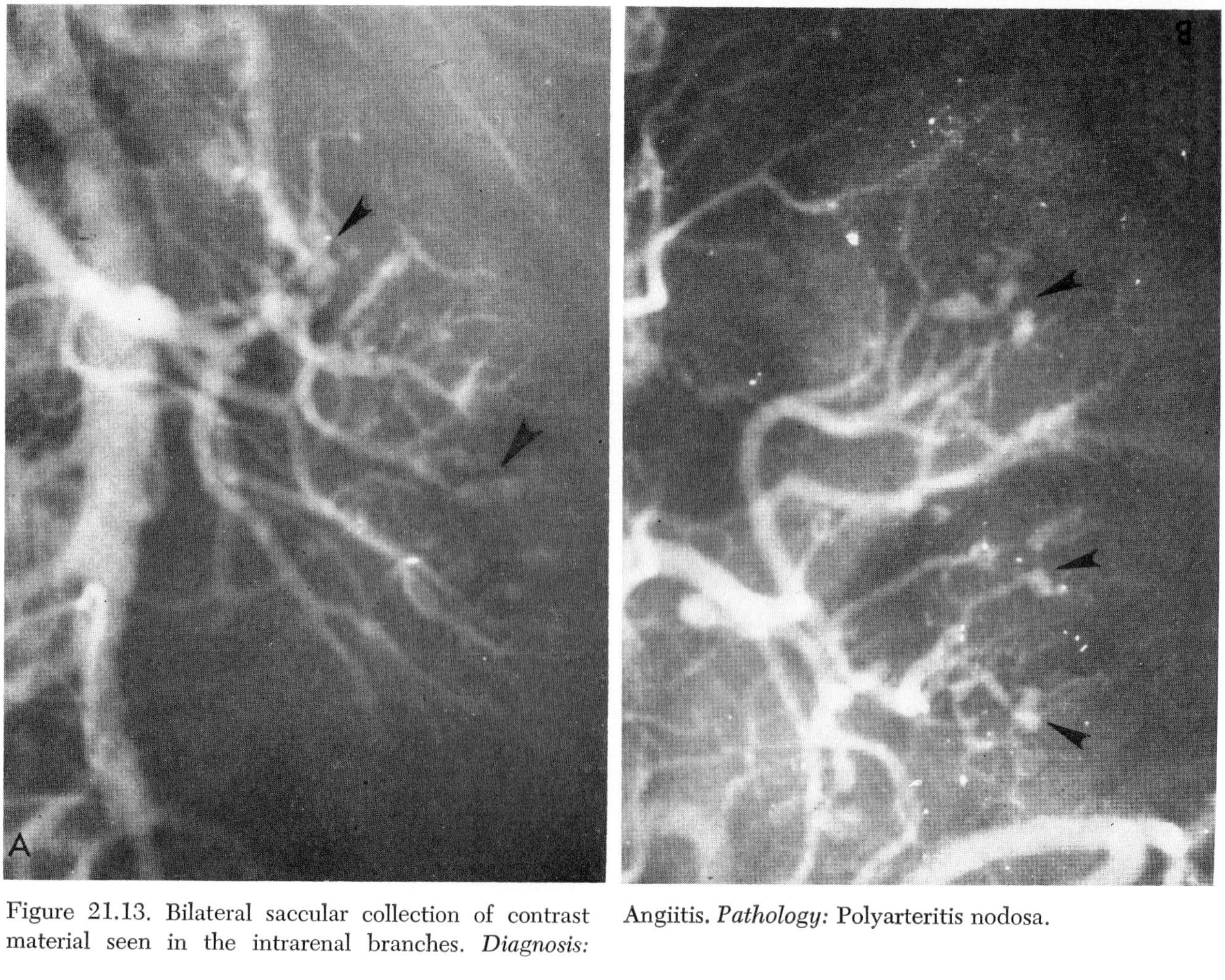

Figure 21.13. Bilateral saccular collection of contrast material seen in the intrarenal branches. *Diagnosis:* Angiitis. *Pathology:* Polyarteritis nodosa.

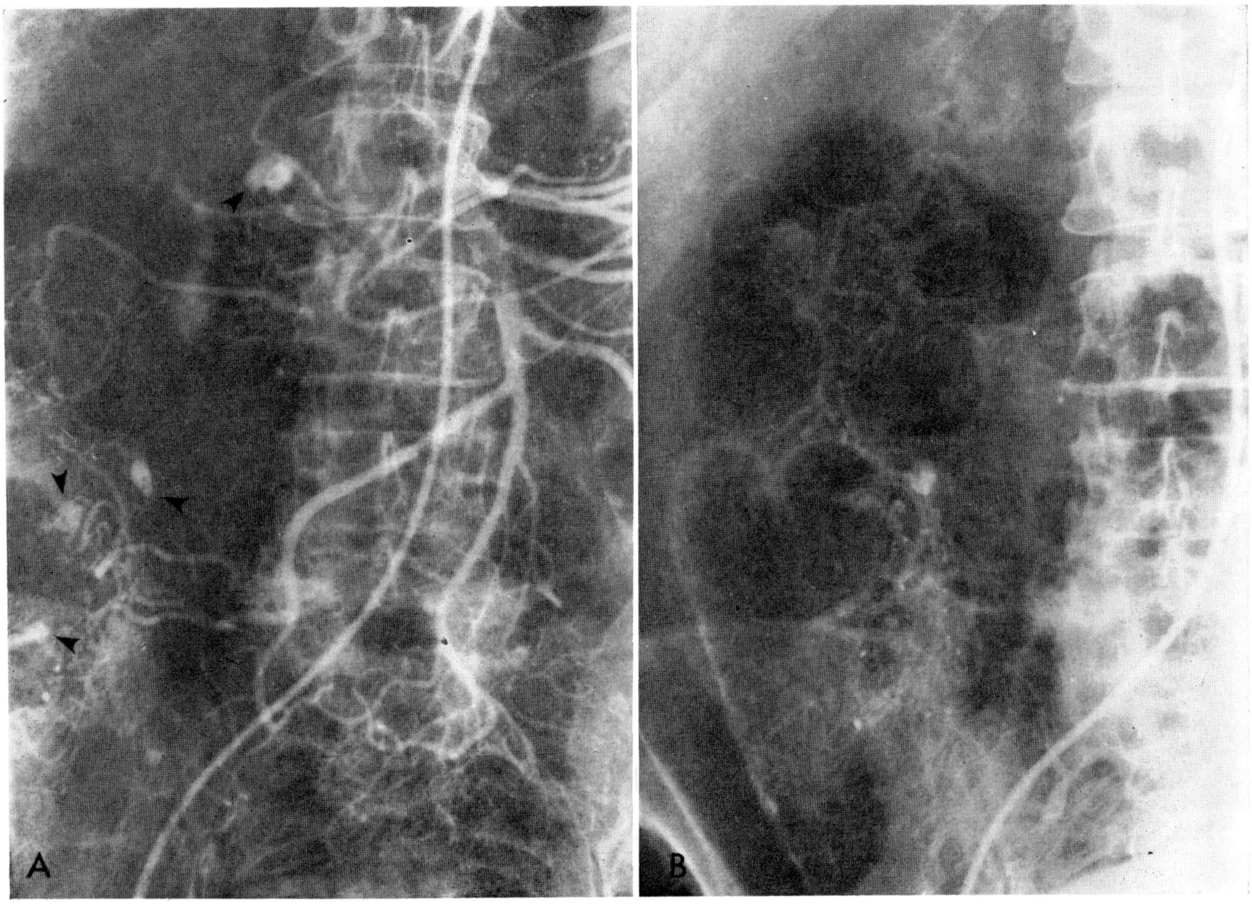

Figure 21.14. Superior Mesenteric Arteriogram. (A) Abnormal collections of contrast material from the terminal branches of the superior mesenteric artery (Arrow) is seen. (B) Venous phase: Abnormal collections are again noted. The patient had Osler Weber Randau syndrome. *Comment:* Note telangiectatic dysplastic vessels.

Necrotizing Diseases

Aneurysms of *medium and small arteries* of the muscular type may develop due to the destruction of the elastic tissue by *fibrinoid necrosis.* There is a greater incidence of involvement of the renal, mesenteric and hepatic vasculature, although almost any vessel may be involved, including the gluteal arteries.[678] These aneurysms may be due to polyarteritis nodosa,[675–677] lupus vasculitis,[615, 674] or drug abuse.[612]

Structural Abnormalities

Dilatation of the vessel, either focal or multifocal, can be due to distortion of the normal medial architecture. This usually is on a congenital basis and may occur anywhere, with a particular affinity for the renal, splenic, and hepatic arteries.[680]

Cystic Medial Necrosis

These aneurysms[516, 679] may be either isolated or associated with arachnodactyly and have a greater predilection for the ascending aorta.

Fragmentation of the Elastic Tissue

These are seen in pseudoxanthoma elasticum[586, 587] or Ehlers-Danlos syndrome.[681, 682] Small aneurysms, angiomatous malformations, or occlusions are rather frequent in these rare clinical curiosities.

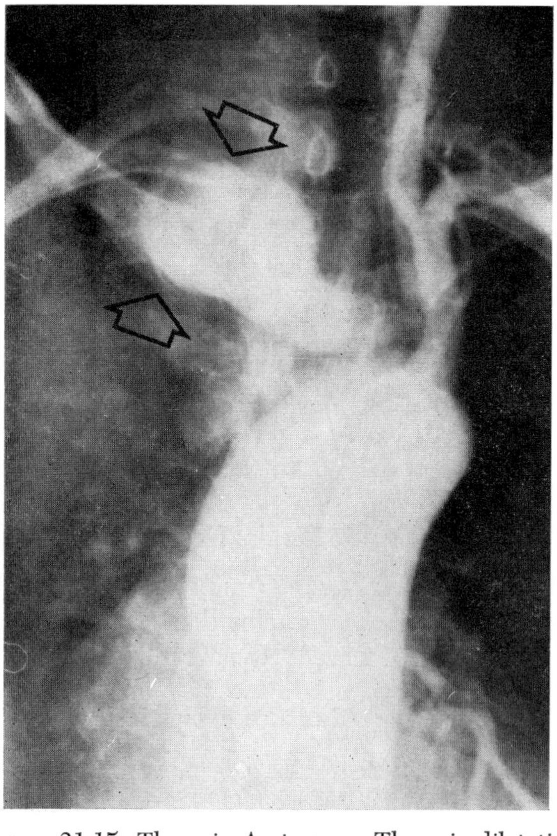

Figure 21.15. Thoracic Aortogram. There is dilatation of the innominate artery. *Diagnosis:* A true aneurysm due to blunt trauma.

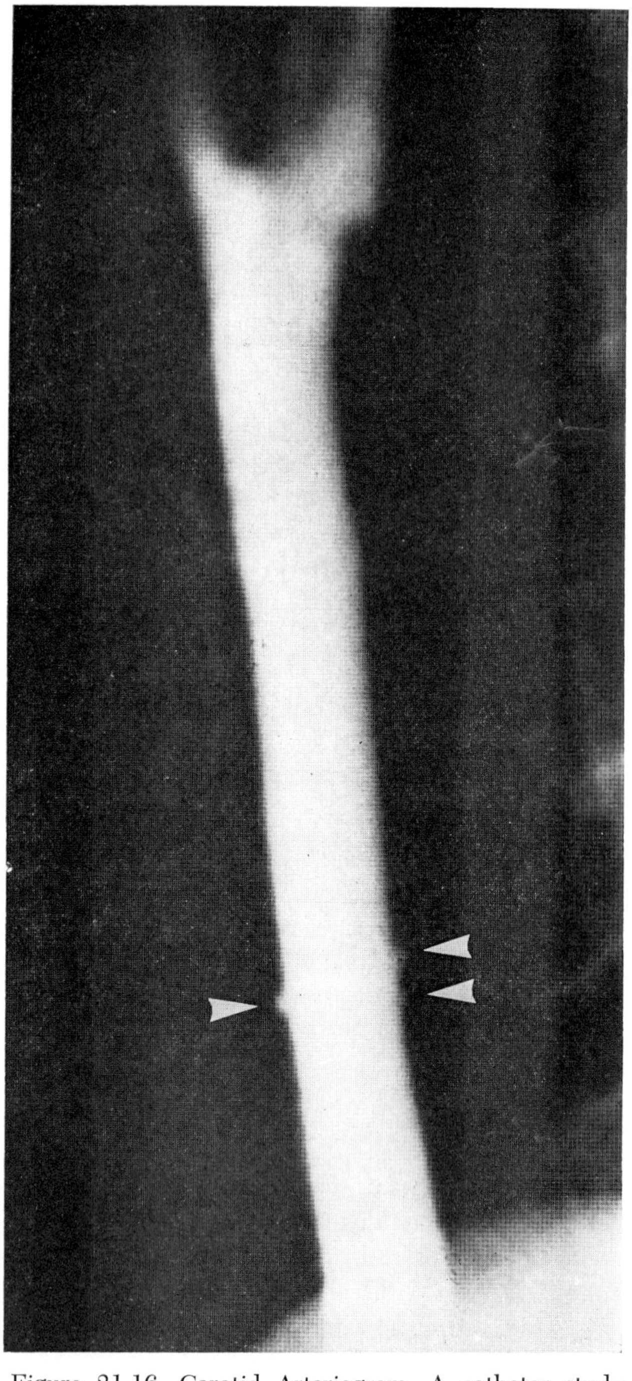

Figure 21.16. Carotid Arteriogram. A catheter study done three days after the percutaneous puncture reveals microaneurysms in the anterior and the posterior walls. The posterior wall was transfixed twice. *Diagnosis:* Microaneurysms. (From Vitek, J. J. Microaneurysms of the carotid artery after non-traumatic percutaneous puncture. *Radiol, 106:*101, 1973. Courtesy of the authors and publishers.)

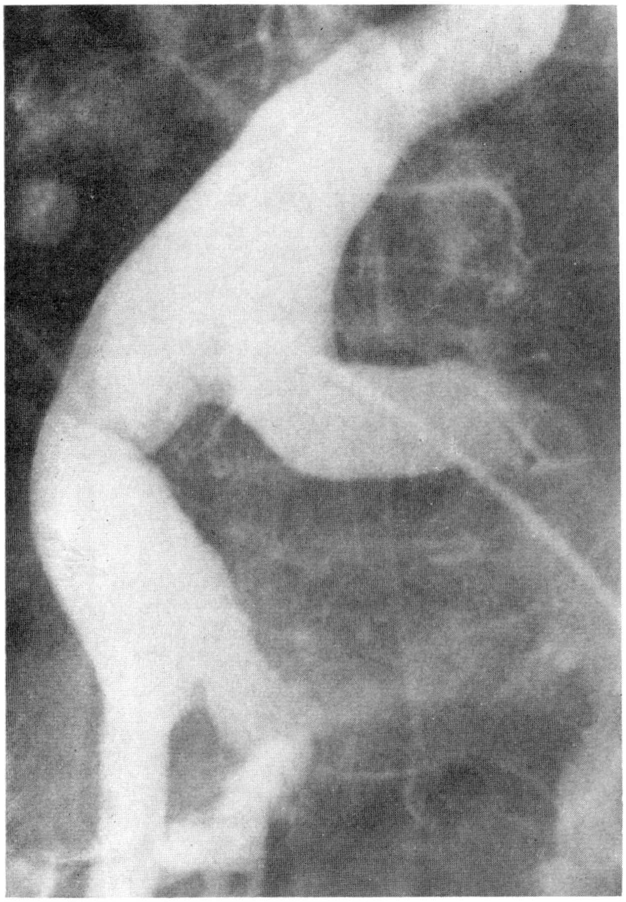

Figure 21.17. Abdominal Aortogram. The distal abdominal aorta and its branches are dilated and tortuous. The patient had signs and symptoms of intermittent claudication. *Diagnosis:* "Ectasia" (arteria dolicho et magna). This is a long name for an age-old process.

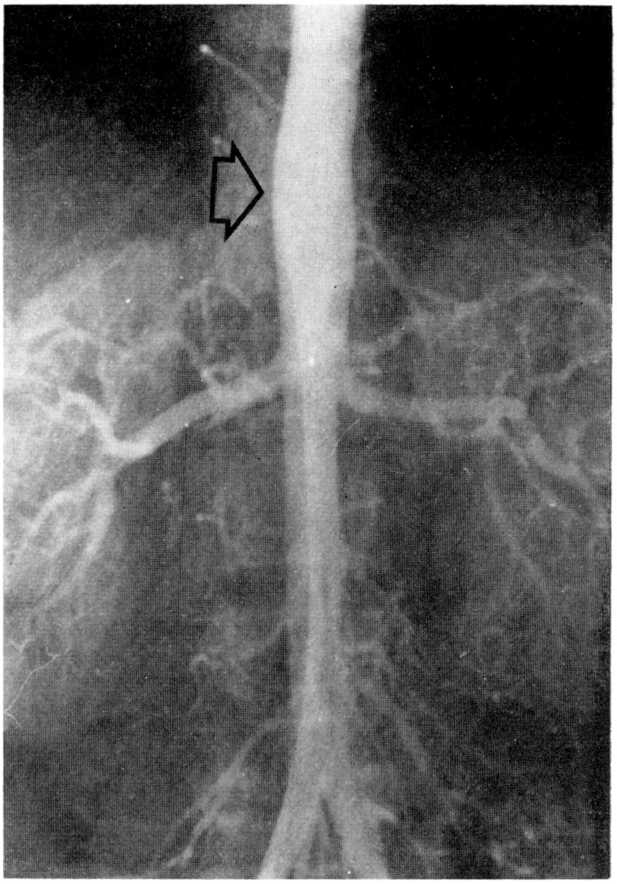

Figure 21.18. Abdominal Aortogram. There is localized distension of the suprarenal portion of the aorta due to injection pressure.

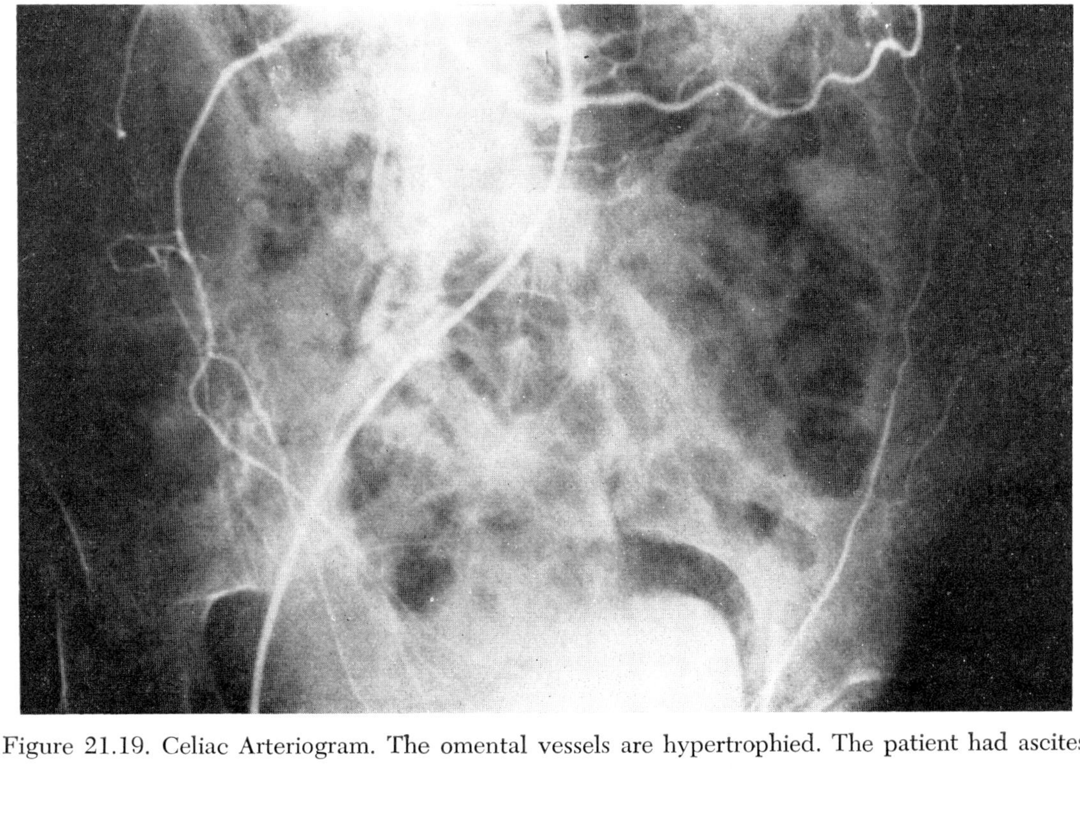

Figure 21.19. Celiac Arteriogram. The omental vessels are hypertrophied. The patient had ascites.

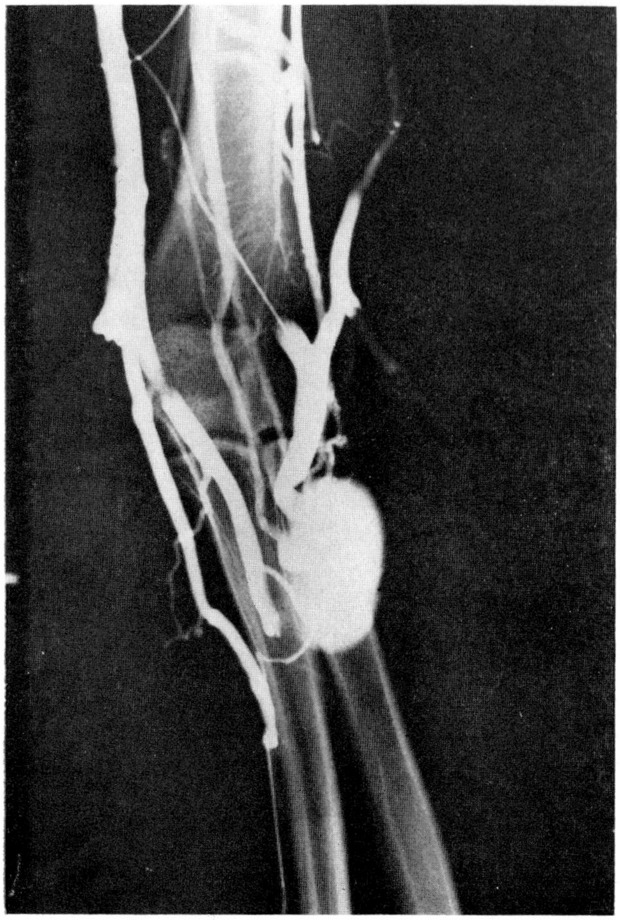

Figure 21.20. Upper Extremity Venogram. A saccular collection of contrast material is perfused by the antecubital vein. *Diagnosis:* Venous saccular aneurysm.

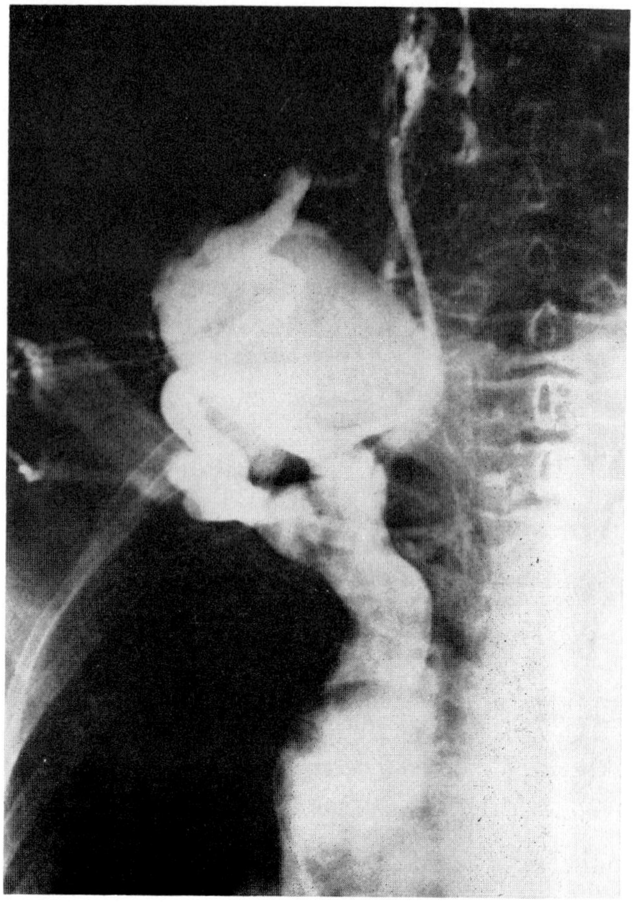

Figure 21.21. Upper Extremity Venogram. Reveals a huge sac filling with contrast at the junction of the subclavian and internal jugular vein. *Diagnosis:* Venous aneurysm.

Abnormal Dilatation of Preexisting Vessels

Telangiectasia may involve the small vessels, capillaries and venules. They are lined only by endothelium.[111] The spectrum of lesions found in this group varies from *dilatation,* either localized or diffuse, to *arteriovenous malformation.* They have no apparent relation to function; characteristically multiple systems are involved with either of the above vascular abnormalities.[683, 684]

Aneurysms of Special Interest

Splenic artery aneurysms,[685–689] due to atherosclerosis, congenital inflammation (pancreatitis), trauma, or portal hypertension are usually located in the main trunk or in the hilar area. They have a greater affection for young females in the twenty to forty age group and for people of either sex over sixty years of age. The aneurysms may rupture spontaneously, due either to increased circulatory blood volume or repeated valsalva maneuvers, particularly in the last trimester of pregnancy.[690] When these aneurysms rupture they may bleed fatally into the peritoneal cavity, retroperitoneum, pancreas, splenic vein, stomach, or colon. Occasionally they may even cause splenic infarction.[691]

Aneurysms of the renal artery[695] are fascinating, particularly if these lesions are associated with renovascular hypertension.[730, 731] Even more fascinating are the roentgenograms if there are multiple aneurysms in the intrarenal vasculature due to necrotizing angiitis.

Popliteal artery aneurysms[692–694] are usually due to atherosclerosis. They have gained importance because of *silent thromboembolic disease* which may develop distal to the aneurysm. In addition there may be spontaneous rupture or extrinsic pressure on important adjacent structures. The aneurysms are usually saccular and single in normotensive patients, and fusiform and bilateral in people with hypertension.

Gastrointestinal tract aneurysms are important if they rupture spontaneously into the gastrointestinal tract causing acute massive bleeding. This is seen with aneurysms of the jejunal,[696] mesenteric[697] and gastric[698, 699] arteries. In addition, they may occur following surgery, or as a result of chronic pancreatitis.[700] *Aneurysms of the hepatic artery* may rupture, causing hemobilia.[672] They may be congenital.[680] They may subsequently thrombose.[701]

Miscellaneous causes of aneurysms include multiple ones due to giant cell arteritis[702] and aneurysms of vascular grafts.[704, 705] Finally, aneurysms may be seen of the persistent primitive sciatic artery, which is a continuation of the internal iliac artery, coursing medial to the femoral artery in the thigh.[703]

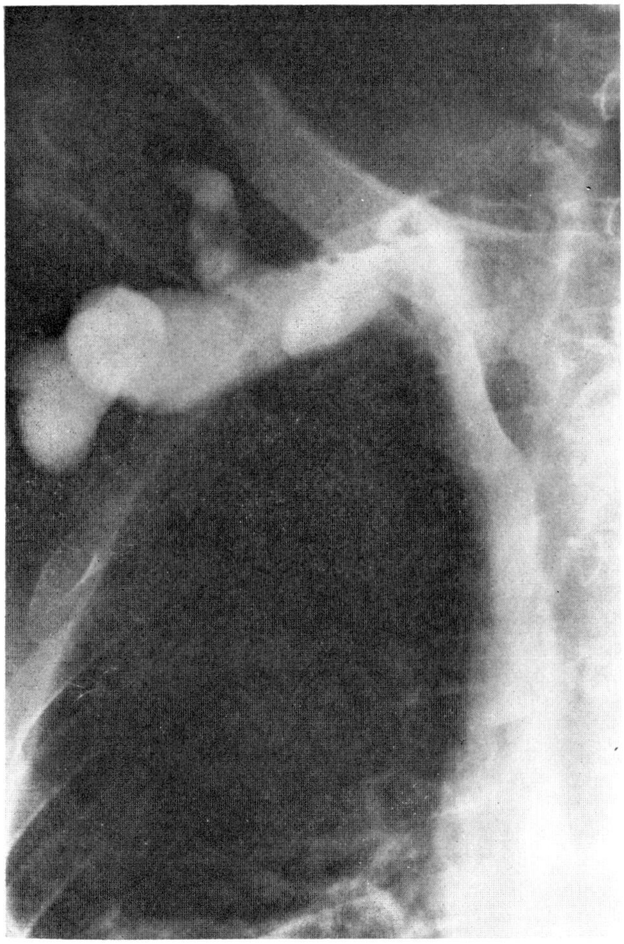

Figure 21.22. Upper Extremity Venogram. Note the marked dilatation of the subclavian vein. *Diagnosis:* Phlebectasia.

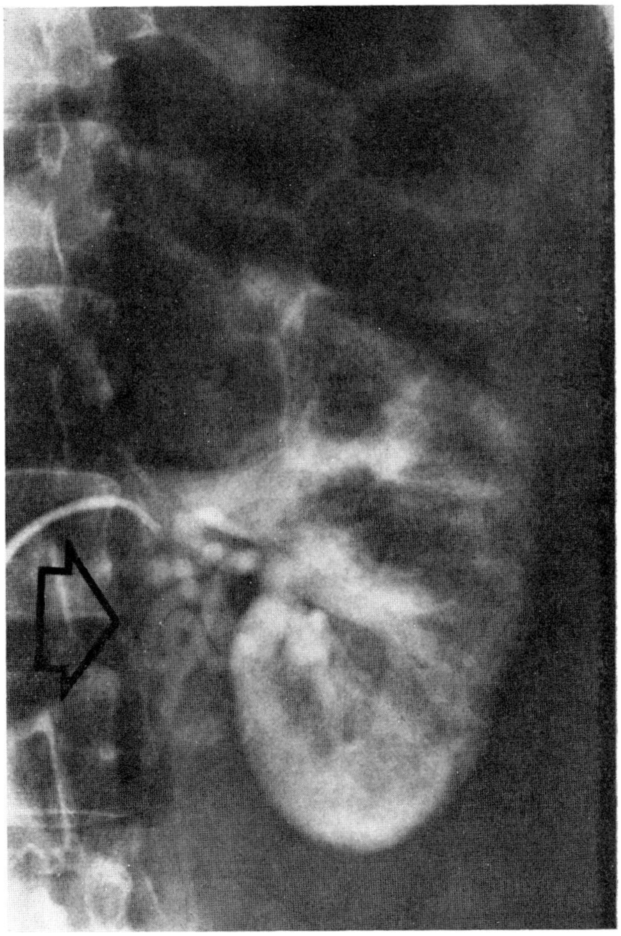

Figure 21.23. Renal Arteriogram—late phase. Tortuous dilated abnormal veins in the left renal pelvic area course towards the retroperitoneum. Notice the lack of perfusion to the upper medial border of the kidney due to another aberrant renal supply to this area. *Comment:* Pelviureteric varices.

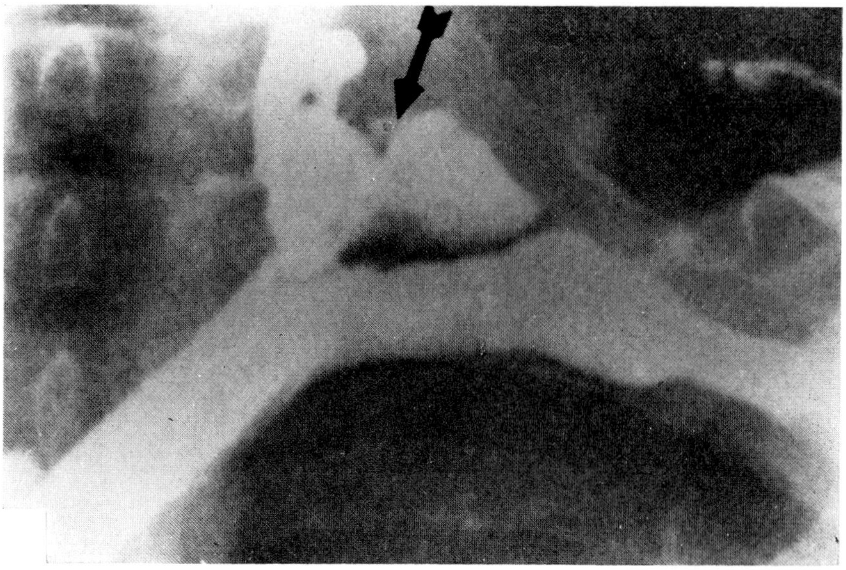

Figure 21.24. Subclavian Venogram. A lobulated sac connected with the subclavian vein opacifies to its entirely during a valsalva maneuver. This fifty-six-year-old man had a swelling in his neck. *Diagnosis:* Persistent jugular lymph sac. (From Steinberg, I. Roentgen diagnosis of persistent jugular lymph sac. *Radiol, 82:*1022, 1964. Courtesy of the author and publishers.)

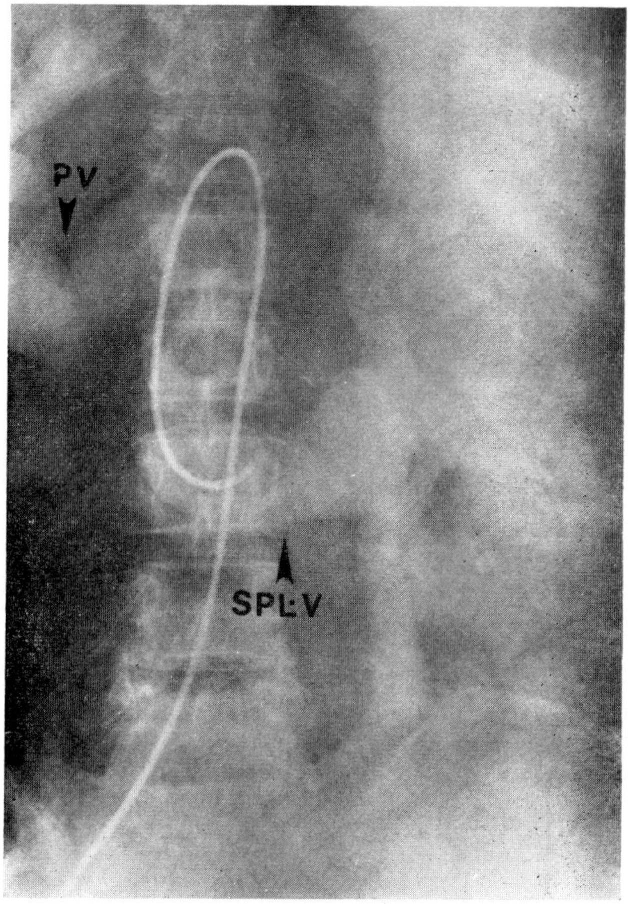

Figure 21.25. Splenic Arteriogram—venous phase. The spleen is enlarged and both the splenic (Spl. V.) and portal (P.V.) veins are dilated. *Comment:* Dilatation of the veins due to increased drainage from an enlarged spleen.

Excessive Flow

Diffuse dilatation of a regional arborization invariably occurs if there is undue increase in flow in that circulation for a long period of time. This may be a compensatory phenomena as demonstrated by *collateral vessels.* Compensatory changes are also seen in the hepatic artery in patients with *cirrhosis* and decreased portal venous inflow, as well as in the renal artery when there is *compensatory hypertrophy of a kidney.*[1482] Dilatation may occur when there are excessive demands created by increased metabolic needs, as seen with very vascular *benign* or *malignant lesions.* Ipsilateral dilatations of the ovarian artery may be seen in ectopic gestations. It may also be due to *decreased peripheral resistance* at various levels as seen in precapillary arteriovenous shunting of sufficient magnitude.

VEINS

The usual lesion in *venous dilatation* is related to abnormalities of the wall, with *loss of elastic tissue* and *proliferation of connective tissue.*[577, 706] The important areas of abnormality are in the *gastrointestinal tract* since chronic bleeding may be the result. The causes of venous dilatation in general may be congenital, aging changes, increased flow, or increased hydrostatic pressure. Localized congenital dilatation may involve the jugular vein,[706, 707] the superior vena cava,[708] azygos vein,[709] femoral vein[710] (which may present as a hernia), antecubital vein, portal vein,[711] or pulmonary vein.[712, 713] Diffuse congenital dilatation is seen as diffuse phlebectasia of the limbs or other areas.[714, 715] Localized[108, 579] and diffuse[577, 716] dilatations due to aging usually are related to loss of elastic tissue with replacement by fibrous tissue.

Venous dilatation due to increased hydrostatic pressure is seen in the lower extremity veins and with pelvic varicosities,[717] particularly those in the scrotal,[385] vulvar,[718] or broad ligament[719] areas. In constrictive pericarditis and cardiac failure there may be marked dilatation of the inferior vena cava resulting in a *mega cava.*[354]

Venous dilatation due to increased flow is best seen in collateral veins which dilate very easily because of poor tissue support. At the same time, they are exposed to high pressure. The *rate of flow* in these dilated veins, such as esophageal varices, is higher than that in the dilated veins produced by purely increased hydrostatic pressure that occurs in lower extremity veins.[720] Examples of dilatation also include dilated azygos or hemiazygos veins in inferior or superior vena caval obstruction.[721] Other examples include dilated left intercostal vein due to obstruction of the superior vena caval system[722] or dilated esophageal veins due to superior vena caval obstruction.[723, 724] Venous dilatation may occur due to arteriovenous communications, causing increased flow, decreased velocity and increased lateral pressure. This produces dilatation and thinning of the wall (Bernoulli phenomena), an example of which is renal vein dilatation with hypernephromas.[725] Aneurysms of the inferior vena cava may result after portocaval shunts.[729] Other isolated dilatations (varices) have been described in the colon[726] and stomach,[727] and in the mesentery with rupture.[728]

CHAPTER 22

NARROWING

The narrowing of a vessel may be *smooth* or *irregular; concentric* or *eccentric; focal* or *multifocal; functional* or *organic; intermittent* or *permanent* and involve short or long segments. *With few exceptions, the lesions which cause narrowing of a vessel have the potential to cause gradual and complete occlusion.*

The angiographic appearance of a narrowed vessel depends on the *integrity of the intimal surface*. The type of narrowing also depends on the *status of the elastica* of the media. If the elastica is destroyed in a patchy manner, then areas of narrowing alternate with areas of dilatation. The length of the narrowing depends on either the diffuse or patchy type of distribution of the pathologic process. The extent of encroachment upon the lumen is reflected in the caliber of the patent lumen. The circumferential extent of the lesion, eccentric or concentric, depends on the involvement of either a part or the entire circumference of the wall. Unlike multidirectional pressure on the vessel, unidirectional extrinsic pressure on the vessels does cause eccentric areas of localized sharp narrowing.

FUNCTIONAL

Spasm

Spasm of a vessel causes *smooth concentric narrowing of variable lengths* of a single vessel or multiple branches.[780–783] Smooth muscle of the arterial wall has an inherent ability to contract. This is purely myogenic in nature and due to mechanical stimulation, resulting in the sustained contraction of the smooth muscle. The maintenance of spasm is not dependent on nervous factors to any demonstrable measure. The stimulation is mediated by a *sudden stretch of the wall* as with a foreign object, or by a sharp rise in the intravascular pressure. It is usually provoked in *medium size arteries* which have a significant amount of muscle in the wall. It rarely occurs in the vessels of elderly patients because of fibrosis of the medial layer. Neither does it occur in large elastic arteries. It is more *common in the brachial and femoral* arteries than in the axillary or subclavian arteries and in upper rather than in lower extremity veins. The tendency to develop spasm is *inversely proportional to the diameter*

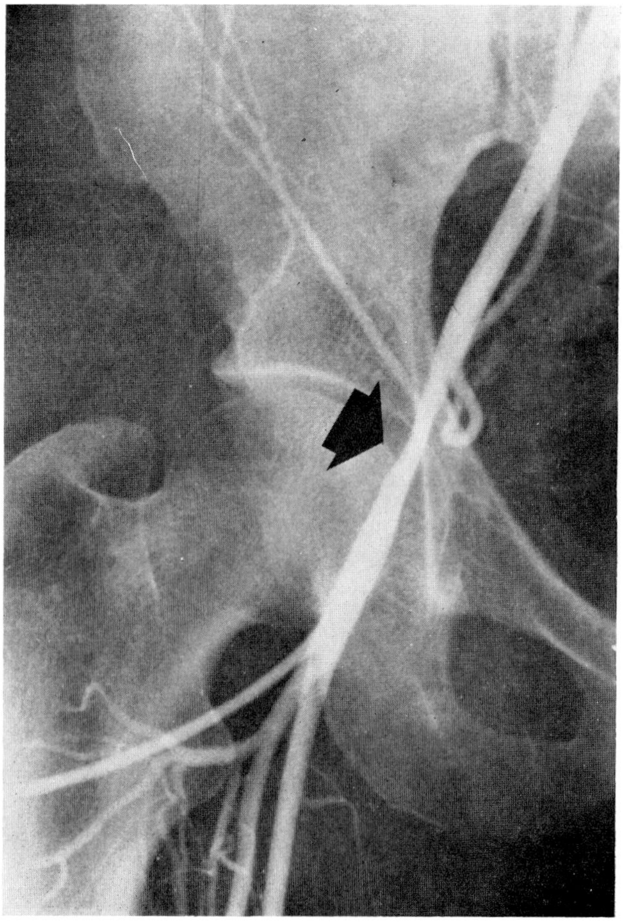

Figure 22.1. Femoral arteriogram reveals a segment of smooth narrowing (Arrow). *Diagnosis:* Arterial spasm induced by the catheter.

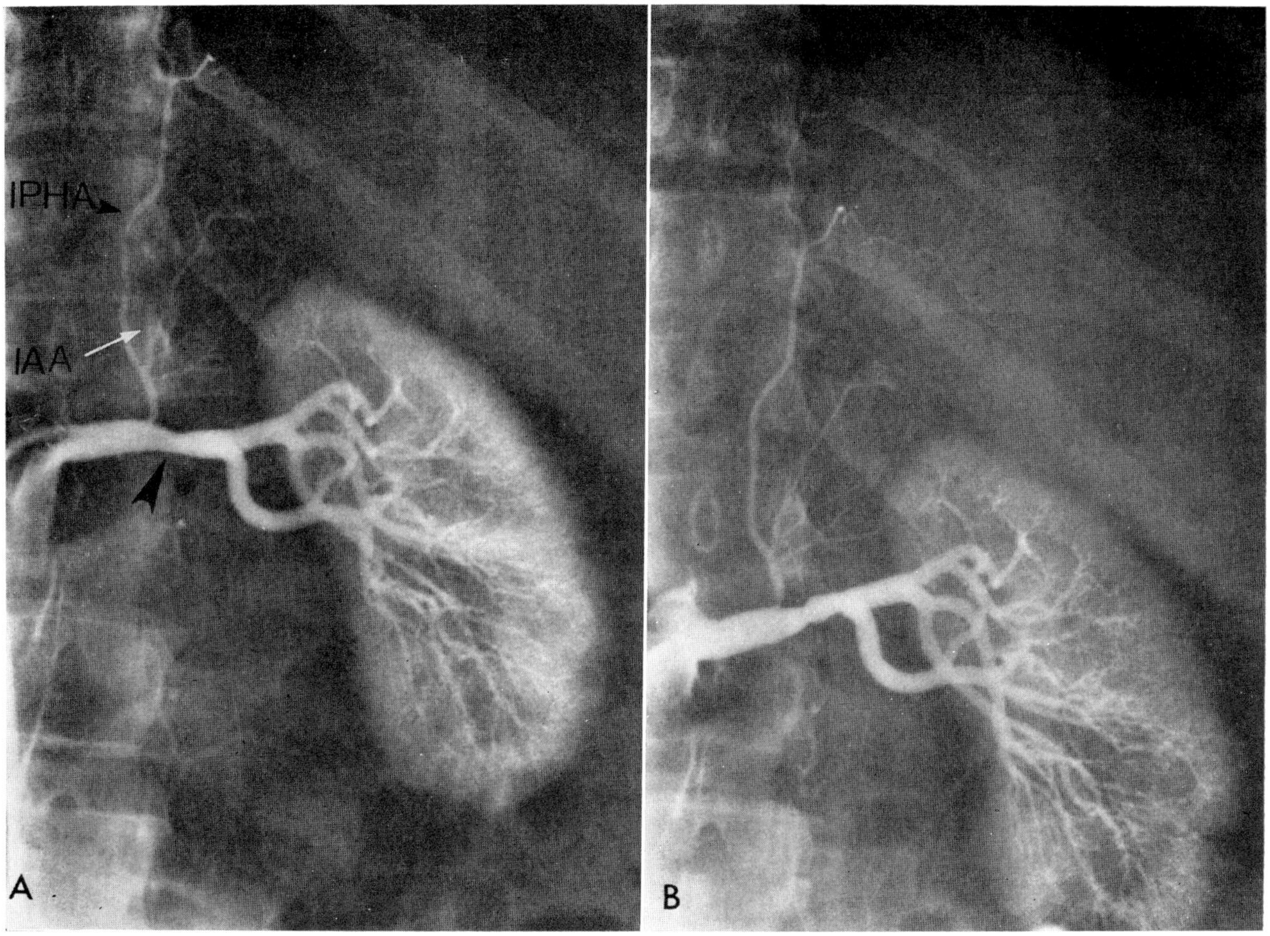

Figure 22.2. Renal Arteriogram. (A) There is mild, smooth narrowing of the midrenal arterial segment (Arrow Head) with good filling of the inferior phrenic artery arising from the renal artery (I.P.H.A.) and giving origin to the inferior adrenal artery (I.A.A.). (B) A repeat catheterization of the same artery reveals more narrowing in the same area with better filling of the inferior phrenic artery and the adrenal arteries. *Diagnosis:* Spasm of the renal artery due to catheterization, probably due to too much manipulation.

of an artery and the age of the individual. It is more common in women, with a higher incidence in individuals with Raynaud's phenomenon.[784-786] Etiologies of spasm include foreign body irritation (needles, guide wires and catheters), blunt trauma, inflammation of an adjacent vein. Vascular spasm of an arborization is due to shock, drugs, as a hemostatic mechanism, and the ever-present miscellaneous causes.

Irritation by Foreign Bodies

Smooth, *concentric narrowing* of various lengths is related to the stimulation from a catheter, needle, guide wire, etc. The incidence of spasm is *directly proportional* to the diameter of the catheter used, duration of the manipulation of the wire or catheter, and/or the emotional status of the individual. It is *inversely proportional* to the diameter of the vessel and the age of the patient. Even elderly patients are not immune from developing spasm of the visceral branches, the left gastric, hepatic, or splenic arteries, even though the peripheral arteries at the puncture site appear to be immune. The diagnosis is made by location of the spasm at the tip of the catheter and also by demonstration of stasis of injected contrast material distal to the tip of the catheter. *The recognition of spasm warns one to withdraw*

(Text continues on page 264)

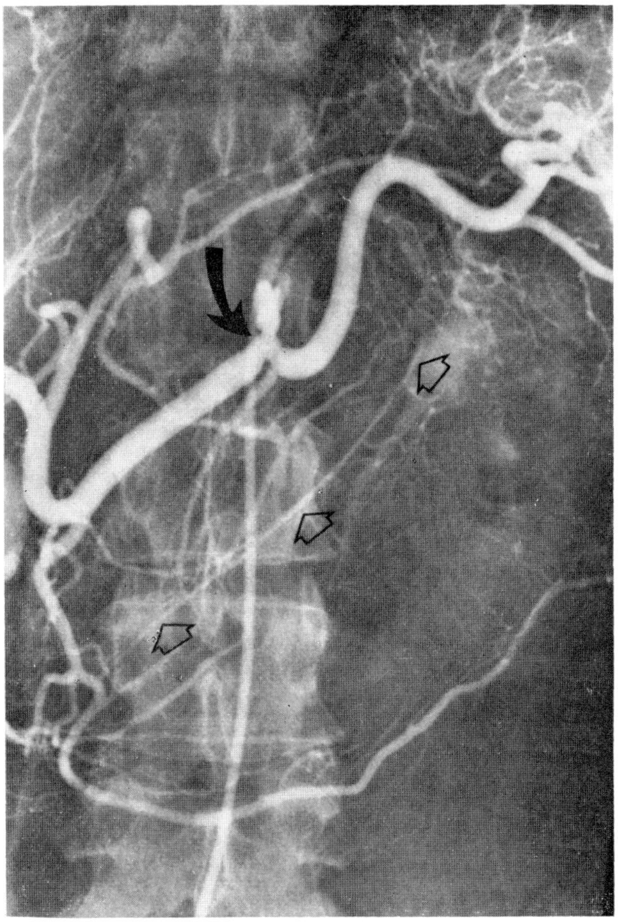

Figure 22.3. Celiac Arteriogram. There is smooth concentric narrowing of the celiac axis (Arrow). There is a good demonstration of the transverse pancreatic artery (Blank Arrow). *Diagnosis:* Spasm due to catheter irritation.

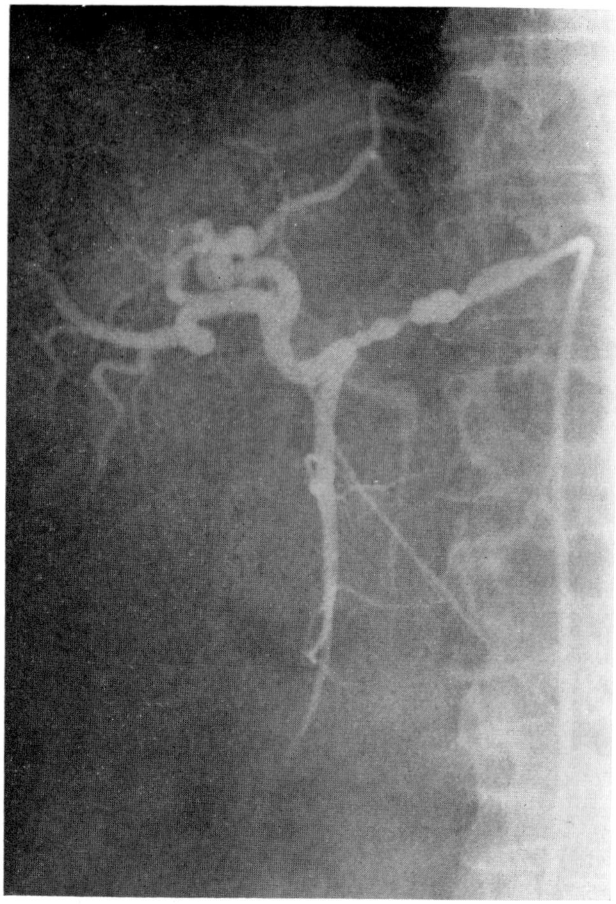

Figure 22.4. Hepatic Arteriogram. The areas of narrowing and dilatation of the main hepatic artery are due to catheter-induced spasm.

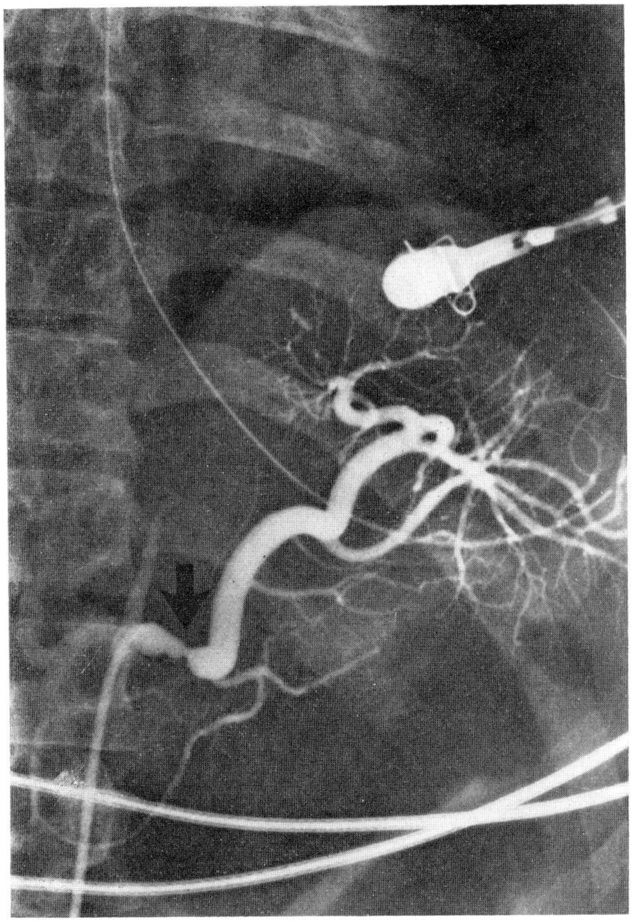

Figure 22.5. Splenic Arteriogram. There is smooth concentric narrowing of the proximal splenic artery. *Diagnosis:* Spasm due to irritation by the catheter.

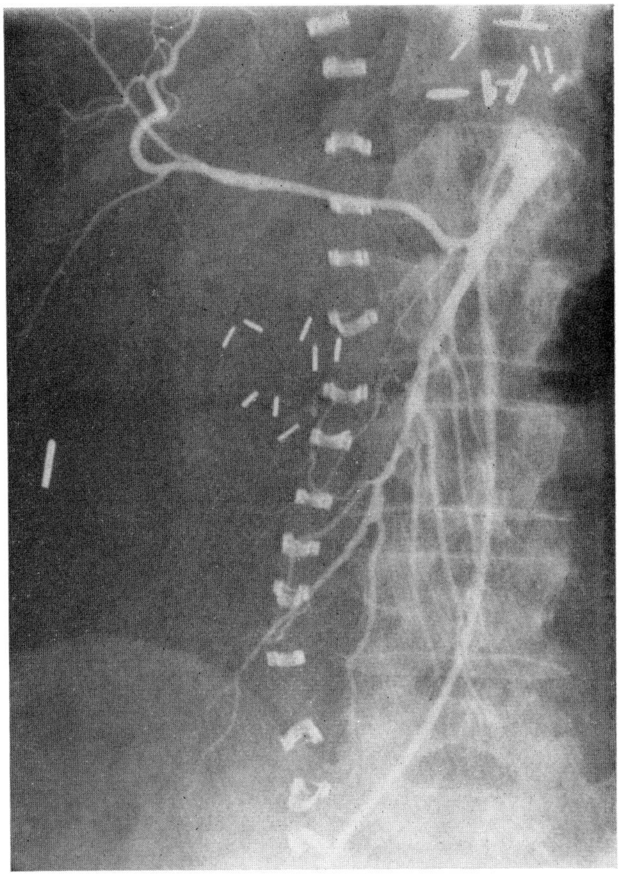

Figure 22.6. Superior Mesenteric Arteriogram. Notice marked narrowing of the main trunk of the superior mesenteric artery as well as the replaced hepatic artery arising from the superior mesenteric artery. This old man was in cardiac arrhythmia and congestive heart failure. *Diagnosis:* Persistent mesenteric vasoconstriction.

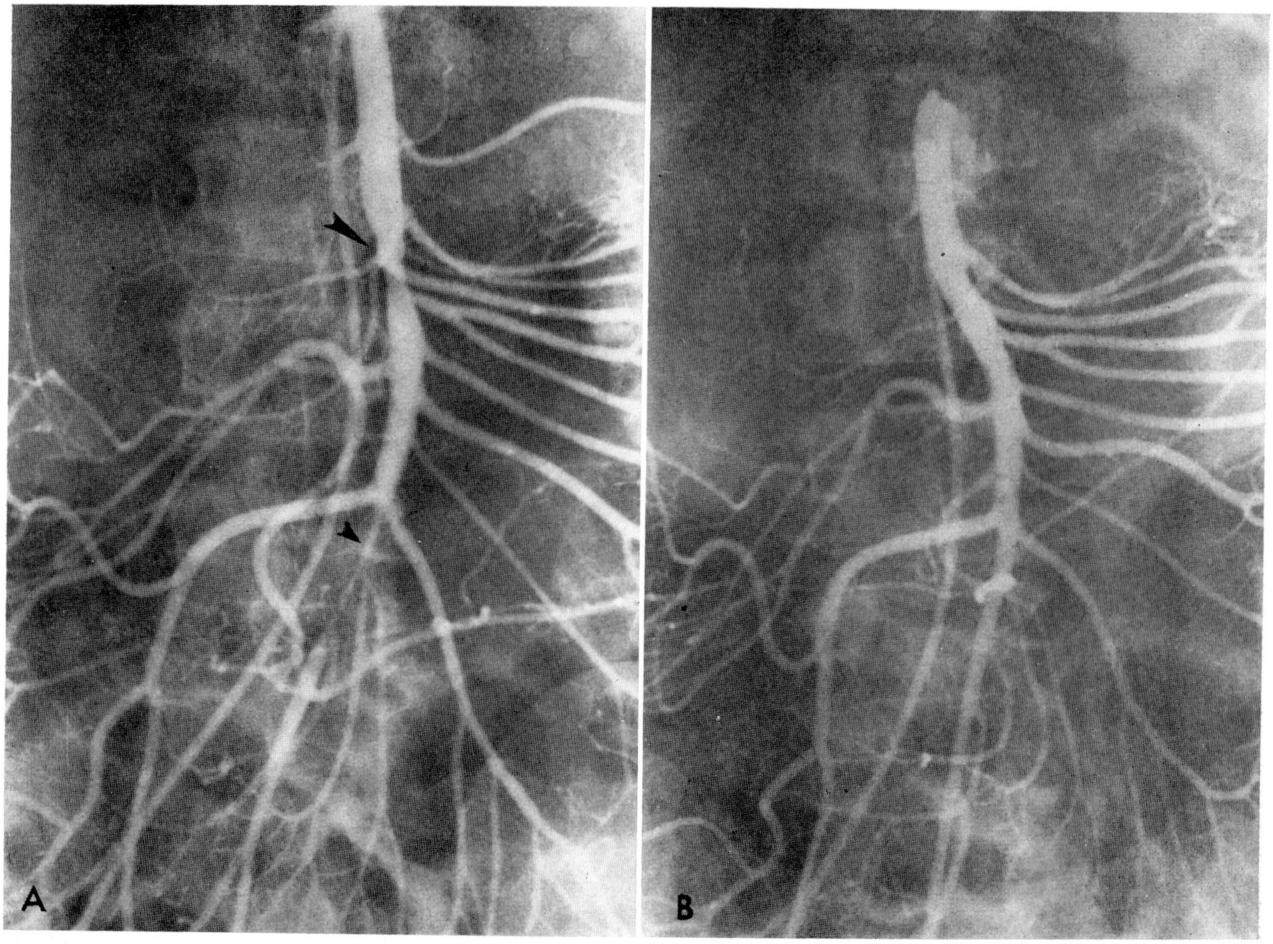

Figure 22.7. Superior Mesenteric Arteriogram. (A) There is smooth narrowing of the proximal portion of the superior mesenteric trunk (Arrow) and also major ileal branch (Arrow). (B) Repeat superior mesenteric arteriogram with prescoline: The narrowing has disappeared. *Comment:* Catheter irritation and proximal spasm. The cause for the spasm of the iliac branch is not clear.

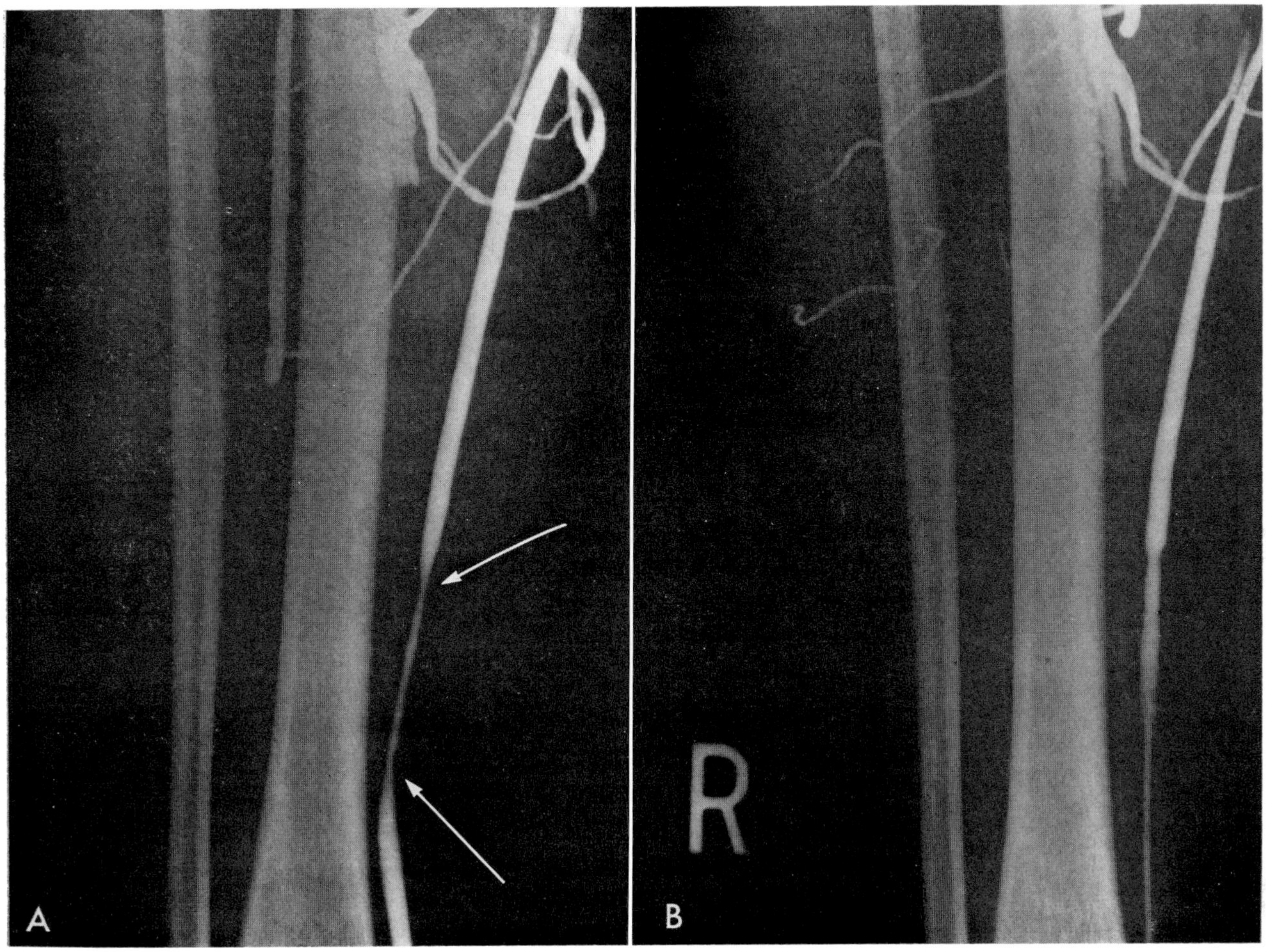

Figure 22.8. Lower Extremity Phlebogram. (A) There is segmental smooth narrowing of the superficial vein. (B) The narrowing is relieved. *Comment:* Venospasm.

Figure 22.9. Right Common Iliac Venogram. Smooth narrowing of the common iliac vein occurs at the tip of the catheter. *Comment:* Jet collapse of the vein due to injection pressure.

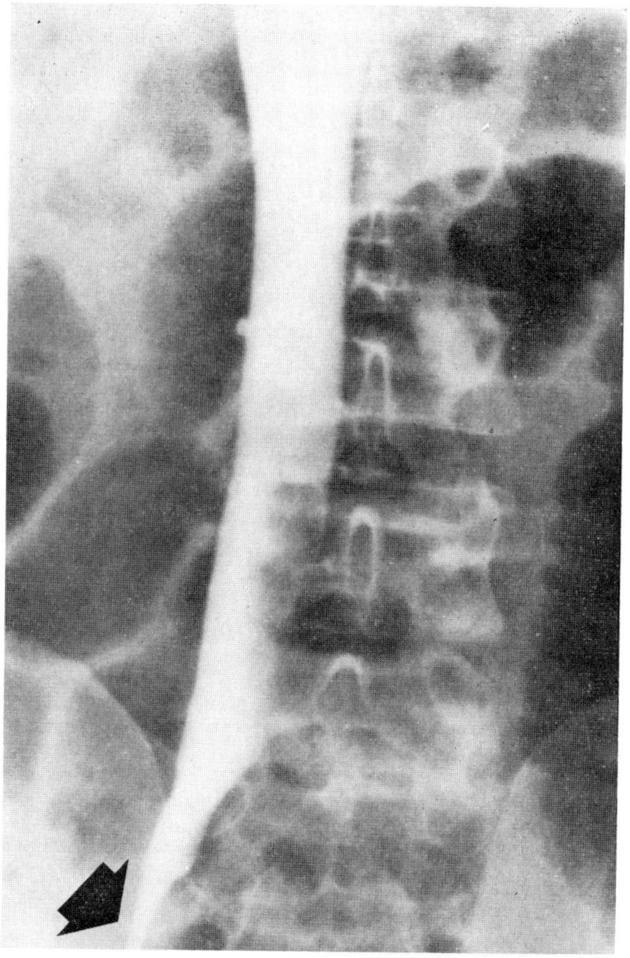

Figure 22.10. Femoral Arteriogram. (A) There is smooth elongated narrowing of the distal superficial femoral and proximal popliteal artery (Arrowhead). (B) A repeat angiogram six hours later is normal. *Diagnosis:* Arterial spasm due to trauma.

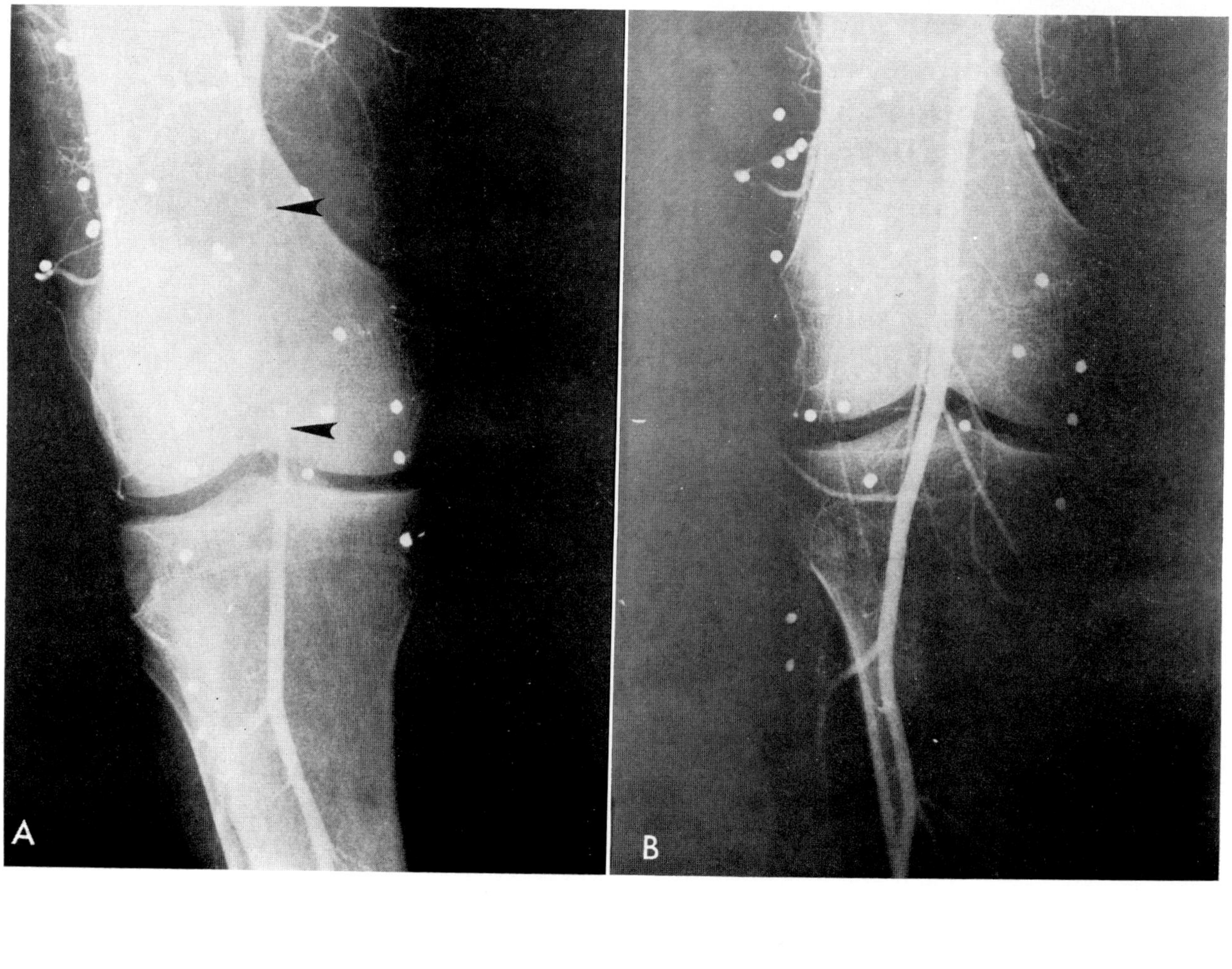

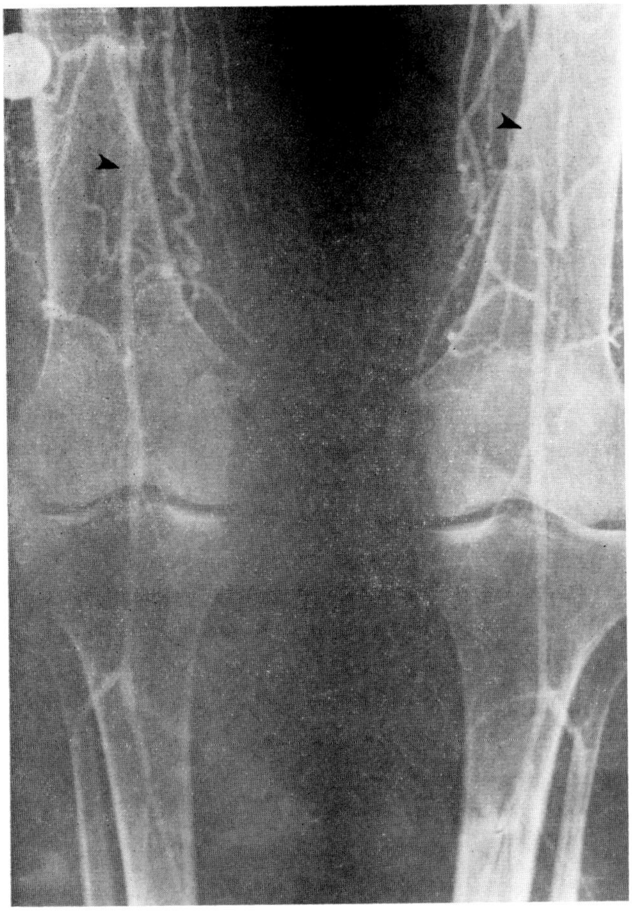

←

Figure 22.11. Bilateral Femoral Arteriograms. Smooth severe narrowing of the superficial femoral arteries and (Arrow) dilated tortuous corkscrew collateral branches are seen. This patient was receiving ergot medication for migraine headache. *Diagnosis:* Marked vascular spasm due to the medication.

Figure 22.12. Superior Mesenteric Arteriogram. (A) Reveals multiple segments of smooth narrowing of the branches of the superior mesenteric artery (Arrows). In a young female who was receiving methysergide maleate (Sansert®) for headaches. (B) Same, after stopping the medication reveals disappearance of the narrowing of the vessels. *Diagnosis:* Drug-induced spasm. (From Buenger, Richard E., and Hunter, James A. Reversible mesenteric artery stenoses due to methysergide maleate, *JAMA, 198:*558, 1966. Courtesy of the authors and the publishers.)

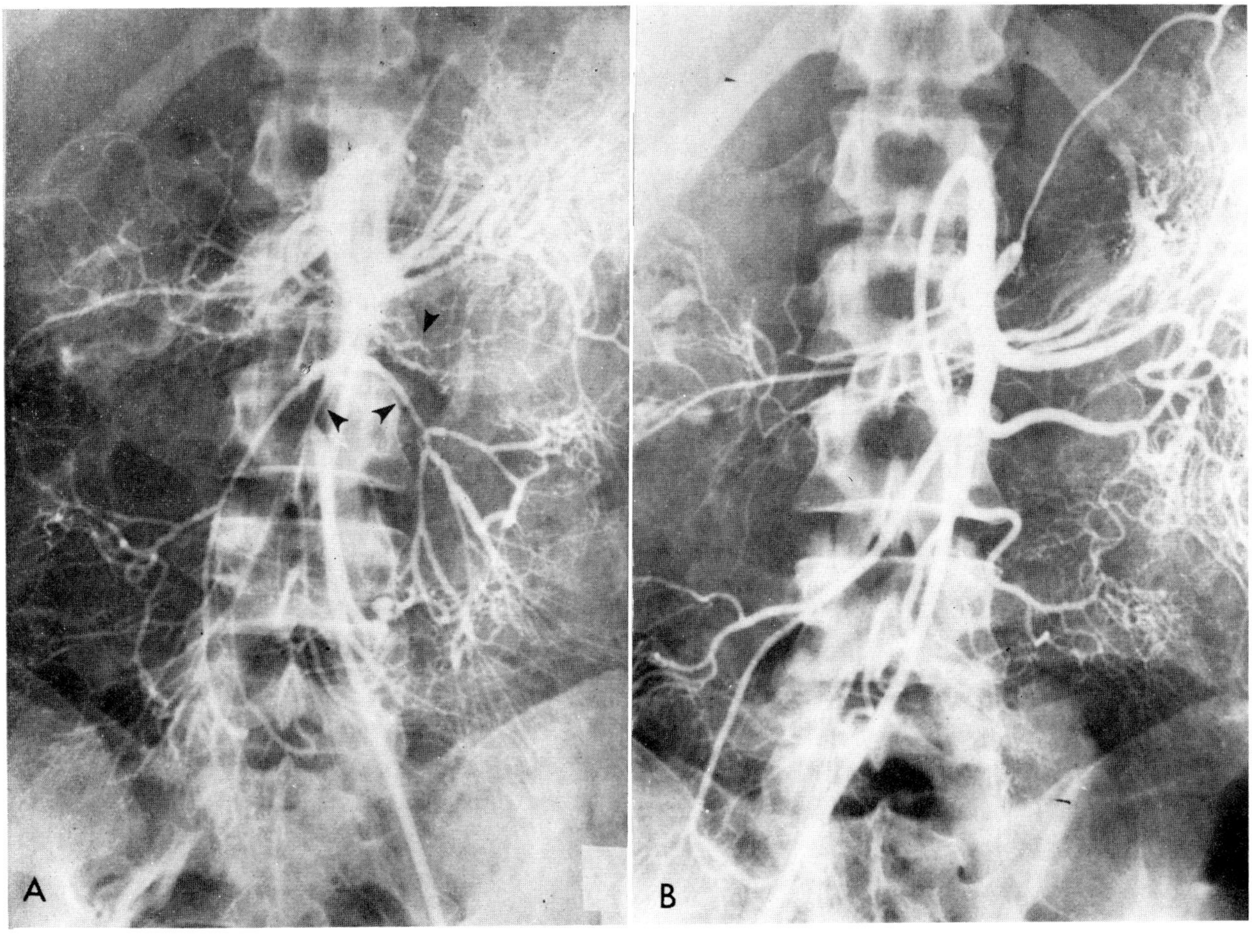

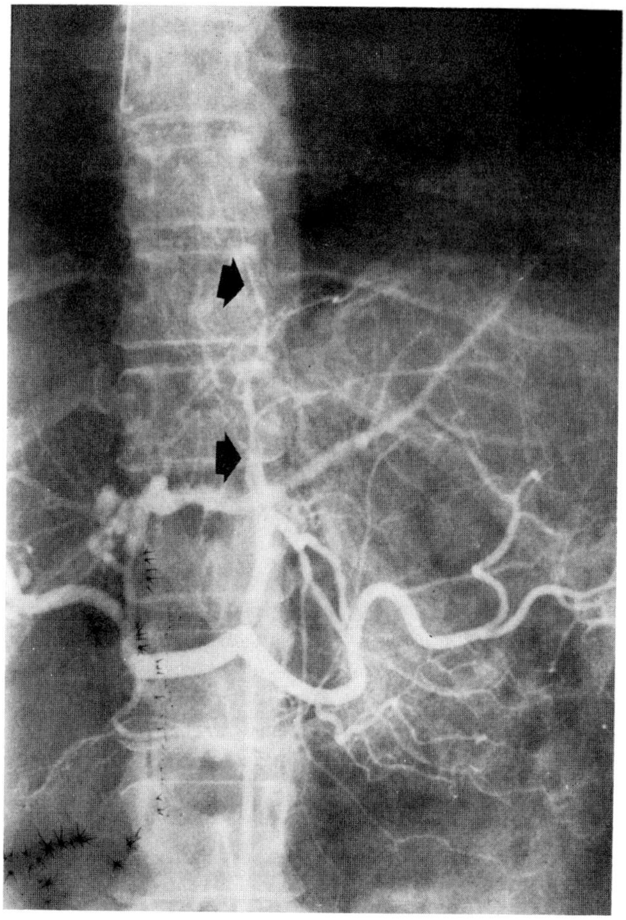

Figure 22.13. Celiac Arteriogram. This patient was known to have esophageal varices which were actively bleeding. The esophageal branches of the left gastric artery are irregular and narrowed. *Comment:* There is spasm of the arteries in the area of bleeding. This is similar to intracranial aneurysmal bleeding with spasm of those adjacent arteries.

the catheter immediately away from that branch to prevent localized regional ischemia. This is especially true in end artery circulation found in the renal or cerebral arteries. In such a situation profound damage can be done if contrast is injected distal to the area of spasm.[856] An awareness that such lesions are functional avoids embarrassing false diagnosis. A repeat examination after withdrawal of the catheter into the parent branch may reveal the true nature of the lesion. If not, a post-Prescoline angiogram may be of some help (Figs. 22-1 to 22-8).

Blunt Trauma

Smooth narrowing of varying length occurs in the vicinity of trauma.[780–783] The relatively exposed position of extremity vessels makes them the frequent victims of traumatic spasm. This spasm may persist from twenty minutes to twenty-four hours after injury and, in extreme cases, may even cause occlusion. It is very intense when there is associated intimal damage with intraluminal clot formation or extravasation of blood into the vessel wall. The direct application of a 2.5% solution of papaverine in the periarterial tissue is more effective in obtaining sustained relaxation, even after withdrawal of application. A forceful, local intravascular injection of normal saline may also help (Fig. 22-10).

Inflammation

Inflammation such as thrombophlebitis of adjacent veins[787] may cause either myotonic or reflex spasm of the associated arteries. This may involve the popliteal[789] or brachial[788] artery.

Vascular Occlusion

Smooth angiospasm may occur after the occlusion of the main stem of the artery. With venous occlusion there is marked arterial spasm which is sustained through a considerable period of time. This may persist even after relief of the venous occlusion. In arterial occlusion there is both arterial and venous spasm.[795]

Shock

Vascular spasm related to shock or trauma to the autonomic nervous system is not an uncommon clinical entity.[780, 790] "Tension in the walls of the vessel must be less than the hydrostatic pressure exerted by the column of blood; otherwise the vessel will collapse. When the vasospasm exceeds the local blood pressure, the artery occludes."[791, 792] Diffuse angiospasm of major and smaller branches of the splanchnic circulation is a common event in shock occurring as a compensatory, homeostatic mechanism. This takes place during states of hemorrhagic, traumatic or cardiogenic shock.[775, 793, 794] Per-

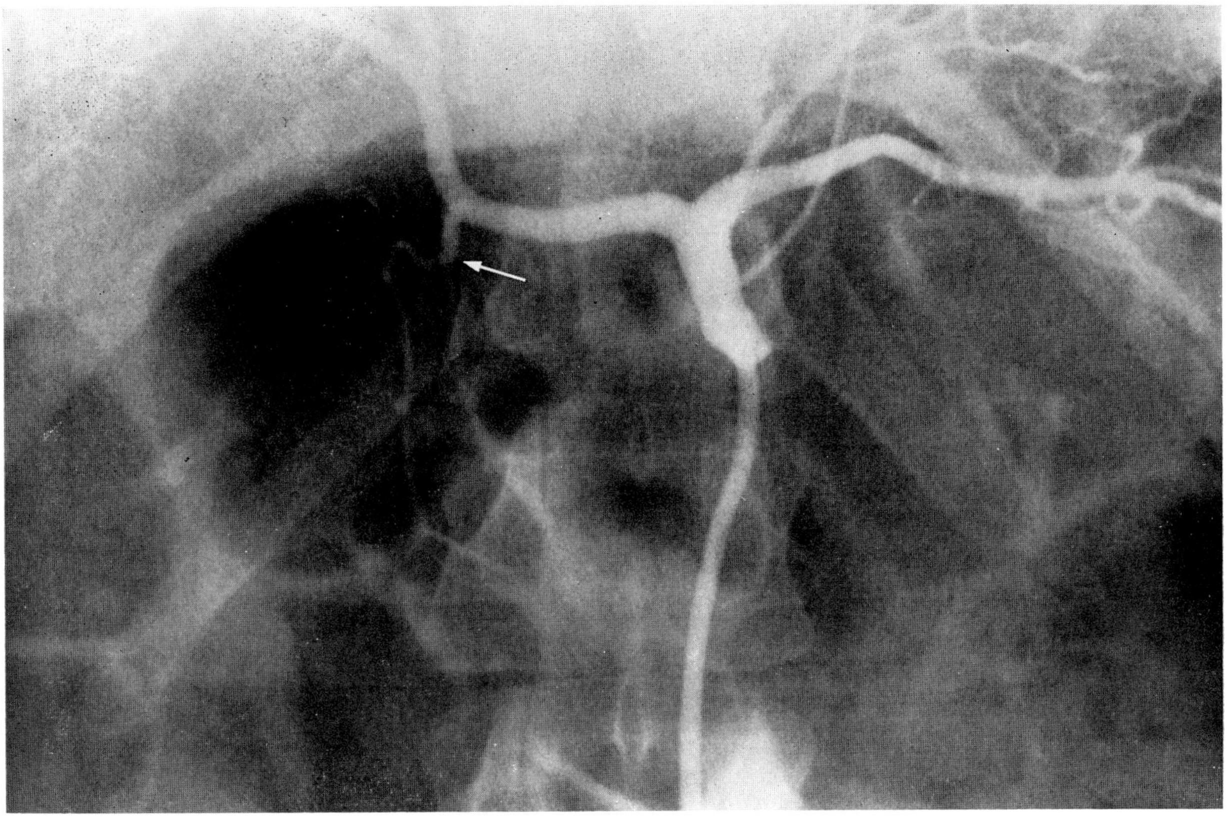

Figure 22.14. Celiac Arteriogram. Smooth narrowing of the gastroduodenal artery is seen in a patient with upper gastrointestinal hemorrhage. The superior mesenteric arteriogram did not fill the gastroduodenal artery. *Comment:* Spasm of the gastroduodenal artery probably due to hemorrhage in the vicinity. *Gastroscopy:* Confirmed hemorrhagic duodenitis.

sistent mesenteric vasoconstriction is an obvious major factor in the development of bowel necrosis.[132]

Drugs

In addition to the popular vasoconstrictors such as *vasopressin* and *epinephrine* which are used for intraarterial infusion to arrest gastrointestinal bleeding, such drugs as levarterenol,[132, 796] digitalis,[797, 798] methysergide maleate,[799] may cause vasoconstriction of the splanchnic vasculature. The *ergot*[800] group of drugs deserves special mention as they are powerful vasoconstrictors. They may even cause damage to the endothelium with stasis and thrombosis of the affected vasculature. They cause bilateral *fairly symmetrical smooth narrowing* of lower extremity vessels.[801] Even the major arteries, the aorta,[800] iliac[802] and carotid arteries[803] are not immune from the vasospastic effect of ergot medication (Figs. 22-11, 22-12).

Hemostatic Mechanisms

Spasm may be demonstrated in a bleeding artery or in the vicinity of a bleeding site. Cervical internal carotid artery spasm due to subarachnoid hemorrhage,[804] spasm of the left gastric artery due to variceal bleeding from the esophagus, and spasm of the gastroduodenal artery and its branches in hemorrhagic duodenitis are examples of this phenomena (Figs. 22-13, 22-14).

Miscellaneous

Angiodyskinesia,[805] a phenomenon caused by a disturbance in the normal hemodynamic regulatory mechanism that normally provides adjustments to the increased venous pressure in

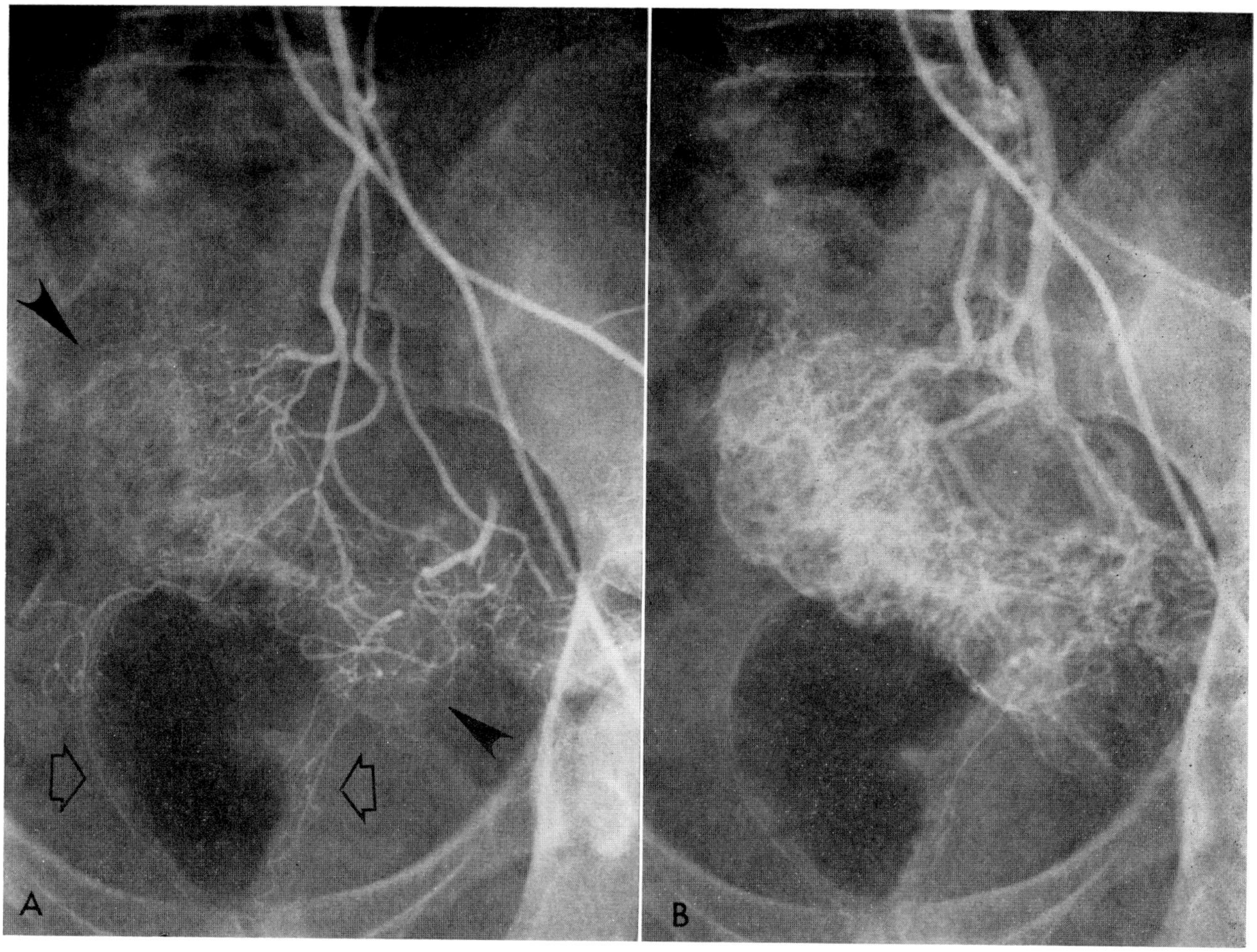

Figure 22.15. Inferior Mesenteric Arteriogram. (A) Arterial phase: There is tapering and narrowing of branches of the rectum (Arrow) compared to the perfusion of the sigmoid colon (Arrow Head). (B) Venous phase: There is lack of mucosal stain and venous opacification in the rectum and intense opacification of the sigmoid colon, mucosa and the other veins. This patient had intracavitary radium insertion five days prior to the examination. *Comment:* Radiation induced spasm?

the lower extremities, produces arterial spasm and early venous return. Arteriospastic phenomenon of the extremities[806] is characterized by intermittent or permanent smooth narrowing of the small arteries of the extremities. This may cause ischemia without organic occlusion of the vessels.

ORGANIC DISORDERS OF THE VESSEL WALL

1. Hypoplasia: Elongated areas of smooth tubular narrowing.
2. Hyperplasia: Smooth narrowing of variable lengths, single or multiple vessels.
3. Inflammation: Smooth narrowing of single or multiple vessels.
4. Metabolic (atherosclerosis): Patchy in its distribution. The narrowing may be concentric, eccentric, smooth or irregular, involve single or multiple vessels, and short or long segments.
5. Atrophy (disuse): Uniform smooth narrowing of the entire vessel and its arborization.
6. Narrowing due to extrinsic causes:

Encasement and infiltration present as *smooth narrowing* of single or multiple vessels of variable length, as *torsional narrowing, sawtooth narrowing,* or *irregular serpigenous narrowing. Extrinsic compression* may be of localized nature, giving sharp narrowing of a short segment, or a torsional effect, or elongated smooth narrowing, and is usually *eccentric.*

Congenital Hypoplasia

This is characterized by smooth *uniform narrowing* of a variable length. There is usually no significant histologic abnormality in the vessel wall. It has been demonstrated in the aorta,[412] femoral arteries,[807] and celiac and mesenteric stenosis associated with supravalvular aortic stenosis.[850] The same effect is achieved if there is an insult to the vessel during its growth as seen in aortic hypoplasia due to irradiation[814] (Fig. 22-16).

Hyperplasia of the Components of the Vascular Wall

Nonspecific proliferation of the intima with increased connective tissue accumulation of elastic and collagenous tissues in the media is seen in abdominal aortic coarctation. *Smooth narrowing* in the aorta starts above or below the level of the celiac artery and usually terminates above the level of the inferior mesenteric ar-

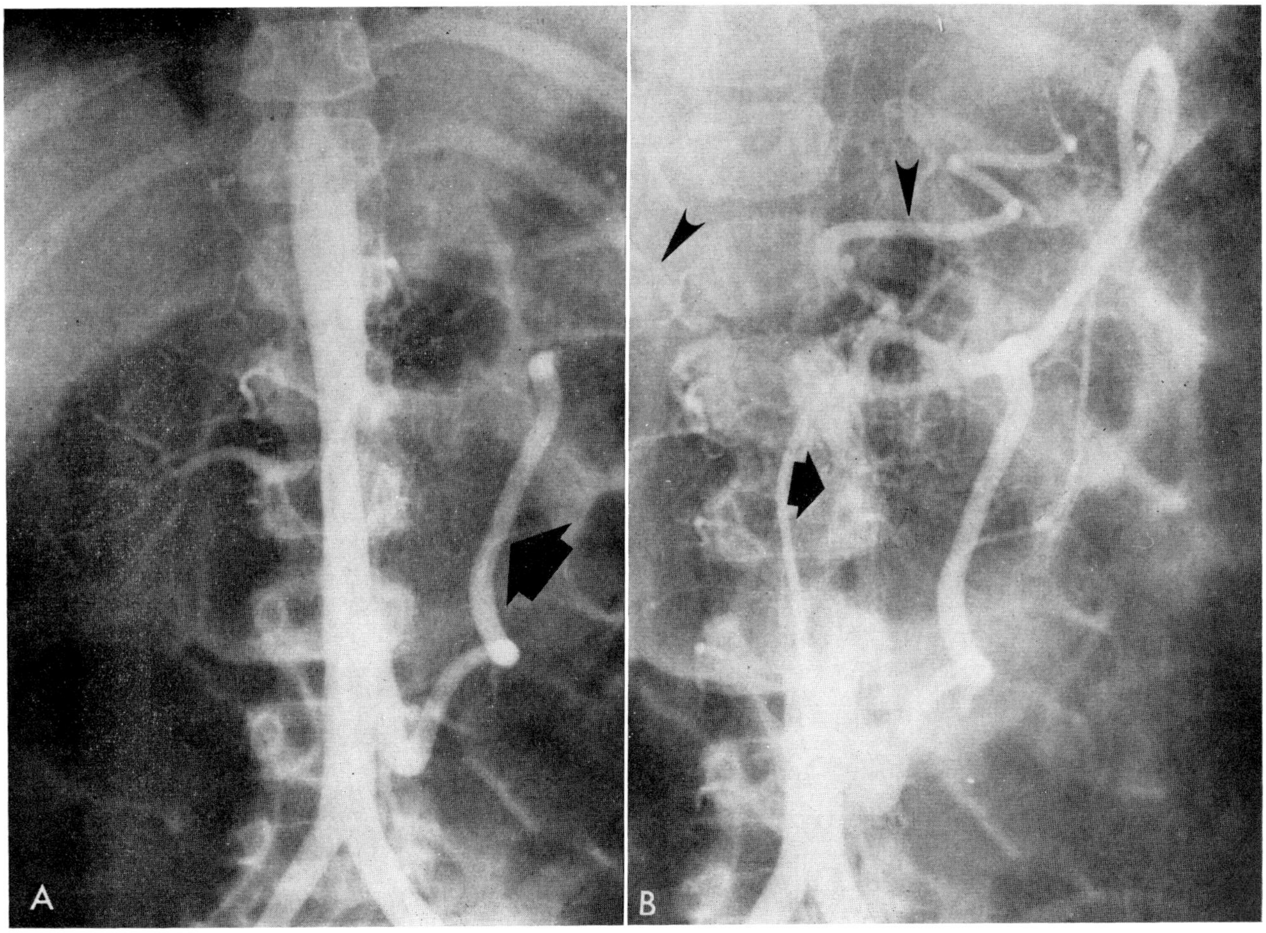

Figure 22.16. Flush Aortogram. (A) Smooth narrowing of the midabdominal aorta, nonvisualization of the left renal artery and a very prominent dilated branch coursing towards the splenic flexure arising from the inferior mesenteric artery (Arrow) are present. (B) Late arterial phase: The same branch fills the superior mesenteric artery (Arrow) and perfuses the branches of the celiac artery (Arrow Head). This twelve-year-old patient had hypertension. *Diagnosis:* Hypoplastic abdominal aorta with occlusion of the left renal, celiac and superior mesenteric arteries with perfusion to the superior mesenteric artery from the marginal artery.

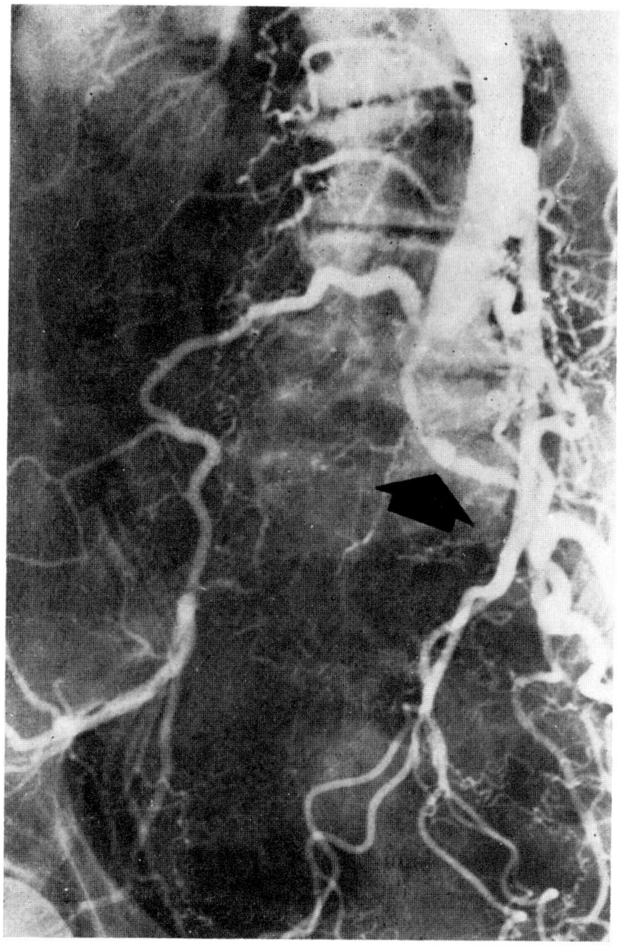

Figure 22.17. Pelvic Arteriogram. There is smooth narrowing (Arrow) of the distal abdominal aorta. The patient was seventy years old. *Diagnosis:* Aortic thrombosis. Leriche syndrome?

tery. Though the visceral arteries are involved along the way, there is usually no visceral manifestation. The renal artery ostia are also frequently involved.[808–810, 812]

Smooth, uniform narrowing is caused by intimal fibroplasia, fibromuscular hyperplasia, adventitial or periarterial fibroplasia. These lesions are very common in the renal arteries, particularly in the distal two-thirds and may even involve the branches. It is rare in the extra renal arteries. In addition, intimal fibroplasia has been described involving the abdominal aorta[629] with hypertension, perimuscular fibrosis of the renal arteries in hypertension,[811] isolated periarterial fibrosis of the femoral arteries,[813] and superior mesenteric artery (Figs. 22-25, 22-37).

Coarctation of the aorta is a sharply localized area of narrowing with a localized deformity of the aortic media. This occurs at the junction of the aortic arch and the descending aorta. A curtain-like infolding of the vessel wall toward the lumen is seen in the aorta, sparing the inferior aspect.[412]

Miscellaneous Causes of Narrowing

Mucoid cystic degeneration of the arterial wall, especially of the adventitia, can cause smooth concentric narrowing of a vessel. This is frequently found in the younger population, affecting the popliteal artery.[815] Neurofibromatous tissue in the wall of a vessel may cause

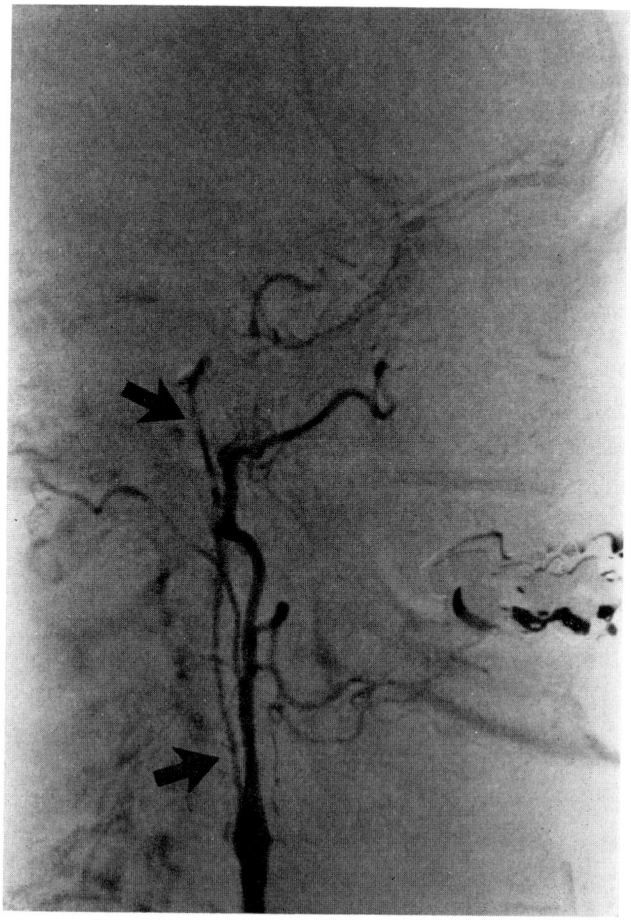

Figure 22.18. Carotid Arteriogram. There is smooth narrowing of the internal carotid artery. This young female had cerebral symtoms. *Radiographic Diagnosis:* Arteritis. No further confirmation obtained.

smooth concentric narrowing, not only due to the tumor tissue itself, but also to associated intimal and medial fibrous proliferation. This has been seen in the renal artery with hypertension, as well as in the aorta.[816–818]

ENCASEMENT AND INFILTRATION

A schirrous invasive process, whether benign or malignant, can cause narrowing of a vessel by either wrapping the vessel with schirrous tissue or by direct infiltration. Infiltrating cellular malignant tumors can achieve the same results. Schirrous reaction due to pancreatic lesions, either pancreatitis or malignancy, is probably the most common, frequent example seen in clinical angiography. The *smoothness or the irregularity* of the narrowed vessel depends on the uniformity of fibrous encasement, the aggressive behavior of the schirrous stroma, the diameter of the vessel and its physiological status (artery or vein). The *smaller the caliber of the vessel* in the intrinsic vasculature of the organ, the *greater the varieties and types of narrowing.* This includes smooth, irregular, torsional, and sawtooth narrowing, and even occlusion. The larger the caliber of the vessel, the more advanced must be the disease to produce the above varieties of narrowing (Fig. 22-22).

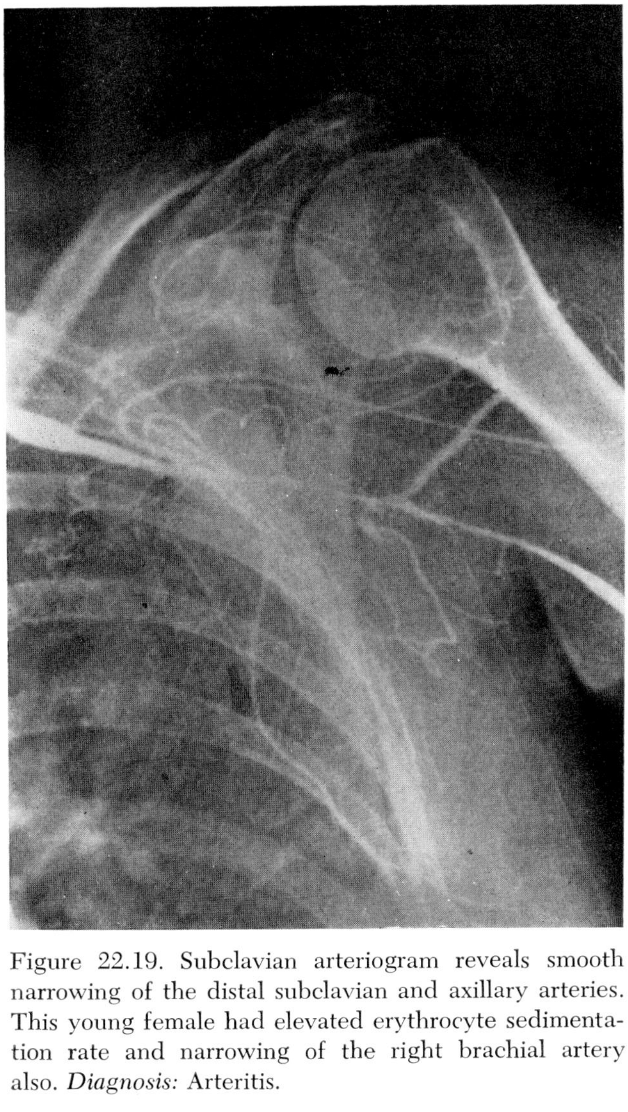

Figure 22.19. Subclavian arteriogram reveals smooth narrowing of the distal subclavian and axillary arteries. This young female had elevated erythrocyte sedimentation rate and narrowing of the right brachial artery also. *Diagnosis:* Arteritis.

Pancreas

Adenocarcinoma of the pancreas is usually a dense, *schirrous tumor* with irregular, indistinct margins due to infiltration and retraction of associated tissues.[1371] Two thirds of them are in the head, and the remaining one-third in the body and tail.[1235] Carcinoma of the uncinate process,[1380] a hook-like posterior extension of the head of the pancreas tucked between the superior mesenteric artery and the aorta, usually invades the dorsal pancreatic artery before it invades the superior mesenteric or middle colic arteries (Figs. 22-24, 22-26, 22-27).

Angiographically,[1375–1377] *encasement and occlusion* of the regional vessels are the most frequent manifestations of these tumors. The encasement may be in the form of sawtooth, irregular, torsional, or smooth narrowing. The encasement and/or occlusion may be of the intrinsic pancreatic vessels and the adjacent extrinsic vessels such as the celiac artery, superior mesenteric artery and their branches, or the splenic, portal, or superior mesenteric veins. A *dilated gallbladder,* if present, aids in establishing the presence of obstructive jaundice. If major vessels are involved, such as the gastroduodenal, superior mesenteric, or hepatic arteries, or superior mesenteric or portal veins, it may suggest that the lesion is inoperable.[1381] The anatomic extent of the lesion is usually greater than that demonstrated at angiography. The diagnosis of pancreatic carcinoma is *limited angiographically*[1372–1374] by the following diseases which may mask or mimic a malignancy (Figs. 22-39, 22-43 to 22-46).

Atherosclerosis of the pancreatic[1378] and other adjacent vessels, penetrating gastric ulcers with encasement due to periarterial fibrosis, chronic pancreatitis with vascular occlusion (usually venous), and associated arterial atherosclerosis. Mimicking carcinomatous invasion are atherosclerotic occlusion of the celiac and mesenteric arteries with tortuous collaterals, other retroperitoneal tumors which infiltrate into the pancreatic branches, such as reticulum cell sarcoma[1379] or other malignancies about the head of the pancreas such as carcinoma of the ampulla of Vater, common bile ducts, or primary duodenal carcinoma.

Renal Transitional Cell Carcinoma

These tumors arise from the draining structures of the kidney and are usually less expansive and more invasive than hypernephromas, presenting as infiltrating, or schirrous, or epidermoid tumors.[1403] On rare occasions they can be expansile, poorly differentiated and vascular. *Infiltration and total occlusion of the regional vasculature* are the usual angiographic findings. If the adjacent renal parenchyma is invaded, the tumor may stimulate abundant neoplastic vascular response[1404–1406] (Figs. 28-45, 28-46).

Gallbladder

Carcinomas of the gallbladder are usually infiltrating, resulting in a small or normal sized gallbladder.[111, 1214] On occasion it may be enlarged, particularly if there is mucoid excretion or purulent material in the gallbladder. *Occlusion or encasement* of the regional vessels is common. Infiltration of even the superior mesenteric artery or portal vein is not unusual in extensive lesions. Neovasculature in the liver suggests extension into that organ.[1382–1385]

Cholangiocarcinoma

Infiltrating malignant tumors are more common than fungating lesions.[1214, 1383, 1386] *Irregular encasement* of the vessels is the result of these more invasive and less expansive tumors. When extensive, the exact site of origin cannot be determined angiographically. Infiltration into the right lobe of the liver is not unusual in extensive disease. Unlike hepatomas, these cholangiocarcinomas tend to involve women more than men.

Stretching and Encasement of Vessels in Benign Lesions

Benign lesions which can cause *desmoplastic reactions* include retroperitoneal fibrosis, mesenteric fibromatosis due to Gardner's syndrome,[819] familial polyposis,[820] and mesenteric panniculitis.[821, 822] Severe desmoplastic reactions are also caused by carcinoid tumors, especially in the ileocecal area. This is associated with vascular encasement and irregular areas of narrowing. Penetrating gastric ulcers, because of fi-

(Text continues on page 274)

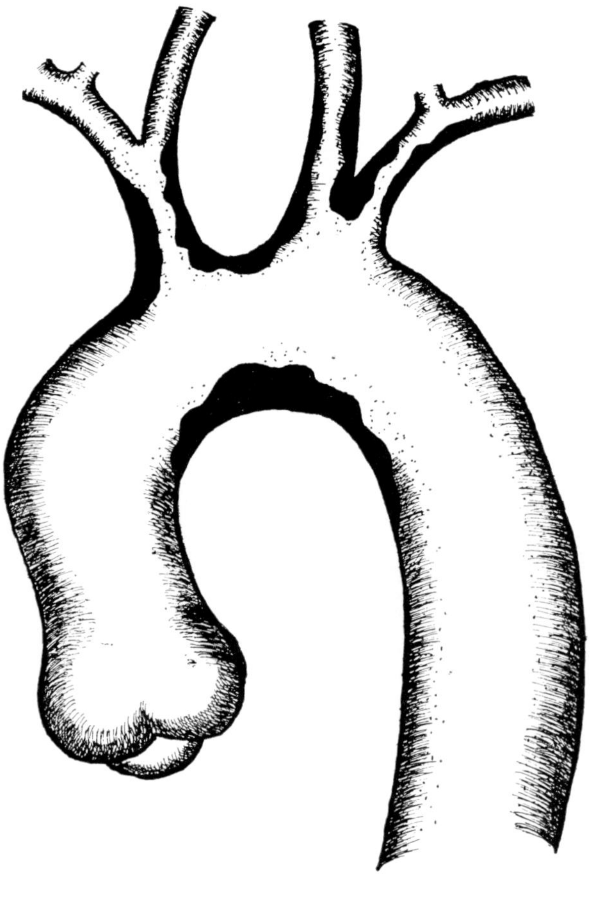

A

Figure 22.20 A

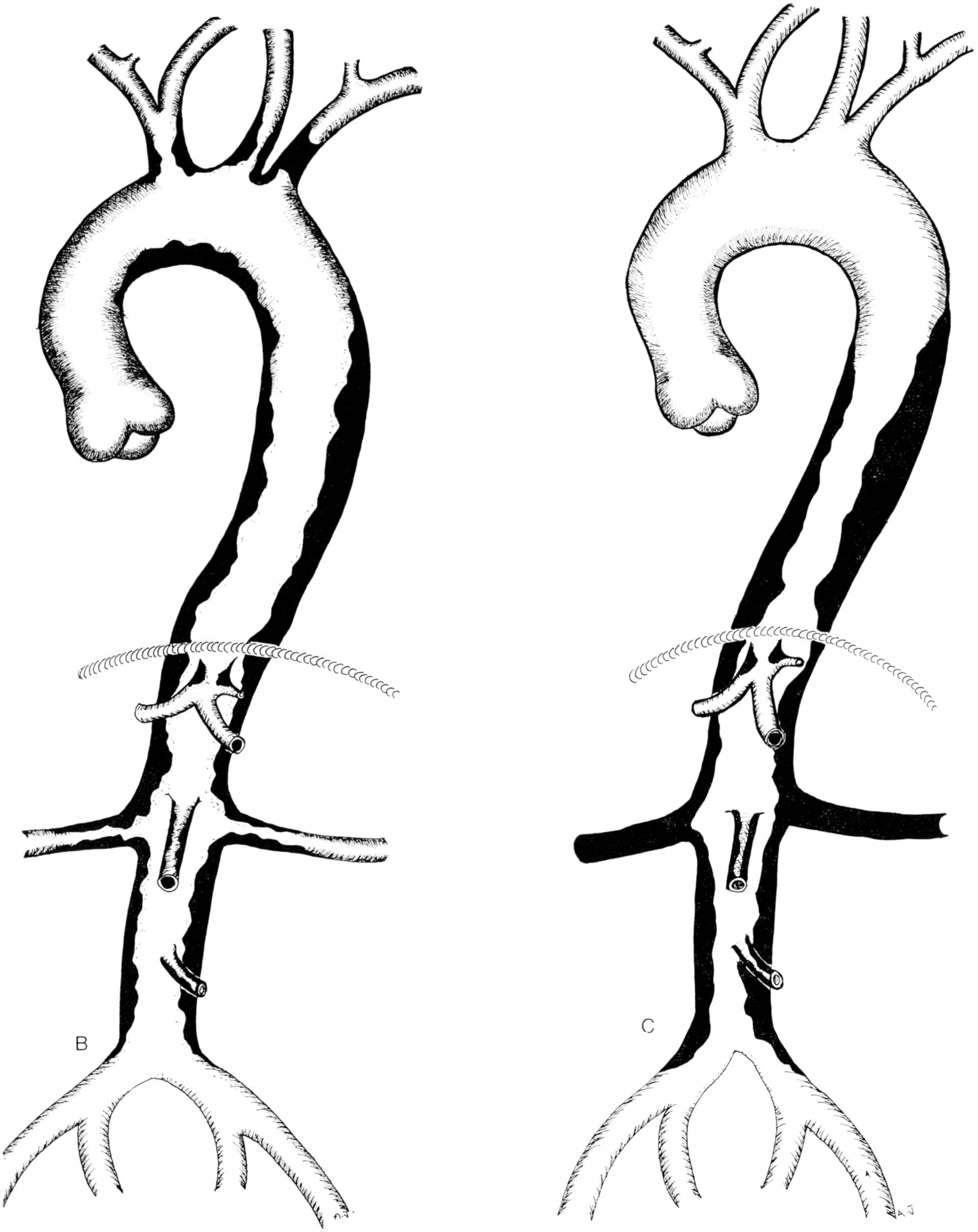

Figure 22.20 *(Continued)*. Varying involvement of aorta and its branches by aortitis.

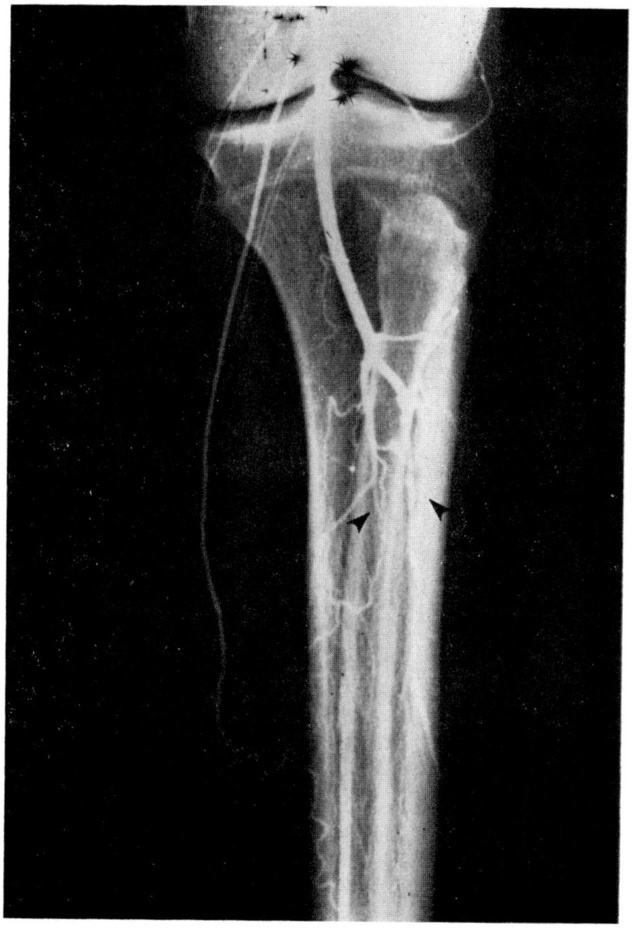

Figure 22.21. Femoral Arteriogram. There is smoothly tapered occlusion of all the branches of the popliteal trifurcation. The remainder of the artery has a smooth configuration. The same findings were present in the opposite extremity. The patient was a young man. *Diagnosis:* Thromboangiitis obliterans.

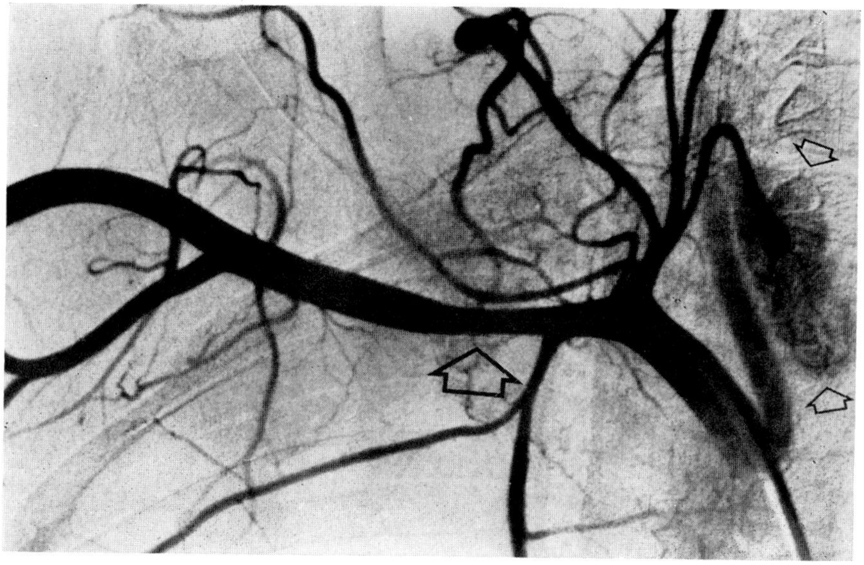

Figure 22.22. Right Subclavian Arteriogram. There is a localized smooth narrowing of the right subclavian artery (Large Arrow). Incidentally, seen is a stain of the thyroid gland (Small Arrow) in a patient with Pancoast tumor. *Diagnosis:* Pancoast bronchogenic carcinoma infiltrating the wall of the subclavian artery.

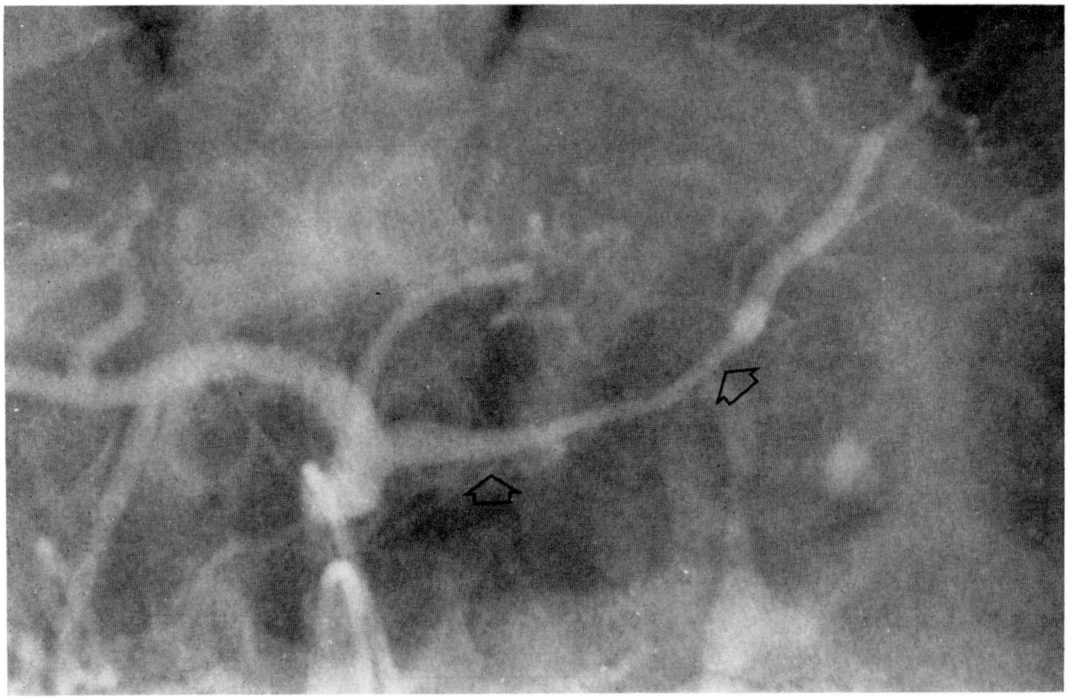

Figure 22.23. Simultaneous Celiac and Superior Mesenteric Angiograms. There is smooth narrowing of the midportion of the splenic artery (Arrow). The patient was a known alcoholic. *Diagnosis:* Pancreatitis. A differential diagnosis would include benign versus malignant pancreatic process. Other retroperitoneal lesions may encase the splenic artery.

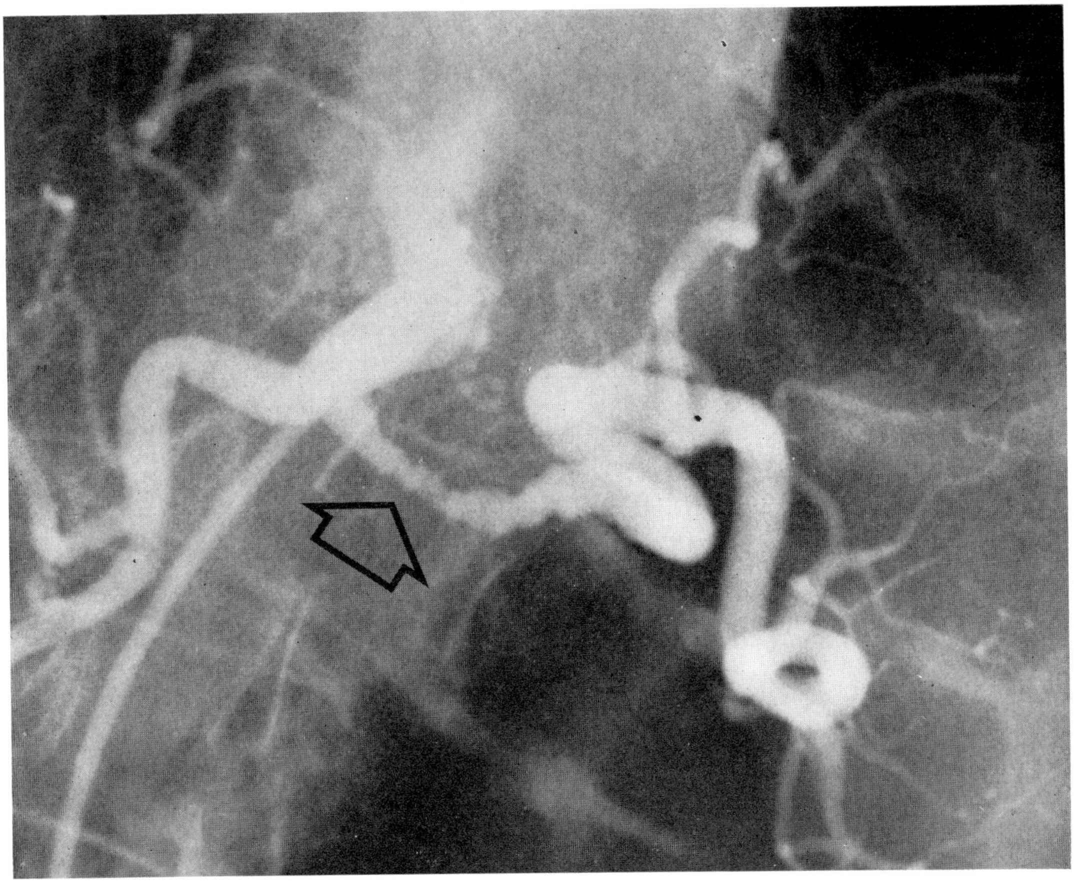

Figure 22.24. Celiac arteriogram reveals serrated irregular narrowing of the main trunk of the splenic artery. This patient has backache and weight loss. *Diagnosis:* Carcinoma of the pancreas. *Surgery:* Confirmed an inoperable carcinoma of the pancreas. (Courtesy of Dr. H. Qazi, St. Lukes Hospital, Racine, Wisconsin.)

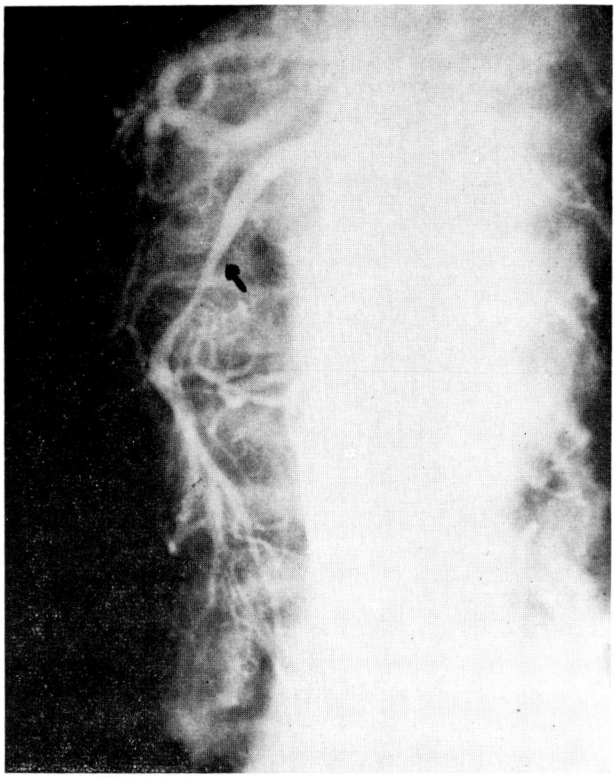

Figure 22.25. Aortogram (cross-table). Reveals smooth narrowing of midsuperior mesenteric artery. *Pathology:* Periarterial fibrosis.

brotic reaction, can cause encasement with smooth or irregular areas of narrowing.[111, 823]

Retroperitoneal Fibrosis

This disease of unknown etiology causes a nonspecific, nonsuppurative inflammation of the fibro fatty tissue within the retroperitoneal space extending to Gerota's fascia superiorly and to the pelvis inferiorly.[1343–1345] In many cases it extends to the mediastinum. There is gradual compression and involvement without invasion of the retroperitoneal tubular structures such as the ureters, veins and arteries. The lesion may be diffuse or segmental, unilateral or bilateral.

Carcinoid

This fascinating tumor,[1387, 1392] which acts as a missing link between benign and malignant neoplasms, deserves to be labelled *a malignant neoplasm in slow motion.* The incidence of occurrence increases from the duodenum to the terminal ileum. The slow rate of local spread and distal metastasis characterize the life cycle of this tumor. Angiographically, *encasement,* either irregular or smooth, or *occlusion* of the small or major branches of the superior mesenteric arteries can be demonstrated because of the associated, severe desmoplastic reaction[1390] caused by carcinoids within the mesentery. The extent of fibrosis, when present, may even reach the retroperitoneal area as well.[1391] Retraction of the fibrotic mesentery causes stellate crowding of the mesenteric branches coursing in the layers of the mesentery. Narrowing of the major branches may suggest lymphnodal extension of the lesion. These findings, though suggestive of an illeocecal carcinoid, are *not pathognomonic,* as more or less similar findings may be given by desmoplastic disorders which can induce fibrosis and retraction of the mesentery. This is seen in retractile mesenteritis or fibromatosis due to Gardner's syndrome or familial polyposis.[819–822] One of the interesting findings with ileocecal carcinoid tumors is the comparative hypovascularity, or even avascularity of the primary lesion. However, their metastatic lesions in the liver or primary carcinoids of the stomach[1394] or bronchus[1395] are very vascular. This is probably due to *strangulation of their own blood supply* by the induced fibroplastic reaction of the mesentery. The popular clinical carcinoid syndrome[1396] rarely occurs without metastasis to the liver. Primary lesions of the ileocecal area tend to metastasize more frequently to the liver.[1388, 1389] Their association with other primary malignancies[1387] or their ability to induce hypertension in individuals with preexisting renal disease[1393] always places carcinoid tumors in the range of the clinical spotlight (Fig. 22-48).

Inflammatory Disorders of the Vessel Walls Causing Narrowing

These diseases include *necrotizing angiitis, arteritis, and thromboangiitis obliterans.* Dur-

(Text continues on page 282)

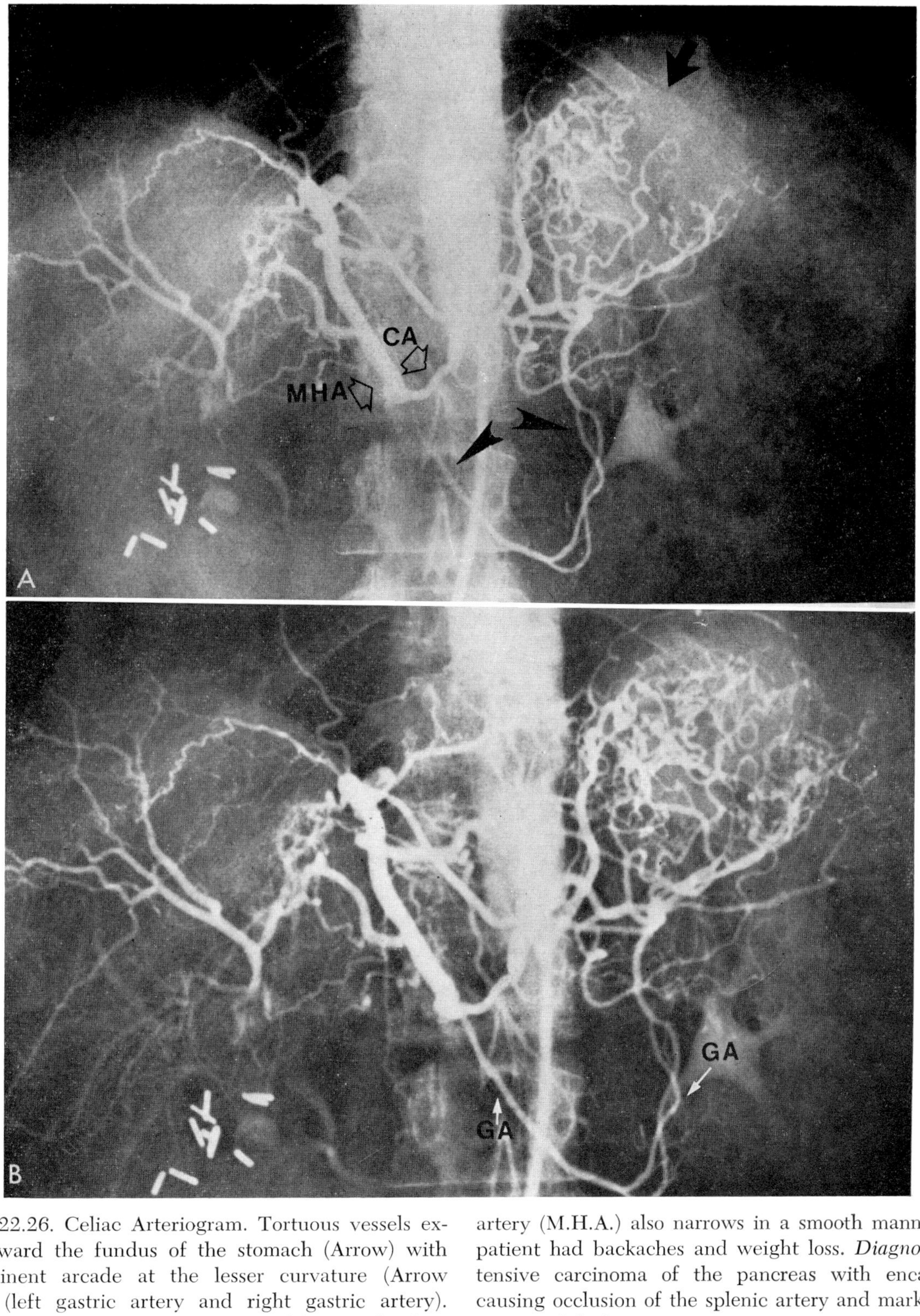

Figure 22.26. Celiac Arteriogram. Tortuous vessels extend toward the fundus of the stomach (Arrow) with a prominent arcade at the lesser curvature (Arrow Head); (left gastric artery and right gastric artery). The celiac artery (C.A.) tapers smoothly just distal to the origin of the left gastric artery. The main hepatic artery (M.H.A.) also narrows in a smooth manner. The patient had backaches and weight loss. *Diagnosis:* Extensive carcinoma of the pancreas with encasement causing occlusion of the splenic artery and marked narrowing of the hepatic artery.

Figure 22.27. Superior Mesenteric Arteriogram—venous phase. There is smooth narrowing of the portal vein. The patient had painless jaundice. *Diagnosis:* Encasement due to a malignant pancreatic neoplasm. *Surgical Diagnosis:* Inoperable pancreatic carcinoma.

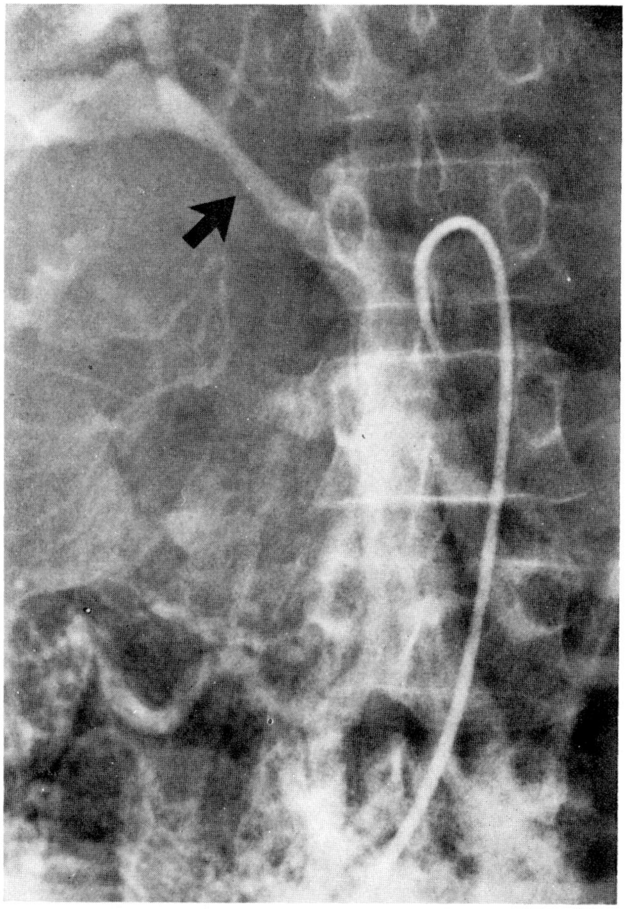

Figure 22.28. Inferior Vena Cavagram. (A) A.P. projection: Tortuous vertebral venous plexus are visualized (Arrow) but no visualization of the upper portion of the inferior vena cava. There are tortuous dilated abnormal veins (Arrow). (B) Lateral projection: Smooth narrowing of the inferior vena cava (Arrow) is seen. The patient has lupus erythematosus. *Diagnosis:* Thrombosis of the inferior vena cava with possible recanalization. *Pathology:* Thrombosis of the renal vein with extension into the inferior vena cava and recanalization of the cava.

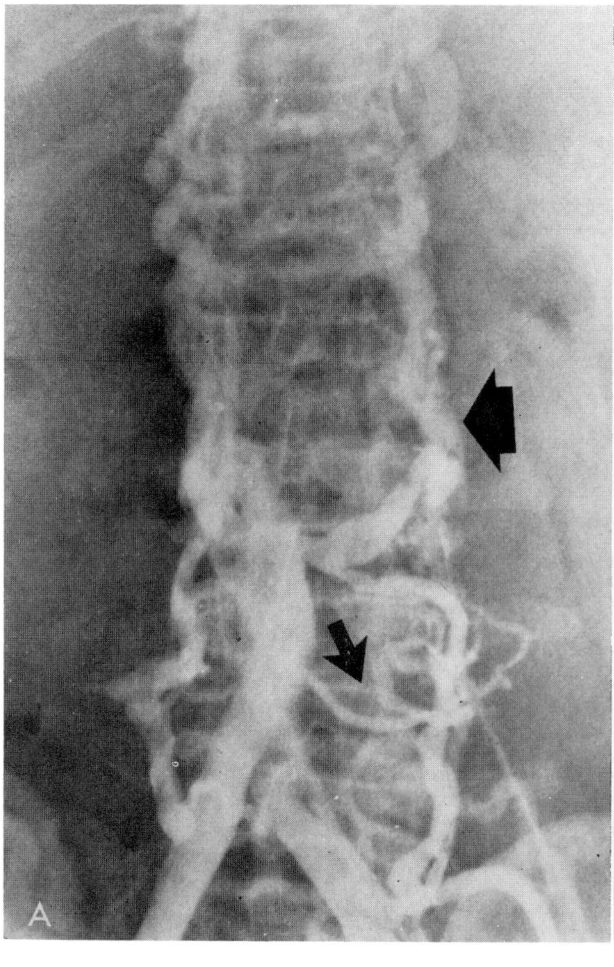

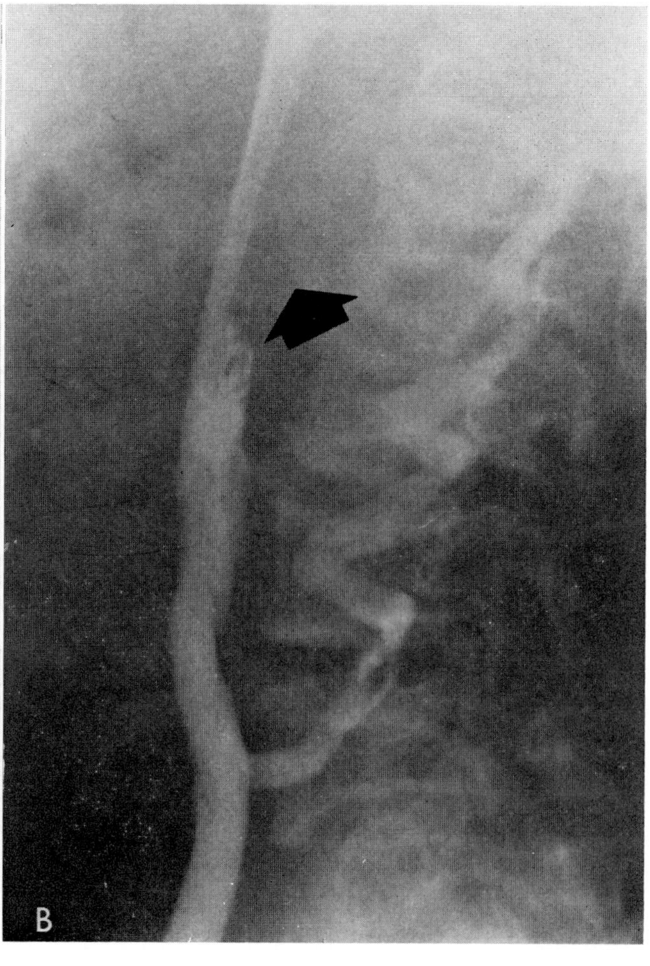

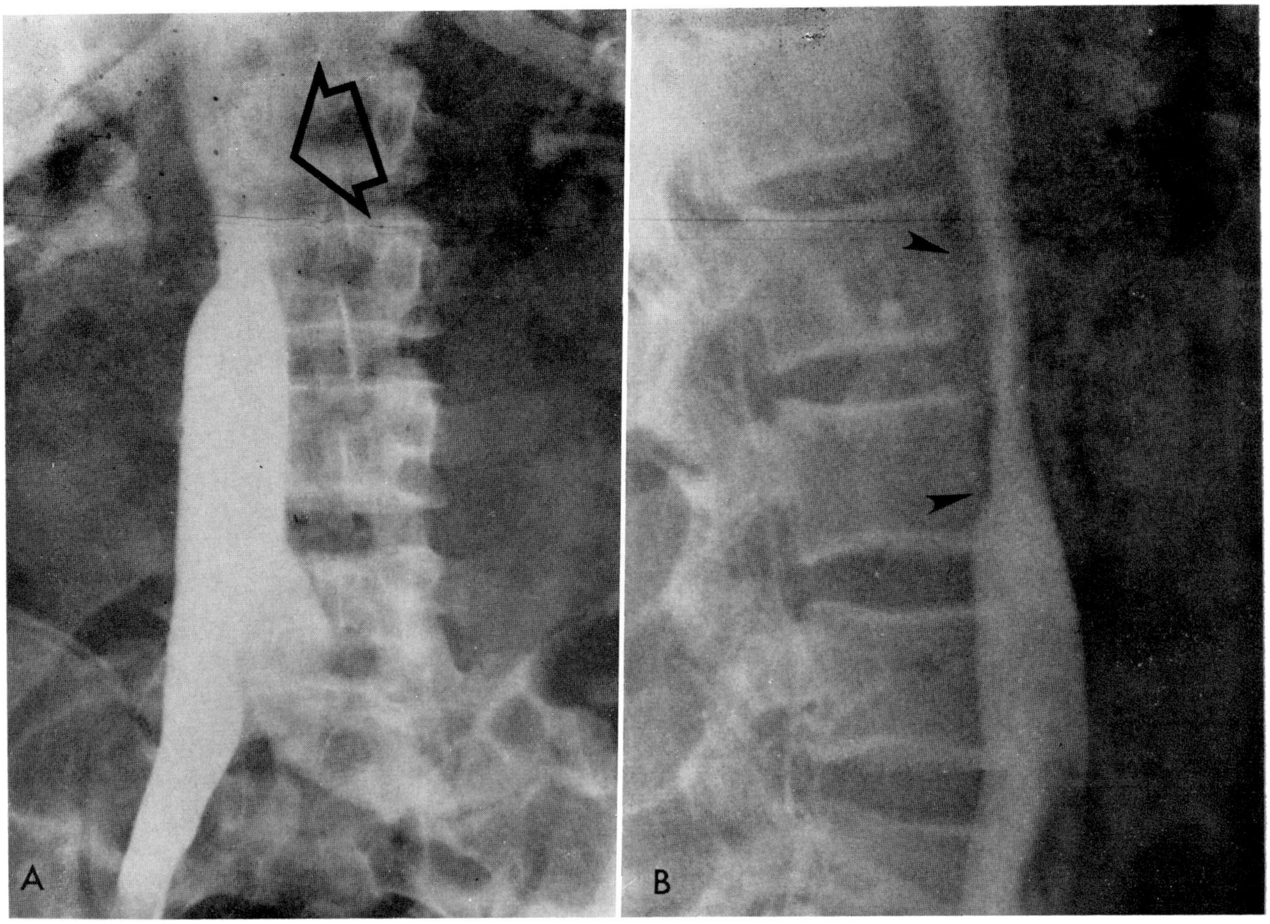

Figure 22.29. Inferior Vena Cavagram. (A) A.P. projection: There is a sudden change in the caliber of a portion of the inferior vena cava. (B) Lateral projection: Again a concentric narrowing of the same segment of inferior vena cava (Arrow) is revealed. This patient had penetrating trauma due to a bullet. *Diagnosis:* Perivenous hematoma with secondary compression.

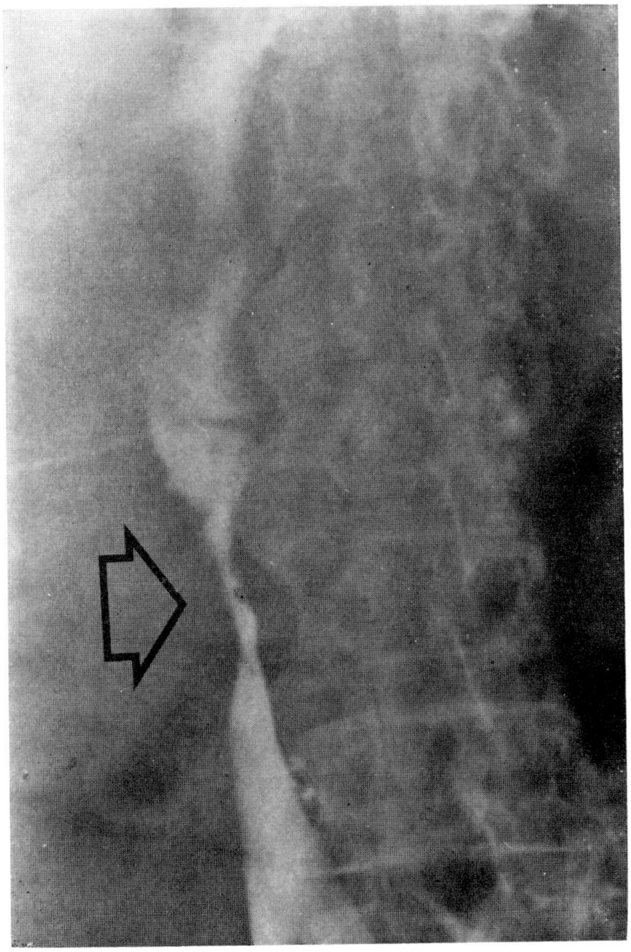

←

Figure 22.30. Inferior Vena Cavagram. Marked concentric narrowing of a segment of the inferior vena cava (Arrow) is seen. Notice the marked osteophytes at the same level. *Diagnosis:* Marked narrowing of the inferior vena cava due to extrinsic pressure by osteophytes causing perivenous fibrosis. *Autopsy:* Confirmed the radiographic impression at a later date.

Figure 22.31. Superior Vena Cavagram (subtraction film). There is marked narrowing of the superior vena cava with irregularities of the walls (Arrow) and marked narrowing of the right innominate vein (I.V.). This patient had a right paratracheal mass. *Diagnosis:* Infiltration of the superior vena cava due to a malignant mass. *Pathology:* Bronchogenic carcinoma.

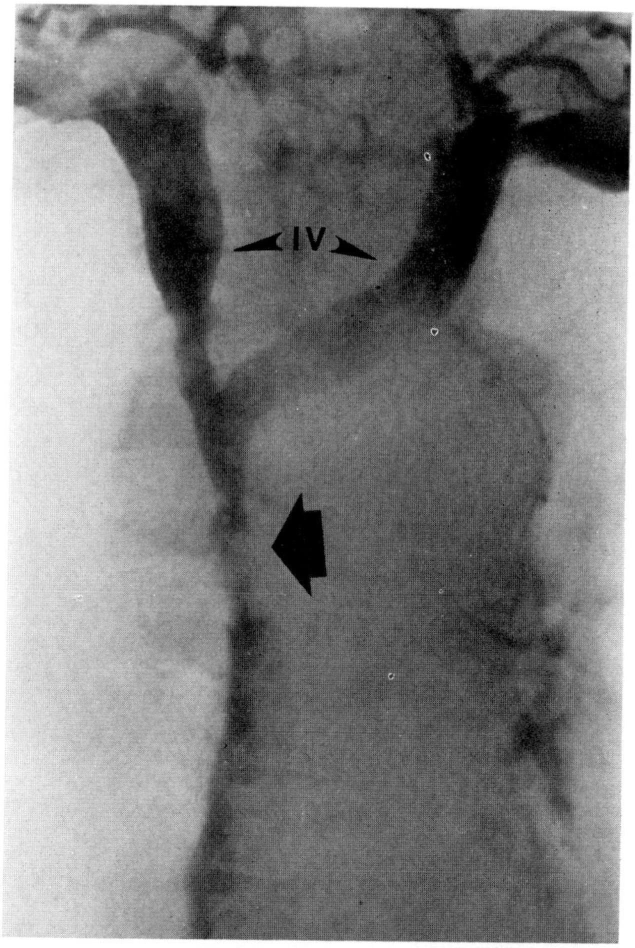

Figure 22.32. (A) Flush abdominal aortogram: There is concentric narrowing of the proximal abdominal aorta and the origin of the left renal artery (Arrow). A prominent tortuous vessel is seen along the projection of the pancreatic arcade. (B) Lateral projection: The celiac axis is not seen. *Diagnosis:* Atherosclerotic narrowing of the aorta at the level of the celiac axis origin. There is collateral circulation (pancreaticoduodenal arcade) from the superior mesenteric artery which fills the celiac axis.

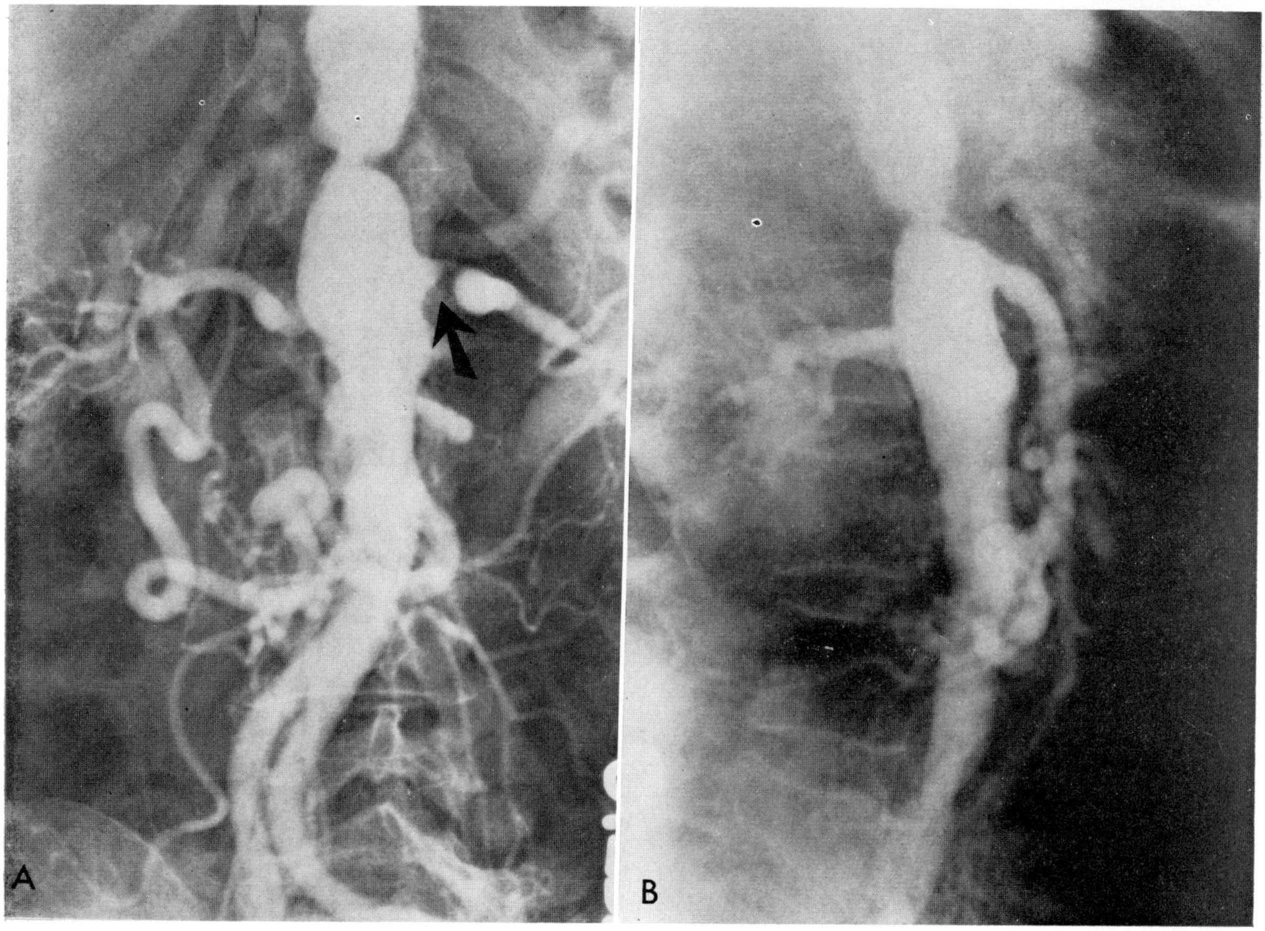

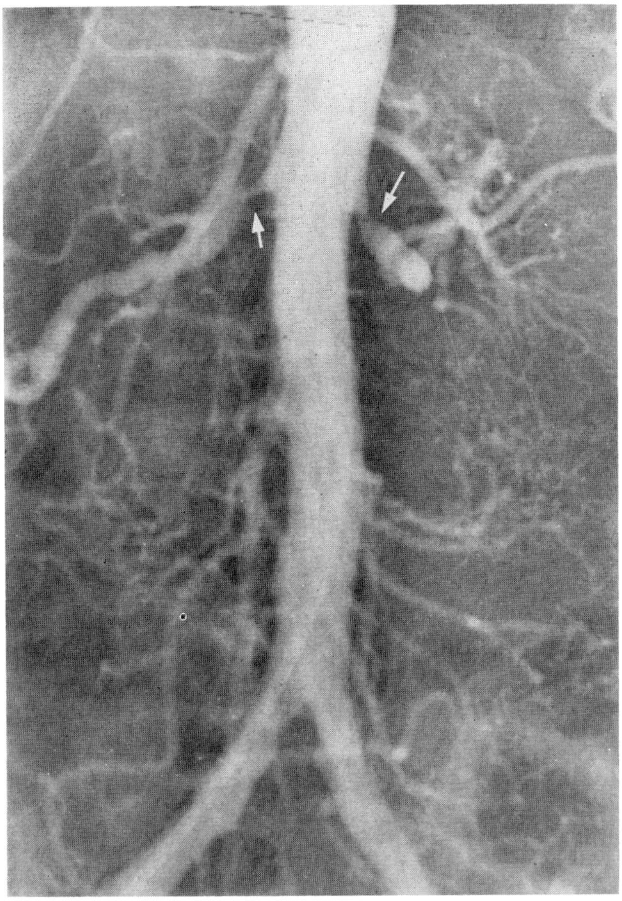

←

Figure 22.33. Abdominal Aortogram. The renal arteries (Arrow Head) are narrowed in a concentric manner. There are luminal irregularities of the contrast filled aorta. The patient is fifty-seven years old and without hypertension. *Diagnosis:* Atherosclerosis of the abdominal aorta with atherosclerotic narrowing of the renal arteries.

Figure 22.34. Renal Arteriogram. (A) Left renal arteriogram: A smooth localized concentric area of narrowing in the midrenal artery is revealed. (B) Right renal arteriogram: The same findings are in the midportion of the right renal artery. The flush aortogram revealed the same findings. The patient had hypertension. *Diagnosis:* Stenosis of both renal arteries. Hyperplastic diseases like adventitial or intimal hyperplasia versus atherosclerotic narrowing. *Surgery:* Atherosclerotic narrowing.

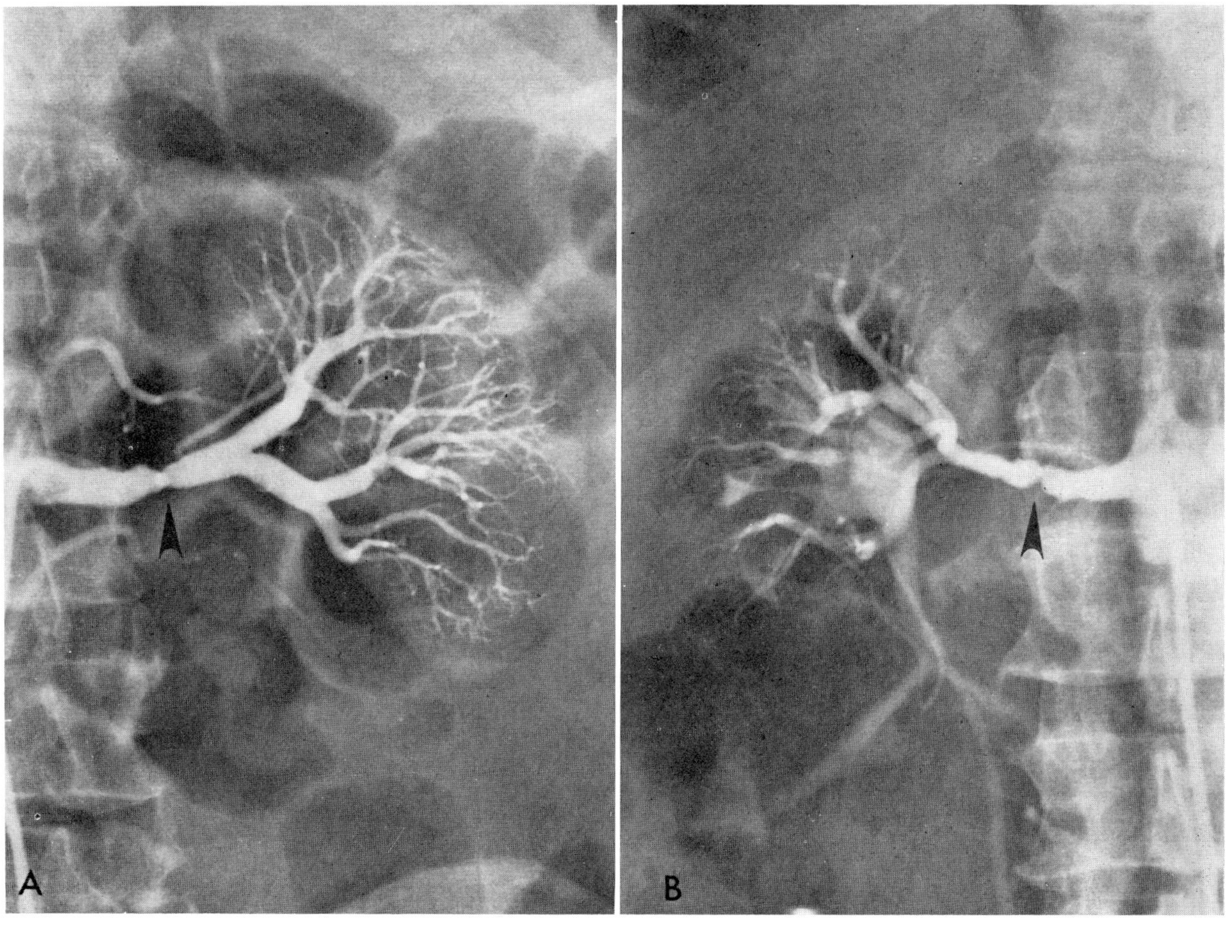

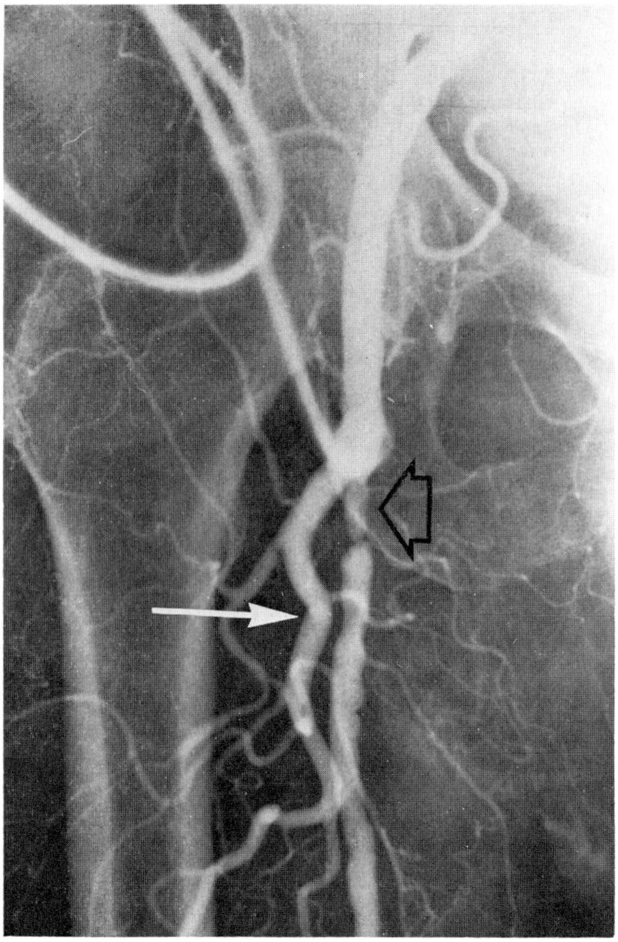

Figure 22.35. Femoral Arteriogram. There are irregular areas of narrowing in the superficial femoral artery (Blank Arrow). No abnormalities of the deep femoral artery (White Arrow) are seen. This sixty-five-year-old patient had symptoms of intermittent claudication. *Diagnosis:* Atherosclerosis of the superficial femoral artery which spares the deep femoral artery.

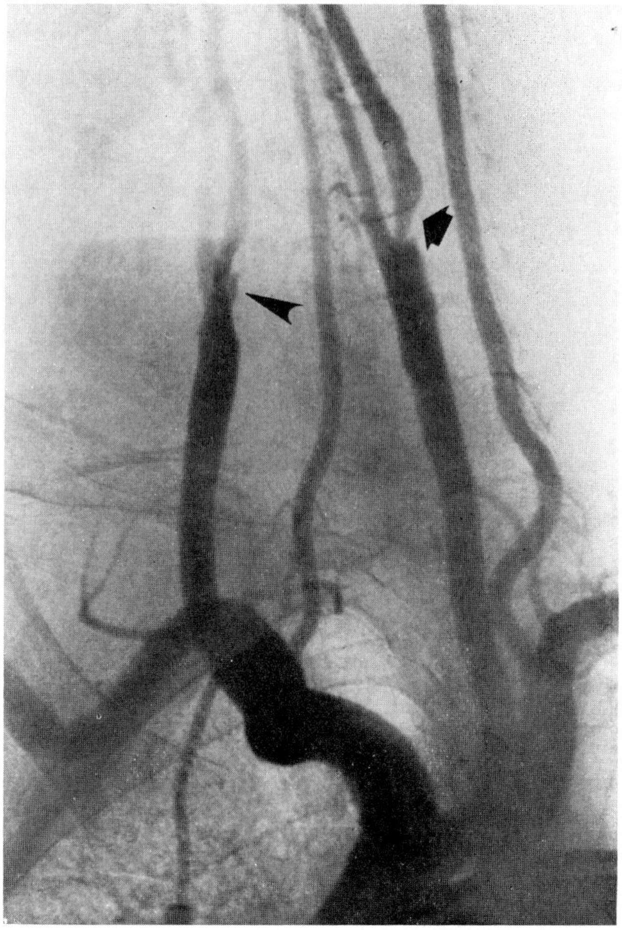

Figure 22.36. Aortic Arch Angiogram (L.A.O.). There is concentric narrowing of the proximal left internal carotid artery (Arrow) and eccentric narrowing of the proximal right internal carotid artery with an extra collection of contrast (Arrow Head). This sixty-eight-year-old woman had repeated attacks of transient ischemic episodes. *Diagnosis:* Atherosclerotic narrowing of the left internal carotid artery. Atherosclerotic ulcer of the right internal carotid artery.

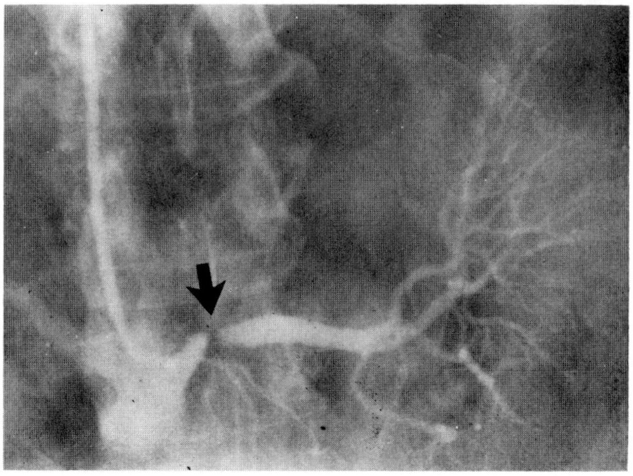

Figure 22.37. Renal Arteriogram. Extreme concentric narrowing of the very proximal portion of the right renal artery occurs in a young patient with a history of hypertension. *Diagnosis:* Severe stenosis of the renal artery due to hyperplastic disorders like intimal hyperplasia or subadventitial hyperplasia. *Pathology:* Intimal hyperplasia.

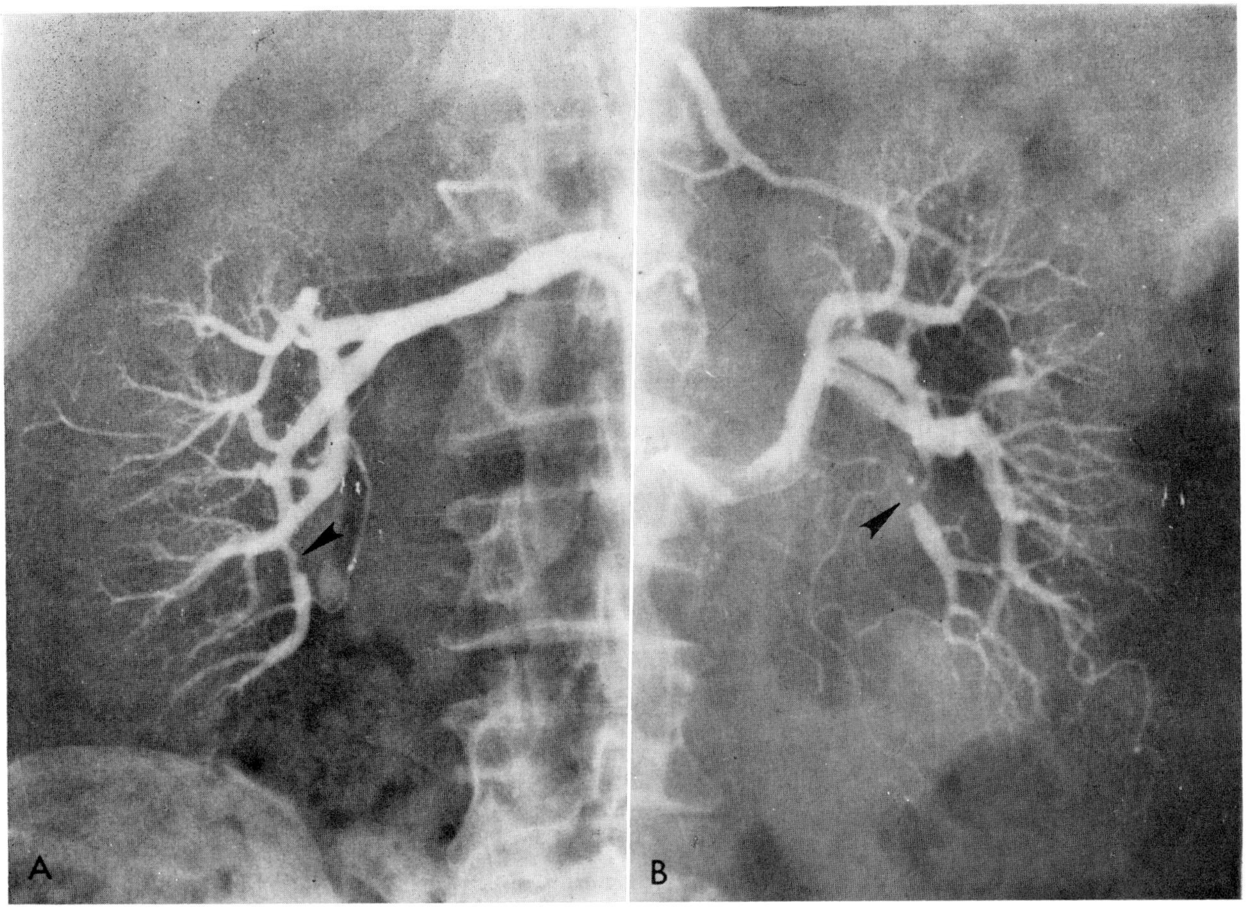

Figure 22.38. Renal Arteriogram. (A) On the right side note the eccentric irregular narrowing of the intrarenal branch occurs (Arrow). Notice also the smooth concentric narrowing at the very proximal renal artery at the tip of the catheter. (B) On the left side there is severe concentric smooth narrowing of the intrarenal branch (Arrow). Note atherosclerotic narrowing of the intrarenal branches. The concentric narrowing at the tip of the catheter was not seen on the flush aortogram suggesting catheter irritation and spasm.

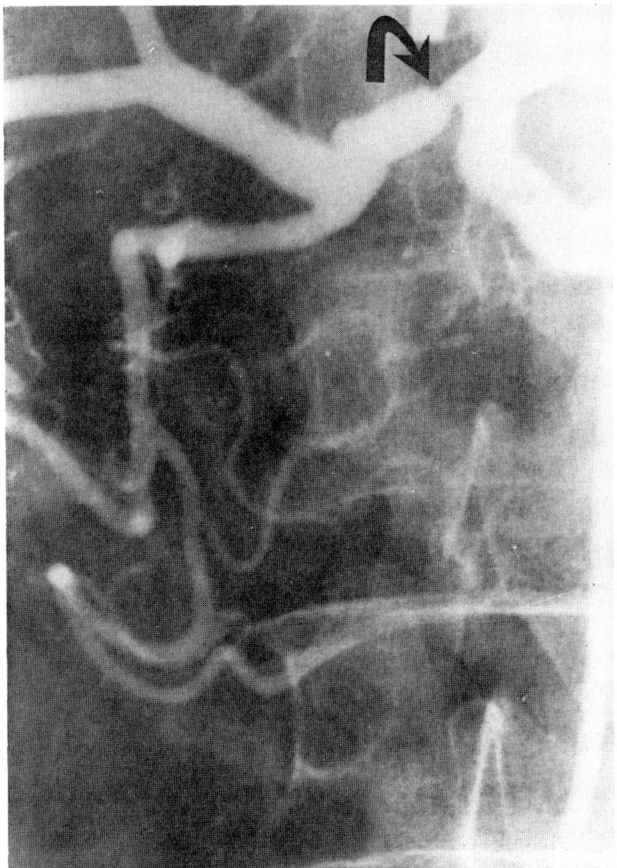

←

Figure 22.39. Celiac Arteriogram. There is smooth concentric narrowing of the main hepatic artery (Arrow) in a patient with backache and weight loss. *Diagnosis:* Encasement due to an invasive scirrhous carcinoma of the pancreas.

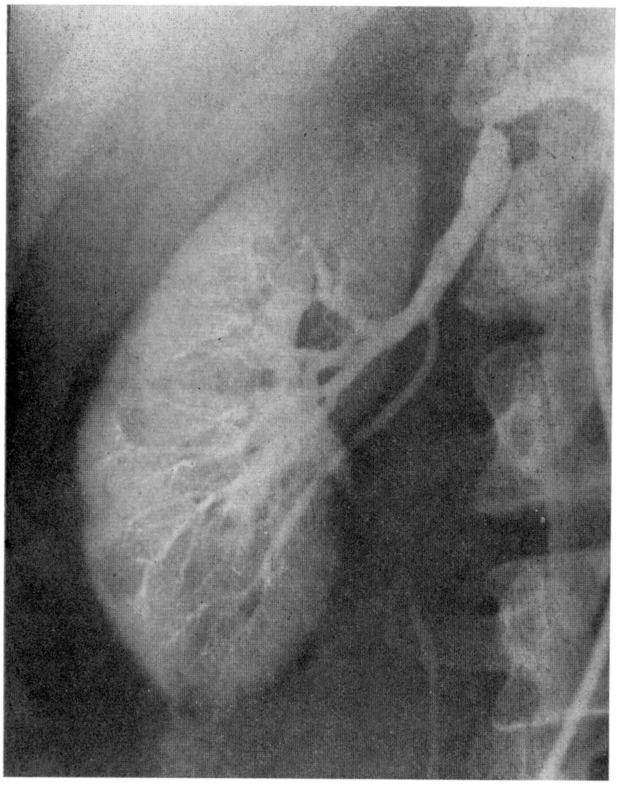

Figure 22.40. Selective renal arteriogram reveals marked narrowing of the main trunk as well as post-stenotic dilatation in a young woman with recent onset of hypertension. *Diagnosis:* Fibromuscular dysplasia. *Pathology:* Intimal hyperplasia.

ing some phases in their life cycles, these diseases may show *smooth narrowing* of the lumen due to intimal proliferation, or organized thrombi (arteritis or thromboangiitis obliterans), or due to acute inflammatory edema and exudate, as is seen in necrotizing angiitis. Though necrotizing angiitis primarily involves the medium sized vessels and the intrinsic vessels of an organ, such as kidney or liver, or an arborization such as the mesenteric vasculature, large vessels cannot escape involvement from secondary narrowing. This is seen in lupus vasculitis of the aorta.[660] *Arteritis,* an exceptional inflammatory disorder, can involve not only the branches of the aorta, but the aorta itself (Figs. 22-18 to 22-20).

Thromboangiitis obliterans[425, 825, 826] is an inflammatory disease causing segmental involvement of the arteries and veins. This is shown as smooth narrowing and gradual obliteration of the vessels. It usually affects *both lower legs distally with proximal progression and no evidence of skip areas.* This lack of skip area is in contradistinction to atherosclerosis. Very rarely visceral branches[848] may be affected by this disorder by way of smooth narrowing and gradual obliteration of the vessel lumen. Even vessels such as the aorta[827] or pulmonary arteries[828] are not immune from this disease (Fig. 22-21).

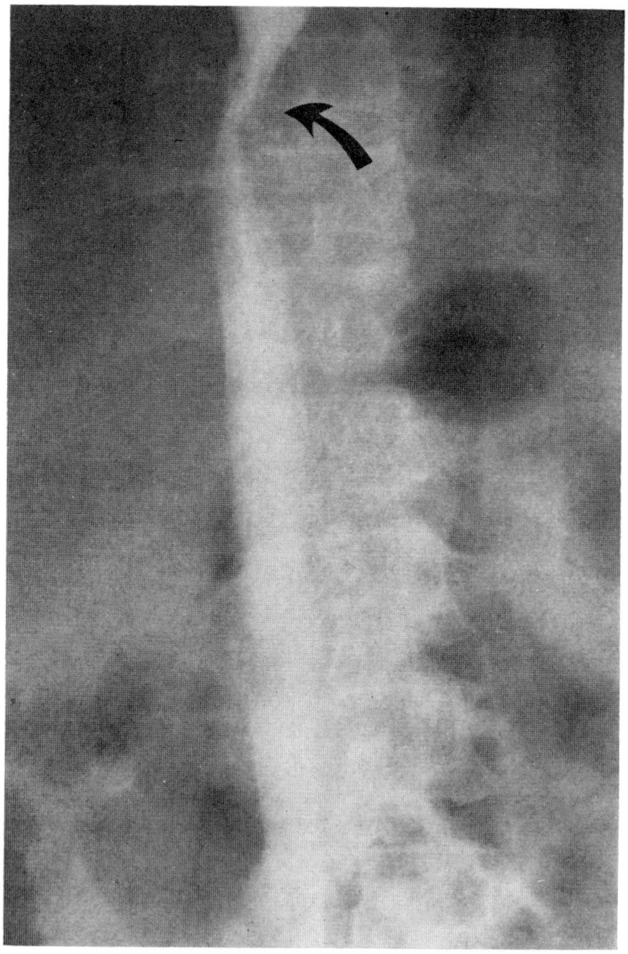

Figure 22.41. Inferior Vena Cavagram. There is smooth narrowing of the inferior vena cava at its junction with the right atrium. This patient had massive ascites. *Comment:* Such narrowing in patients with abdominal ascites is not uncommon.

Metabolic Narrowing (Atherosclerosis)

Complications of atherosclerosis are probably the most common disorders causing *patchy, diffuse, irregular or smooth areas of narrowing.* Most of the involvement is in the *elastic conducting arteries.* Involvement of the *distributing arteries* occurs in the *most proximal* portion very close to the orifices, as in the celiac, superior and inferior mesenteric and renal arteries. *Involvement of only the distal ramifications of these distributing arteries, without evidence of proximal disease, or involvement of other conducting arteries, should make one skeptical about the lesion being due to atherosclerosis rather than due to infiltration or encasement.* In order of frequency the celiac, superior and inferior mesenteric, splenic, gastroduodenal, and superior hemorrhoidal arteries may be involved by atherosclerosis causing stenosis. Extreme cases may even involve pancreatic vessels[862] (Figs. 22-33 to 22-36 and 22-38).

Extrinsic Compression of a Vessel

This may be caused by muscles, tendons, arteries, fascia, crura, nerve roots, osseous structures, etc.

Thoracic Outlet Compression Syndrome

This is a complex consisting of neural, arterial and venous disorders of the upper extremity related to extrinsic compression of these structures.[829] Narrowing of the *subclavian artery* may be achieved in a purely mechanical way when the arm is held in an unnatural position, or in the presence of anatomic abnormalities in the thoracic outlet. The injury to the subclavian artery, vein, or brachial plexus can occur from pressure, stretching or friction.

Posterior compression occurs from a cervical rib, fibrous band or the scalenus medius muscle. Pressure from anterior structures is caused by the scalenus anterior muscle, clavicle and the costoclavicular ligament. In the *axilla,* pressure is caused by the pectoralis minor muscle at the coracoid process and the sling formed by the two heads of the median nerve and the head of the humerus.

Structural changes that can occur in the sub-

(Text continues on page 290)

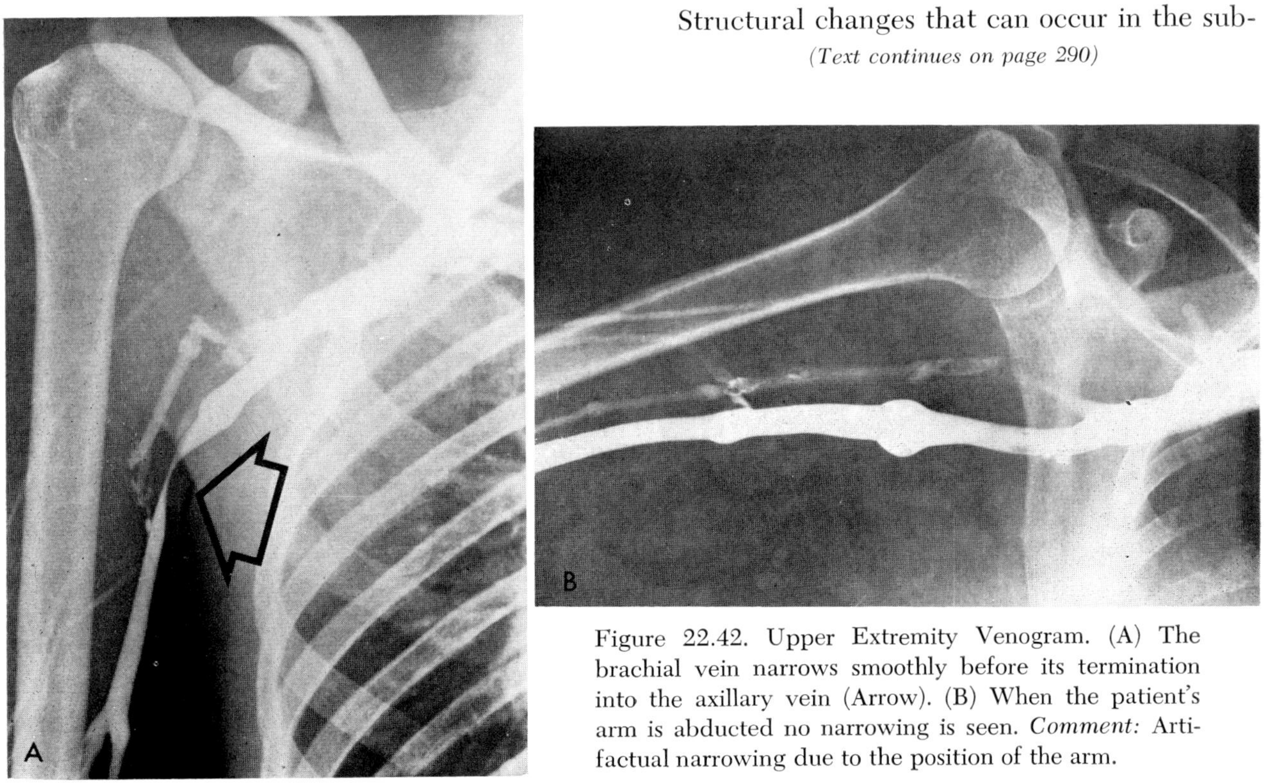

Figure 22.42. Upper Extremity Venogram. (A) The brachial vein narrows smoothly before its termination into the axillary vein (Arrow). (B) When the patient's arm is abducted no narrowing is seen. *Comment:* Artifactual narrowing due to the position of the arm.

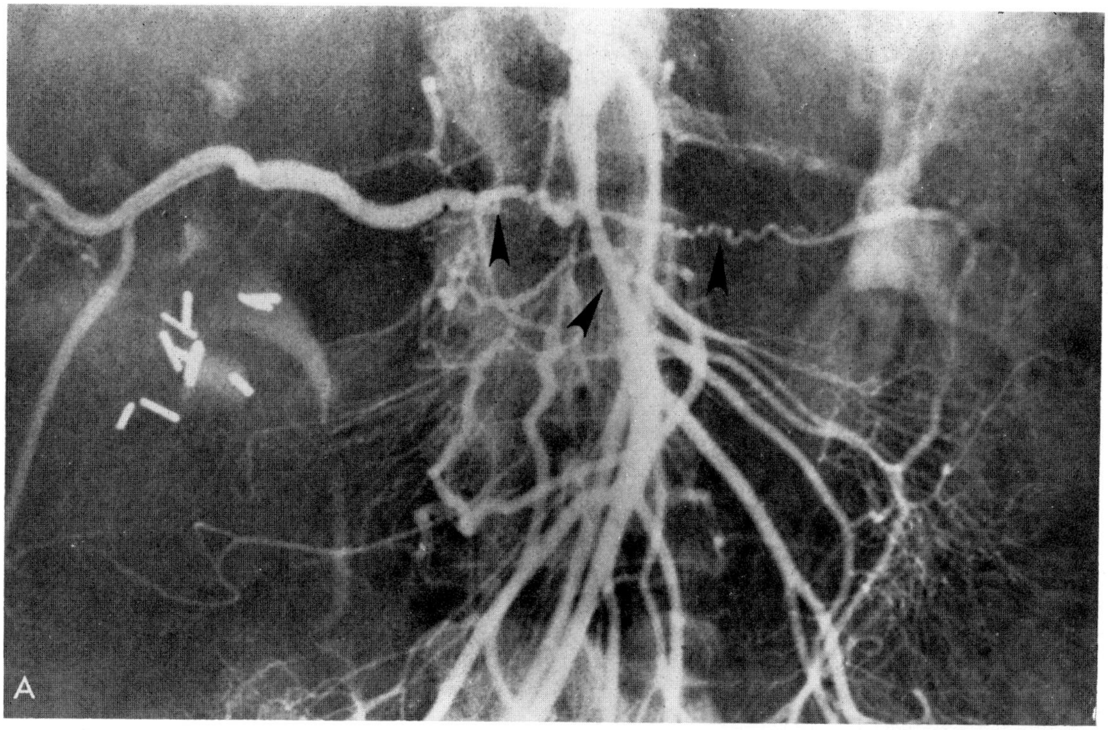

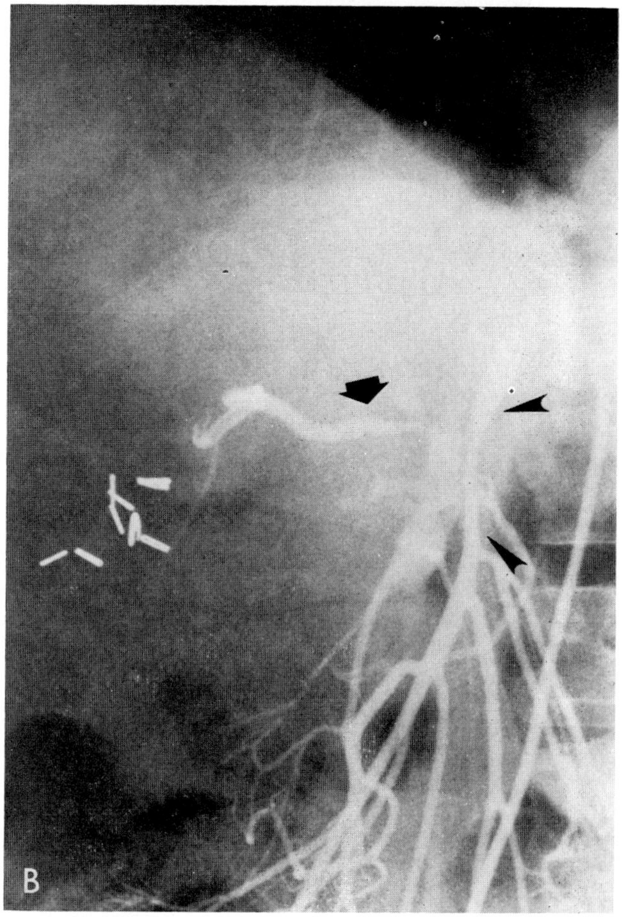

Figure 22.43. Superior Mesenteric Arteriogram. (A) There is smooth narrowing of the proximal superior mesenteric artery (Blank Arrow), tortuous proximal small branches (Arrow Head), acute angulation and abrupt narrowing of the replaced hepatic vessels with segmental corkscrew (Large Arrow) appearance. (B) A right posterior oblique view reveals the superior mesenteric artery (Arrow Head) and right hepatic artery (Arrow). The patient had weight loss and painless jaundice. *Diagnosis:* Extensive carcinoma of the pancreas with encasement of a small, a medium and a large vessel.

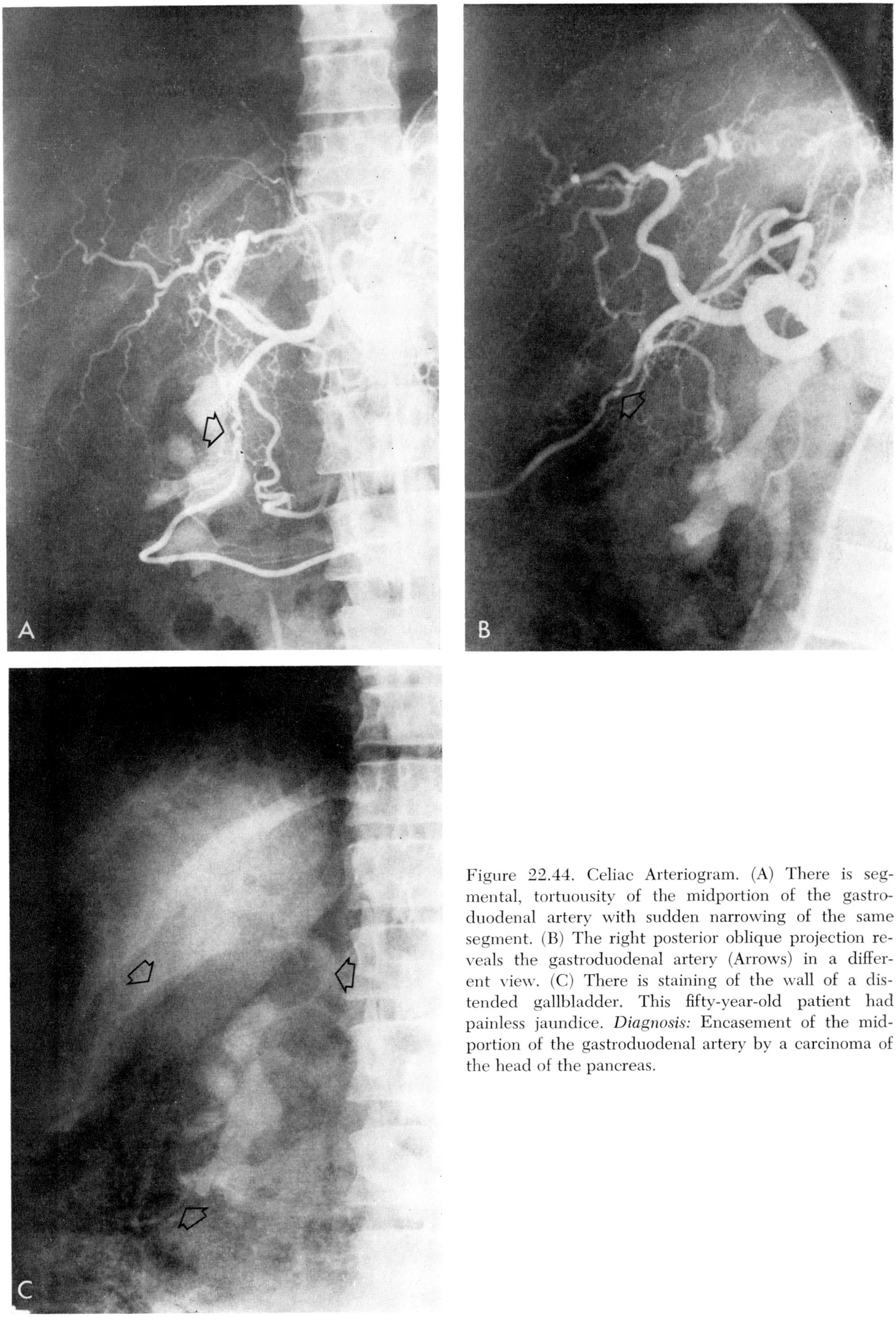

Figure 22.44. Celiac Arteriogram. (A) There is segmental, tortuousity of the midportion of the gastroduodenal artery with sudden narrowing of the same segment. (B) The right posterior oblique projection reveals the gastroduodenal artery (Arrows) in a different view. (C) There is staining of the wall of a distended gallbladder. This fifty-year-old patient had painless jaundice. *Diagnosis:* Encasement of the midportion of the gastroduodenal artery by a carcinoma of the head of the pancreas.

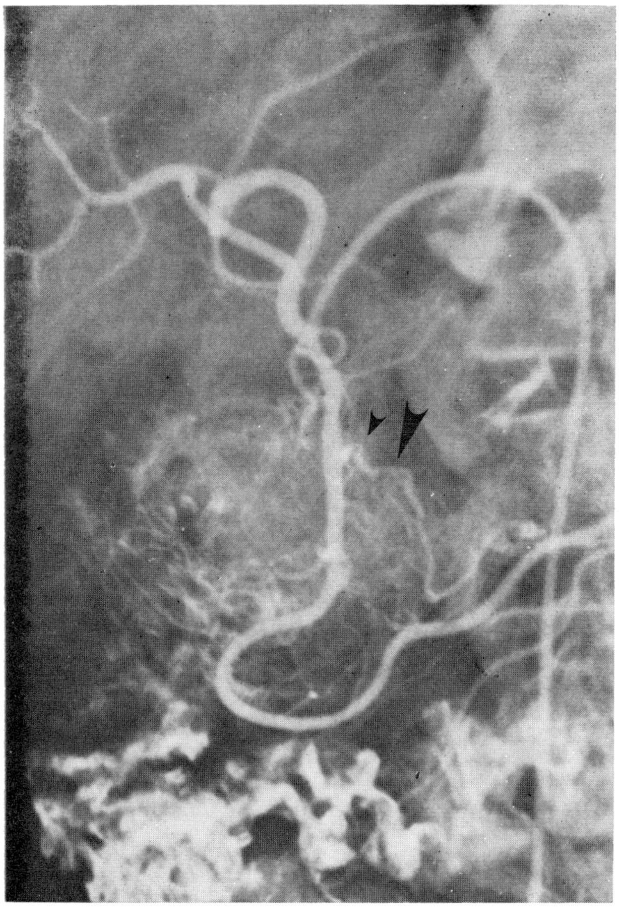

Figure 22.45. Gastroduodenal Arteriogram. There are abrupt angulations of the pancreatic branch from the gastroduodenal artery (Arrow). The patient had painless jaundice. *Diagnosis:* Pancreatic carcinoma causing encasement.

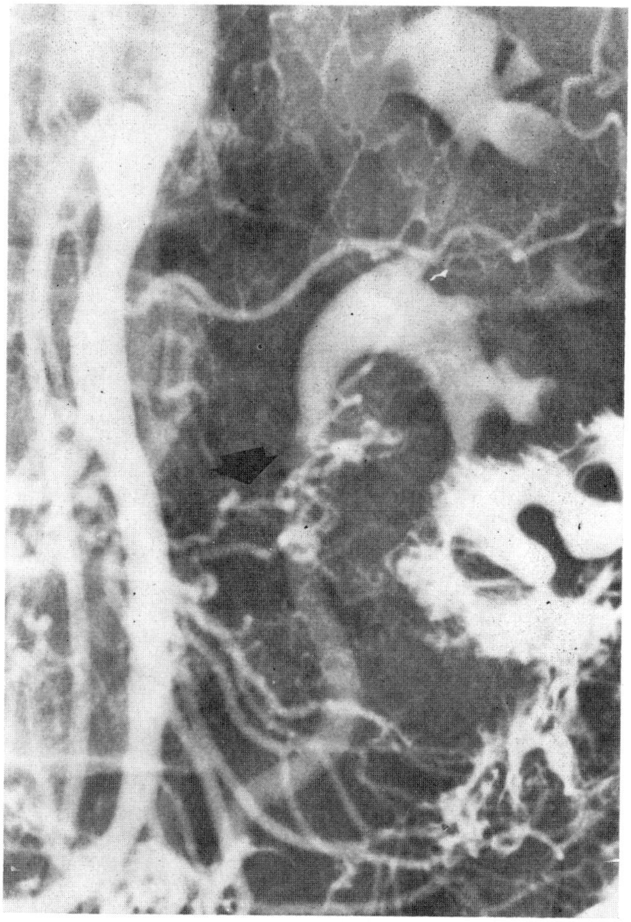

Figure 22.46. Superior Mesenteric Arteriogram. (A) Arterial phase: There are acute angulations and segmental torsions of the small branches of the superior mesenteric artery (Arrow). *Diagnosis:* Encasement of vessels from an invasive scirrhous process. Most likely carcinoma of the pancreas. *Pathology:* Pancreatic carcinoma.

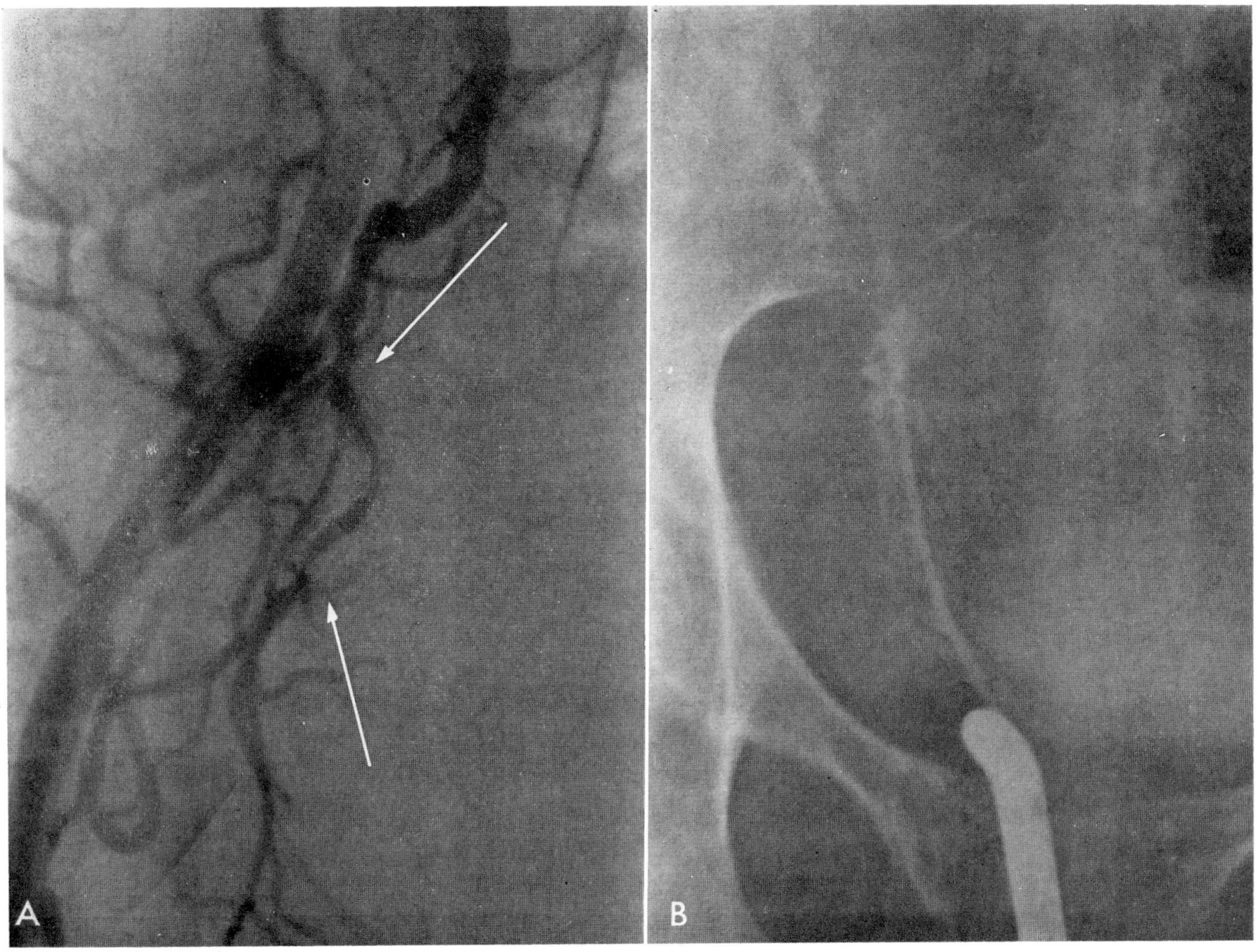

Figure 22.47. Pelvic Arteriogram. (A) There is irregular narrowing of the proximal internal iliac artery. (B) Remnant of the right ureter with filling defects. The patient had previous surgery for a transitional cell tumor of the right proximal ureter. *Diagnosis:* Encasement of the proximal internal iliac artery due to transitional cell tumor implant in the remnant of the ureter.

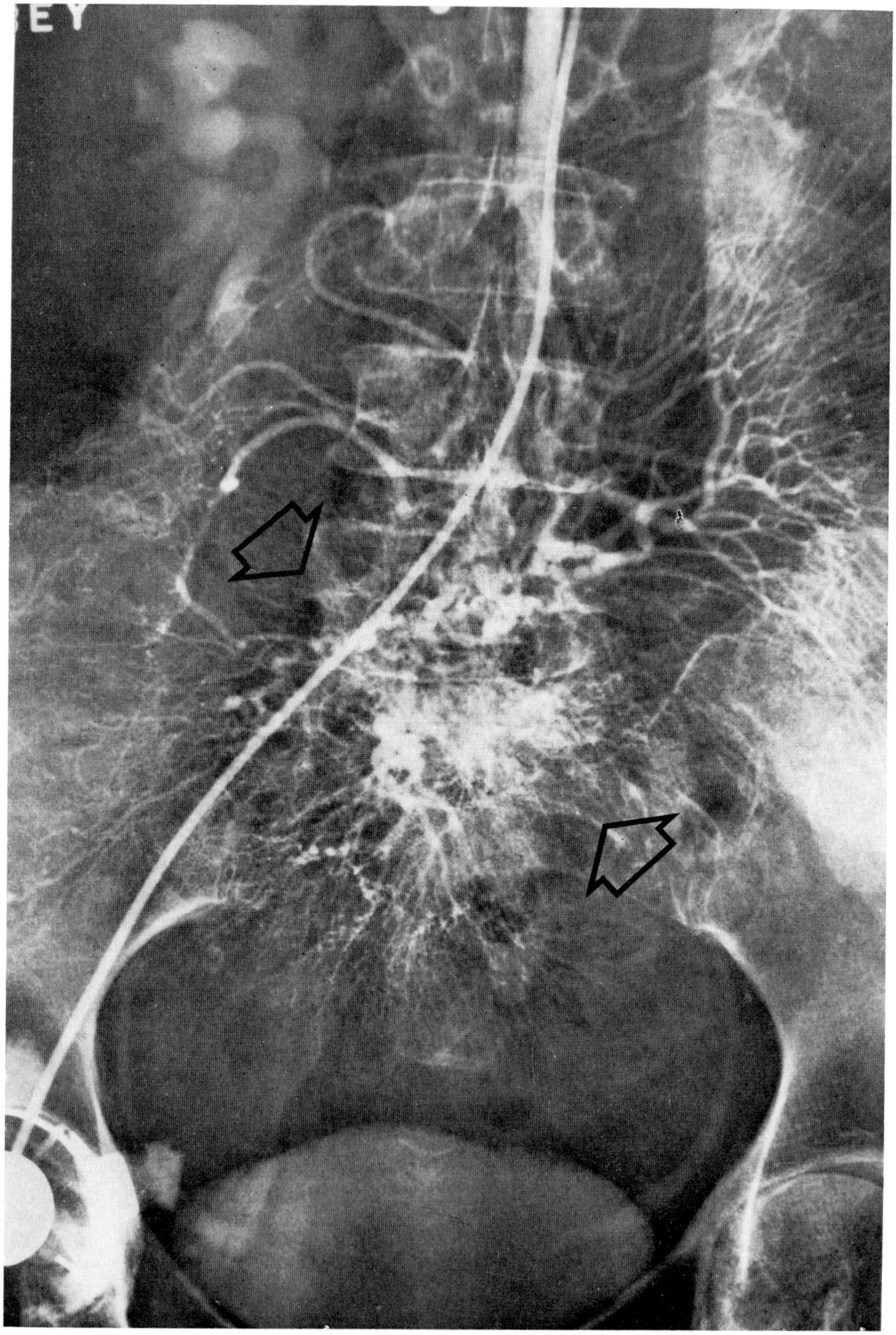

Figure 22.48. Superior Mesenteric Arteriogram. Tortuous narrowing of the main jejunal and iliac branches with comparatively diminished pefusion to those segments of the bowel. Tethering of all the branches in this area (Arrow) is present. This patient was known to have a carcinoid syndrome. *Comment:* Encasement of jejunal iliac branches due to fibrosis caused by the carcinoid tumor. *Differential Diagnosis:* Retractile mesenteritis and severe desmoplastic reaction of the mesentery due to Gardner's syndrome, Peutz-Jeghers syndrome and radiation.

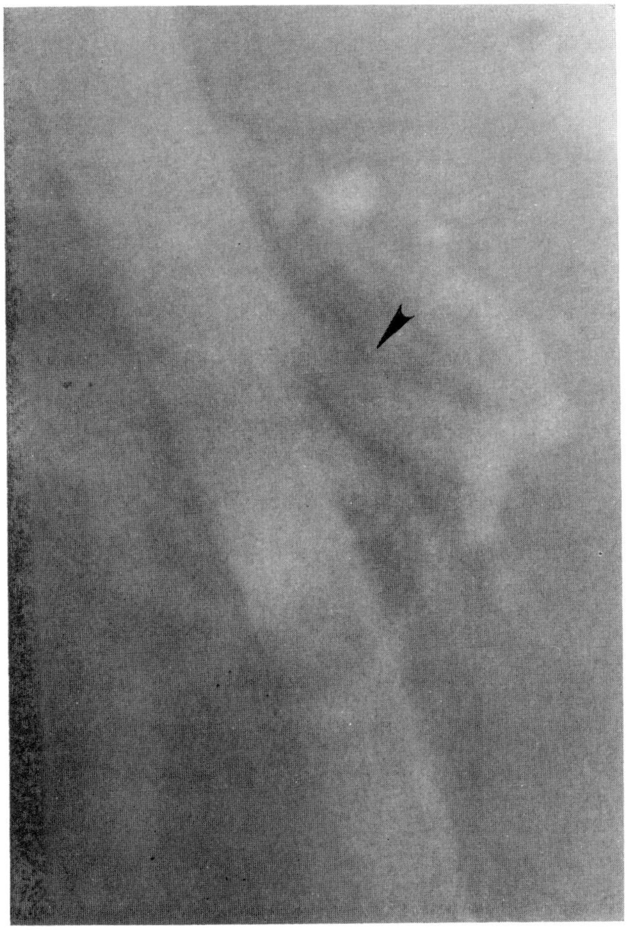

Figure 22.49. Cross-table Lateral Abdominal Aortogram. The very proximal celiac artery is eccentrically narrowed in a young patient and varies in different phases of respiration. *Diagnosis:* Arcuate ligament of the diaphragm causing intermittent pressure on the celiac axis.

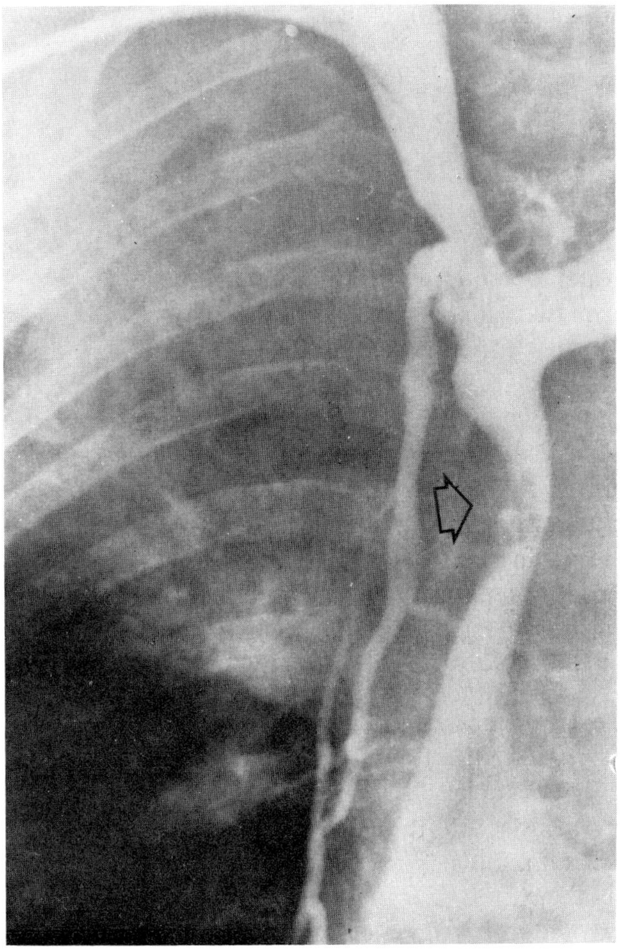

Figure 22.50. Superior Vena Cavagram. Notice the eccentric compression and irregularity of the right lateral wall of the superior vena cava and changes in the lung. *Diagnosis:* Bronchogenic carcinoma with infiltration into the wall of the superior vena cava.

clavian arterial wall include narrowing, arterial thrombosis, and proximal or distal embolization.[830, 831] Of interest is the fact that *extrinsic vascular compression in these areas is not unusual in asymptomatic normal individuals as well*[867] (Figs. 23-15 to 23-17).

Vertebral Artery Compression

Sudden rotation or extension movements of the head or neck may cause narrowing or obliteration of the vertebral artery. This may be due to tendons arising from the C 6 vertebral rim which are part of the *longus colli or scalenus anticus muscle*.[832] The inferior thyroid artery and scalenus anticus muscle may compress an anomalous vertebral artery arising from the posterolateral aspect of the subclavian artery in relation to the thyrocervical artery.[833] Finally, compression may be due to redundant cervical fascial bands.[834] The clinical manifestations become obvious if the contralateral vertebral artery is hypoplastic (Fig. 24-38).

Popliteal Artery Entrapment

The popliteal artery may be *entrapped by the medial head of the gastrocnemius muscle*.[660, 835, 836] The artery *loops* around the medial head with or without *smooth narrowing* or even *occlusion*. This is usually seen in young individuals with *intermittent claudication*. It may be a bilateral phenomenon. The same picture may be caused by a fibrous band in the vicinity of the knee joint.

Miscellaneous Causes

Adrenal tissues acting as a ring causing renal artery compression[837] or neurofibrous tissue compressing the celiac axis are unique because of their rarity.[849]

Compression Caused by the Crura of the Diaphragm or Its Median Arcuate Ligament

These structures may cause *eccentric narrowing* of the superior surface of the *celiac artery* during deep expiration. It may disappear or decrease in severity during inspiration. On occasion complete occlusion may occur on deep expiration.[838, 839] This is caused by a low median arctuate ligament of the diaphragm rather than a high origin of the celiac artery. This is more common in endomorphs, mesomorphs and females.[317] In extreme cases the origin of the superior mesenteric artery may also be involved.[840] The *functional significance* of such narrowing is *debatable* with strong arguments for or against its relationship to symptoms[840–847] (Fig. 22-49).

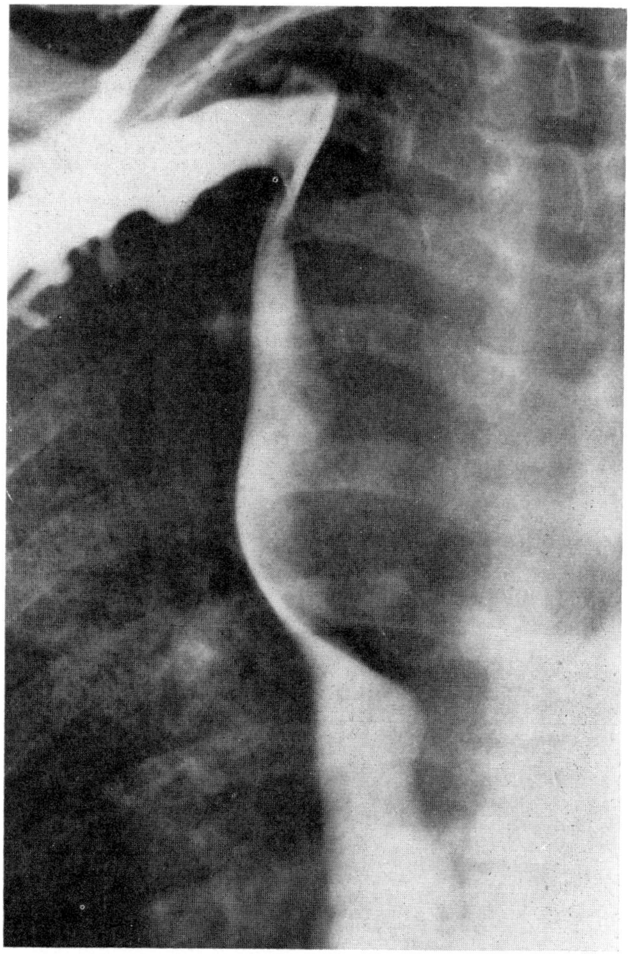

Figure 22.51. Superior Vena Cavagram. There is marked eccentric narrowing of the superior vena cava. Notice the soft tissue mass in the right paratracheal area. *Diagnosis:* Marked superior vena caval narrowing by a bronchogenic carcinoma.

Narrowing Caused by Disuse Atrophy

Like any other tubular viscus, the vessel may also diminish in its caliber *as a response to the*

(Text continues on page 298)

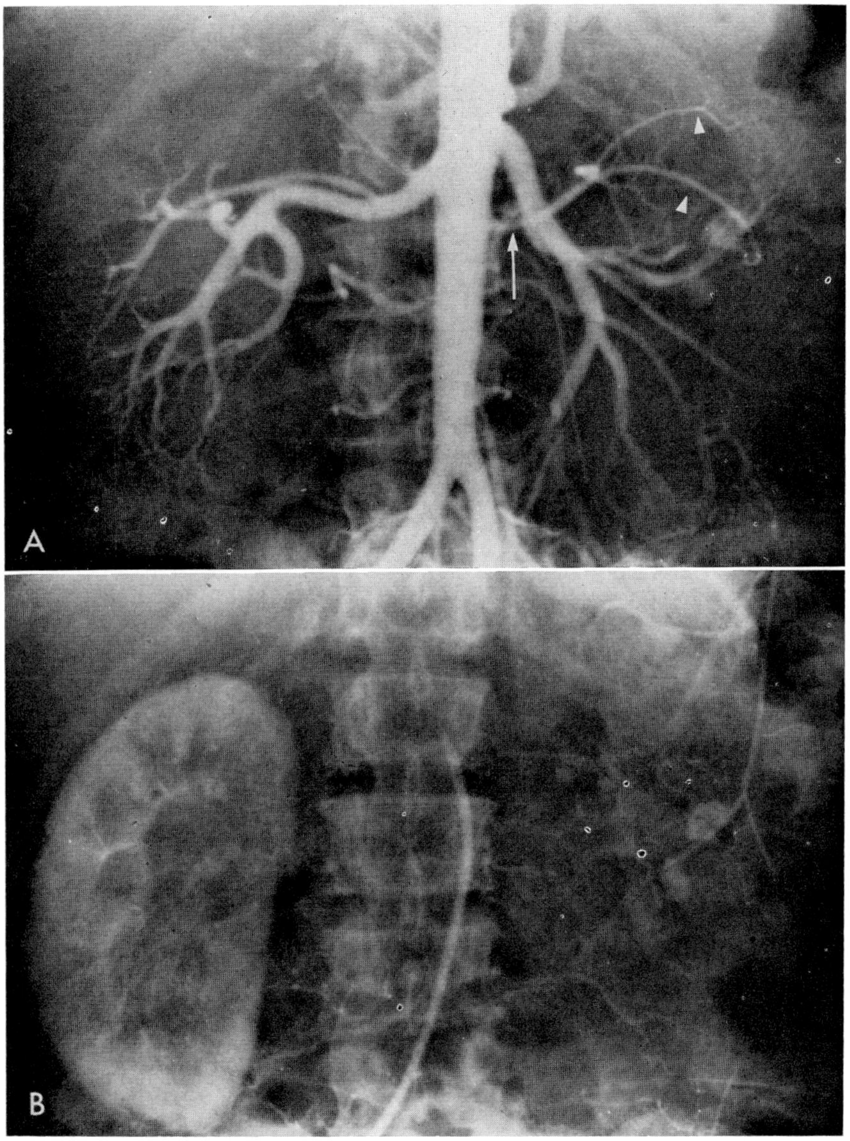

Figure 22.52. Flush Arteriogram. (A) Arterial phase: Marked thinning of the left renal artery occurs (Arrow), with thinning, stretching and deviation of the intrarenal branches. (B) Parenchymal phase: A poor nephrogram occurs on the left side. *Diagnosis:* Atrophy of the renal artery because of marked hydronephrosis of four to five months duration.

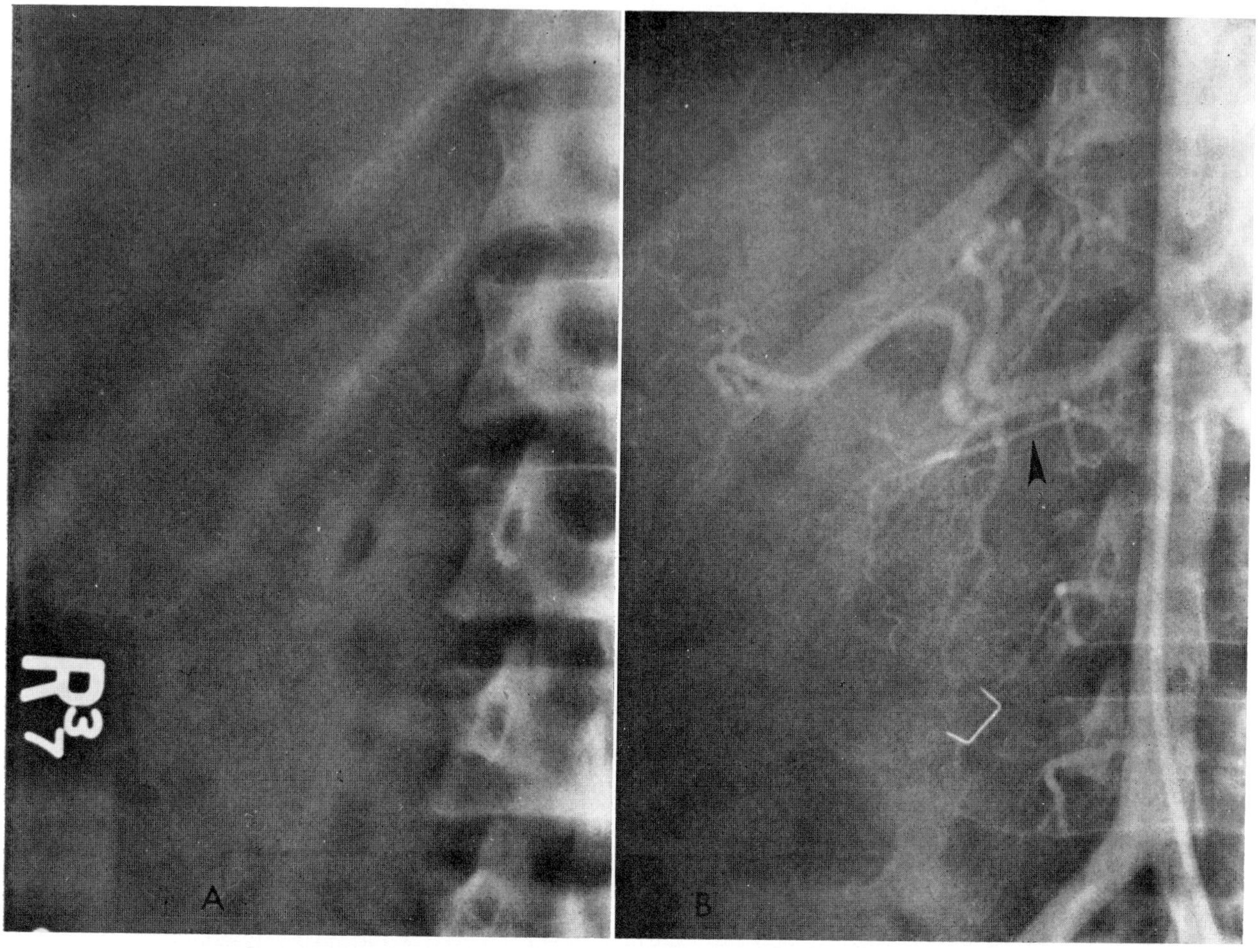

Figure 22.53. (A) Nephrotomogram: There is a nonfunctioning right kidney with an abnormal collection of gas in the retroperitoneal area. (B) Flush Aortogram: A tiny smooth main renal artery with sparse intrarenal branches (Arrow) is seen. *Diagnosis:* Nonfunctioning right kidney with a phlegmon and perinephric abscess. *Pathology:* Confirmed the diagnosis.

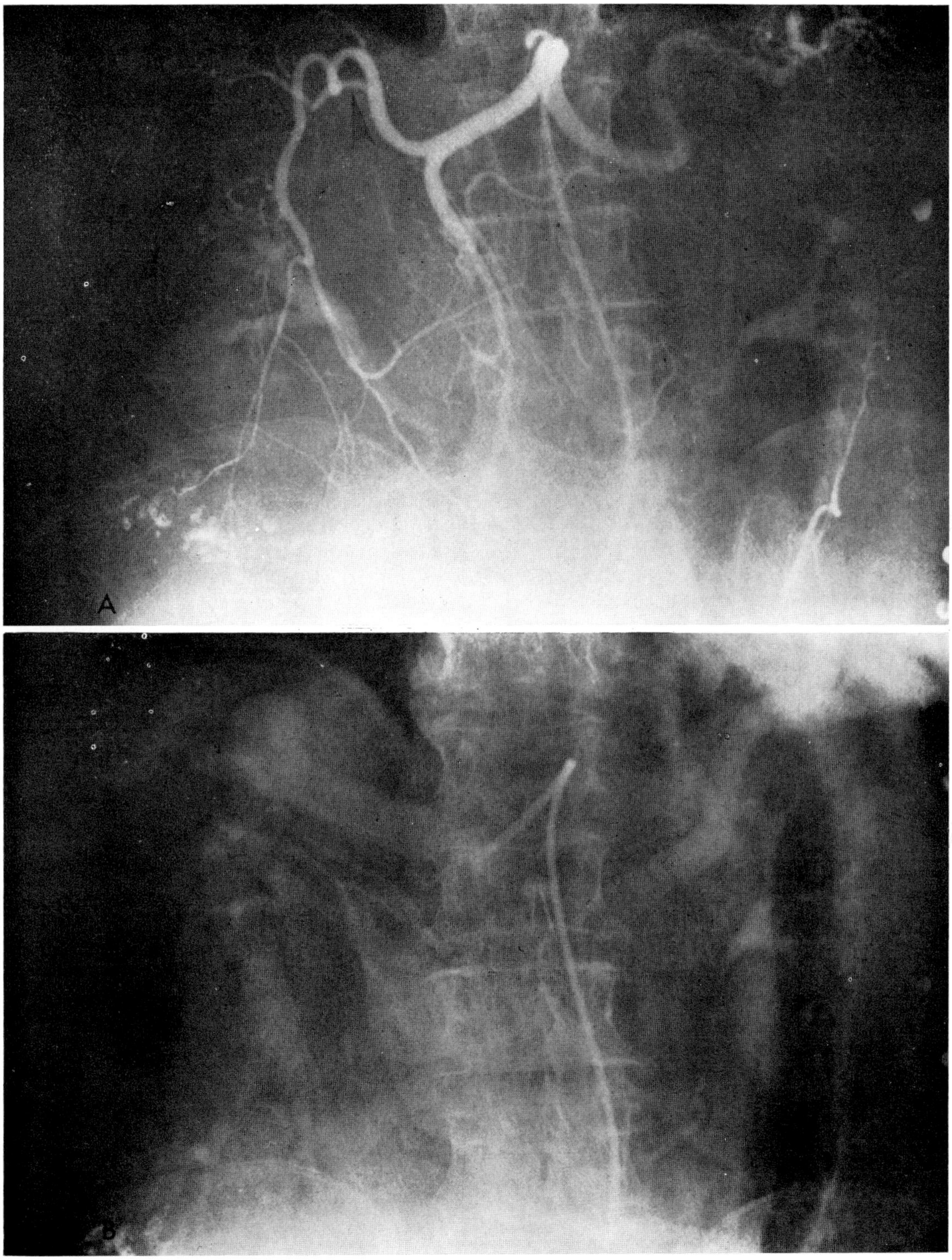

Figure 22.54 A and B

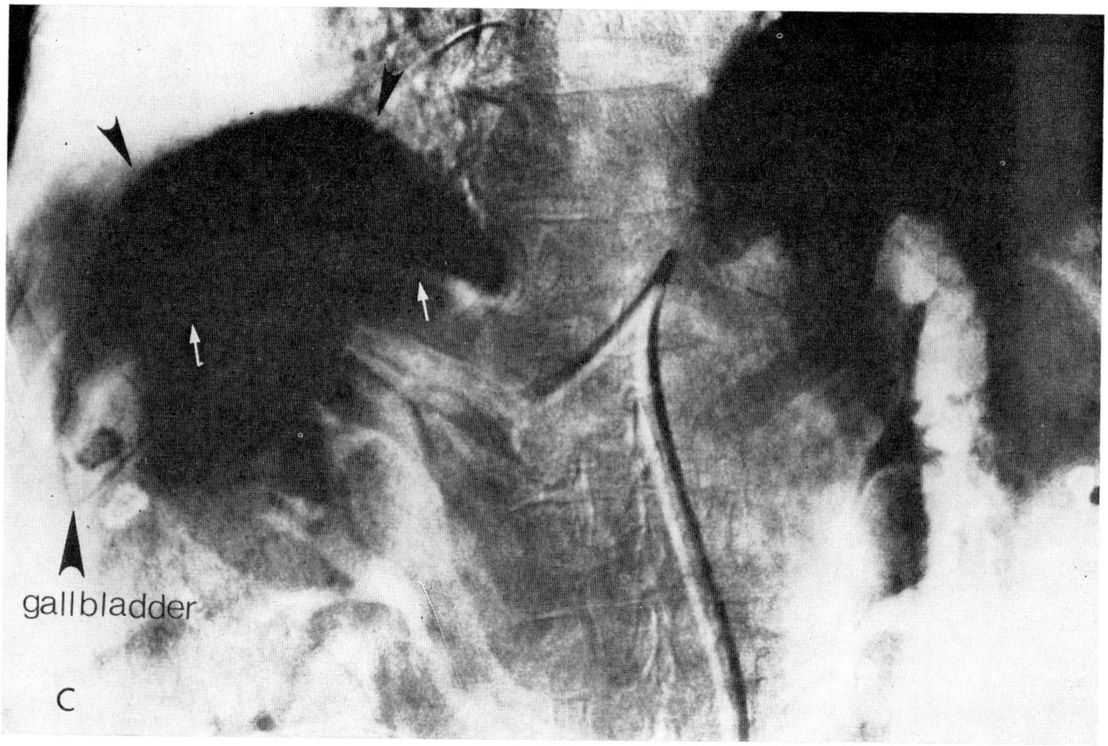

Figure 22.54. Celic Arteriogram. (A) Arterial phase reveals a small right hepatic artery (Arrow), and a prominent left hepatic artery with change in its course. The intrahepatic branches of the right lobe are crowded, and there is stretching of the vessels of the left lobe. (B) Late phase reveals a high gallbladder with a stone in it and the portal venous radicles. (C) Subtraction film reveals staining of the shrunken right lobe of the liver (Arrows). Isotope liver scan revealed normal uptake from the enlarged left lobe and no uptake from the small right lobe. *Diagnosis:* Atrophy of the right lobe of the liver. Compensatory hypertrophy of the left lobe.

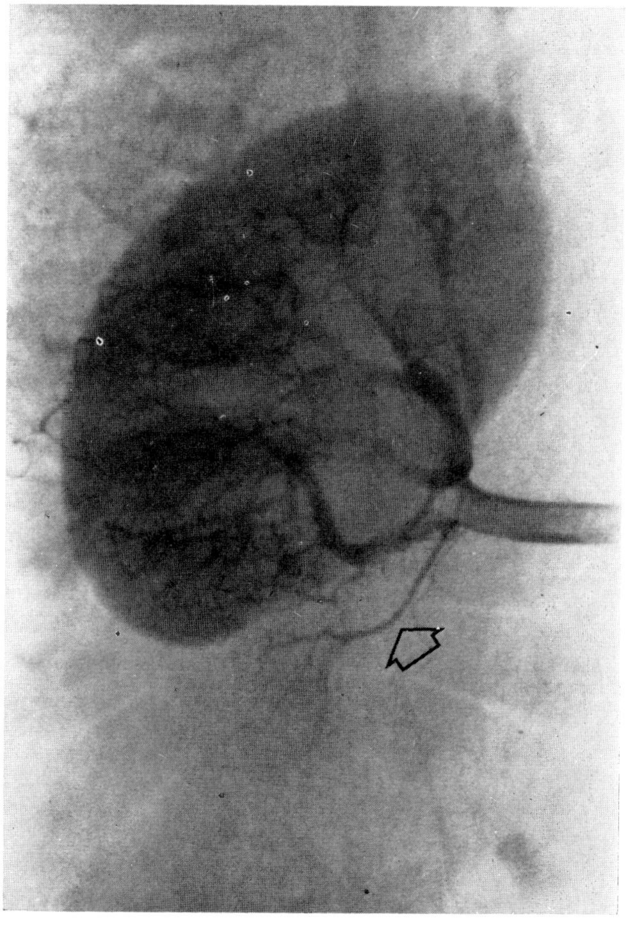

Figure 22.55. Renal Arteriogram (subtraction). A small artery perfuses the inferior pole of the kidney (Arrow) in a patient who had trauma to that flank with hematuria years ago. *Radiological Diagnosis:* Post traumatic atrophy? (Courtesy of Dr. T. Grant, St. Vincent Hospital, Toledo, Ohio.)

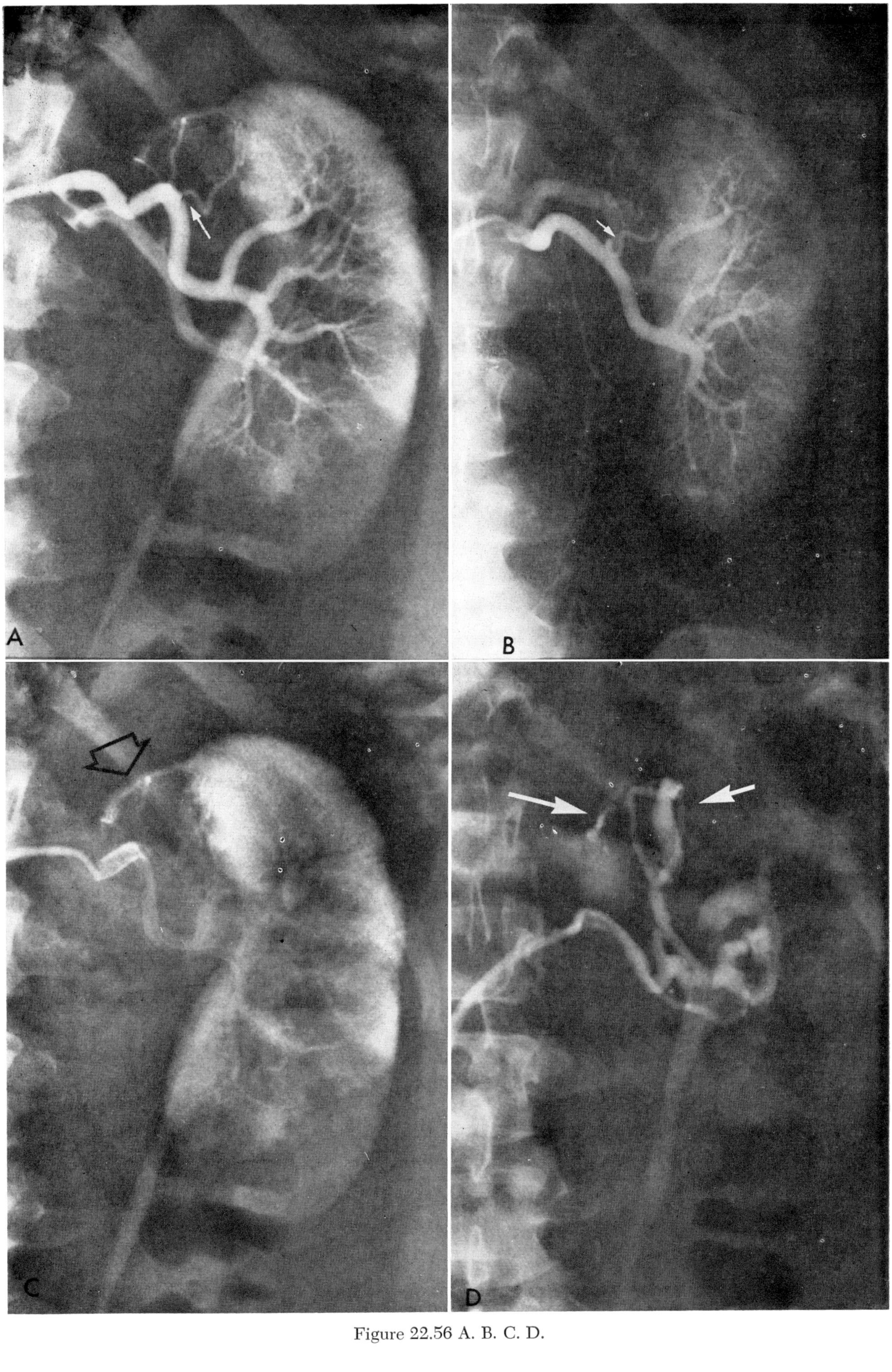

Figure 22.56 A. B. C. D.

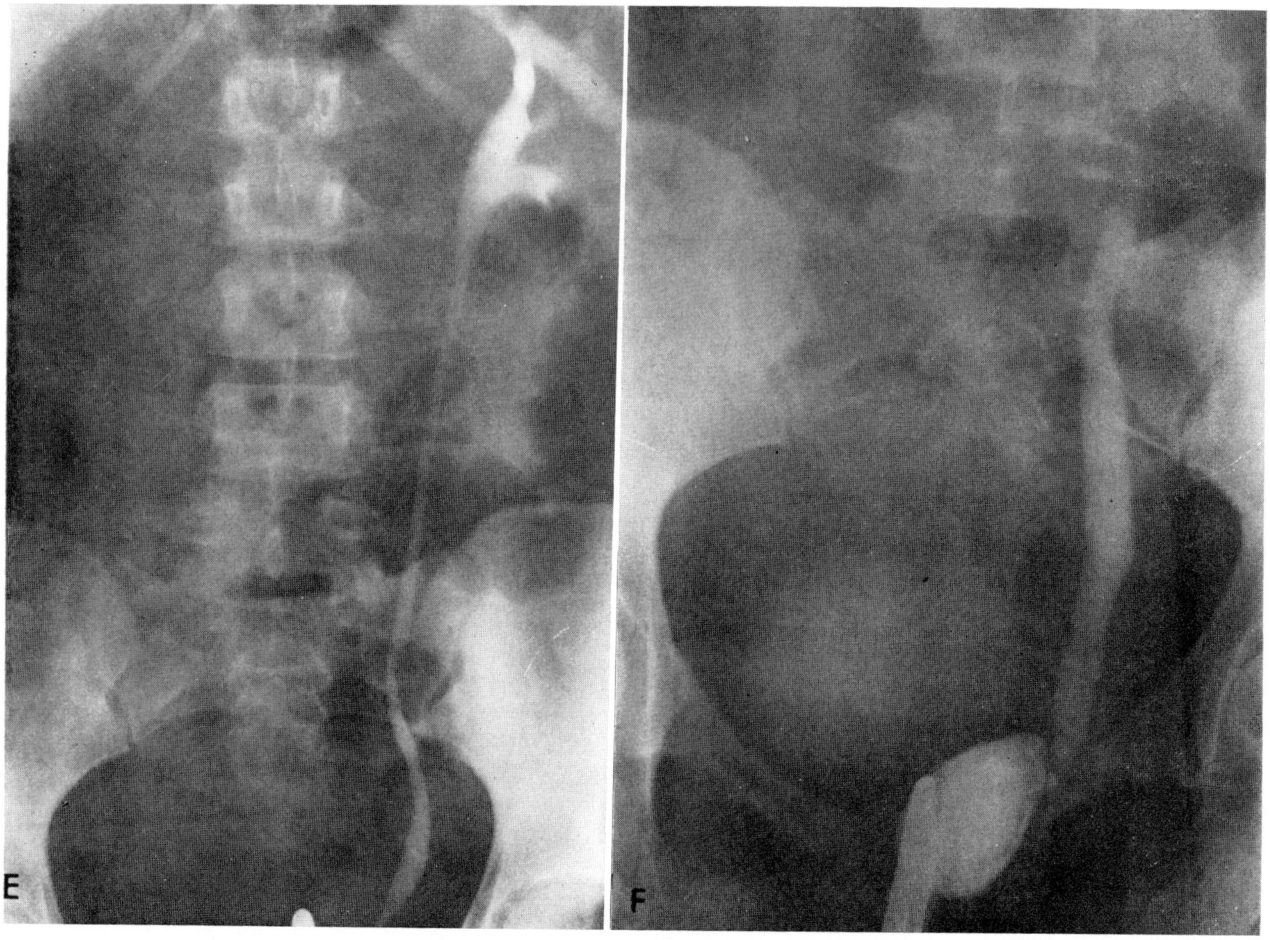

Figure 22.56. Renal Arteriogram. (A,B) Reveals early bifurcation of the renal arteries. There are fine symmetrical branches arising from both the divisions of the renal arteries coursing towards the medial portion of the kidney. (C) Opacification of the wall of a cystic type of mass. (D) Renal venogram reveals the venous drainage of this cystic structure. (E) Retrograde pyelogram reveals incomplete number of calyces and at the same time, note the laterally placed ureter. (F) Catheterization of an abnormally located ureteral orifice reveals another dilated ureter. *Diagnosis:* Duplicated kidney with hydronephrosis of the duplicated upper collecting system draining into an ectopic orifice.

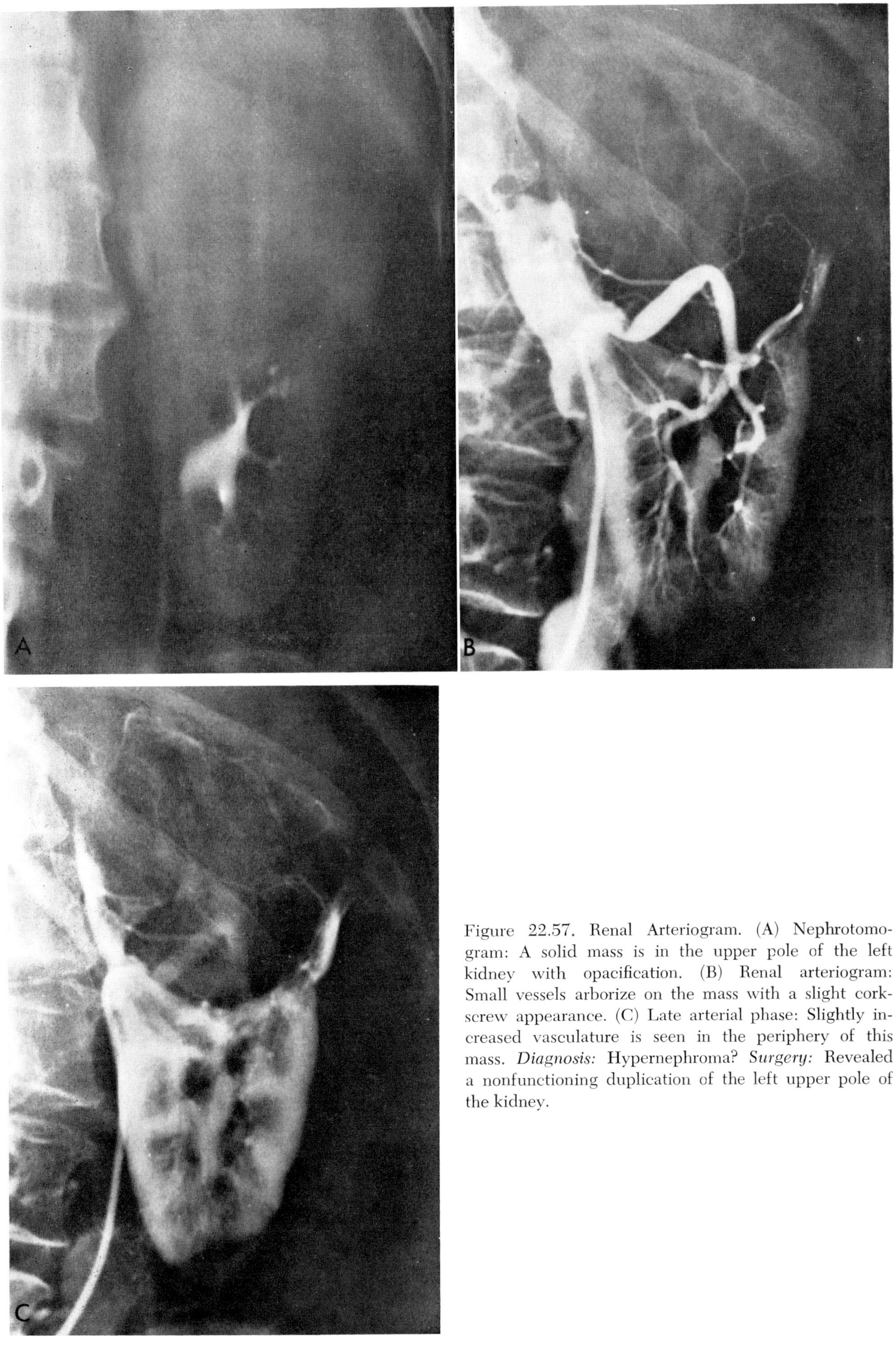

Figure 22.57. Renal Arteriogram. (A) Nephrotomogram: A solid mass is in the upper pole of the left kidney with opacification. (B) Renal arteriogram: Small vessels arborize on the mass with a slight corkscrew appearance. (C) Late arterial phase: Slightly increased vasculature is seen in the periphery of this mass. *Diagnosis:* Hypernephroma? *Surgery:* Revealed a nonfunctioning duplication of the left upper pole of the kidney.

amount of blood flowing through it. This, of course, is a secondary reflection on the vessel, either due to *decreased metabolic needs* of the organ or *long-standing interference* in that segment of circulation (Figs. 22-52 to 22-57).

These findings are best exemplified in the *renal* vasculature and its response to changes in the kidney. A decrease in the caliber of the renal artery of nearly 50 or 60 percent is a common finding in *hydronephrosis* of the kidney. When the cause of the hydronephrosis is relieved, within ten days of occurrence, then the renal artery may regain its original caliber. The degree of recovery of the artery decreases with an increase in the duration of the hydronephrotic change. The probability of no recovery at all if the obstruction is not relieved within thirty to forty days after onset[886–888] is very high. So-called *atrophic pyelonephritis* may also reveal elongated narrowing of the artery. This sometimes spares the renal artery orifice from being narrowed.

The Functional Significance of Narrowing

Arterial stenosis does not reduce flow and distal pressure until a *critical degree of stenosis* is attained.[852–855] After this point there is a precipitous fall in flow and pressure even with minimal increments of the stenosis. The critical amount of stenosis depends upon the flow velocity and characteristics of that artery. There is a critical mean velocity flow at which even small degrees of further stenosis will cause significant changes in pressure and blood flow. The *percentage reduction of blood flow depends not only on the percent of stenosis but also on the length of stenosis.* Hypotension, hypovolemia or transient increase in demand from the organ may change an insignificant narrowing to a significant one. Organ systems which have different peripheral vascular resistance have their own characteristic, critical stenosis.

A 1 cm long stenosis with even 50 percent reduction of lumen may not change blood flow or pressure. In some arteries, even 80 percent reduction of the luminal diameter may still maintain undiminished flow. Beyond these points a minimal increase in severity of the stenosis causes a greater fall in pressure and flow. Experimentally, the amount of critical stenosis causing pressure drop varies, depending on the circulatory bed. The *critical percent of occlusion* of the lumen is 30 percent for the coronary arteries, 82 percent for the renal arteries, 95 percent for the femoral and iliac arteries, and 74 percent for the carotid arteries.

The Functional Hemodynamic Significance of Stenosis

The functional significance of an anatomic narrowing is not established by angiography alone. In certain areas, criteria have been established to prove the functional significance of a narrowed vessel (renal artery). In some, such as the mesenteric or the peripheral extremity arteries, strong clinical findings coupled with angiographic findings are used to evaluate the lesion. Furthermore, establishing the presence of a hemodynamically significant occlusion does not assure that a cure may be obtained after correction of the anatomic lesion. This is due to other numerous related factors. *The endless quest for knowledge is only exceeded by the labyrinth of the human body. It should be sought after, but may never be found.*

Renal Artery Stenosis

The frequency of renal artery narrowing increases with age even in people with normal blood pressure. *Demonstration of a unilateral or bilateral stenosis may not always bear a direct relationship to the associated hypertension,* especially in patients over fifty years of age.[857] The kidney perfused by a stenotic renal artery may be completely innocent, but its colleague, the contralateral kidney which is perfused with normal-looking vasculature, may actually be involved by intrarenal small vessel disease. In such a situation removal of the kidney on the stenotic side would actually be hazardous.[277, 858, 859] The *hemodynamic significance of renal artery stenosis* in relationship to the existing hy-

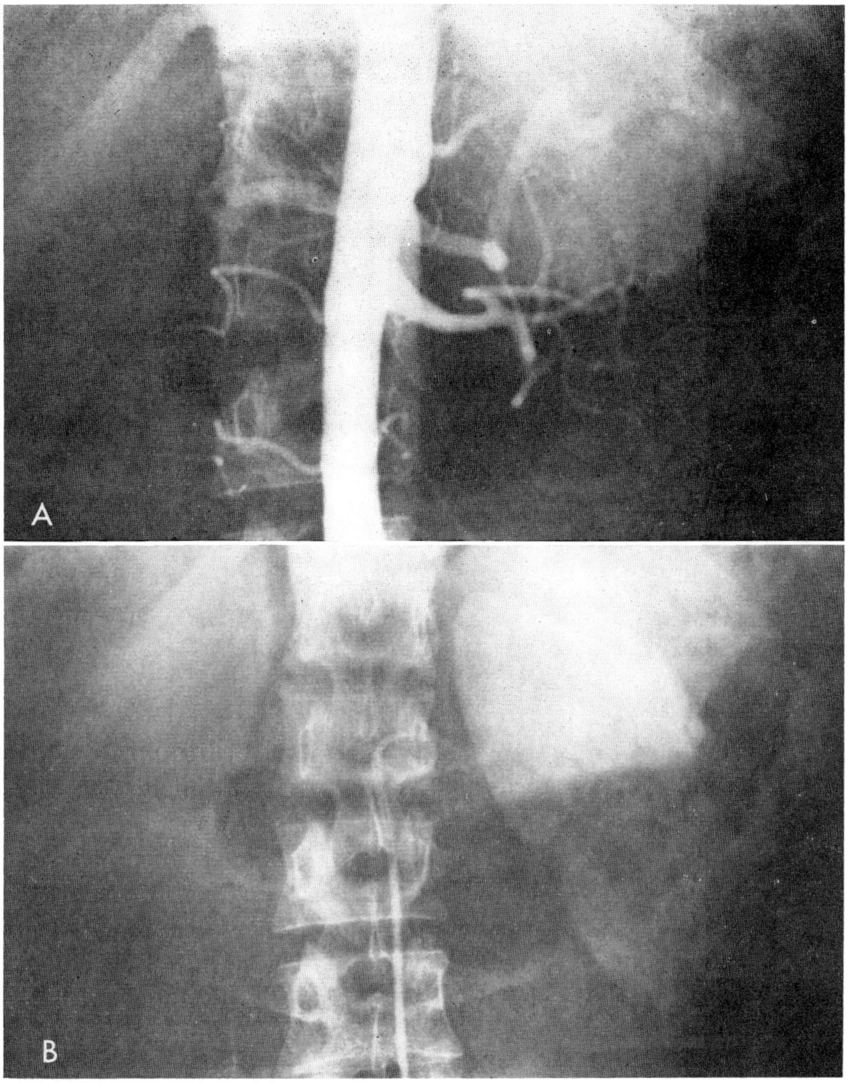

Figure 22.58 A, B *(Continued on next page)*

pertension may be further evaluated through (1) presence of collateral vessels and the direction of flow within them,[465] (2) presence of significant pressure gradient[497, 861] and (3) estimates of the percentage of critical stenosis, quantitative studies[860] and selective renal venous sampling for renin levels.[29, 33]

Mesenteric Vascular Stenosis (Abdominal Angina)

To warrant a diagnosis of visceral angina,[865] two of the three visceral arteries should be narrowed. If a single vessel is involved by stenosis, it is usually the celiac. The inferior mesenteric artery is the second most frequently narrowed or occluded vessel.[863, 864] This is especially true in elderly patients. When both the celiac and superior mesenteric arteries are narrowed, flow from the celiac to the mesenteric circulation occurs at the cost of a diminished gastric blood flow.[851] Corrective therapy should be instituted only in a very few selective cases with convincing symptoms after excluding other intraabdominal abnormalities as a cause of the symptoms. If not, many patients may return after surgical correction with their preoperative symptoms.[866]

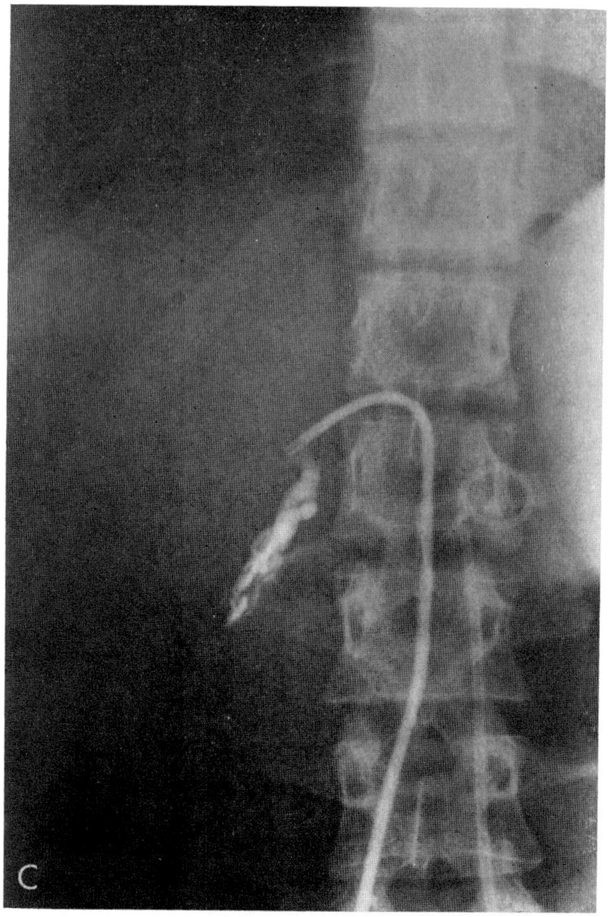

Figure 22.58. (A) Flush arteriogram: The right renal artery does not visualize. (B) Parenchymal phase: No nephrogram on the right side. (C) Renal venogram: A nubbin of viable renal tissue without function is seen in a patient who had hypertension.

Venous Narrowing

The pliable veins which lack significant pulsation and have insignificant internal pressure are even *more susceptible to external influences* as a cause of narrowing than the arteries. As such it is very difficult to assess whether narrowing is due to extrinsic pressure from a pathologic process, either benign or malignant, or due to direct infiltration. If the vein is completely thrombosed, then the etiology is not apparent either. This is due to the fact that the thrombosis may have been due to compression, stasis or direct infiltration from fibrous or inflammatory tissue or tumor. In certain clinical situations *two entirely different processes may have the same end result.* Thus the splenic vein may be narrowed or occluded by either pancreatitis or malignancy. The superior vena cava may be narrowed from malignant tumor or fibrosing mediastinal disorders (Figs. 22-31, 22-50, 22-51).

Intermittent Venous Narrowing

This is a commonly observed clinical finding during angiography related to contraction of the muscles and tendons or due to mechanical factors such as jet collapse. Right common iliac artery may compress the left common iliac vein, causing unilateral edema.[869] A tortuous

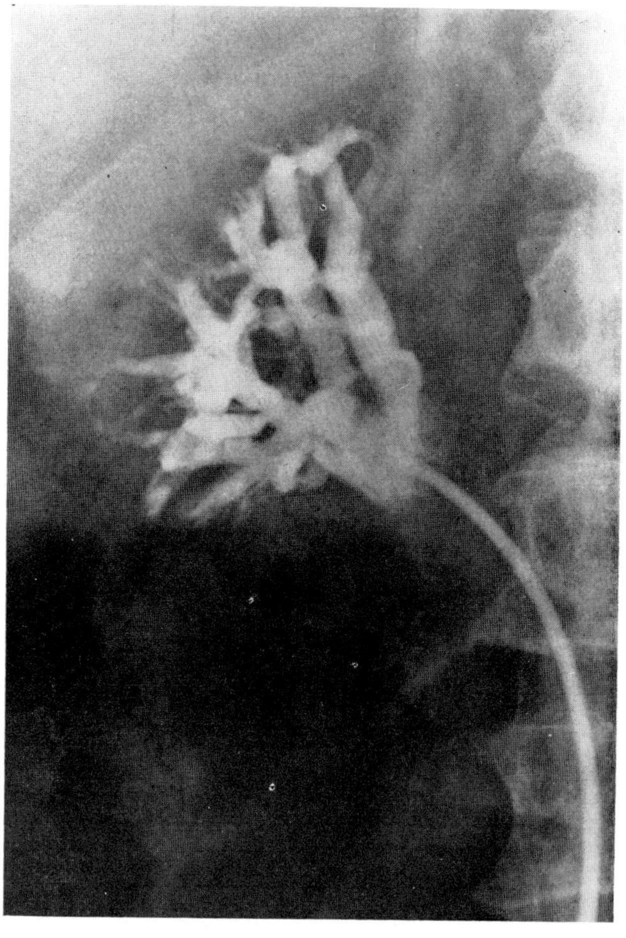

Figure 22.59. Right Renal Venogram. There is crowding of the intrarenal vasculature, dilatation of the intrarenal veins and no peripheral filling in a patient who had hypoplastic nonfunctioning kidney on the right side.

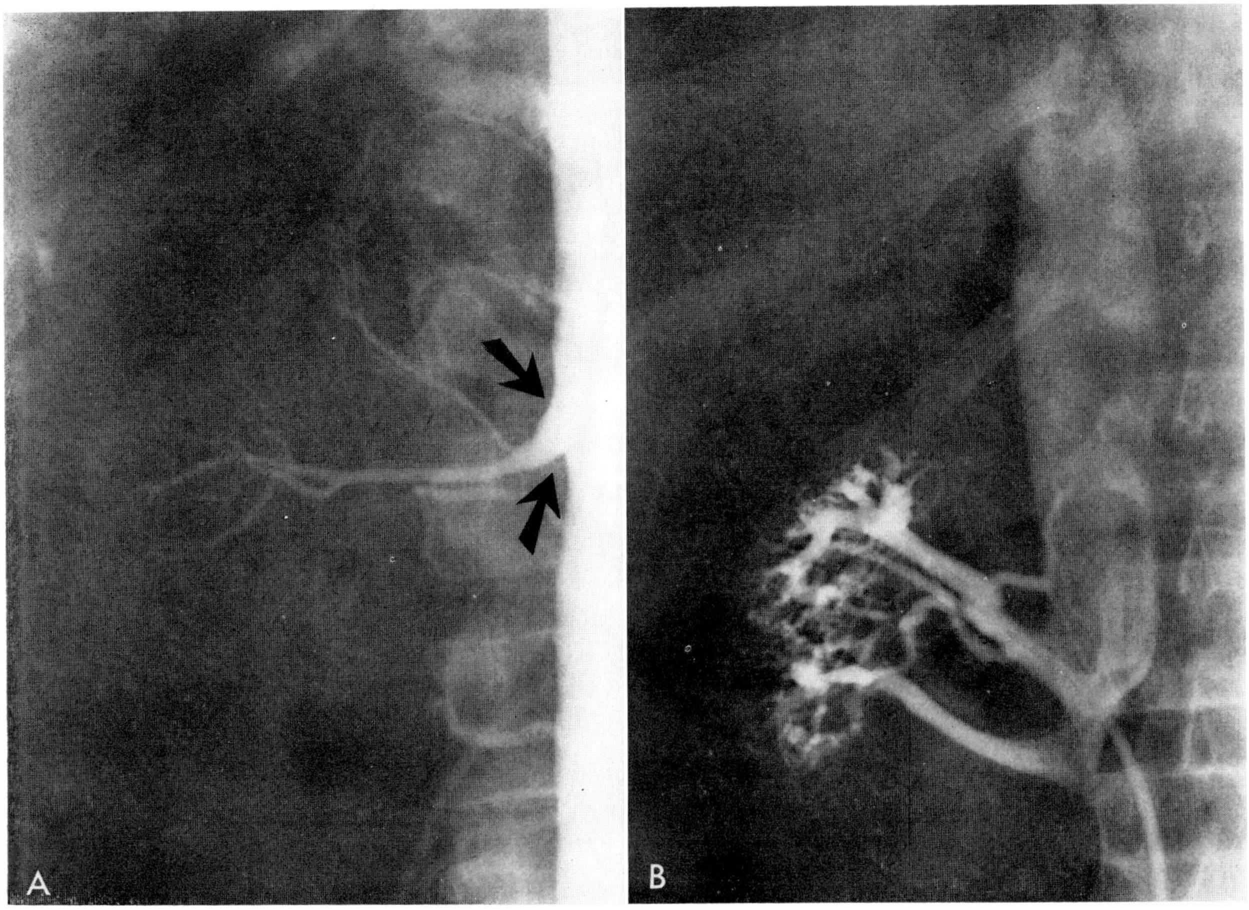

Figure 22.60. (A) Flush arteriogram: Marked thinning of the distal right renal artery occurs with a normal orifice. (B) Venogram: A small kidney is seen with crowding of the intrarenal branches. *Comment:* Possible atrophic pyelonephritis versus hypoplastic kidney.

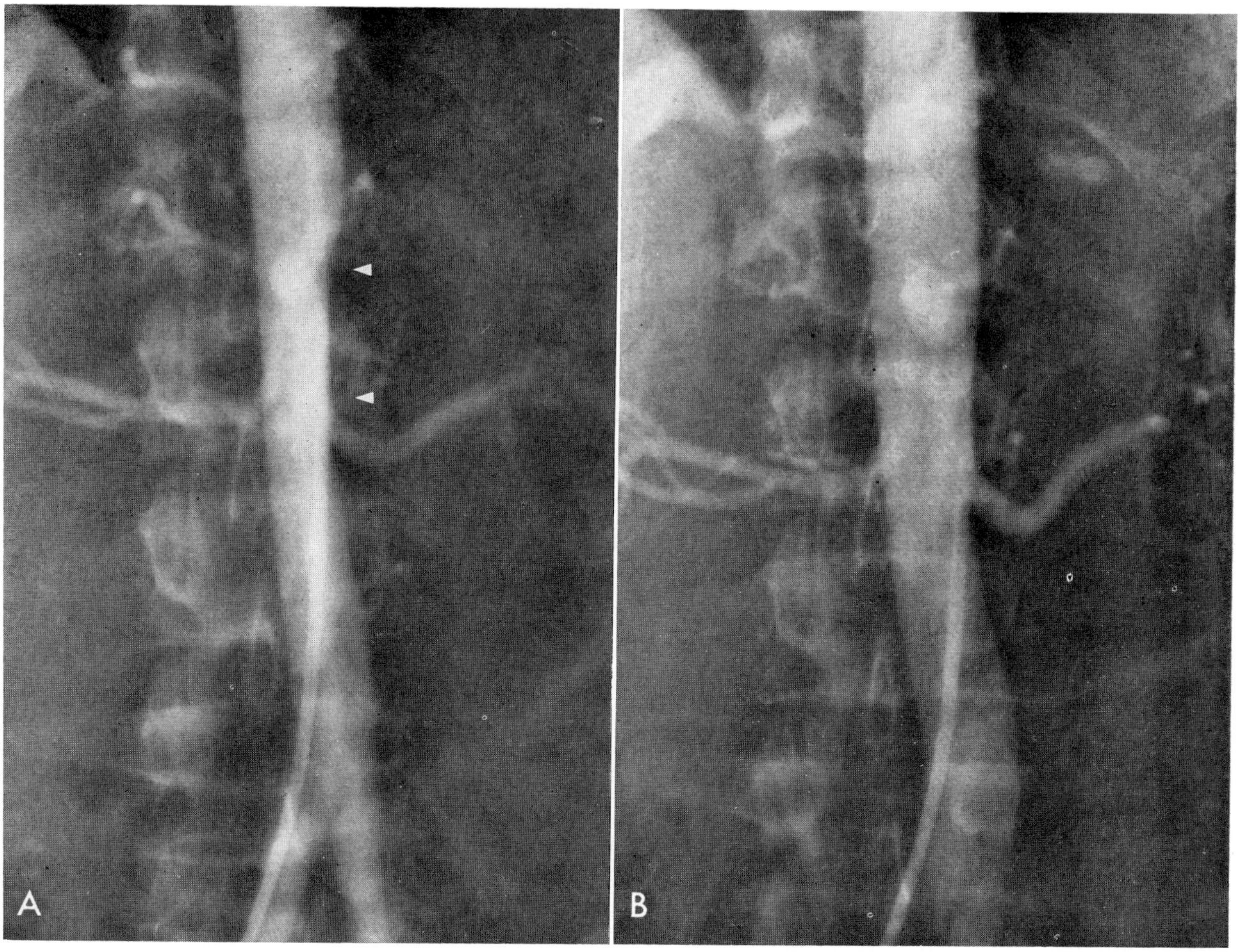

Figure 22.61. Abdominal Aortogram. (A) There is smooth narrowing of the midabdominal aorta during a Valsalva maneuver. (B) No Valsalva maneuver. *Diagnosis:* Compression by diaphragmatic crura?

aorta may compress the left innominate vein in patients in congestive heart failure.[873] Intermittent narrowing or obstruction of the subclavian vein may occur from the thoracic outlet structures.[870–872] In certain clinical situations associated with other findings, narrowing of a vein may be of diagnostic value. As an isolated finding, however, the diagnostic value is debatable.

The *femoral vein* may be narrowed by endometriosis[874] and hernial protrusions,[875] causing cyclic narrowing, or narrowing during straining. Masses in the liver,[876] pregnancy,[877] a cirrhotic liver,[879–881] acute abdominal distension,[878] may cause narrowing of the *inferior vena cava* at varying levels. Narrowing, or splaying of the *left renal vein* may aid in the diagnosis of pancreatic[390] or other retroperitoneal masses. Sharp localized narrowing of the inferior vena cava may be caused by coarctations.[882, 883] Elongated areas of narrowing may be due to congenital[884] abnormalities of the iliac vein. This may lead to growth disturbances. Narrowing may also be caused by retroperitoneal or mediastinal fibrosis in individuals with arteritis of the aorta or its branches[885] which may also affect the superior or inferior vena cava. Recanalization and organization of a thrombus may cause either elongated areas of narrowing in any vein or circumferential stenosis more commonly seen in the pulmonary veins.[868]

CHAPTER 23
NARROWING AND DILATATION

THE PRESENCE of narrowing and dilatation in the same or different vessels is actually a reflection of the disease process which has the

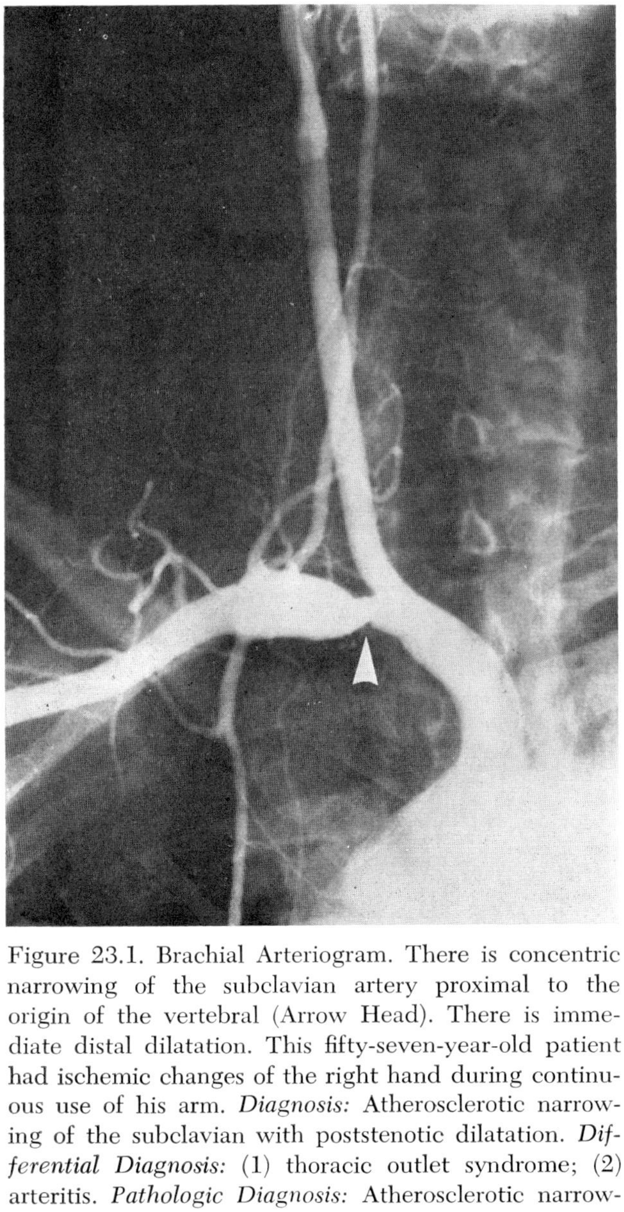

Figure 23.1. Brachial Arteriogram. There is concentric narrowing of the subclavian artery proximal to the origin of the vertebral (Arrow Head). There is immediate distal dilatation. This fifty-seven-year-old patient had ischemic changes of the right hand during continuous use of his arm. *Diagnosis:* Atherosclerotic narrowing of the subclavian with poststenotic dilatation. *Differential Diagnosis:* (1) thoracic outlet syndrome; (2) arteritis. *Pathologic Diagnosis:* Atherosclerotic narrowing.

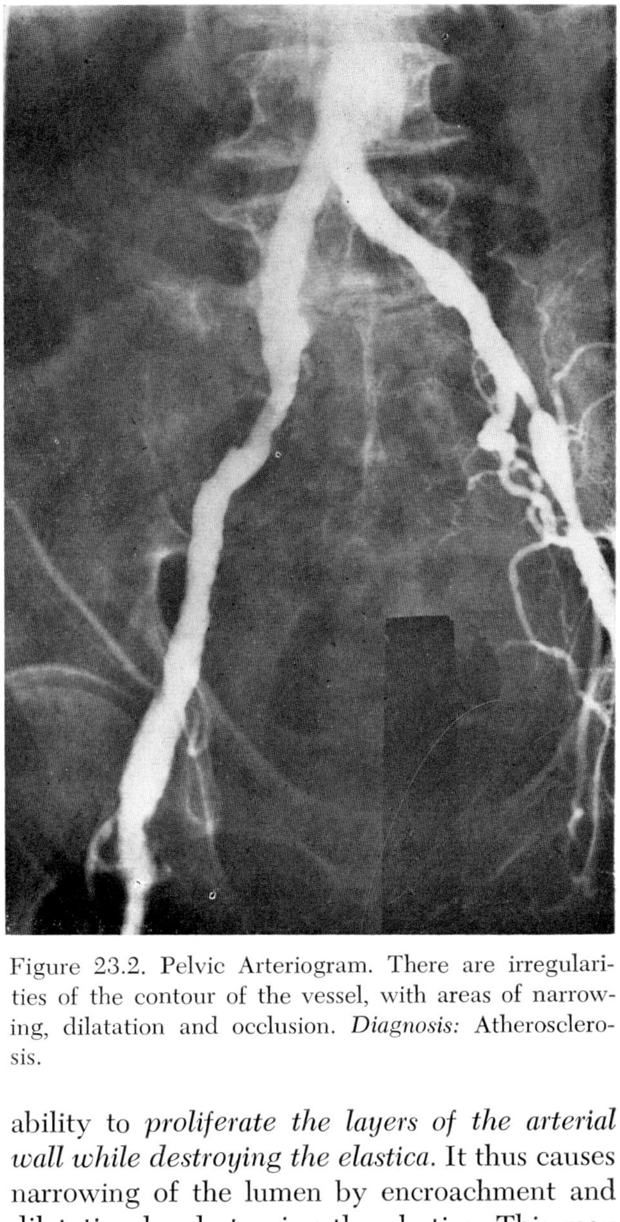

Figure 23.2. Pelvic Arteriogram. There are irregularities of the contour of the vessel, with areas of narrowing, dilatation and occlusion. *Diagnosis:* Atherosclerosis.

ability to *proliferate the layers of the arterial wall while destroying the elastica.* It thus causes narrowing of the lumen by encroachment and dilatation by destroying the elastica. This may be limited to a focal area of *narrowing and dilatation* as seen in stenosis with poststenotic dilatation. It may be seen as *alternating areas of*

(Text continues on page 308)

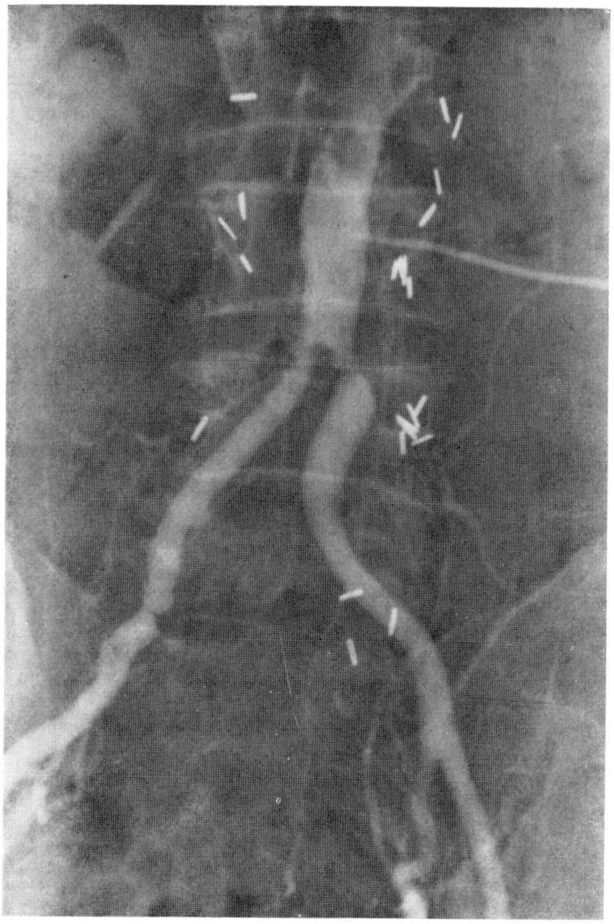

Figure 23.3. Translumbar Abdominal Aortogram. There is narrowing of the proximal left common iliac artery with a distal area of dilatation. The artery appears smooth on the side distal to this point. *Diagnosis:* Atherosclerotic narrowing of the artery with poststenotic dilatation. Does the stenosis protect the distal left vessel from developing atherosclerosis?

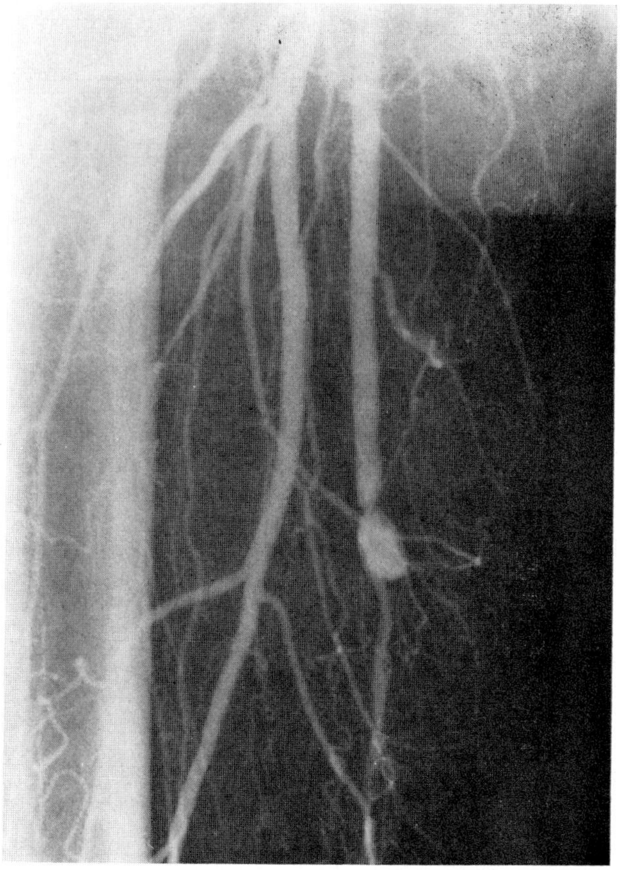

Figure 23.4. Femoral Arteriogram. There is narrowing of the superficial femoral artery, with poststenotic dilatation and occlusion. *Diagnosis:* Atherosclerotic vascular disease.

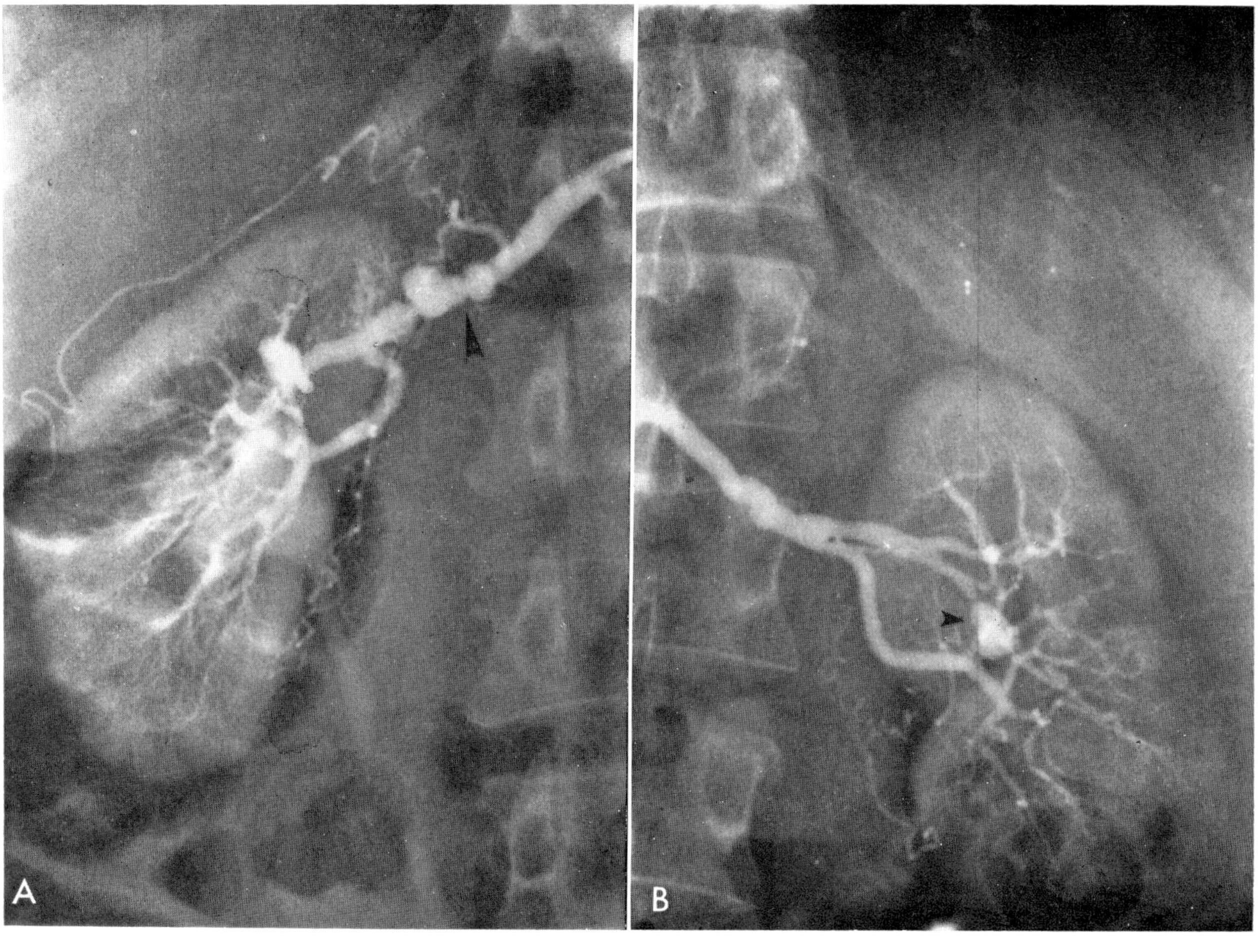

Figure 23.5. Renal Arteriogram. (A) Renal arteriogram: There are areas of dilatation and narrowing. Notice the good filling of the capsular and peripelvic vessels. (B) Renal arteriogram (other side): Slight dilatation and narrowing of the midrenal artery is seen. A localized, well-circumscribed collection of contrast within the (Arrow) renal parenchyma is seen in a thirty-five-year-old female with hypertension. *Diagnosis:* Medial fibroplasia with aneurysms. *Comment:* The increased filling of the perinephric vasculature is due to partial obstruction of the main renal stem.

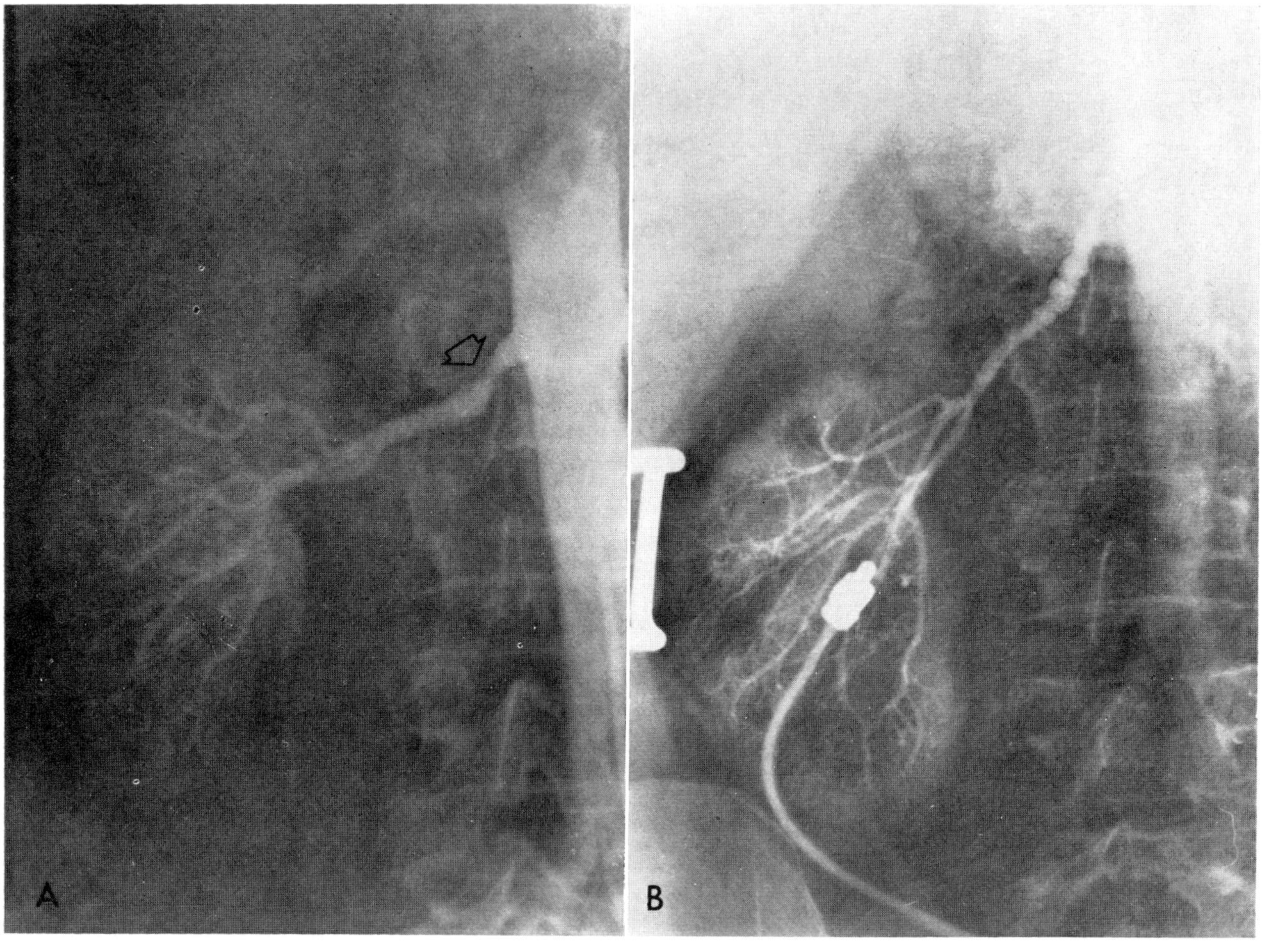

Figure 23.6. Flush Aortogram. (A) Arterial phase: Concentric narrowing of the right proximal renal artery with distal dilatation is seen. (B) The same artery was injected after stretching the kidney during surgery. This reveals multiple areas of narrowing and dilation. This young female had hypertension. *Diagnosis:* Medial fibroplasia with aneurysmal dilatation. Pathology confirmed the diagnosis. *Comment:* Advantage of stretching the renal arteries.

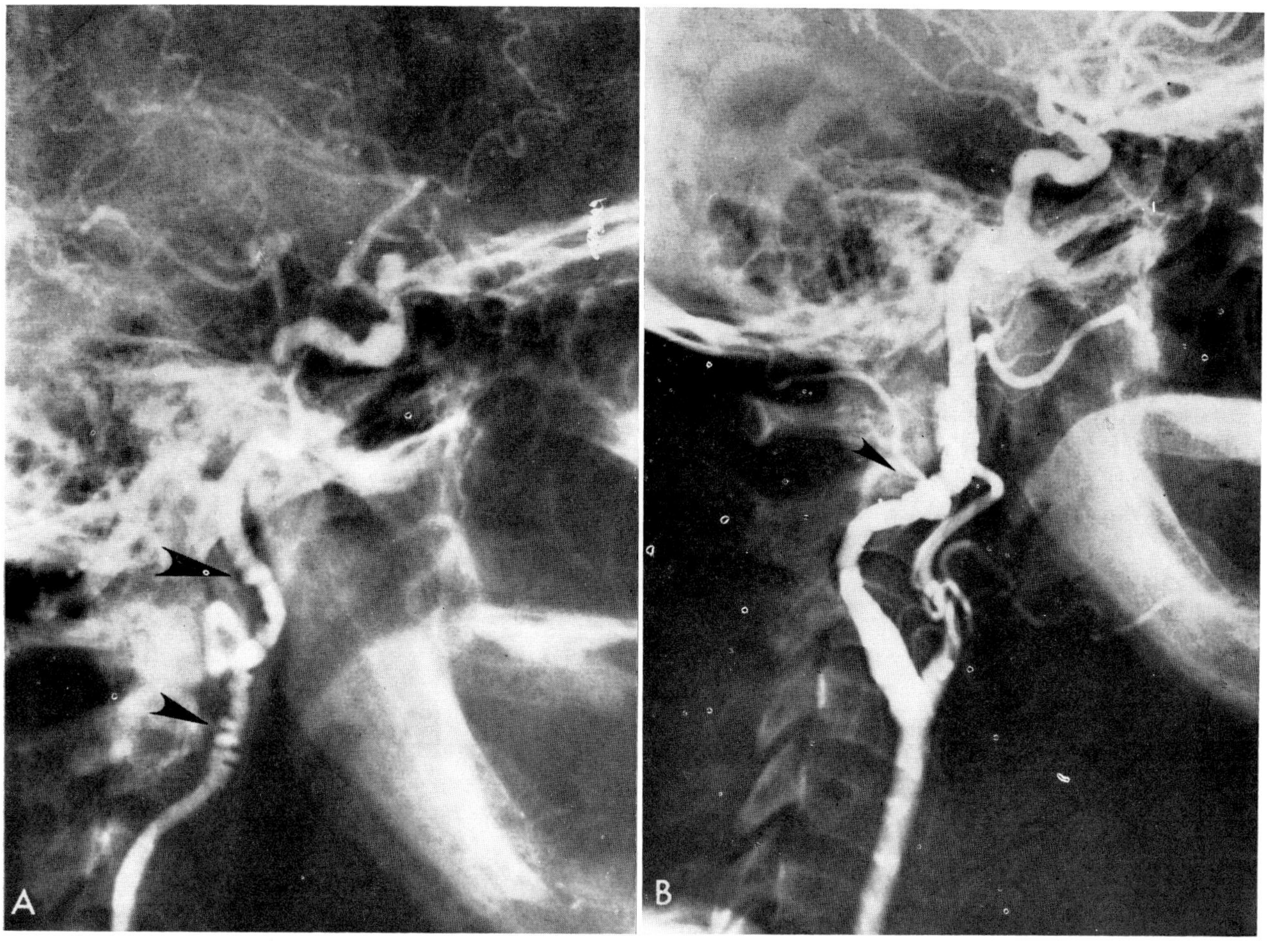

Figure 23.7. Common Carotid Arteriogram. (A) Left side: Cervical part of the internal carotid artery has areas of alternating narrowing and dilatation. (B) Right side: The findings are the same; however, the dilatation is more pronounced. This forty-seven-year-old patient had nonspecific cerebral symptoms. *Radiographic Diagnosis:* Medial fibromuscular hyperplasia with aneurysms.

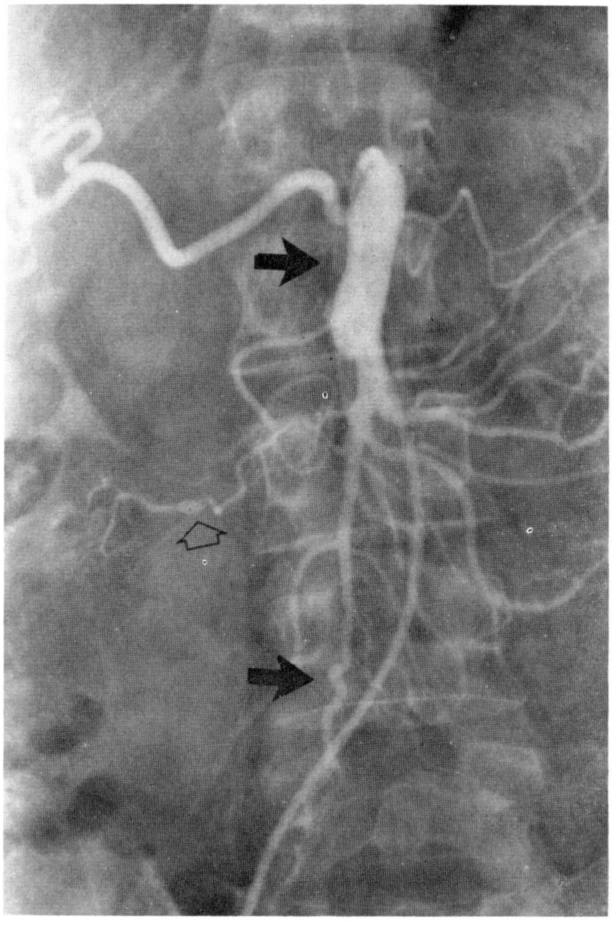

←

Figure 23.8. Superior Mesenteric Arteriogram. Fusiform dilation of the very proximal superior mesenteric artery (Arrow) and localized dilatation of the proximal branch of the superior mesenteric artery (Arrow Head) are present. *Diagnosis:* Fibromuscular hyperplasia.

narrowing and dilatation as in medial fibroplasia with aneurysms, subadventitial fibroplasia or stationary waves, and atherosclerosis, necrotizing angiitis, or arteritis.

SINGLE AREA OF NARROWING AND DISTAL DILATATION

This is seen as *focal stenosis* with *poststenotic dilatation.*[889–891] A mass of fluid, when ejected through a constricting area under high velocity, strikes a more slowly moving mass of fluid distal to the stenotic area. This creates high lateral pressure, producing eddy currents of high and low pressure. The repeated impact of this pressure against the elastic wall of the artery over a long period of time is capable of inducing structural fatigue and distension of that wall. This results in poststenotic dilatation. Dilatation may also be due to a drag force, acting to pull the endothelium down the stream of flow.[892] *Poststenotic dilatation usually occurs when the stenosis is of a short segment of arterial wall. It does not occur if the narrow segment is long and gradual.* The tighter the stenotic lesion, the longer the area of poststenotic dilatation.[893] The best example of stenosis and poststenotic dilatation is coarctation of the aorta with its distal area of dilatation. This occurs most often in the thoracic,[412, 894] and less often in the abdominal, aorta[895] Any other cause of localized sharp narrowing may give similar pictures. This may be seen with atherosclerosis, extrinsic vascular compression, thoracic outlet syndrome, etc. (Fig. 23-1).

MULTIPLE AREAS OF SHARP NARROWING AND INTERVENING DILATATION—STRING OF BEADS

The best available example of this abnormality is *medial fibroplasia with aneurysmal dilatations.* One of the noticeable features is the alternating rhythmic pattern of *narrowing due to thick ridges of collagen and muscle,* and *dilatation due to destruction of the internal elastica of the medial layer.* In the group of *intimal hyperplastic diseases,* an aneurysm may be seen if the elastica is disrupted. Though these lesions are very common in the distal two thirds of the renal artery, they may also involve visceral, the internal carotid vertebral, and external iliac arteries.[630, 631] Another fascinating angiographic finding is in the vessels of those individuals with homocystinuria. Here alternating areas of narrowing and dilatation are caused by fibrous intimal proliferation and disruption and fragmentation of the elastica[896] (Figs. 23-5 to 23-9).

Subadventitial hyperplasia manifests itself as alternating areas of narrowing with apparently well-preserved areas of vascular segments in between. This may give the same appearance as above, but *the beads* are *no wider* than the uninvolved proximal segment of the artery. This is usually seen to involve the renal arteries.[632, 633]

Stationary waves give the impression of alternating narrowed and dilated segments of an artery. These waves tend to occur in medium sized arteries. They are more frequently seen when there is distal obstruction or increased resistance to the normal flow of blood. They may be due to the presence of increased velocity of back flow due to distal obstruction under local laminar flow conditions.[897] Another explanation is *ripples* at the contrast blood interphase.[898] And a final explanation relates the waves to a reflection of longitudinal arterial pressure waves at the point of obstruction and amplification of resonance.[899] Be that as it may, when they are seen they should not be mistaken for organic arterial disease. They usually disappear after a repeat study with prior local intraarterial infusion of Prescoline[784] (Fig. 23-11).

RANDOM NARROWING AND DILATATION

This occurs when the same disease *randomly destroys the media* and affects the other layers through *deposition of tissue or patchy areas of inflammation.* Atherosclerosis or hyperplastic disorders cause this type of response. Arteritis or angiitis are causes of inflammatory change. The medium sized and small intrinsic vessels of an organ are usually involved by angiitis or hyperplastic disorders. The large and medium sized vessels, such as the aorta and its branches, are usually involved by atherosclerosis or arteritis (Figs. 23-1 to 23-4 and 23-12 to 23-14).

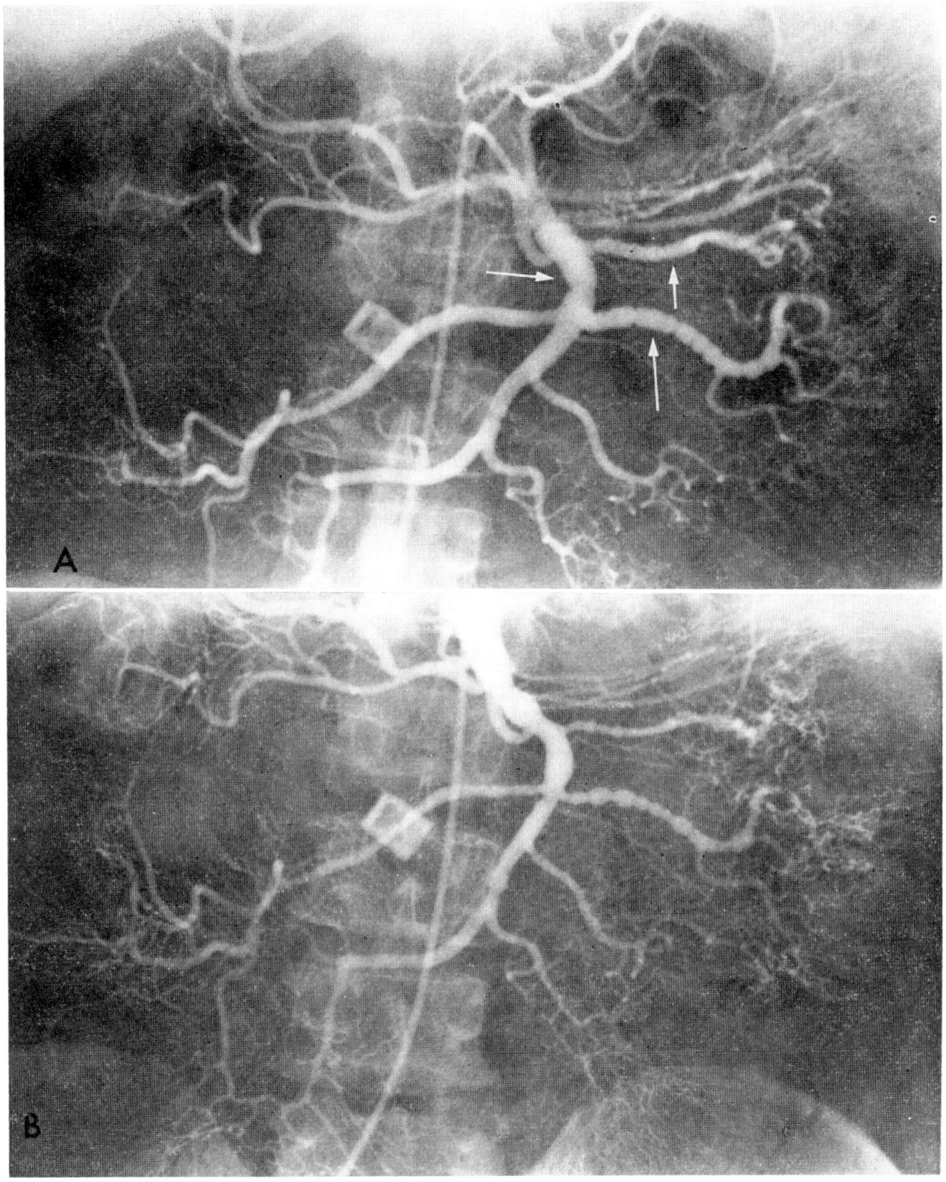

Figure 23.9 A and B *(Continued on the next page)*

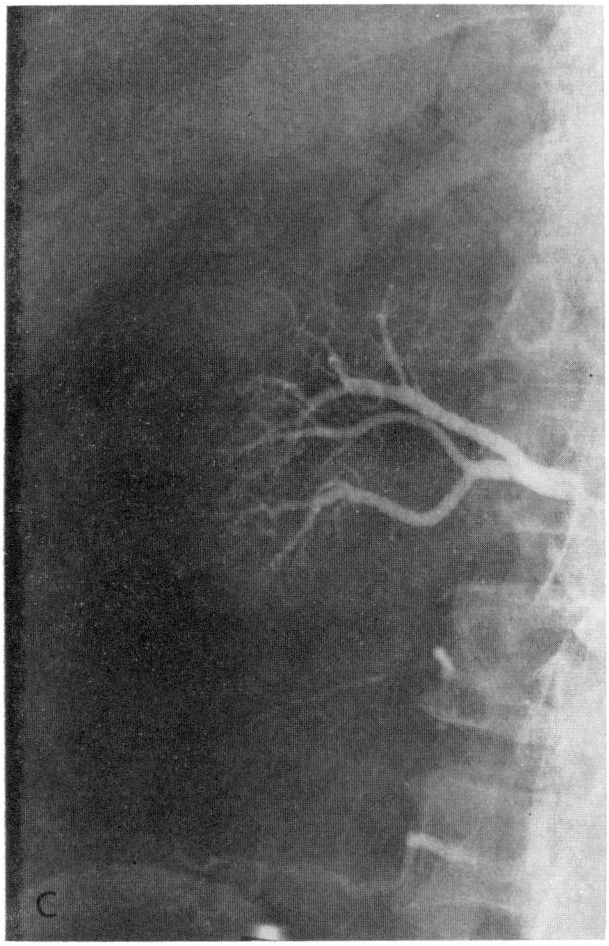

Figure 23.9. Superior Mesenteric Arteriogram. (A) Regular alternating areas of concentric narrowing of the superior mesenteric artery and its branches (Arrow) are seen. (B) Thirty milligrams of prescoline was injected into the superior mesenteric artery. The areas of narrowing increased in severity and the main superior mesenteric artery decreased in its caliber. (C) Renal arteriogram: The same alternate concentric areas of narrowing is noted in the renal artery hilar branches. The patient had renal failure. The same findings were noted in the opposite kidney also. The prescoline was infused with the intention of differentiating between stationary waves and fibromuscular disease, but the arteries exaggerated the manifestations after prescoline infusion. *Diagnosis:* Inconclusive.

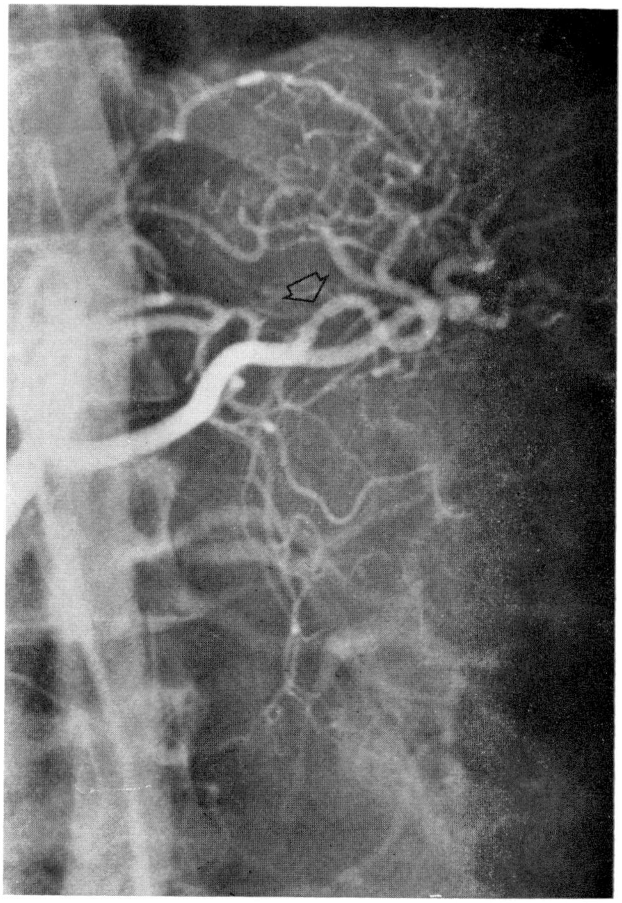

Figure 23.10. Celiac Arteriogram. The splenic artery bifurcation (Arrow) shows alternating areas of narrowing and dilatation. This young man was a known alcoholic with repeated attacks of pancreatitis. *Diagnosis:* Chronic pancreatitis with secondary changes in the splenic artery.

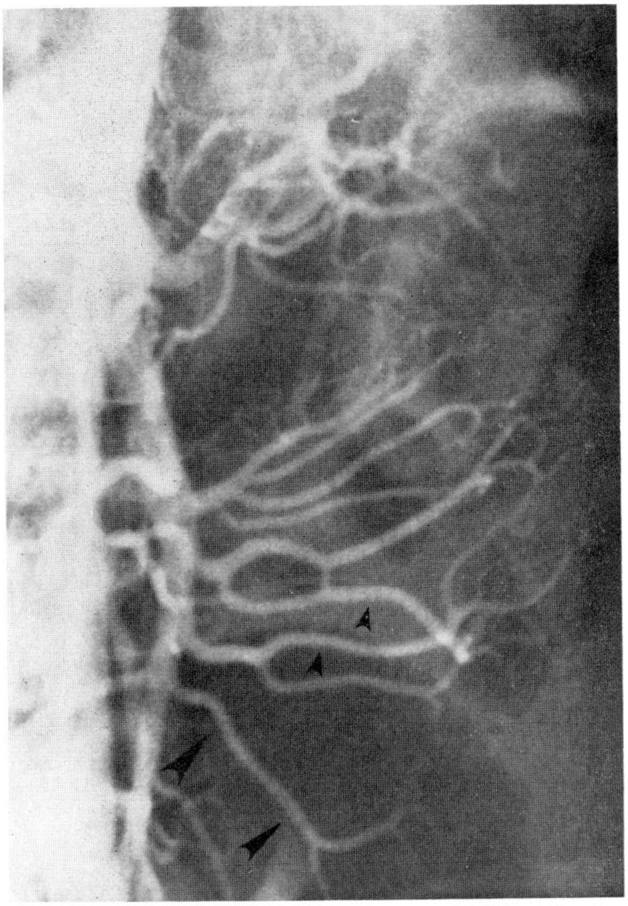

←

Figure 23.11. Superior Mesenteric Arteriogram. There are alternate areas of narrowing and dilatation of the jejunal branches (Arrow). This was not evident in a second examination. *Diagnosis:* Stationary waves.

Figure 23.12. Flush Aortogram. (A) Note the occlusion of the left renal artery with narrowing and dilatation of many of the branches of the superior mesenteric (Arrow Head) and hepatic arterial branches (Arrow Head). (B) Late arterial phase: The same changes are better shown (Arrow Head). *Diagnosis:* Angiitis. *Pathology:* Polyarteritis nodosa.

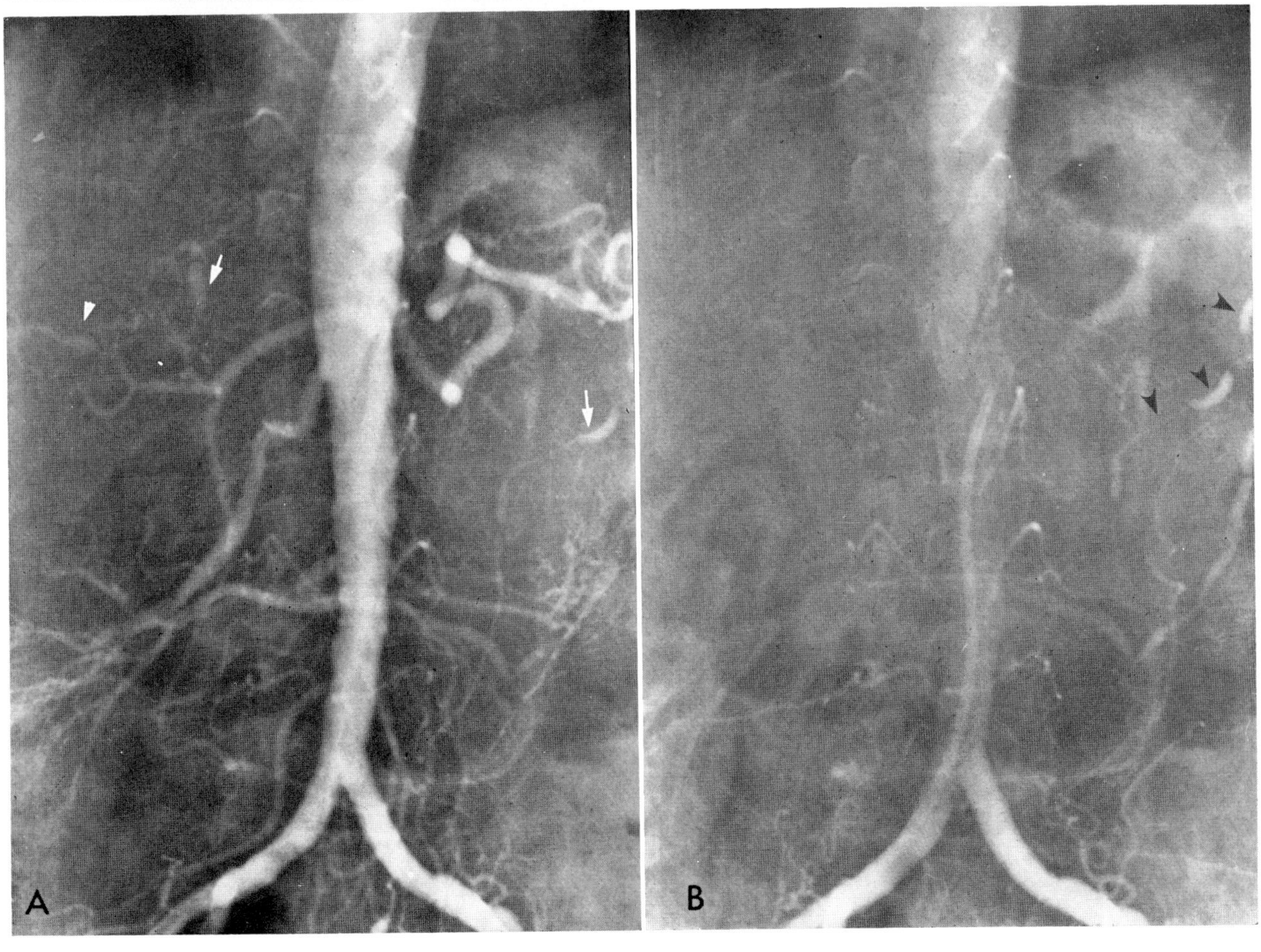

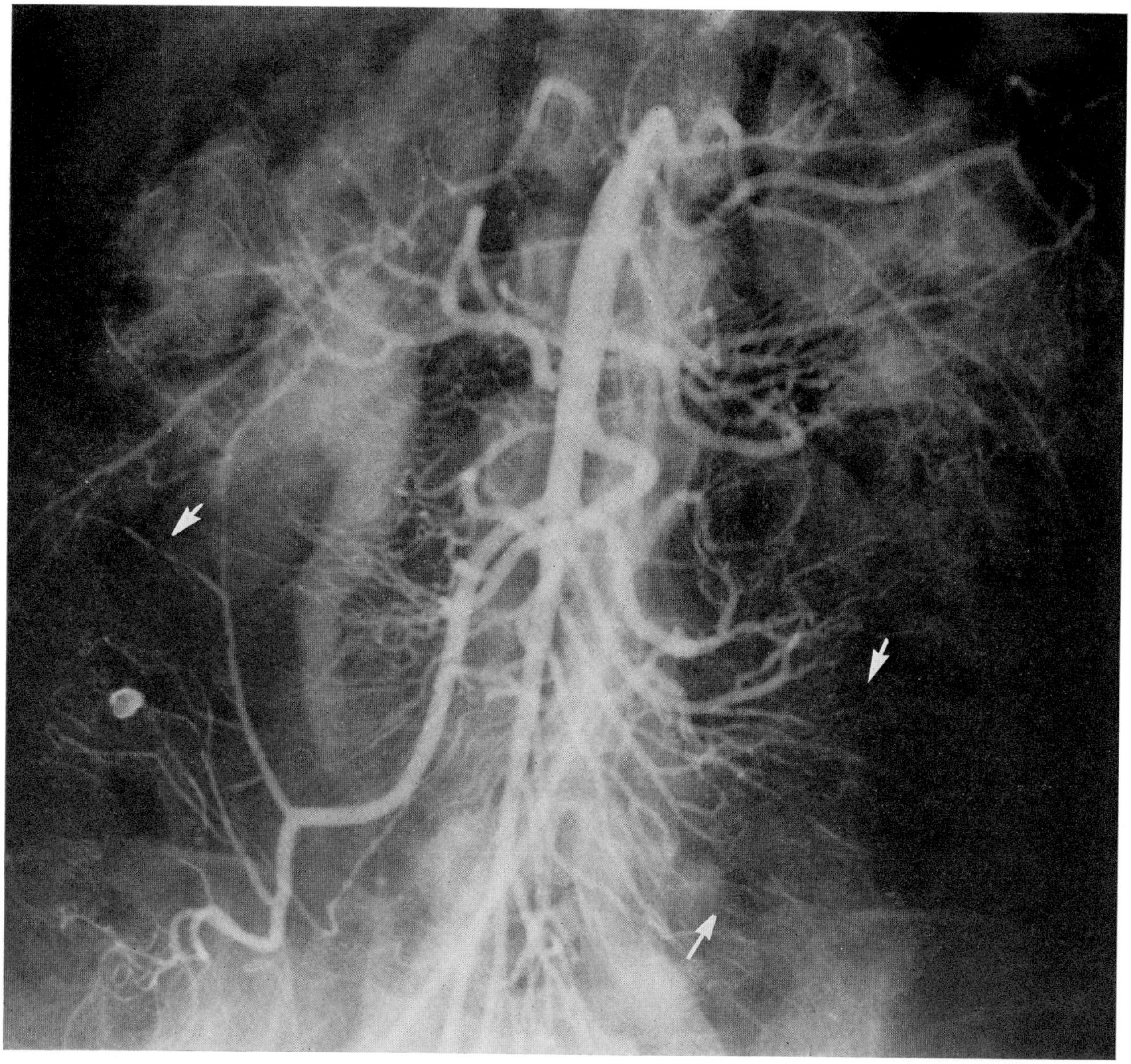

Figure 23.13. Superior mesenteric arteriogram reveals multiple areas of narrowing and occlusions of the branches of the superior mesenteric artery. This young lady has repeated episodes of abdominal pain. *Diagnosis:* Necrotizing angiitis. *Pathology:* Acute phase of polyarteritis nodosa.

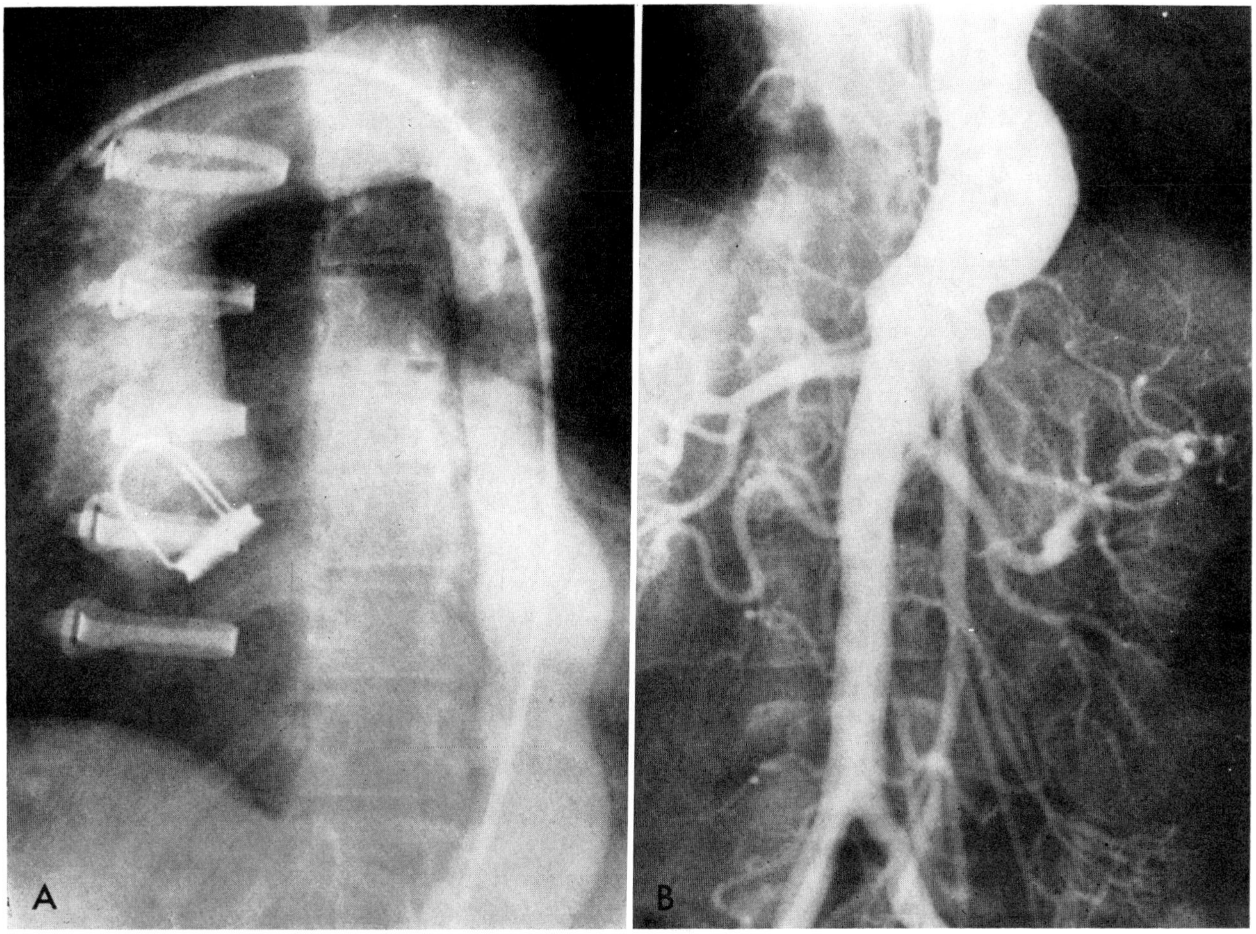

Figure 23.14. Aortic Arch Angiogram. (A) There is segmental narrowing and dilatation. An aortic valvular prosthesis was inserted for aortic insufficiency. (B) Abdominal aortogram: There is dilatation of the distal thoracic aorta. This young woman had an elevated sedimentation rate. *Diagnosis:* Aortitis.

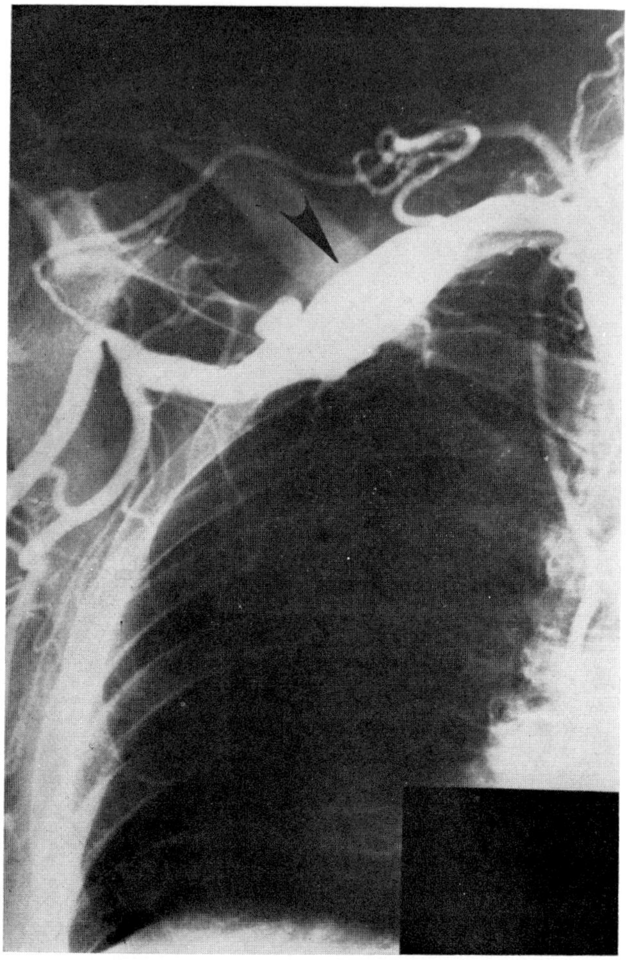

Figure 23.15. Subclavian Arteriogram. There is dilatation of the mid- and distal subclavian artery. The patient had a cold hand. *Diagnosis:* (1) Atherosclerotic aneurysm with mural thrombus and distal embolization, (2) Thoracic outlet syndrome with poststenotic dilatation and distal embolization. *Surgical Diagnosis:* Thoracic outlet syndrome with mural thrombus in the dilated poststenotic segment.

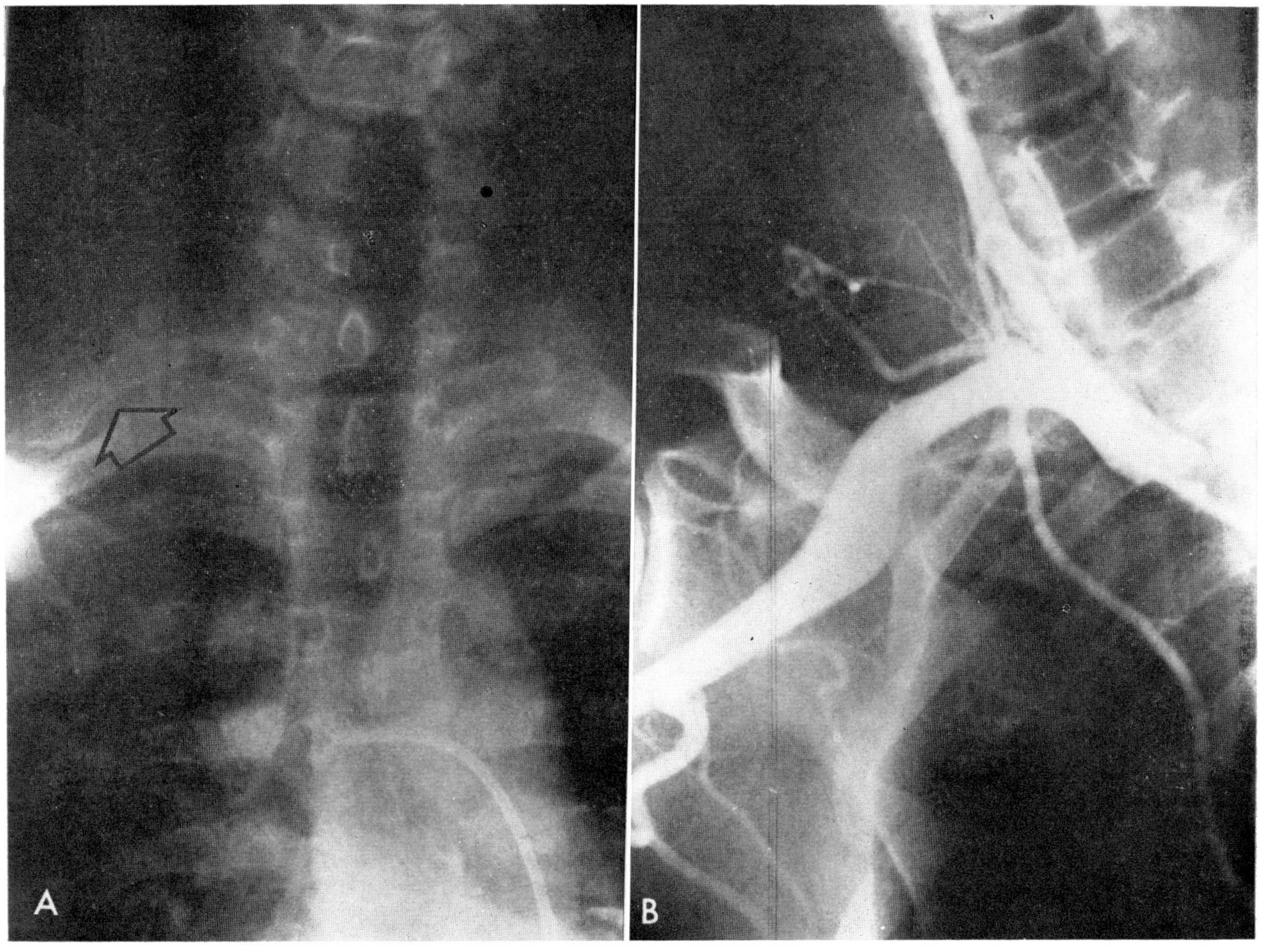

Figure 23.16. Subclavian Arteriogram. (A) There is a cervical rib (Arrow). (B) There is elevation of the right subclavian artery over the rib and dilatation. This patient has ischemic changes in the right hand. *Diagnosis:* Thoracic outlet syndrome with arterial compression and poststenotic dilatation. At surgery a mural thrombus was found in the dilated arterial segment.

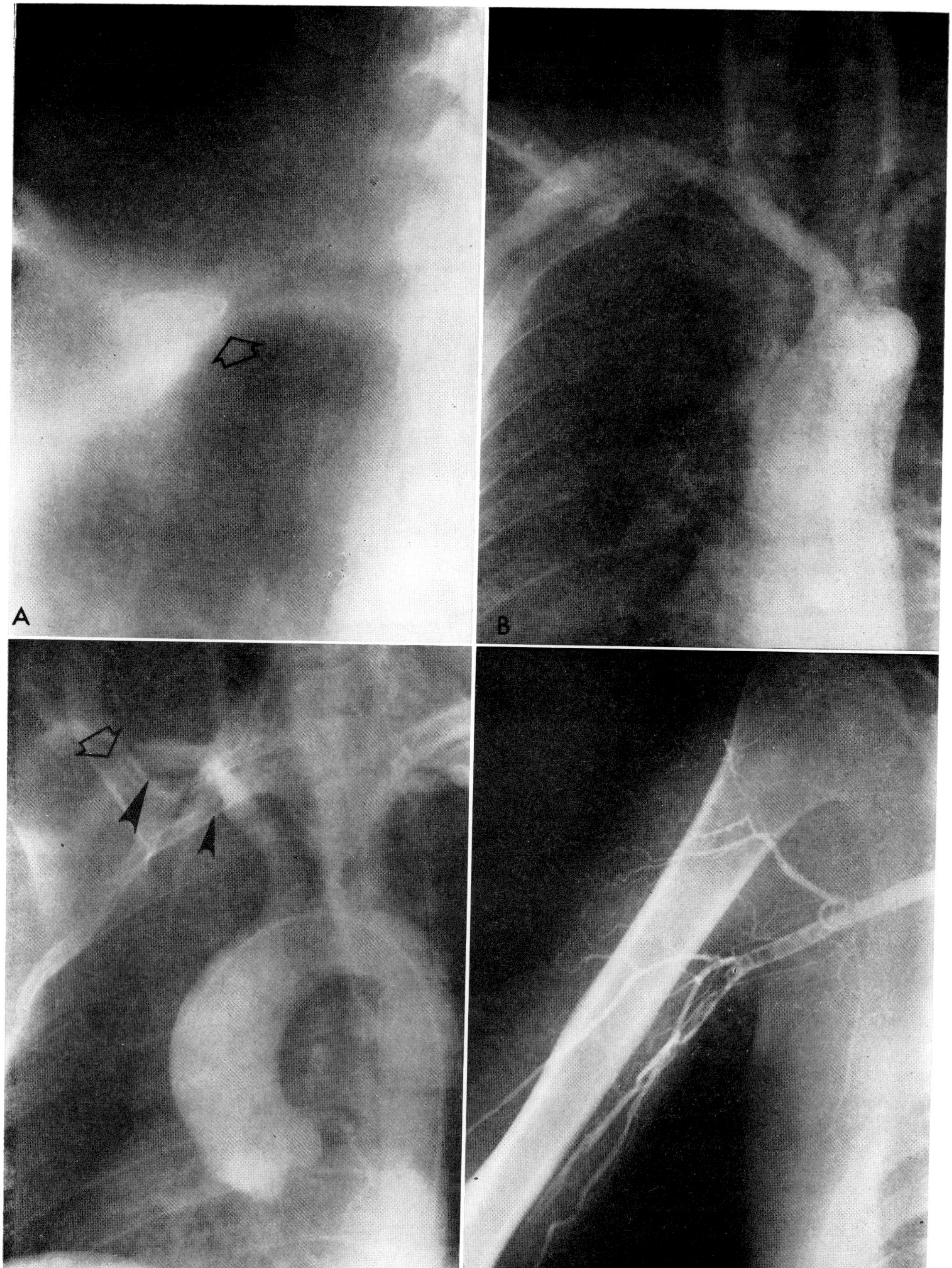
A
B
C
D

←

Figure 23.17. (A) Subclavian Arteriogram. There is a bony abnormality at the midportion of the right first rib (Arrow). (B) Arteriogram: An abnormal cephalad course of the distal subclavian artery with marked fusiform dilatation (Arrow) is seen. (C) Same patient: In the left anterior oblique projection. Inferior marginal irregularities are noted in the area of dilatation (Arrow Head). (D) Right axillary arteriogram: Multiple filling defects in the proximal brachial artery with nonvisualization of its distal course can be seen. This patient presented with a hard supraclavicular mass and nonpalpable right radial pulse. *Diagnosis:* Thoracic Outlet syndrome with poststenotic dilatation because of pressure on the subclavian artery by the bony mass with mural thrombi and secondary distal embolization. *Comment:* Sometimes the mural thrombi may be better shown in an oblique projection.

CHAPTER 24

OCCLUSION

ARTERIAL OCCLUSION

A gradually occluded vessel was narrowed before it was totally occluded.

Injection of contrast into the parent vessel of an occluded vessel reveals *nonfilling of the occluded vessel* provided that no variation of normal is present. If the occluded vessel is intrinsic to the organ, then *stasis* of contrast proximal to the occlusion, *lack of parenchymal stain* in the area supplied by the vessel, or lack of venous opacification depending on the level and extent of occlusion, will occur. In some areas such as the lung or bowel, *hemorrhagic infarcts* are due to arterial or venous occlusion and may be demonstrated by *intense staining* of the infarcted zone.[868, 1047]

A. Embolic occlusion
B. Thrombotic occlusion
   1. Atherosclerosis
      a. Conducting arteries—aorta, iliac, femoral, popliteal, subclavian arteries
      b. Distributing arteries—celiac, mesenteric, renal, profunda femoris
         Occlusion usually occurs close to the origin of these distributing vessels
   2. Arteritis
      a. Takayasu's aortitis. The conducting arteries and branches of the aorta are involved close to their orifices. Usually the distal vessel is spared[627]
      b. Thromboangiitis obliterans.[825, 826] This disease causes bilateral smooth occlusions usually of the lower extremity vessels and then extends in a centripetal manner
   3. Proliferative and hyperplastic disease
      a. Intimal and medial proliferation—abdominal aorta
      b. Intimal hyperplasia—renal and other medium sized arteries

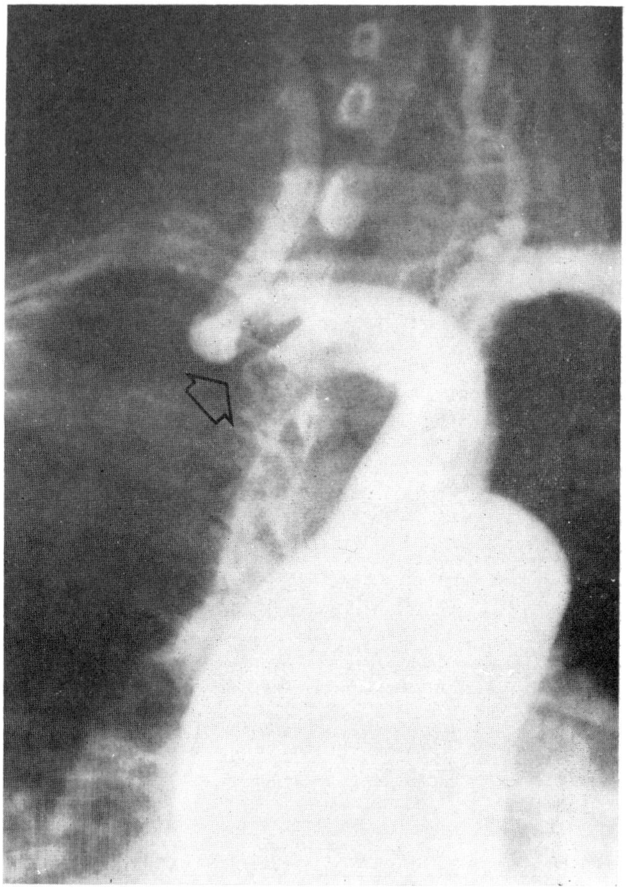

Figure 24.1. Thoracic Aortogram. There is a filling defect in the innominate artery (Arrow) with occlusion of the right subclavian artery. *Diagnosis:* Embolus due to atrial fibrillation.

   4. Necrotizing angiitis—the small intrinsic vasculature of an organ is usually involved
   5. Trauma—thrombosis, laceration, avulsion, and intimal fracture
   6. Catheterization procedures
   7. Dissecting hematomas—occlusion usually occurs in the medium sized vessels
   8. Extrinsic compression
      a. Ligaments—The median arcuate liga-

ment of the diaphragm compressing the celiac or superior mesenteric arteries

b. Diaphragmatic crura—The lateral crura may compress the renal artery

c. Muscles: Scalenus—subclavian artery, pectorialis minor—axillary artery, longus colli—vertebral artery, gastrocnemius (medial head)—popliteal artery[660, 835]

d. Miscellaneous: Aberrant nerve roots —iliac artery,[1037] synovial cysts—popliteal artery,[1038] hemorrhage into the anterior tibial compartment—anterior tibial artery[1039]

9. Infiltrative occlusions
   a. Infiltrating tumors
   b. Desmoplastic lesions—pancreatic carcinoma, pancreatitis, carcinoid, and other desmoplastic processes[111, 819–823, 1041]

10. Miscellaneous
    a. Venous occlusion causing arterial thrombosis[1040]
    b. Mucoid cystic degeneration of the arterial wall—popliteal artery
    c. Radiation thrombosis—femoral[1043] and carotid[660] arteries

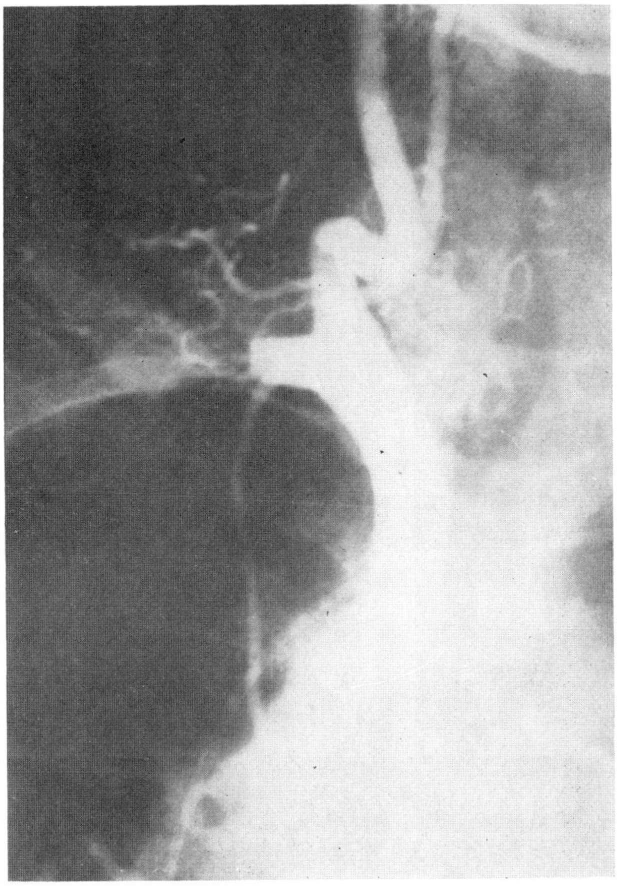

Figure 24.2. Left Subclavian Arteriogram. The left subclavian artery is completely occluded distal to the origin of the vertebral artery. *Diagnosis:* Embolus due to atrial fibrillation.

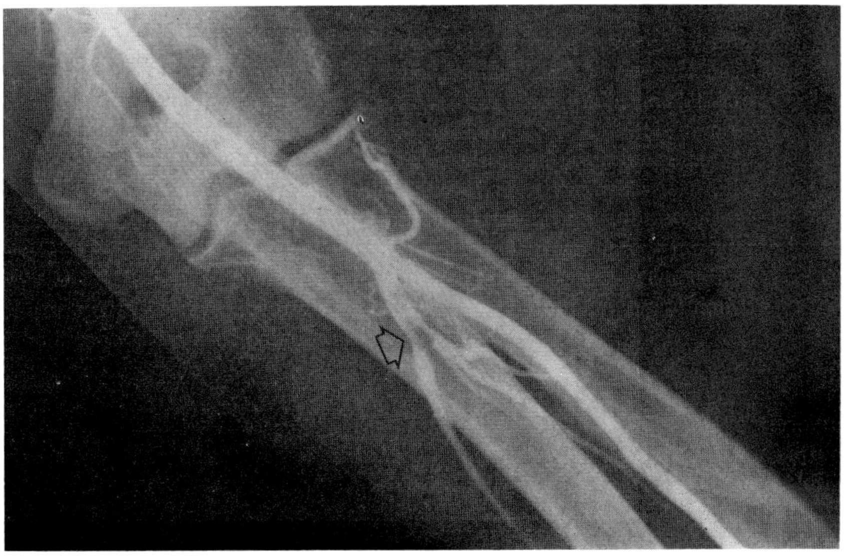

Figure 24.3. Brachial Arteriogram. Filling defects are seen at the origin of the ulnar artery (Arrow). *Diagnosis:* Emboli. The etiology is unknown.

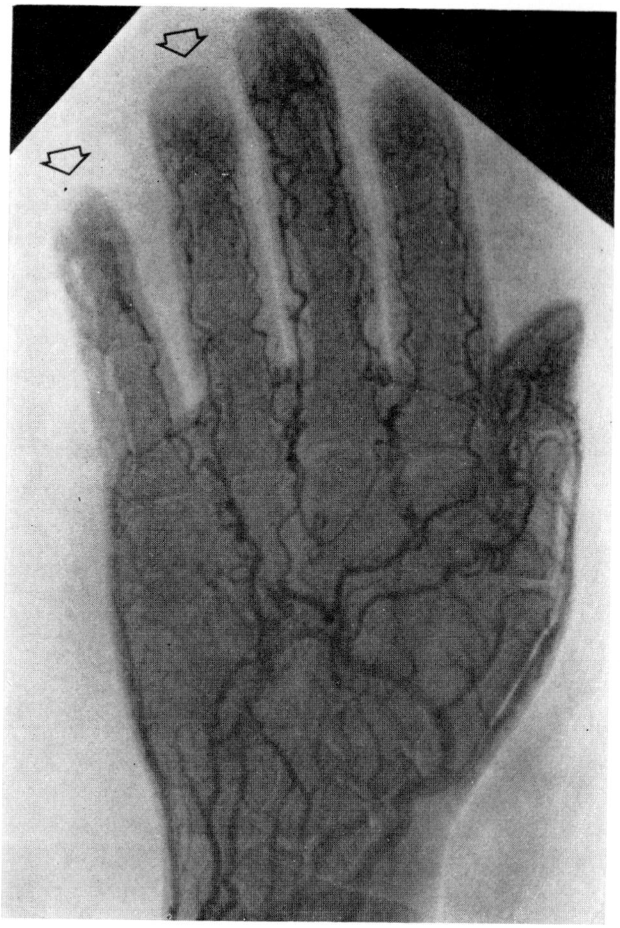

Figure 24.4. Arteriogram of the Hand. The small vessels of the hand supplying the distal fingertips (Arrow) do not visualize. This sixty-year-old patient developed ischemic changes of the fingers following surgery to replace the aortic valve. *Diagnosis:* Atheromatous emboli to the small vessels of the fingers.

d. Sickle cell anemia—posterior tibial artery[1044]
e. Atresia—celiac artery with ulcer-like symptoms[1045]

EMBOLISM

Embolism[920–926] is one of the catastrophic events of the vascular tree. The end result may be fatal to that segment of the circulation, or treatable. The *suddenness of embolism* and *chronicity of thrombosis* presents a contrasting, striking clinical picture. Embolism occurs when a clot or a bit of foreign material is transported by the bloodstream to a segment of the vascular bed. It is brought to a halt in some segment because of its size or consistency, causing obstruction to the arterial tree distal to this point. The *site of impaction* depends on the size and specific gravity of the embolus and the width of the vessel. The tendency of an embolus to halt at an arterial bifurcation, sudden bend, or previously diseased vessel is noteworthy. Emboli lodge in healthy vessels, causing a pulsatile proximal artery and a patent nonpulsatile distal artery. If the main

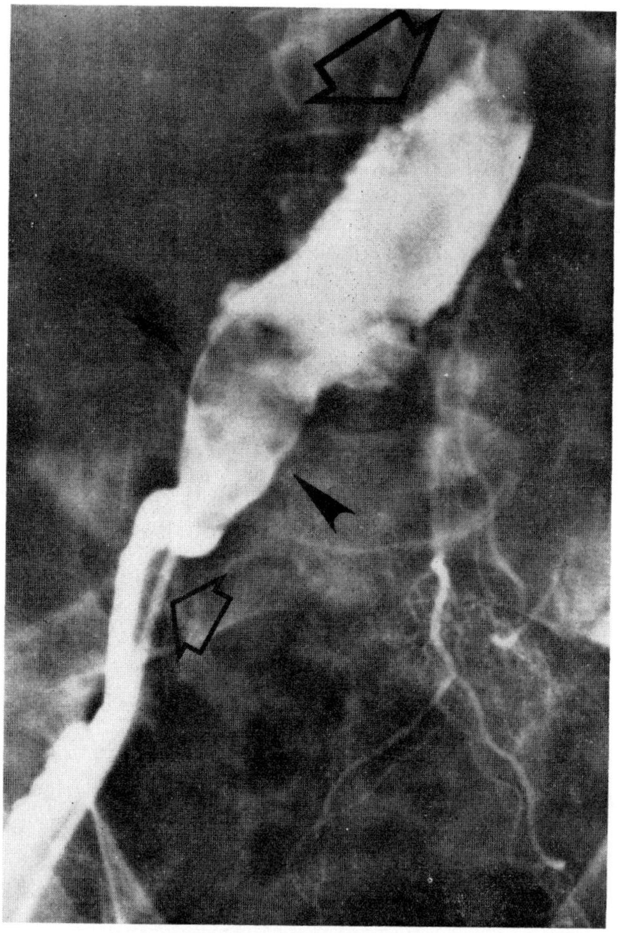

Figure 24.5. External Iliac Arteriogram. There is dilatation of the proximal common iliac artery (Large Arrow) and a filling defect proximal to the external iliac artery (Arrow Head). The catheter appears to be in an extraluminal position (Small Arrow) and the left common iliac and the right internal iliac arteries do not fill. *Diagnosis:* The catheter passes through a thrombus in the external iliac artery and a large thrombus almost occludes the dilated common iliac artery.

channel is occluded and provided with inadequate collaterals, distal thrombosis develops in four to six hours. Extensive distal thrombosis with limited proximal thrombosis is the end result. This is due to the blood flow preventing proximal extension of the thrombus beyond the primary, major collateral.

Emboli may be solid, liquid or gaseous. They may be bacterial vegetations, tumors, masses or bullets. They are usually portions of blood clots derived from a parent thrombus elsewhere. *Ninety percent of all emboli come from the left ventricle of the heart.* They arise from mural thrombi caused by myocardial infarction, fibrillation, subacute bacterial endocarditis, or rheumatic heart disease. An *atheromatous aorta with mural thrombi* also contributes to this clinical catastrophe. In some patients no source of emboli may be identified. Before reaching its final destination, an embolus undergoes oscillation, tumbling, regurgitation and fragmentation.[927] Unlike venous emboli, which travel long distances through vessels which gradually widen, arterial emboli travel shorter pathways as the vascular tree decreases in caliber distally.

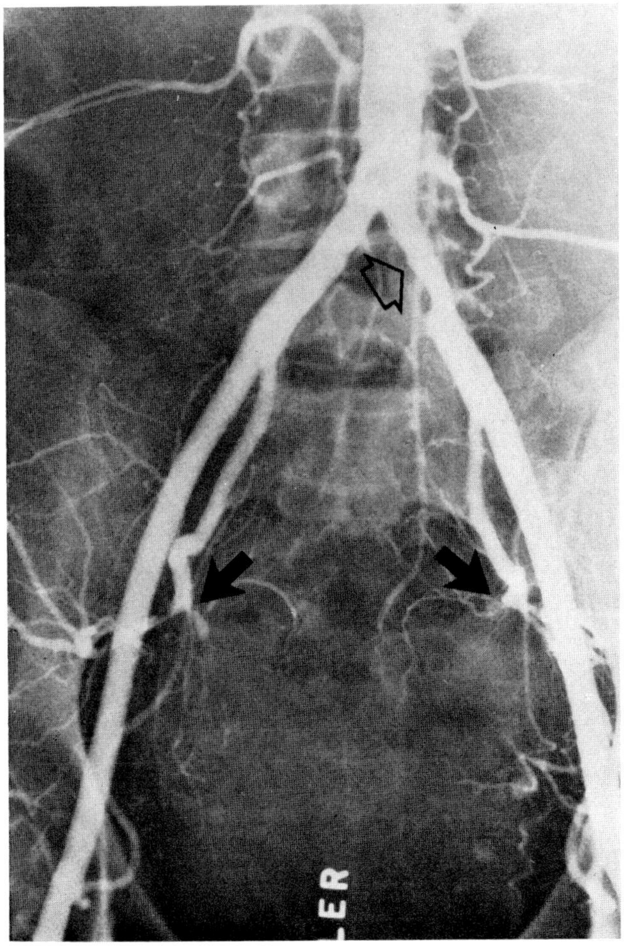

Figure 24.6. Pelvic Arteriogram. There is irregular eccentric narrowing of the left common iliac artery (Blank Arrow) and partial occlusion of the internal iliac artery (Arrow). The patient was sixty years old. *Diagnosis:* Atherosclerosis.

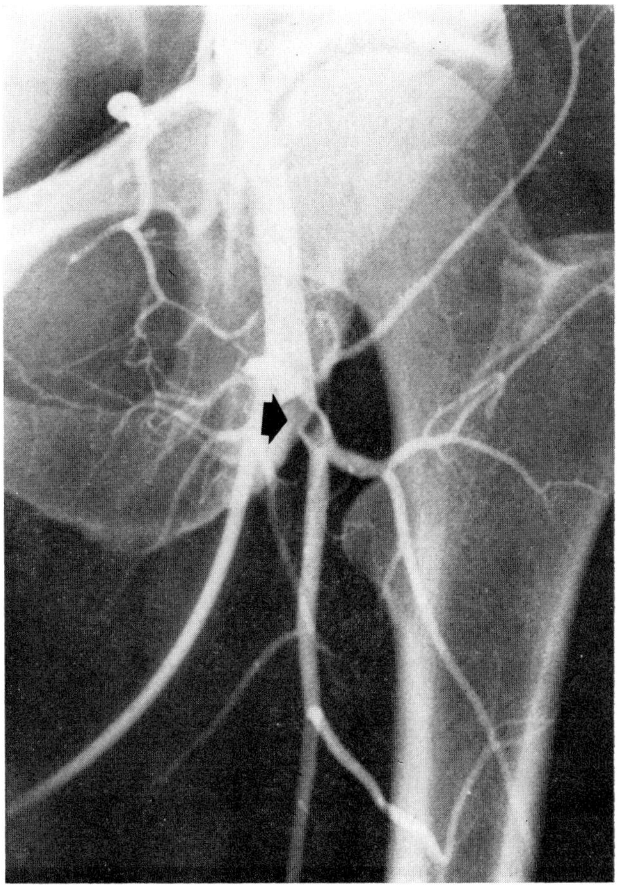

Figure 24.7. Femoral Arteriogram. A filling defect is seen in the main femoral artery with occlusion of the superficial femoral artery. *Diagnosis:* Embolus.

Embolism to the aorta and its peripheral branches is related to the age of the patient and other associated cardiovascular disorders. The older the patient, the greater the incidence of embolism. *The brain, lower extremities, spleen*

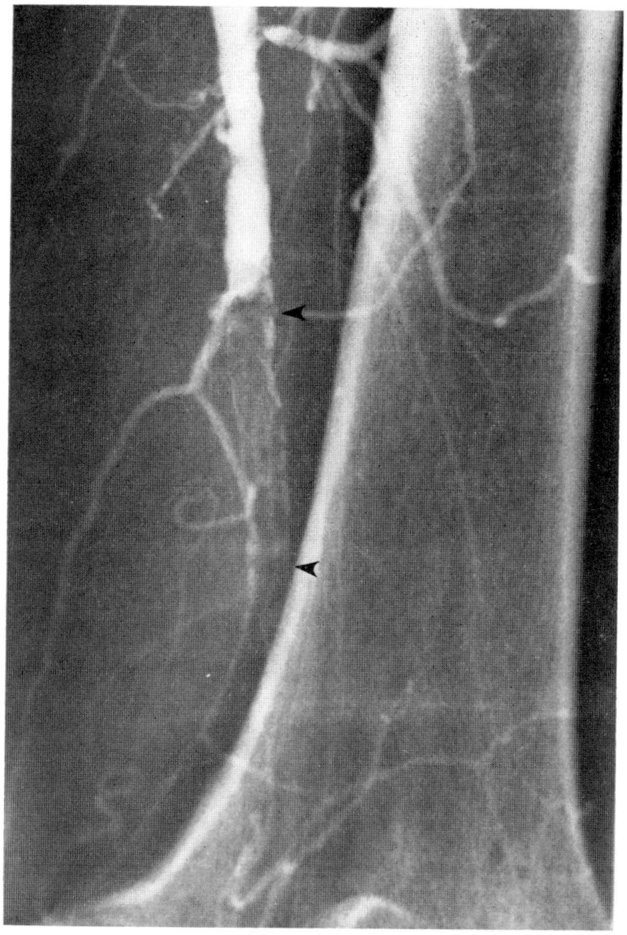

Figure 24.8. Femoral Arteriogram. There is a long filling defect in the distal femoral artery and no visualization of the popliteal artery. *Diagnosis:* Arteriosclerotic thromboembolic disease.

and kidney are frequent victims of embolism. The lower leg vessels, which are actually the bottleneck in the flow of blood from the aorta to the toe, are usually the first to be involved. This is especially true of the posterior tibial artery.

The upper extremity vessels receive less emboli because the solid nature of the embolus with its increased specific gravity traveling in a central or lower portion of the stream tends to bypass the origin of the brachiocephalic vessels. It may also be due to the fact that too large a clot is unable to enter these vessels, while too small a clot may be undetectable clinically (Figs. 24-1 to 24-4).

The *effects of an embolus* on a segment of the circulation are determined by the site of obstruction, spasm of the major vessels, availability of collaterals, distal and proximal extension of thrombosis, and demand of the organ for blood. Unlike emboli to the lungs, those to the systemic circulation always cause infarction of the affected part (Figs. 24-5, 24-7 to 24-9).

Emboli from Atheromatous Ulcers

Emboli are frequent complications of ulcerative atherosclerosis.[928–933] Grumous lipid material is discharged into the vessel lumen, causing roughening of that intimal surface. This predisposes to thrombus formation which can also break loose into the bloodstream. Emboli may originate either in the aorta, large arteries, or even an atheromatous valve ring. The embolic

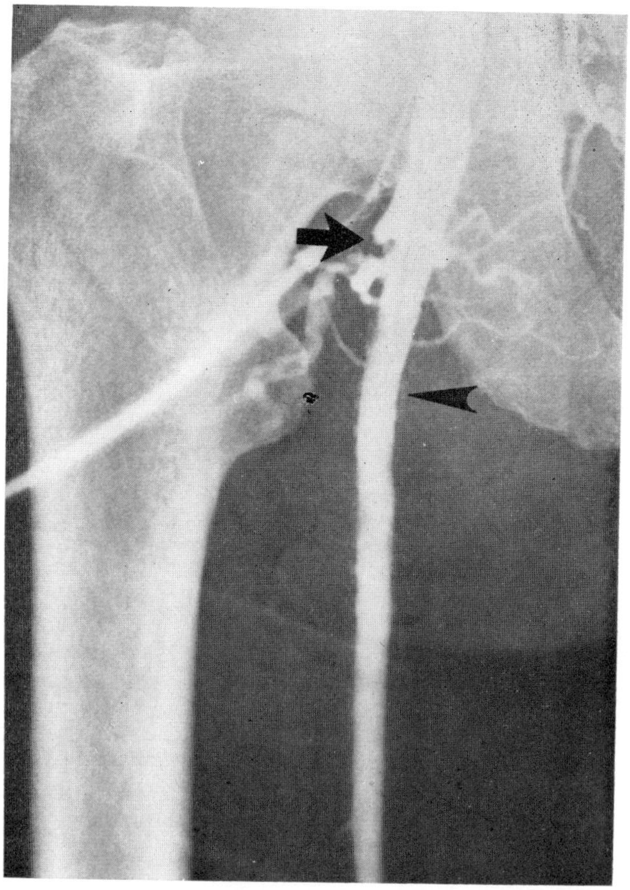

Figure 24.9. Femoral Arteriogram. There is occlusion of the profunda femoris artery due to arteriosclerosis (Large Arrow). This is a rare occurrence. There is calcification of the media due to Monckeberg's medial sclerosis of the superficial femoral artery without encroachment upon the lumen (Arrow Head).

material may be plaques, *cholesterol crystals,* or detached thrombi. The crystals may occlude vessels between 100 and 200 microns in size. Even small and medium sized vessels are not immune from this complication. *Multiple organ involvement* is characteristic, with the kidney, spleen and pancreas having the highest incidence of involvement. Renal failure or onset of hypertension, accentuation of existing hypertension, splenic infarcts, pancreatitis, gastrointestinal bleeding, peripheral gangrene, ischemic bowel disease resembling regional enteritis, and other patterns may resemble the disease picture of subacute bacterial endocarditis, or polyarteritis nodosa.

The added insult of emboli increases the incidence of ischemic necrosis in individuals with already decreased circulation due to associated vascular disease. Livido reticularis and digital infarcts may be the dominant clinical findings. *Renal function should be checked, especially after difficult catheter manipulations in individuals with severe atheromatous disease.*

In the carotid vessels, small ulcers and ulcers filled by thrombus may not be demonstrated angiographically. Most lesions are on the posterior walls of the vessel within 2.5 cm of the bifurcation of the common carotid artery. The base of the ulcer is usually within the contour of the arterial wall[934] (Fig. 22-36).

Emboli from Tumors and Masses

One of the most fascinating angiographic demonstrations of intra-arterial emboli is offered by *myxomas* of the heart. These may fall within the territory of general angiography.

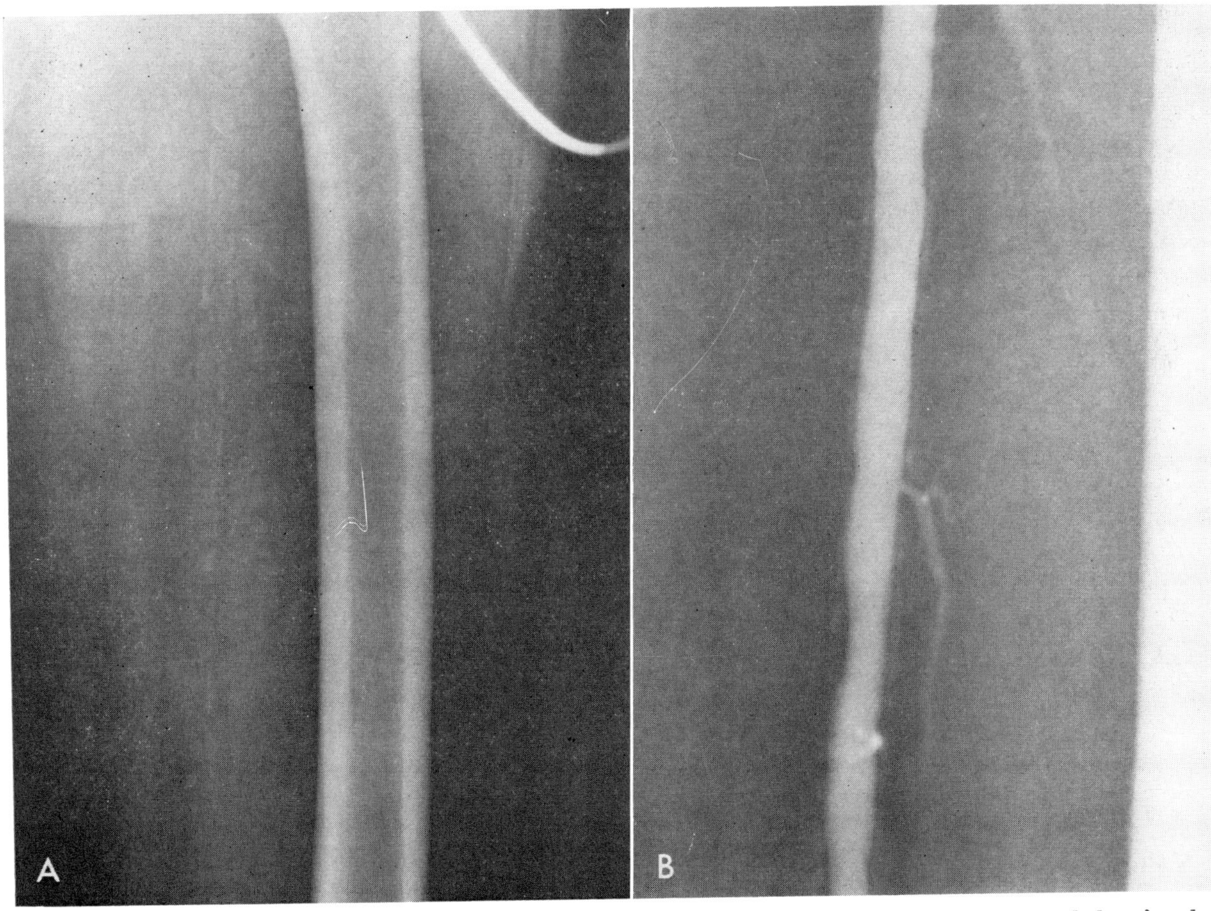

Figure 24.10. Femoral Arteriogram. There is linear calcification adjacent to the intima with no gross irregularities on the intimal surface and distal superficial femoral irregularities. *Diagnosis:* Monckeberg's sclerosis and patchy atherosclerosis.

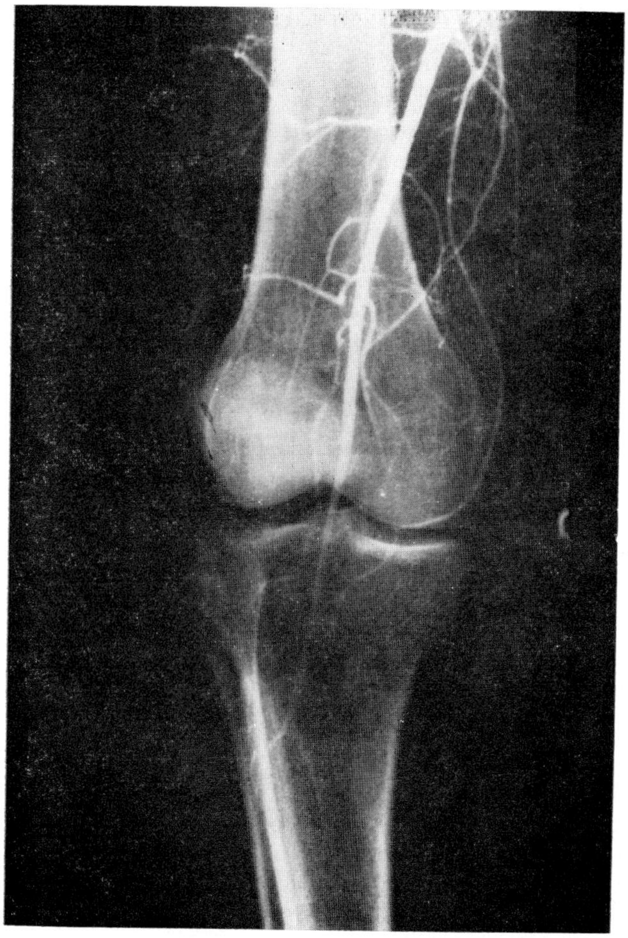

Figure 24.11. Femoral Arteriogram. The popliteal artery is narrowed at its trifurcation. The distal branches do not visualize. *Diagnosis:* Burns of the leg with severe edema causing obstruction.

Occlusion and/or dilatation of the involved vessel occurs because of invasion of the muscularis by tumor tissue, fibroblastic reaction, and destruction of the elastica. False aneurysms are not uncommon. Manifestations may develop even after extirpation of the primary tumor.[962] Emboli from vascular wall tumors (angiosarcomas[963]), osteosarcomas,[964] and even hydatid cysts[965] may make one wonder about the abnormal deviations of nature.

Pulmonary Artery Embolism

A firm angiographic diagnosis must be based solely on the demonstration of *filling defects, cut off, or localized pruning of the arterial tree. Segmental injection of contrast* and *magnification techniques* are crucial in establishing the diagnosis.[935, 938] Pulmonary emboli *decrease* in number and size within twenty-four hours after occurrence. Further reduction occurs in one week, and by the end of a month only minimal traces may be seen.[936, 937] If an embolus is not fragmented and lysed completely, then organization begins with ingrowth of granulation tissue from the walls of the pulmonary vessels. The *residual changes* of such organization include transverse webs, longitudinal

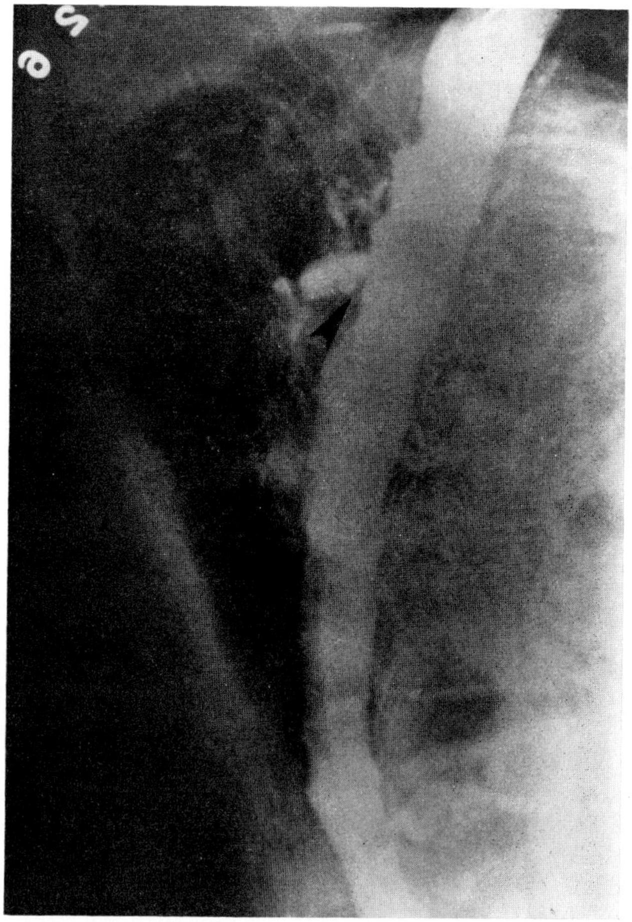

Figure 24.12. Cross-table Lateral Aortogram. There is filling of the superior mesenteric artery trunk with concentric narrowing at its origin (Arrow) and no visualization of celiac axis. This patient has clinical signs and symptoms of abdominal angina. *Diagnosis:* Atherosclerotic occlusion of the celiac and stenosis of superior mesenteric artery orifice.

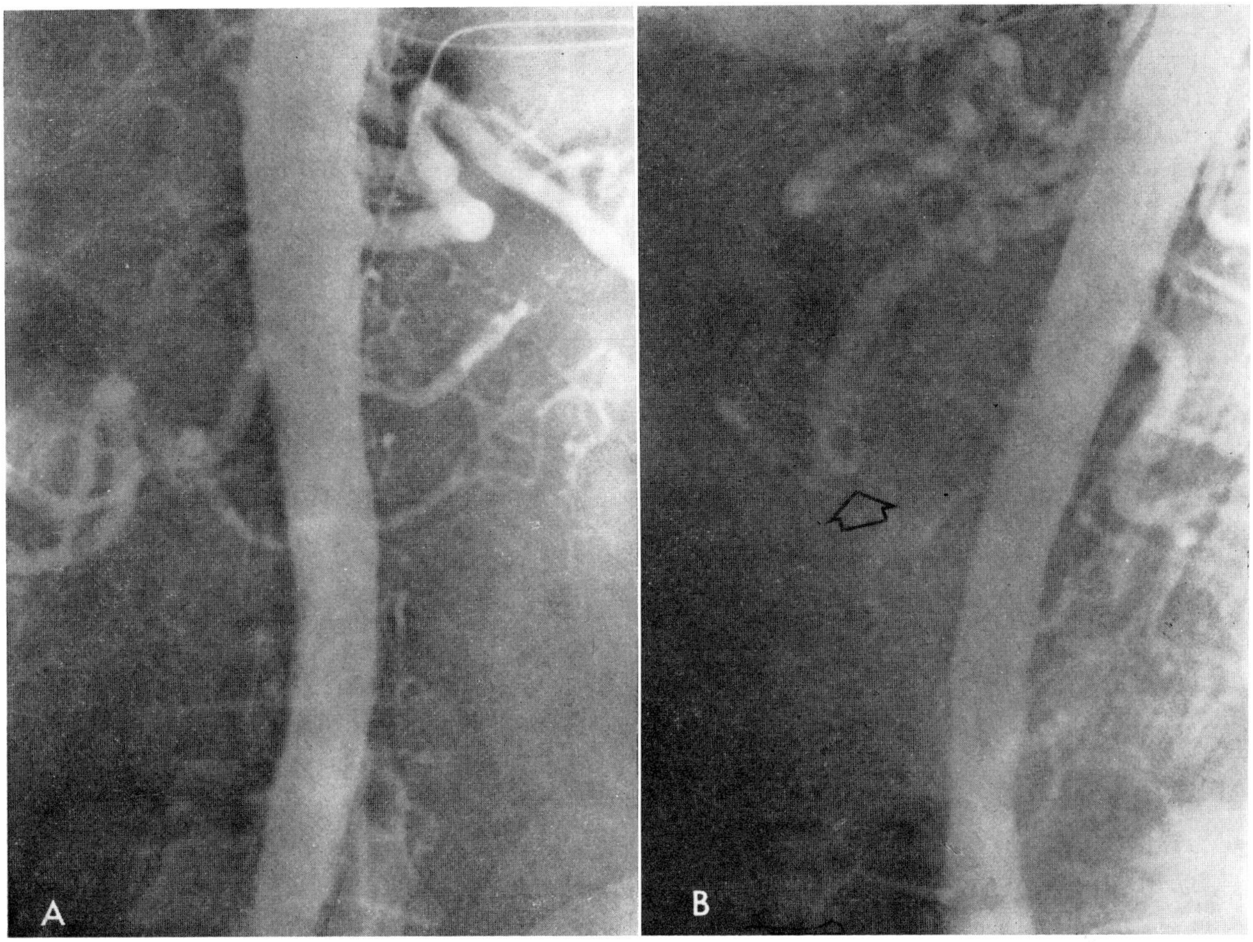

Figure 24.13. (A) Flush aortogram: A conspicuous absence of the superior mesenteric artery branches is noted. (B) Cross-table lateral aortogram: The most proximal segment of the superior mesenteric artery terminates abruptly. *Diagnosis:* Embolic occlusion of the superior mesenteric artery.

channels, eccentric plaques, and circumferential stenosis of small vessels[939] (Figs. 24-15 to 24-17).

Air Embolism and the Lung

Injection of significant amounts of air (1 to 2 cc/kg) into the pulmonary arteries bilaterally causes filling defects in the arteries, abrupt tapering of small vessels, abnormal small vessels, a decrease in the arteriovenous circulation time and oxygen saturation, and an increase in the pulmonary artery pressure. All these findings usually disappear within five to fifteen minutes after injection of air. In unilateral injection the same findings are noted as above except for the absence of filling defects on the contralateral side.[940]

Superior Mesenteric Artery Embolus

The main superior mesenteric artery is almost parallel to the aorta and therefore it is more likely to receive emboli from the heart.[943–947] Emboli to the superior mesenteric artery are twice as *common in men* and may cause occlusion of the main stem or branches, or become superimposed on atheromatous plaques. Associated thrombosis is not usual without underlying vascular disease. If thrombosis occurs, it can be seen as early as two hours following its onset. The embolus may cause

(Text continues on page 329)

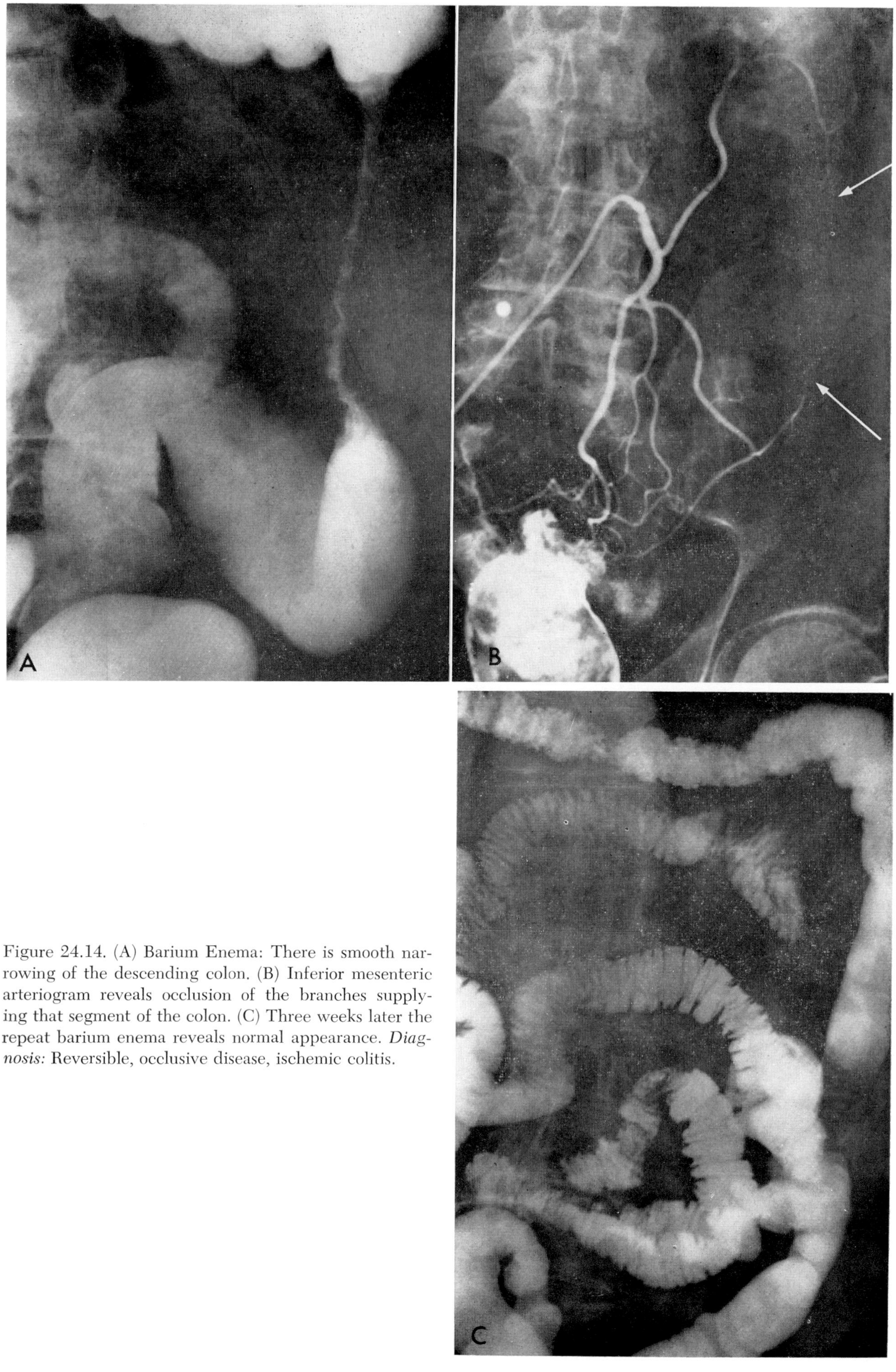

Figure 24.14. (A) Barium Enema: There is smooth narrowing of the descending colon. (B) Inferior mesenteric arteriogram reveals occlusion of the branches supplying that segment of the colon. (C) Three weeks later the repeat barium enema reveals normal appearance. *Diagnosis:* Reversible, occlusive disease, ischemic colitis.

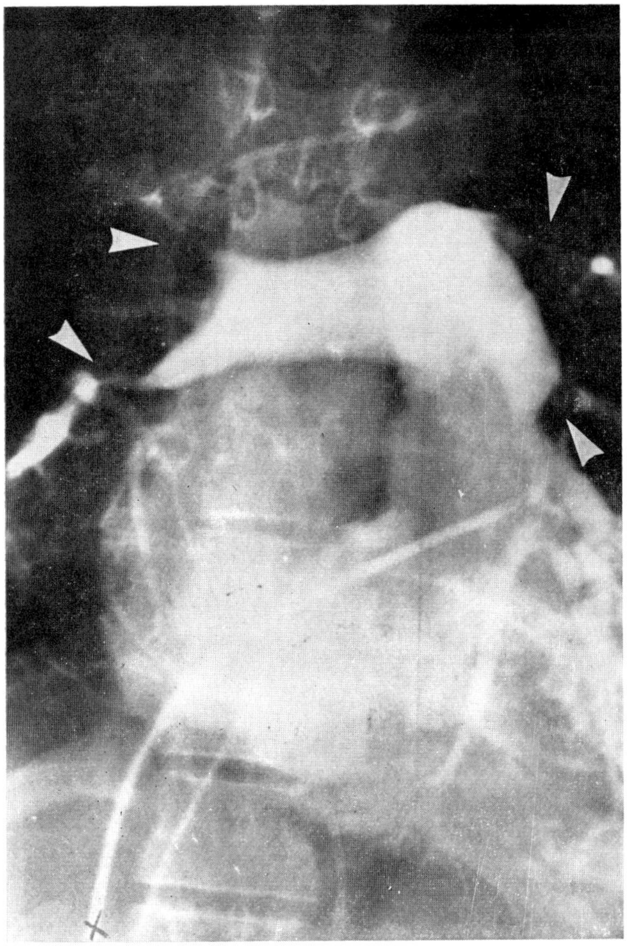

←

Figure 24.15. Pulmonary Arteriogram. A moderately sized filling defect is at the bifurcation of the right main pulmonary artery (Arrow) and within the branches of the left pulmonary artery (Arrow). *Diagnosis:* Multiple massive pulmonary emboli.

Figure 24.16. Pulmonary Arteriogram. (A) There are multiple filling defects in the pulmonary artery branches with a meniscus sign (Arrow). (B) Stasis is seen in right lower lobar branches. *Diagnosis:* Pulmonary emboli.

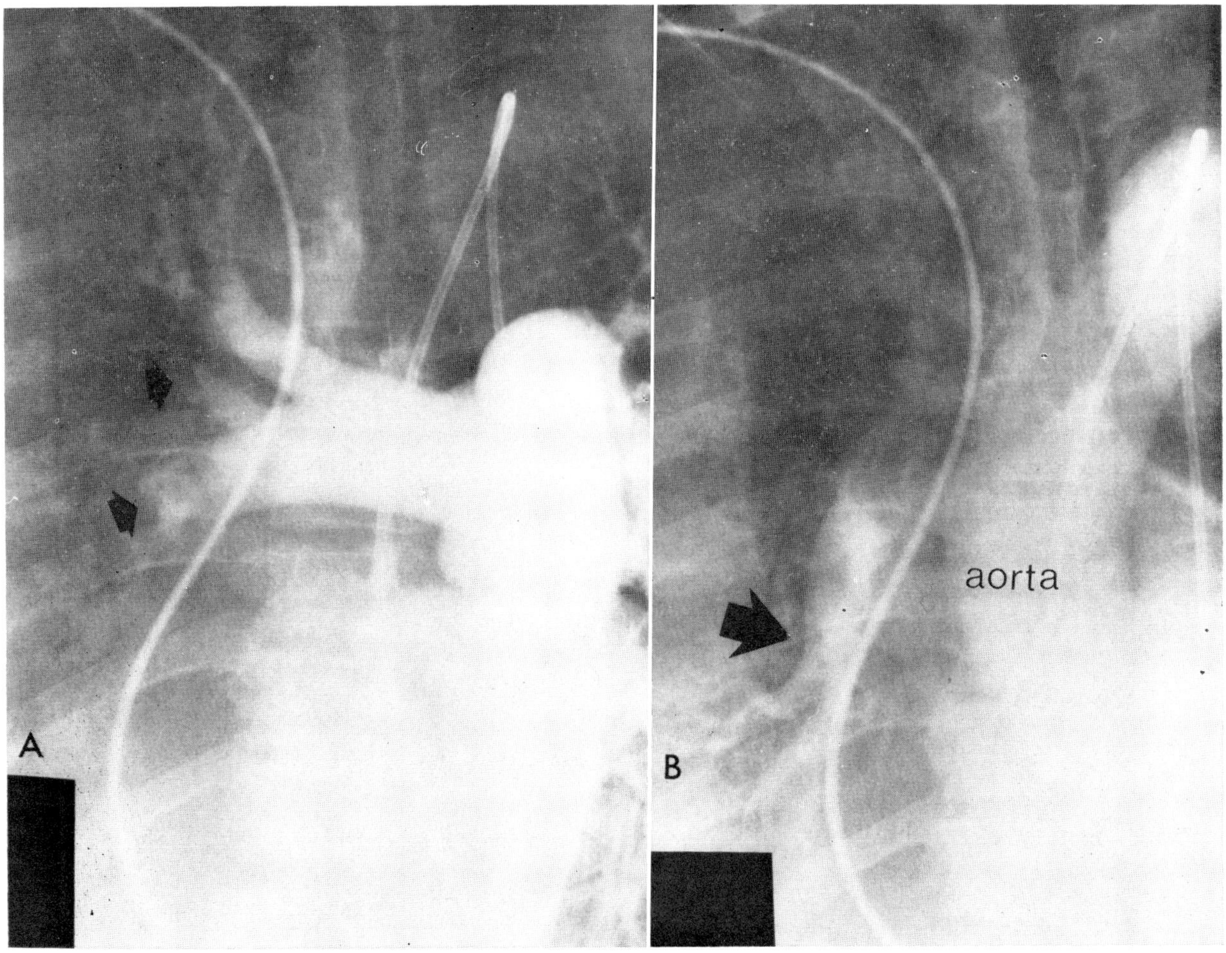

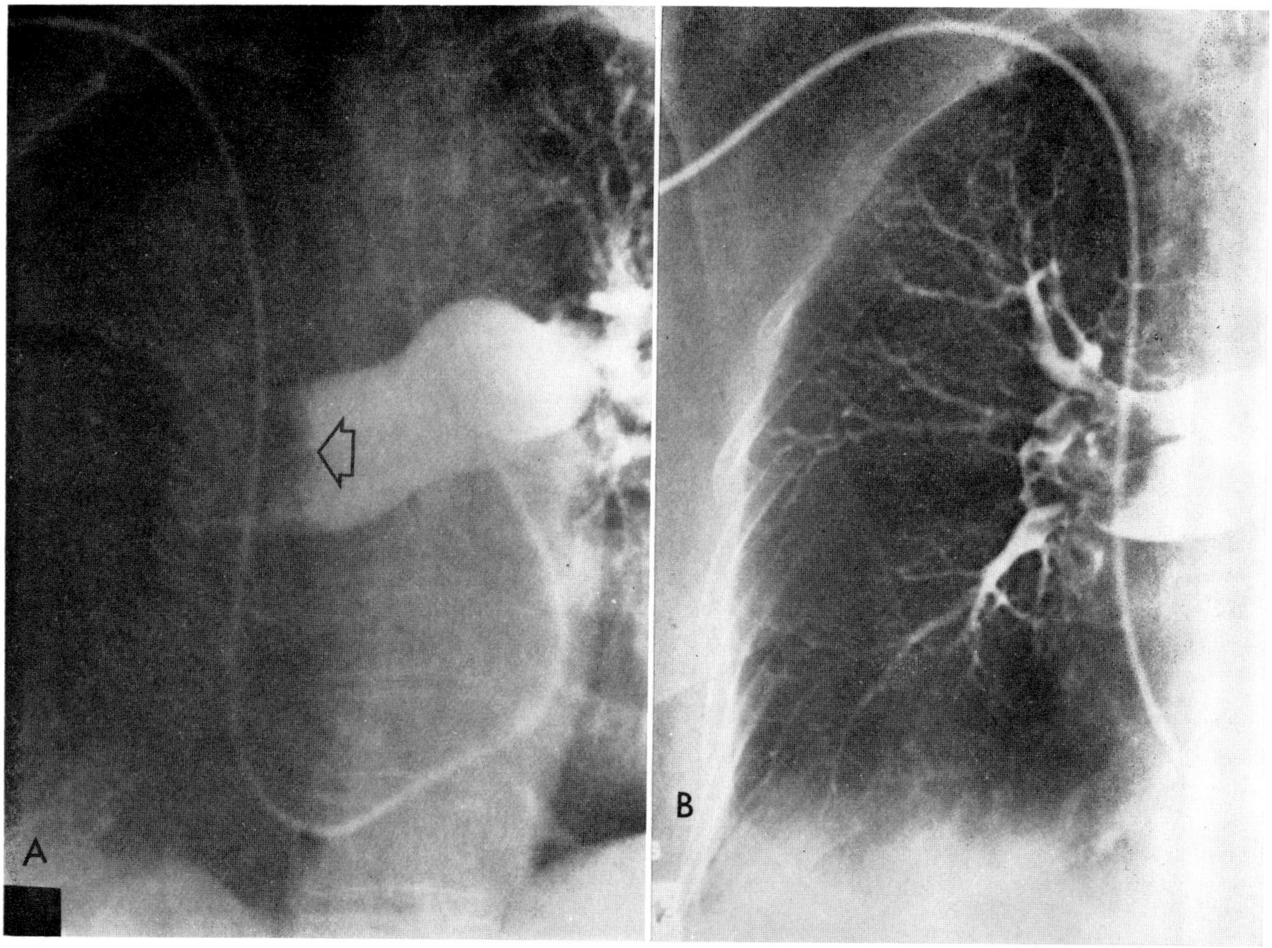

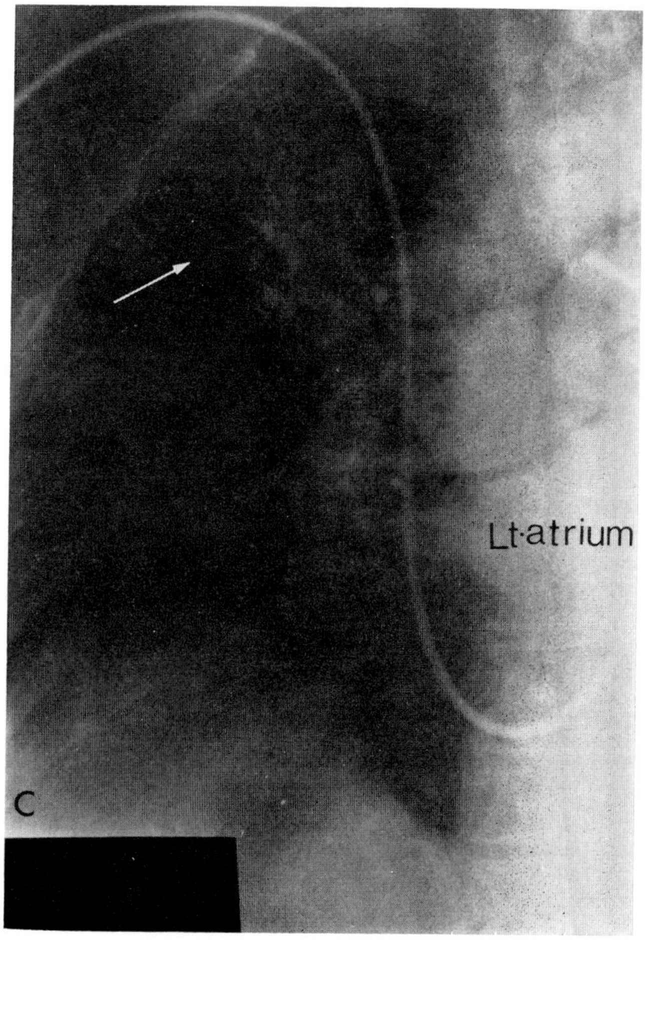

Figure 24.17. Pulmonary Arteriogram. (A) A moderately sized filling defect is in the right main pulmonary artery (Arrow) with lack of perfusion of the majority of the intrapulmonary branches on the same side. (B) A selective injection into the right pulmonary artery reveals the filling defect better. (C) The Levo phase reveals stasis of contrast in the pulmonary arteries on the right side (Arrow), no opacification of the pulmonary veins on the right side. *Diagnosis:* Pulmonary embolus to the right main pulmonary artery.

complete or incomplete infarction. The *critical segment* of the main stem is between the branching of the middle colic artery and the origin of the ileocolic artery. It is noteworthy that *distal to the origin of the middle colic artery, the remaining portion of the superior mesenteric artery actually behaves as an end artery.* Unfortunately, an embolus usually lodges past the origin of the middle colic artery as the main trunk gradually narrows from then on.

The resulting infarction depends on the underlying vascular disease, presence and severity of spasm of other branches, migration and fragmentation of the embolus, and superimposed thrombus with its proximal and distal propagation. *Colonic ischemic necrosis* is often due to occlusion of the small branches, while *small bowel ischemic necrosis* is usually due to the occlusion of the main trunk distal to the origin of the middle colic artery. The effect of acute occlusion of the main trunk of the superior mesenteric artery is often fatal. *Acute occlusion of small branches* may give the clinical appearance of regional enteritis or ulcerative colitis. People with *chronic occlusion* present with pain similar to abdominal angina. In patients with shock and decreased peripheral perfusions, there may be intestinal necrosis resulting from superior mesenteric artery thrombosis.

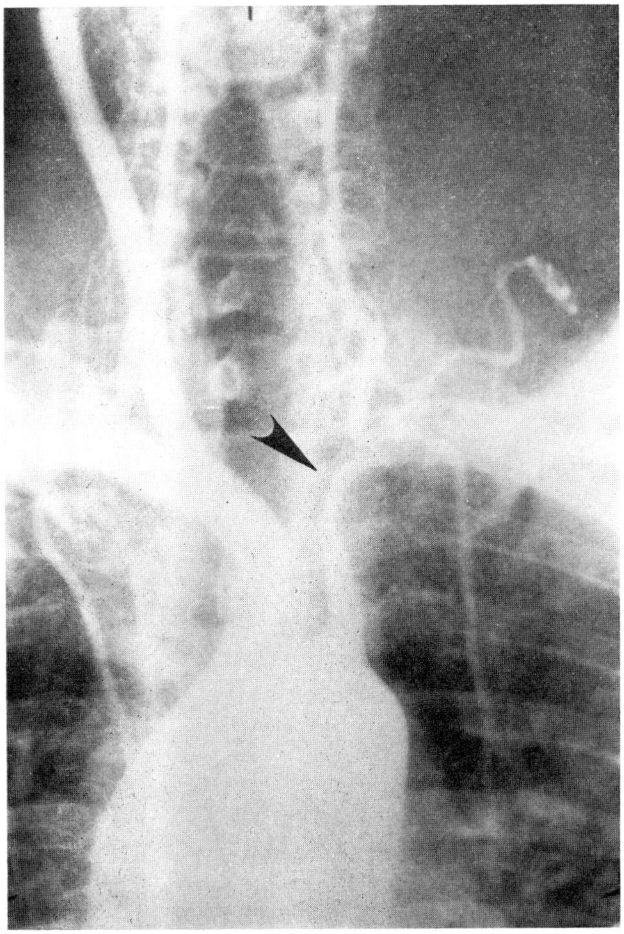

Figure 24.18. Thoracic Aortogram. There is smooth flame-shaped narrowing of the left subclavian artery and total occlusion of the left common carotid artery in a young woman. *Diagnosis:* Takayasu arteritis.

In infants the emboli may arise from the ductus arteriosus, umbilical artery catheterization, or intracardiac surgery.[941, 942] Other causes of superior mesenteric artery occlusion in infants are thrombosis, arteritis or bands.[948]

THROMBUS

Acute arterial thrombosis is the complicated pathologic counterpart of the chronic disease. The underlying lesion of both acute and chronic thrombotic occlusion seems to be the selective *atheromatous* involvement of specific arteries. Unlike embolic occlusion, *thrombotic occlusion occurs in main trunks which have underlying disease.* Thrombotic occlusion is like embolic occlusion in that it is usually segmental with a pulsatile artery proximal and a nonpulsatile artery distal to the occlusion. If there are inadequate collateral vessels, propagation of the thrombus is not unusual.[924]

Acute thrombosis readily occurs in an already diseased vessel provided there are predisposing causes.[966] These *causes* include *increased viscosity of the blood* seen in dehydration due to diarrhea, vomiting, frequent enemas, or diuretics; *increased number of platelets* found in acute hemorrhage, splenectomy, polycythemia or hyperlipemia; or a *decreased perfusion pressure* found in congestive heart failure, cardiac fibrillation, or shock. A thrombus may propagate and enlarge causing obstruction, give rise to an embolus, or it may be removed by fibrinolytic

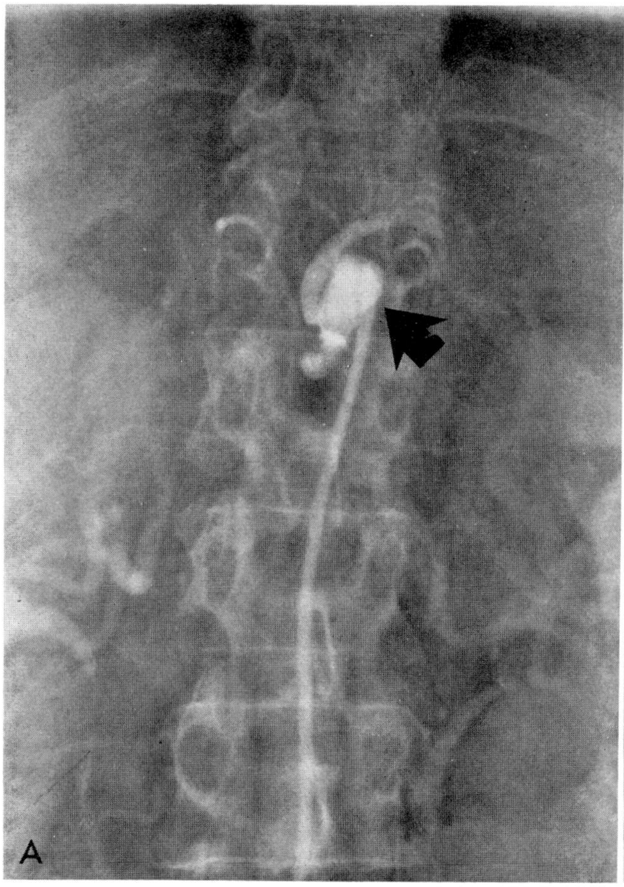

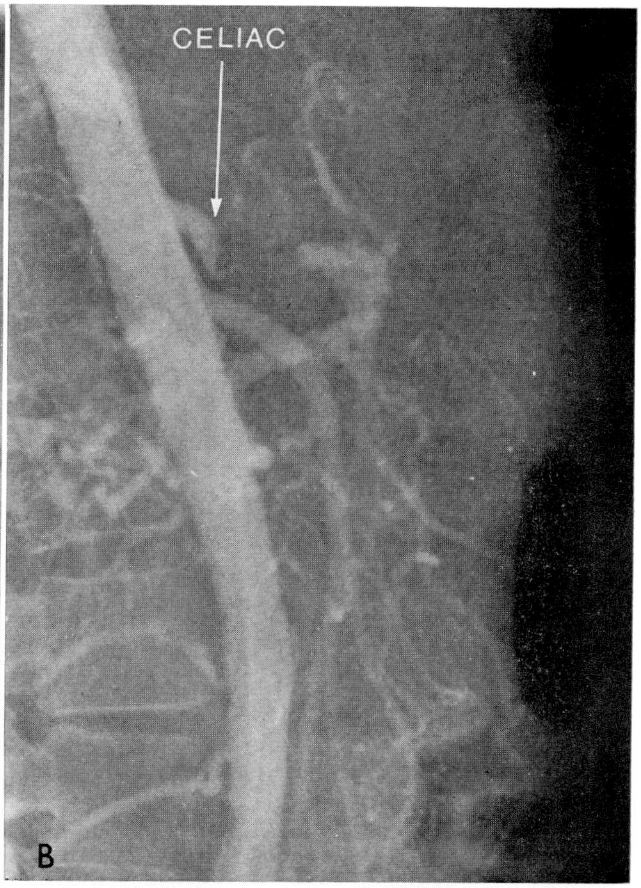

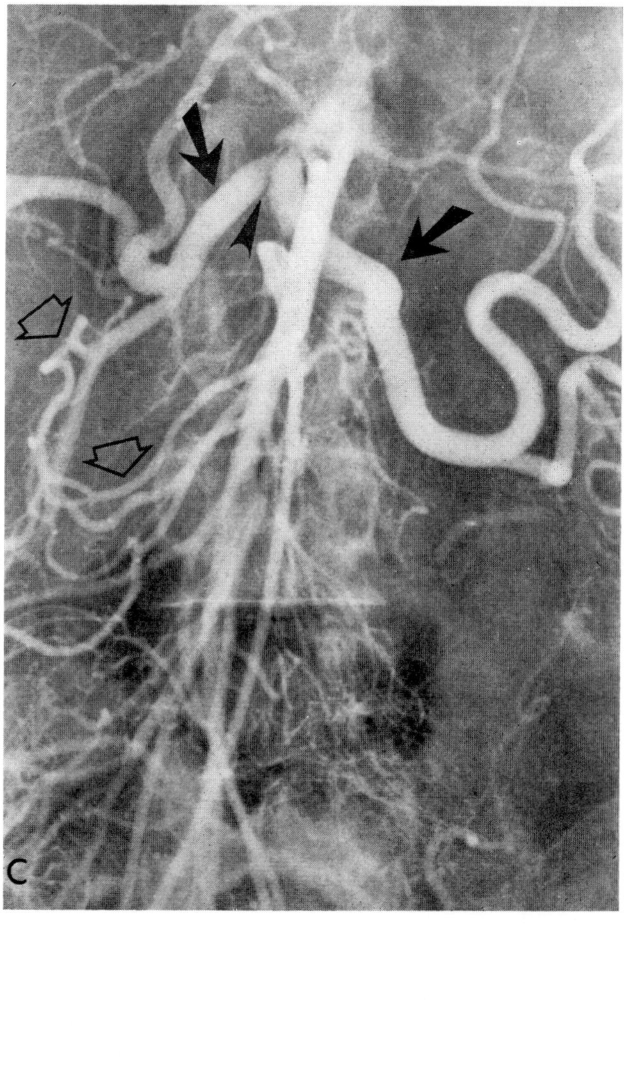

Figure 24.19. (A) The celiac angiogram reveals abrupt termination of the celiac trunk distal to the left gastric artery origin (Arrow). (B) A cross-table lateral aortogram reveals the same findings. (C) A superior mesenteric arteriogram fills the distal part of the celiac (Arrow) branches via the pancreatic arcade (Blank Arrow). A translucent line is seen at the bifurcation of the celiac axis (Arrow Head). *Diagnosis:* Iatrogenic dissection of the celiac axis due to excessive manipulation of the guide wire. There is immediate demonstration of collateral flow.

action, or become organized and recanalized.[111, 967–969] Multiple lesions associated with thrombosis are not uncommon in elderly individuals. Thus, *simultaneous lesions* may be seen at the aortic bifurcation and the femoropopliteal areas. A proximal lesion may be overlooked if the clinical picture is dominated by the distal one.[970] It is very interesting to note that when compared with the lower extremity vasculature,[971] there is decreased incidence of thrombosis of upper extremity arteries due to increased fibrinolytic activity in their walls.

Arterial thrombi form when platelets come into contact with injured surfaces or foreign material such as the catheter. This sets up a chain of events, the end product of which is a dangerous thrombus. Unlike venous thrombi, the role of fibrin is late and less prominent in arterial thrombi. This may explain why substances such as aspirin, which inhibit platelet adhesiveness, are more effective as anticoagulants.[206]

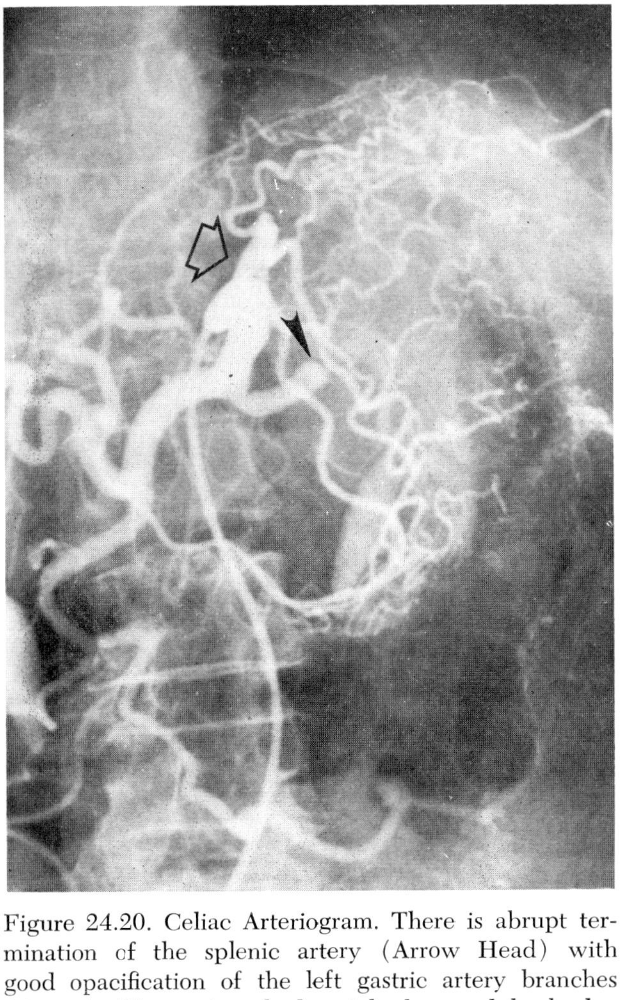

Figure 24.20. Celiac Arteriogram. There is abrupt termination of the splenic artery (Arrow Head) with good opacification of the left gastric artery branches (Arrow). The patient had weight loss and backache. *Diagnosis:* Occlusion of the splenic artery due to infiltration by a scirrhous carcinoma of the pancreas.

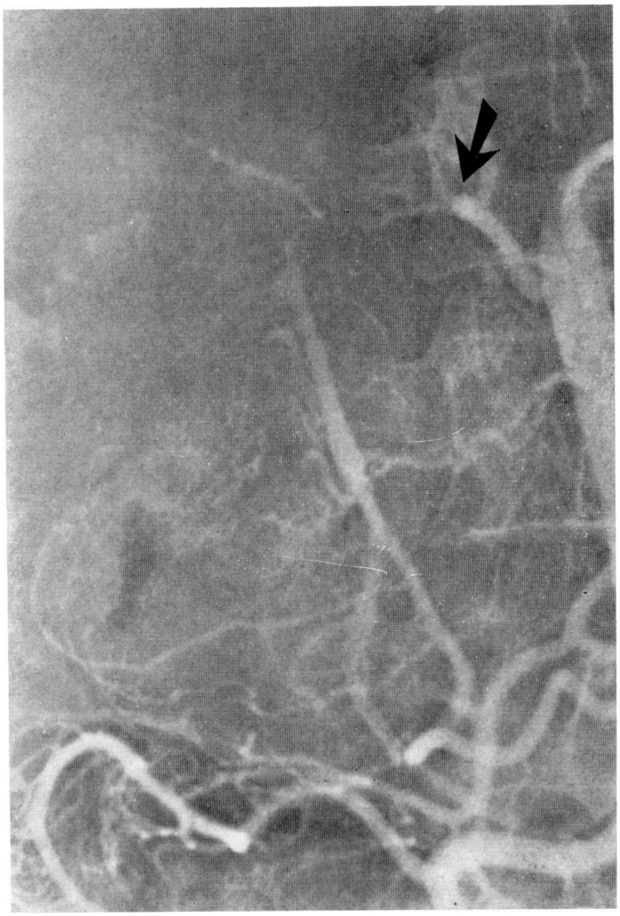

Figure 24.21. Superior Mesenteric Arteriogram. The inferior pancreaticoduodenal artery (Arrow) is occluded. The patient had painless jaundice. *Diagnosis:* Pancreatic carcinoma with encasement and infiltration. *Surgical Diagnosis:* Inoperable pancreatic carcinoma.

Traumatic Vascular Occlusion

An artery may be damaged by contusion, compression, laceration, or complete severance.[532, 661, 904] These may happen after blunt, penetrating or osseous trauma. Occlusion of a vessel after *blunt trauma* may be due to avulsion, thrombosis, or intimal fracture. Sudden stretching and partial fixation of an artery can

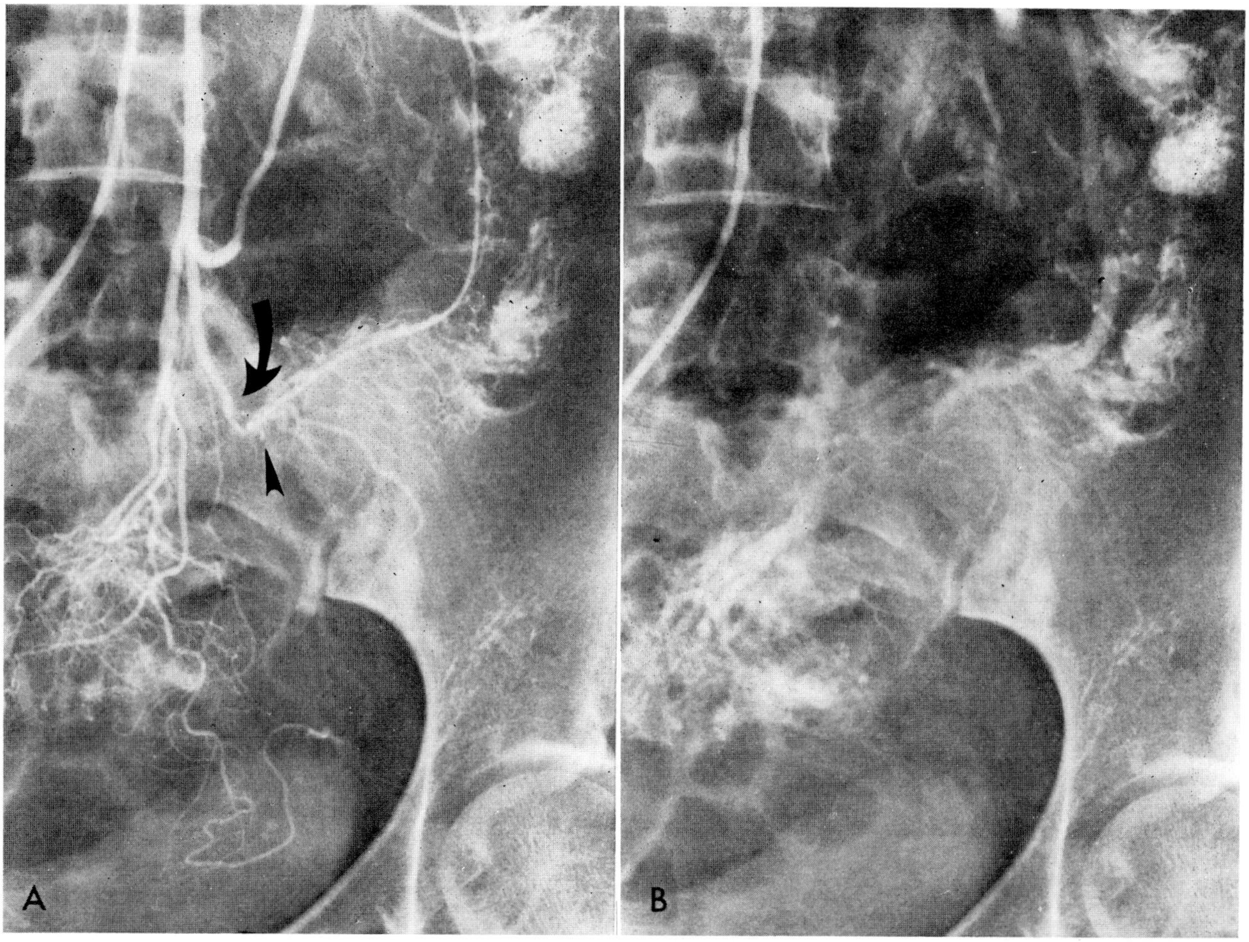

Figure 24.22. Inferior Mesenteric Arteriogram. (A) Early arterial phase: There is lack of arterial perfusion to the midsigmoid colon, sudden amputation of one of the sigmoidal branches (Arrow Head) and sudden change in caliber of the main sigmoidal branch (Arrow). Notice the good opacification of the middle rectal artery coursing towards the internal iliac artery. (B) Venous phase: No venous opacification is seen in the same area. The patient had carcinoma of the sigmoid colon. *Comment:* Occlusion of the sigmoidal arteries and veins due to infiltration by an adenocarcinoma.

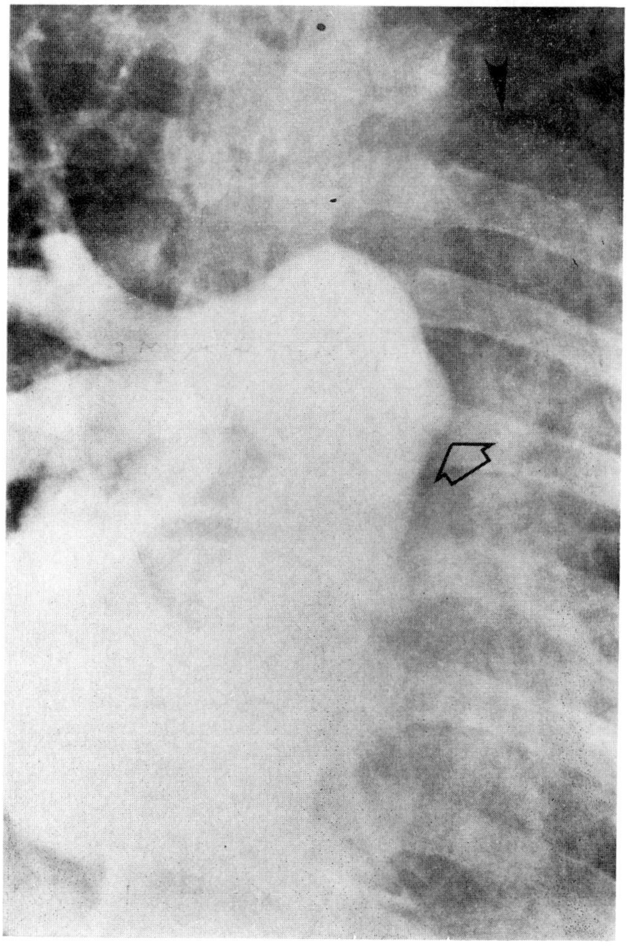

Figure 24.23. Pulmonary Arteriogram. There is a mass (Arrow Head) adjacent to the left pulmonary artery (Arrow) which does not visualize. *Diagnosis:* Infiltrative occlusion of the left pulmonary artery by a malignant mass. *Pathologic Diagnosis:* Bronchogenic carcinoma with total occlusion of the pulmonary artery.

occur with an extreme combination of movements such as extension, rotation and bending, particularly if the artery, like the internal carotid, is close to the bone.[533] This also occurs if there is excessive mobility of an organ with a relatively fixed artery, as seen with the renal artery.[911, 912]

There may be a *latent clinical period after trauma* before the manifestation of symptoms. This is the time necessary for the formation of a thrombus (internal carotid artery[905]). Most often the thrombosis is due to intimal or medial damage and is seen in the aorta,[664] splen-

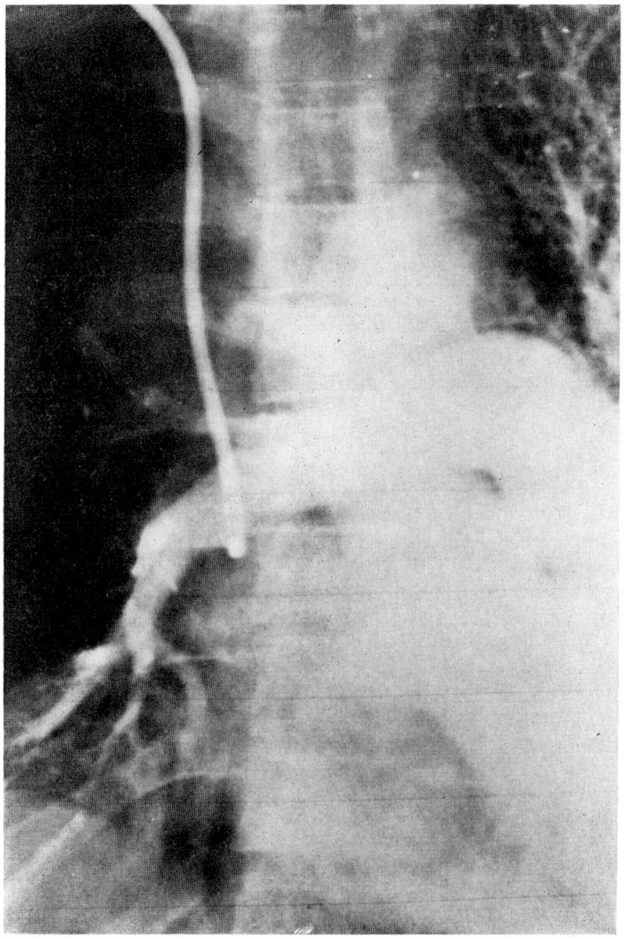

Figure 24.24. Basilic Vein Catheterization. The catheter tip is in the superior vena cava. Pulmonary arterial phase: Shows no visualization of the right middle and upper lobe pulmonary arteries. A paratracheal mass was seen on the chest film. *Diagnosis:* Occlusion of the pulmonary arterial branches on the right side due to infiltration by a bronchogenic malignancy.

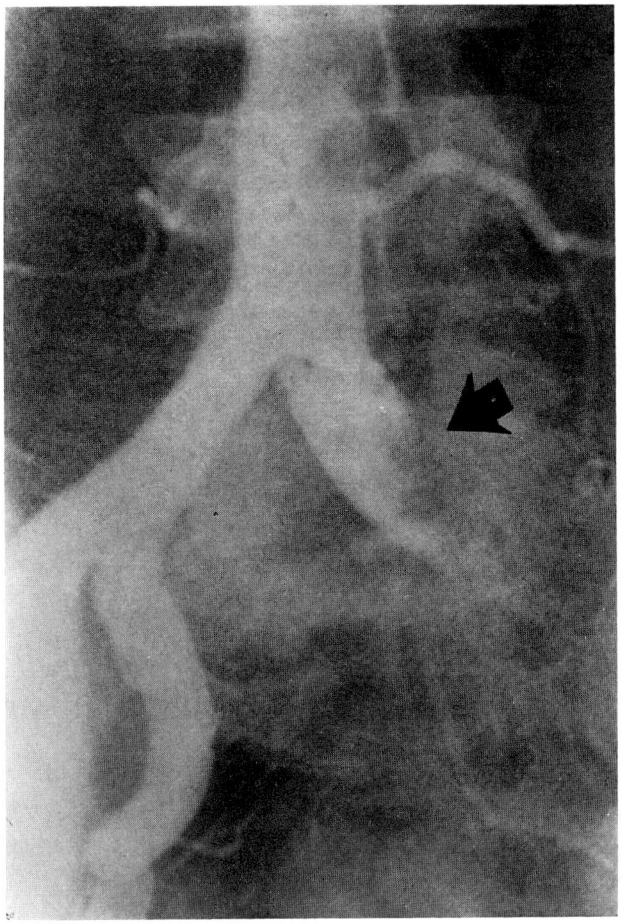

Figure 24.25. Pelvic Arteriogram. Reveals occlusion of the left common iliac artery. This patient had blunt lower abdominal trauma three hours prior to this study. *Diagnosis:* Intimal fracture with total occlusion. Surgery confirmed the radiographic diagnosis.

ic[913] and iliac arteries,[915] inferior vena cava and hepatic veins.[914] *Intimal tears* may act as a valve, curling up to form a plug, predisposing to thrombus formation.[533, 916, 917] The detached intima may also cause intermittent occlusion as seen in the carotid artery.[918] Repeated intimal trauma may also cause thrombosis of the artery. Palmar and digital artery occlusion have been described due to occupational tasks;[660] axillary artery thrombosis has been seen in people who use crutches (Figs. 24-25, 24-27).

Lacerations and avulsions are usually associated with large hematomas. When the artery is completely lacerated, the ends retract into the adjacent muscle, and as a result bleeding usual-

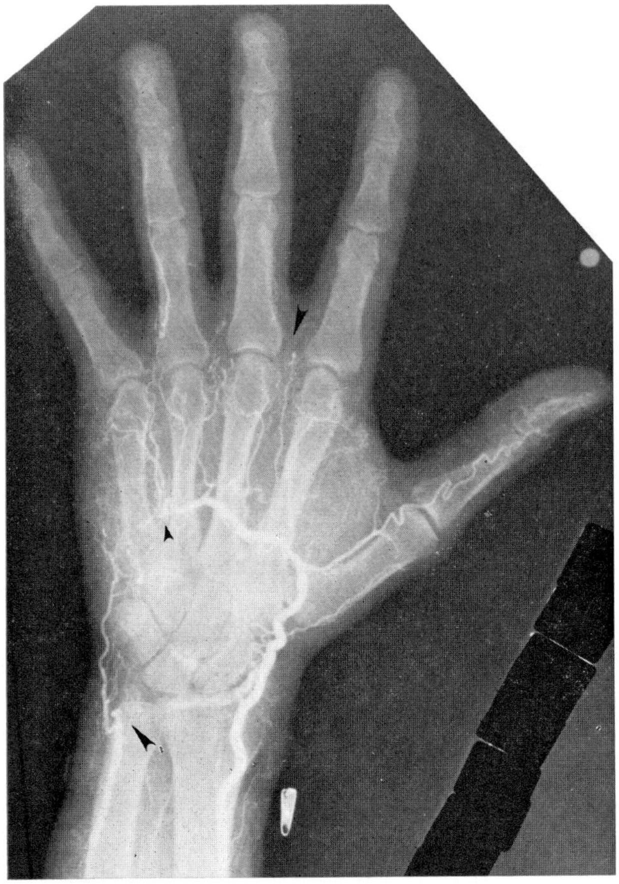

Figure 24.26. Brachial arteriogram reveals occlusion of ulnar artery, and also occlusions of the digital vessels in a young man. *Diagnosis:* Thromboangiitis obliterans.

ly stops and therefore only small hematomas tend to develop. However, partial laceration prevents retraction of the arterial ends into the adjacent tissues resulting in profuse bleeding. Unrepaired lacerations may lead into communicating periarterial hematomas. Thus pseudoaneurysms occur. Occasionally these may be associated with infection and/or subsequent rupture (Fig. 24-28).

Certain types of *osseous trauma* are more frequently associated with vascular injury than others.[421, 906, 910] Apart from arteriovenous fistula, periarterial hematomas or lacerations or total disruptions are not uncommon. Pelvic fractures extending into the sacroiliac joints may damage the common iliac vessel and those extending to the greater sciatic notch may damage the hypogastric vessel.[907] Pubic fractures can affect the obturator artery,[908] and the internal carotid artery may be involved in basal skull fractures.[909] And so on and so forth! Dislocations may have the same effect on adjacent blood vessels too (Fig. 24-30).

Trauma due to a *high velocity missile*[900-903] occurs when it passes through the soft tissues, even if the artery is not directly hit. The missile causes a momentary central cavity within which the artery is stretched, vibrated and thrashed around. This may split the intima,

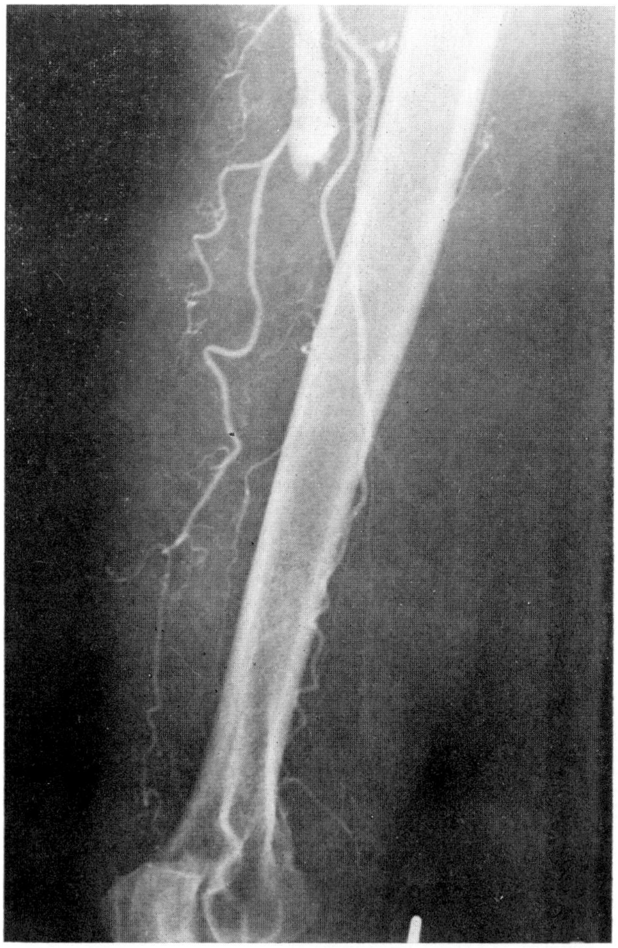

Figure 24.27. Axillary Arteriogram. There is minimal dilatation of the proximal brachial artery and no visualization distally. This patient had been using crutches for eight years. *Diagnosis:* Traumatic (due to crutches) thrombosis of the brachial artery. *Surgical Diagnosis:* Segmental aneurysmal dilatation of the brachial artery with an occluding mural thrombus.

leading to secondary thrombosis, hemorrhage or aneurysms. The generated heat may cause delayed development of hematomas, aneurysms, or arteriovenous fistulae.

Last, but not least, *catheter trauma* may cause a flap valve tear of the intima or arterial spasm; both of which may lead to secondary thrombosis.[919]

OCCLUSIONS OF SPECIFIC ARTERIES

Aortic Arch Vessels and Their Occlusions

The majority of occlusions are due to *atherosclerosis,* but occasionally are due to embolus or trauma.[1031, 1032] The lesions are usually multiple with the length of occlusion being variable. They occur proximally at the origin of the vessels from the arch or distally at their bifurcation, such as seen in the internal carotid artery. Proximal lesions are well localized with patent distant vessels. Distal lesions are rarely localized, and unusual extensions into the distal branches are noted.

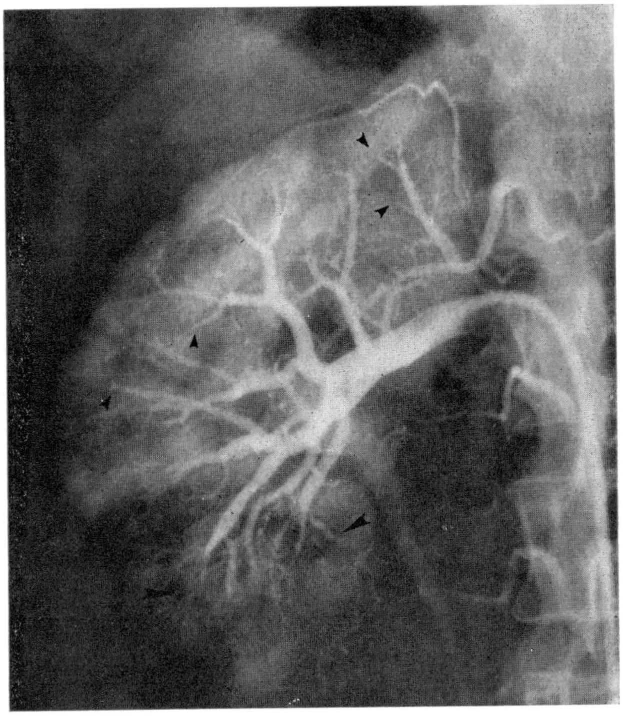

Figure 24.29. Renal arteriogram reveals areas of narrowing and occlusions in a young woman. *Diagnosis:* Necrotizing angiitis. *Pathology:* Acute phase of polyarteritis nodosa.

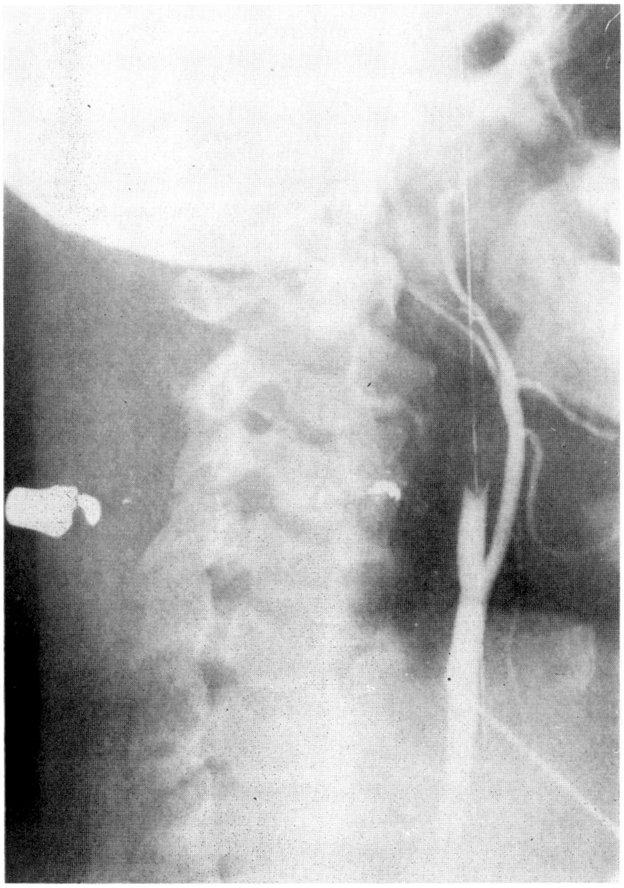

Figure 24.28. Carotid Arteriogram. There is occlusion of the internal carotid artery. *Diagnosis:* Severed artery from a gunshot wound.

Aortic Occlusions

Aortic thrombosis usually stops below the level of the renal arteries, but can be associated with thrombosis of the common iliac arteries as well.[664, 1034] If the thrombosis extends above the level of the renal arteries, there may be associated hypertensive changes.[1035] Apart from atherosclerosis, aortic thrombosis may be caused by mitral stenosis with small repeated emboli,[1036] trauma, or rarely, proximal extension of thromboangiitis obliterans.[827] Acute atherosclerotic aortic thrombosis is an unusual entity which may mimic clinically a saddle embolus[1506] (Fig. 22-17).

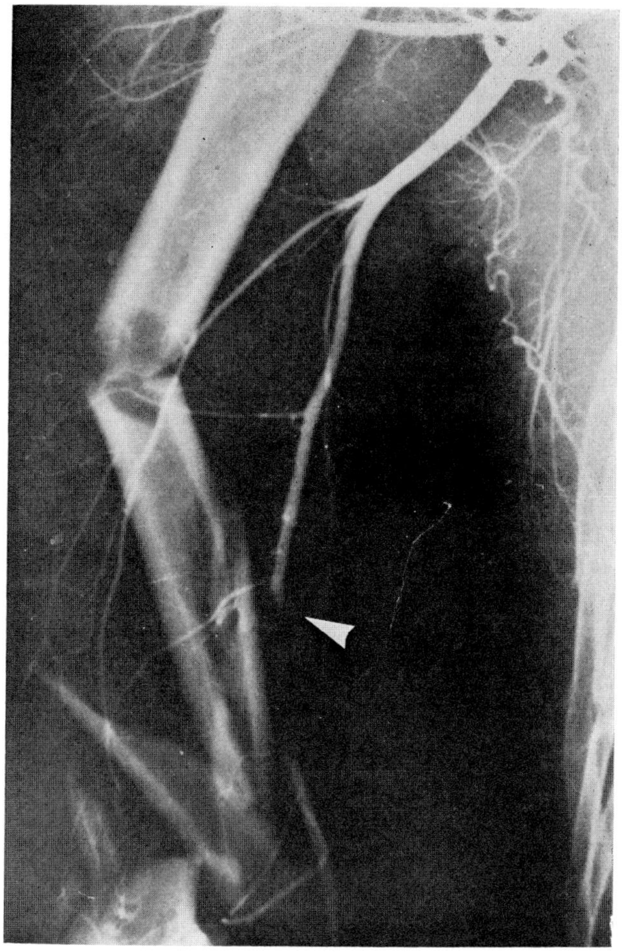

Figure 24.30. Subclavian Arteriogram. There is occlusion of the distal brachial artery with collateral circulation. The humeral shaft is fractured. *Diagnosis:* Osseous trauma causing arterial occlusion.

Occlusions of the Inferior Mesenteric Artery

Spontaneous *acute* inferior mesenteric artery *occlusion is rare* because of the availability of rich collateral blood supplies. Approximately 62 percent of elderly individuals have stenosis or occlusion at the origin of the inferior mesenteric artery. If the superior mesenteric artery is also compromised, and if there are atherosclerotic plaques in the left internal iliac artery orifice, then the inferior mesenteric artery and its dependent vessels are always at the verge of ischemia. This is especially true during operative trauma and catheterization procedures[946, 949, 950] (Fig. 24-14).

Occlusions of the Renal Artery

If circulation to an occluded renal artery is not established within sixty to ninety minutes following occlusion, then necrosis will develop.[951, 952] Experimentally[952] selective renal artery occlusions up to sixty minutes' duration result in only minimal gross and microscopic changes. Bilateral occlusion of the renal artery lasting up to sixty minutes is very critical. If the renal artery is selectively occluded only for thirty minutes, then delayed, sustained hypertension was found. In patients with atheromatous aortas, acute or chronic renal failure is not unusual after abdominal aortic surgery or excessive manipulation of a catheter during angiography. Spontaneous atheromatous emboli causing patchy, ischemic degeneration and spotty atrophy are not uncommon.[953, 954] Catheter emboli to the renal vasculature usually are tokens of poor angiographic techniques with improper irrigation of the catheter.

Hepatic Artery Occlusion

Accidental ligation or occlusion of the hepatic artery[302, 958] may have extreme end results ranging from complete recovery to fatal necrosis.[957] It may be safe to occlude the artery in malignancies[955] of the liver provided the portal vein is patent. Simultaneous occlusion of the hepatic artery and portal vein is definitely fatal. The arterial occlusion is an uncommon complication of catheterization procedures.[956]

Splenic Artery Occlusions

Experimentally the spleen can survive the severe ischemia caused by complete occlusion of its arterial supply.[959] Another interesting finding is the fact that gastric ulcers can infiltrate and occlude the splenic artery.[111, 913]

Cystic Artery Occlusion

Whether occlusion of the cystic artery is due to catheter emboli or thrombosis causing infarction, the *end result is acute cholecystitis.*[960, 961]

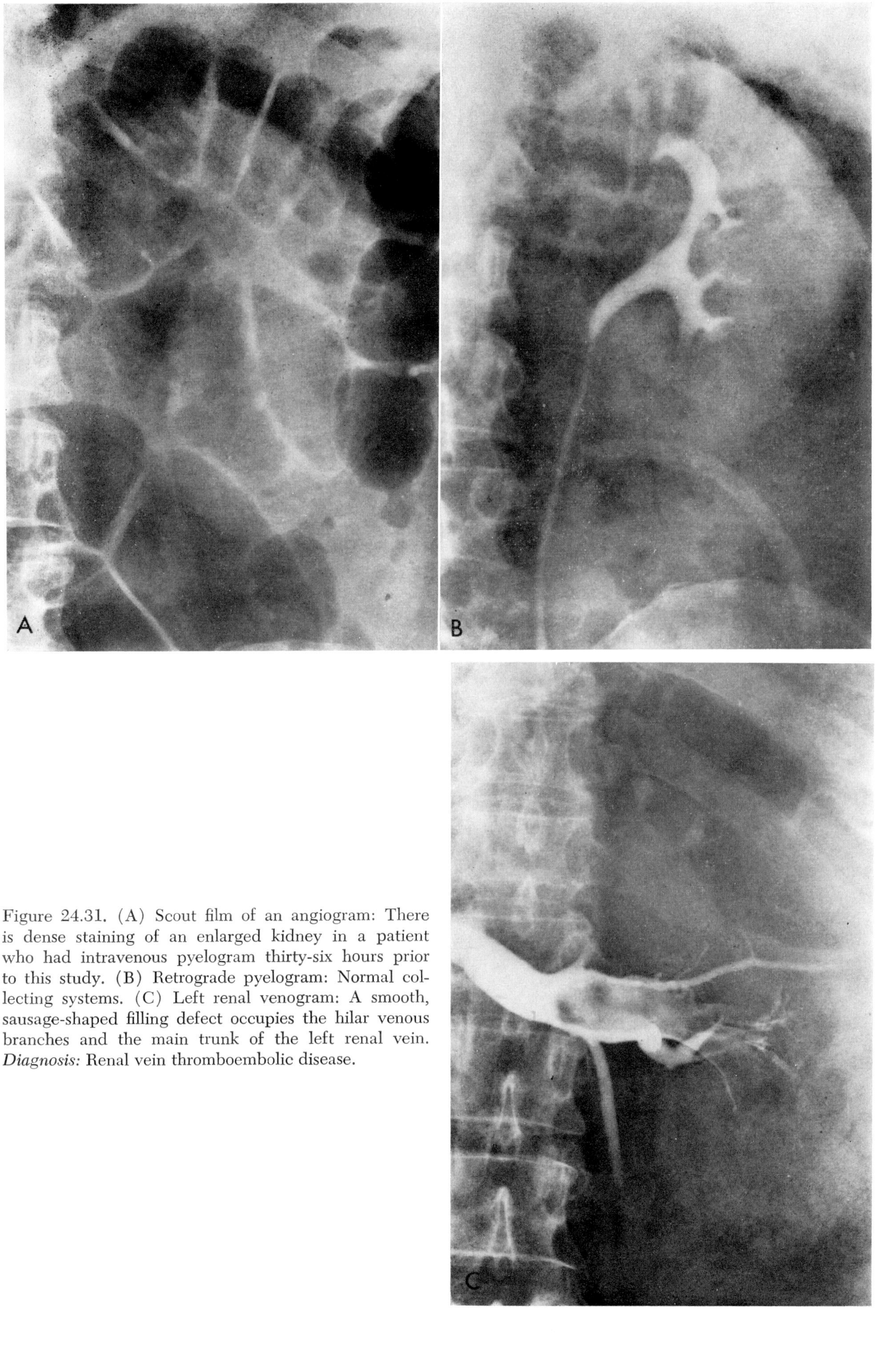

Figure 24.31. (A) Scout film of an angiogram: There is dense staining of an enlarged kidney in a patient who had intravenous pyelogram thirty-six hours prior to this study. (B) Retrograde pyelogram: Normal collecting systems. (C) Left renal venogram: A smooth, sausage-shaped filling defect occupies the hilar venous branches and the main trunk of the left renal vein. *Diagnosis:* Renal vein thromboembolic disease.

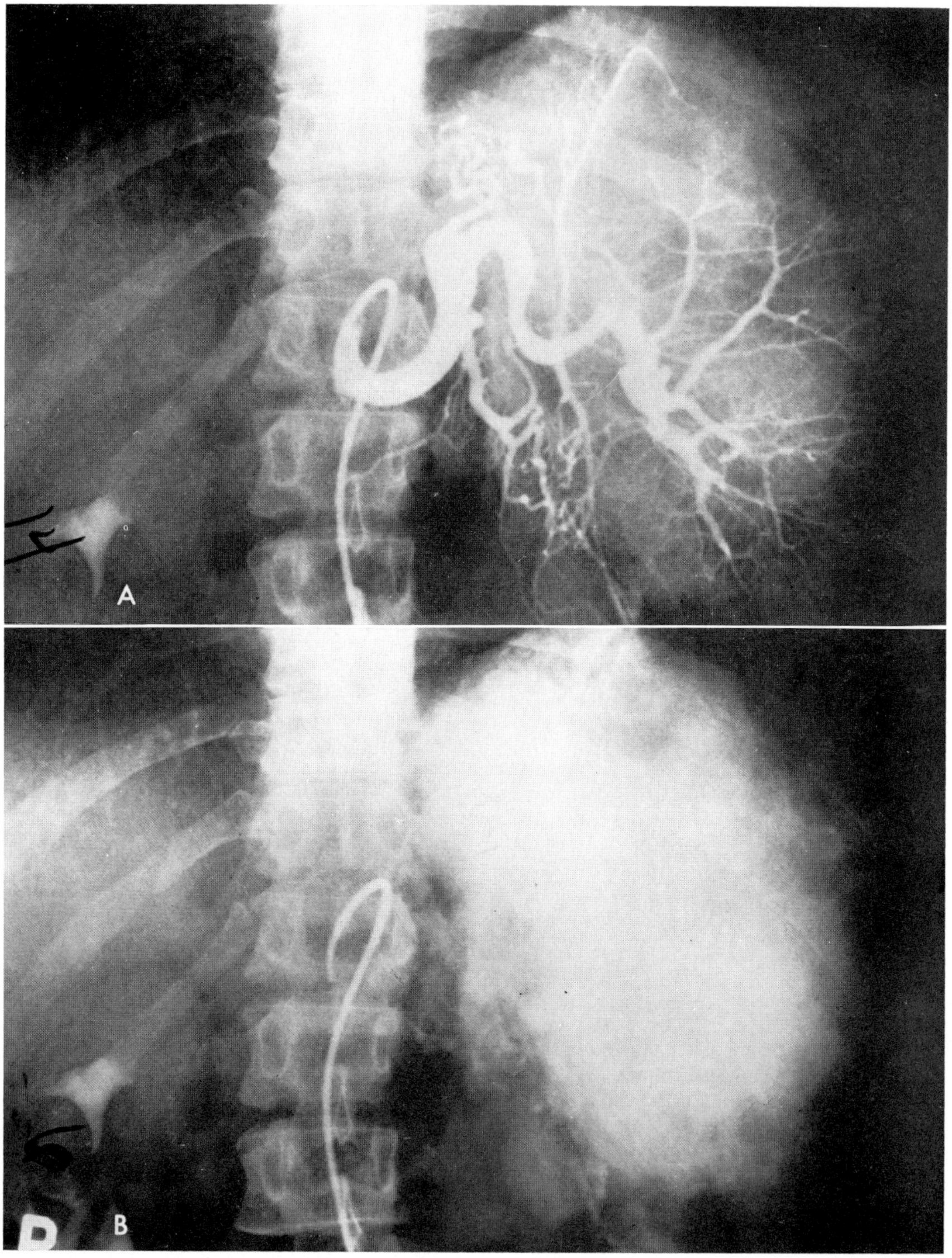

Figure 24.32. Splenic Arteriogram. (A) Arterial phase reveals an enlarged spleen. (B) Venous phase at 14 seconds shows an enlarged spleen with stasis of contrast and nonvisualization of the splenic vein. *Diagnosis:* Splenic vein thrombosis. *Pathology:* Etiology undetermined.

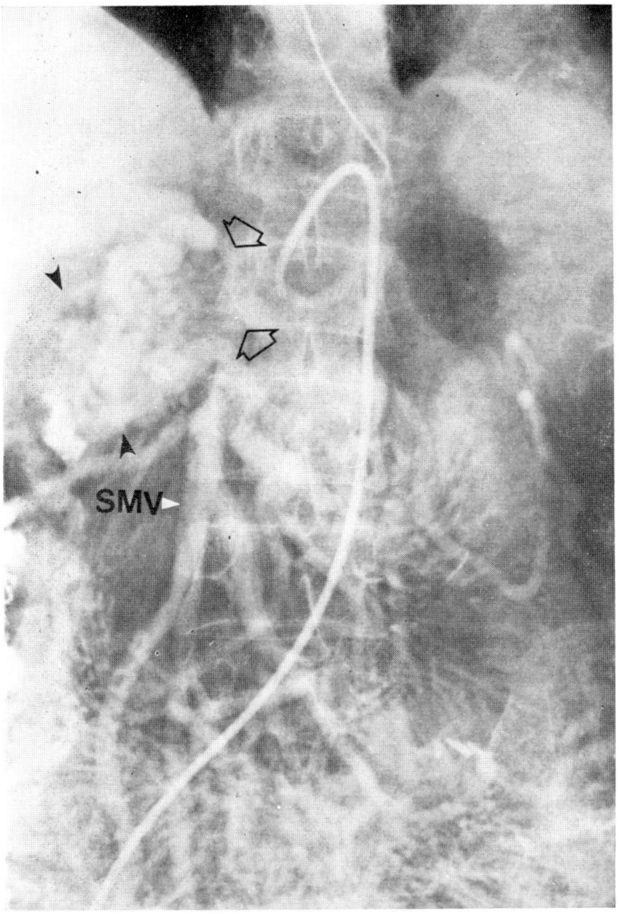

←

Figure 24.33. Superior Mesenteric Arteriogram—venous phase. Superior mesenteric vein (S.M.V.). There is no filling of the portal vein near the porta hepatis (Arrow), numerous as well as tortuous dilated veins near the porta hepatis (Arrow Head). This patient had painless jaundice. *Diagnosis:* Pancreatic carcinoma with encasement and occlusion of the portal vein with collateral circulation along the porta hepatis.

Figure 24.34. Celiac Arteriogram—venous phase. There are numerous veins coursing along the curvatures of the stomach (Arrows) and also another vein paralleling the vertebral column (I.M.V.). There is nonfilling of the proximal portal vein. This patient was suspected to have cancer of the pancreas. *Diagnosis:* Infiltrative occlusion of the proximal portal vein due to pancreatic carcinoma with secondary collateral circulation via gastric epiploic veins and the inferior mesenteric vein.

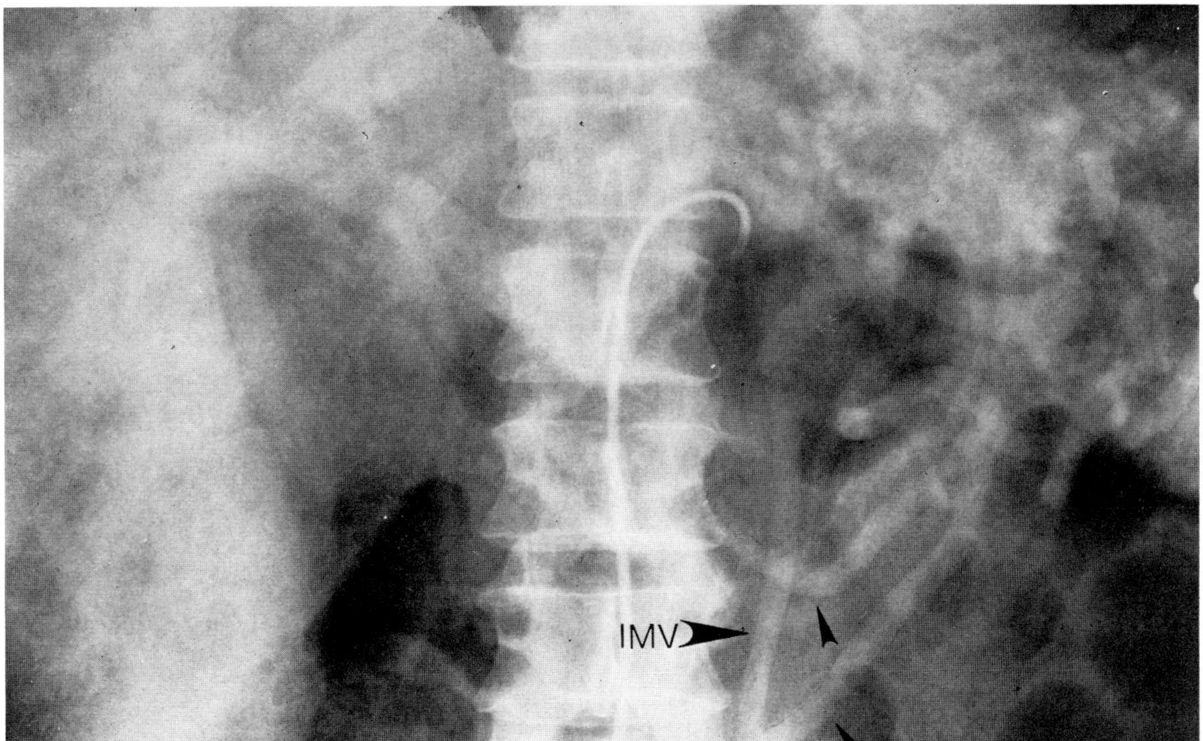

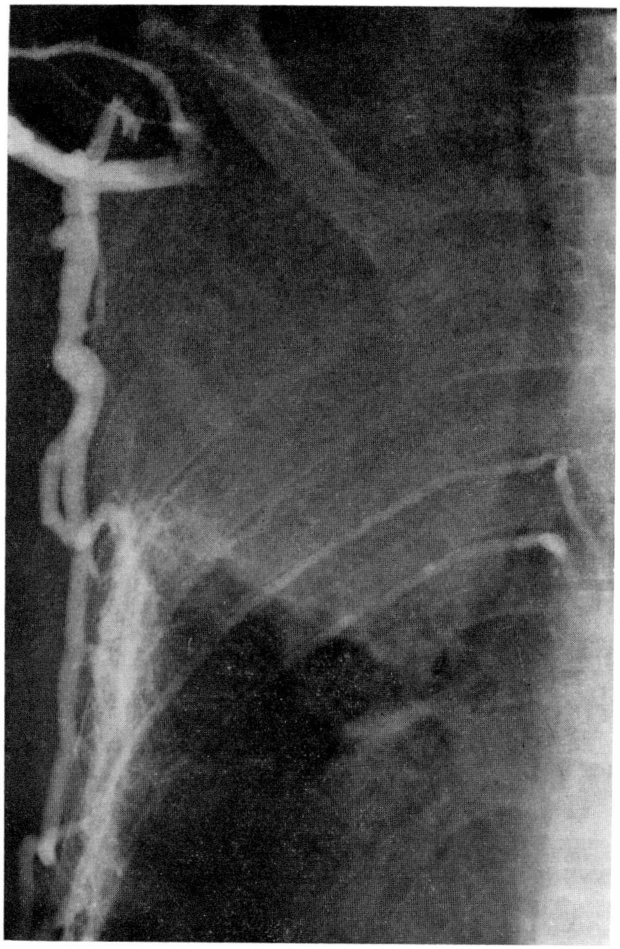

Figure 24.35. Superior Vena Cavagram. There is complete occlusion of the subclavian and innominate veins with collateral circulation via the lateral thoracic and intercostal veins to the azygous vein. *Comment:* Obvious malignant destruction of the rib cage due to a bronchogenic carcinoma and secondary occlusion of all the veins.

Lower Extremity Occlusions

In order of frequency[641] they involve the femoral, popliteal, aorta, and external iliac arteries. They may be *long*[478] *occlusions,* extending 20 cm or more, *or short,* 1 to 10 cm. *Long occlusions* may involve the entire superficial femoral artery, superficial femoral and popliteal arteries, or total popliteal artery occlusion. Collateral circulation is better developed in long superficial femoral artery occlusion and occurs via the deep femoral artery. In contrast femoropopliteal occlusions have poor collateral circulation as does total occlusion of the popliteal artery. *Short occlusions* involve the superficial femoral artery at the adductor (Hunter's) canal, or the popliteal artery above the knee. Popliteal artery occlusion is common in its proximal and mid one-third. The distal portion is usually free of disease for a long time. External iliac lesions are either at, or beyond, the origin of the internal iliac arteries.[1030] Occlusion of peripheral extremity arteries is a frequent manifestation of atherosclerosis, even in young working people.[1033]

VENOUS OCCLUSION

The collapsible, nonpulsatile veins with sluggish circulation are more *highly vulnerable to*

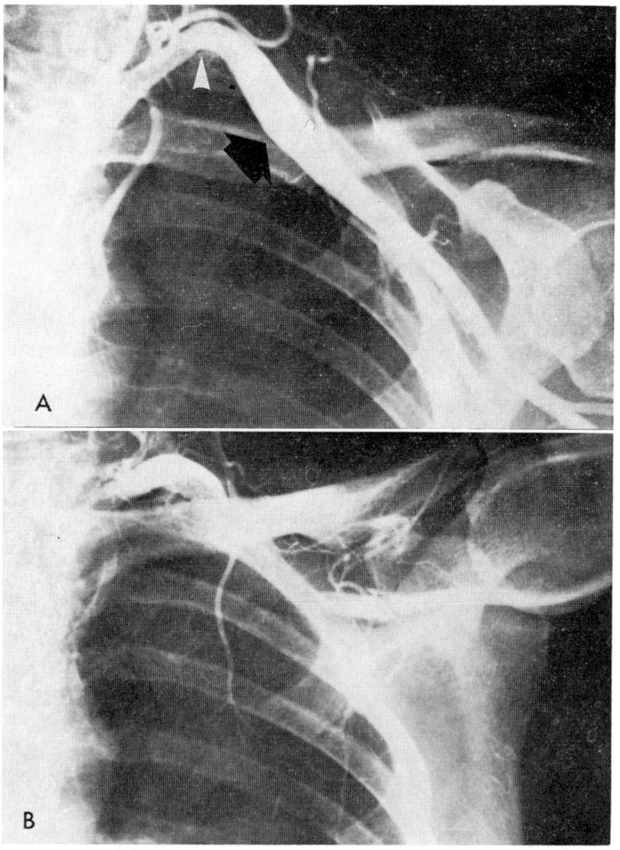

Figure 24.36. Subclavian Arteriogram. (A) When the arm is in neutral position there is normal flow through the artery. The artery is elevated over the cervical rib (Arrow Head) and there is poststenotic dilation distally (Arrow). (B) With the arm in a stress position there is occlusion of the subclavian artery and filling of the axillary artery via collaterals. *Diagnosis:* Thoracic outlet syndrome.

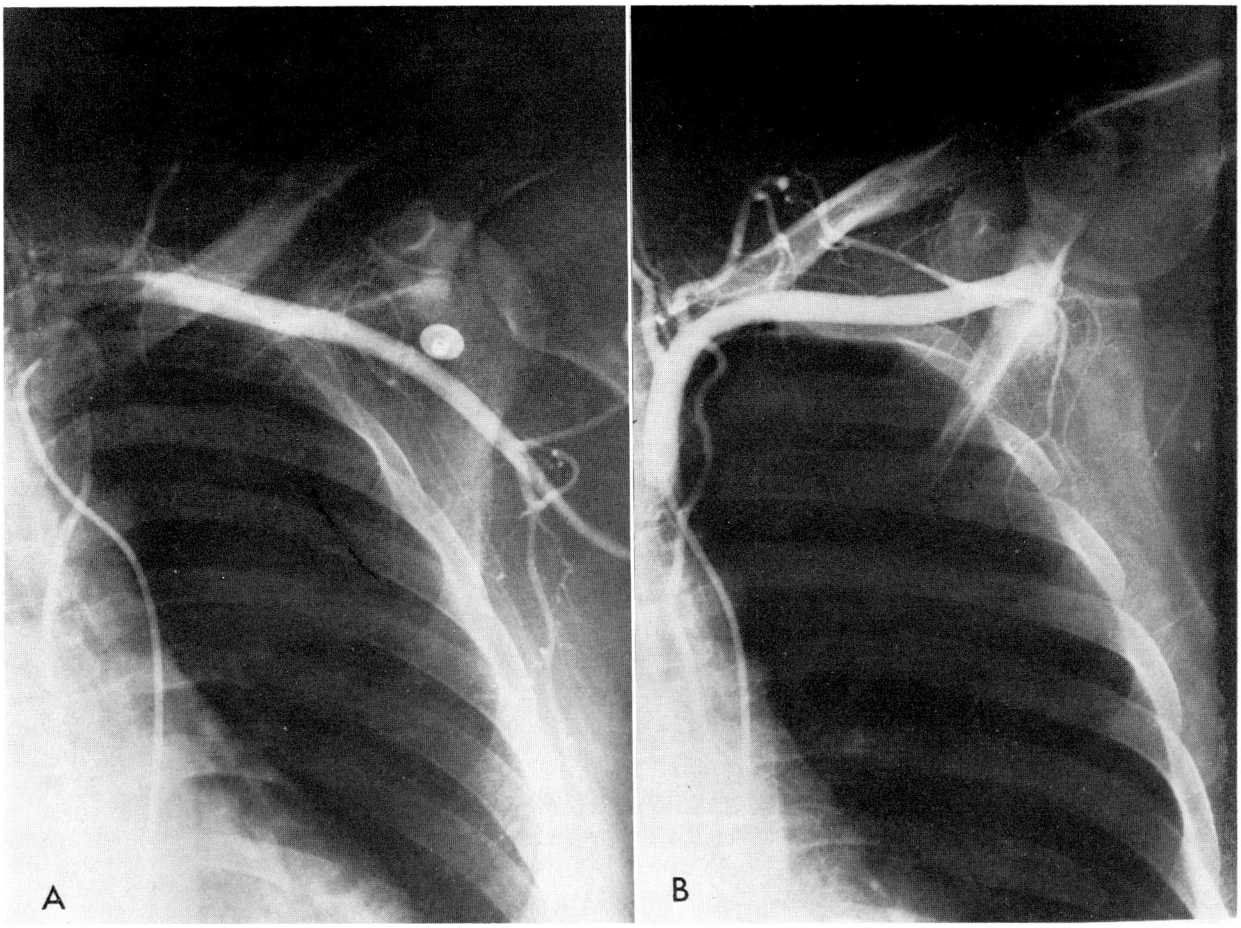

Figure 24.37. Left Subclavian Arteriogram. (A) In a neutral position no abnormality is seen. (B) During hyperabduction a sharp cut off of the axillary artery at the level of the head of the humerus is seen in a patient who had manifestations in the right upper extremity. Incidentally, the right subclavian arteriogram was negative. *Diagnosis:* Angiographically hyperabduction syndrome. Clinical significance?

occlusion than are the arteries. Thrombotic occlusion[972] may be due to change in the viscosity of the blood, structural changes in the vascular wall, or stasis due to extrinsic compression or intrinsic abnormalities. The thrombi that form in the sluggish venous circulation resemble a blood clot. These thrombi are composed of red blood cells held together by a luxurious fibrin network. That is why heparin and oral anticoagulants which block fibrin formation are effective in preventing the formation of venous thrombi.[206]

Tumoral thrombi belong to a separate group as they are more common in the renal and hepatic, portal veins and the inferior vena cava. They provide an easy pathway for the growth of hypernephromas, hepatomas and pancreatic carcinomas.[1046] Some veins, including the splenic and lower extremity veins, are more prone to extrinisic pressure, stasis and thrombosis. Others are more prone to infection and occlusion, such as the portal vein and its tributaries and the pelvic veins (Figs. 28-104 to 28-106).

Infiltrative Occlusions

Malignant masses can effortlessly swallow a vein by direct infiltration (superior vena cava and other veins), or by the desmoplastic reaction they can create (pancreatic carcinoma, carcinoid). The same results can be achieved by invasive fibrosing processes such as idiopathic fibrosis[1012] and fibrosing mediastinitis.[989] Thus

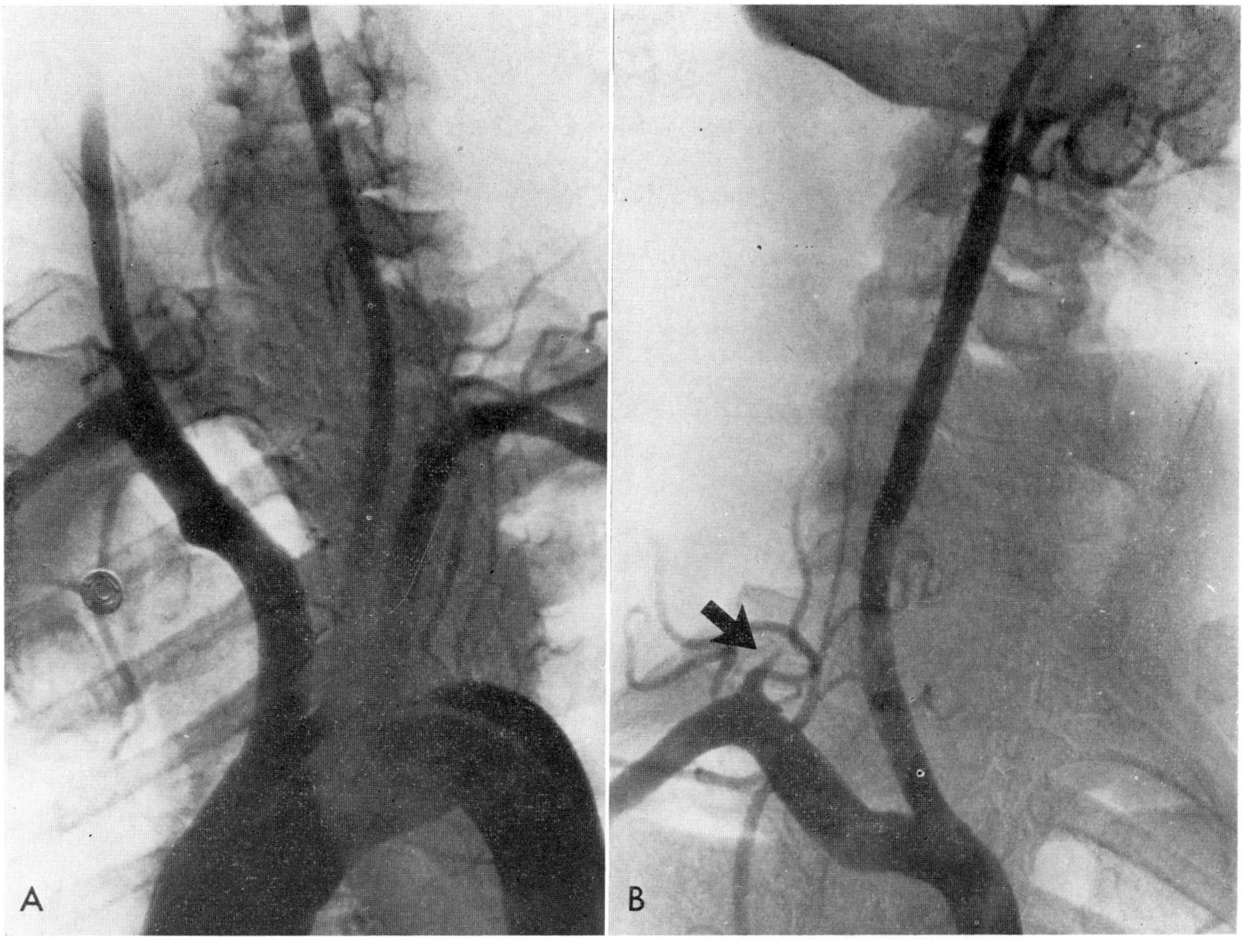

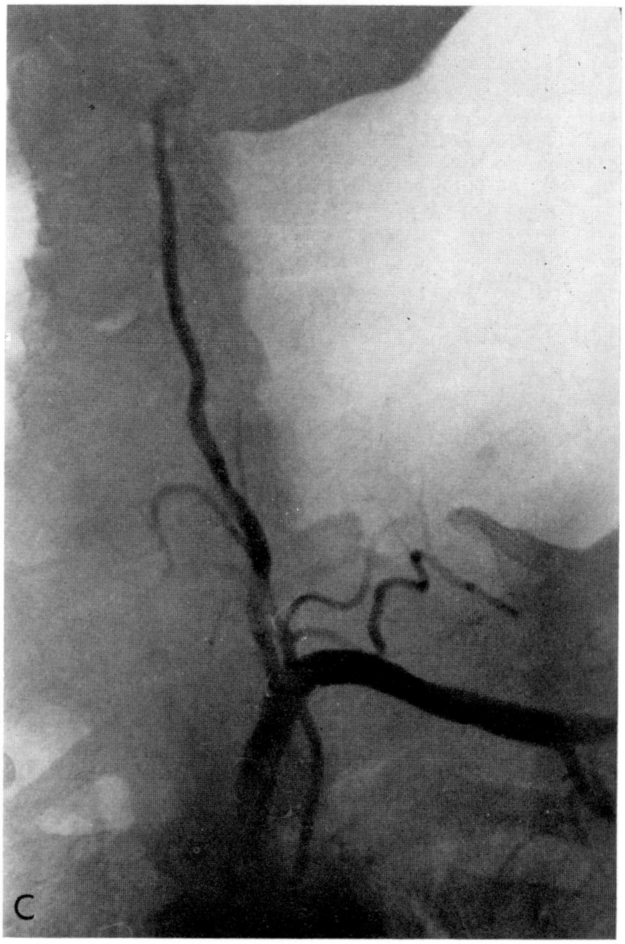

Figure 24.38. (A) Aortic arch arteriogram (left anterior oblique projection) with the patient's head turned to the right. There is no filling of the vertebral arteries. (B) Innominate arteriogram: There is occlusion of the right vertebral artery distal to its origin (Arrow). (C) Left subclavian arteriogram: The head is in an A.P. position. There is good filling of the left vertebral artery. The patient complained of total blindness when turning his head to the right. *Diagnosis:* Arteriosclerotic occlusion of the right vertebral artery. Intermittent occlusion of the left by longus colli and scalenous muscles.

it is understandable that venous occlusion due to benign or malignant lesions may be difficult to differentiate without other circumstantial evidence (Figs. 24-32 to 24-35).

Functional occlusion, another cause of non-visualization of a patent vein, poses a problem of establishing the anatomical patency of that vein (Figs. 24-41, 24-42).

Radiographic Findings with Venous Occlusion

If the vein draining a solid organ is occluded, a characteristic pattern is seen which is similar for different solid organs and other structures. When contrast is injected intraarterially the contrast material stays within the parenchyma of the organ, causing an *intense prolonged stain* of the parenchyma (nephrogram, hepatogram, etc.). The intensity and duration of the stain depends on the acuteness of the onset of thrombosis, whether it is incomplete or complete occlusion and the availability of collateral venous drainage. If the veins are completely occluded due to an acute process, obviously no draining veins are seen, and there is an intense prolonged parenchymal stain. If it is gradual and complete or incomplete, the parenchymal stain may not be that intense or prolonged because of the development of collateral drainage. The associated *congestion and edema* of the parenchyma uniformly *stretches the intrinsic arterial vasculature* in a diffuse manner, but the vessels maintain their normal arboriz-

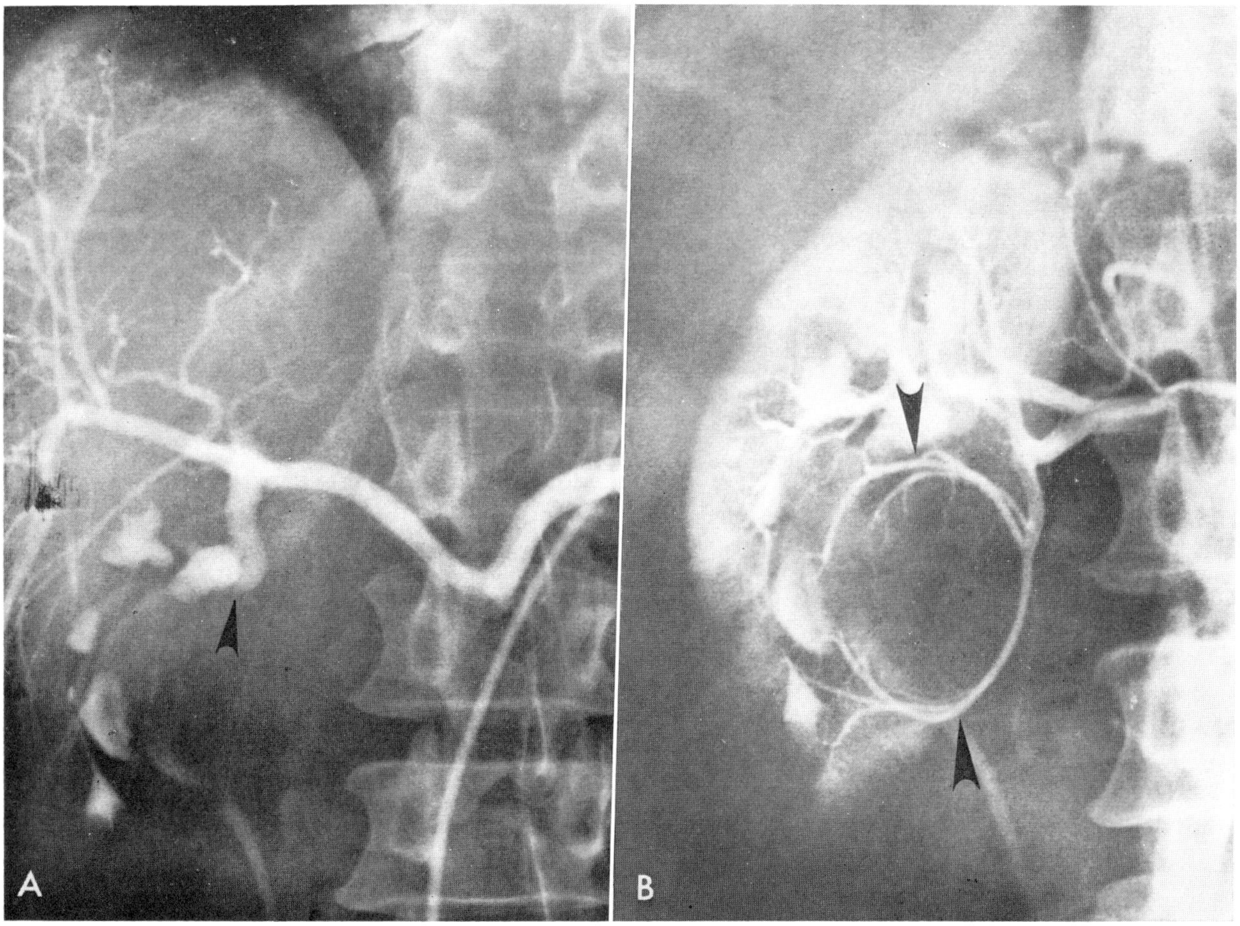

Figure 24.39. Celiac Arteriogram. (A) The proximal gastroduodenal artery (Arrow) terminates abruptly. (B) A renal arteriogram in the same patient reveals deviation and stretching of the lower pole vessels in a circumferential manner (Arrow). *Diagnosis:* Extrinsic pressure on the gastroduodenal artery by renal cyst causing occlusion.

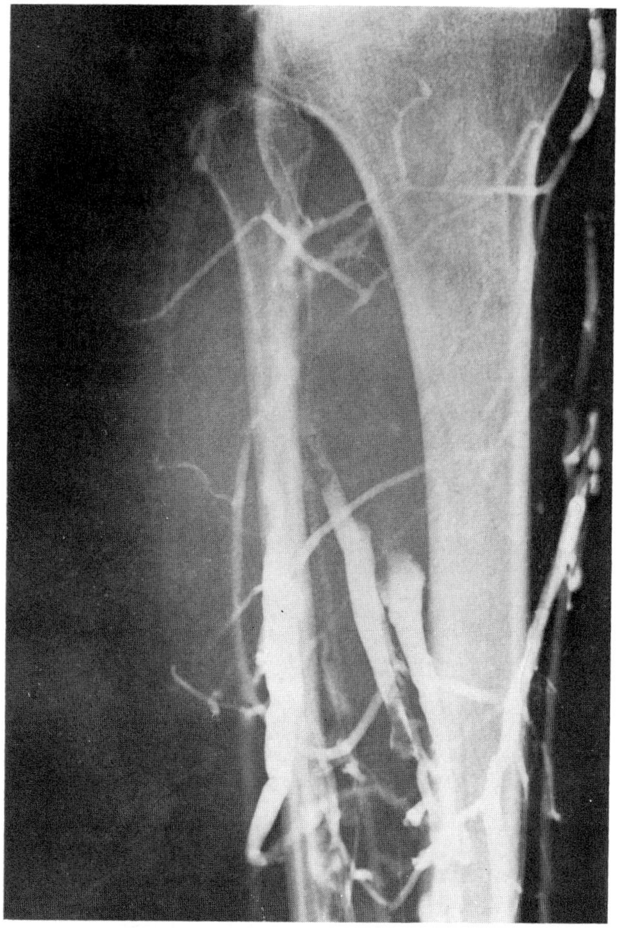

Figure 24.40. Leg Venogram. The deep calf veins are not filled and there is deviation of some of the veins. There are small filling defects noted in one of the veins (Arrow) in a patient who was diagnosed clinically as thrombophlebitis. Upon repeated questioning, he disclosed a history of trauma six weeks prior to the study. *Diagnosis:* Hematoma causing extrinsic compression on the veins. *Comment:* Other deep, soft tissue masses in the extremities may have an identical clinical presentation.

ing pattern. The normal arborization may be deviated at certain areas if there are associated intraparenchymal, subcapsular or periparenchymal hemorrhages. In extreme cases of congestion and edema there may be sparse filling of the peripheral small arterial branches due to increased resistance. If there is associated necrosis, extravasation of contrast into the wall or into the lumen of the viscus, such as bowel, may occur.[1014–1016]

For the best opacification of an abnormal venous pattern, if the ostia are patent and accessible, a direct injection of contrast into the desired vein is the most desirable approach. If the ostia are also occluded, then a direct parenchymal injection, if feasible, will aid in better opacification of the abnormal venous anatomy.

ORGANIZATION AND RECANALIZATION OF A THROMBUS

Organization and recanalization are two different, independent healing processes.[111, 967–969] The former is just a healing process, and the latter is an attempt by nature to reestablish the circulation through the thrombus. Organization proceeds at a constant rate in a healthy vessel. There are factors which influence canalization of thrombi in veins, but not atherosclerotic thrombi in the arteries. When a thrombus becomes organized, the intravascular mass is populated by fibroblast and capillary channels to become a vascularized connective tissue mass. During recanalization, the capillary channels may anastomose together to provide new channels through which blood may flow. The thrombus may eventually be incorporated into the vessel wall as a fibrous lump or thickening. Full recanalization occurs within eight to twelve months. Fissures and channels between the vessel wall and clot occur, partly because of shrinkage of the clot and recanalization. Thickening of the vascular intima and fibrin deposits in the clot cause longitudinal negative shadows as seen roentgenographically.[982] *The radiographic findings* which result from residual organized emboli are transverse webs, eccentric plaques, and circumferential stenosis[868] (Fig. 25-56).

THROMBOSIS OF SPECIFIC VEINS

Renal Vein Occlusion

This is most common in children under one year of age. The thrombi may arise in the small venules and extend toward the hilar veins. They may also arise in the main renal vein and then extend toward the small veins or in the large branches themselves. In adults thrombi may arise from the inferior vena cava or gonadal veins and extend into the renal veins. Primary causes of renal vein thrombosis[973–977] are suppurative renal lesions, trauma, dehydration, membranous proliferative glomerulonephritis, and lipoid nephrosis (Fig. 24-31).

Tumor thrombi may arise from hypernephromas extending into the renal vein. *Metabolic* causes of thrombosis include diabetes mellitus, lupus erythematosus, amyloidosis, eclampsia of pregnancy, and multiple myeloma. Chemicals causing thrombosis include heavy metal poisoning. Mechanical causes of thrombosis involve inferior vena caval obstruction, from adjacent masses extrinsic to the vein, or constrictive pericarditis (Figs. 28-104, 28-105).

Acute complete renal vein occlusion causes marked congestion, hemorrhagic infarcts, retroperitoneal hemorrhage, and if the kidney survives, eventually atrophy. Acute incomplete occlusion causes mild congestion of the kidney and venous collaterals with gradual return to good function. Gradual, complete or incomplete occlusion demonstrates a little or no renal congestion with return to good function with the help of venous collaterals. The increase in the size of the swollen kidney occurs within twenty-four hours, reaching a peak at one week. Then there is gradual decrease in size over the next one to two months, producing atrophy of the parenchyma and a thin renal artery. *The radiographic findings* in complete venous occlusion include poor filling of the stretched vessels with stasis and a prolonged nephrogram. There is also marked swelling of the medullary pyramids. In partial occlusions, only collateral venous drainage may be demonstrated without other abnormalities[978–981] (Fig. 25-63).

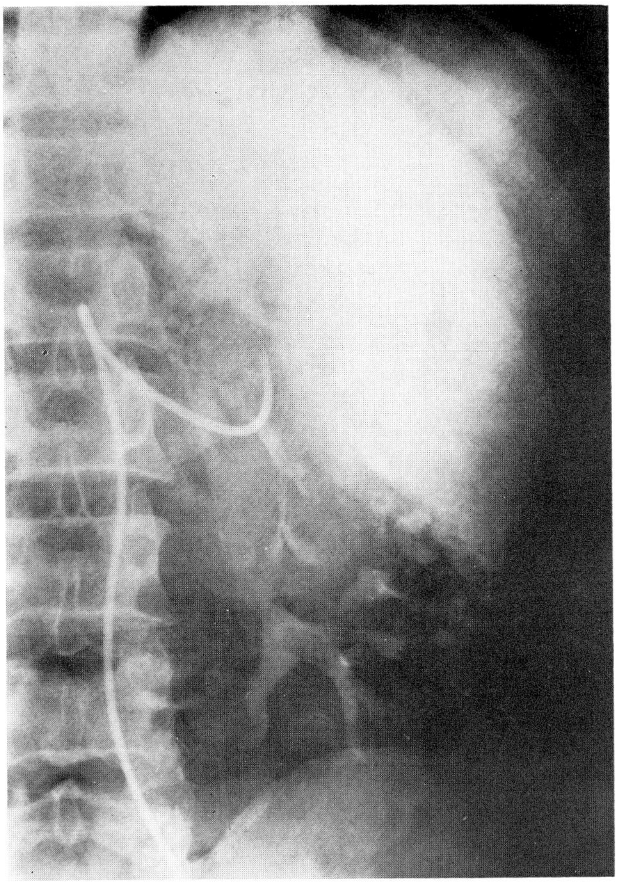

Figure 24.41. Splenic Arteriogram—venous phase: The spleen is enlarged with intense, persistent homogenous staining and no visualization of the splenic vein. There are dilated abnormal veins at the inferior pole of the spleen. This patient was a chronic alcoholic. *Diagnosis:* Splenic vein thrombosis or nonvisualization due to marked increase in portal pressure (portal hypertension) and functional occlusion of the splenic vein. *Surgical Diagnosis:* The splenic vein was patent suggesting nonvisualization due to functional occlusion and hepatofugal flow.

Hepatic Vein Occlusions

Thrombosis of the small and medium sized veins with patent ostia is known as Budd-Chiari's syndrome. Occluded ostia with distended intrahepatic veins is called Chiari's disease.[982] *Budd or Chiari, the blessed liver is provided with poor venous detours.* Injection of contrast into the hepatic artery reveals *stretching* and *bowing* of the arterial branches with *stasis.* There is a prolonged hepatogram and delayed reversal of flow in the portal and collateral veins.[484] Selective hepatic vein injection reveals a *spider web* abnormality due to intrahepatic collateral circulation.[484, 485] Intraparenchymal injection of contrast[499, 500] into the liver shows the flow of contrast from one occluded hepatic vein to an unoccluded one via sinusoids or lymphatics. Apart from the previously mentioned general causes of thrombosis[983] hepatic vein occlusion may occur with primary obliterative endophlebitis localized to the small hepatic veins.[984] If the inferior vena cava becomes oc-

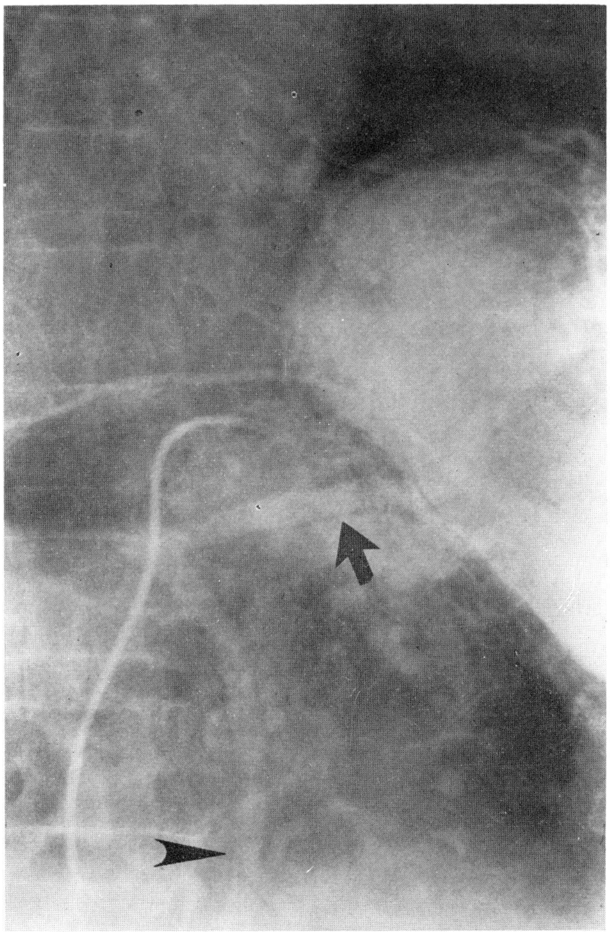

Figure 24.42. Splenic Arteriogram. The venous phase shows dense opacification of the spleen and of the splenic vein (Arrow). There is retrograde filling of the interior mesenteric vein (Arrow Head) and no filling of the portal vein. The patient was known to have portal hypertension. *Diagnosis:* Portal hypertension with hepatofugal flow and no visualization of the portal vein. This is probably due to back pressure and drainage of the contrast via collaterals. At autopsy the portal vein was patent.

cluded, then secondary hepatic vein thrombosis may occur. Causes of inferior vena caval occlusion include thrombi, tumors from the kidney, adrenal gland, pancreas, lung, liver, and caval wall invading the cava, webs, diaphragms, membranes and stenosis. In addition, trauma[914] endogeneous toxins, senecio poisoning, or liver masses such as hematomas[560] and tumors may all occlude the hepatic veins at different levels (Figs. 25-47 to 25-49).

Superior Vena Caval Occlusion

Because of the close relationship of this great venous conduit to the right main stem bronchus and lymph nodes which receive drainage from both lungs, it is in a vulnerable position to be involved by primary cancers of the lung, particularly those which are anaplastic.[985] Lymphomas, granulomatous diseases such as tuberculosis and histoplasmosis, mediastinal fibrosing processes,[989] aortic aneurysms, and ventriculo-atrial shunt catheters[987] and transvenous cardiac pacemakers[988] all compete to involve the superior vena cava[986, 990] (Figs. 25-59 to 25-61).

The primary lung cancers may prove inoperable if they involve the major veins of the mediastinum, pericardium, or the pulmonary arteries close to their origins.[991, 992]

Inferior Vena Caval Occlusion

The inferior vena cava can be affected by thromboembolic disease in its *lower one-third* below the renal veins.[486, 489] In its *middle third* it may be involved by neoplasms of the adjacent organs—kidneys, adrenals and pancreas. Extrinsic pressure against the inferior vena cava from hepatic masses or lymph nodes, or direct extension of thrombi from the hepatic veins involve the *upper one-third.* On rare occasions retroperitoneal fibrosis, trauma, tumors of the caval walls, and congenital membranes at the junction of the right atrium and inferior vena cava may cause occlusion of this vein. *Spurious obstructions* due to shunting of blood through vertebral and azygos systems is not an uncommon finding in crying infants, or during unintentional Valsalva maneuvers. In the presence of abdominal masses this may add to the confusion and even suggest a false diagnosis of occlusion[1021] (Figs. 25-50 to 25-53).

Subclavian Vein Occlusion

Apart from direct invasion by malignant tumors of the lung, the subclavian vein and its tributaries may be involved by traumatic injuries to the clavicle[993] effort or unusual position of the extremities[994] and after radical mastectomy. The diaphragms[1007] and hypertrophied valves[1008] may also act as obstructing lesions. After radical mastectomy the subclavian vein and its tributaries may be entrapped by scar tissue or involved by thrombophlebitis, recurrent tumor, or radiation. They frequently recover after symptomatic treatment.[995, 996] On rare occasions spasm and edema of the pectoralis minor may cause obstruction of the axillary vein without thrombosis.[1005] Thoracic outlet structures may do the same to the subclavian vein, without thrombosis[1006] (Fig. 25-62).

Portal Vein Occlusion

Acute complete occlusion is rare and usually due to splenectomy or polycythemia. Death may result due to massive infarction of the small bowel.[642] If there is no associated cirrhosis, collateral veins may develop rapidly.[997] Acute occlusion of one branch of the portal vein is not fatal, as the ischemic segment atrophies with survival of the bile ducts, reticulo-endothelial cells, and connective tissue. The unaffected lobe hypertrophies.[302] Common causes of obstruction include thrombosis resulting from bland or septic thrombi,[998] dehydration,[999] suppurative pylephlebitis,[1001] and polycythemia.[1002] Cholangiocarcinoma and pancreatic carcinomas may also infiltrate and occlude the vein. After a variable period of time, recanalization and collateral venous flow occurs. The prognosis may be poor in extrahepatic obstruction because of the small caliber of the portal vein available for shunting procedures, and also because of extension of thrombus into the splenic vein.[1004] In long-standing cases,[301, 1000, 1003] injection of contrast into the hepatic artery reveals increased hepatic vasculature in a small liver with the vasculature on occasion resembling angiomatoid type of vessels (Fig. 25-37).

Superior Mesenteric Vein Occlusion

All or any segment of the superior mesenteric vein may be involved in occlusion.[1009–1011] The incidence of occlusion is more common in the superior than the inferior mesenteric vein. Occlusion of mesenteric vasculature, either arteries

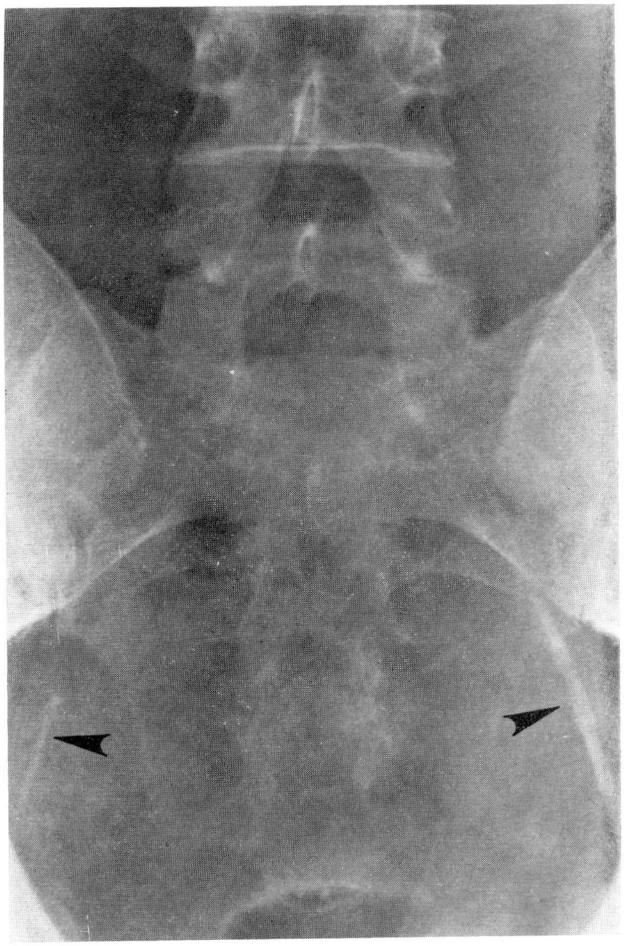

Figure 24.43. Thrombosed calcified common iliac veins.

or veins, causes hemorrhagic infarcts in the bowel within eighteen hours.[111] Extrinsic compression or involvement by malignancies or mechanical bowel obstructions; phlebitis from appendicitis, enteritis, colitis or peritonitis; surgical trauma; stasis from portal vein thrombosis or cirrhosis; increased viscosity of the blood seen during dehydration, polycythemia, or leukemia; fibrosing processes either idiopathic[1012] or carcinoid; vasoconstrictor infusion[110] may all cause occlusion. Oral contraceptives are also included.[1013] Injection of contrast into the superior mesenteric artery reveals reflux of contrast into the aorta, spasm of its branches, sparse opacification of the peripheral branches, and stasis within the arteries. Intense and prolonged opacification of thickened bowel wall, occasional intraluminal extravasation, and *spiking* due to extravasation of contrast into the wall because of mucosal necrosis and transmural infarction may occur.[1014–1016]

Splenic Vein Occlusion

This celebrated vein of the left upper quadrant provides a great amount of diagnostic information because of its close relation to the pancreas and frequent involvement by either benign[1017, 1018] or malignant pancreatic lesions.[913] Trauma does not spare the splenic vein either. The strength of diagnostic information dwindles down if there are associated diseases. For example, in the same individual, atherosclerosis of the splenic artery and chronic pancreatitis occluding the splenic vein, may add to the confusion. Acute obstruction causes engorgement of the spleen with eventual decrease in arterial flow and decrease in the size of the spleen[1019] (Figs. 25-34 to 25-36).

Pulmonary Vein Obstruction

An astute clinical radiologist can suspect and diagnose obstruction of the pulmonary vein by chronic fibrosing mediastinitis, causing recurrent pulmonary edema[1020] on the plain chest films alone.

The Deep Veins of the Lower Extremity and Their Occlusion

In *acute thrombosis* the deep crural veins under the inelastic crural fascia cannot be demonstrated because of increased subfascial pressure related to edema.[1022–1024, 1507] Therefore, the blood is driven to the superficial veins via the perforators, causing translucent defects in the superficial veins—*the knot hole phenomena.* With *subacute occlusion,* once the edema subsides, the thrombi in the deep veins may be well demonstrated angiographically. During the first week the thrombus appears loose; embolization is common during this time. After a few weeks the thrombus becomes adherent and retracts. At this point recanalization begins and continues for several months. In the general population the usual involvement is of the deep calf veins. There is increased incidence of involvement of the iliofemoral segment in women using oral contraceptives.[1029] Paraplegics,[1027] especially of a flaccid type, have a high incidence of venous occlusion in the thigh, then in the legs and then in the pelvis. Hemiplegics[1028] develop silent thrombosis of the deep veins of the involved side. *Pseudobstruction* of the popliteal vein by the plantaris muscle during extension[1026] or various types of false defects (filling defects, occlusions, valveless veins) due to contraction and relaxation of the calf muscles[1025] are not unusual.

FUNCTIONAL OCCLUSION

The low pressure antegrade flow of a venous stream can be easily arrested and even reversed if it is exposed to increased resistance due to high grade obstruction or to an opposing high pressure stream. Such a vein may not be opacified by contrast in an antegrade manner. This suggests occlusion in spite of anatomic patency of that vein. For example: Severe portal hypertension with reversal of flow in the portal vein[1182] causes nonvisualization of the patent portal and/or splenic vein after injection of contrast into the splenic artery or splenic parenchyma. Another example is an arteriovenous fistula in other circulatory units achieving the same (Figs. 24-41, 24-42).

CHAPTER 25

COLLATERAL CIRCULATION

Recognition of the presence of a collateral vessel is more important than finding a name for it.

The presence of a collateral vessel may *signify* the functional importance of an anatomic lesion as in renal artery stenosis. It may be the *clue* to the presence of vascular occlusion of the median unpaired branches of the aorta (celiac, superior mesenteric artery, inferior mesenteric artery) whose origins are not visualized in the frontal projection. And it may *aid* in finding a solution for an obscure intracranial disorder (subclavian steal). *To avoid errors,* however, the *bidirectional flow* in the intercommunications of the subdivisions of a single vascular complex such as the splanchnic circulation must be recognized. The retrograde flow in some circulatory units may be caused by (1) high injection pressure, (2) positioning of the part (extending the head for the vertebral artery), (3) increased intrabronchial pressure, (4) injection at the site of the origin of a potential collateral vessel, or (5) injections of large volumes of contrast at high flow rates. Retrograde flow may also be due to excessive demands from another organ. This is seen in the siphonage phenomena associated with arteriovenous fistula, or in cirrhosis of the liver, and in general with tumors.

Each vascular bed has its own characteristic response to acute or chronic occlusion of its major arterial supply. The efficiency varies from excellent in some vascular units to poor in end units. It may be totally inadequate, relatively inadequate under certain clinical conditions, or reasonably adequate in restoring the circulation. Sometimes the death of one member of a paired organ is preferable to its ischemic viability. Many organs are introverts in their vascular supply; occlusion jeopardizes their vitality. *Developmental variations* may determine the number of vessels available for collateral flow due to either the absence of some vessels or the lack of the usual intercommunicating pathways. Such lack of intercommunicating paths in some is manifested by the *susceptibility of junctional zones* at the splenic flexure of the colon, the rectum, or the duodeno-jejunal junction. Mediocre communication in physiologically different, diverse systems such as the liver, lung or heart, although angiographically impressive, may not be of practical functional significance.

The number and size of communicating channels proximal and distal to an occlusion, the pressure gradient, the duration of occlusion, and the metabolic demands of that organ all decide the available number of collateral vessels. Unlike normal blood flow, collateral flow responds qualitatively, but not quantitatively. In simple ligation there are better collaterals than in a vessel with thrombosis, because the thrombosed vessel usually has associated disease in its tributary branches as well. Associated spasm may influence the efficiency of functional collaterals. Occlusion of a wide collateral channel may be more dangerous than the occlusion of a small, ineffective vessel. This is seen with occlusions of the deep femoral artery along with femoral artery occlusions, or occlusion of the subscapular artery with the occlusion of the axillary artery.[421]

Some circulatory units such as the kidneys and the heart are *end artery type* and therefore lack communication between major vessels. Short, wide vessels with parallel courses are efficient in the formation of collaterals; transverse branches perform poorly in developing collateral flow. Thus the brachial artery with its

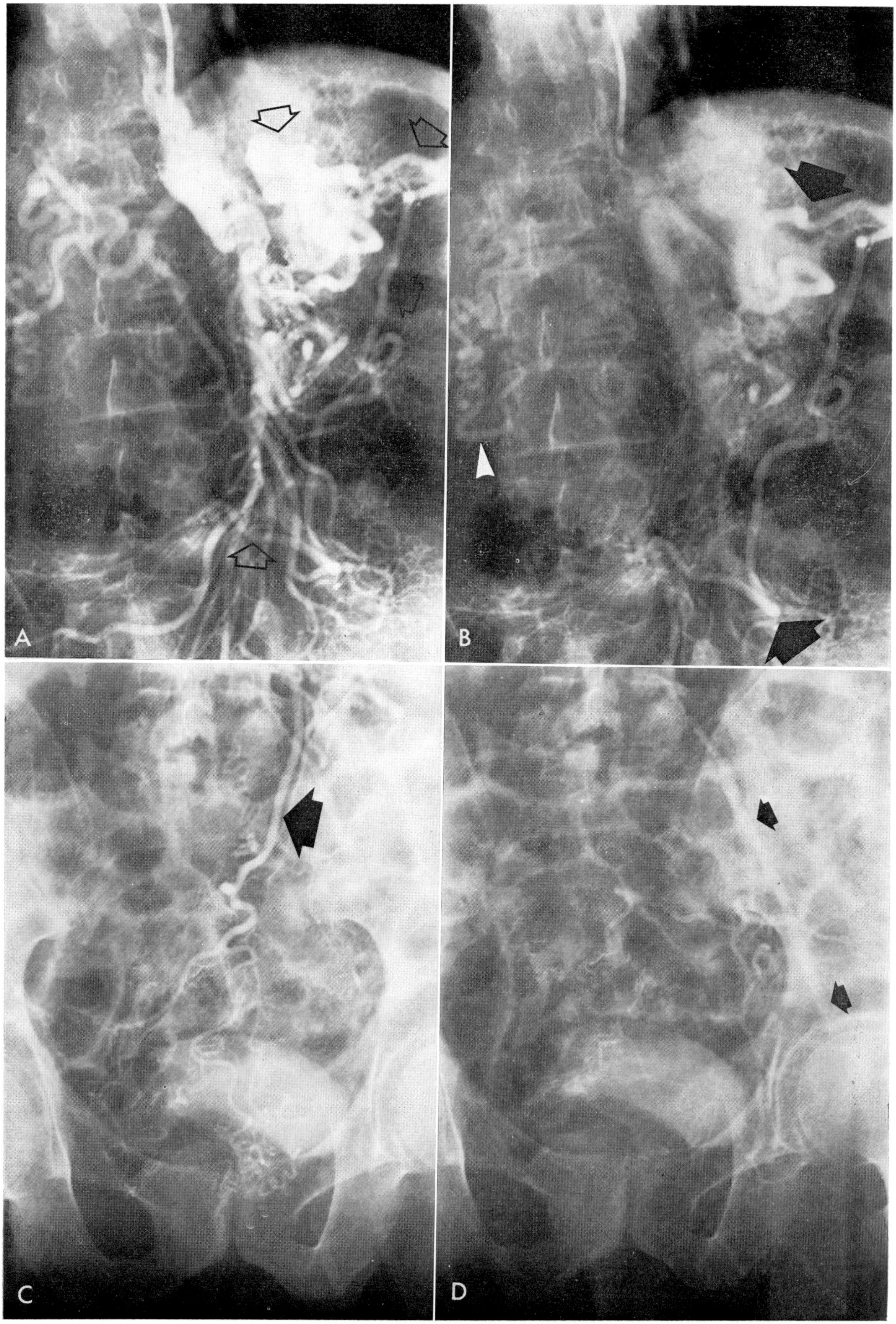
A
B
C
D

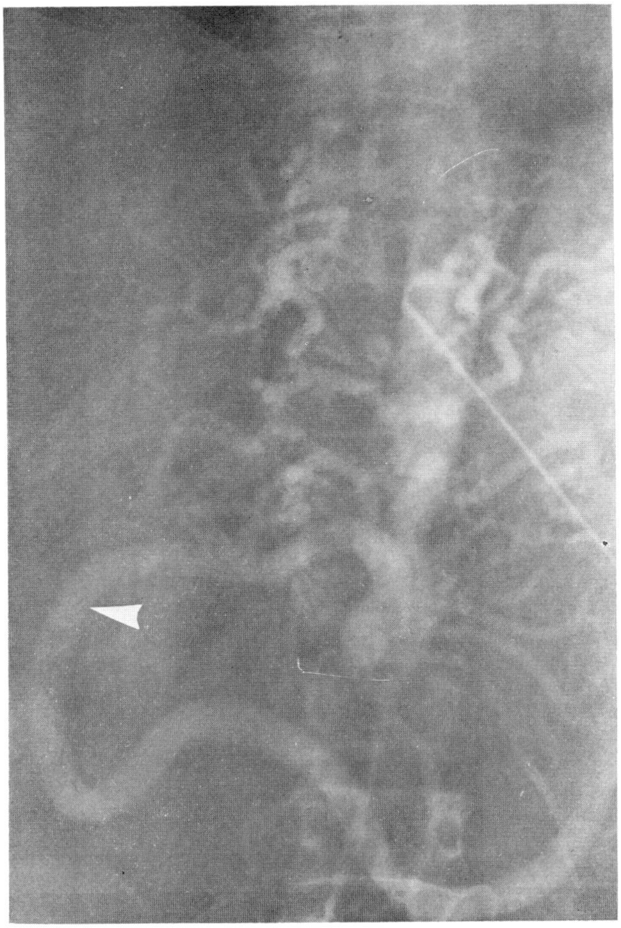

Figure 25.2. Translumbar Aortogram. Nonvisualization of the aorta distal to the superior mesenteric origin. A very prominent, dilated, tortuous vessel arising from the proximal superior mesenteric artery courses towards the splenic flexure (Arrow Head) with very prominent tortuous subcostal vessels. *Diagnosis:* Thrombotic occlusion of the aorta with collateral supply from the middle colic via the marginal artery and the subcostal vessels.

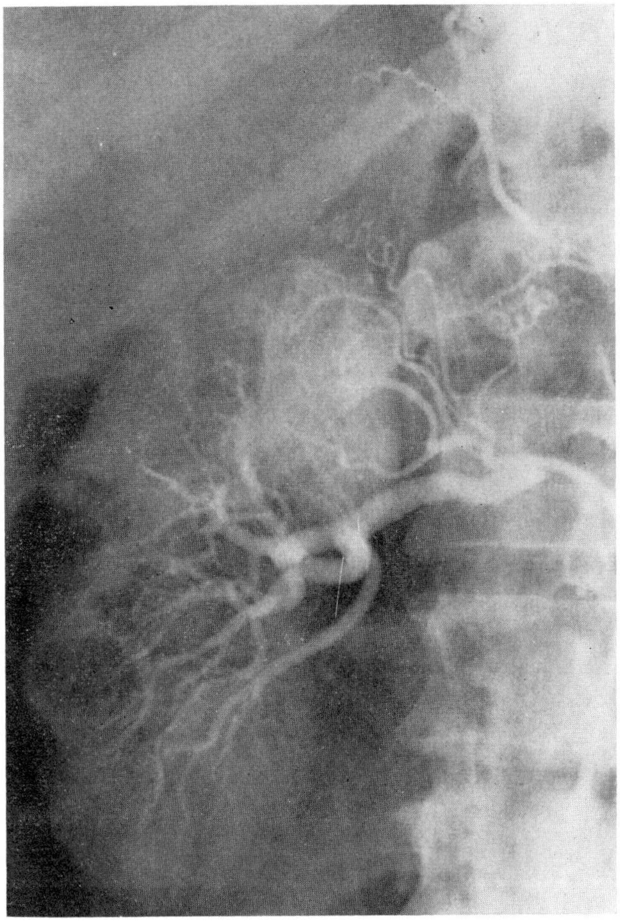

Figure 25.3. Renal Arteriogram. The catheter tip is engaged in a small vessel which gives branches to the kidney, adrenal gland and renal capsular vessel. At the same time, notice retrograde filling of the right inferior phrenic artery. *Comment:* Renoadreno capsular vessel.

←

Figure 25.1. Abdominal Aortogram. The study was done via a left axillary approach. (A) The aorta does not fill below the origin of the superior mesenteric artery. A very prominent collateral (marginal artery) (Arrow) arises from the superior mesenteric artery. (B) Late arterial phase: The same collaterals (Arrow) fill the inferior mesenteric artery. Also seen are collaterals from the celiac crossing the pancreas (Arrow Head). (C) There is good perfusion of the inferior mesenteric artery from the collateral vessel. (D) The external iliac artery fills via the hemorroidal vessels. This seventy-year-old patient's symptoms were claudication before defecation. *Diagnosis:* Aortic thrombosis with the marginal artery supplying the inferior mesenteric artery and the lower extremities.

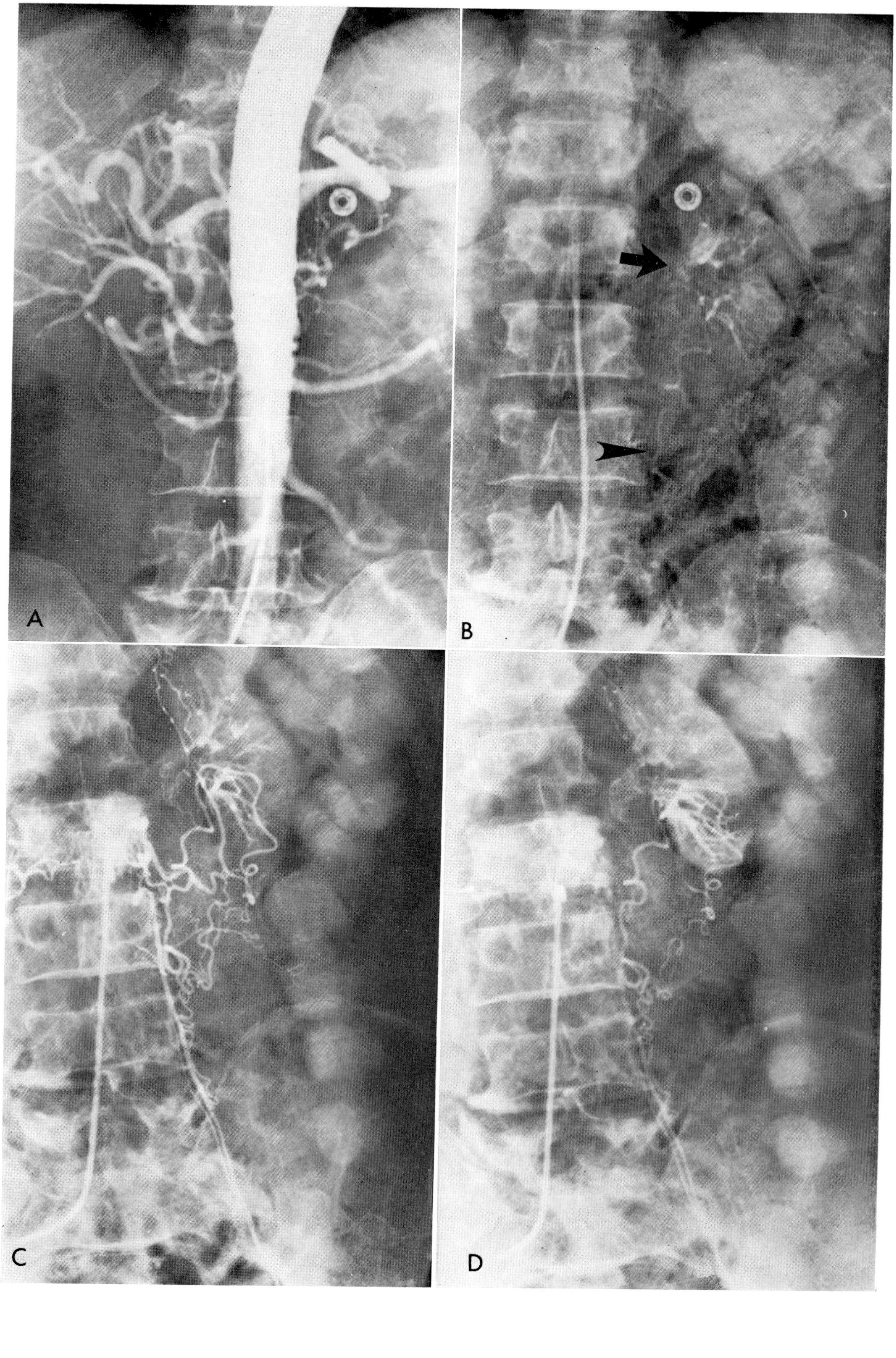
A
B
C
D

longitudinal branches performs quite differently from the transverse branches of the popliteal artery. The higher the level of obstruction, the better the collaterals which are formed. When obstruction occurs in the capillaries the death of that part of the organ, while small, is definite. Muscular bed arterial branches are good collateral vessels, but the same muscle is supplied with insignificant collaterals.[101, 422, 423, 425–427]

Structure

Collateral vessels are preexisting pathways. They are branches of large- and medium-sized arteries with thick muscular walls which have gaps in the internal elastic lamina giving them their characteristic and unmistakable *corkscrew* appearance.

The Stimulus

Collaterals develop due to a *pressure gradient* across the occlusion.[430, 431] The transformation of high end pressure in the parent artery into lateral pressure directed into its branches produces increased flow through the collaterals. *The presence of the pressure gradient and the visualization of the collaterals may suggest the functional significance of the anatomic lesion.*[428] Arteriovenous fistula are probably the greatest stimuli to the formation of collaterals.[429] The collateral vessels cease to function when the pressure gradient is eliminated after the restoration of the blood flow through the narrowed or occluded vessel. Demand for collateral vessel formation may not exist if mild stenosis causes an insufficient pressure gradient. However, the pressure gradient may be increased through exercise which increases the metabolic needs of the tissue. Unfortunately this is not the situation in end artery organs such as the heart or kidneys.[425]

In long-standing occlusions some collaterals become large and some may regress. Remarkably, atherosclerosis spares the collateral vessels.[425, 426] The onset of collateral blood supply does not eliminate the systemic manifestations produced by the ischemia of the organ, as in renal artery stenosis or occlusion with hypertension.[432] Incomplete restoration or reconstitution of the arterial flow is associated with incomplete disappearance of collateral vessels. A bypass autograft functions at 15 percent less efficiency than a normal intact artery, but 10 percent better than a reconstructed femoral artery.[433]

←

Figure 25.4. (A) Flush arteriogram: The left renal artery does not visualize. (B) Parenchymal phase: Tortuous vessels in the left paravertebral area (Arrow Head) fill the intrarenal branches (Arrow). (C) Selective lumbar arteriogram: This shows the retroperitoneal paravertebral tortuous branches filling the intrarenal branches. (D) Late phase: Better filling of the intrarenal branches noted. *Diagnosis:* Atherosclerotic occlusion of the left renal artery with collateral circulation via periureteral, peripelvic and pericapsular arteries.

ARTERIAL COLLATERAL CIRCULATIONS

Coarctation of the Thoracic Aorta

Almost all of the vessels proximal to the obstruction try to overcome the compromise in the caliber of this great vessel. The subclavian and intercostal arteries are the major ones which work to carry the load through their connections with the branches of the internal mammary artery anteriorly and along the chest wall vessels. It is also carried around the scapula and spinal cord, across the thyroid, and laterally via the lateral thoracic artery.[435, 436]

Abdominal Aortic Collaterals

Dramatic interconnections can occur between the three subunits of the splanchnic visceral complexes as they try to bypass the occluded site. The internal iliac and pudendal arteries, and the parietal vessels in the posterior and anterior abdominal walls also try their best to circumvent the occlusion.

Occlusion of the aorta *between the celiac and superior mesenteric* arteries results in the celiac artery perfusing the superior mesenteric artery via the pancreatico-duodenal vessels. In turn, the superior mesenteric artery perfuses the inferior mesenteric via the marginal artery and the inferior mesenteric artery perfuses the lower extremities via the rectal vessels.

(Text continues on page 363)

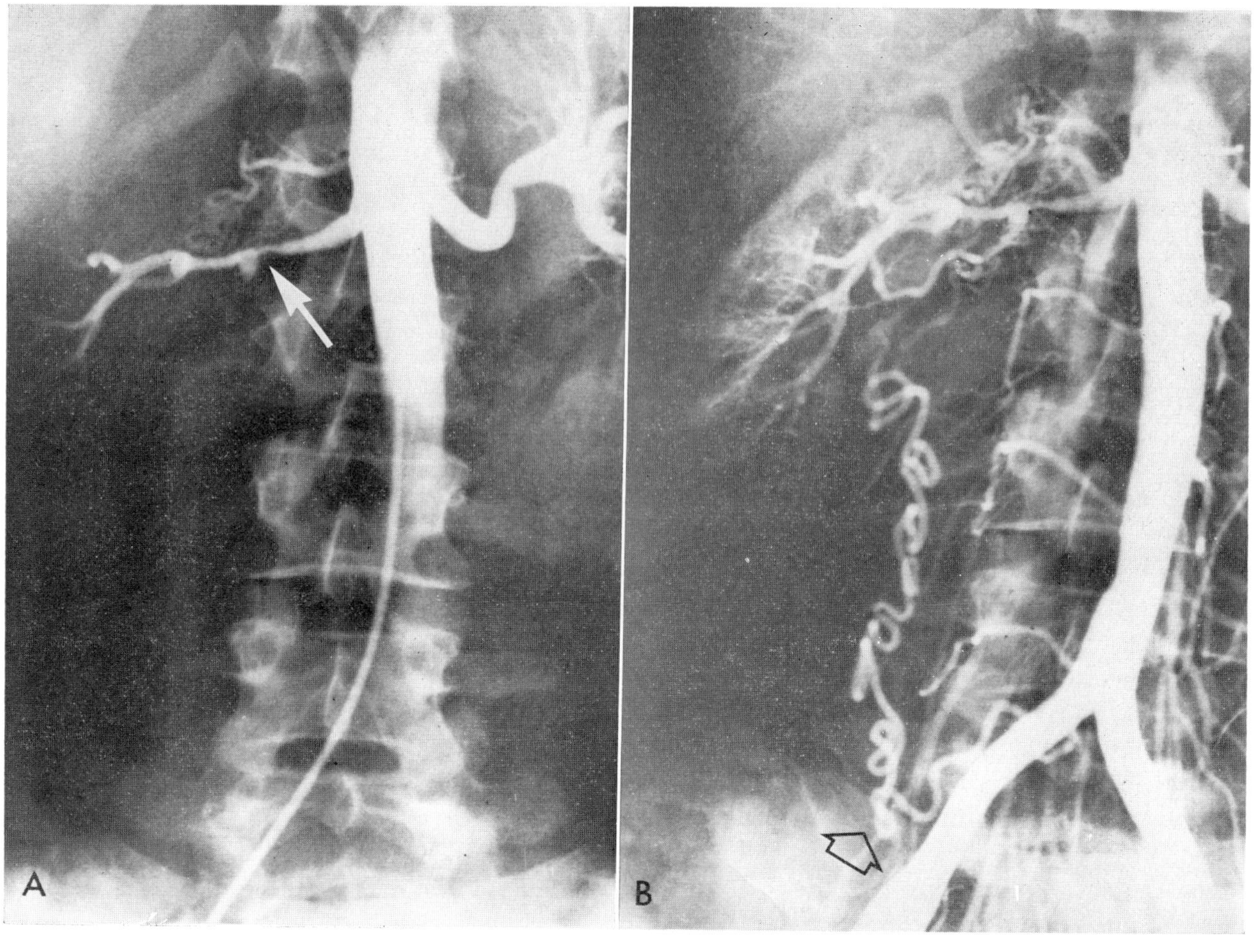

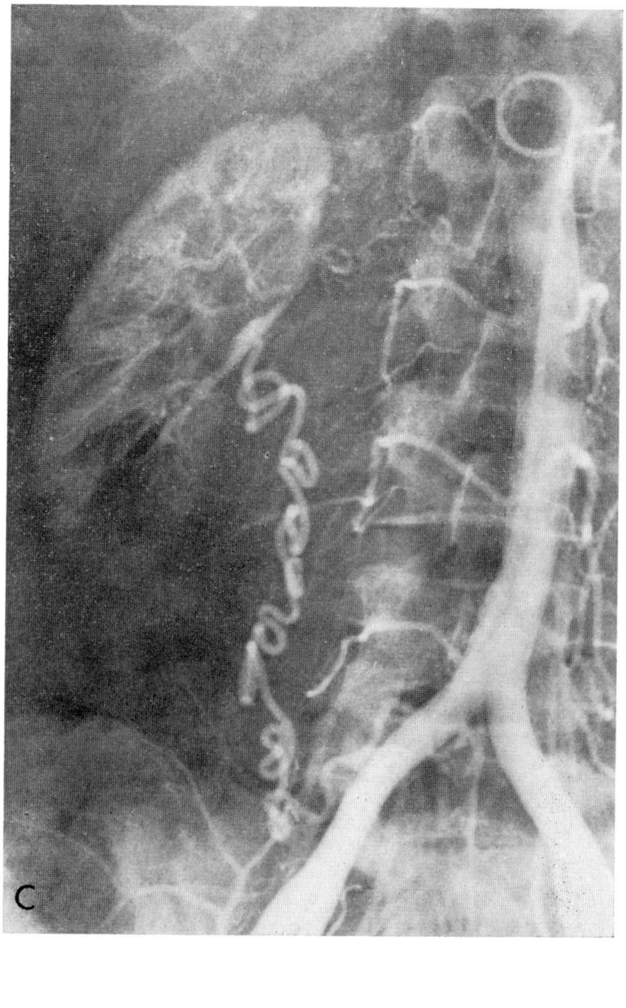

Figure 25.5. Flush Aortogram. (A) Early arterial phase: There is smooth narrowing of the right renal artery in its midportion with a slight saccular dilatation (Arrow). A prominent lumbar artery at L1 with abnormal tortuous vessels is seen. (B) Midarterial phase: A very prominent tortuous vessel arises from the common iliac and courses along the right ureter to perfuse the intrarenal vasculature (Arrow). Notice more branches from the same lumbar artery. (C) Late arterial phase: There is better filling of the tortuous vessel along the right ureter perfusing the renal hilar branch in a young individual with hypertension. *Diagnosis:* Hyperplastic disease of the right renal artery, either intimal or adventitial type. Very prominent ureteral artery and lumbar collaterals supplying the renal vasculature. *Pathology:* Intimal hyperplasia. (Courtesy of Dr. D. Sloan, Michael Reese Hospital, Chicago.)

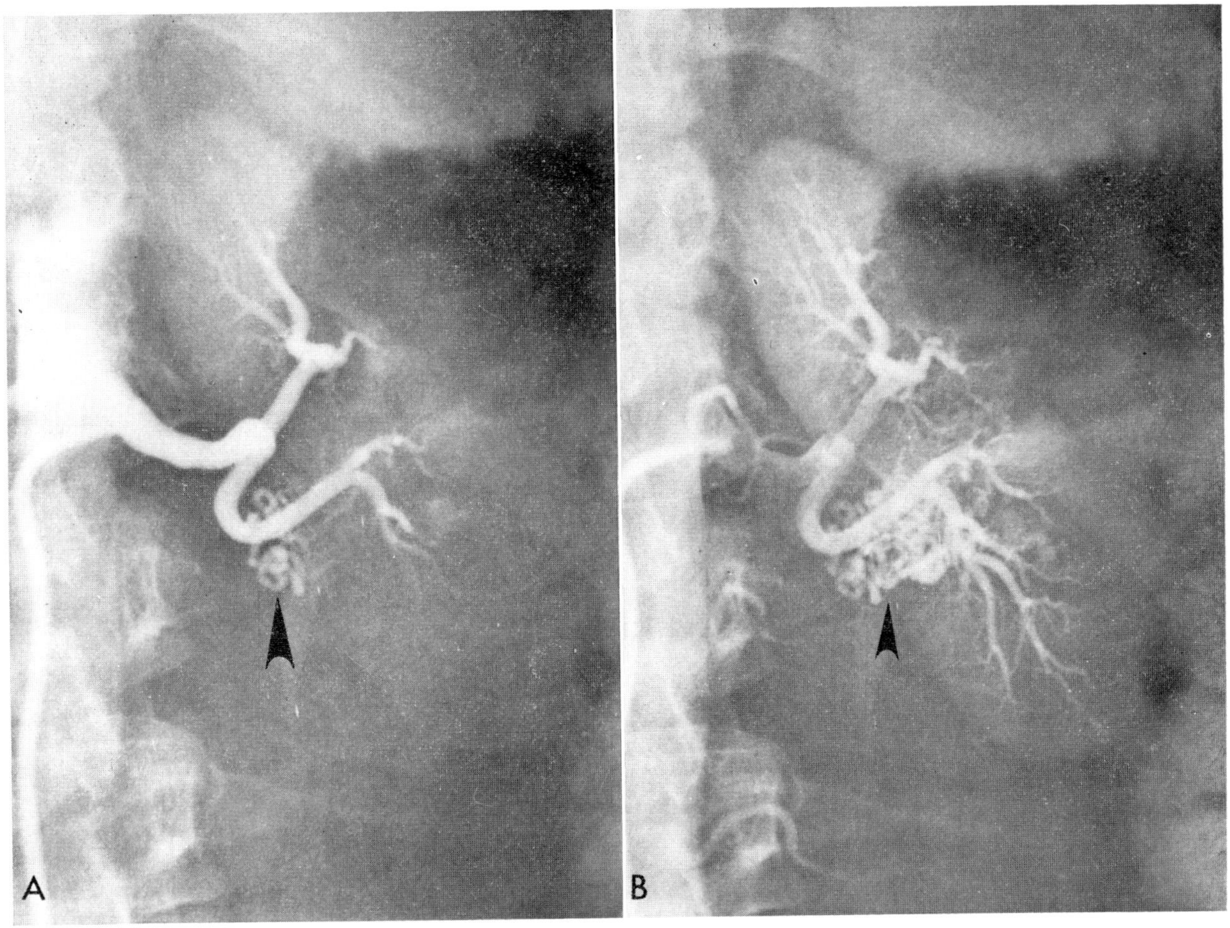

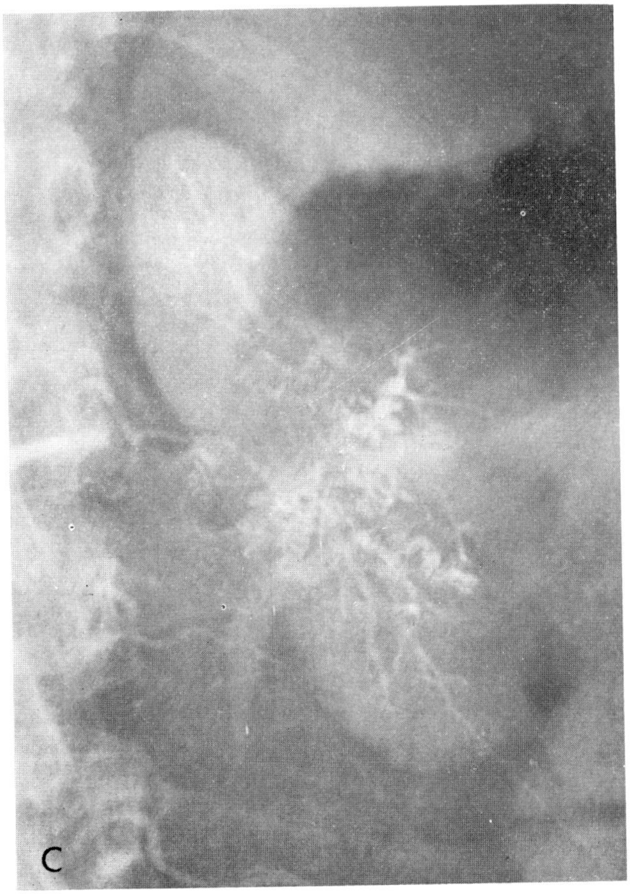

Figure 25.6. Renal Arteriogram. (A) Early arterial phase: Very tortuous arterial branches arise from the renal hilar branch. (B) Midarterial phase: The same tortuous branches increase. There is lack of arterial perfusion to the midportion of the kidney. (C) Late arterial phase: Partial delayed perfusion occurs to this segment of the kidney by these collaterals. This patient had hypertension. *Diagnosis:* Occlusion of the dorsal branch of the renal artery with renal hilar collaterals perfusing the corresponding segments of the kidney.

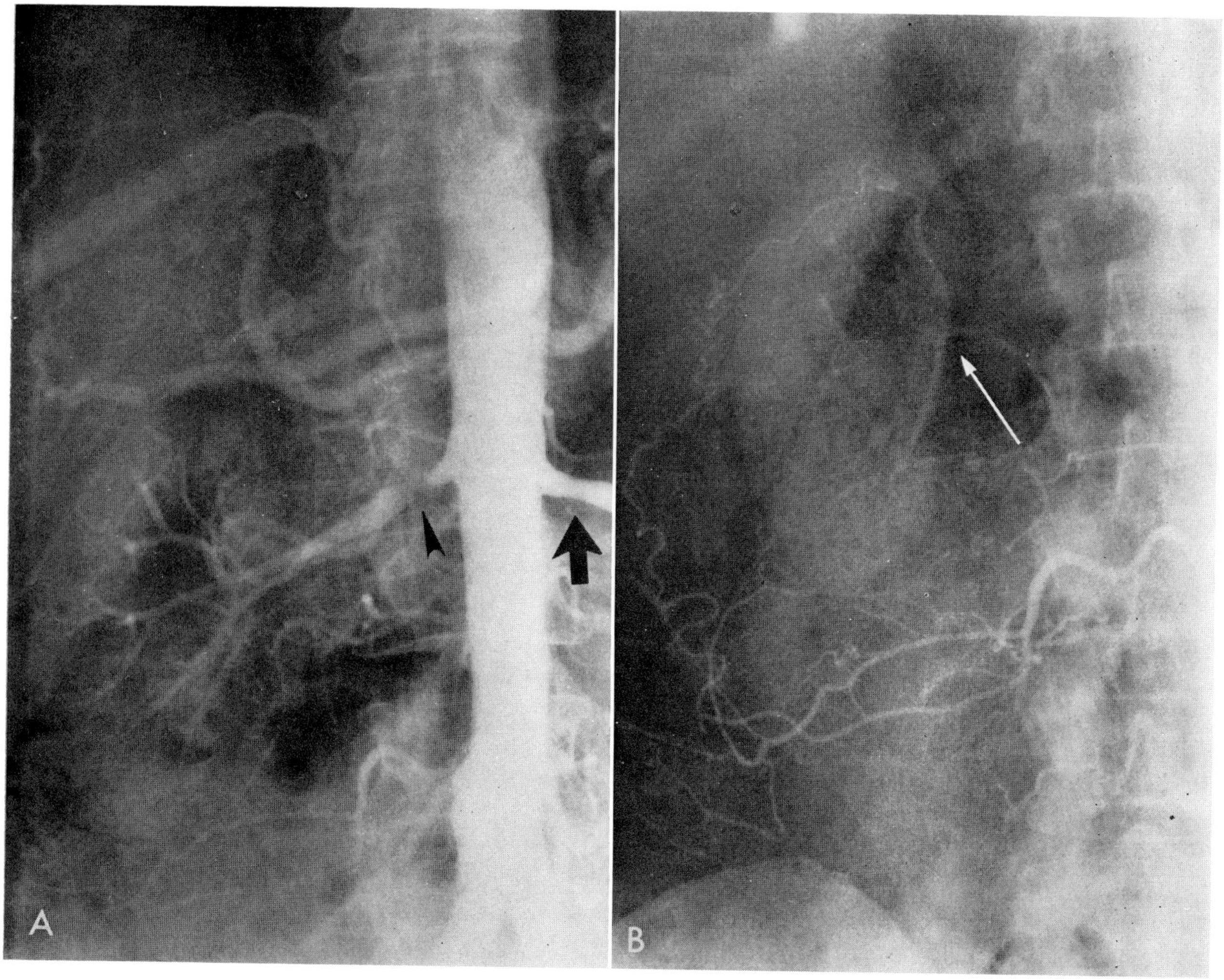

Figure 25.7. (A) Flush aortogram: There is extreme narrowing of the proximal right renal artery (Arrowhead) and minimal narrowing of the proximal renal artery on the left side (Arrow). (B) Selective lumbar arteriogram—same side: Retroperitoneal vessels communicate with the renal capsular vessel perfusing the renal artery (Arrow). *Diagnosis:* Marked stenosis of the right renal artery and minimal stenosis of the left renal artery probably due to atherosclerosis. Retroperitoneal collaterals perfused by the lumbar artery carries blood via the capsular artery to the renal artery.

→

Figure 25.8. Flush Aortogram. (A) The right renal artery does not visualize. A prominent vessel arises from the last lumbar artery. (B) Midarterial phase: The same tortuous vessel from the lumbar artery courses towards the renal artery (R.A.). (C) Note the small kidney with a poor nephrogram. *Diagnosis:* Atherosclerotic occlusion of the right renal artery causing a shrunken kidney because of underperfusion. The viability is maintained by periureteral collaterals supplied by the lumbar artery.

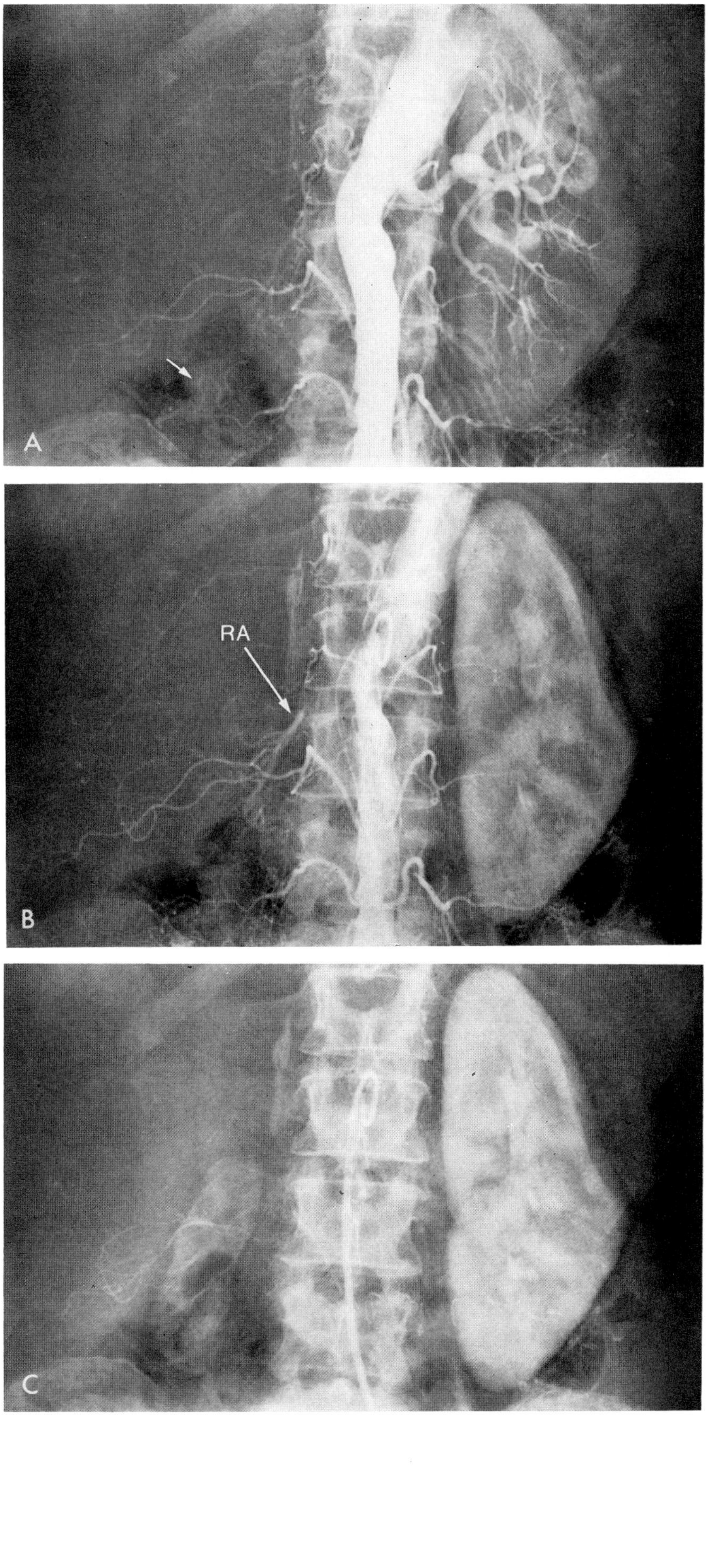
A
RA
B
C

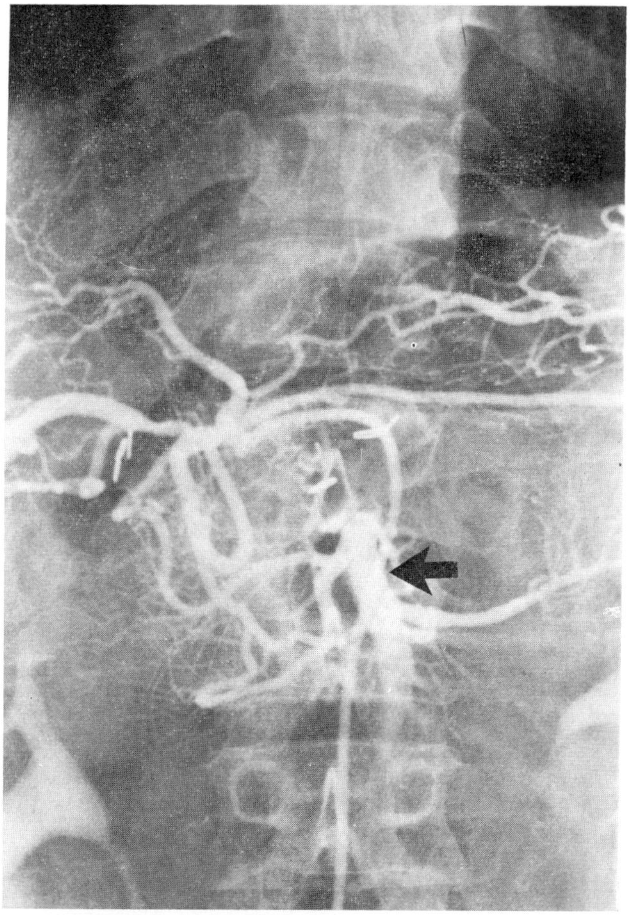

Figure 25.9. Hepatic Arteriogram. There is opacification of a patent superior mesenteric artery (Arrow) filled via the pancreatic arcade. *Comment:* Filling of the superior mesenteric artery, or celiac artery via existing intercommunicating channels (pancreaticoduodenal vessels) may occur under normal conditions also.

Figure 25.10. (A) Superior mesenteric arteriogram: There is opacification of the hepatic artery (Arrow) via vessels along the course of the pancreas (Arrow Head). (B) Celiac arteriogram: The celiac axis is patent. *Comment:* This demonstrates another normal vascular intercommunicating pathway between the superior mesenteric and the celiac arteries.

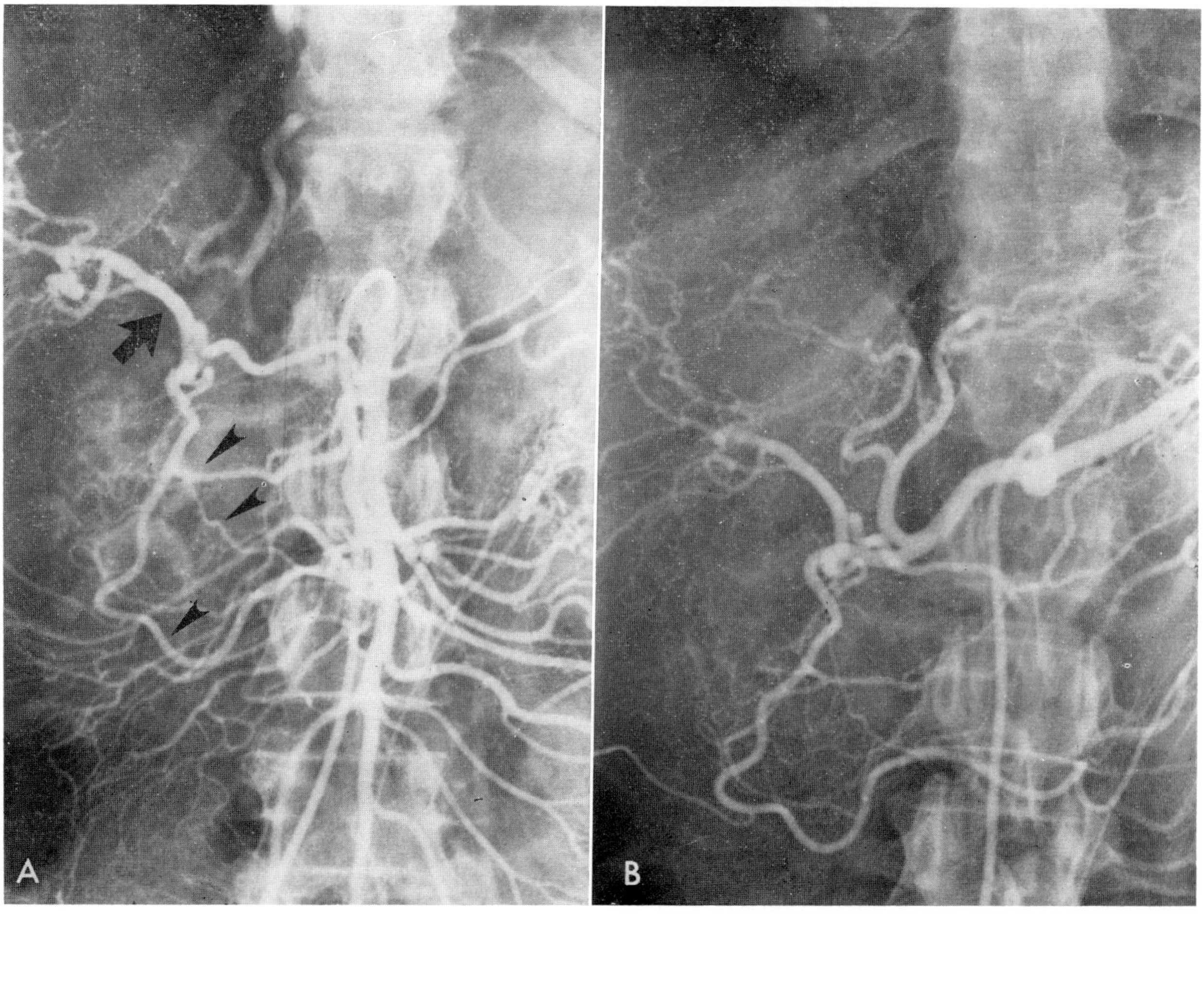

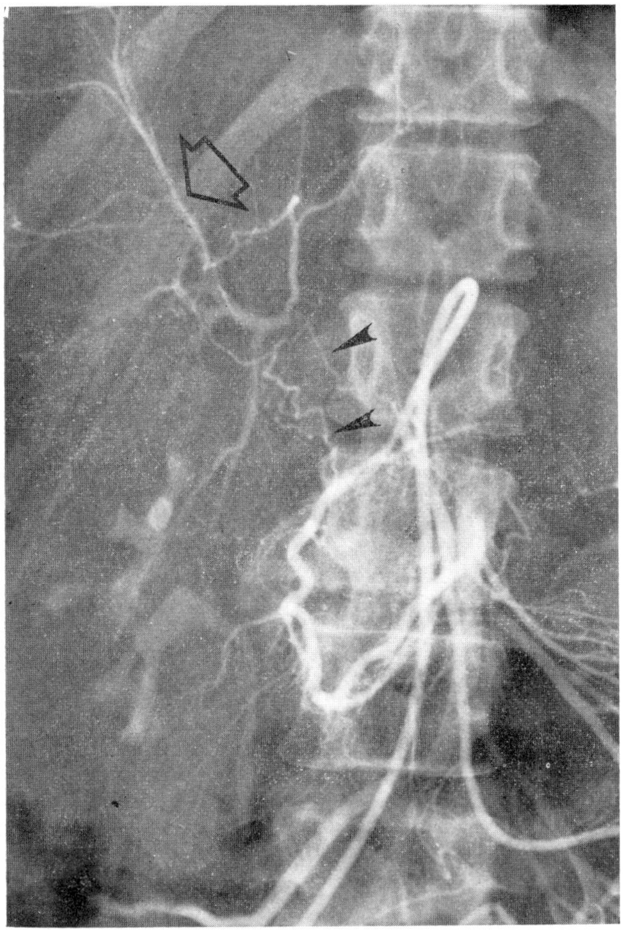

←

Figure 25.11. Gastroduodenal Arteriogram. There are small filliform vessels (Arrow Head) from the gastroduodenal opacifying the hepatic arcade (Blank Arrow). *Diagnosis:* Preexisting collateral communications.

Figure 25.12. Left Gastric Arteriogram. There is flow of contrast from the left gastric arterial branches (Blank Arrow) along the lesser curve of the stomach perfusing the right gastric artery (Arrow). This in turn opacifies intrahepatic branches (Arrow Head). *Comment:* This is a potential route of collateral circulation.

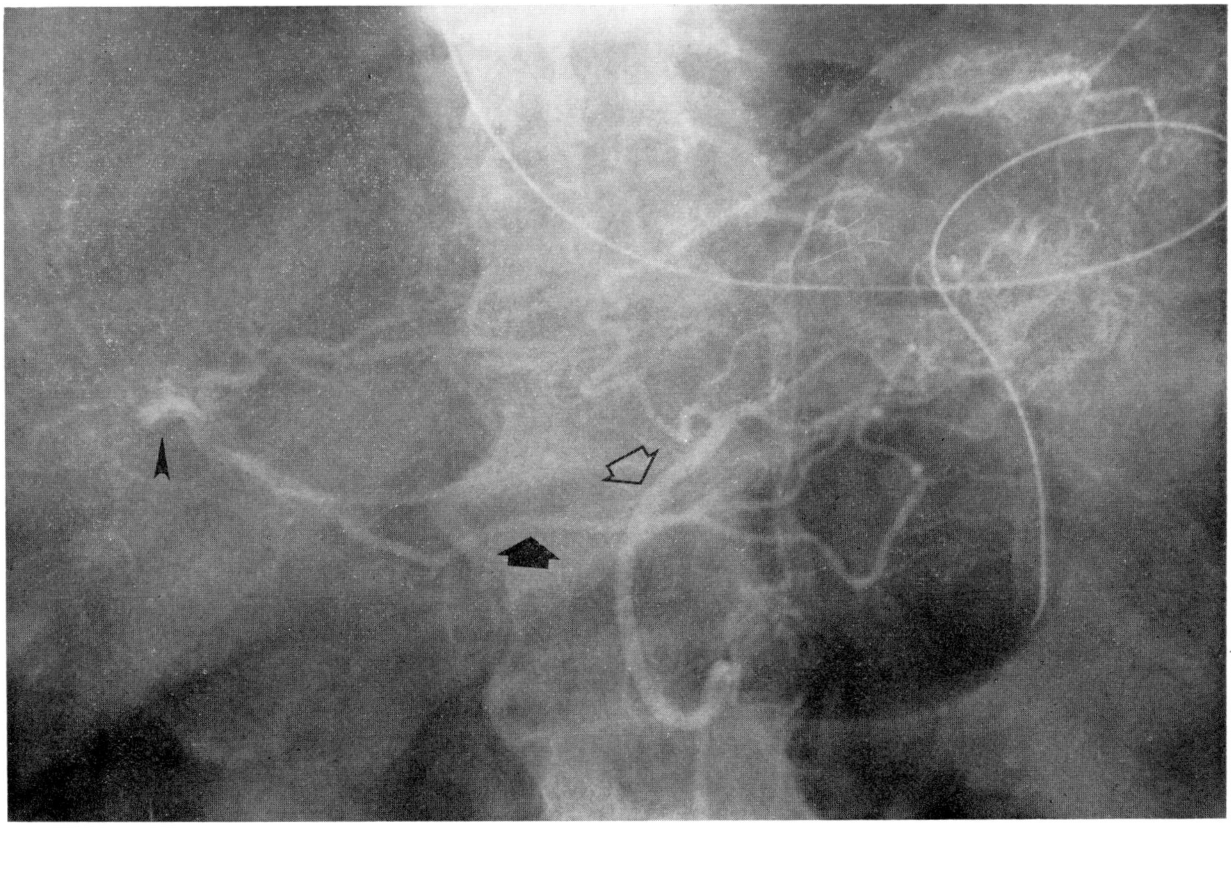

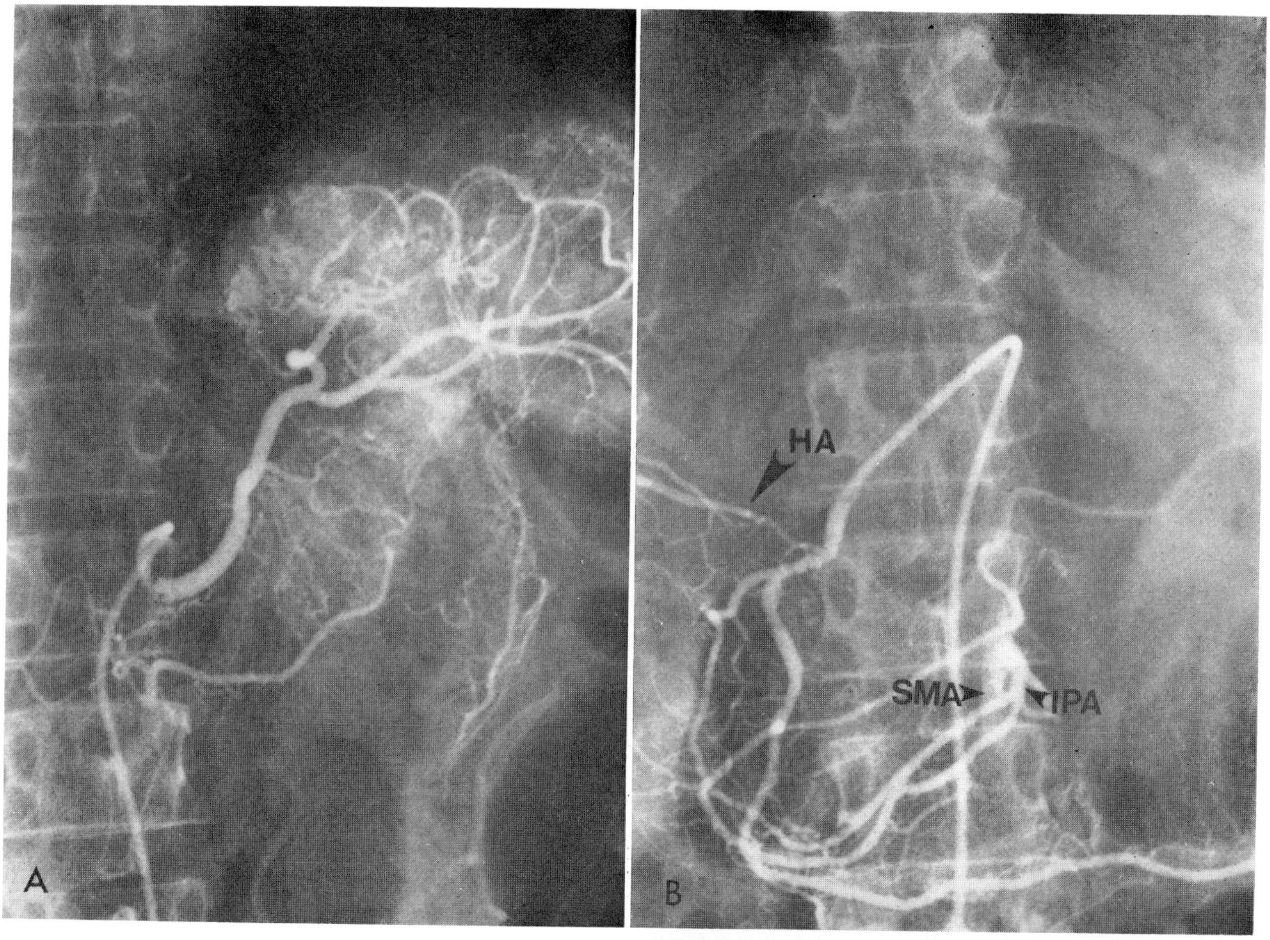

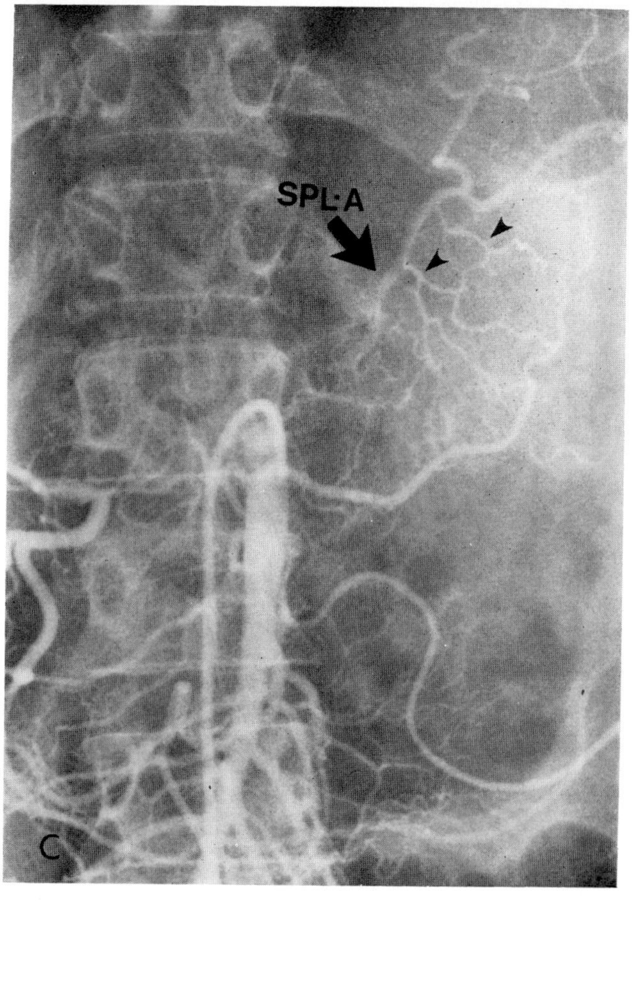

Figure 25.13. (A) Splenic arteriogram: The pancreatic branches fill from the splenic artery. (B) Gastroduodenal arteriogram: Small hepatic branches are seen (H.A.): There is good filling of the superior mesenteric artery via the pancreatic arcade through a prominent inferior pancreaticoduodenal artery (I.P.A.). (C) Superior mesenteric arteriogram: The splenic artery fills via the pancreatic arcade (Arrow Head), and the hepatic artery fills via the gastroduodenal artery. *Comment*: Bidirectional flow in these subdivisions of splanchnic circulatory unit is common.

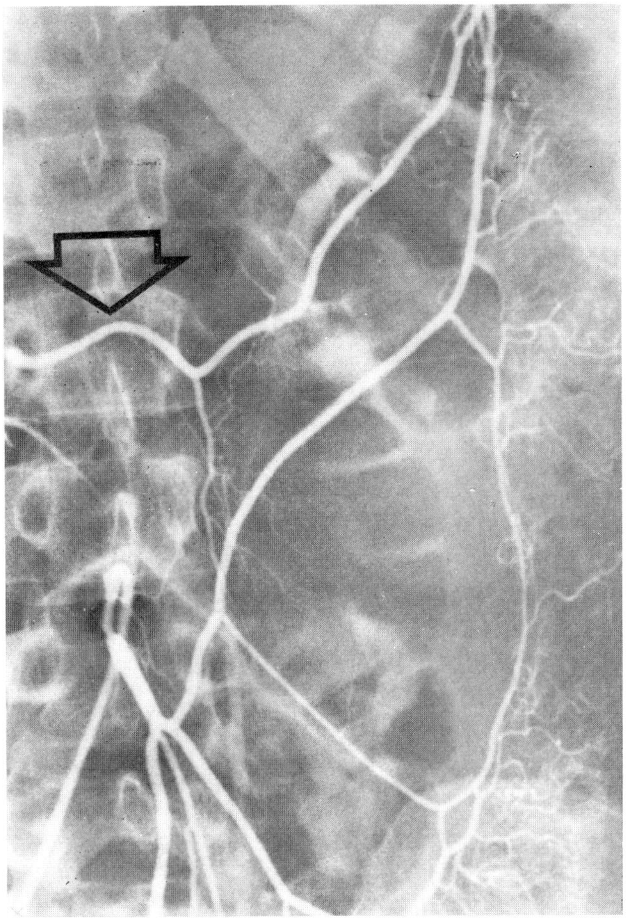

Figure 25.14. Inferior Mesenteric Arteriogram. Notice reflux of contrast into the middle colic artery (Arrow) via the ascending branch of the left colic artery. *Comment:* This existing intercommunication has good potential for bidirectional flow.

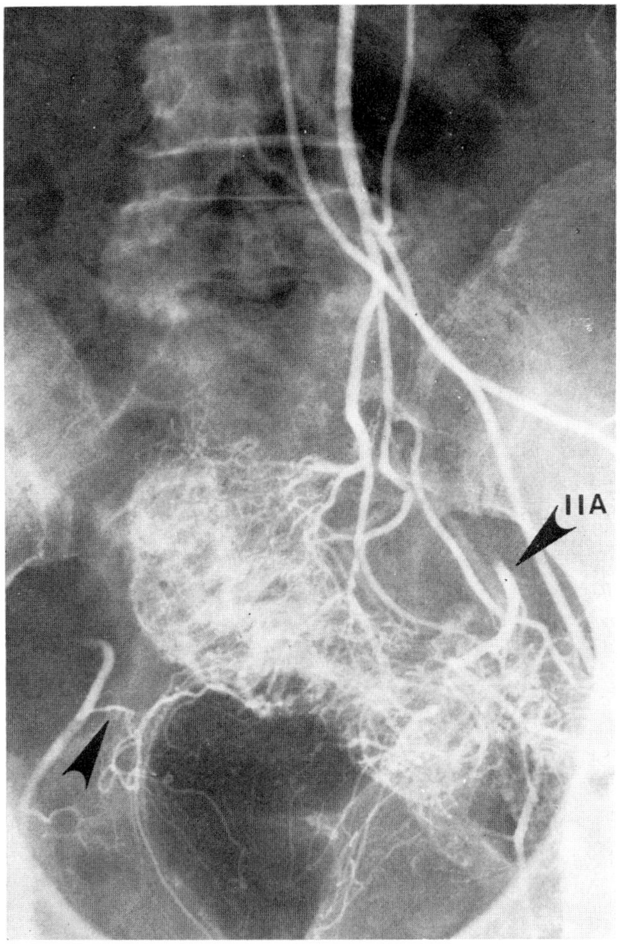

Figure 25.15. Inferior Mesenteric Arteriogram. Retrograde opacification of the internal iliac arteries (I.I.A.) via middle rectal arteries (Arrow). *Comment:* Intercommunication between the systemic and mesenteric circulation is a potential bidirectional collateral channel.

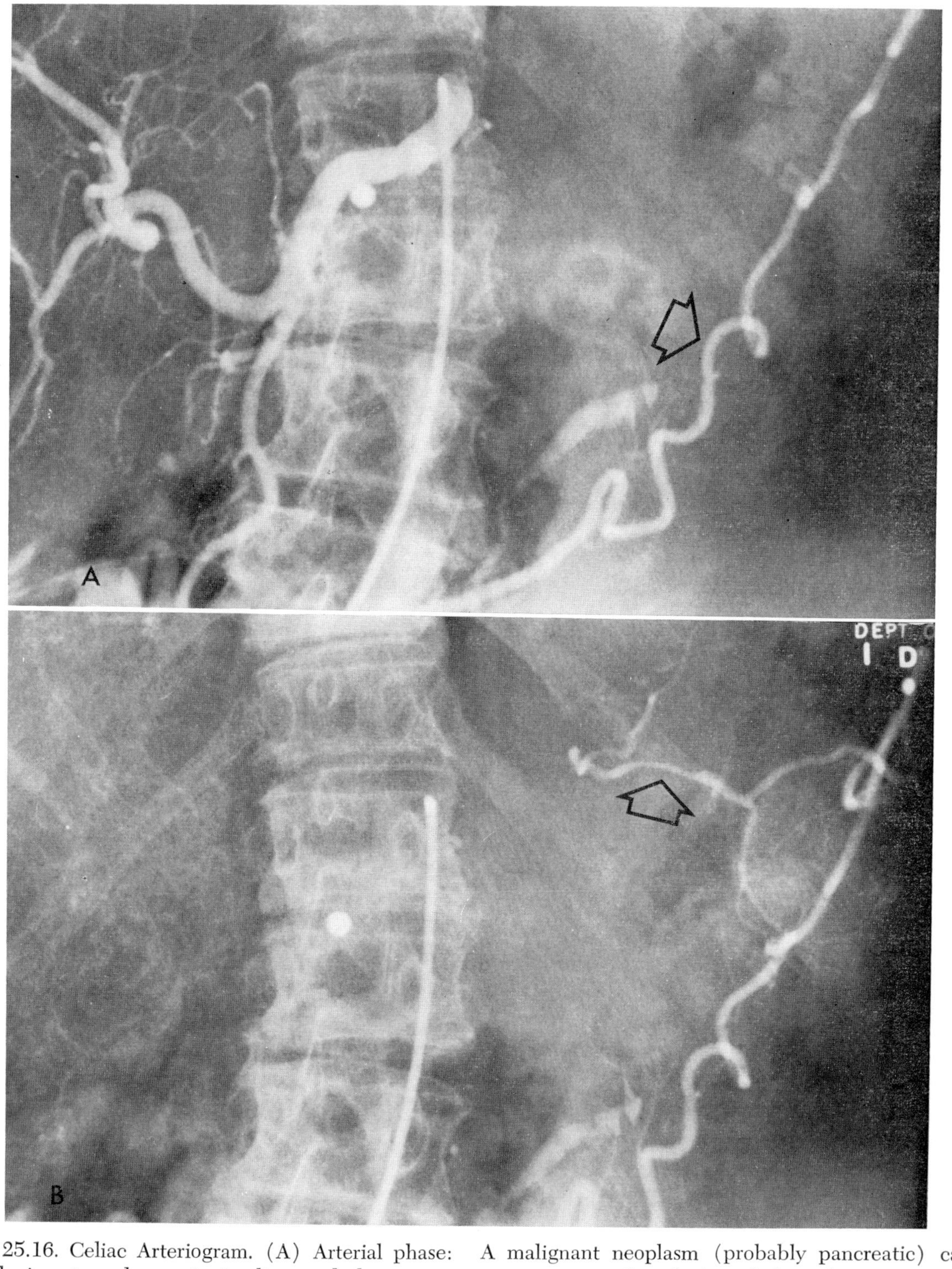

Figure 25.16. Celiac Arteriogram. (A) Arterial phase: The splenic artery does not visualize, and the gastroepiploic artery (Arrow) is prominent. (B) Late arterial phase: An irregularly narrowed vessel (Arrow) fills. The patient had backache and weight loss. *Diagnosis:* A malignant neoplasm (probably pancreatic) causing encasement and occlusion of the splenic artery. There is collateral flow from the gastroepiploic to the distal splenic artery. *Pathologic Diagnosis:* Inoperable pancreatic carcinoma.

Occlusion of the aorta *between the superior and inferior mesenteric artery* results in perfusion of the inferior mesenteric artery by the superior via the marginal artery. Again, the inferior mesenteric artery supplies the lower extremities via the rectal vessels (Figs. 25-1, 25-2).

Occlusion of the aorta *below the inferior mesenteric artery* results in perfusion of the lower extremity vessels via the rectal plexus with the supply coming from the inferior mesenteric artery. From the rectal plexus, blood reaches the internal iliac artery and finally the external iliac artery.

The Renal Artery and Its Collaterals

The development of the collaterals due to renal artery stenosis plays a vital part in preserving viable nephrons, thereby preventing total infarction. This underperfused, viable renal tissue may be responsible for the increase in blood pressure.

The *presence of collaterals* strongly indicates the functional significance of the anatomic lesion. The collaterals are not seen if there is no pressure gradient.[428, 463, 464] A humoral factor may be involved.[1494] The development of collateral circulation will not decrease the developed hypertension[432] once it has developed. The collaterals may revert high renin rations of 1.4 to 1, so that the ratio will be less than 1.4.[29]

These collateral vessels are preexisting vessels with a potential for rapid functioning when and if needed.[465, 466] These preformed channels provide only 5 percent of the total renal flow after acute occlusion; they are not modified by contralateral nephrectomy.[1493] The kidney, lying in the retroperitoneal bed and surrounded by numerous small vessels, has ample opportunities to receive inadequate perfusion from all of them. Capsular, periureteric, peripelvic, inferior adrenal, lumbar, intercostal, gonadal, and internal iliac arteries all participate in supplying collateral flow. This is further reinforced by the adipose renal capsular artery and its anastomosis with the retroperitoneal plexus of Turner.[370, 468, 469] If there is a dual blood supply to the kidney, it favors the formation of intrarenal collaterals about the pericalyceal network, perforating capsular arteries and the vasa rectae[467] (Figs. 25-4 to 25-8).

Splanchnic Collaterals

The celiac, superior mesenteric, and inferior mesenteric arteries constitute a single vascular unit which may allow bidirectional flow through intercommunications. The two significant intercommunications are at the head of the pancreas via the *pancreatico-duodenal vessels* and along the margin of the colon via the *marginal artery.* These intercommunications are also blessed with two areas of *reinforcement;* one at the level of the thoracic diaphragm via the *inferior phrenic artery,* the other at the level of the pelvic diaphragm via the *rectal plexus of internal iliac* and internal pudendal vessels.[470, 471] The most noteworthy feature of this entire circulation is the tremendous adaptability to *give* and also to *take* within itself and with the systemic circulation. Even if occlusion of all three arteries occurs, the inferior phrenic, adrenal arteries and bare area of the liver supply the celiac artery; the retroperitoneal plexus of Turner supplies the superior mesenteric artery; the rectal plexus perfuses the inferior mesenteric artery.[472–474] The neglected adipose tissue arteries, which are the branches of the superior mesenteric and inferior mesenteric arteries to the mesenteric fat, are also good collaterals in drastic situations[470] (Figs. 25-9 to 25-21).

Even under acute conditions the occurrence of a vascular steal within this circulation is unlikely unless the flow through both the celiac and superior mesenteric arteries is compromised. When both are narrowed, flow from the celiac to the mesenteric circulation occurs at the cost of decreased gastric blood flow.[851]

Hepatic Collaterals

Because of the multiplicity of the variations, the arterial supply to the liver is extremely unpredictable. Relatively few vessels may be available when there is ligation; many of the avail-

(Text continues on page 379)

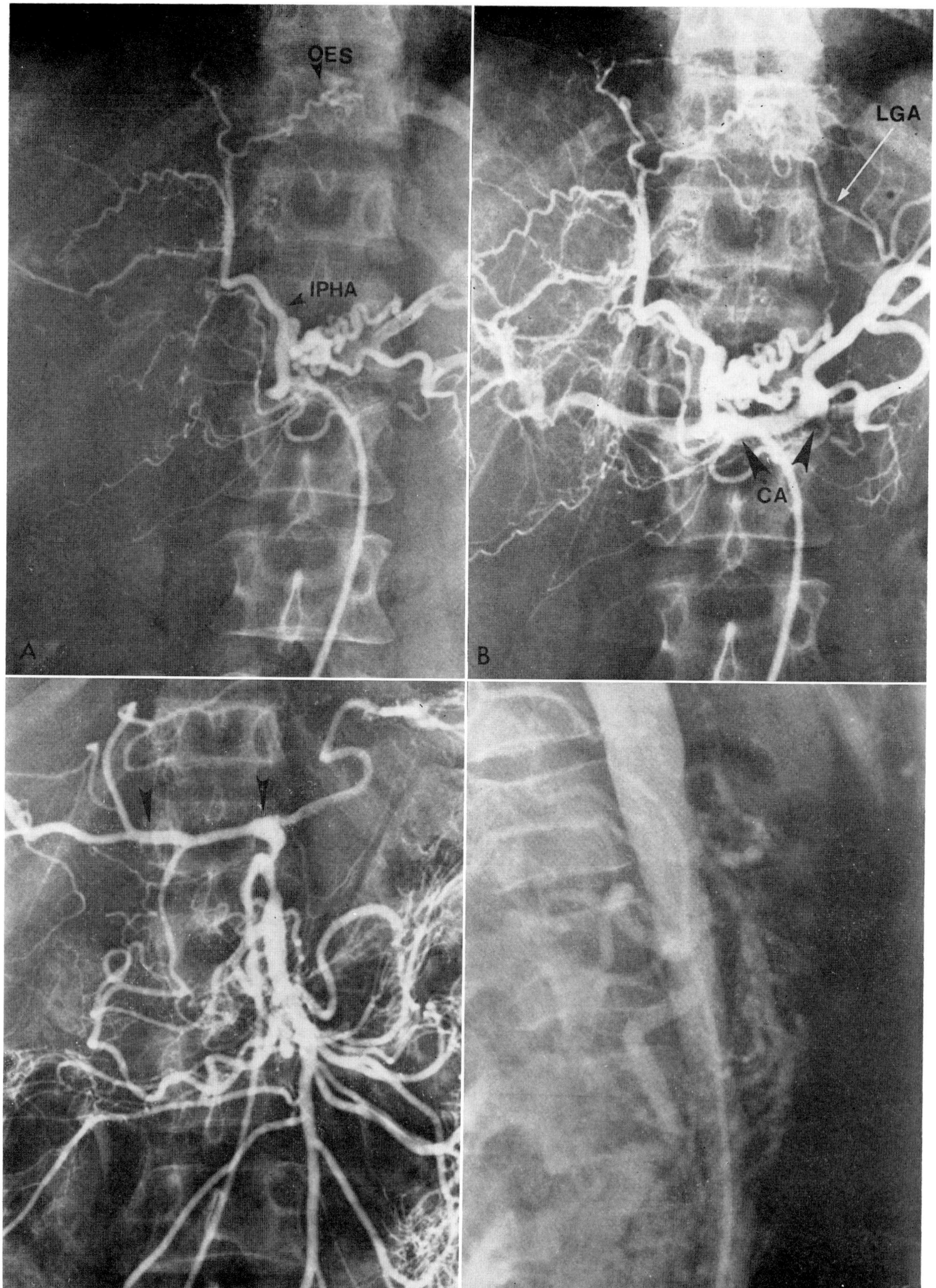
OES
IPHA
A
LGA
CA
B
C
D

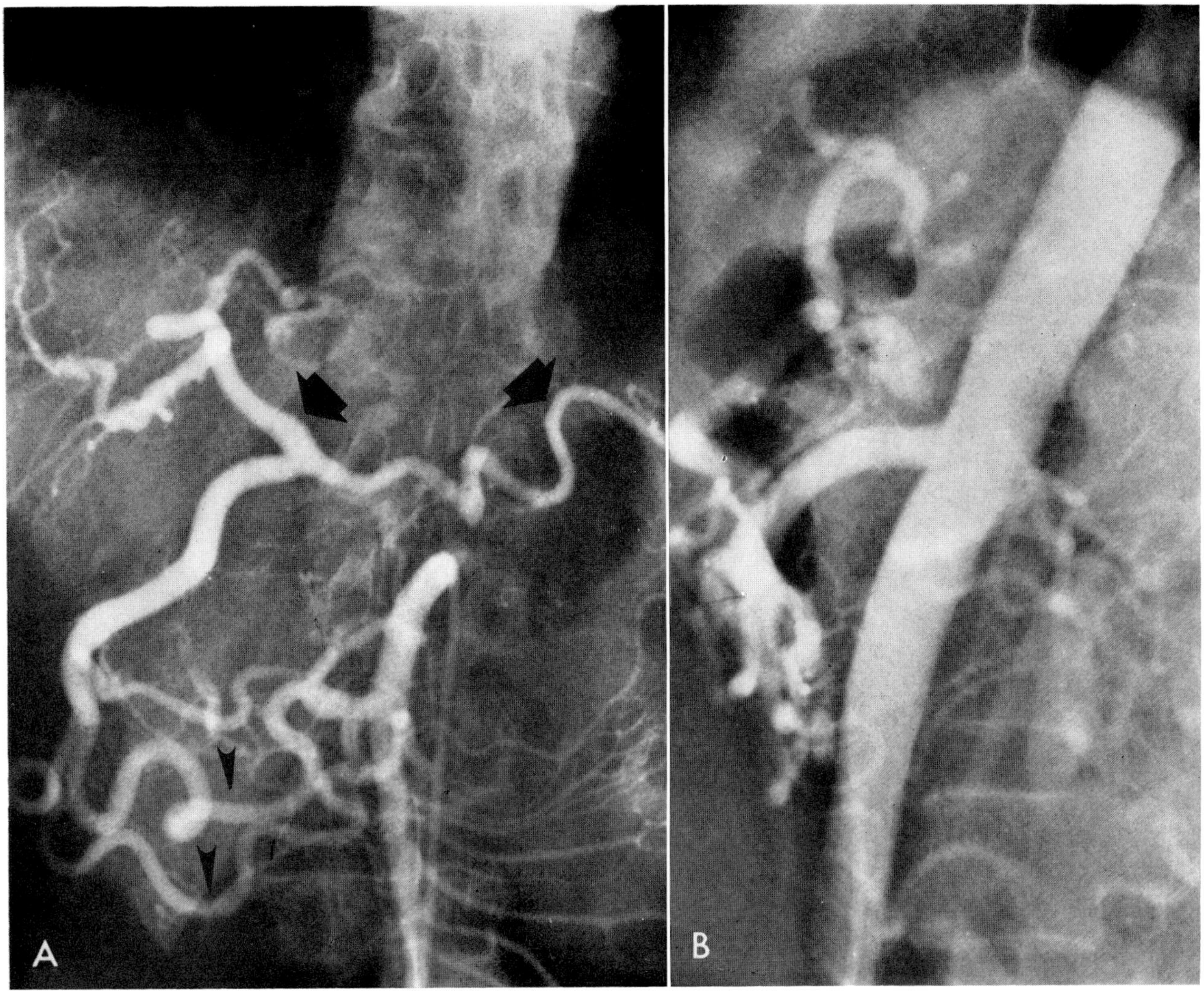

Figure 25.18. Superior Mesenteric Arteriogram. (A) There are tortuous dilated vessels (Arrow Head) from the superior mesenteric artery coursing along the duodenal sweep. These perfuse the hepatic (Arrow) and splenic (Arrow) arteries in a retrograde fashion. (B) A cross-table lateral aortogram: The celiac axis is not seen. The superior mesenteric artery origin is seen, however. The patient was a sixty-year-old with weight loss and backache. *Diagnosis:* Inoperable carcinoma of the body of the pancreas causing occlusion of the celiac axis due to encasement. The perfusion of the celiac branches was via inferior pancreaticoduodenal arteries.

←

Figure 25.17. *Right Inferior Phrenic Arteriogram.* (A) A prominent inferior phrenic artery (I.P.H.A.) fills the celiac axis (C.A.) via collaterals going from the esophageal branches (O.E.S.) to the left gastric artery (L.G.A.) and other collaterals. (B) The *midarterial phase* shows further filling of the celiac artery and its branches. *Superior mesenteric arteriogram.* (C) The celiac branches (Arrow) fill from the superior mesenteric arterial branches via the pancreatic arcade. (D) A *cross-table lateral aortogram.* Celiac axis does not visualize and there is narrowing of the proximal superior mesenteric trunk. This woman had postprandial abdominal pain. Of interest was reproduction of her identical abdominal pain during perfusion of the superior mesenteric artery with contrast. *Diagnosis:* Atherosclerotic occlusion of the celiac artery and atherosclerotic narrowing of the proximal superior mesenteric artery. Prominent collateral vessels arise from the inferior phrenic and superior mesenteric arteries. After surgery the patient had total relief of her abdominal pains and gained weight.

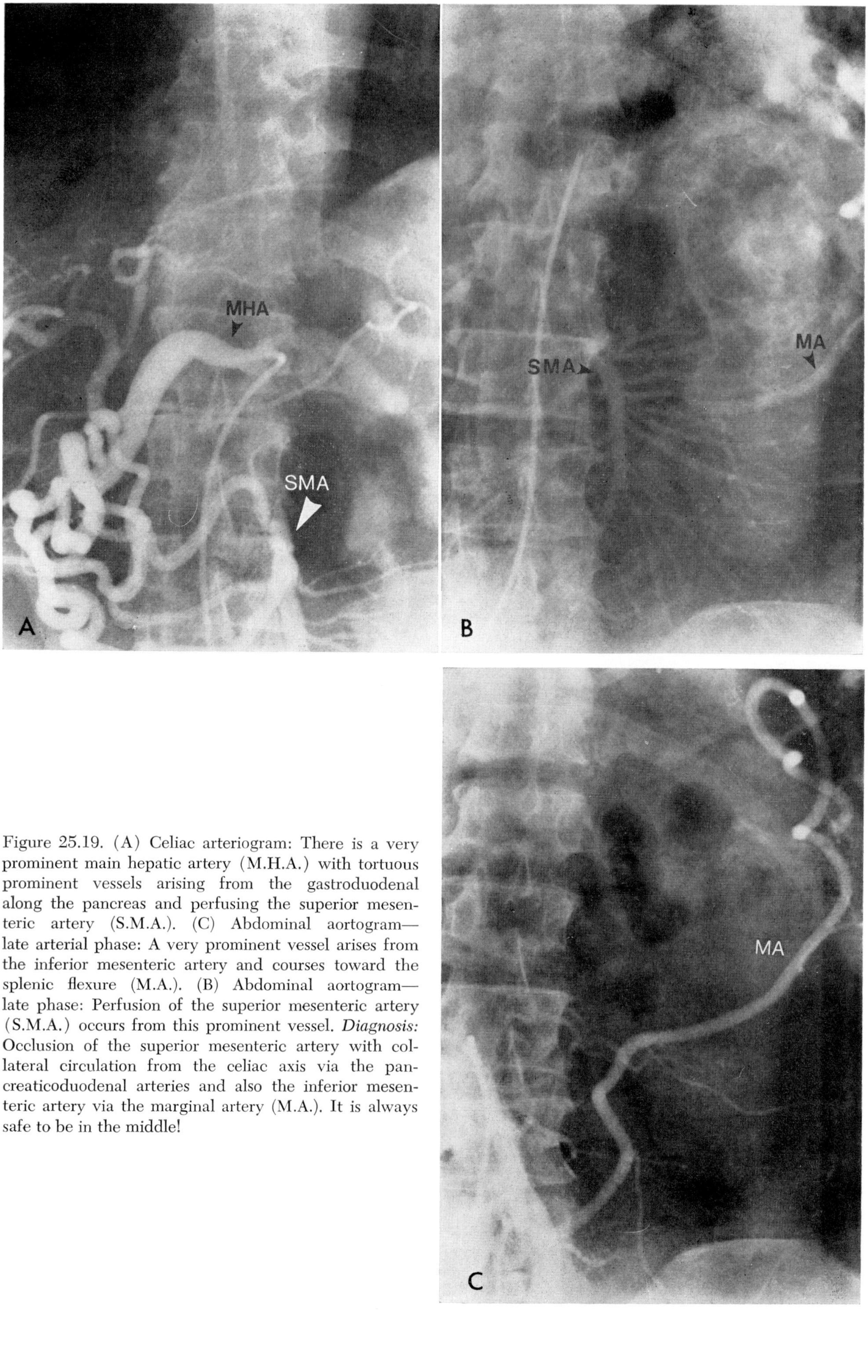

Figure 25.19. (A) Celiac arteriogram: There is a very prominent main hepatic artery (M.H.A.) with tortuous prominent vessels arising from the gastroduodenal along the pancreas and perfusing the superior mesenteric artery (S.M.A.). (C) Abdominal aortogram—late arterial phase: A very prominent vessel arises from the inferior mesenteric artery and courses toward the splenic flexure (M.A.). (B) Abdominal aortogram—late phase: Perfusion of the superior mesenteric artery (S.M.A.) occurs from this prominent vessel. *Diagnosis:* Occlusion of the superior mesenteric artery with collateral circulation from the celiac axis via the pancreaticoduodenal arteries and also the inferior mesenteric artery via the marginal artery (M.A.). It is always safe to be in the middle!

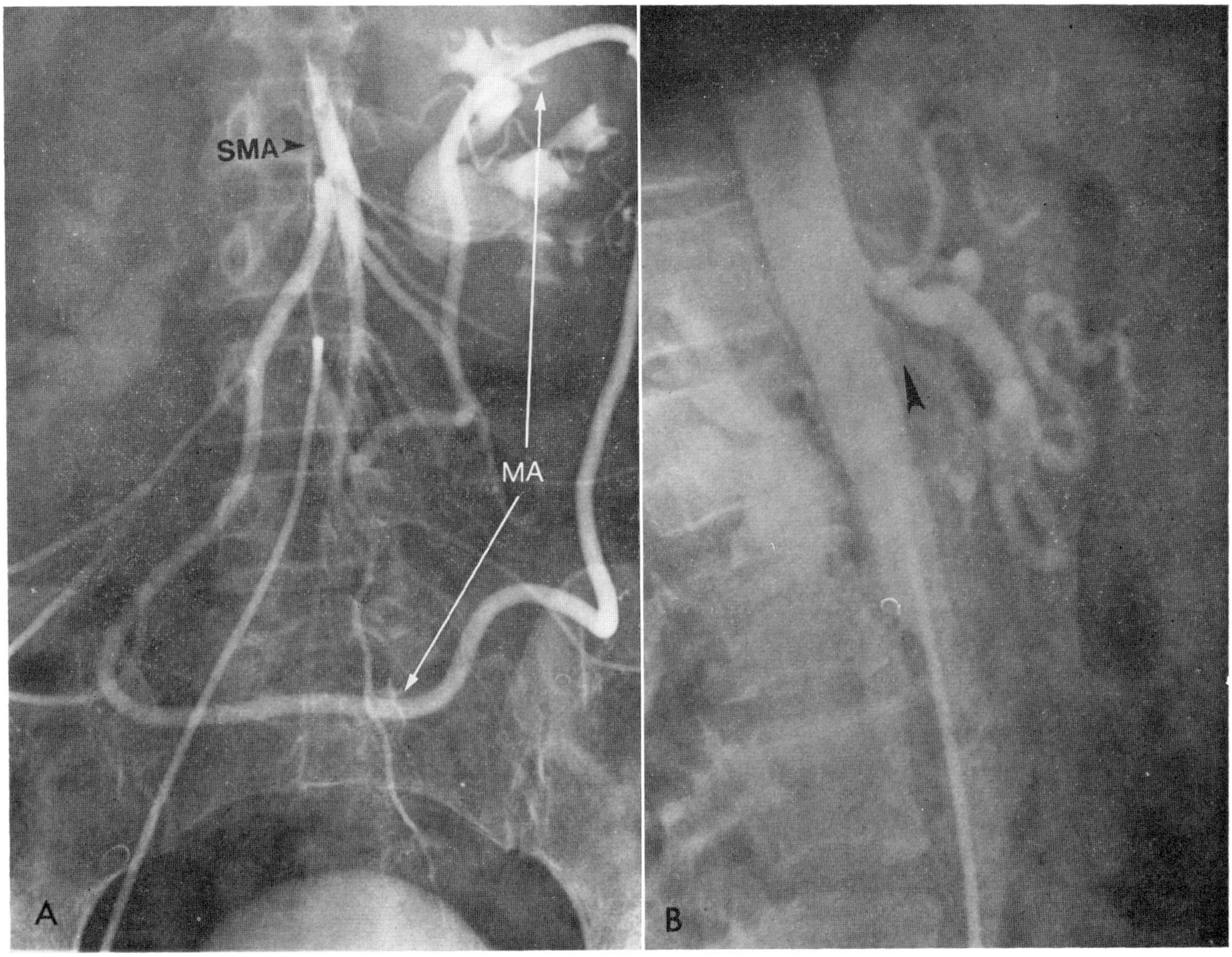

Figure 25.20. Selective Inferior Mesenteric Arteriogram. (A) A very prominent, tortuous branch along the colonic border courses towards the superior mesenteric artery (M.A.) with good opacification of the superior mesenteric artery (S.M.A.). (B) Cross-table lateral aortogram: marked concentric narrowing of the very proximal superior mesenteric artery (Arrow) is present. *Diagnosis:* Marked stenosis of the proximal superior mesenteric artery with good perfusion from the inferior mesenteric artery via the marginal artery.

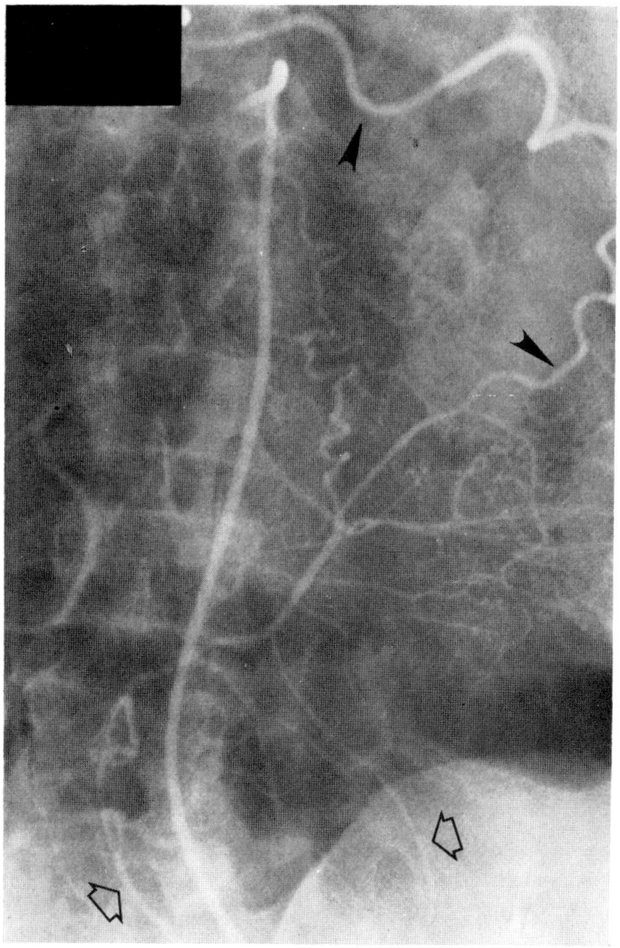

Figure 25.21. Superior Mesenteric Arteriogram—late arterial phase. There is good filling of the marginal artery (Arrow Head) perfusing the branches of the inferior mesenteric artery (Arrow) in a patient who had an aortic graft with surgical ligation of the inferior mesenteric artery. *Diagnosis:* Collateral circulation to the inferior mesenteric artery after surgical ligation.

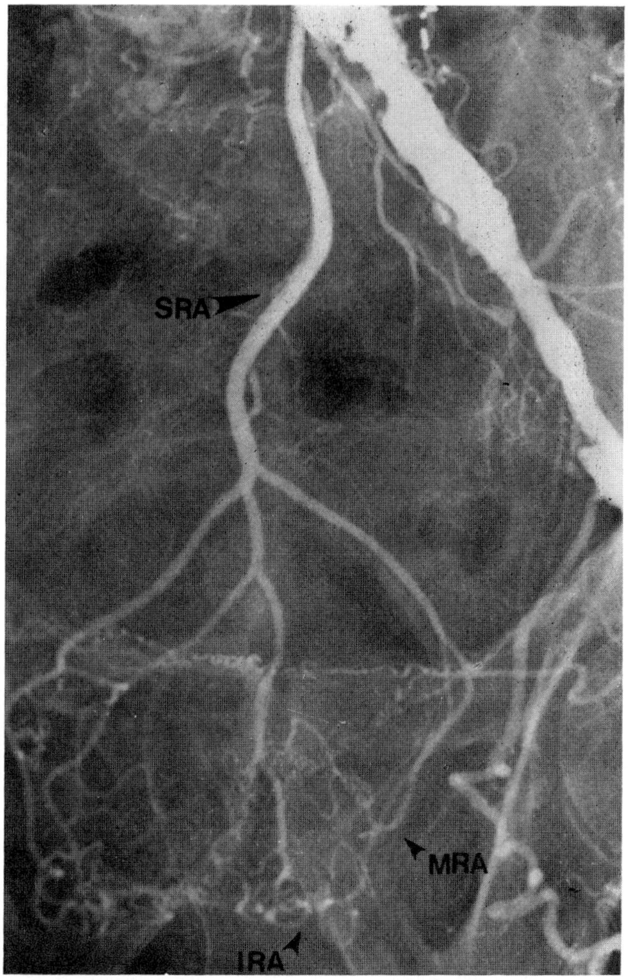

Figure 25.22. Translumbar Aortogram. Note the occlusion of the right common iliac artery, severe atherosclerosis of the left common iliac artery and external iliac artery and occlusion of the left internal iliac artery. Superior rectal artery (S.R.A.) with very prominent superior rectal branches is present. Middle rectal branches (M.R.A.) inferior rectal branches (I.R.A.). *Comment:* Severe arteriosclerosis of the abdominal aorta and occlusion of the above mentioned vessels, is seen. Very good opacification of the rectal plexus is noted.

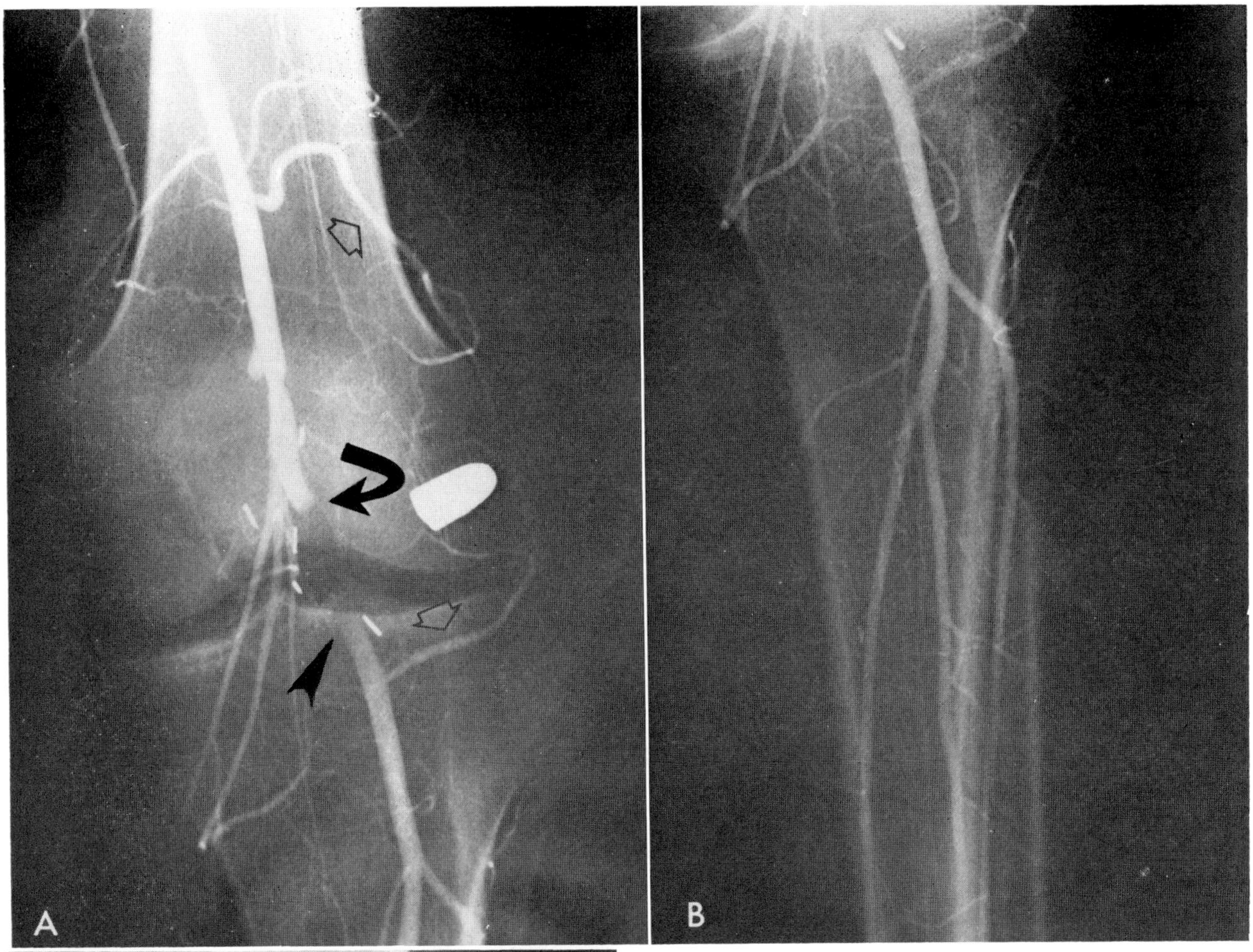

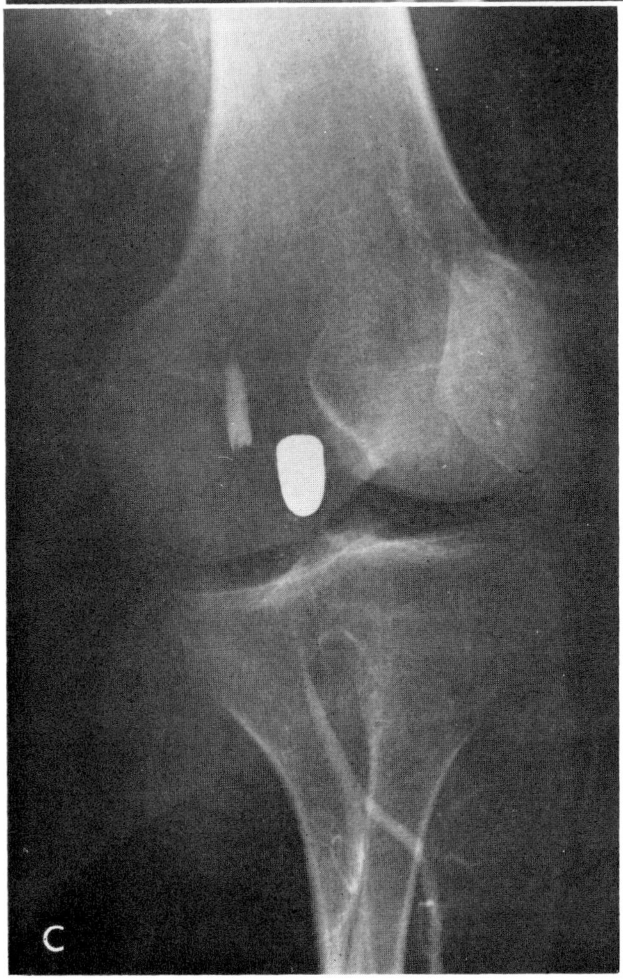

Figure 25.23. Femoral Arteriogram. (A) Abrupt termination of the proximal popliteal artery (Curved Arrow) with good filling of the distal popliteal artery (Arrow Head) via collateral vessels (Blank Arrow) is seen. Notice the bullet. (B) Very good filling of the popliteal artery and its branches via collaterals. This young patient had a recent gunshot wound. (C) Notice the stasis in the proximal popliteal artery. *Diagnosis:* Post-traumatic laceration of the artery with thrombosis. *Comment:* Very good collateral formation by-passing the occlusion in a young patient with otherwise normal vessels.

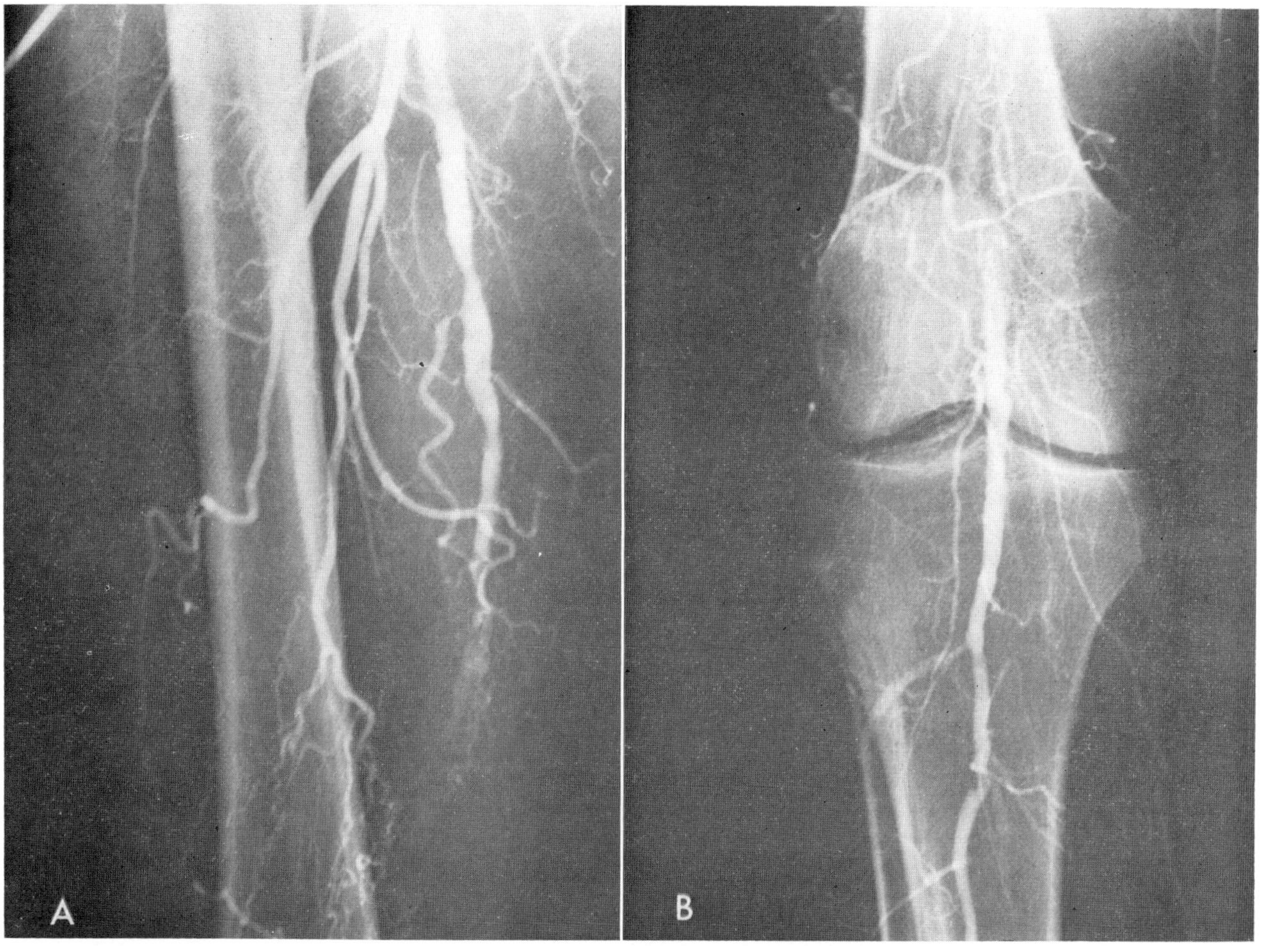

Figure 25.24. Femoral Arteriogram. (A) Alternate areas of irregular narrowing of the superficial femoral artery with termination at the adductor canal level is seen. There are very prominent tortuous, dilated, corkscrew branches from the deep femoral artery. (B) There is good filling of the popliteal artery via the collateral branches. *Diagnosis:* Atherosclerotic occlusion of the distal superficial femoral artery with moderate collateral circulation to the popliteal artery.

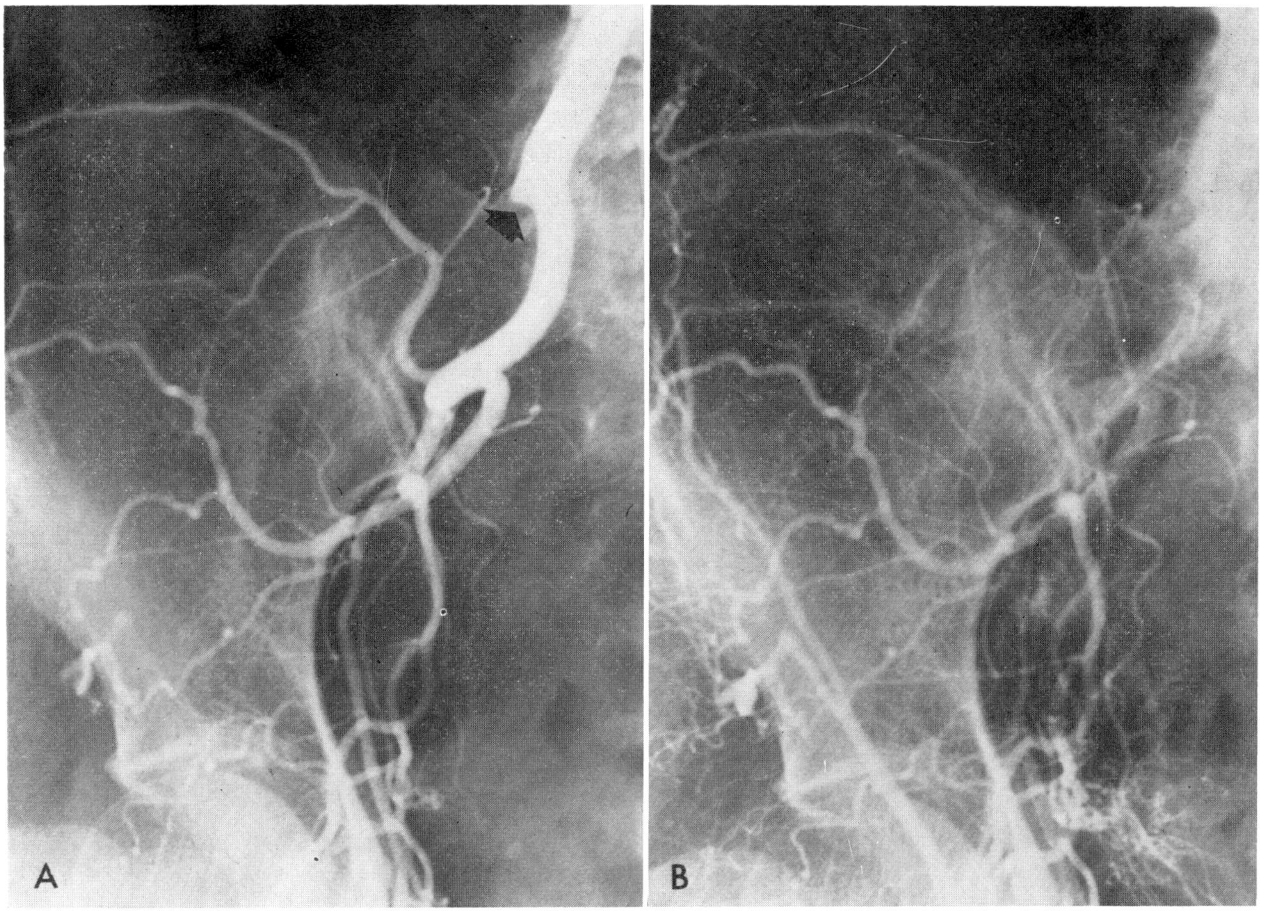

Figure 25.25. Right Common Iliac Arteriogram. (A) There is occlusion of the external iliac artery (Arrow) with collaterals originating from the internal iliac artery at the level of the gluteus maximus muscles. (B) Late phase: Reveals good collaterals. ***Diagnosis:*** Inadvertent surgical ligation of the right external iliac artery with development of good collateral flow.

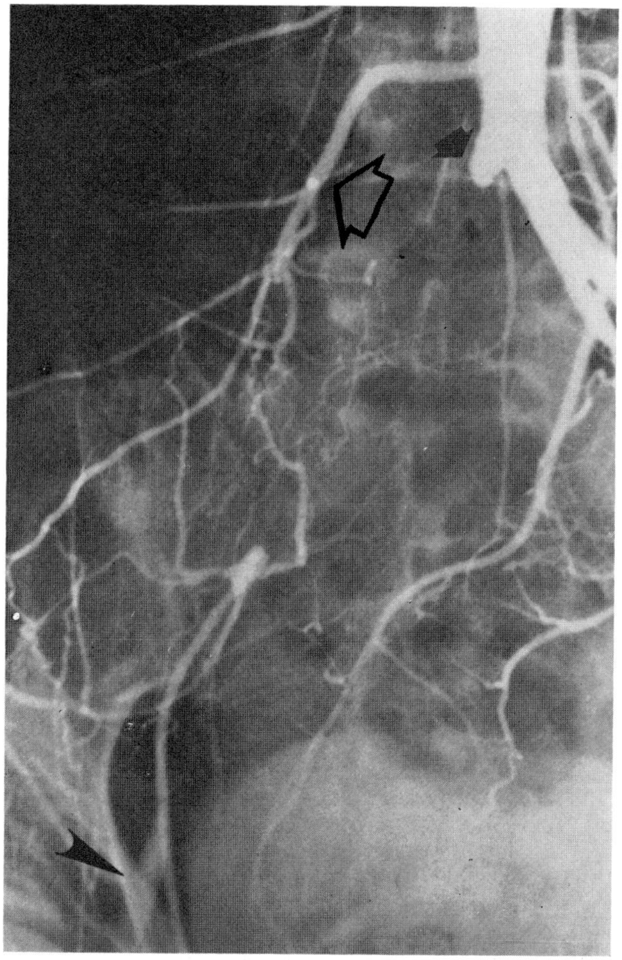

Figure 25.26. Pelvic Arteriogram. The right common iliac artery (Arrow) does not fill but the external iliac artery (Arrow Head) fills via prominent collaterals from the lumbar artery (Blank Arrow). *Diagnosis:* Atherosclerotic occlusion of the right common iliac artery.

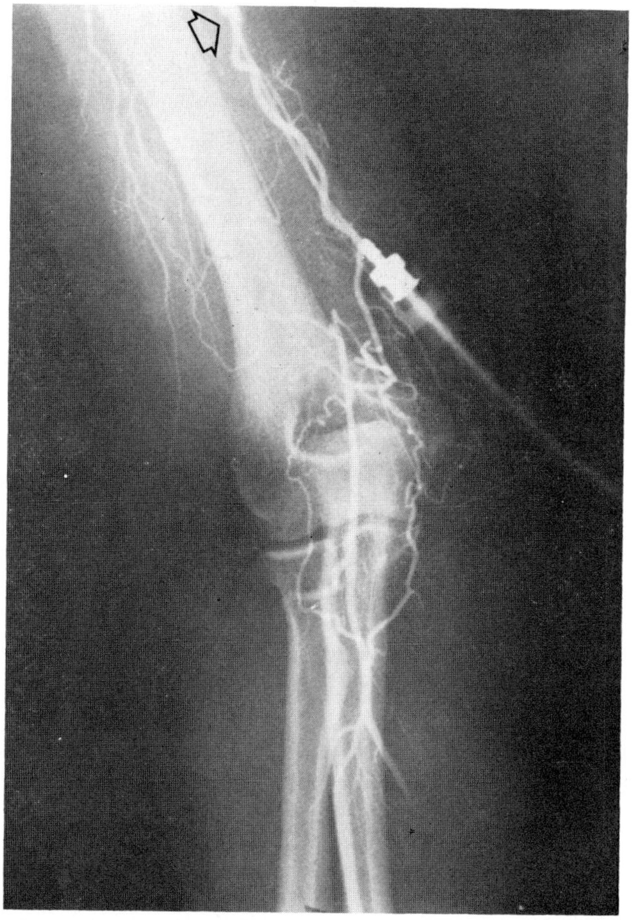

Figure 25.27. Brachial Arteriogram. There is occlusion of the distal brachial artery (Arrow) with collateral circulation trying to by-pass the occluded site. *Diagnosis:* Occlusion due to prior cutdown and arteriotomy.

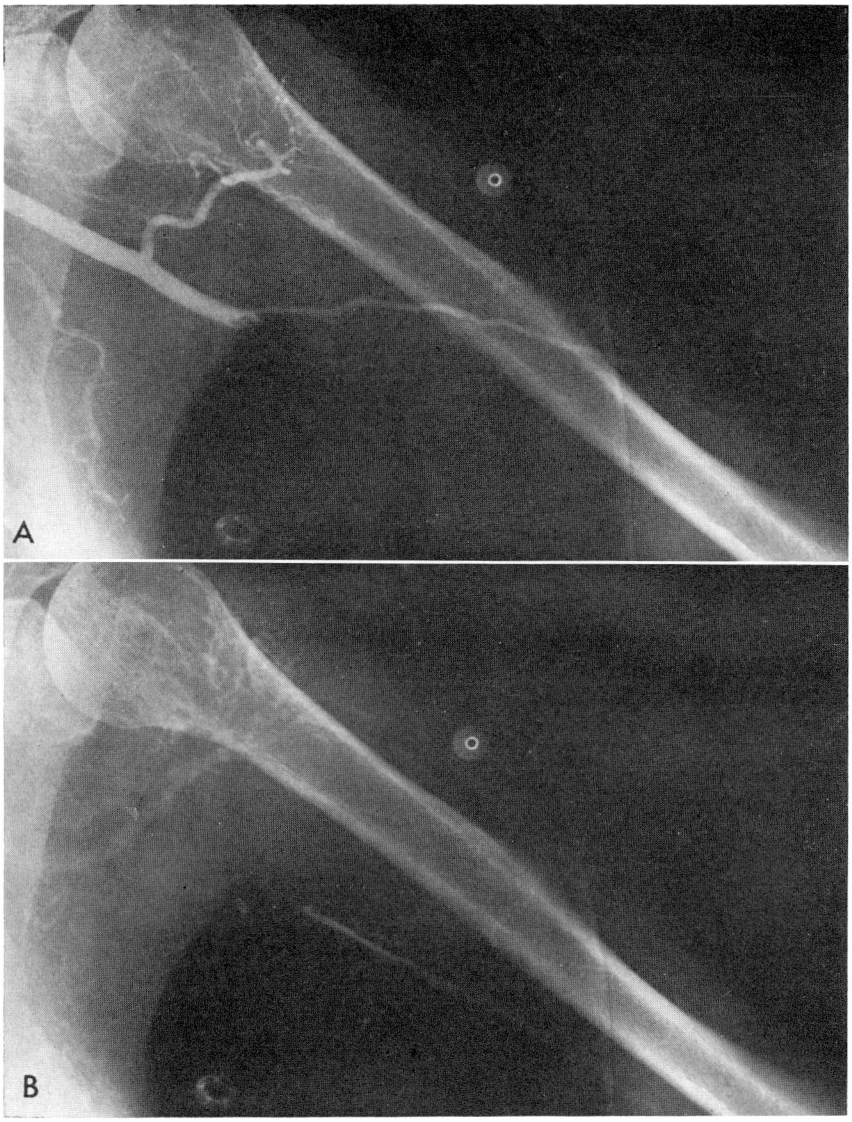

Figure 25.28. Brachial Arteriogram. (A) Early phase: Note the abrupt termination of the brachial artery with a filling defect and a prominent proximal collateral. (B) Late phase: The distal brachial artery fills via this collateral. *Diagnosis:* Embolus to brachial artery probably from a mural thrombus in the heart.

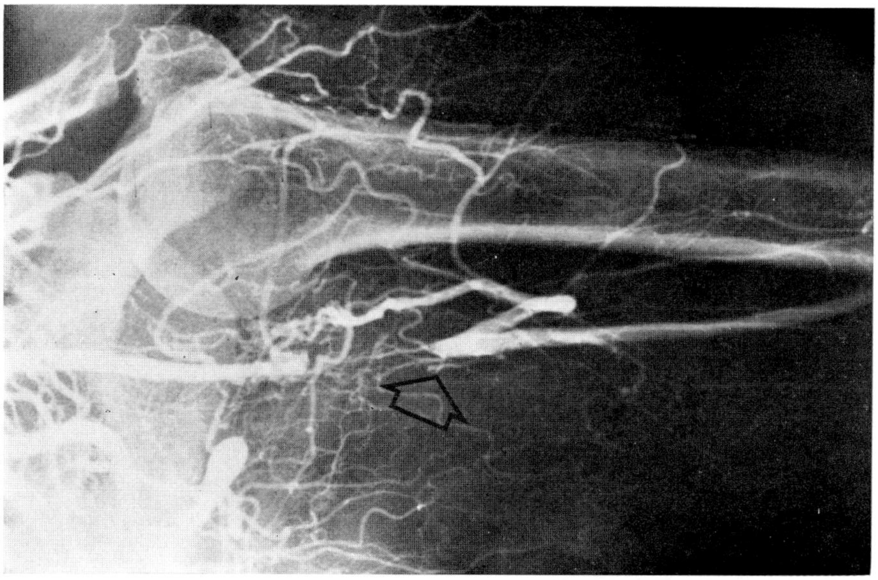

Figure 25.29. Left Subclavian Angiogram. The proximal brachial artery does not visualize; however, there is good filling of the distal brachial (Arrow) via collaterals. *Diagnosis:* Postcatheterization thrombosis.

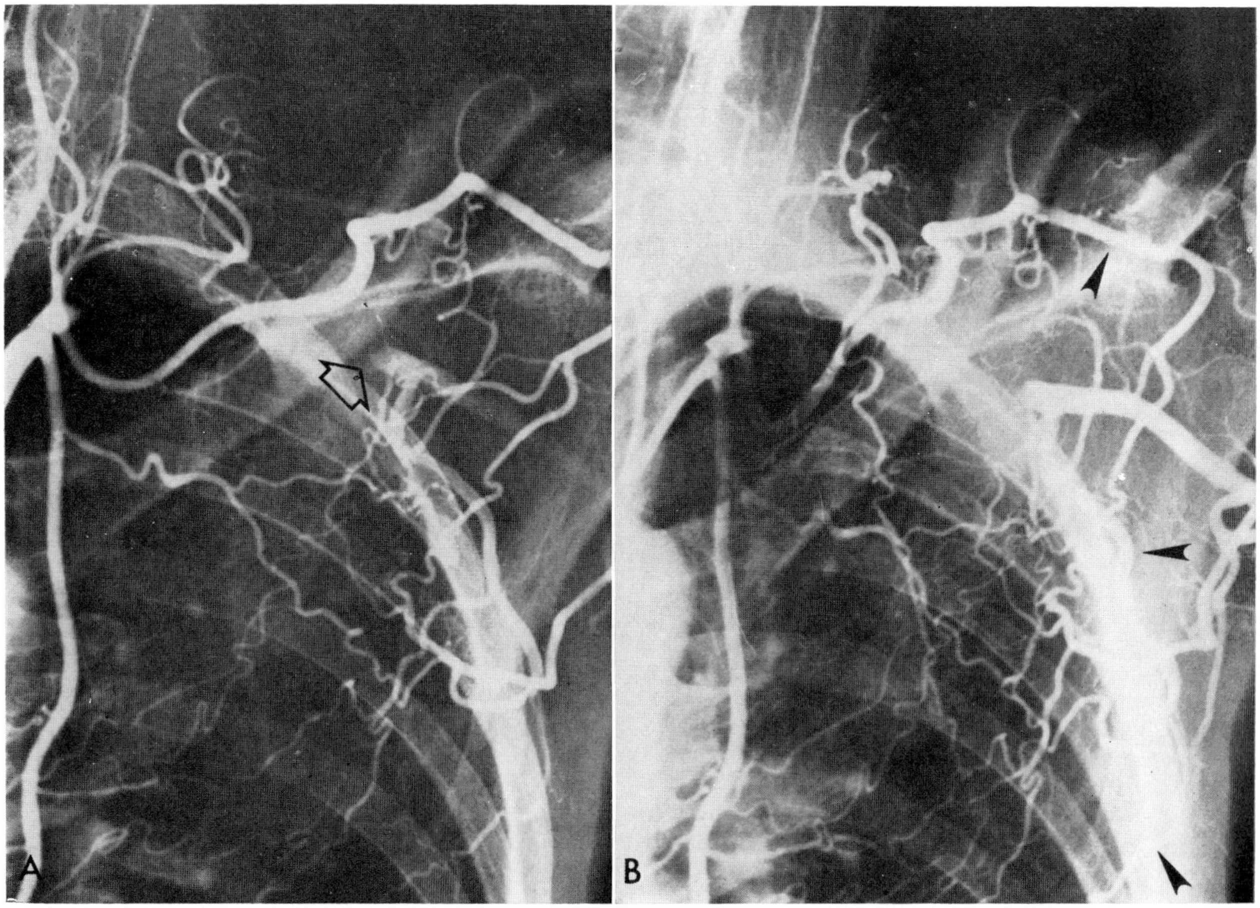

Figure 25.30. Subclavian Arteriogram. The subclavian artery does not visualize, but there is good collateral flow to the axillary artery (Arrow). *Diagnosis:* Traumatic thrombosis of the subclavian artery. The trauma occurred three months prior to the angiography.

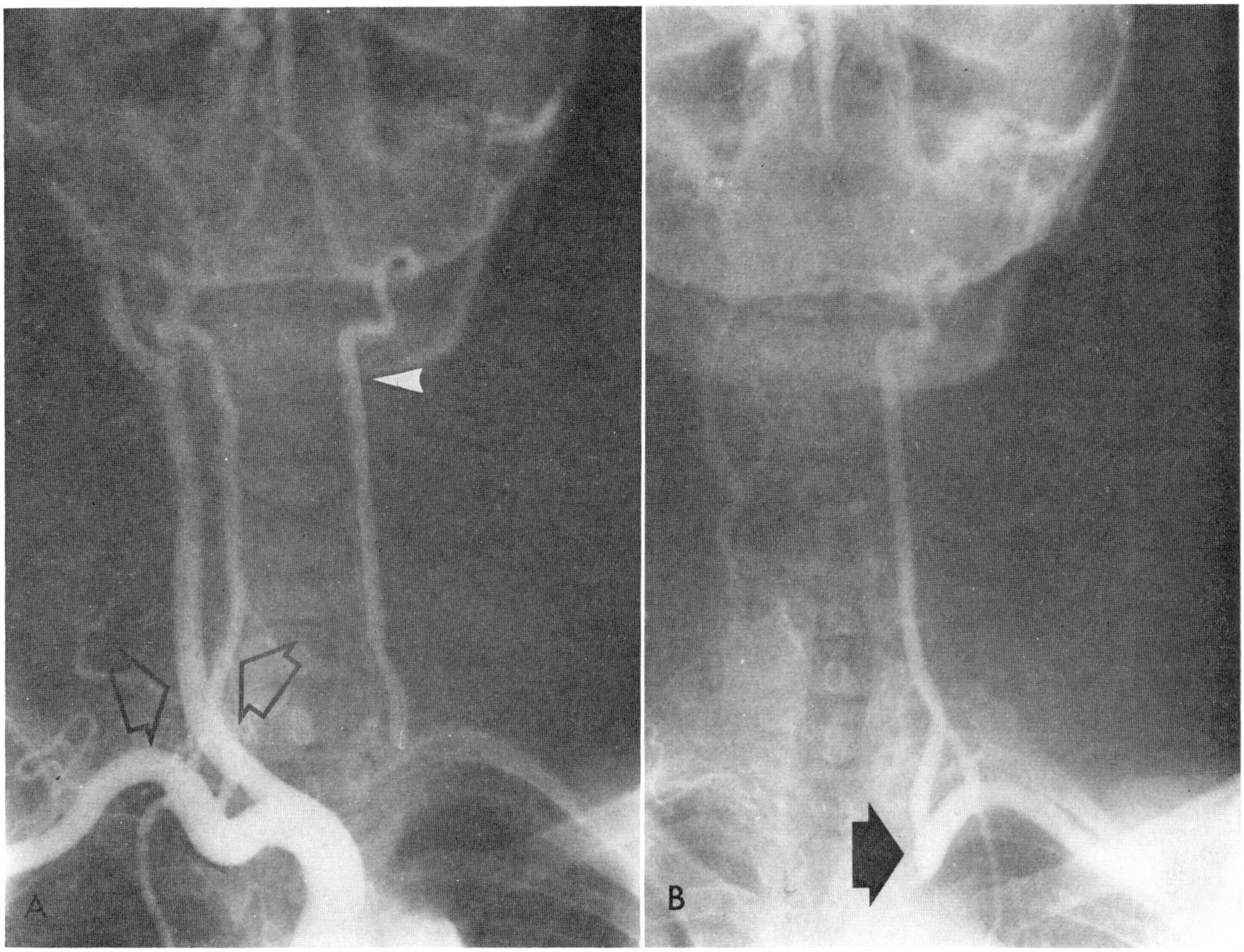

Figure 25.31. Innominate Arteriogram. (A) There is filling of the right common carotid artery, right vertebral artery (Arrow) and visualization of the left vertebral artery (Arrow Head) via the basilar artery. (B) Late arterial phase: There is good opacification of the left vertebral artery and the subclavian artery with a proximal abrupt termination (Arrow). *Diagnosis:* Subclavian steal due to atherosclerotic occlusion of the left proximal subclavian artery.

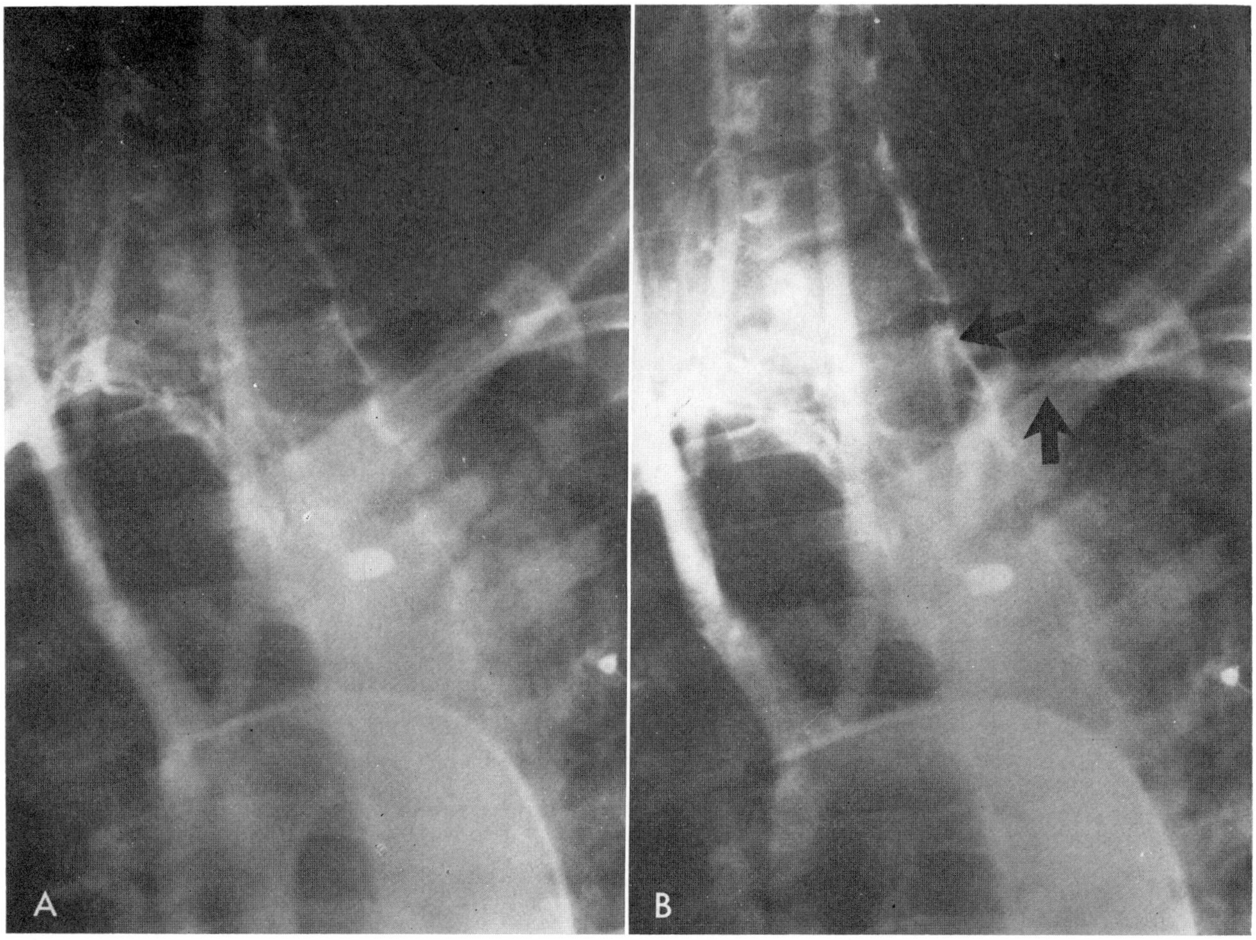

Figure 25.32. Aortic Arch Angiogram—(L.A.O. projection). (A) The left subclavian artery does not fill. (B) There is delayed filling of the left subclavian artery via the vertebral. Note the metallic, bullet-like density. *Diagnosis:* Traumatic subclavian artery occlusion with collaterals via the vertebral. "Traumatic subclavian steal."

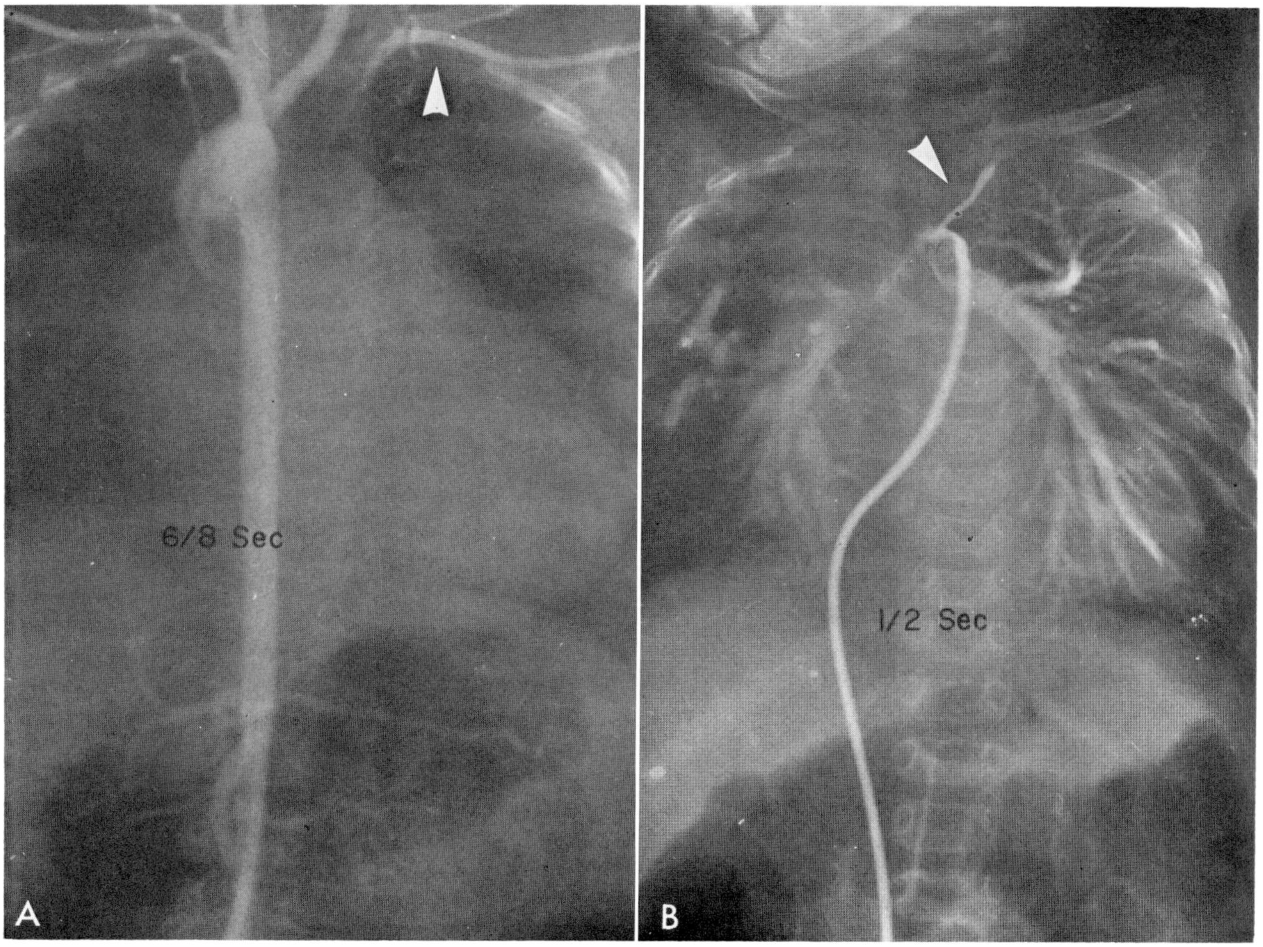

Figure 25.33. Aortic Arch Angiogram. (A) A right-sided aortic arch with no filling of the left subclavian artery from the arch: It is filling from the collaterals across the neck. (B) A pulmonary arteriogram shows the origin of the left subclavian artery. *Diagnosis:* Isolated origin of the left subclavian artery in a patient with a right sided aortic arch. Another steal.

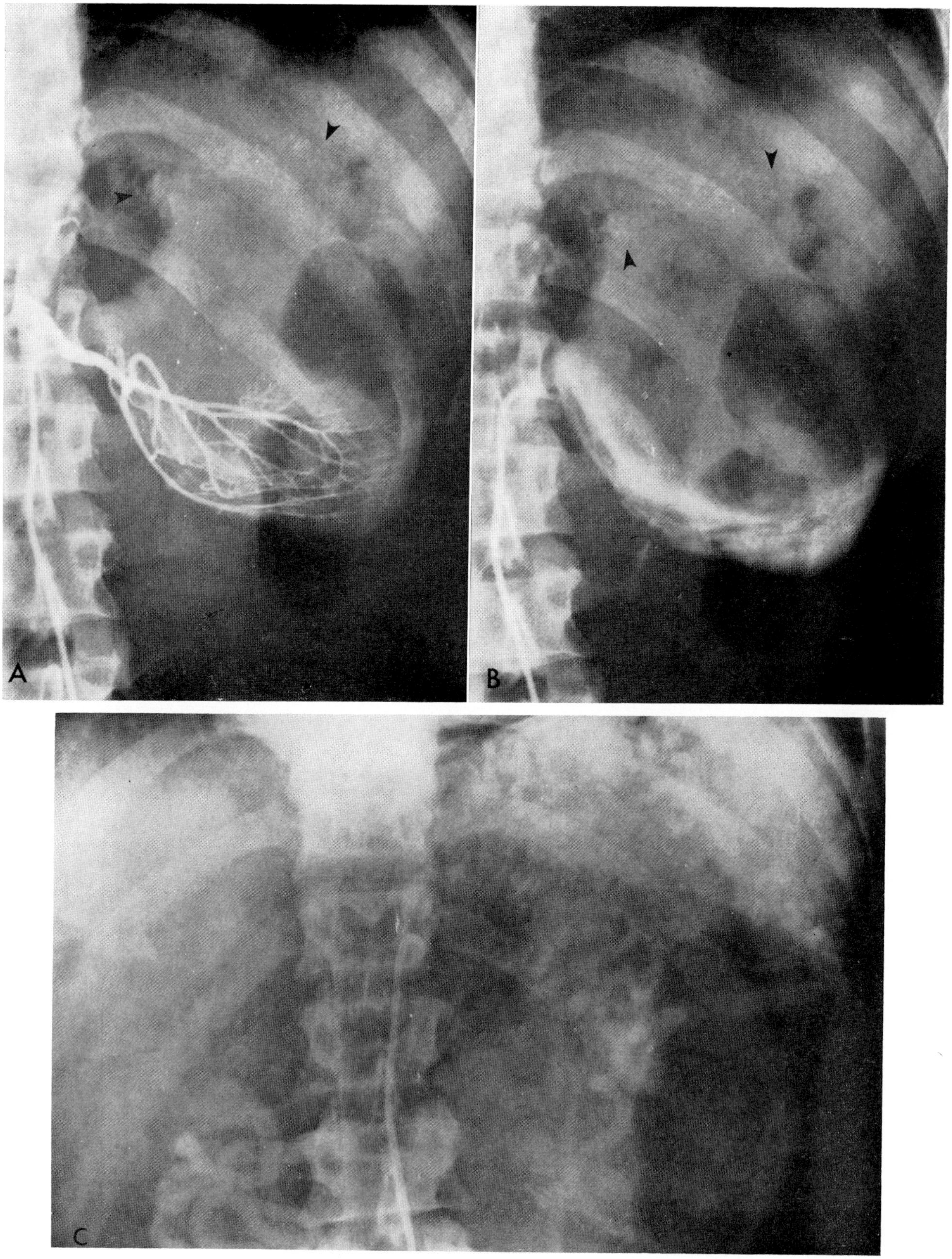

Figure 25.34. (A) Selective renal arteriogram: Partial perfusion of the distorted kidney occurs. (B) Parenchymal phase: A moderately sized filling defect within the renal parenchyma with secondary compression of the opacified renal parenchyma is seen. Notice the faint calcific densities (Arrow). (C) Late phase of the splenic arteriogram: Very prominent tortuous collateral veins are present along the lesser and greater curvature of the stomach and omentum. *Diagnosis:* A pseudocyst of the pancreas with invasion of the kidney and splenic vein thrombosis.

able collaterals are small and insignificant.[365] As a result *occlusion of the hepatic artery may be fatal in some but not in others.*

The hepatic circulation supplies *an end artery organ,* as there is no intrahepatic communication between the right and left hepatic arteries. There is an avascular plane between the right and left lobes of the liver. A good attempt at collateral flow is made by the replaced hepatic artery, vessels of the greater and lesser curvature of the stomach, vessels of the hepatic capsule (inferior phrenic and intercostal arteries), and through the arteries of the ligaments of the liver and pancreatic arcade.[475–477]

Lower Extremity Collaterals

Collateral circulation via the deep femoral artery is excellent when long segments of the superior femoral artery are occluded.[478] In total femoropopliteal occlusion there is very poor collateral circulation. In total popliteal occlusion also the collateral circulation is extremely poor.

The Steals

Certain vascular units or hypervascular lesions in general can *siphon* blood from the adjacent available vascular conduits either for their existence or because of their opportune location. Such lesions obviously deprive the primary circulation of its regular quota of blood. In addition, however, there is insufficient contribution to the interposed parasitic circulation also. The clinical effects of such an unwelcome, obligatory sharing are due to the ischemic effects on both the primary and the parasitic circulation. Because of this decrease in blood supply, the underperfused organs are vulnerable. The siphonage is due to maintenance of circulation to a vital organ whose primary vascular supply is terminated, excessive demands from a metabolically superior lesion (tumor), or decreased resistance causing shunting (arteriovenous fistula).

Subclavian Steal

Discrete localized obstruction of the subclavian artery, proximal to the origin of the vertebral artery, causes decreased flow to that arm, low pressure distal to the obstruction, retrograde flow down the collateral channels into the subclavian artery beyond the obstruction, and associated ischemic changes in the limb or the brain.[454–456] A pressure gradient of 20 mm of Hg is needed before any reversal of flow in the ipsilateral vertebral artery can occur. A brachial artery pressure difference of 20 mm Hg is compatible with the diagnosis of subclavian steal.[437] *The steal may be unilateral or bilateral,*[445] *and may or may not be associated with symptoms.*[446] Exercising the arm may cause a reversal of flow in case a neutral study does not demonstrate a reversal.[447] A favorable response to surgical treatment is suggested if the cerebral manifestations are eliminated by inflating a blood pressure cuff on the arm to the level of systolic blood pressure.[448] The total decrease in cerebral blood flow with only a subclavian steal is 10 to 20 percent. *Subclavian steals per se may not produce any intracranial manifestations.* If, however, the steal is associated with occlusion of the other intracranial vessels, further decreases in the flow may cause cerebral manifestations.[451–453]

While *atherosclerosis is the most common cause* for the occlusion of a subclavian artery, other causes may produce the same findings. These include atresia of the subclavian artery,[438] embolus to the subclavian artery,[439] blunt trauma,[440] and postsurgical thrombosis (Blalock-Taussig procedures),[441] tumor thrombus,[442] Takayasu's arteritis,[442] pseudocoarctation with kinking of the subclavian artery,[443] and a right sided aortic arch with isolation of the left subclavian artery.[444]

The *collaterals*[447, 449, 450] appearing after the occlusion of the subclavian artery proximal to the origin of the vertebral artery depend on the patency of the collateral vessels and anatomic configurations and variations. The collateral routes are from the contralateral vertebral artery via the basilar artery; the external carotid to the vertebral artery via the occipital and muscular branches respectively, the muscular branches of the neck vessels (costocervical,

(*Text continues on page 385*)

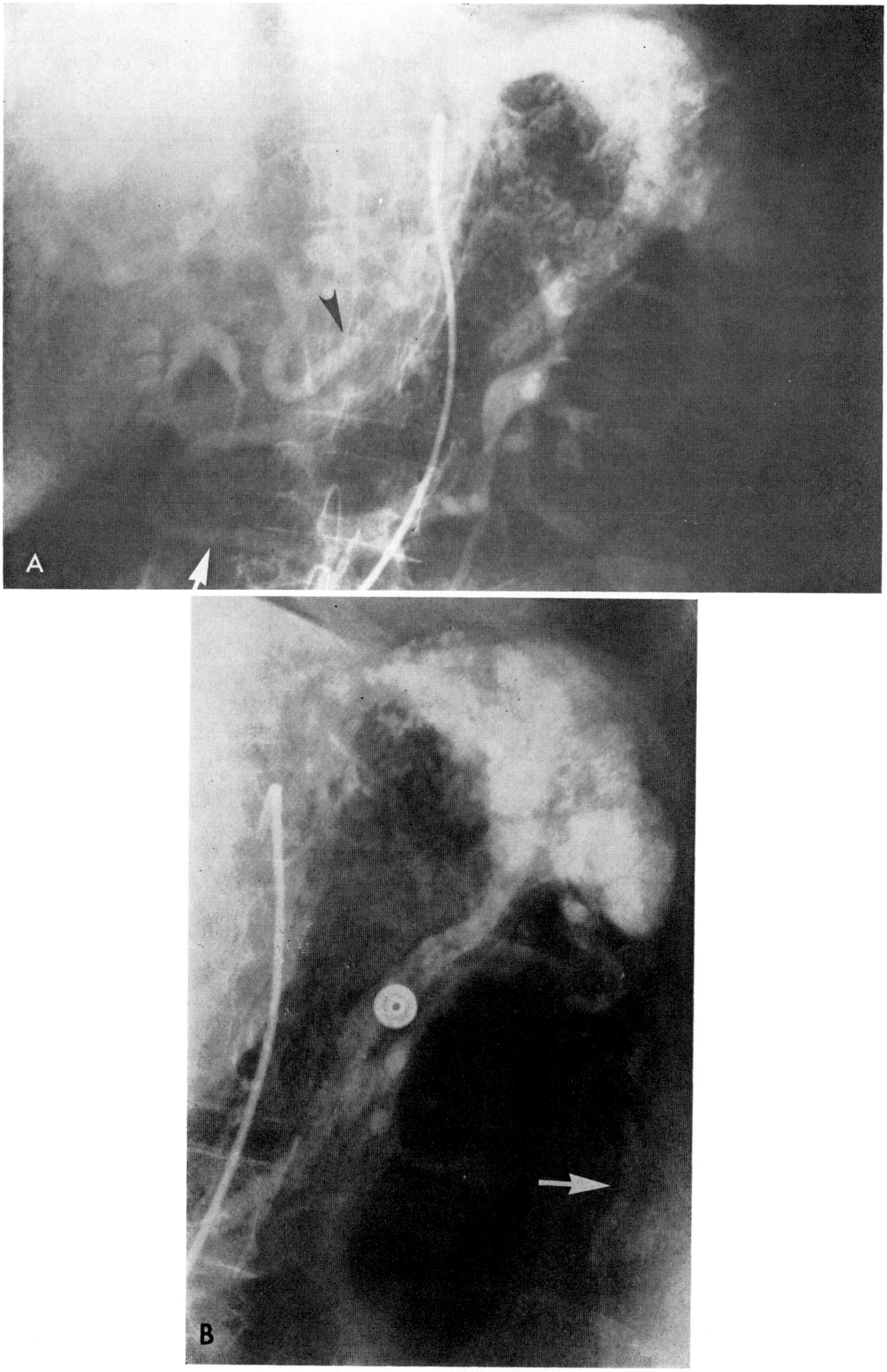

Figure 25.35 A and B

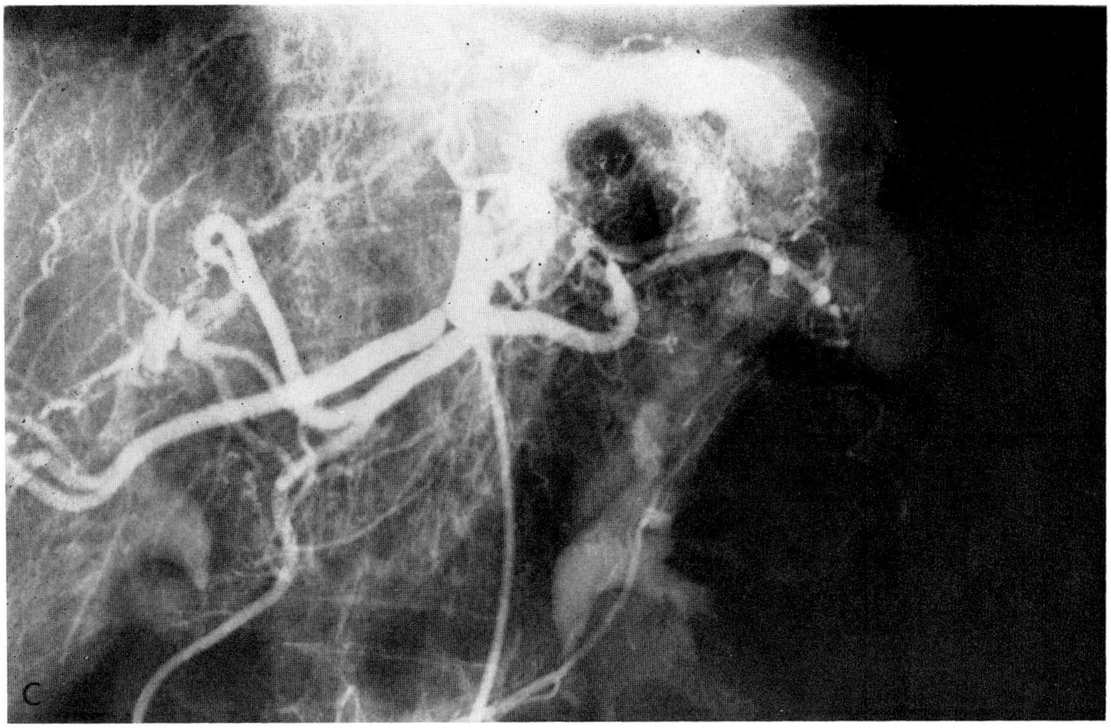

Figure 25.35 (A) Venous phase of celiac arteriogram reveals prominent veins along greater and lesser curvatures of the stomach, opacifying the portal vein. (B) Close up of the left upper quadrant reveals tortuous fundal and omental veins. (C) Celiac arteriogram of the same patient. *Diagnosis:* Splenic vein thrombosis due to pancreatitis.

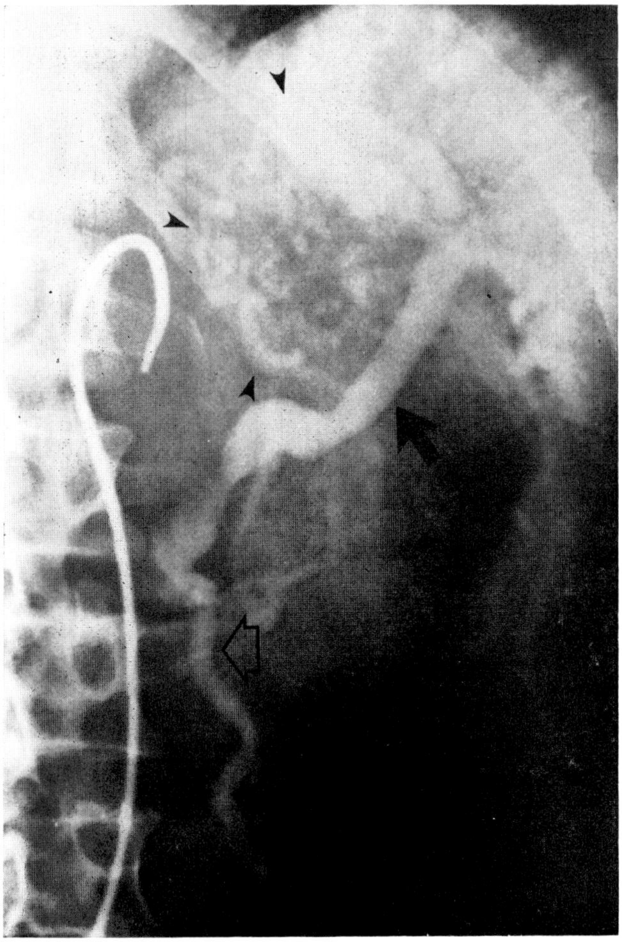

Figure 25.36. Celiac Arteriogram—venous phase. Tortuous veins are seen at the fundus of the stomach (Arrow Head). There is no visualization of the portal venous circulation beyond the splenic vein (Arrow). The patient had weight loss and backache. *Diagnosis:* Carcinoma of the body of the pancreas with occlusion of the splenic vein due to encasement. Collateral drainage bypassed this obstruction.

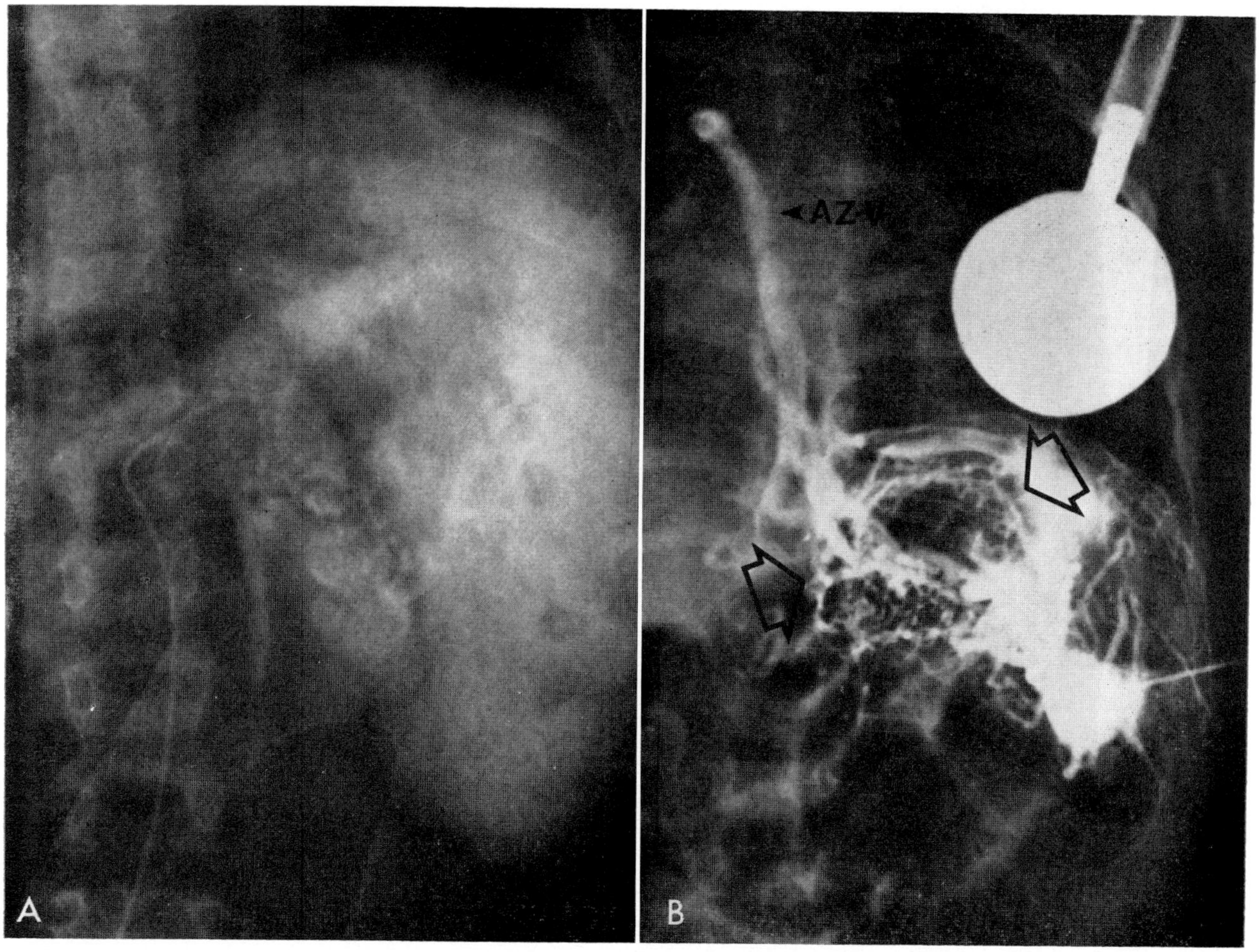

Figure 25.37. (A) Celiac arteriogram: The spleen is enlarged and the splenic vein is not seen. This twelve-year-old patient had esophageal varices. (B) Percutaneous splenoportogram (ten years prior to the preceding examination). Tortuous fundic collaterals (Arrow) fill the azygos vein (AZ.V.) via the esophageal and paraesophageal veins. *Diagnosis:* Splenic and portal vein thrombosis with collateral drainage into the azygos vein via esophageal varices.

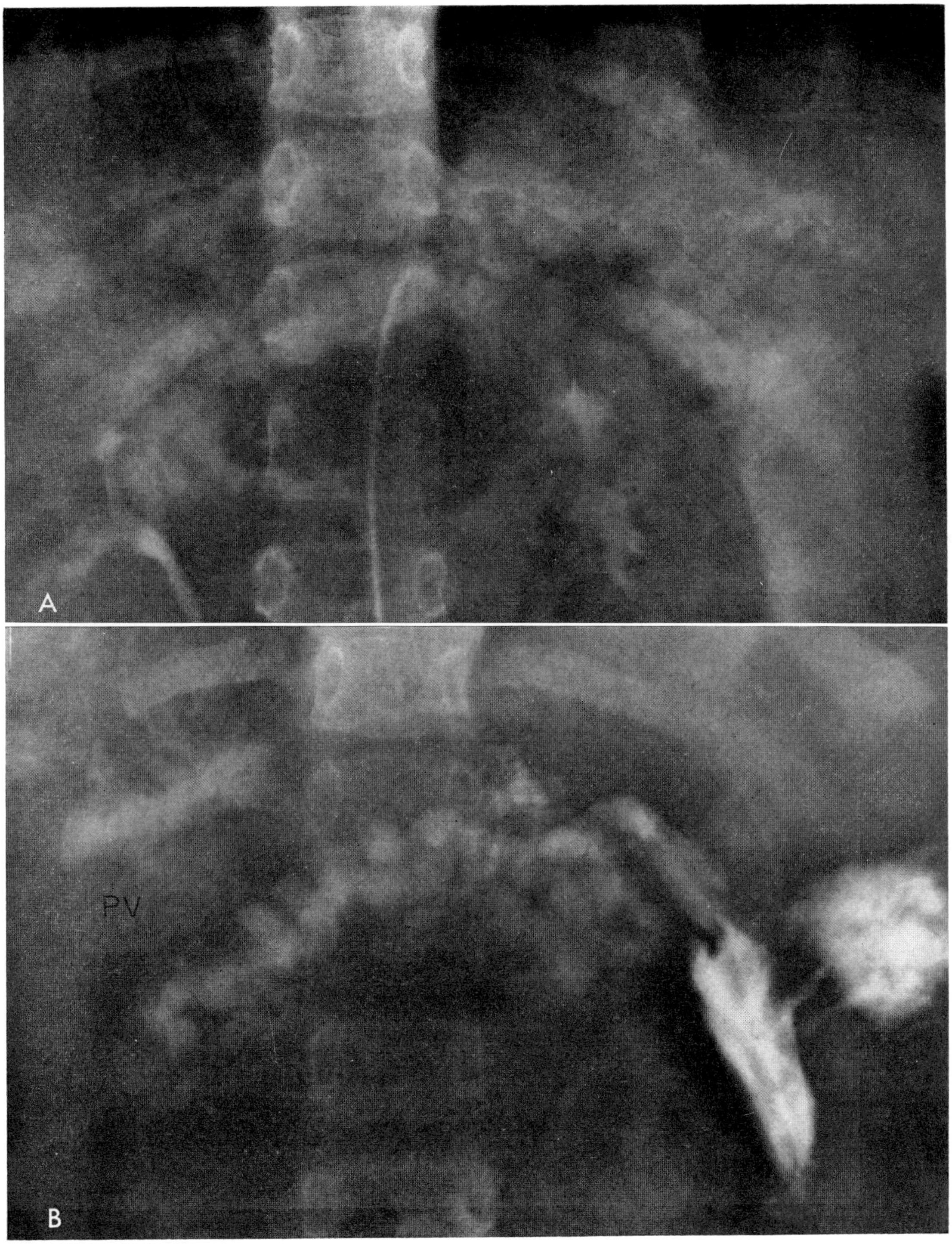

Figure 25.38. (A) Celiac arteriogram—venous phase: The spleen is enlarged and the splenic vein is not seen. (B) Percutaneous splenoportogram: Numerous tortuous veins are seen filling the portal vein (P.V.). This young patient had esophageal varices. *Diagnosis:* Portal vein thrombosis with hepatopetal collaterals.

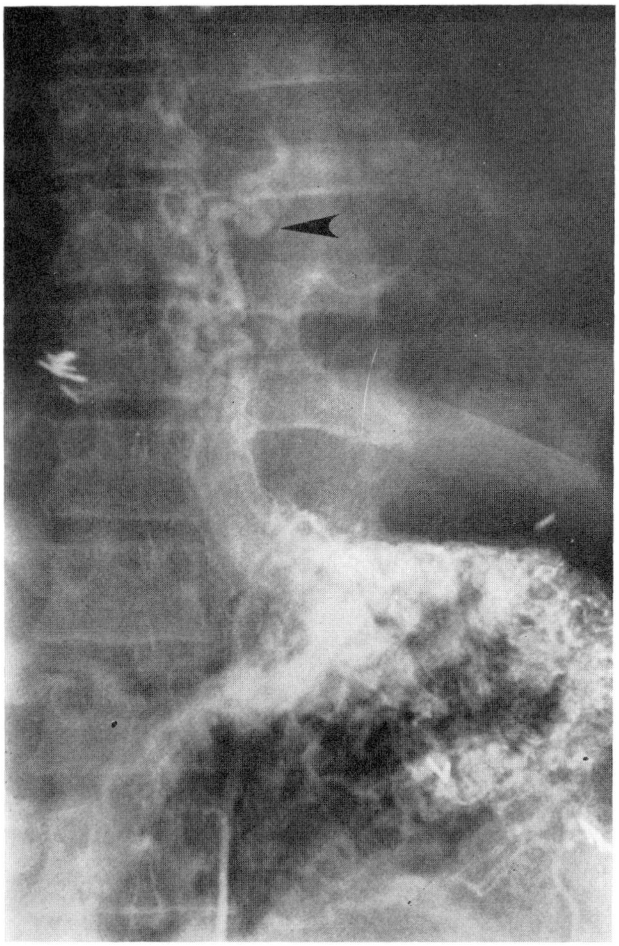

Figure 25.39. Left Gastric Arteriogram. There are dilated tortuous veins coursing toward the esophagus. The patient was known to have had alcoholic cirrhosis. *Diagnosis:* Esophageal varices.

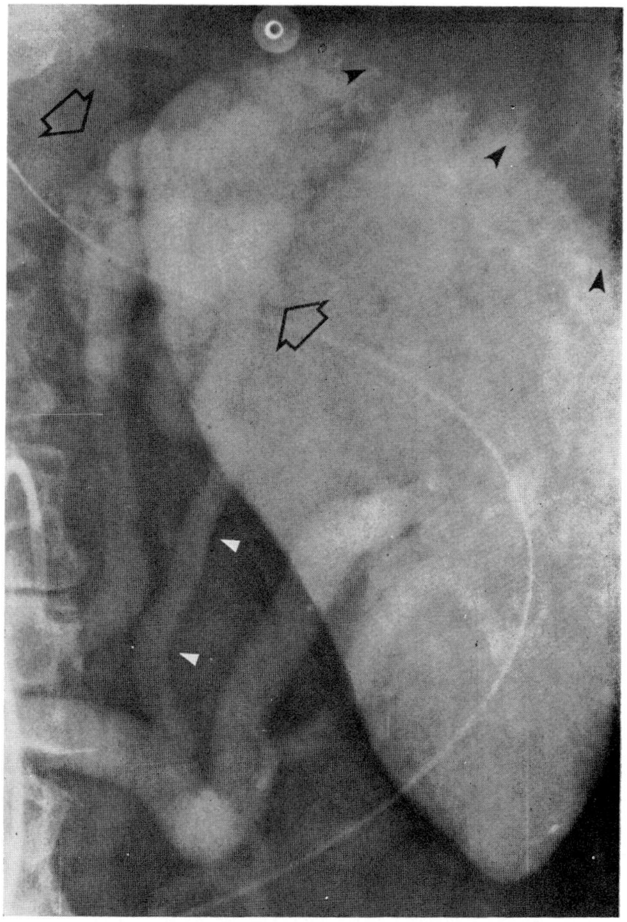

Figure 25.40. Splenic Arteriogram—venous phase: There are tortuous dilated veins (Blank Arrow) in the gastric fundus which are drained by the left gastric vein (Arrow Head). Incidentally seen is splenomegaly and infarcts (Arrow Head). The patient had portal hypertension. *Diagnosis:* Splenomegaly with infarcts. Gastric varices due to portal hypertension.

thyrocervical, vertebral), and across the midline at the level of the thyroid gland. Variations which modify the presence or absence of cerebral symptoms include direct origin of the vertebral artery from the aortic arch and asymmetry in the size of vertebral arteries. Total extra cerebral collateral supply from the thyrocervical, costocervical, and internal mammary arteries may maintain sufficient pressure to prevent siphonage of the blood from the brain to the arm. *Reversal of flow*[270, 457] in the vertebral artery may occur even without any occlusion of the subclavian or innominate arteries. This is due to various factors such as increased intrabronchial pressure or the injection of a large bolus under high pressure near the orifice of the vertebral arteries. Positioning of the head also influences the reversal of flow in a normal vertebral artery (Figs. 25-31 to 25-33).

Innominate Steal

The collaterals, trying to bypass the occluded innominate artery, are more complicated and are associated with significant hemodynamic imbalance than that with isolated subclavian artery occlusions.[458, 459]

Aorto-iliac Steal

Patients having major vascular occlusion of the splanchnic system or of the lower extremity vessels are susceptible to moderate or severe bowel ischemia when they undergo *abdominal aortic surgery or high ligation of the inferior mesenteric artery.*[460, 461] This is due to previous occlusion of the inferior mesenteric artery from atherosclerotic disease, compromise of other collaterals, or damage to vessels during surgery, ligation of the inferior mesenteric artery with congenital absence of collateral vessels, or postoperative dehydration or hypotension causing thrombosis of the critical arteries.

Renal Splanchnic Steals

Diversion of the blood flow to the occluded celiac artery via the capsular and inferior phrenic artery may cause deprivation of perfusion to the kidney.[282] This in turn causes hypertension related to renal ischemia.

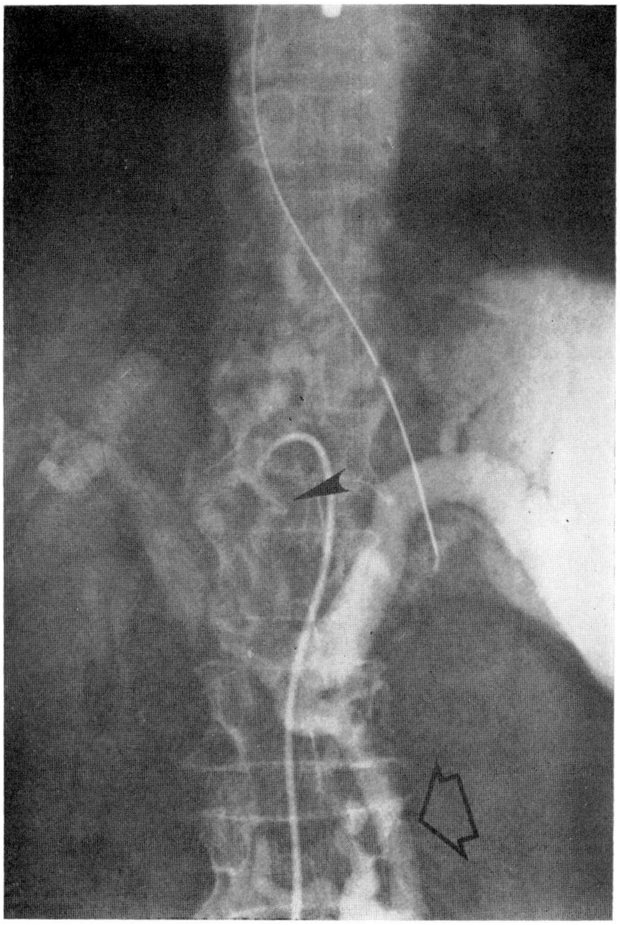

Figure 25.41. Celiac Angiogram—venous phase. There is reflux of contrast into a tortuous collateral vein. The patient was known to have portal hypertension. *Diagnosis:* Portal hypertension with varices.

Hepatic Steal

Excessive demands from the hepatic vascular bed due to arteriovenous fistula, vascular tumors, or cirrhosis of the liver may siphon blood from the superior mesenteric artery via the pancreatic arcade.[302]

Tumor Steal

Vascular thyroid adenomas stealing blood from the carotid artery may cause transient cerebral ischemic attacks.[462]

(*Text continues on page 395*)

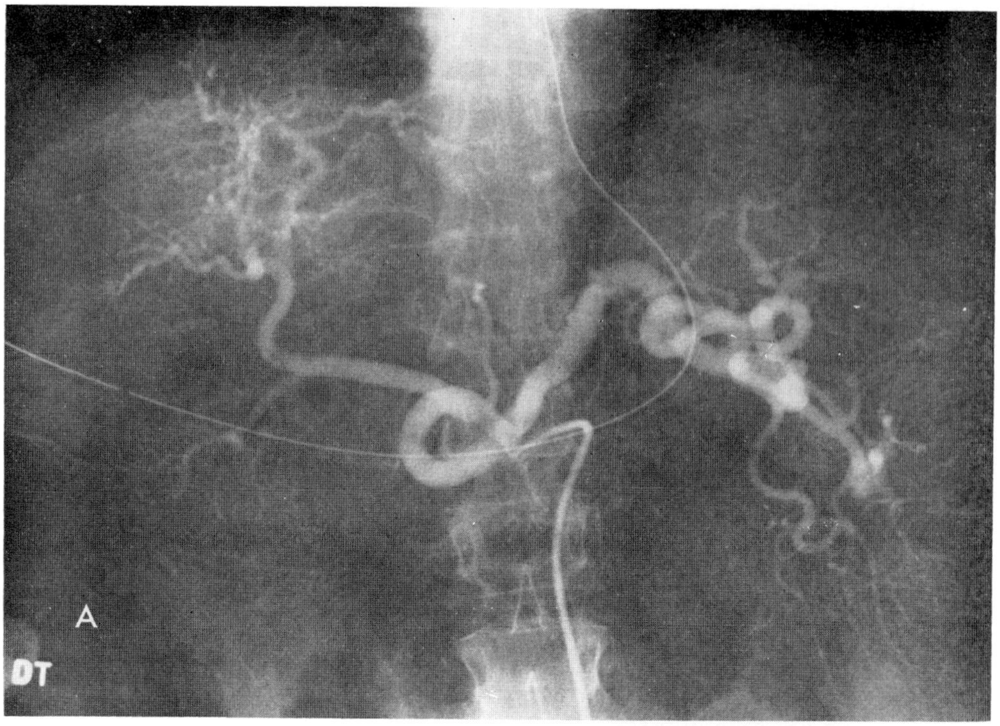

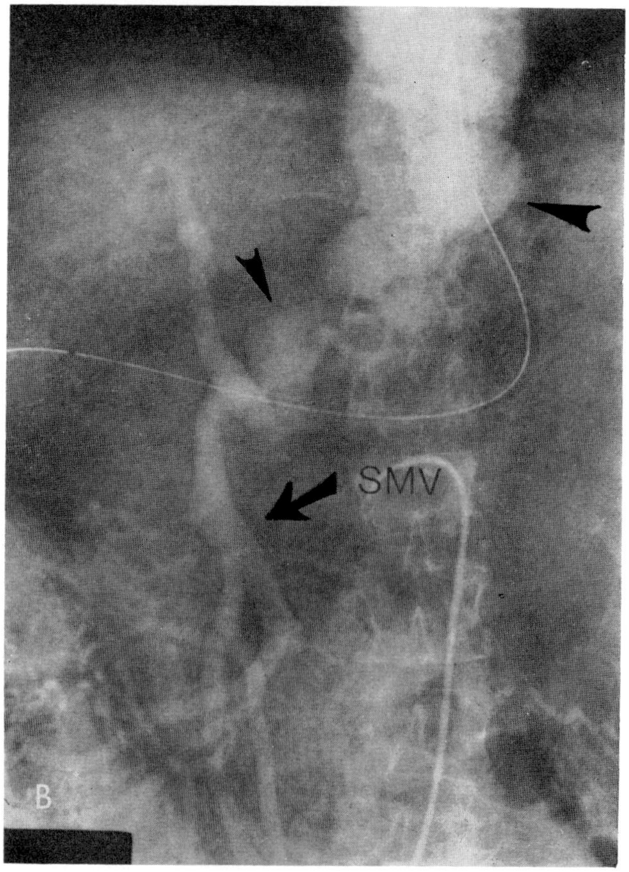

Figure 25.42. (A) Celiac arteriogram reveals a small liver with corkscrew intrahepatic branches. (B) Superior mesenteric arteriogram—venous phase: Abnormal huge veins traversing towards the esophagus. Notice the change in the course of the portal vein due to a shrunken liver. *Diagnosis:* Cirrhosis of the liver. Portal hypertension and varices.

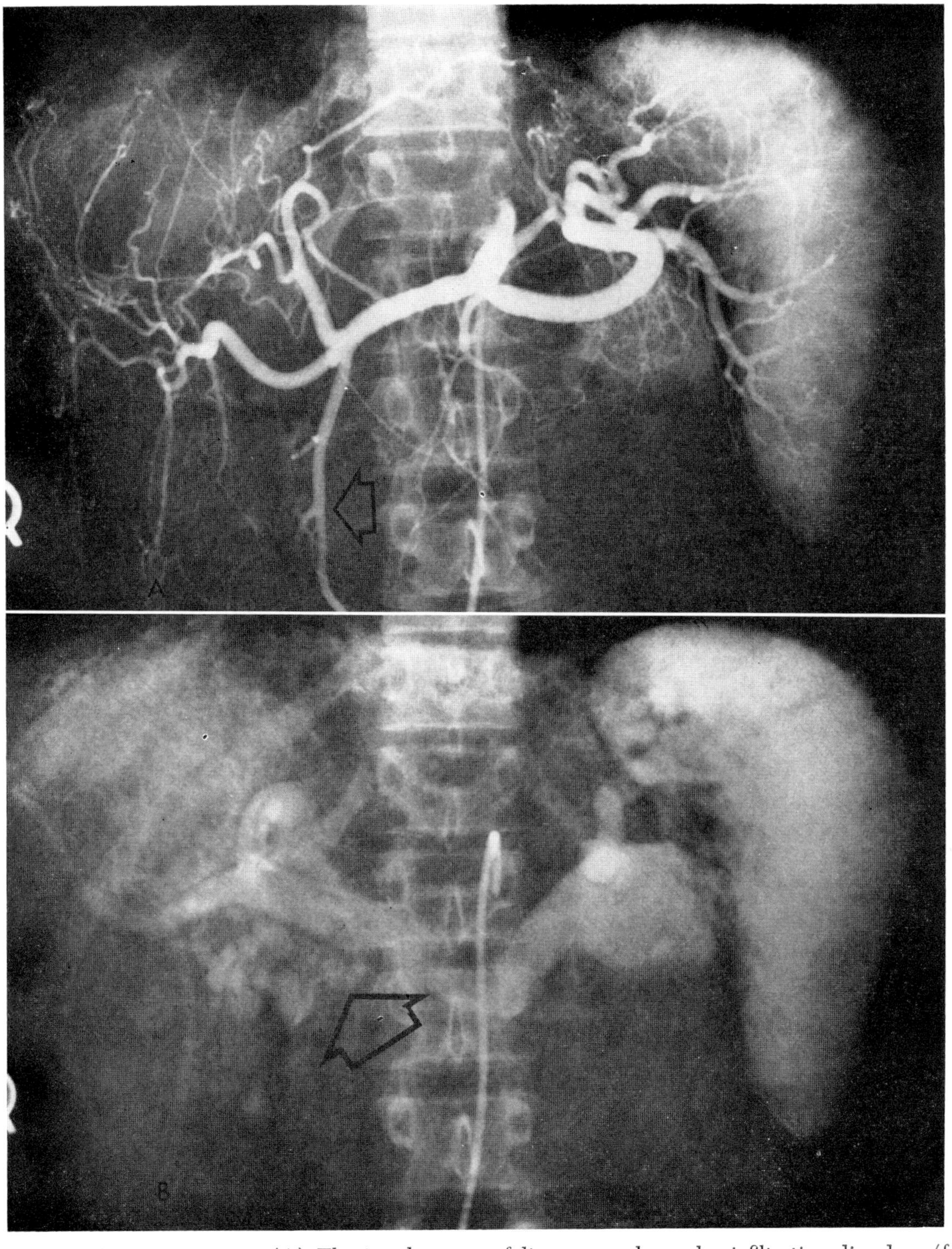

Figure 25.43. Celiac Arteriogram. (A) The intrahepatic arteries are stretched and the course of the gastroduodenal artery (Arrow) is widened. (B) Tortuous veins (Arrow) are seen at the portahepatis. Faint opacification of the liver parenchyma with infiltration of liver parenchyma by infiltration disorders (fat, sarcoid, amyloid, etc.). *Diagnosis:* Portal hypertension of unknown etiology. *Liver Biopsy:* Sarcoidosis with portal hypertension.

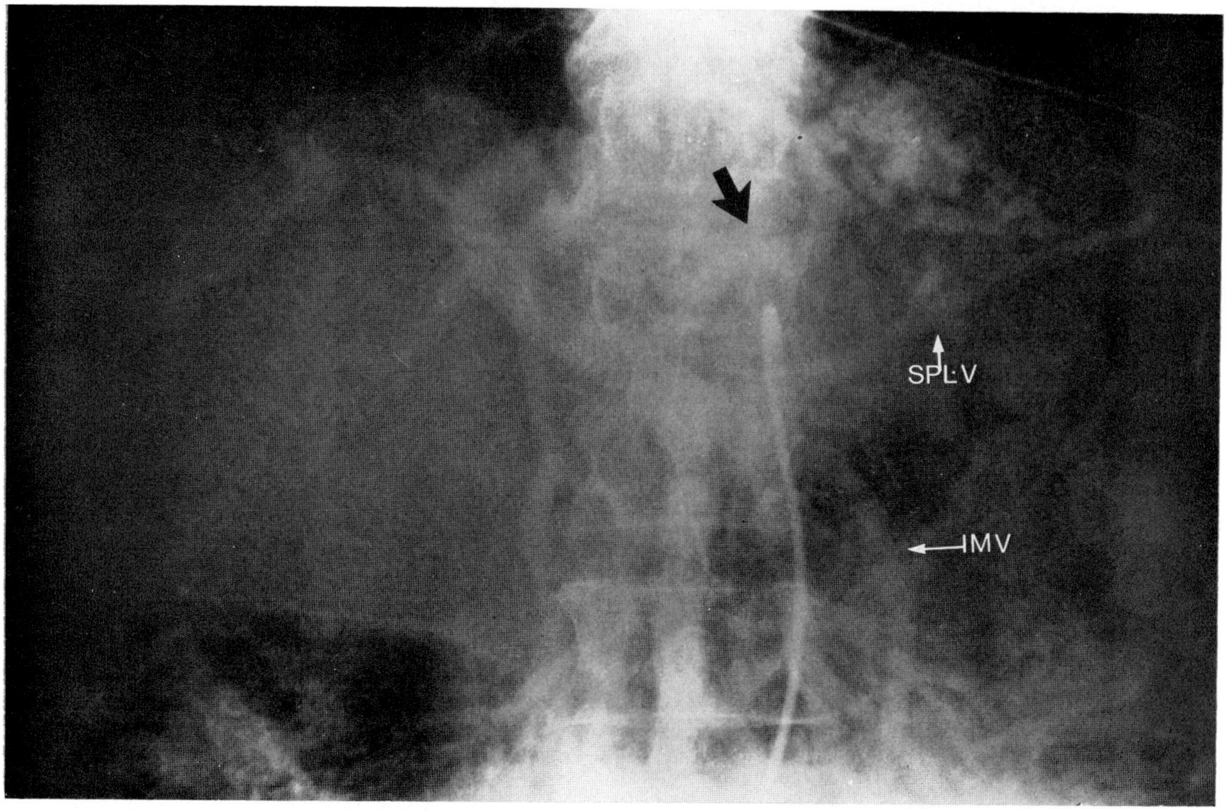

Figure 25.44. Postprescoline Superior Mesenteric Venogram. There is visualization of the inferior mesenteric vein (I.M.V.), splenic vein (Spl. V.) and tortuous dilated veins draining towards the fundus of the stomach and esophagus (Arrow). *Diagnosis:* Marked portal hypertension with appreciable hepatofugal flow via collaterals. This causes underperfusion of the intrahepatic portal venous radicles.

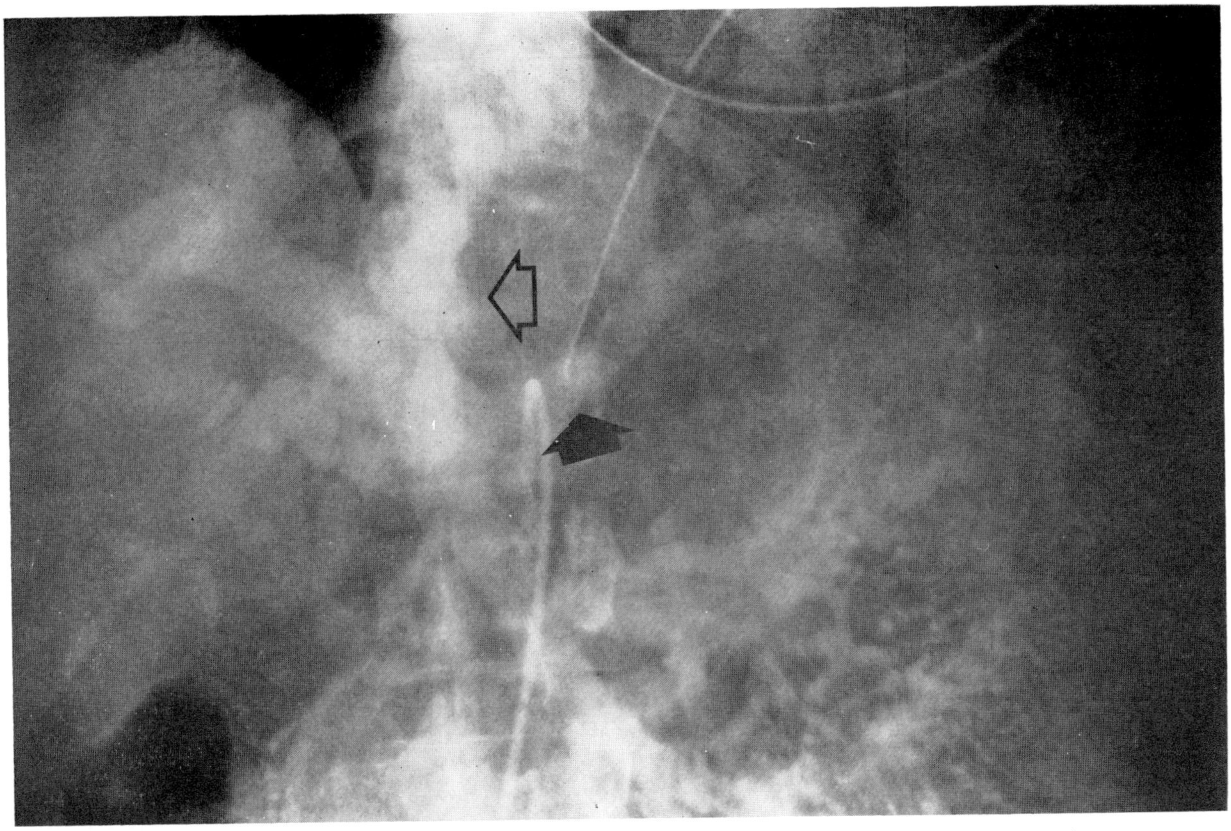

Figure 25.45. Superior Mesenteric Arteriogram—venous phase. Tortuous dilated abnormal vessel coursing towards the esophagus (Blank Arrow) is seen. Another opacified vessel courses towards the spleen (Arrow), and the intrahepatic portal venous radicles do not fill. *Diagnosis:* Portal hypertension with collateral circulation towards esophageal veins and reflux into the splenic vein. There is marked hepatofugal flow and no filling of the intrahepatic portal venous radicles.

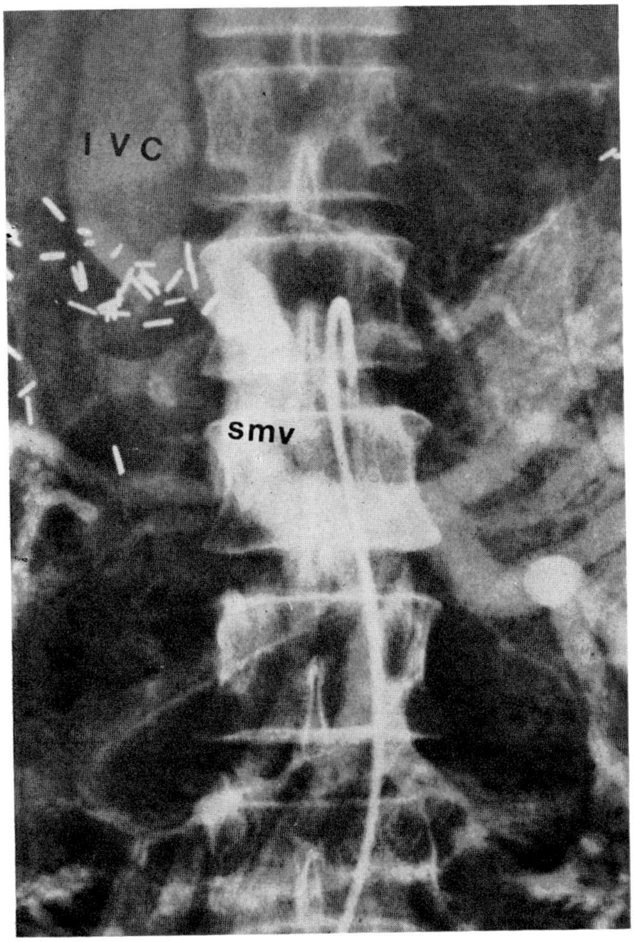

← Figure 25.46. Superior Mesenteric Arteriogram. The venous phase shows opacification of the superior mesenteric vein (S.M.V.) and the inferior vena cava (I.V.C.). The patient has a patent portacaval shunt.

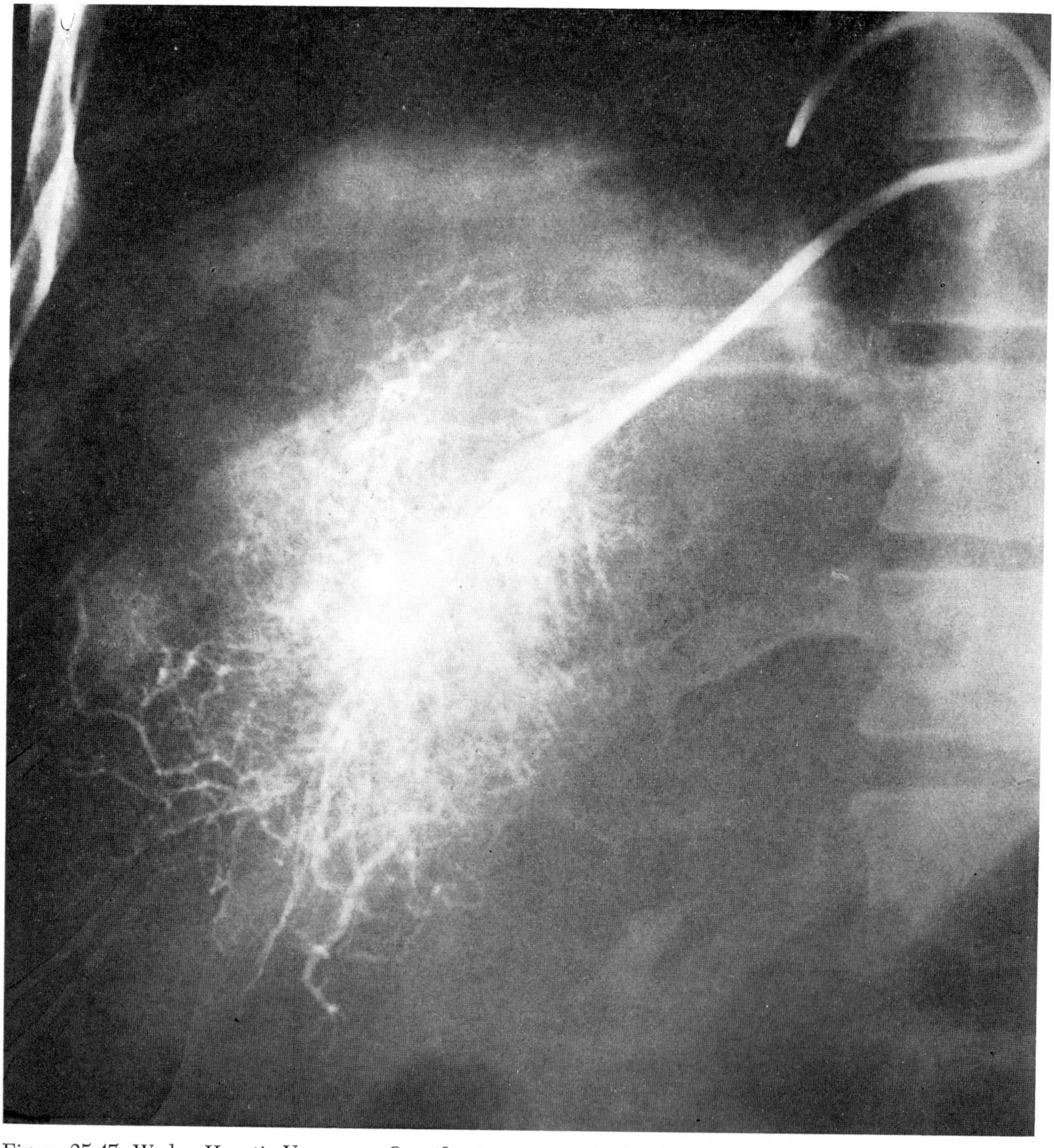

Figure 25.47. Wedge Hepatic Venogram. Opacification of fine veins is revealed with a web-like pattern. The hepatic and portal veins are not opacified. Nor is the hepatic vein that engages the catheter opacified. *Diagnosis:* Budd-Chiari syndrome. (From Kreel, L., Freston, J. W., and Clain, D. Vascular radiology in the Budd-Chiari syndrome. *Br J Radiol, 40:*755. Courtesy of the authors and publishers.)

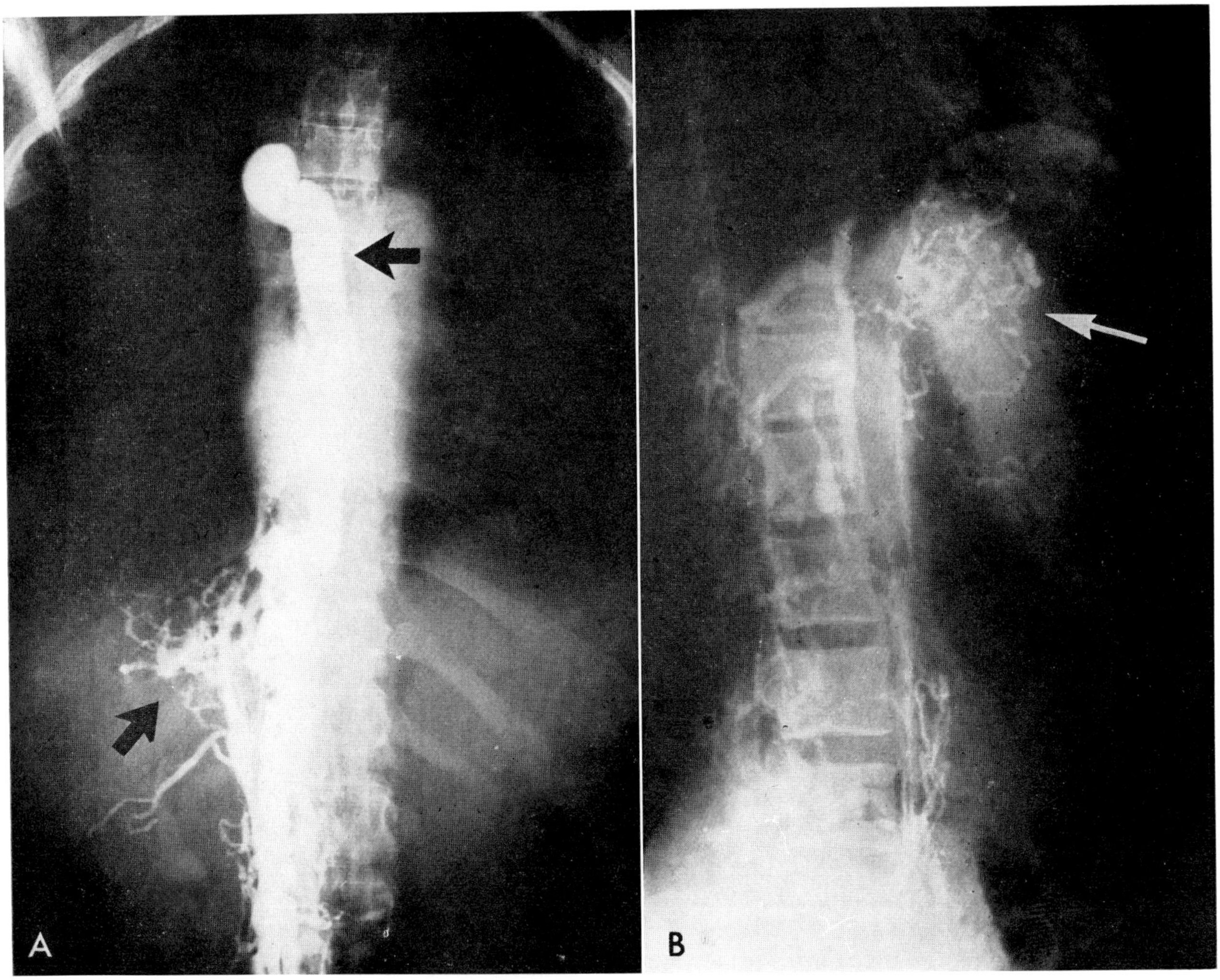

Figure 25.48. Inferior Vena Cavogram. (A) Frontal projection. (B) Lateral projection. The inferior vena cava is completely occluded except for the extremely narrowed hepatic segment. Most of the contrast drains through the azygos vein (Arrow). There is retrograde filling of a coarse network of collaterals into the hepatic parenchyma (Arrows). *Diagnosis:* Budd-Chiari syndrome. (From Deutsch, V., Rosenthal, T., Adar, R., and Mozes, M. Budd-Chiari syndrome. *Am J Roentgen, 116:*430, 1972. Courtesy of the authors and publishers.)

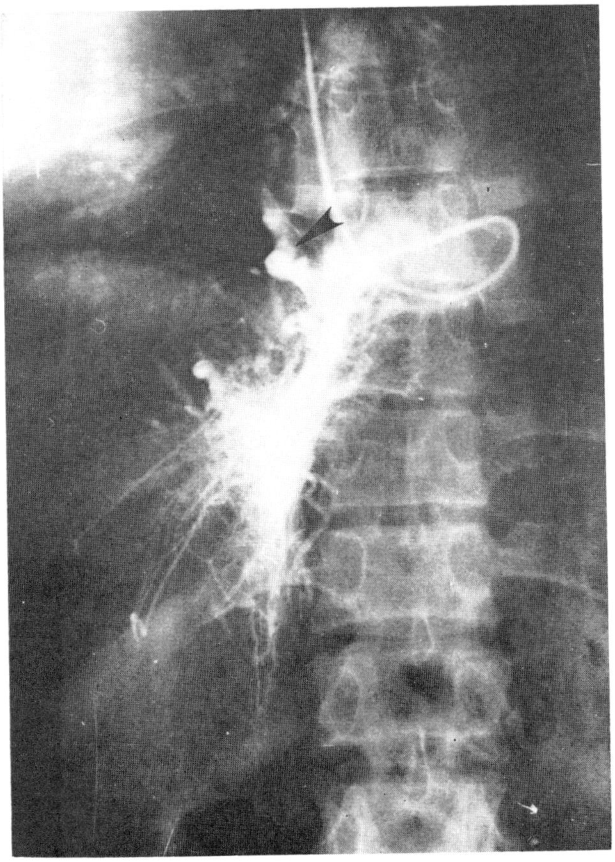

←

Figure 25.49. Hepatic Venogram. The catheter was forced into a partially occluded hepatic vein. The injected contrast flows into the coarse intrahepatic venous collaterals and from there into larger collaterals draining into the azygos system (Arrow). *Diagnosis:* Budd-Chiari syndrome. (From Deutsch, V., Rosenthan, R., Adar, R., and Mozes, M. Budd-Chiari syndrome. *Am J Roentgen, 116:*430, 1972. Courtesy of the authors and publishers.)

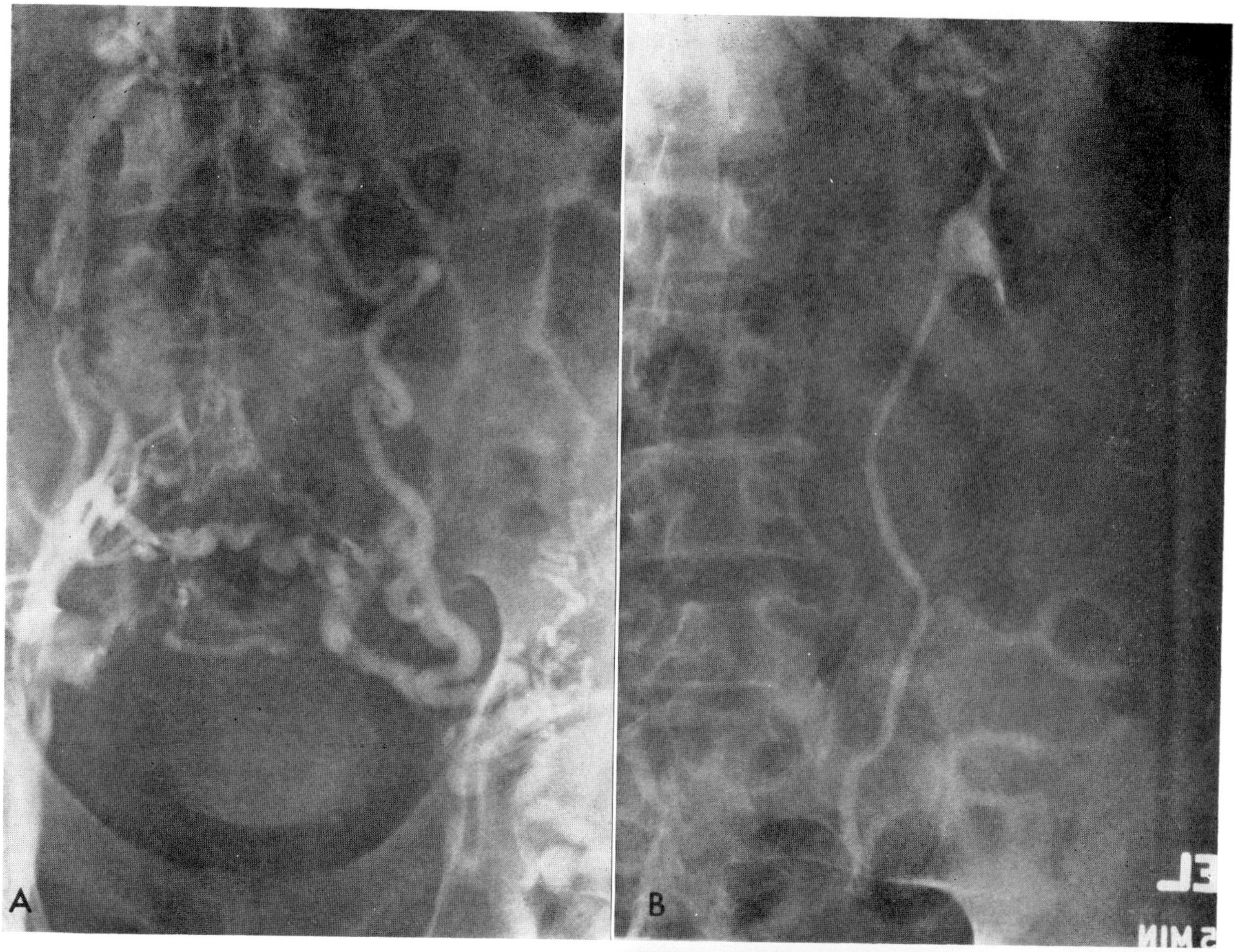

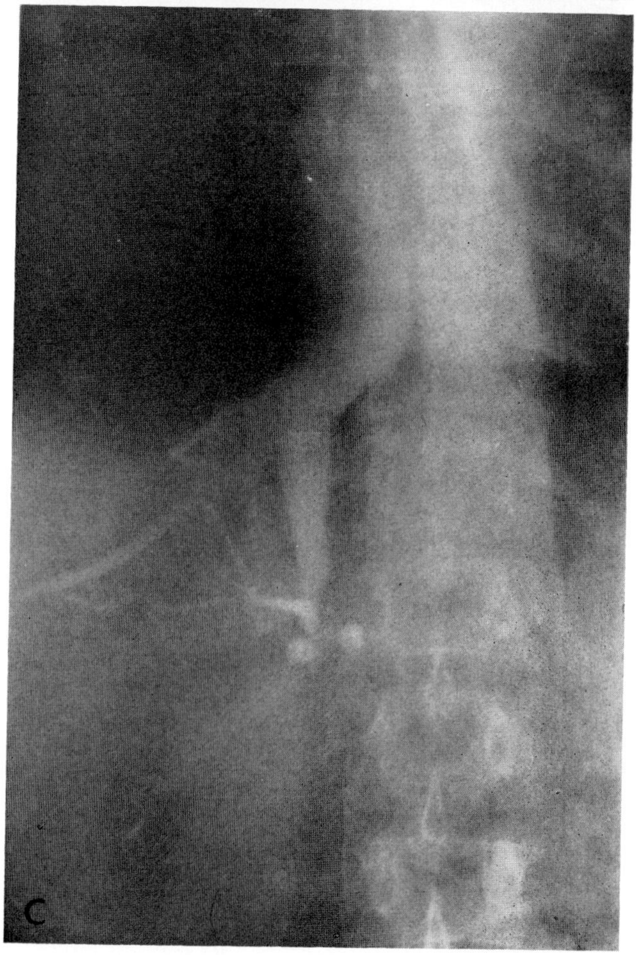

Figure 25.50. Inferior Vena Cavagram. (A) Numerous dilated tortuous veins are seen with no opacification of the inferior vena cava. (B) Intravenous pyelogram: Notice the deviation of the ureter. This patient had edema of the legs for the last eight years. (C) Inferior vena cavagram via the jugular vein: There is a smooth narrowing of the hepatic portion of the inferior vena cava. *Diagnosis:* Idiopathic inferior vena caval thrombosis.

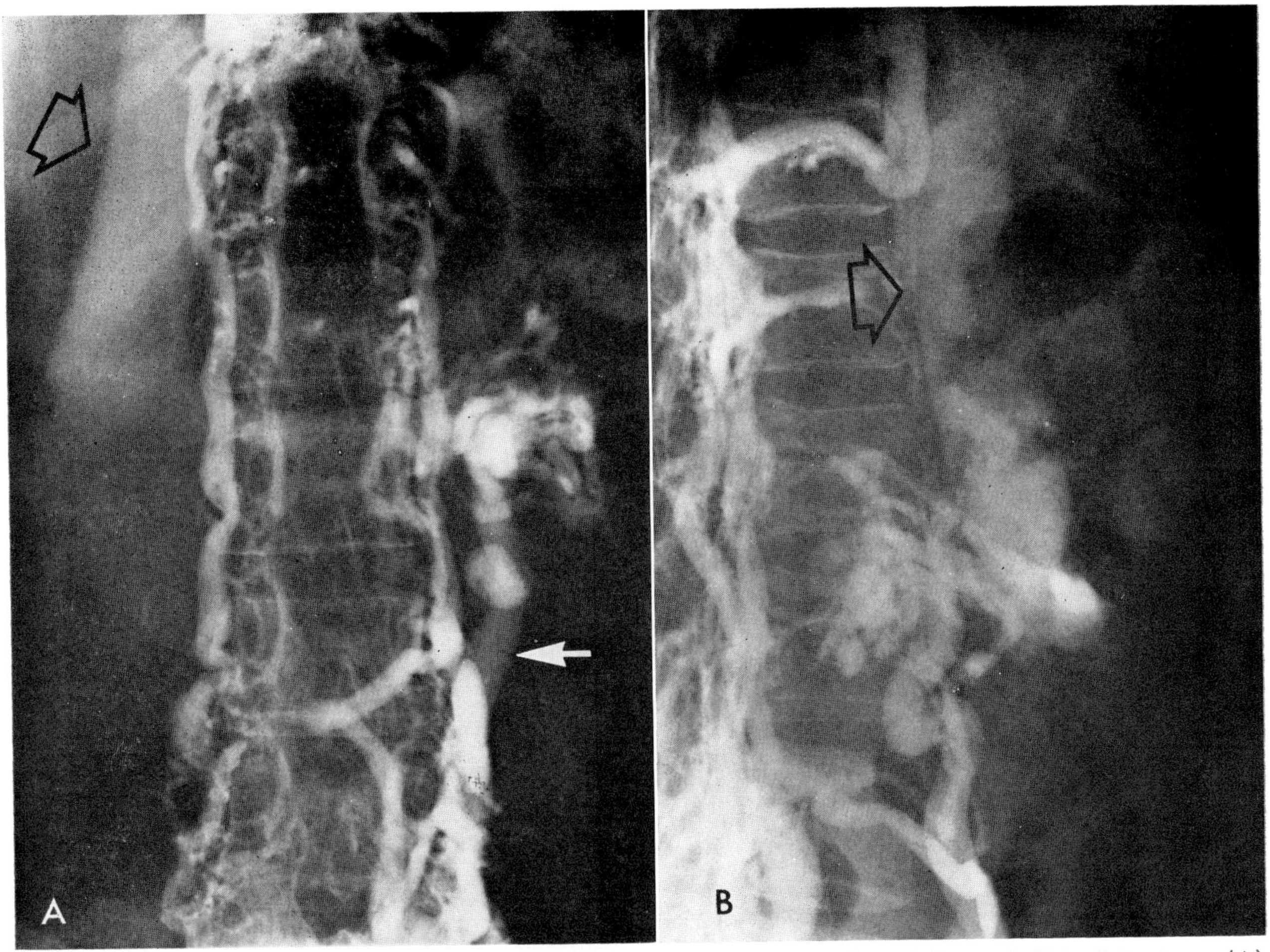

Figure 25.51. Bilateral Femoral Vein Injections. (A) anterior, (B) lateral projections. There is nonvisualization of the infrarenal portion of the inferior vena cava. The renal segment and the suprarenal segments of the inferior vena cava are demonstrated (Arrow). A huge collateral vein (ovarian vein) (White Arrow) joins the left renal vein. *Diagnosis:* Inferior vena caval obstruction due to lymph node masses (lymphoma).

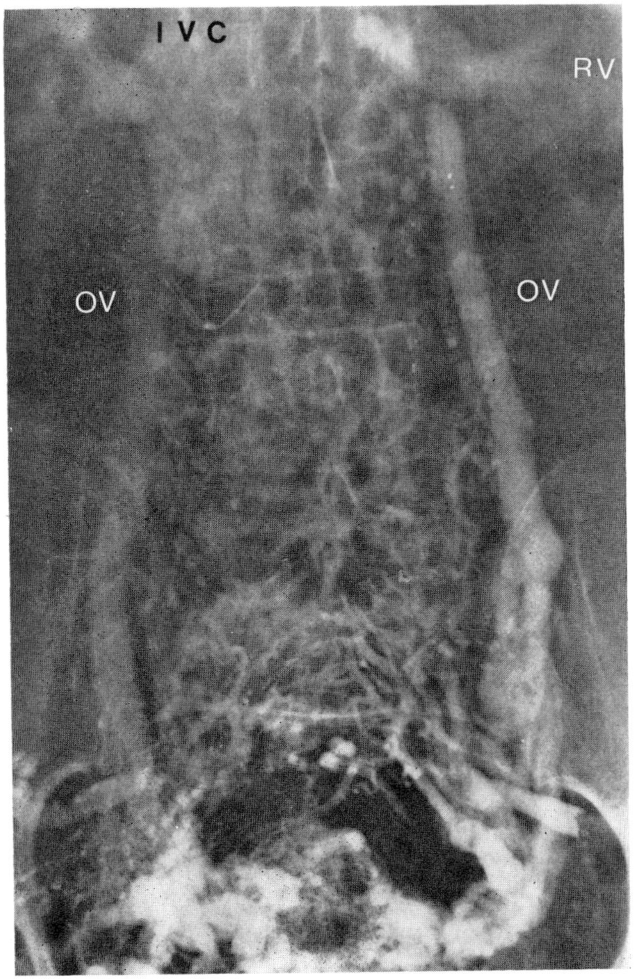

←

Figure 25.52. Inferior Vena Cavagram. Notice the umbrella in the inferior vena cava. Very tortuous dilated uterine veins and the ovarian pedicular veins carry the contrast via huge ovarian veins to the inferior vena cava on the right side and the renal vein on the left side. Notice the proximal opacification of the inferior vena cava (I.V.C.). *Comment:* Inferior vena caval thrombosis with collateral circulation via the ovarian veins. Such huge ovarian veins can carry an embolus.

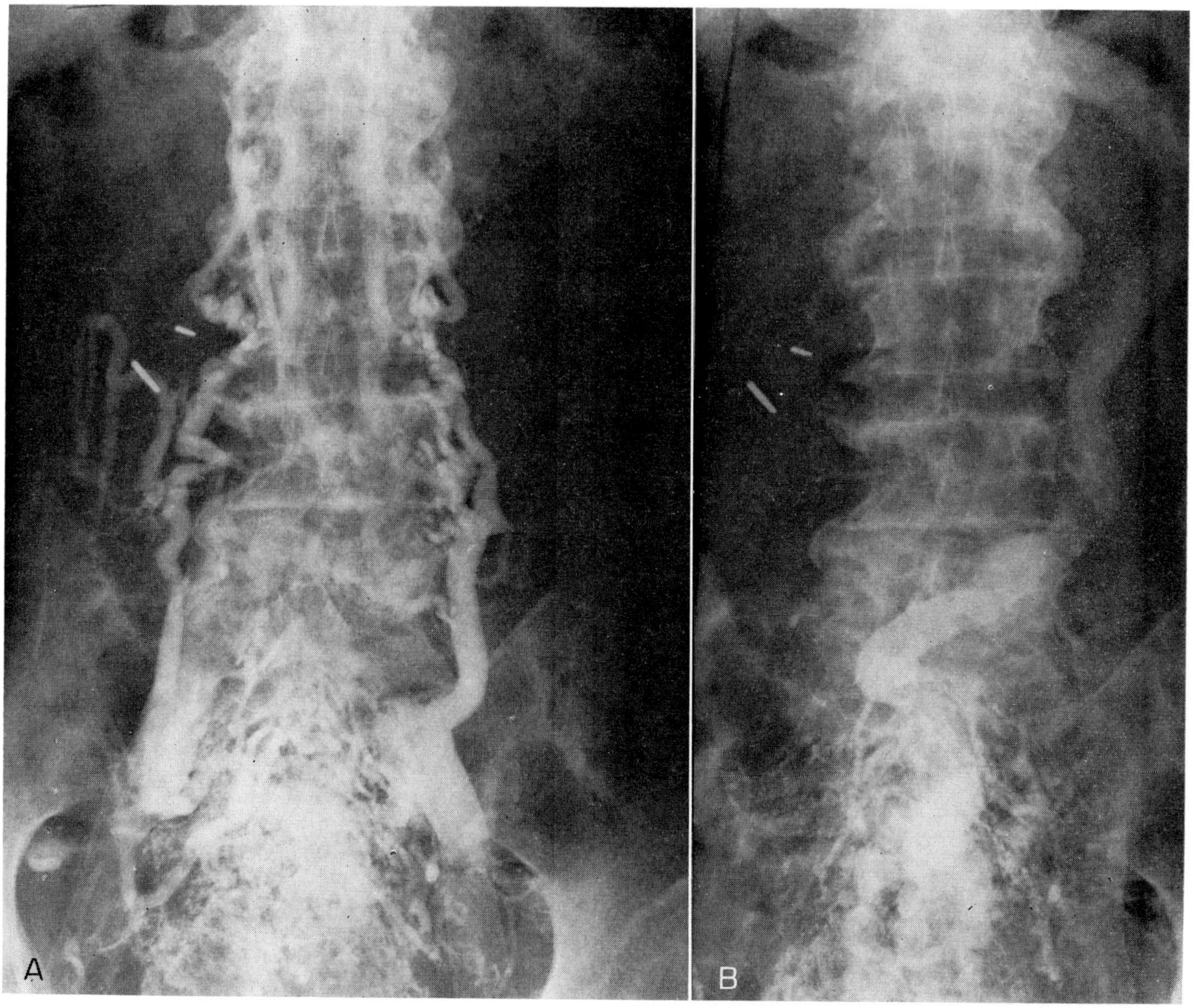

Figure 25.53. Inferior Venacavagram. (A) Note the opacification of paravertebral veins and rectal veins, but no opacification of the inferior vena cava. (B) Late phase: A very prominent vein courses towards the epigastrium. *Diagnosis:* Inferior vena caval occlusion due to involvement by a renal transitional cell carcinoma with collateral circulation via the rectal veins and inferior mesenteric vein.

VENOUS COLLATERAL FLOW

To avoid catastrophes, a change in the venous outflow from a viscus must be reflected in the arterial input. In other words, an increased arterial input should be accompanied by increased venous drainage and, conversely, a decrease in venous outflow should be immediately followed by a decrease in arterial perfusion. Fortunately, multiplicity of veins and their free anastomoses allows less interference with drainage after venous occlusion. But this is not a universal situation. Because of their exceptional importance, if the portal, mesenteric, renal or hepatic veins are occluded, the result is gross interference with drainage of blood and subsequent necrosis. The vena cava, popliteal and axillary veins belong to the middle group. Like arteries, venous thrombosis causes more occlusion and is less easily compensated by collaterals than just simple ligation. The orientation of valves in the veins prevents an anastomosing channel from functioning as a collateral until dilatation of the vein results in incompetency

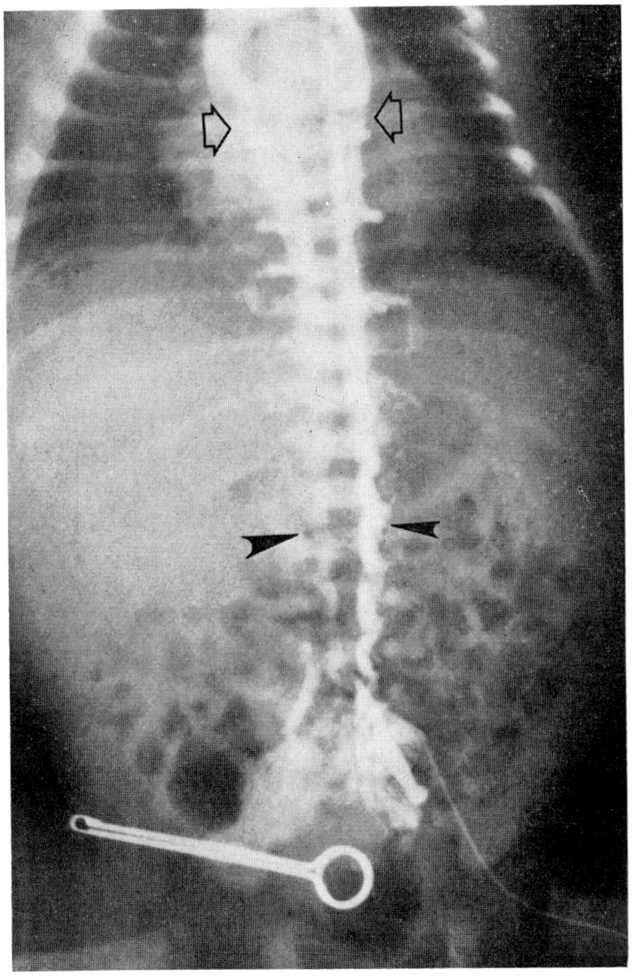

Figure 25.54. Inferior Vena Cavagram. There is good opacification of the paravertebral veins (Arrow Heads), azygous veins (Blank Arrows) and no visualization of the inferior vena cava. (The study was done while the patient was sleeping under the influence of sedatives.) *Diagnosis:* Inferior vena caval thrombosis with collateral circulation via the vertebral venous plexus and the azygous veins. *Comment:* The same appearance can be seen in a normal patient who performs a Valsalva maneuver either because of crying or increased straining.

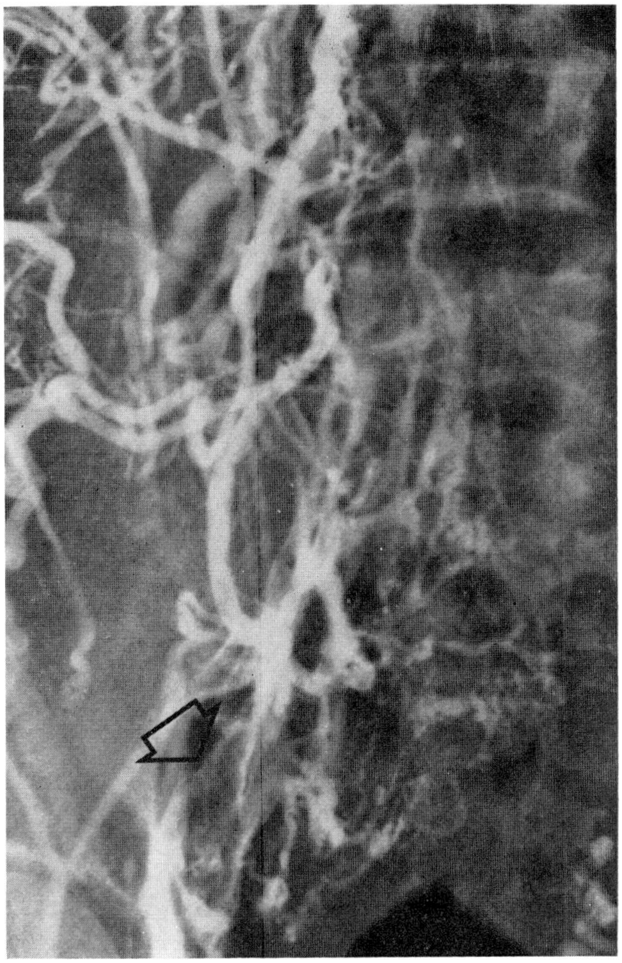

Figure 25.55. Femoral Venogram. Very tortuous prominent abnormal veins are opacified. A filling defect is in the lumen of the right common iliac vein. *Diagnosis:* Extensive thrombosis of the right common iliac vein with marked collateral circulation.

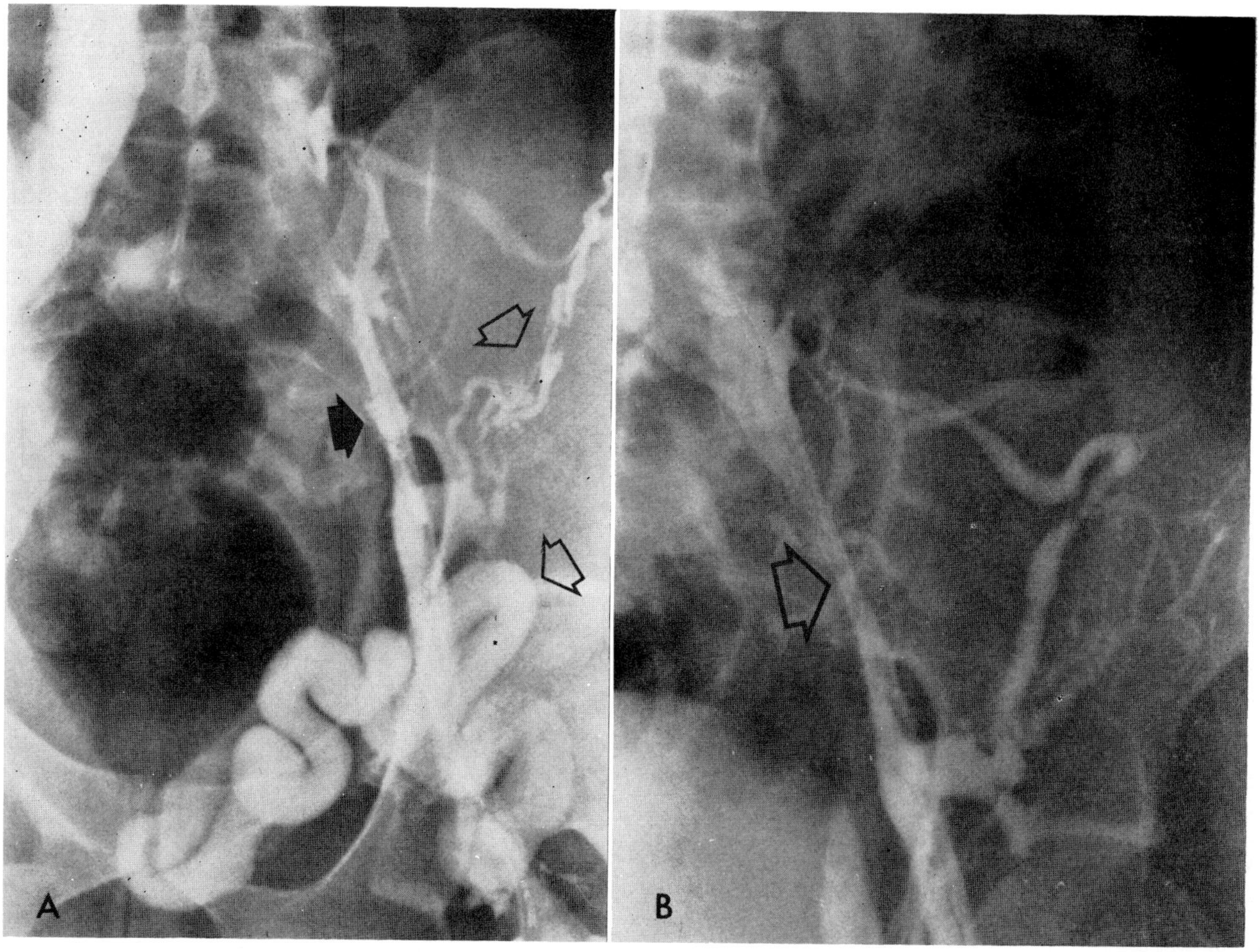

Figure 25.56. Left External Iliac Venogram. (A) Very tortuous dilated veins course towards the symphysis pubis (Blank Arrow) with narrowed external iliac vein (Arrow) tortuous other veins (Blank Arrow). (B) Marked narrowing of the left external iliac vein is seen with a linear translucent filling defect. This patient had blunt trauma to the lower abdomen three years prior. *Diagnosis:* Posttraumatic thrombosis of the left common iliac vein with recanalization and associated collateral venous drainage.

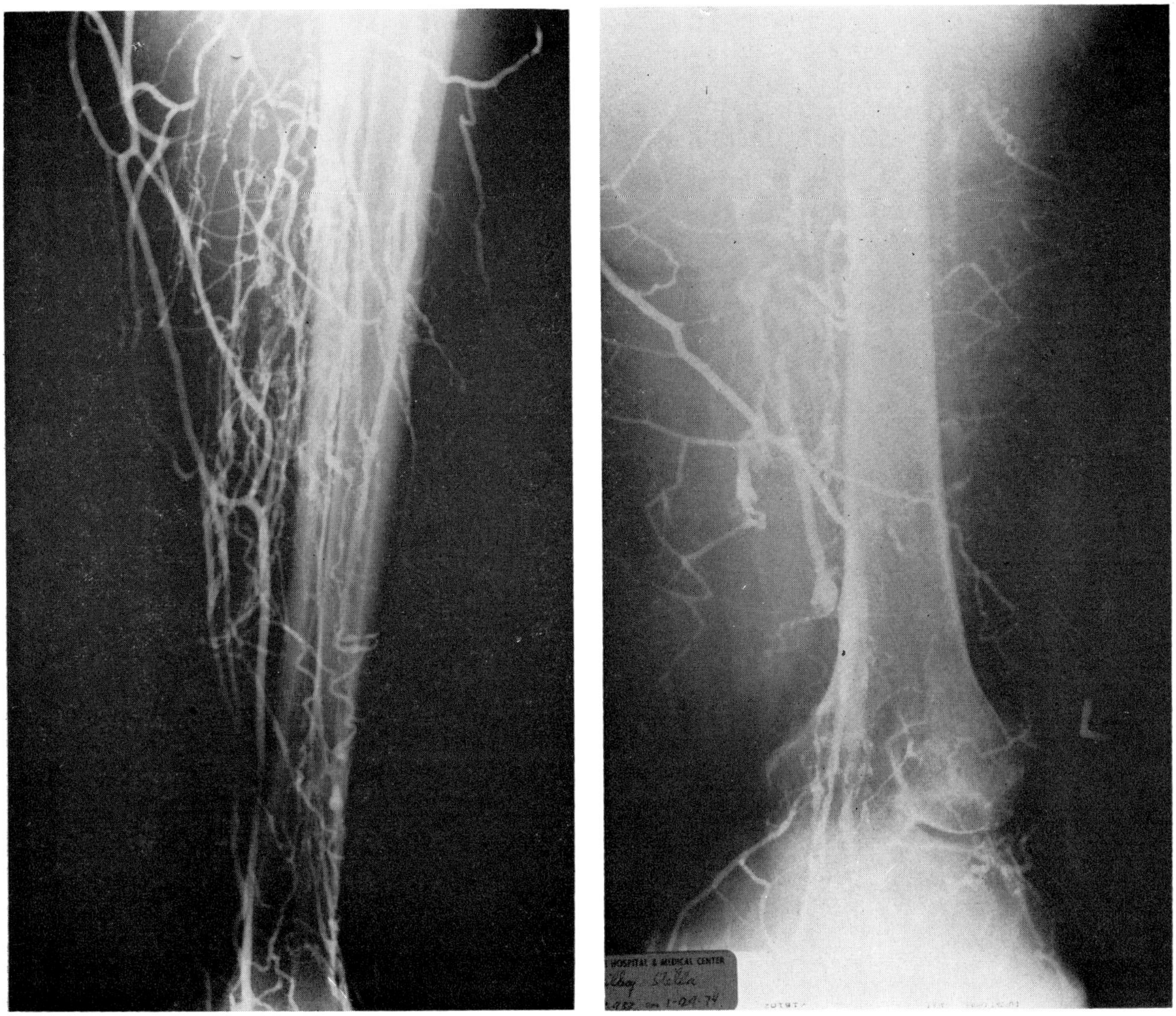

Figure 25.57 A and B. Lower Extremity Venogram. Numerous dilated veins are seen with no visualization of the deep venous system. *Diagnosis:* Acute thrombosis of the deep venous system with collateral circulation.

of the valves.[422] The size of a venous collateral may not mean that it is an efficient conduit, as an unsupported vein can readily undergo dilatation.[434] The same dilated vein may carry recurrent emboli through its lumen. This is seen with a persistent left inferior vena cava, dilated ovarian, or ascending lumbar veins.

Porto-systemic Communication

These communications preexist normally.[434, 479] If necessity arises, blood may flow in either direction as these veins are valveless. The flow may be toward (hepatopetal) or away (hepatofugal) from the liver. The connections occur where the *absorbing epithelium becomes protective,* such as the distal esophagus (coronary veins to esophageal veins), or at the anus (rectal veins). They may occur at the site of *obliterated embryological circulations* such as the falsiform ligament as a remnant of the paraumbilical vein. Connections develop at all points in the abdomen where the gastrointestinal tract, *its appendages or glands originating from it* become *retroperitoneal or adhere to the abdominal walls.* This occurs in the duodenum, colon, small bowel, rectum, spleen, pan-

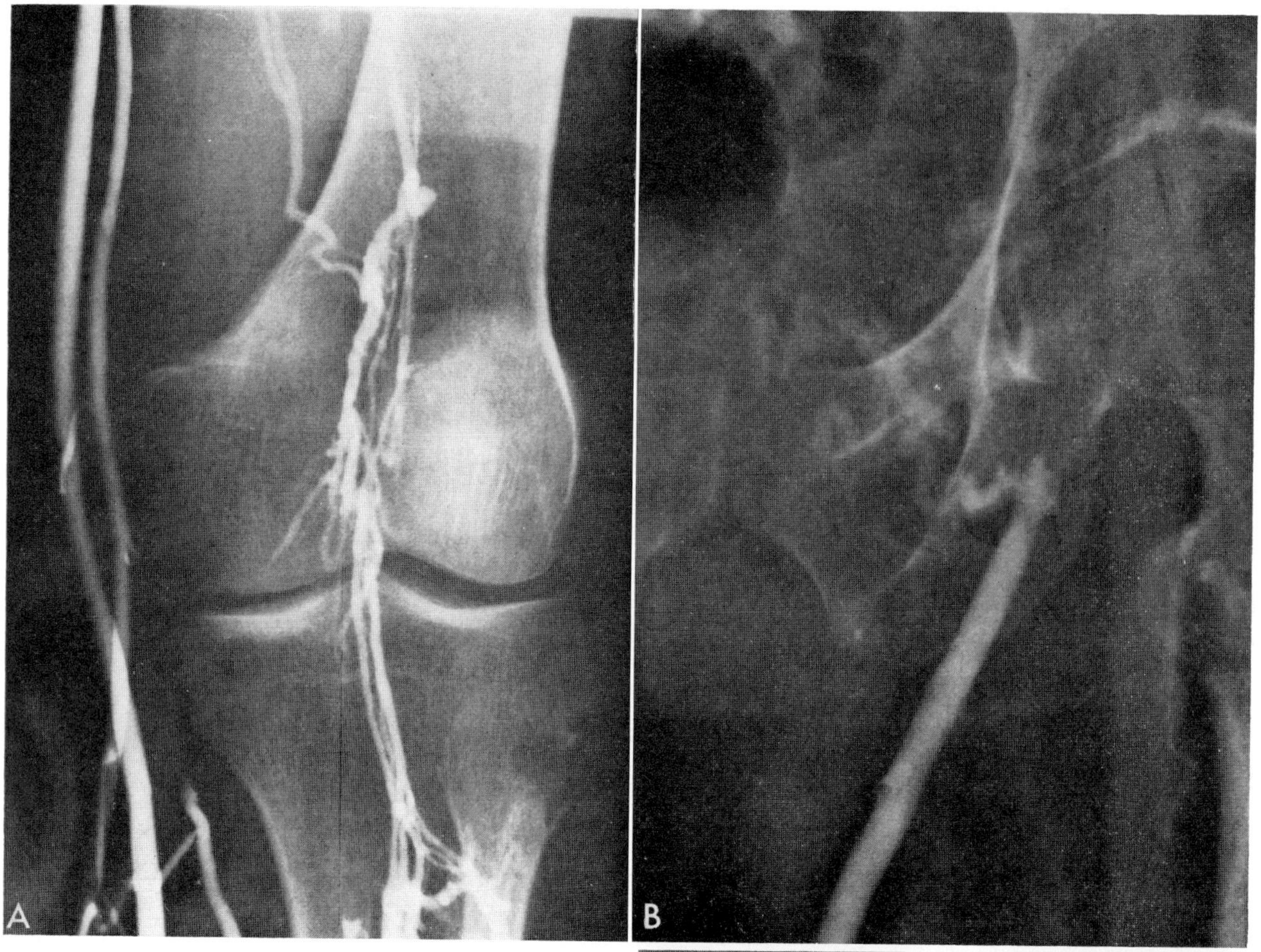

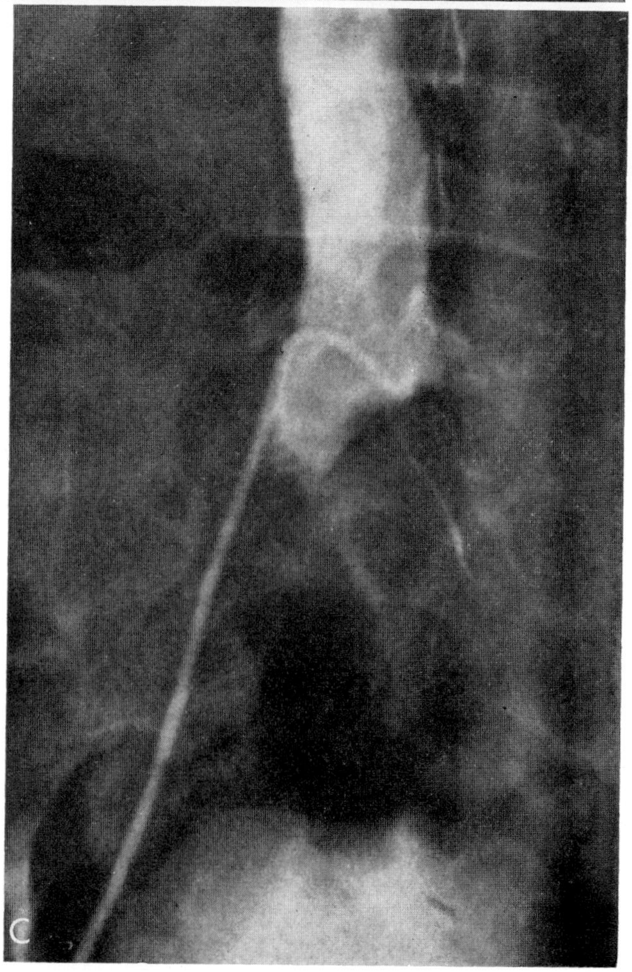

Figure 25.58. Lower Extremity Venogram. (A) No visualization of the deep veins. Small channels are carrying the contrast. Note the superficial veins. (B) A very prominent superficial vein leads into another tortuous vein without visualization of the femoral vein. (C) Right femoral vein catheterization reveals nonvisualization of the left common iliac vein. *Diagnosis:* Extensive thrombosis of the deep veins of the entire left lower extremity. The proximal extent of the thrombus is near the junction of both common iliac veins.

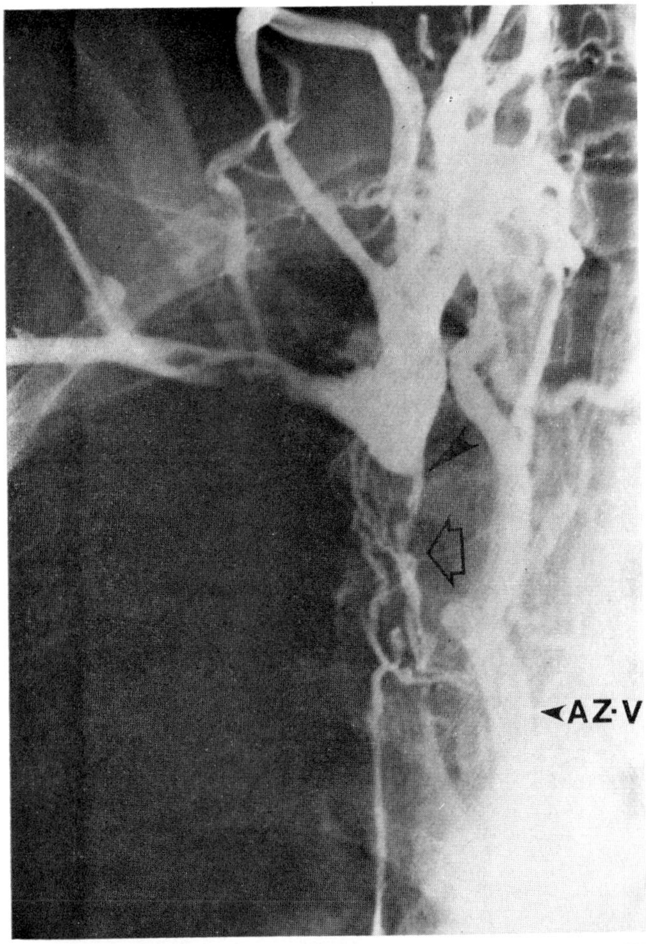

←

Figure 25.59. Superior Vena Cavagram. There is smooth tapering with complete interruption of the right innominate vein (Arrow Head), opacification of very abnormal tortuous prominent veins (Arrow) and opacification of the azygous vein (AZ.V.). The patient had a right paratracheal mass. *Diagnosis:* Occlusion of the superior vena cava by bronchogenic cancer with collateral circulation via the azygous vein.

Figure 25.60. Superior Vena Cavagram. (A) Numerous dilated veins are seen and the superior vena cava is not visualized. Filling defects are in the innominate vein (Arrow). (B) A little later there is good filling of the pericardiacophrenic veins. This patient had a bronchogenic carcinoma. *Diagnosis:* Occlusion of the superior vena cava due to infiltration by a malignant tumor. Clots appear in the innominate veins. Collateral circulation is seen along the pericardiac and anterior chest wall veins.

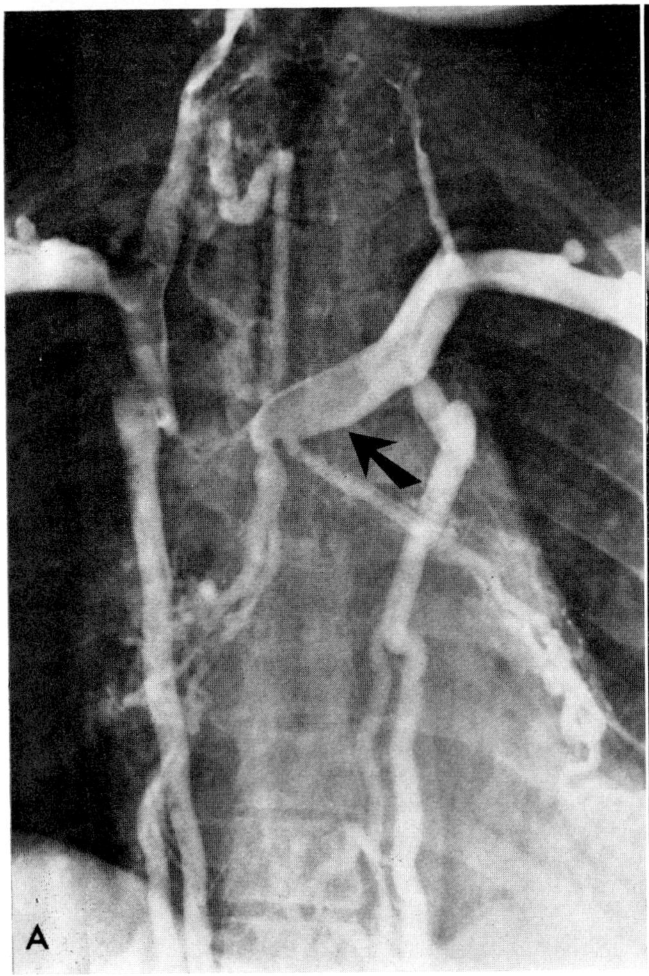

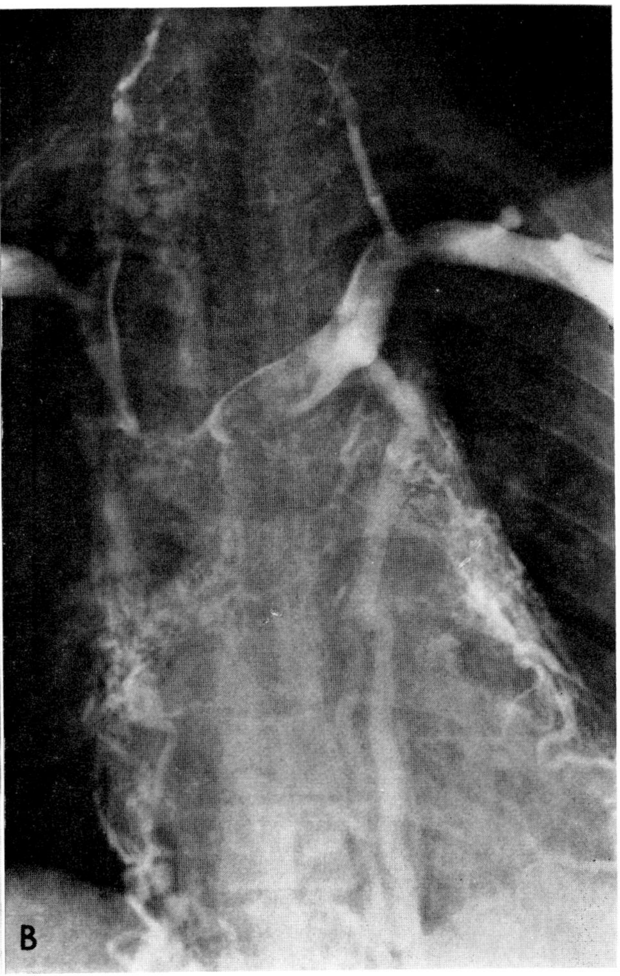

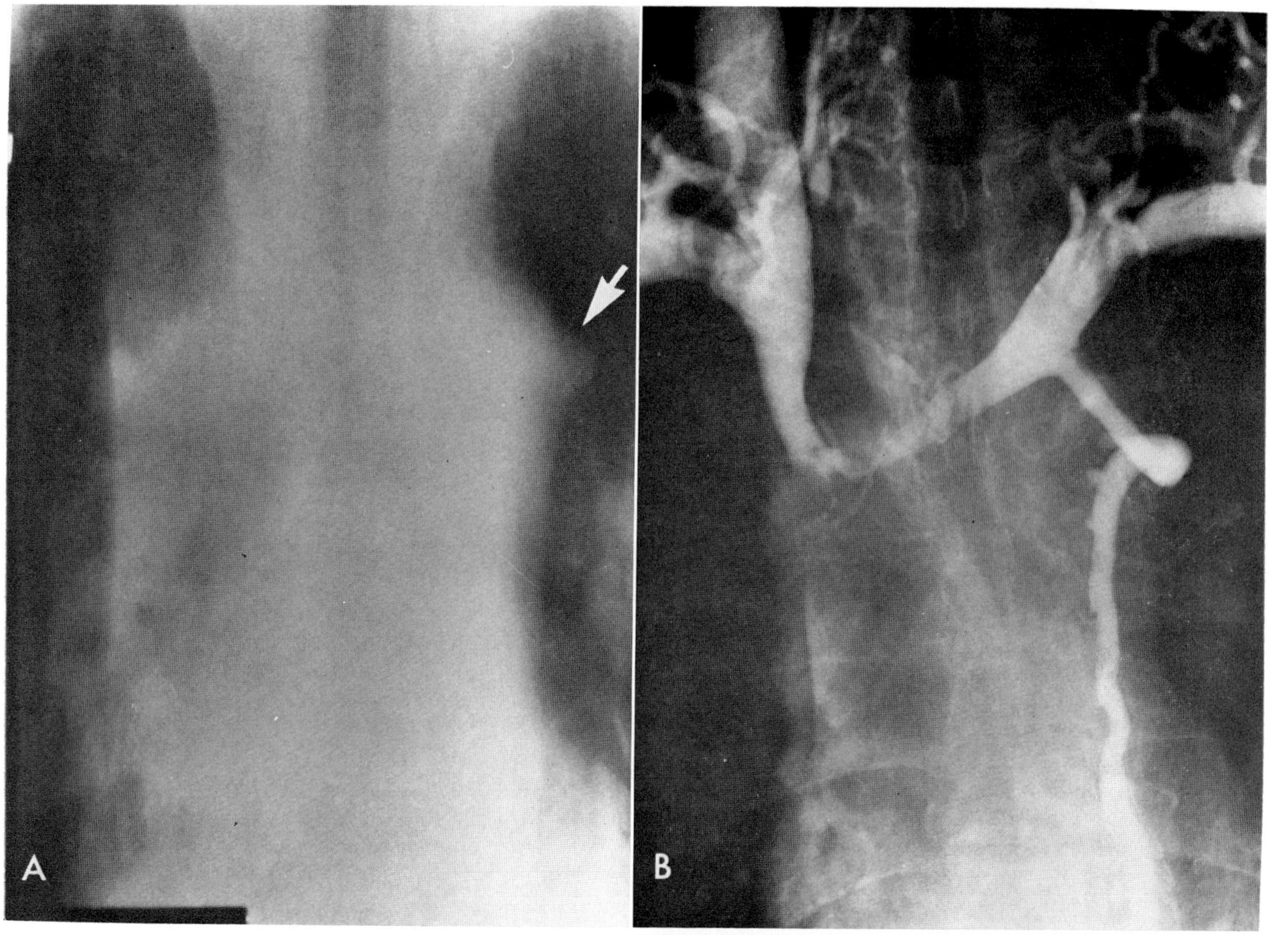

Figure 25.61. (A) Tomograms of the mediastinum reveal a nipple-like shadow adjacent to the aortic knob. (B) Superior vena cavagram reveals nonfilling of the superior vena cava and narrowing of the innominate veins (Arrow). A very prominent collateral vein (Arrow Head) gives the nipple-like shadow seen on the tomograms. The patient had bronchogenic carcinoma in the right lung. *Diagnosis:* Tumor infiltration of great veins and occlusion of the superior vena cava. Note prominent left superior intercostal vein causing the nipple-like shadow.

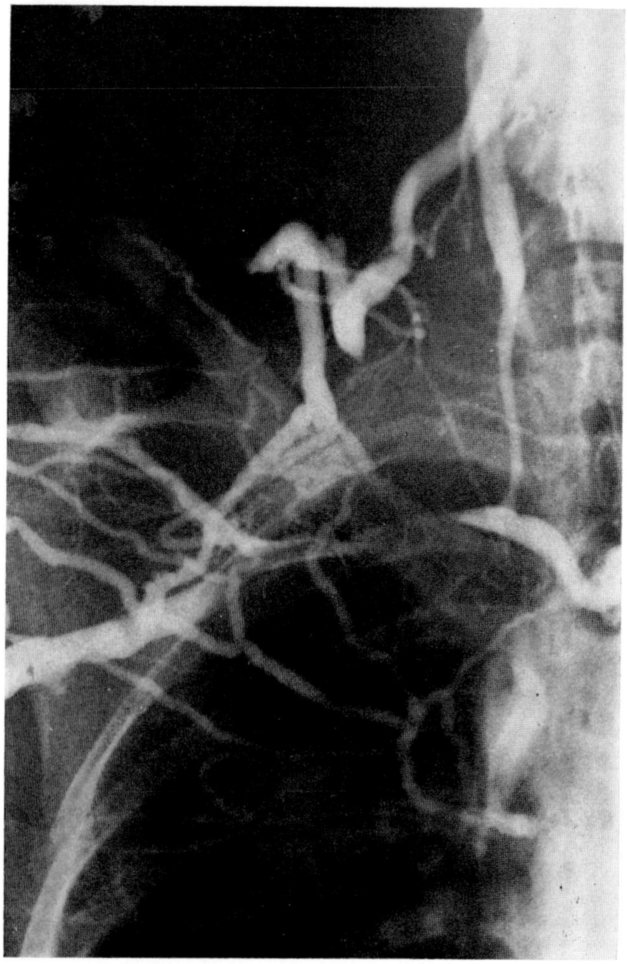

Figure 25.62. Upper Extremity Venogram. The subclavian vein does not fill. Other tortuous dilated veins are opacified. This patient used her arm excessively two days prior to the examination. *Diagnosis:* Effort thrombosis of the subclavian vein.

creas, omentum, and with the veins of Reitzius and Sappey.[434, 479] Finally, collaterals occur at abnormal terminations of a major segment of the portal vein with the systemic circulation.

When the *portal vein* is occluded, the coronary vein (left gastric vein) is usually the first to become dilated. This is followed by the appearance of the short gastric and inferior mesenteric veins.[480] The paraumbilical veins are used more frequently with portal vein obstruction than with obstruction of the inferior vena cava. Obstruction to venous flow is greater with portal cirrhosis than with extrahepatic portal obstruction. In extrahepatic blockage of the portal venous system without associated intrahepatic obstruction, the collaterals which try to bypass the obstruction to carry blood *toward the liver* are the deep cystic veins, epiploic veins of the omentum, veins in ligaments, veins in the wall of the common bile duct, paraumbilical veins, and diaphragmatic veins.[364]

Unusual, fascinating, preexisting portosystemic communications are not uncommon.[481] Portopulmonary shunts occur via the coronary vein to the esophageal veins and then to the inferior pulmonary veins. Blood may be shunted from the splenic to the left renal vein, from the gastric to the left adrenal veins, and from veins of the terminal ileum to the right ovarian plexus veins. Unusual spread of metastasis through these routes may not be uncommon during reversal of flow.

The presence of collateral vessels implies portal hypertension,[297, 302, 1188, 1190] though it may be present without collaterals. Portal venous stasis does not occur with just portal hypertension, but only after formation of the collaterals. As the collaterals grow larger, greater amounts of blood are diverted through them and may increase to 87 percent of the flow. This, however, may not diminish the portal hypertension (Figs. 25-37 to 25-46).

Splenic Vein Collaterals

Portoportal and portosystemic communications help bypass splenic vein obstruction. The *veins* along the *curvatures of the stomach* and short gastric veins carry blood to the portal system beyond the obstruction. Collaterals carry blood *around the esophagus* to the systemic circulation. The veins along the greater and lesser curvatures of the stomach and the epiploic veins are more frequently available for collateral flow in splenic vein obstruction than in obstruction of the portal venous system. Development of these collaterals are probably the second most common cause of variceal bleeding in patients without obvious liver disease[482, 483] (Figs. 25-34 to 25-36).

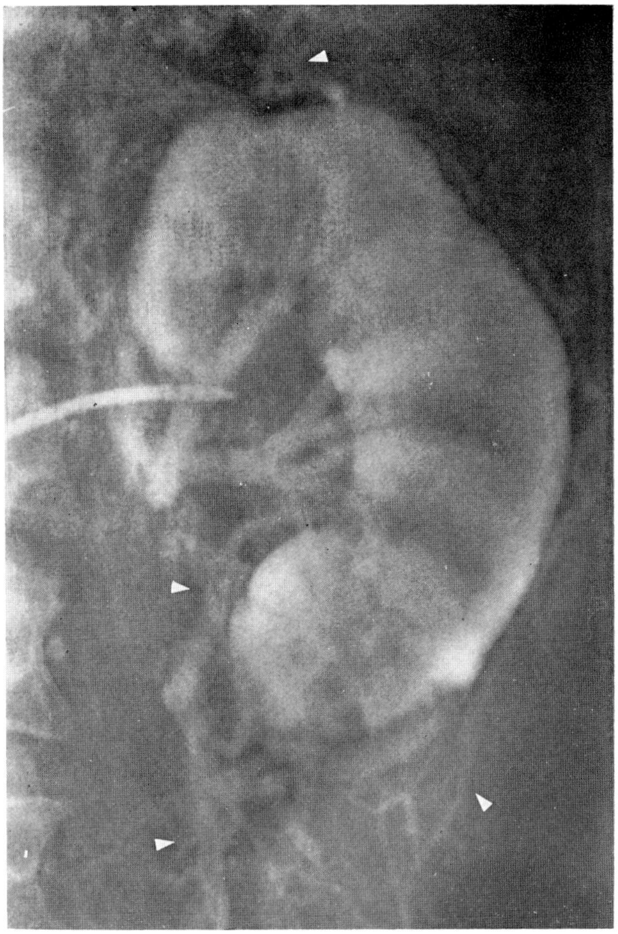

Figure 25.63. Renal Arteriogram—venous phase. No filling of the left main renal vein and abrupt termination of the renal vein branches at the renal hilus. Dilated tortuous veins are in the perinephric area (Arrow) in the renal pelvic area (Arrow) and in the retroperitoneal area. *Diagnosis:* Renal vein thrombosis with collateral venous drainage. *Pathology:* Pancreatic cyst causing left renal vein thrombosis.

Hepatic Vein Collaterals

Poverty amidst plenty. Because the hepatic

veins are so close to the termination of the inferior vena cava and within the reaches of the right atrium, they lack interspersed major tributaries between themselves and the cava.[434, 484, 485] When obstructed, the hepatic sinusoids dilate as they try to overcome the comparatively higher pressure in the portal venous circulation. This venous system is truly at a handicap as it works to overcome both the obstruction and the higher pressure in the portal venous system. Though collaterals are available, they are useless because of their small number and caliber. The *inefficient collaterals* include the capsular veins, diaphragmatic veins, veins in the hepatic ligaments, veins in adhesions, and the hepatic lymphatics. Effort is spent trying to convert the *portal vein to an efferent channel* via the hepatic sinusoids, which occurs only at the expense of the splanchnic circulation. If only a *segmental hepatic vein* is occluded, then the blood may bypass into another unoccluded hepatic vein via the hepatic sinusoids or lymphatics[499, 500] (Figs. 25-47 to 25-49).

Renal Vein and Its Collaterals

If the renal vein is obstructed, the venous companions of the renal collateral arterial supply help to drain the venous backlog. Veins of the perirenal fat and their anastomoses with the subcapsular veins of the kidney and uretral veins assist in drainage. The adrenal, gonadal and lumbar veins, and their connection with the capsular and subcapsular veins of the kidney[492] also supply significant collateral pathways (Fig. 25-63).

Inferior Vena Caval Collaterals

The most fascinating feature of obstruction of this great venous conduit is the *spectrum of clinical manifestations* related to the obstruction of its lumen at different levels.[486–489] The obstruction may jeopardize the outflow of the involved organs. In *infrarenal caval obstruction,* the renal veins remain patent. The collaterals proceed through the left gonadal vein to the left renal vein which in turn empties into the cava. In *middle caval obstructions* at the level of the renal vein, connections between the cava and portal venous system are encouraged through the liver and hepatic veins. If the cava is occluded *above the level of the renal veins,* the major anastomoses develop from the portal and inferior vena cava to the superior vena caval system. The routes can be *central, intermediate, superficial and portal.* The central route is from the iliac vein to the ascending lumbar vein to the vertebral vein to the azygos vein to the cava distal to the obstruction. The intermediate route is from the gonadal and ureteric vein to the left renal and azygos systems. The superficial route involves the abdominal wall veins, the portal route is via the umbilical and rectal veins. The ascending lumbar veins are the earliest and most constant collateral vessels. The vertebral plexus are immediately available but inefficient, while the superficial veins develop over a long period of time.

The ascending lumbar and ovarian veins enlarge to remarkable size with less thrombotic interference than other veins, but with a higher risk of transporting emboli. The presence of a persistent left inferior vena cava is a blessing but a great threat to transporting embolus if the right inferior vena cava has been plicated for the prevention of pulmonary emboli (Figs. 25-50 to 25-56).

Lower-Extremity Venous Collaterals

Femoropopliteal occlusions cause minimal embarrassment of the venous drainage due to the efficient flow via the deep femoral vein.[490] Femoral occlusions have little venous insufficiency due to good return via the deep femoral vein. Iliofemoral occlusions have a high incidence of venous insufficiency because the small, less direct collaterals are inefficient. The efficiency is increased as the valves become incompetent (Figs. 25-57, 25-58).

Superior Vena Cava and Its Collaterals

When the superior vena cava is obstructed, the collaterals develop between the superior and inferior vena cava posteriorly via the azygos and vertebral veins, anteriorly via the veins of the chest and abdominal wall, and across the mid-line by the cervical veins, azygos, hemiazygos and vertebral veins[491] (Figs. 25-59 to 25-62).

CHAPTER 26
EXTRAVASATION

The angiographic extravasation of contrast is actually the clinical counterpart of bleeding. Extravasation of contrast may occur into the wall of the blood vessel, the perivascular space, the lumen of a viscus, ducts, or cavity, or the parenchyma of an organ, muscle or tumor.

EXTRAVASATION INTO THE VESSEL WALL

Extravasation of contrast may occur into the media of a vessel wall[501] (dissecting hematoma), into the periatheromatous cleavage plane,[502] and rarely into the adventitia.[503]

Dissecting Hematomas

This is produced by the penetration of the circulating blood into the substance of the wall of a vessel with subsequent extension of the effused blood for variable distances between the layers.[501] The *aorta* is the most common artery involved, but any artery, including the perforating arteries of the brain, may be affected. Soon after the initiation of the process, propagation occurs. It is primarily distal to the perforating site, but may rarely extend proximally. *Medial degeneration*[504] of the arterial wall is the important prerequisite. Though the medial cleavage precedes the hemorrhage, the cleavage may be present without blood in the dissected plane. This itself may be fatal due to occlusion of the vessels.[505] Hypertension and strain from exercise may be the precipitating factors. Atherosclerosis does not predispose to dissection, but is coincidental.[504]

The dissection may involve[506] the entire aorta, its branches, and may cause aortic insufficiency. It may be limited to the ascending aorta only or may start distal to the left subclavian artery and extend into the descending aorta for varying lengths. If the primary tear is close to the heart, this favors lengthy or wide dissection and a fatal outcome. The junction of the aortic arch with the ascending and descending aorta is subject to great strain, suggesting that these areas are more susceptible to the initiation of a hematoma. The *tears in the intima* may be transverse, longitudinal or oblique.[501] The limited extension of the dissection into the branches of the aorta is due to their muscular nature. The exception to this occurs in the more elastic iliac arteries.[507]

The *false sac*[501] formed in the wall of the vessel communicates with the original lumen through one or several ruptures of the inner layer of the wall. The sac may rupture into the exterior as well. On rare occasions it may remain as a hematoma in the wall. The rupture into the arterial lumen enables endothelialization of the walls of the sac through which blood circulates. Sometimes the sac may become obliterated, which is the rationale for medical management.[510] Internal or external rupture may occur because of excessive bulging of the sac, thereby obliterating the true lumen and further increase in the size of the sac. This process is expedited if there are zones of resistance offered by obstruction, origin of a branch or, sharp curves with associated degenerative changes in the wall.

Healed Dissecting Hematoma

This term is applied when the dissection has an entry from and an exit into the true lumen.[501] This sac becomes lined with endothelium; *it is an imperfect cure of nature to the problem, without restoration of normal function.* However, the above conditions are the prerequisites to survival as they prevent fatal rup-

(Text continues on page 410)

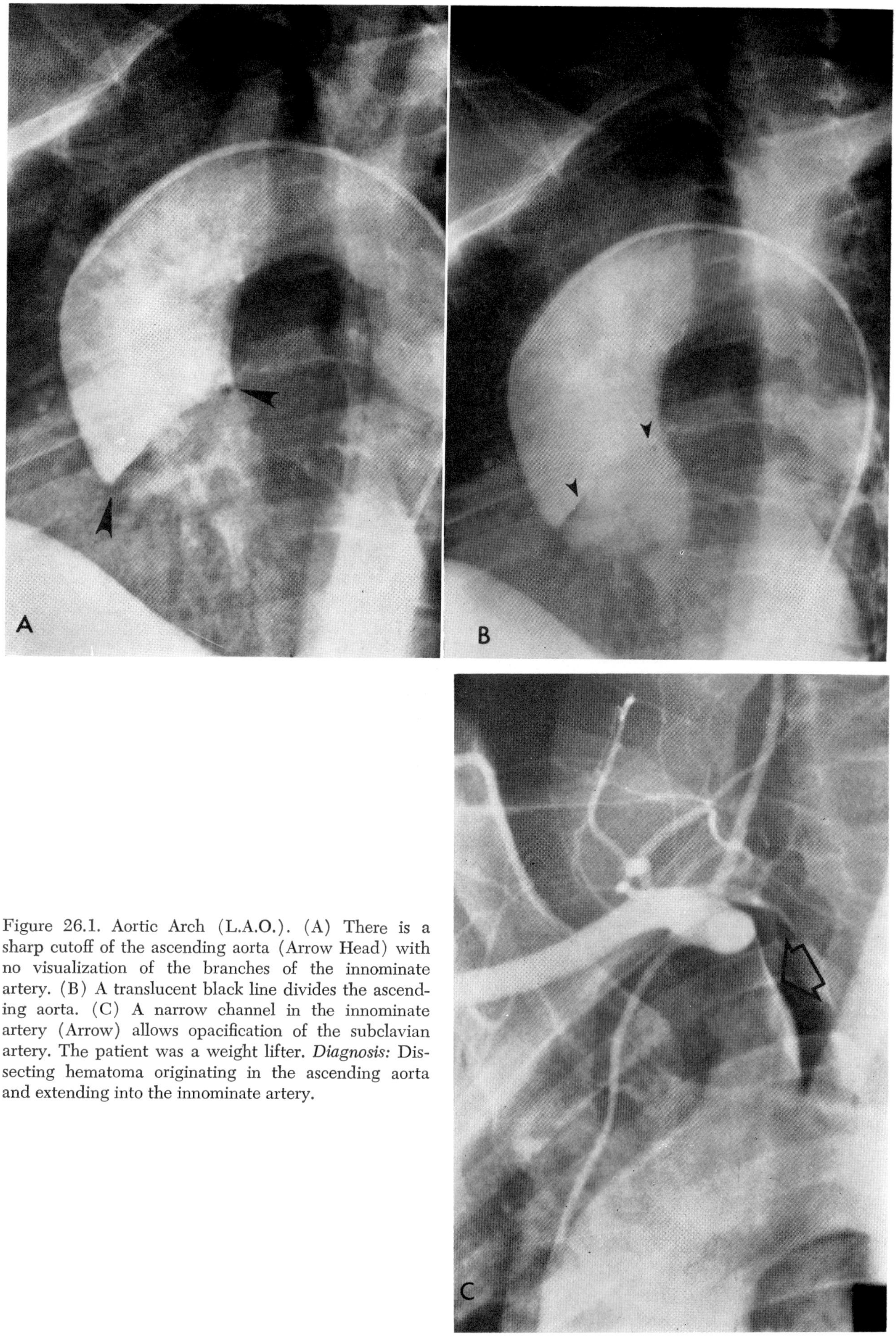

Figure 26.1. Aortic Arch (L.A.O.). (A) There is a sharp cutoff of the ascending aorta (Arrow Head) with no visualization of the branches of the innominate artery. (B) A translucent black line divides the ascending aorta. (C) A narrow channel in the innominate artery (Arrow) allows opacification of the subclavian artery. The patient was a weight lifter. *Diagnosis:* Dissecting hematoma originating in the ascending aorta and extending into the innominate artery.

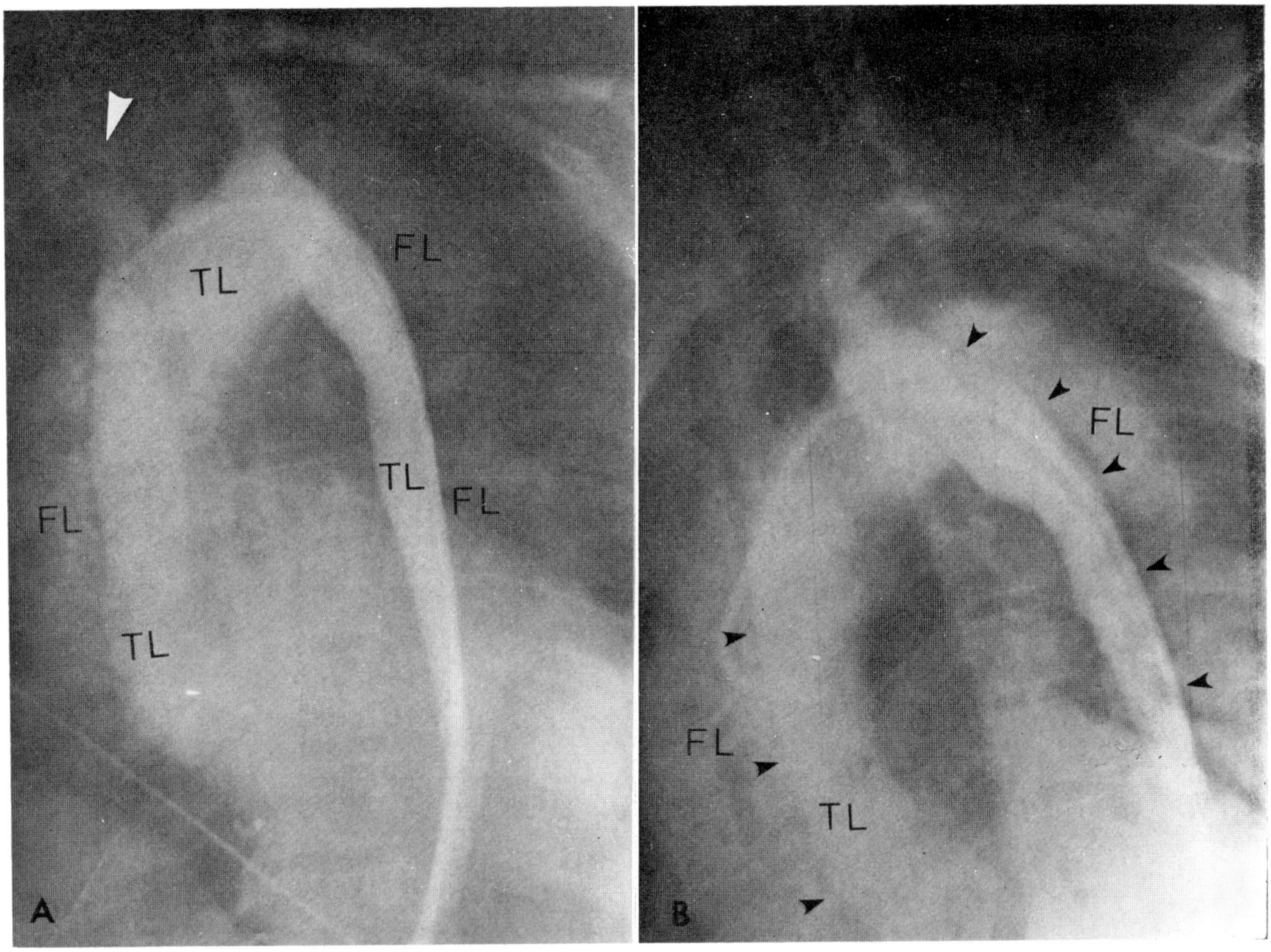

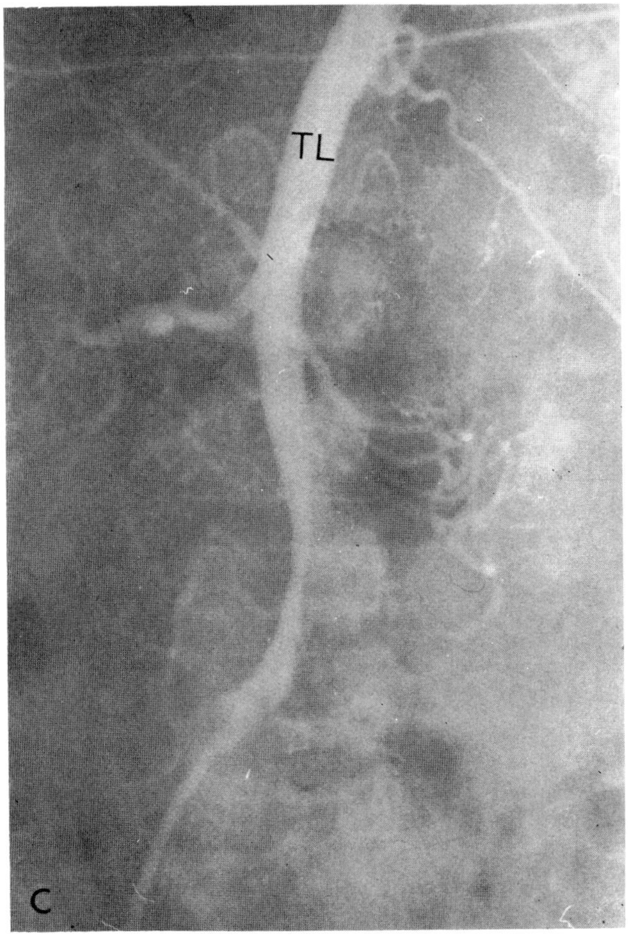

Figure 26.2. Aortic Arch Angiogram. (A) There is a dense compressed column of contrast (true lumen) (T.L.), a transected appearance of the innominate artery (Arrow Head) and no visualization of the left common carotid artery. (B) A second lumen (false) is faintly opacified (F.L.) separated by a thin, lucent line (intimal reflection) (Arrow Head). (C) There is a spiral narrowed column of contrast in the abdominal aorta (true lumen). The left renal artery, left-sided lumbar arteries and aortic bifurcation do not visualize. *Diagnosis:* Dissecting hematoma of the aorta starting at the aortic valve and extending to the abdominal aortic bifurcation.

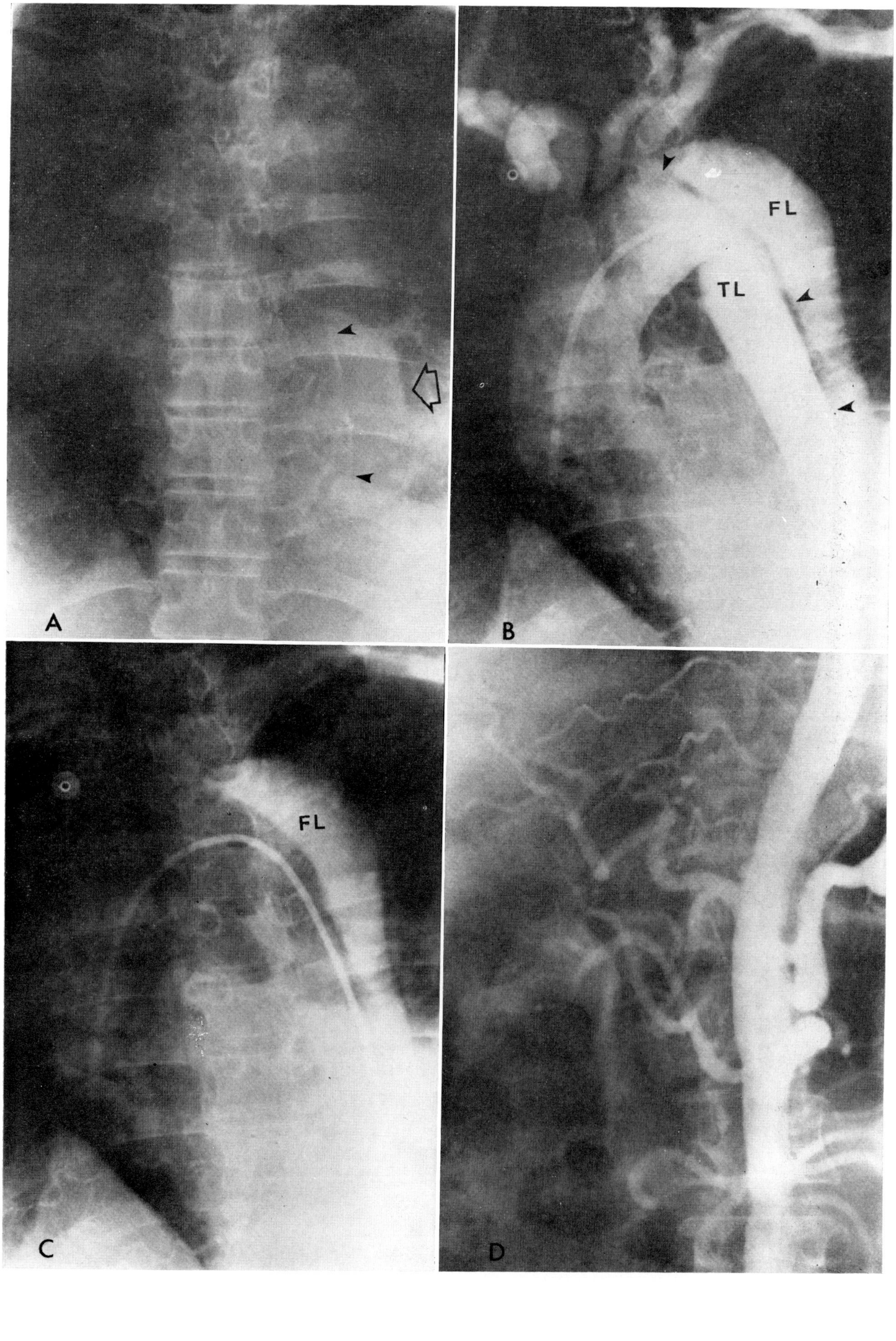
A
FL
TL
B
FL
C
D

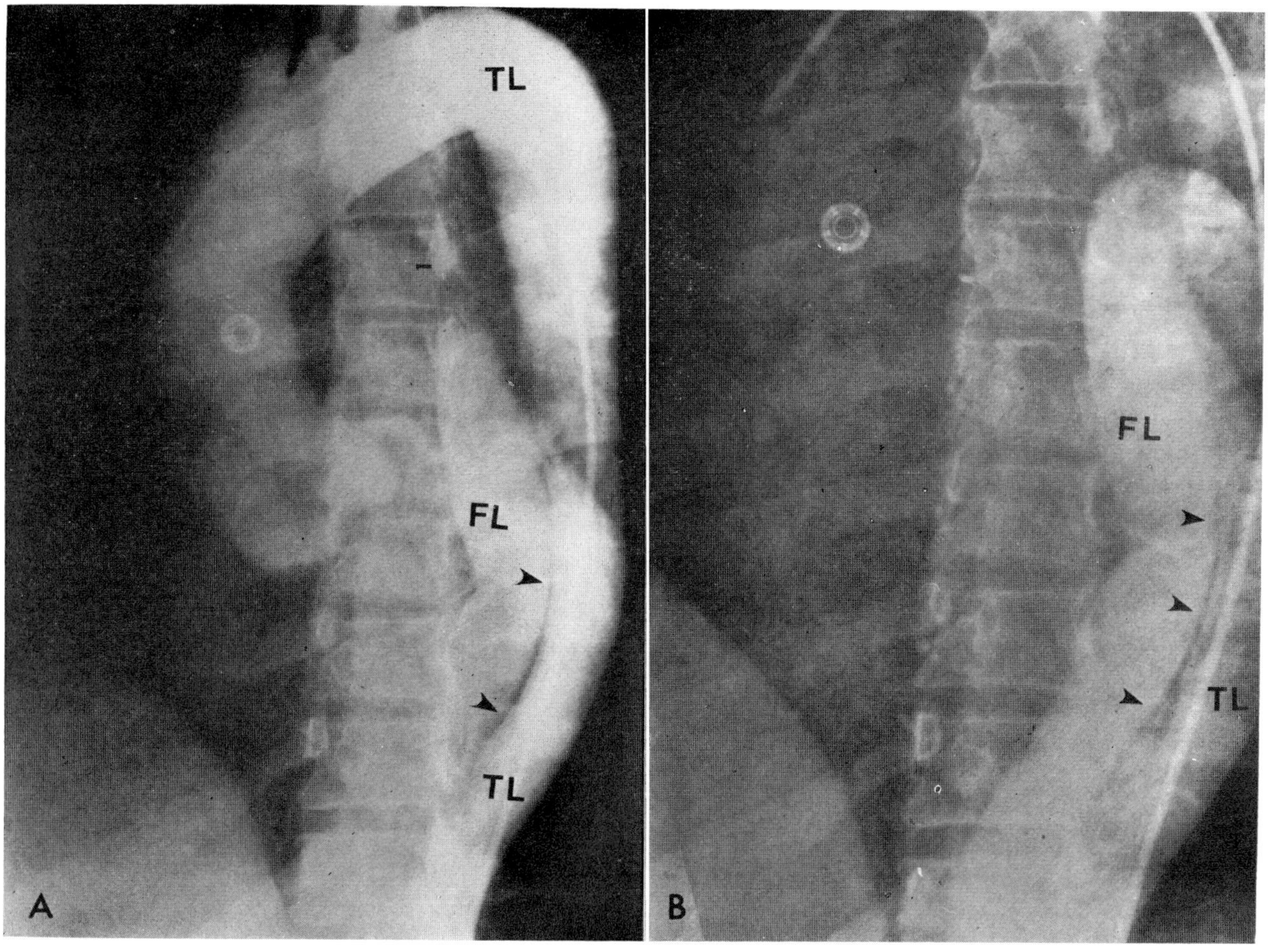

Figure 26.4. Aortogram. (A) Early aortographic phase: There are two longitudinal columns of contrast material (false and true lumens) with a translucent line separating them (Arrow Head). (B) Late arterial phase: Both lumens are well opacified. *Diagnosis:* Extravasation into the aortic wall causing a dissecting hematoma. *Comment:* The false lumen in this particular case is on the right side. However, most occur on the left side.

←

Figure 26.3. (A) Plain chest film reveals undue separation of the intimal calcification (Arrow Head) from the wall of the aorta (Arrow). (B) Aortic arch injection reveals two columns of contrast; the false (F.L.) and true lumens (T.L.) separated by the deflected intima (Arrow). (C) Late phase reveals stasis of contrast in the false lumen. (D) Abdominal aorta of the same reveals nonfilling of the left renal artery, the intercostal and lumbar arteries on the left side. *Diagnosis:* Dissecting hematoma of the aorta originating distal to the take-off of the left subclavian artery and extending distally to the abdominal aorta.

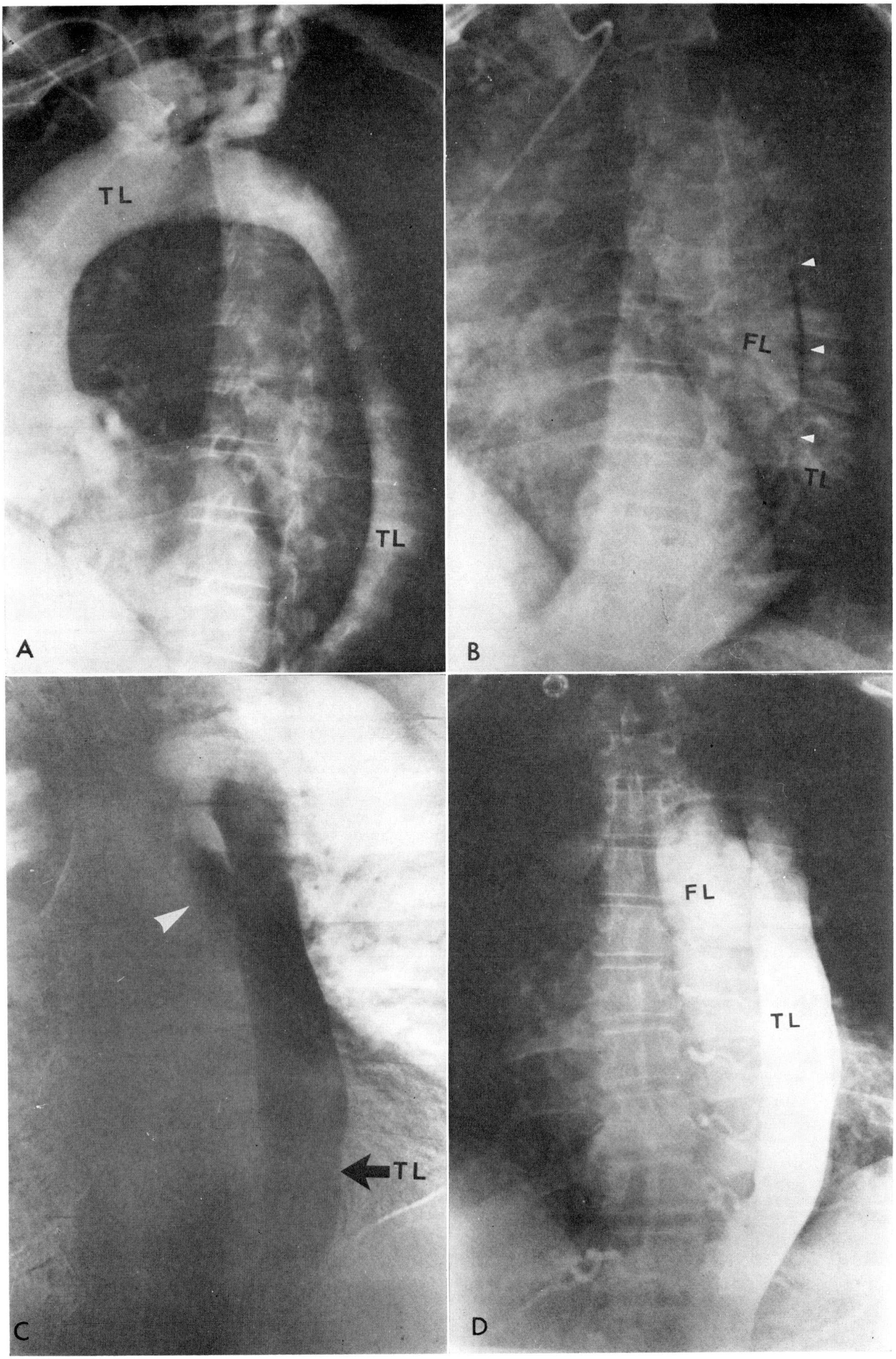

TL
TL
A
FL
TL
B
TL
C
FL
TL
D

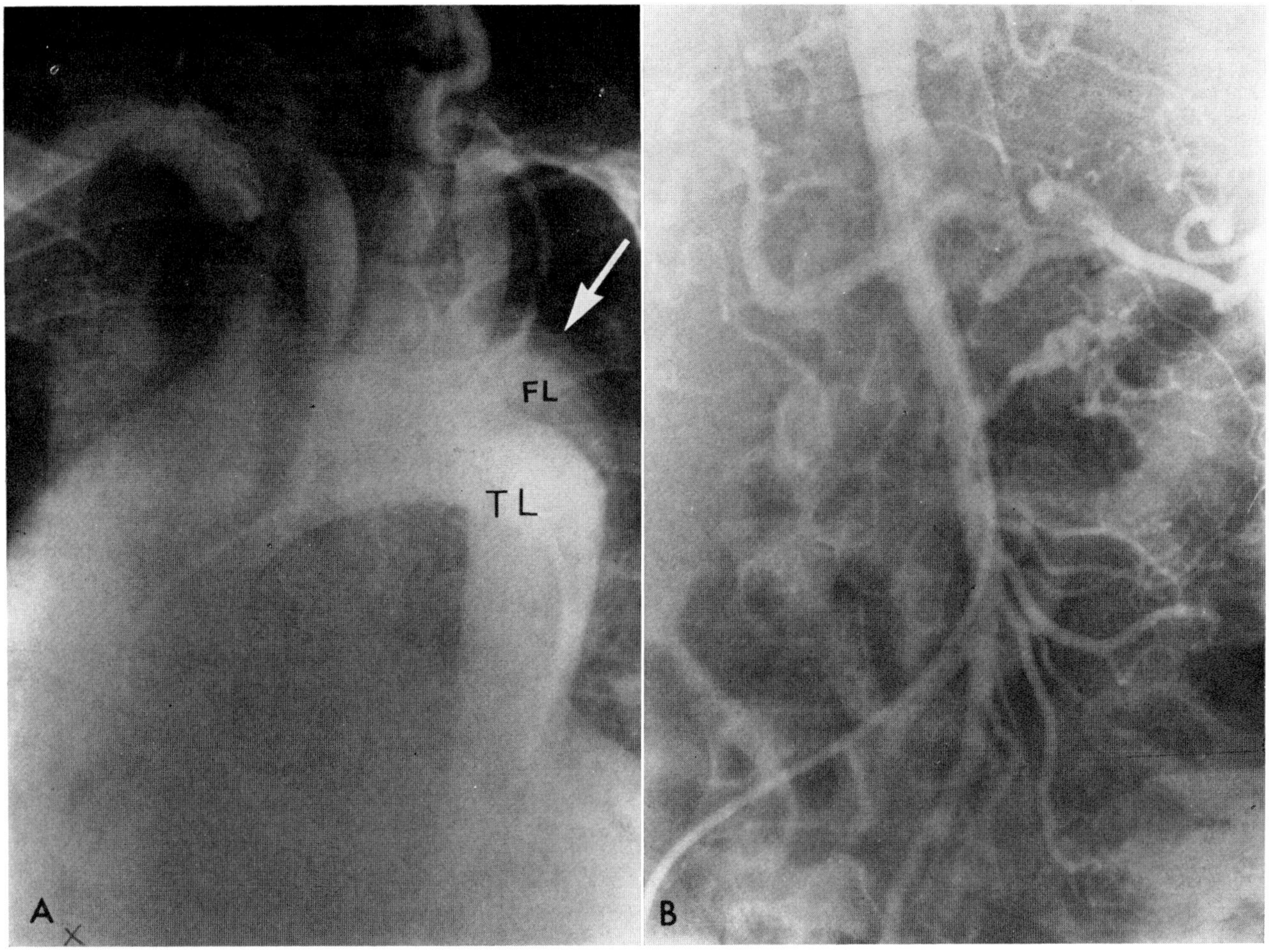

Figure 26.6. Aortic Arch Angiogram (A.P.). (A) A dense column of contrast in the aorta (T.L.) is separated from the aortic contour (Arrow). A defect at the branching of the innominate artery is seen, with filling of the proximal right subclavian artery. A thin column of contrast is seen in the left subclavian artery. (B) Neither the right renal artery or right side lumbar arteries fill. *Diagnosis:* Dissecting hematoma of the ascending aorta extending into the cephalic vessels and extending down to the abdominal aortic bifurcation with a very small, true lumen. (True lumen (T.L.), False lumen (F.L.))

Figure 26.5. Aortogram. (A) Early aortographic phase: Note the marked smooth narrowing of the descending thoracic aorta (true lumen, T.L.). (B) Late aortographic phase: Two longitudinal columns of contrast are separated by a translucent line (intima) (Arrow Head). (C) Subtraction A.P. aortogram: early extravasation of the contrast material from one column to the other (Arrow Head). (D) Better filling of the second column (false lumen, F.L.) and no filling of the right-sided intercostal arteries. *Diagnosis:* Extravasation into the wall of the aorta causing a dissecting hematoma. *Comment:* Unlike a common dissecting hematoma, in this particular case, the false lumen is on the right side.

ture of the arterial wall.[511–513] Death may occur due to rupture of the hematoma into the pleural cavity, pericardium, or the mediastinum. Development of aortic valvular insufficiency or obstruction of a major arterial branch[501, 509] may also result in a fatal outcome.

Reduction of the blood supply to an area by compression of a normal lumen occurs through distension of the false lumen. This decreases the blood supply to that organ, locally or diffusely at varying levels, and is reflected in various clinical manifestations.[508] Spontaneous abdominal aortic dissections are rare but can occur.[514]

The *causes* of dissection can include medial necrosis either idiopathic[515] or due to Marfan's syndrome.[516] It may be due to methonium therapy,[517] cannulation during cardiopulmonary bypass,[518] giant cell mesoaortitis,[519] blunt trauma to the thoracic[520] and abdominal aorta,[521] or catheterization procedures.

(Text continues on page 419)

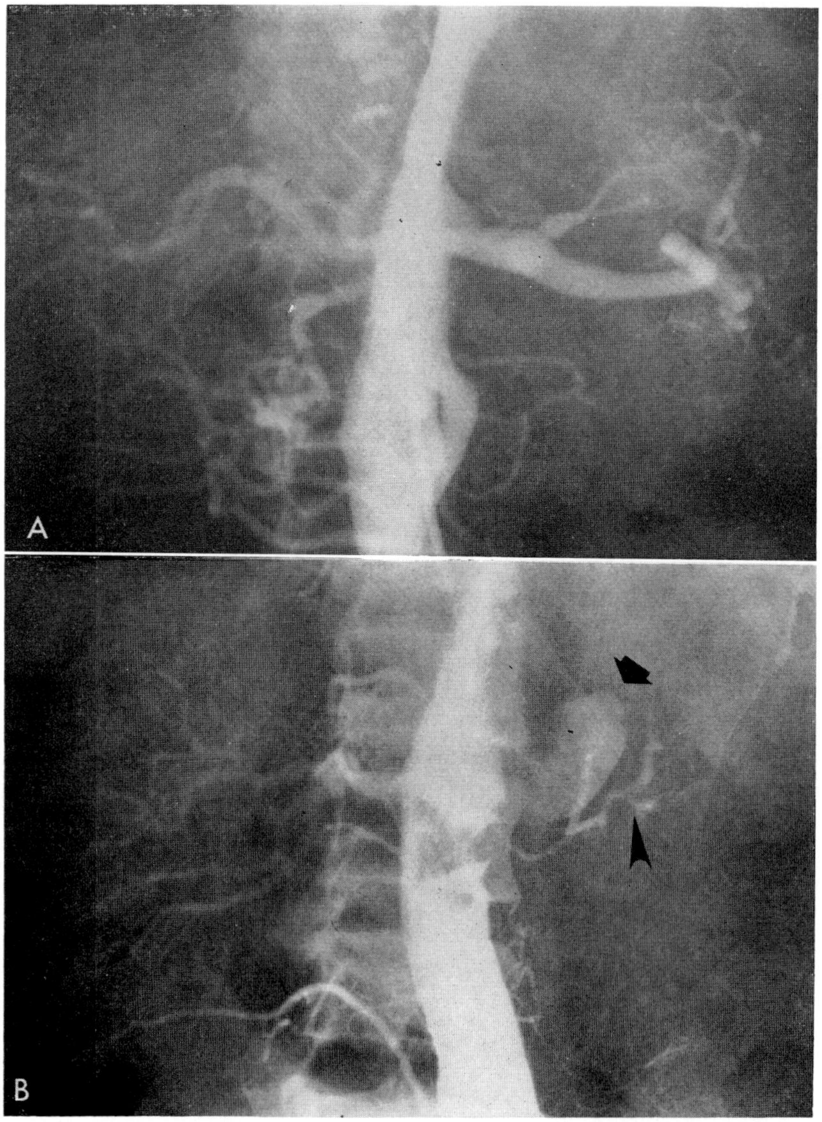

Figure 26.7. Abdominal Aortogram. (A) There is narrowing of the distal thoracic aorta and no filling of the left renal artery. (B) A sac-like collection of contrast is seen along the course of the left renal artery (Arrow). There is minimal filling of the intrarenal branches (Arrow). *Diagnosis:* Dissecting aneurysm of the thoracic aorta which is extending into the left renal artery.

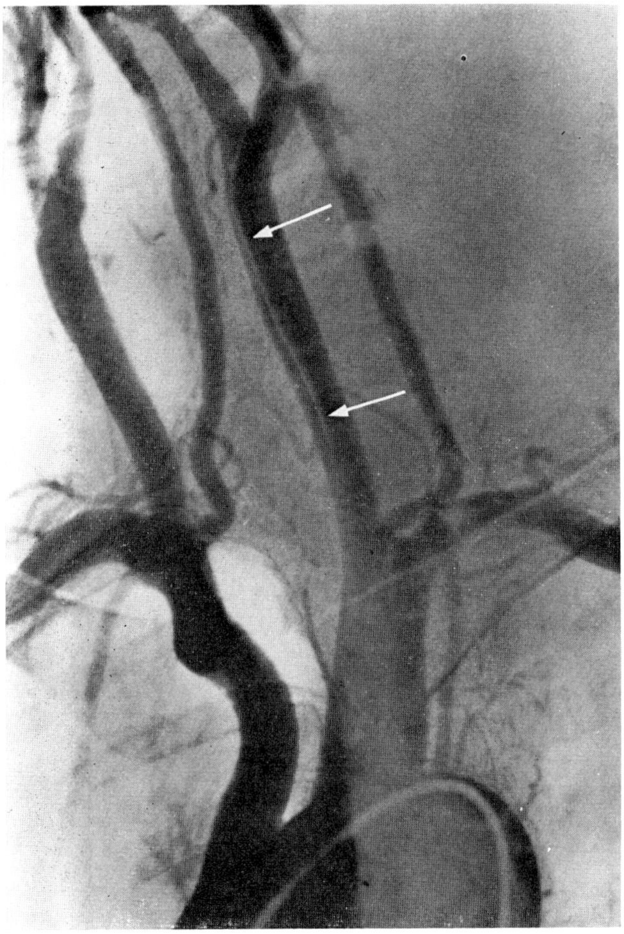

Figure 26.8. Aortic Arch Angiogram (left anterior oblique projection-subtraction films). There is a linear, white line in the main channel of the left common carotid artery (Arrow). *Diagnosis:* Spontaneous dissection of the left common carotid artery.

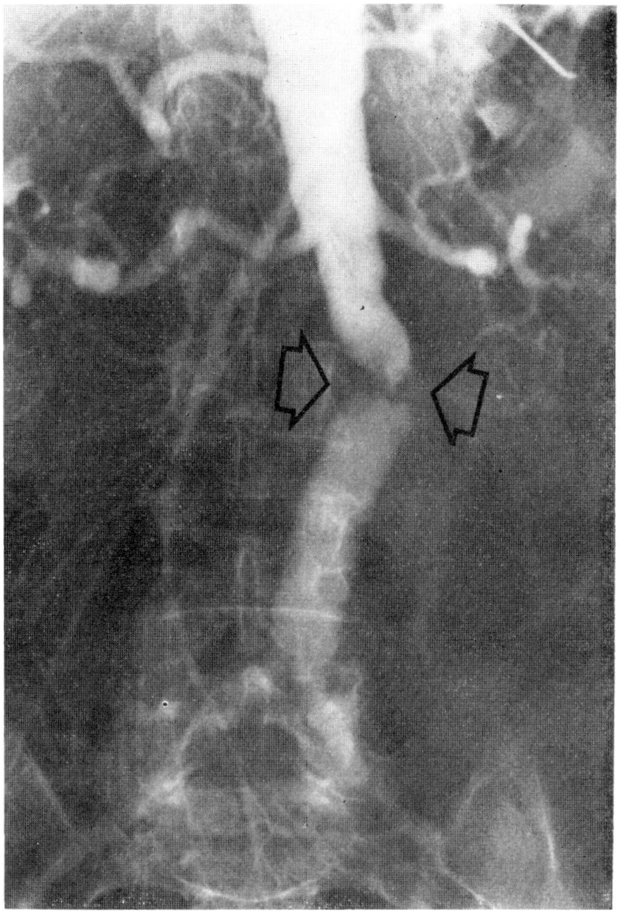

Figure 26.9. Abdominal Aortic Angiogram. The infrarenal portion of the aorta is narrowed at the anastomotic site of an abdominal aortic graft (Arrow). *Diagnosis:* Thrombosis of the anastomotic site. *Surgical Diagnosis:* Dissecting hematoma at the anastomotic site.

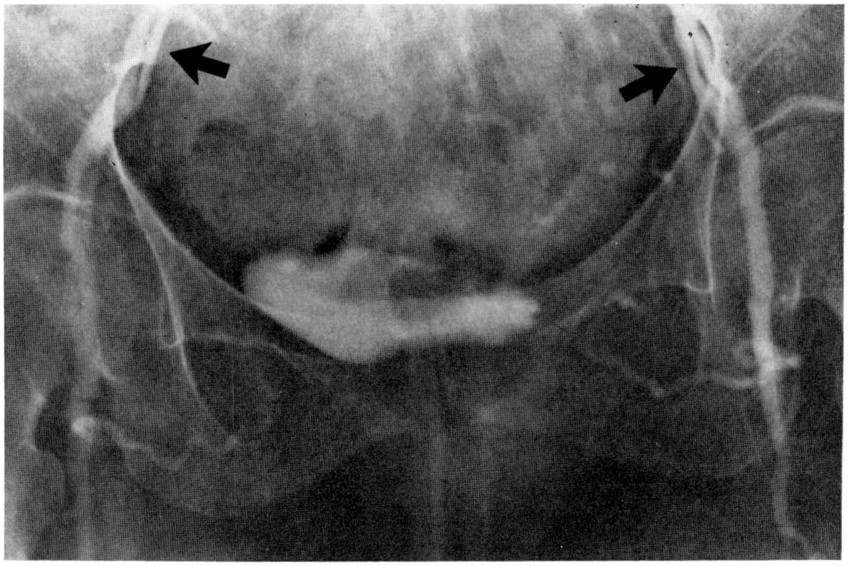

Figure 26.10. Pelvic Arteriogram. This study was done via an axillary approach. There are translucent lines (Arrow) in the external iliac arteries. This patient had bilateral arterial manipulation with a Fogerty catheter. *Diagnosis:* Subintimal dissections.

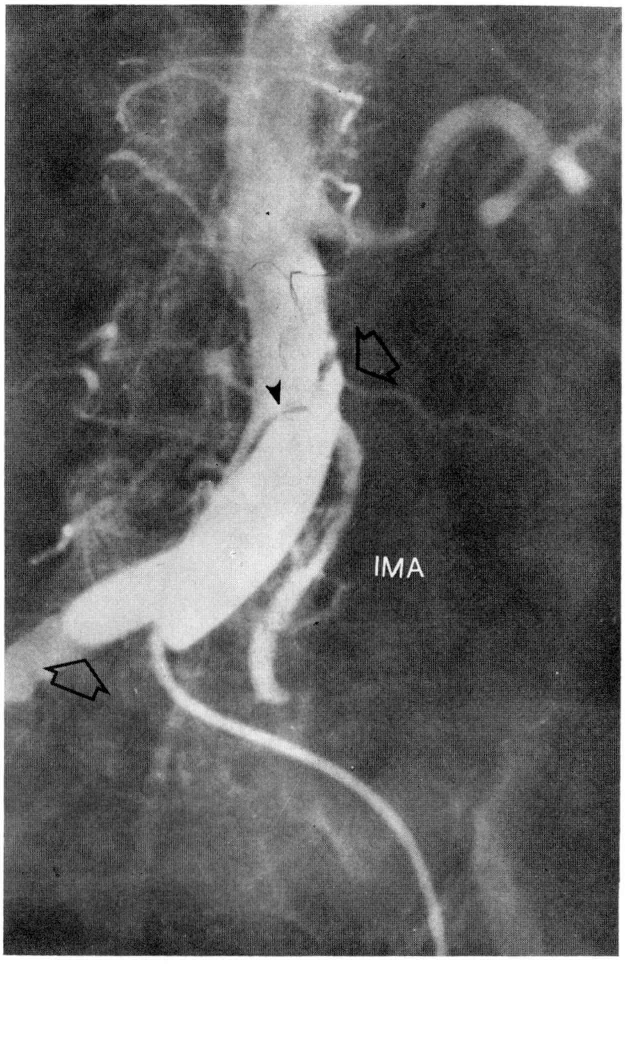

Figure 26.11. Inferior Mesenteric Arteriogram. Note the dense opacification of a segment of aorta (Arrow). The black line is due to intimal deflection (Arrow Head). There is opacification of the proximal inferior mesenteric artery. *Comment:* An attempt to catheterize an inferior mesenteric artery in a very atherosclerotic aorta resulted in subatheromatous injection with partial dissection of the aorta. Fortunately, the patient had no untoward effects.

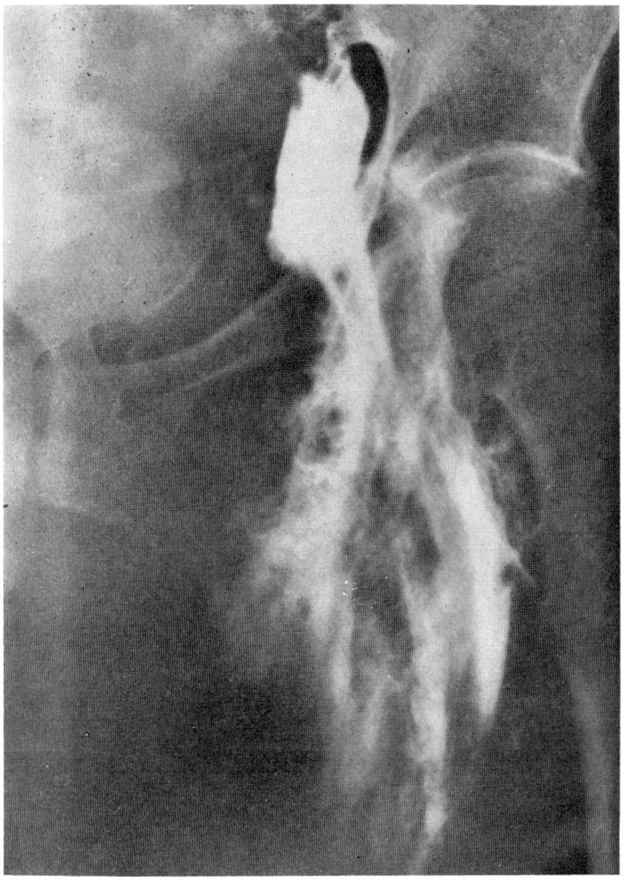

Figure 26.12. Femoral Arteriogram. Note the periarterial extravasation of contrast material due to improper placement of the needle tip.

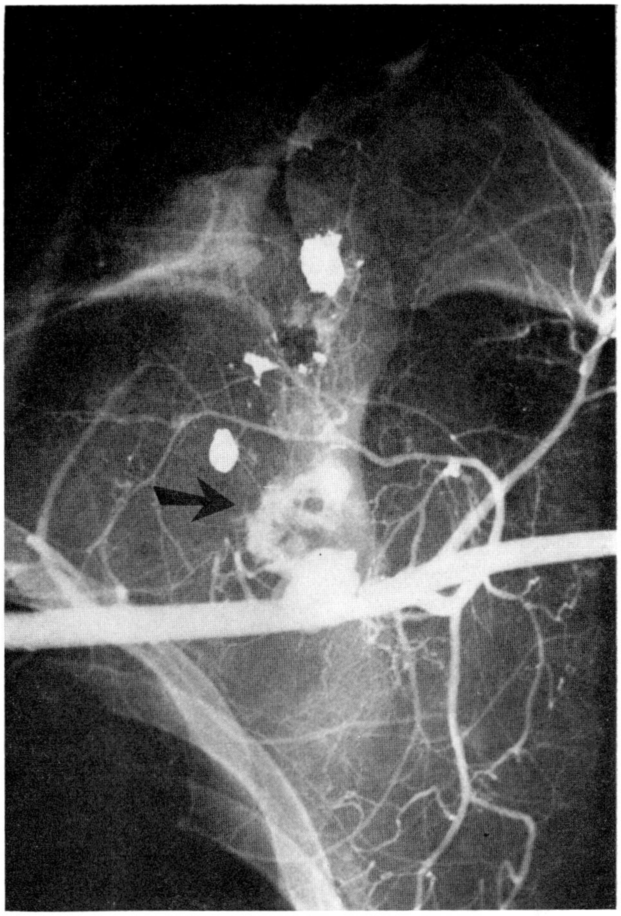

Figure 26.13. Subclavian Arteriogram. Reveals an area of saccular collection of contrast and an area of amorphous collection. Please notice the bullet. *Diagnosis:* Traumatic periarterial extravasation.

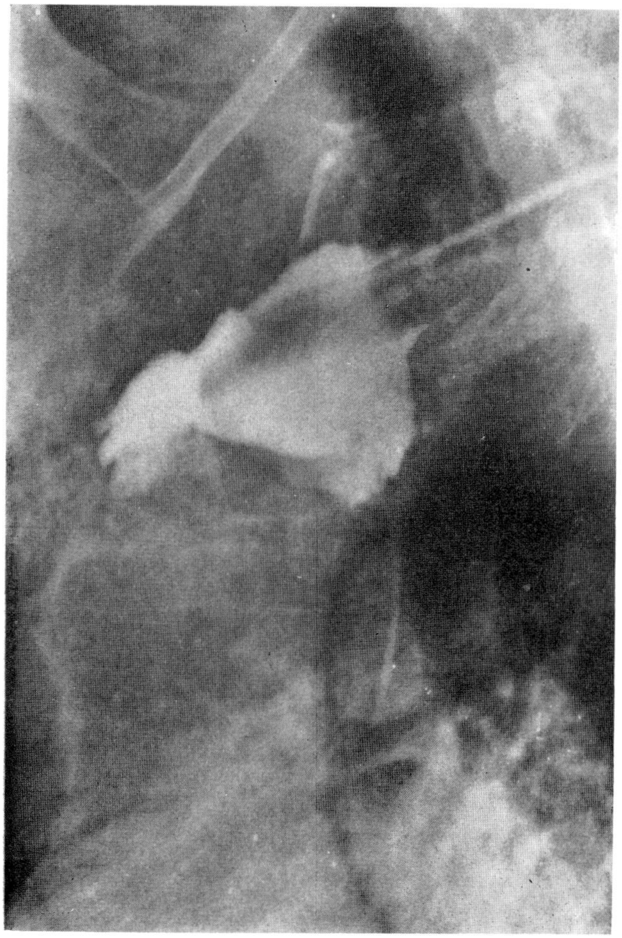

Figure 26.14. Catheter in the Innominate Vein. There is an abnormal perivenous collection of the contrast material. *Comment:* Subadventitial and perivenous extravasation of the contrast probably due to catheter whipping. This blunt end N.I.H. catheter had side holes.

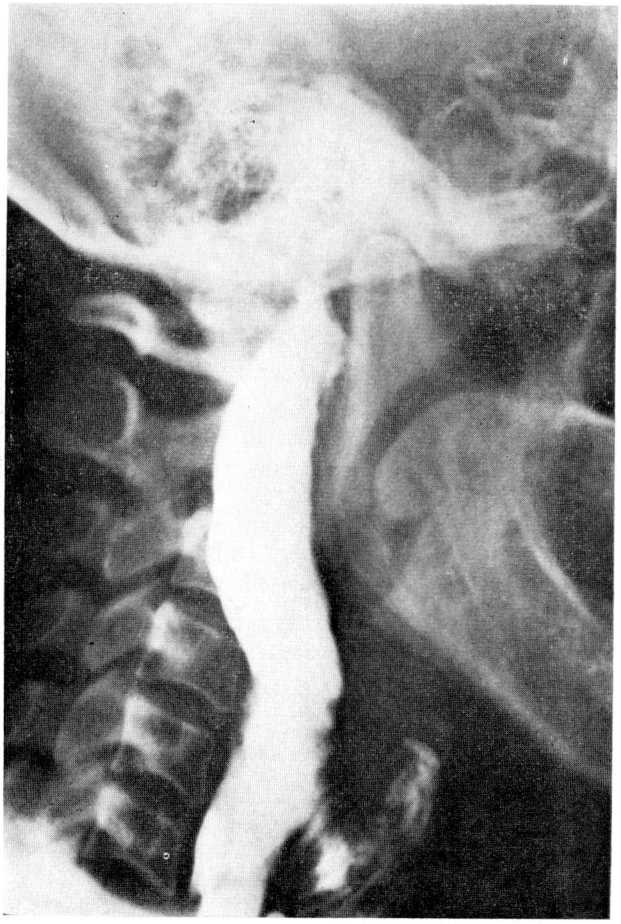

Figure 26.15. Carotid Arteriogram. There is extravasation of contrast material into the carotid sheath. *Diagnosis*: Improper placement of the needle.

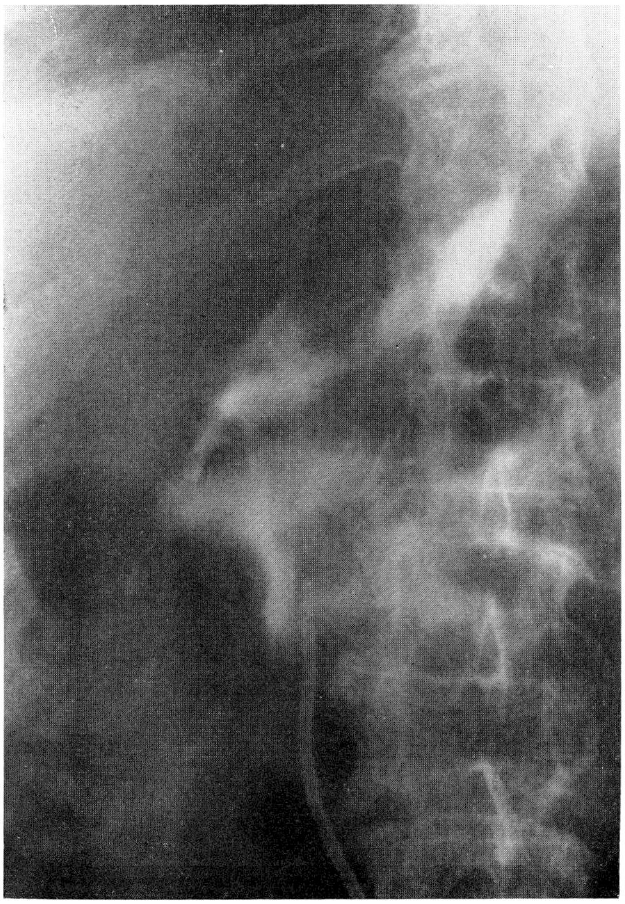

Figure 26.16. An irregular amorphous collection of contrast material is in the right paravertebral area. Notice the catheter which was originally placed in the right renal vein. *Comment:* Perforation of the renal vein from the catheter during injection causing retroperitoneal extravasation of the contrast material.

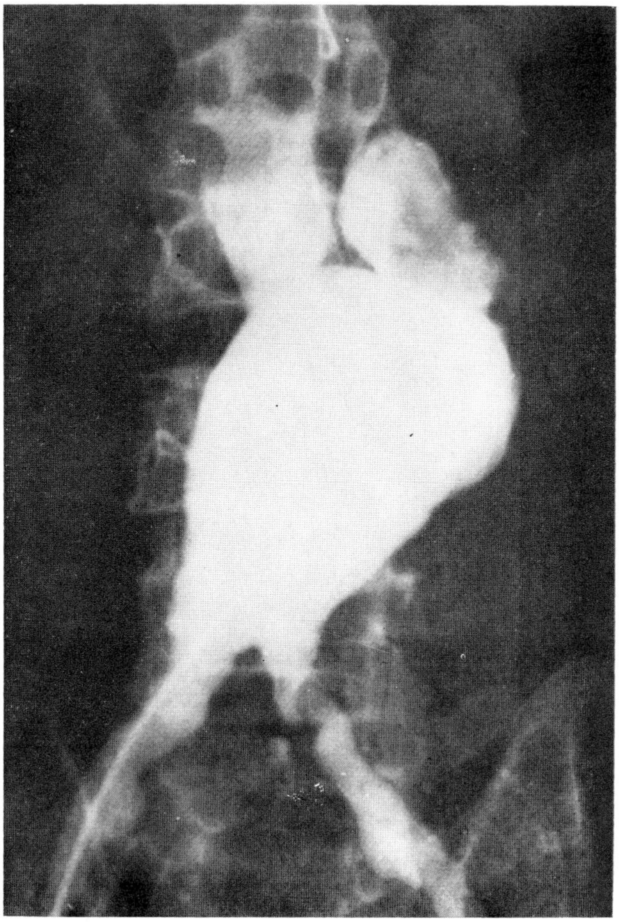

Figure 26.17. Abdominal Aortogram. Reveals a saccular collection of contrast and an area of amorphous collection. *Diagnosis:* Leaking abdominal aortic aneurysm.

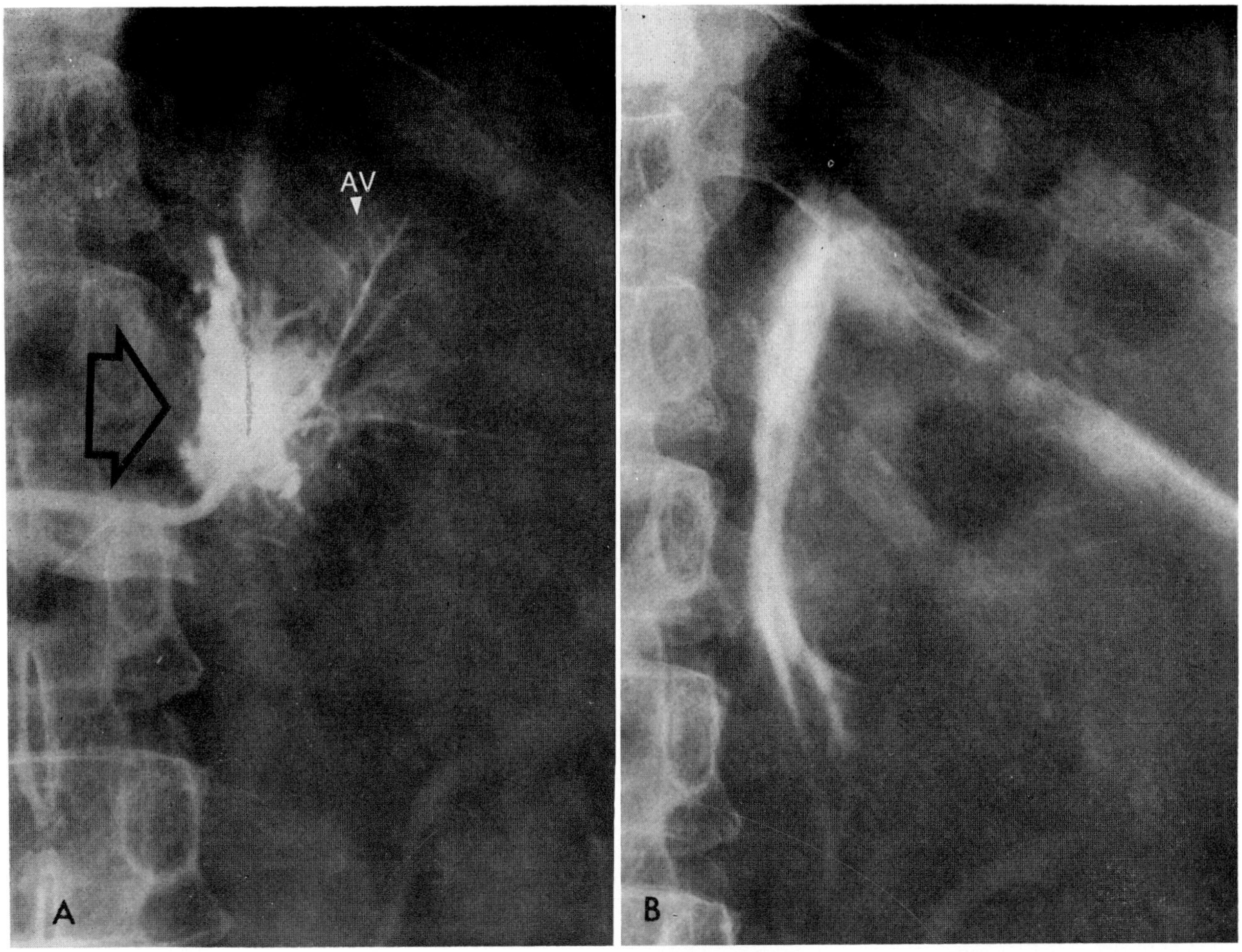

Figure 26.18. Left Adrenal Venogram. (A) There is a periadrenal amorphous collection of contrast material (Arrow) about the adrenal venous system (A.V.). (B) Late phase: This collection of contrast material diffuses around the periadrenal area. *Comment:* Retroperitoneal periadrenal extravasation because of impaction of the catheter tip in the vein and excessive pressure during injection. (Courtesy of T. Grant, Toledo, Ohio.)

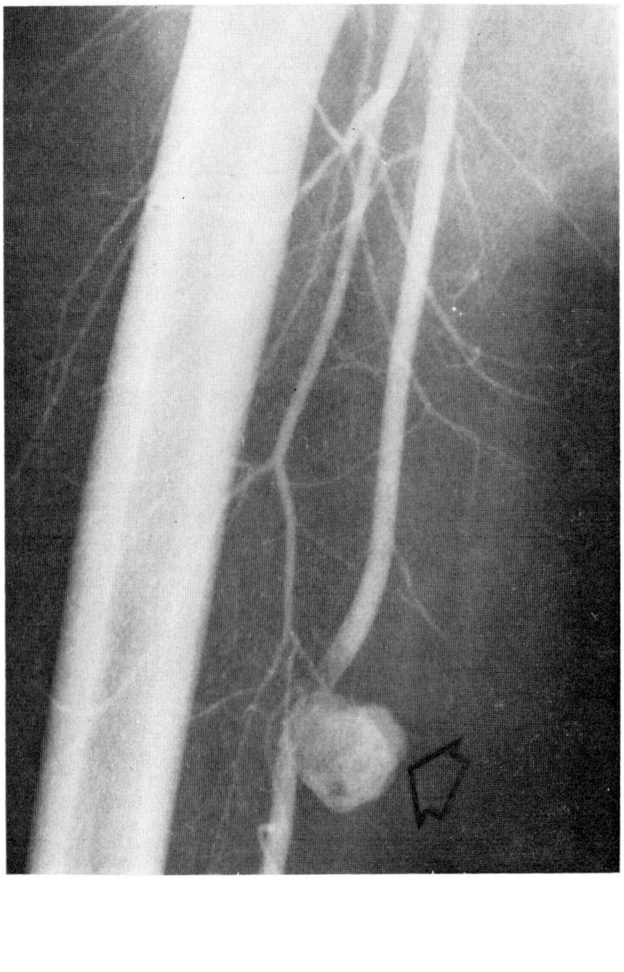

Figure 26.19. Femoral Arteriogram. There is a saccular periarterial collection of contrast. *Diagnosis:* Superficial femoral pseudoaneurysm due to a stab wound.

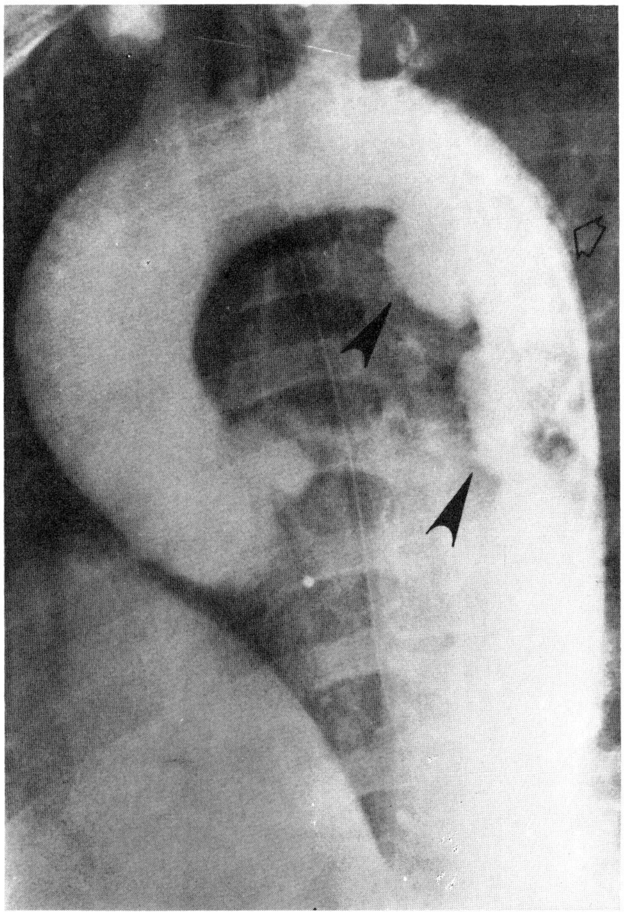

Figure 26.20. Aortogram. Irregularities in the aortic contour (Blank Arrow) and two collections of contrast material beyond the aortic wall (Arrow Head). This patient met with an automobile accident. *Diagnosis:* Periaortic extravasation of the contrast material due to aortic laceration.

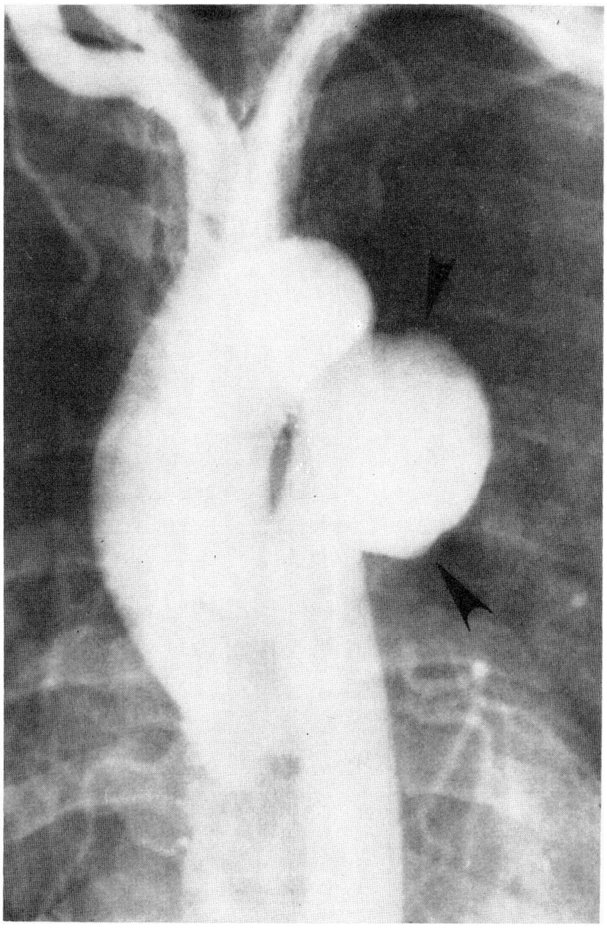

Figure 26.21. Thoracic Aortogram. Periaortic saccular collection of contrast which is distal to the origin of the left subclavian artery. *Diagnosis:* Pseudoaneurysm due to blunt chest trauma.

Figure 26.22. Superior Mesenteric Arteriogram. There is periarterial collection of contrast material coming from the ileac branches. This patient had regional enteritis and resection of the bowel with postoperative bleeding. *Diagnosis:* Extravasation of contrast at the anastomotic site.

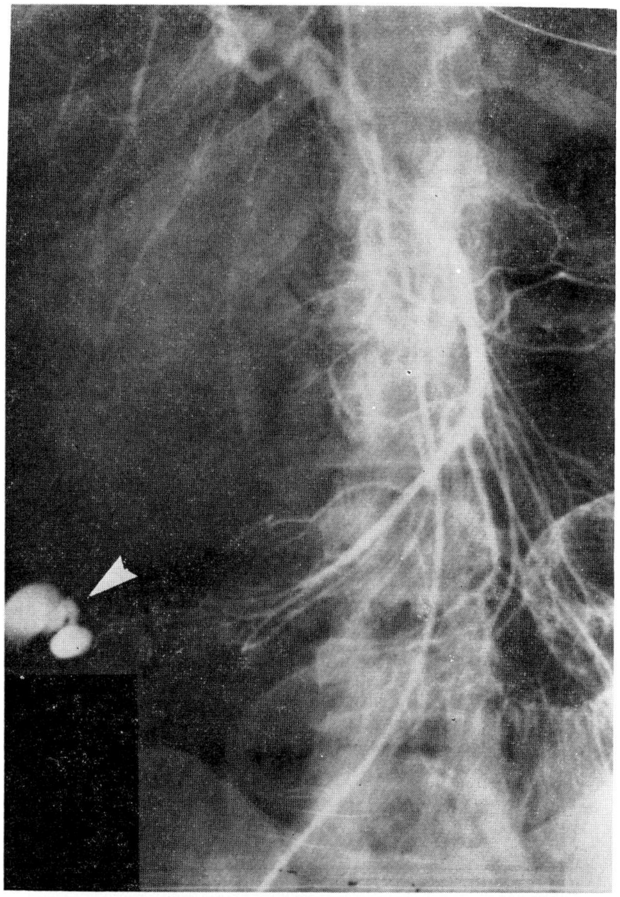

Figure 26.23. Superior Mesenteric Arteriogram. Areas of narrowing and dilatation are seen in the distal portion of the middle colic artery branch (Blank Arrow) as well as oval-shaped collections of contrast material at the termination of this artery (Arrow). This patient was known to have pancreatitis. *Diagnosis:* Encasement of the middle colic artery due to pancreatitis and fibrosis with digestion of the artery by trypsin causing a pseudoaneurysm.

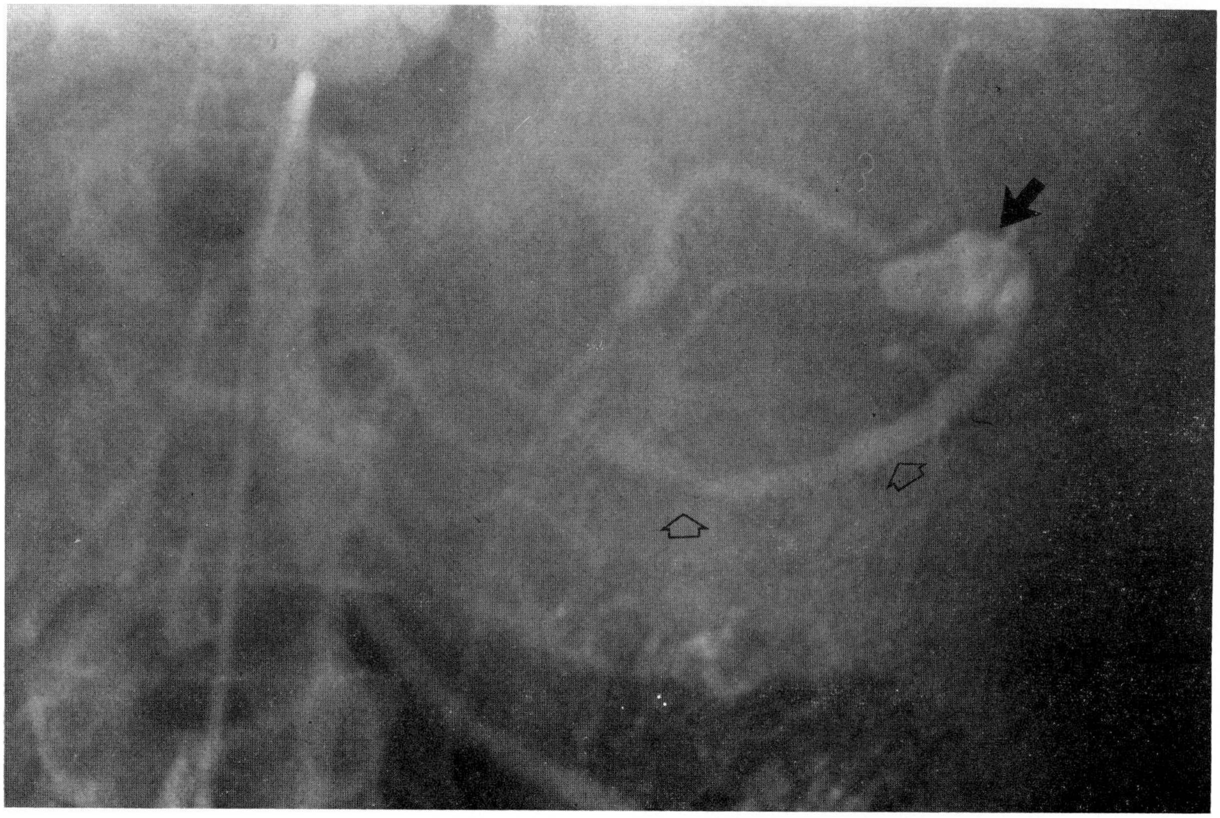

Angiographic Findings

The *deflected intima* is demonstrated as a lucent line which may be parallel to, spiral, or even transverse in relation to the long axis of the vessel. This is the vital radiographic finding for establishing a diagnosis of a dissecting hematoma. *Oscillation* of this line during systole and diastole aids the angiographer in identifying this line with confidence. On occasion, unusual tears of the intima may be difficult to demonstrate. *Failure to visualize the paired aortic branches* such as the intercostal, lumbar and renal arteries on the side of the false lumen adds strong supportive evidence for the diagnosis. Identification of the presence and location of the false sac helps in mapping out the abnormal anatomy. The most *common locations of a false aneurysmal sac*[522, 523] are anterior and to the right in the ascending aorta, posterior and superior in the aortic arch, posterior and lateral to the true lumen in the lower thoracic aorta, spiral at the level of the diaphragm, posterior and lateral in the abdominal aorta, and usually spiral in the iliac arteries.

When *contrast* is injected it *stays longer within the false sac than in the true channel.* The blood pressure in this false sac is lower than that in the true channel. The Sinus of Valsalva is not opacified if only the false lumen is perfused with contrast material. Accidental injection of a large bolus of contrast into the false

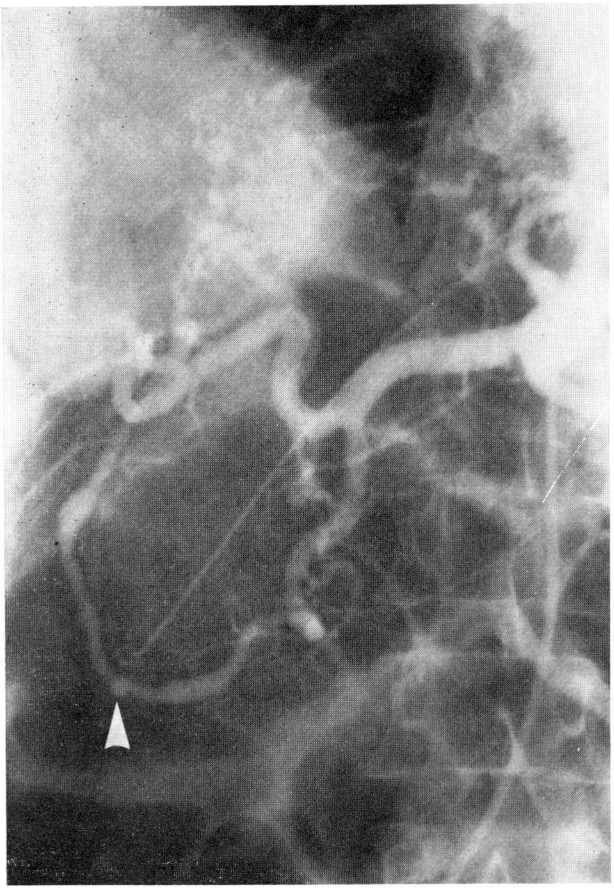

Figure 26.24. Celiac Angiogram. There is a saccular dilatation (Arrow), narrowing and subsequent dilatation of the distal gastroduodenal artery. The patient had hematemesis. *Diagnosis:* A penetrating duodenal ulcer causing encasement of the gastroduodenal artery and formation of a pseudoaneurysm.

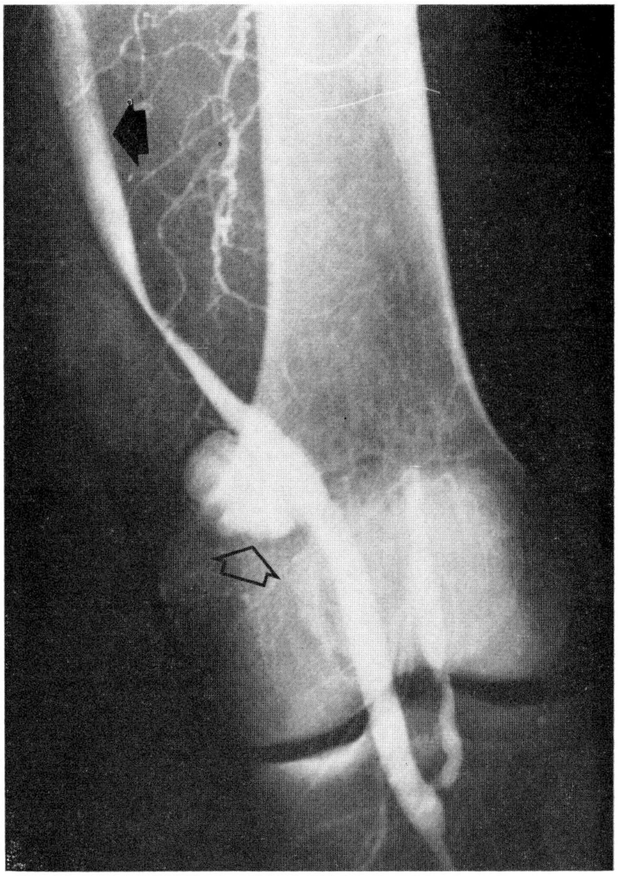

Figure 26.25. Femoral Arteriogram. There is a by-pass graft for the superficial femoral artery (Arrow). There is perivascular collection of the contrast material (Blank Arrow). *Diagnosis:* Pseudoaneurysm of the graft.

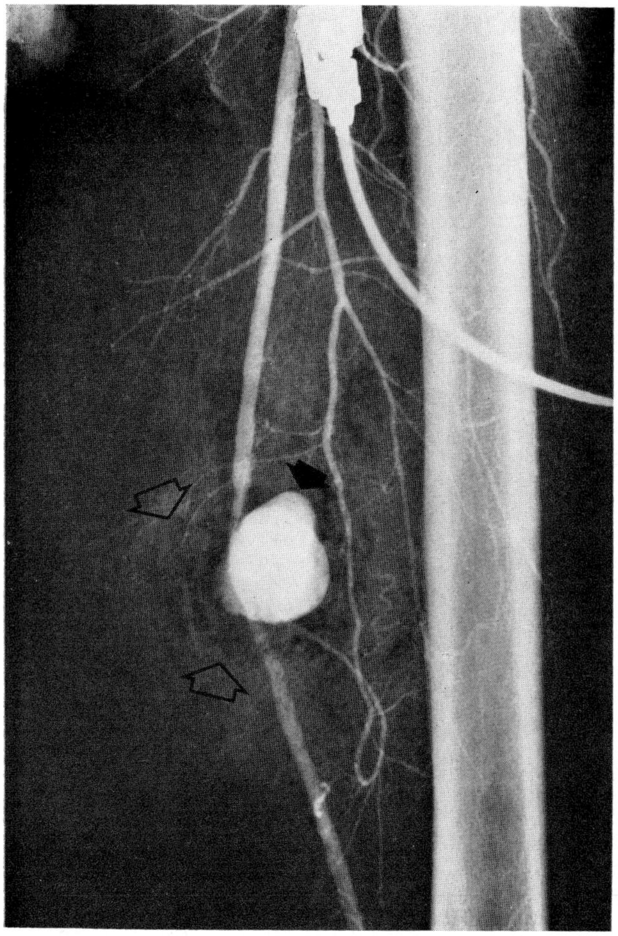

Figure 26.26. Femoral Arteriogram. Notice the mottled lucency (Blank Arrow) and saccular collection of the contrast material with secondary compression of the superficial femoral artery (Arrow). *Diagnosis:* Mycotic pseudoaneurysm.

lumen may symptomatically simulate the original clinical event. A *clotted false lumen*[522] may show ulcer-like projections due to intimal defects leading into the clotted channel. To depend on the thickness of the aortic wall[524, 525] as a diagnostic sign may mislead one because the same radiographic findings are seen with sclerosing aortitis, clotted fusiform aneurysm, excessive periaortic fat or water density masses such as blood, pleural effusions, or tumors adjacent to the aortic wall. Awareness of the possibility of faint opacification of the false lumen or simultaneous dual opacification of both channels will prevent the angiographer from overlooking an existing dissection.

The majority of aortic dissections *extend into the left renal artery* because of the usual location of the false lumen slightly to the left of the posterior lateral aspect of the true lumen in the abdominal aorta. The right renal artery is involved only when the dissection is extensive. If the origin of the left renal artery is from the anterolateral aspect of the aortic circumference, it may escape involvement from the dissection.[526]

The usual site of *subintimal hemorrhage during angiography* is into the periatheromatous cleavage plane.[502] This is an easy route for the development of catheter-induced dissection. It is not an uncommon event if there is excessive manipulation of the guide wire or catheter

(Text continues on page 434)

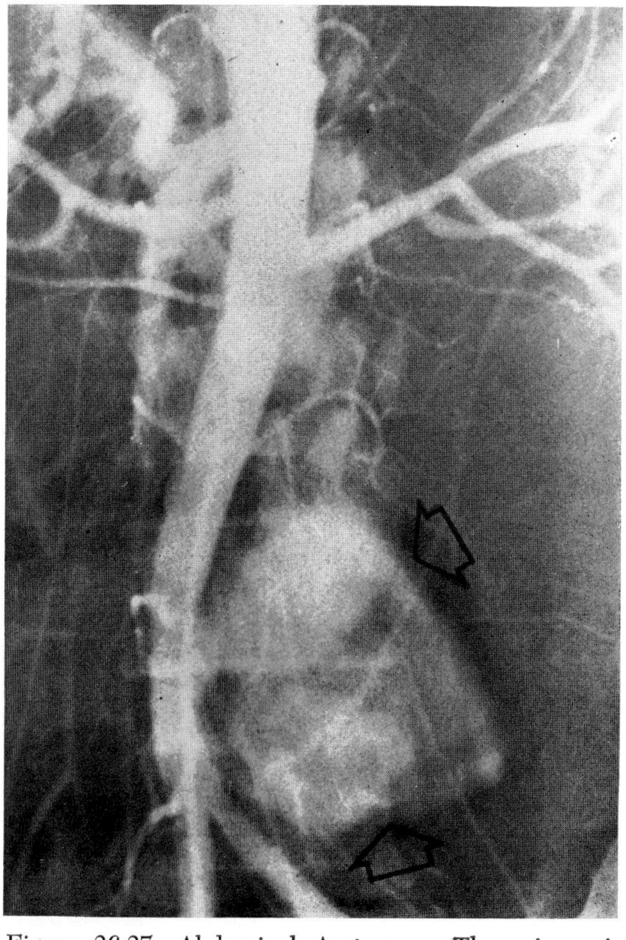

Figure 26.27. Abdominal Aortogram. There is periaortic collection of contrast into a large cavity. This patient had septicemia. *Diagnosis:* Mycotic abdominal aortic pseudoaneurysm.

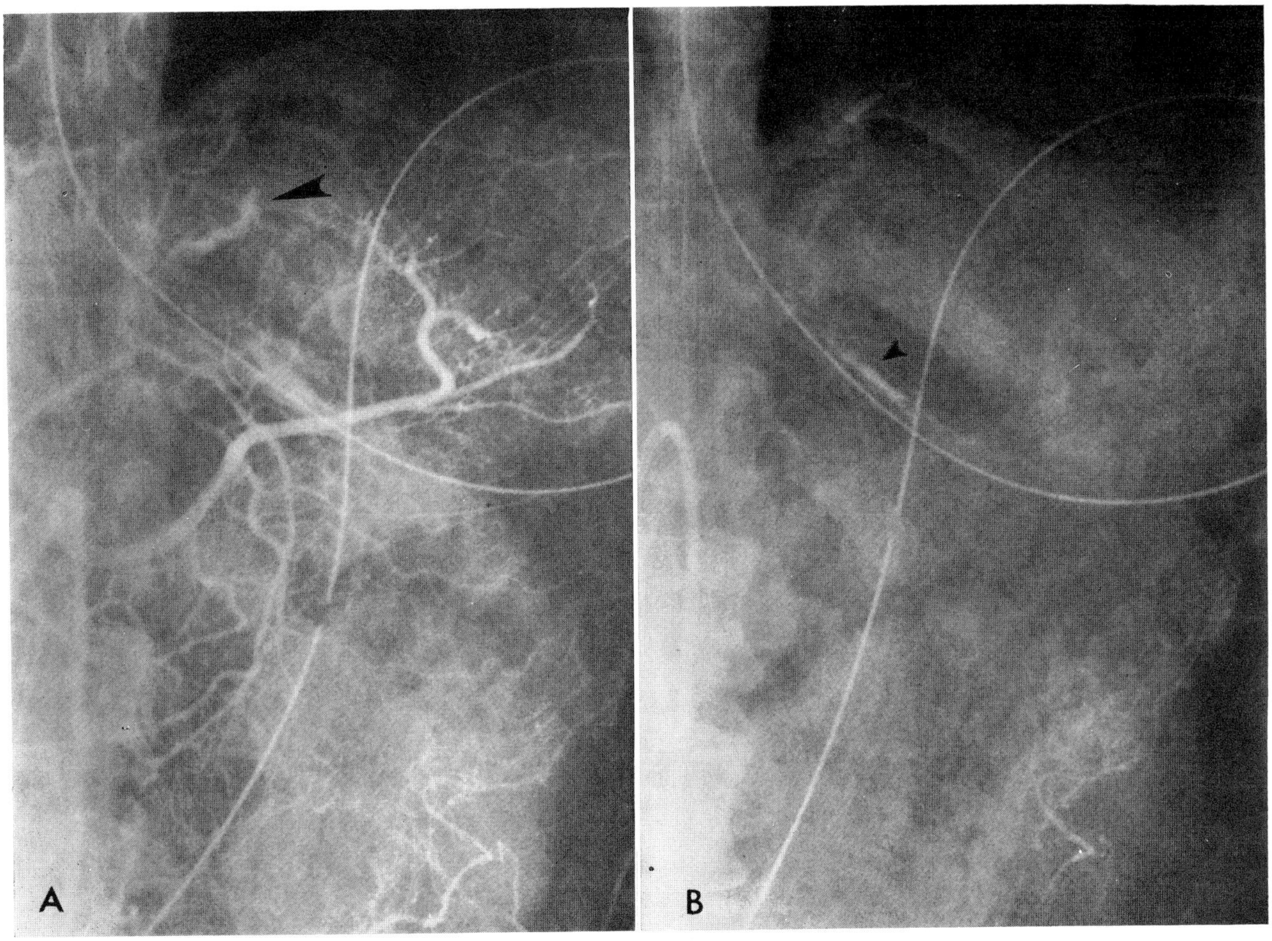

Figure 26.28. Celiac Angiogram. (A) The early phase reveals an abnormal collection of contrast material near the left gastric artery branches (Arrow). (B) The late phase reveals dispersion of this contrast into the lumen of the fundus of the stomach (Arrow). *Diagnosis:* Extravasation due to bleeding from the left gastric artery (Mallory-Weiss syndrome).

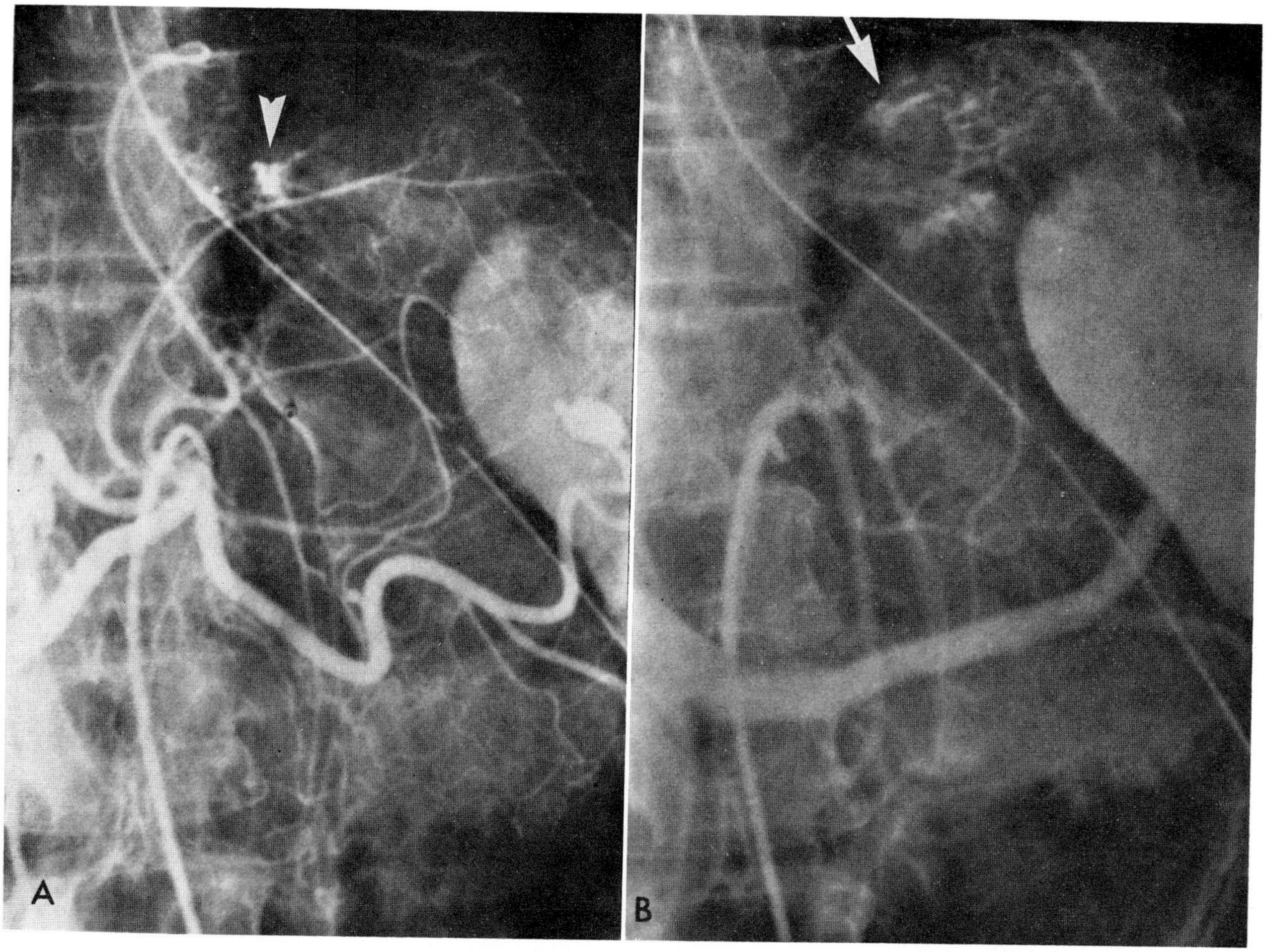

Figure 26.29. Celiac Arteriogram. (A) Arterial phase: periarterial collection of contrast from the left gastric artery branches (Arrow). (B) Parenchymal phase: This collection of contrast (Arrow) persists. The patient had hematemesis. *Diagnosis:* Bleeding into the lumen of the distal esophagus (Mallory-Weis syndrome).

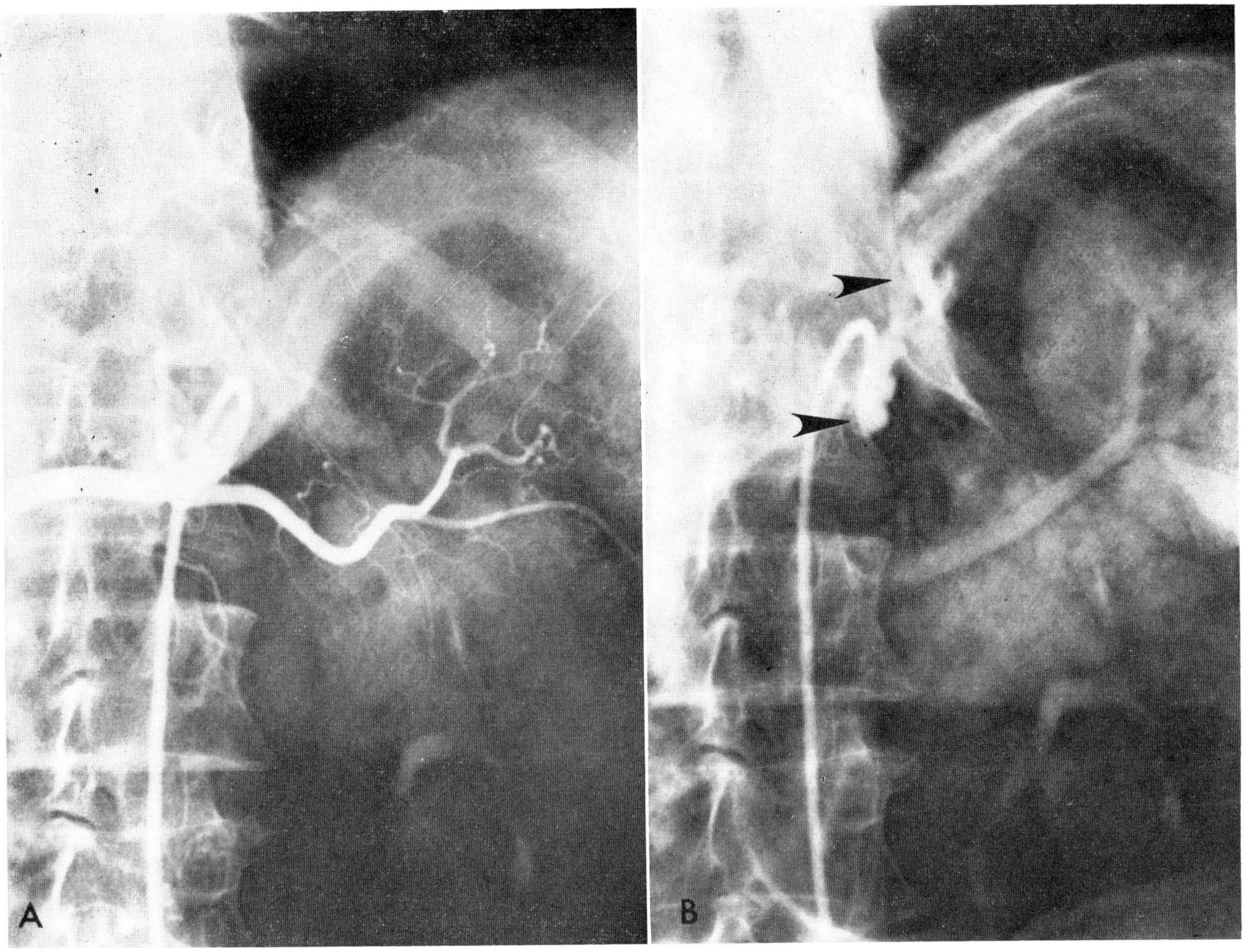

Figure 26.30. Celiac Arteriogram. (A) Arterial phase: No abnormalities are seen. (B) Venous phase: Contrast collects (Arrow) in the vicinity of the proximal portion of the lesser curvature. The patient was a chronic alcoholic with a clinical diagnosis of esophageal variceal bleeding. *Diagnosis:* Bleeding into the stomach from the left gastric artery, bleeding probably caused by an ulcer. *Surgical Diagnosis:* Bleeding ulcer in the lesser curvature of the stomach.

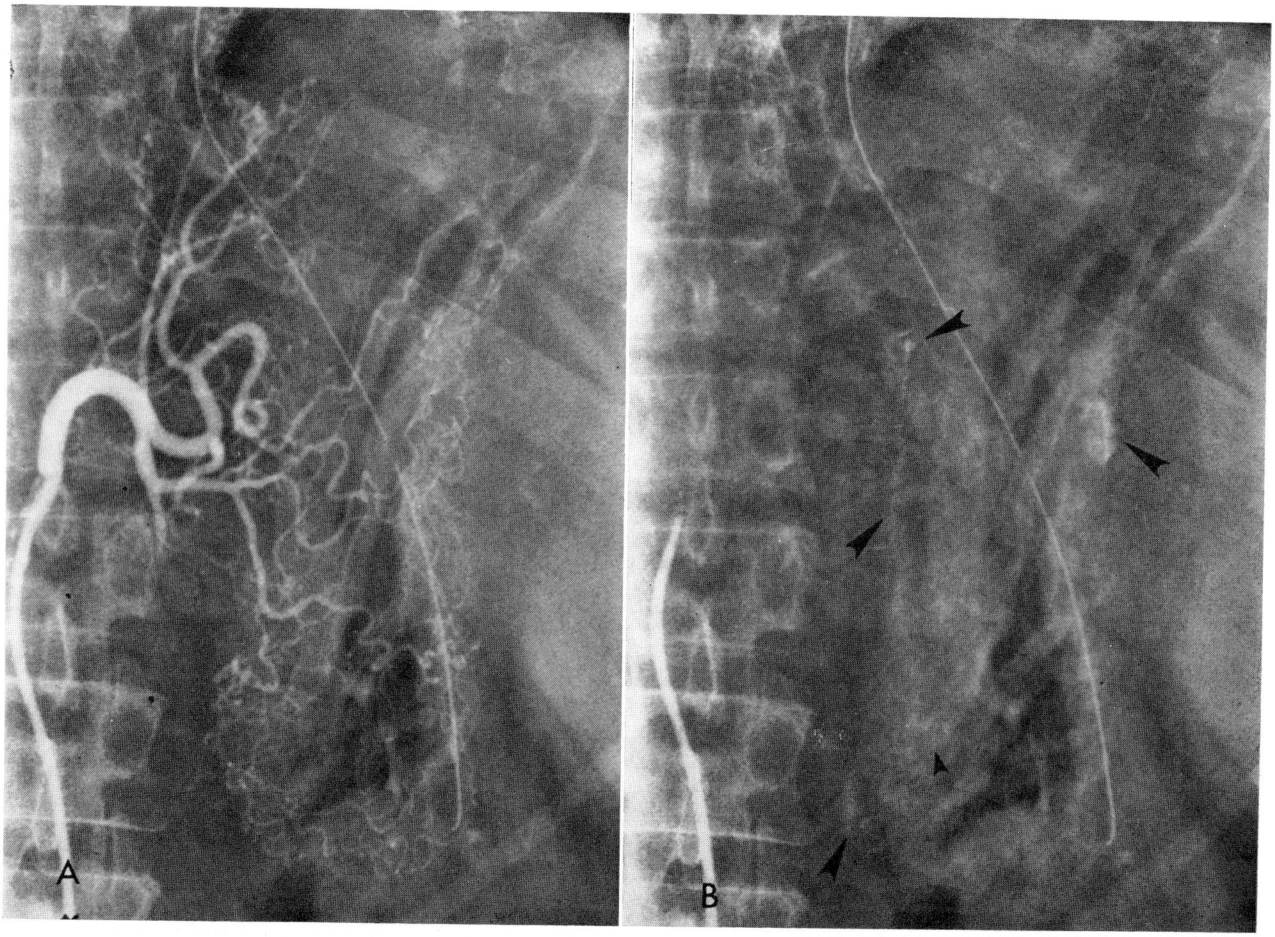

Figure 26.31. Left Gastric Arteriogram. (A) Arterial phase: No apparent abnormality is seen. (B) Late phase: There is intense staining of the gastric mucosa and multiple streaky entravasations. The patient had hematemesis following a bout of heavy alcoholic consumption. *Diagnosis:* Hemorrhagic gastritis. This was confirmed at gastroscopy.

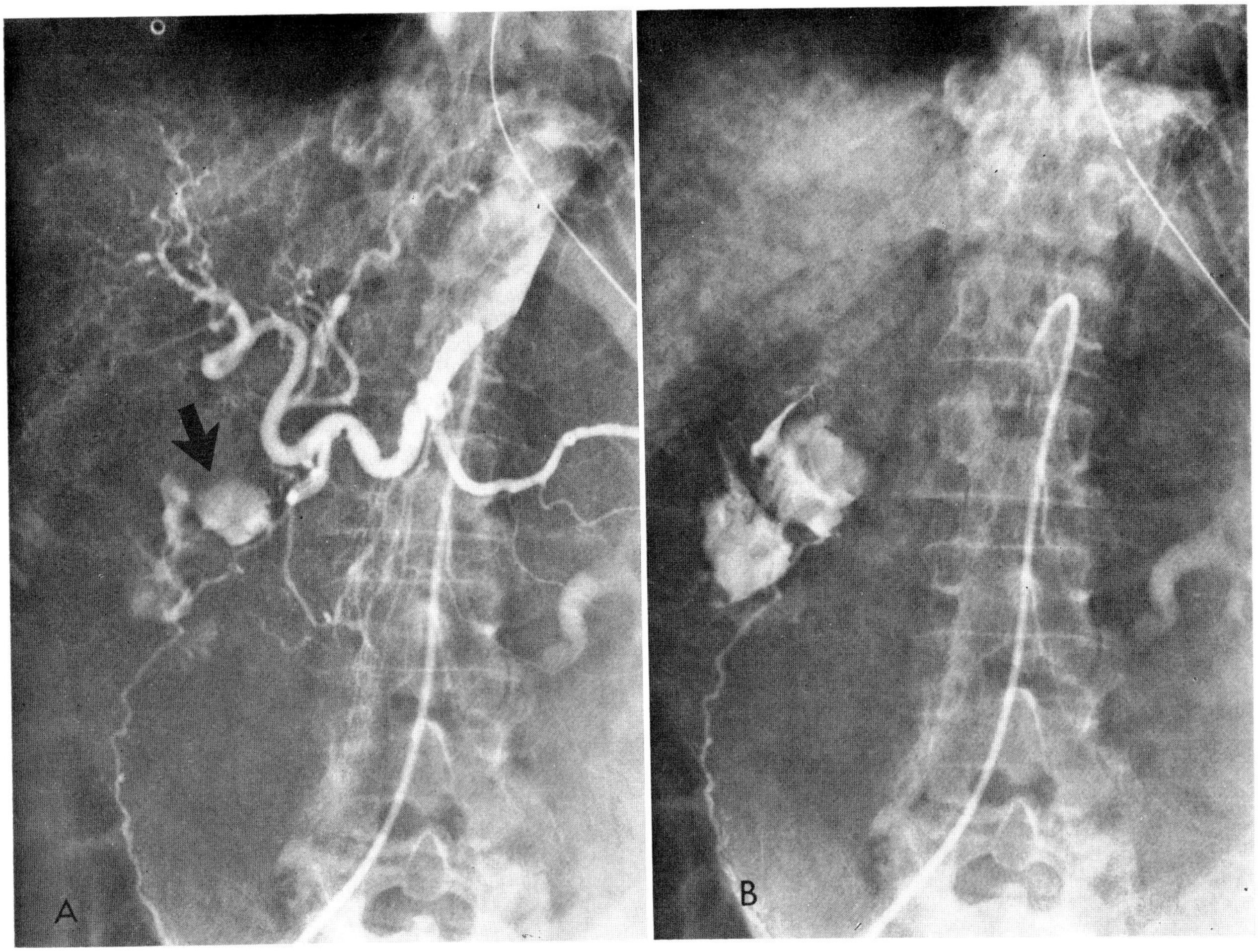

Figure 26.32. Celiac Arteriogram. (A) There is an irregular collection of contrast from the proximal branch of the gastroduodenal artery (Arrow) in the vicinity of the duodenal bulb. (B) This collection persists beyond the venous phase. The patient had acute hematemesis. *Radiographic Diagnosis:* Extravasation of contrast from a bleeding duodenal ulcer. Confirmed at surgery.

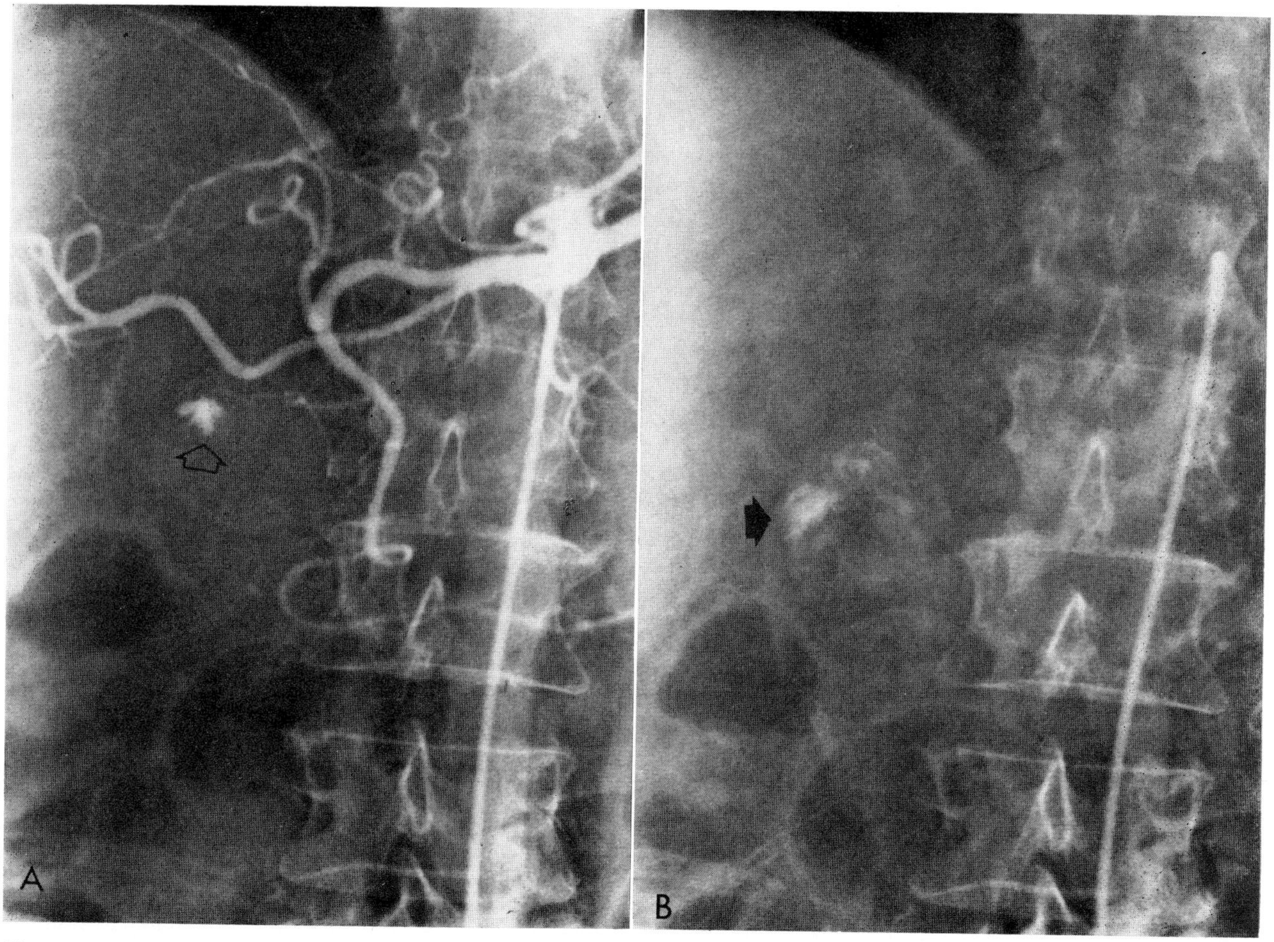

Figure 26.33. Celiac Arteriogram. (A) Arterial phase: There is periarterial collection of contrast from a prominent branch of the gastroduodenal artery (Arrow). (B) Late phase: This contrast persists and outlines the duodenal mucosa. This 67-year-old man began bleeding following a gastrectomy for a duodenal ulcer. *Diagnosis:* Postoperative bleeding from a recurrent ulcer or perhaps a slipped ligature. *Surgery:* Slipped ligature.

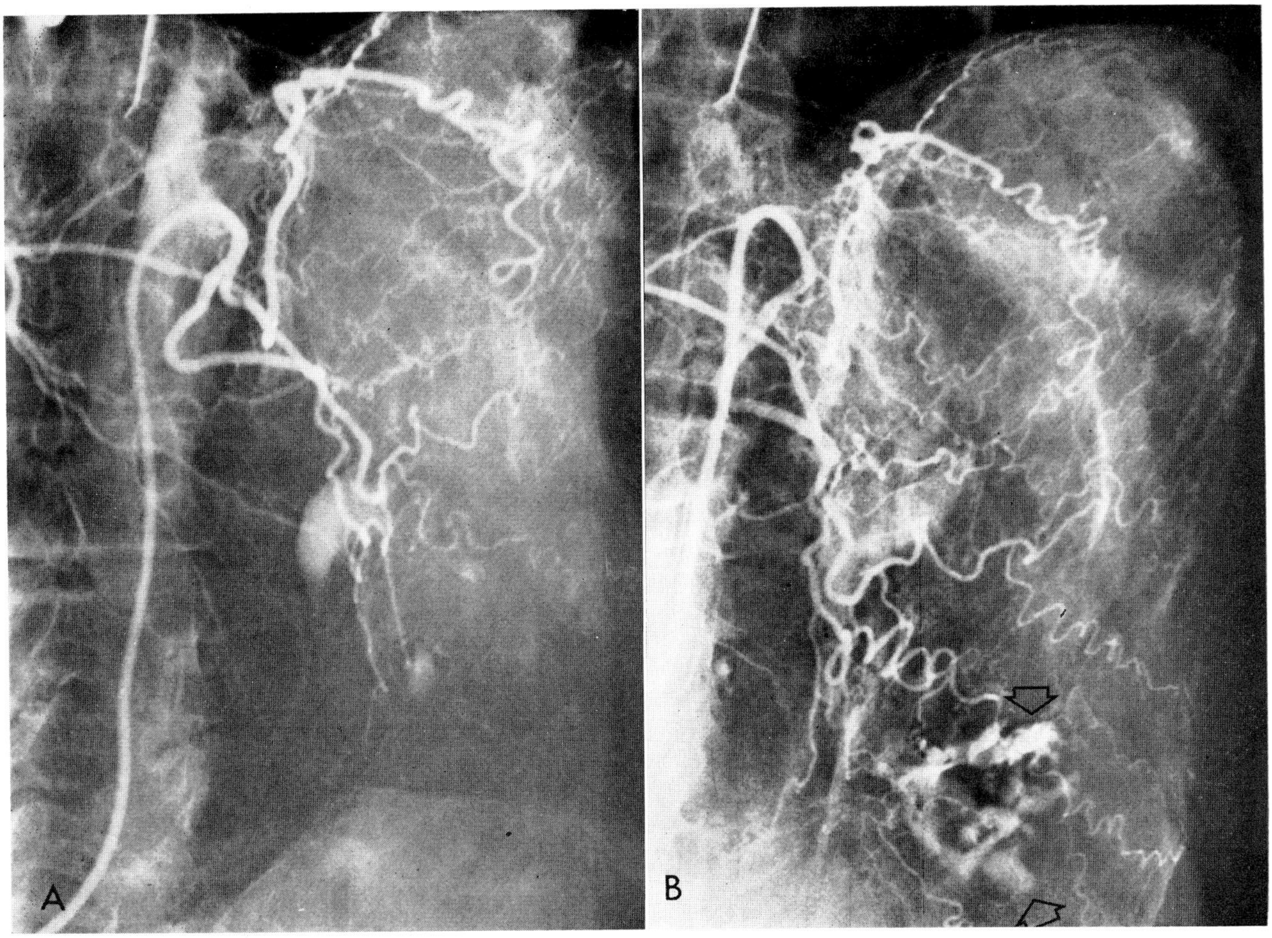

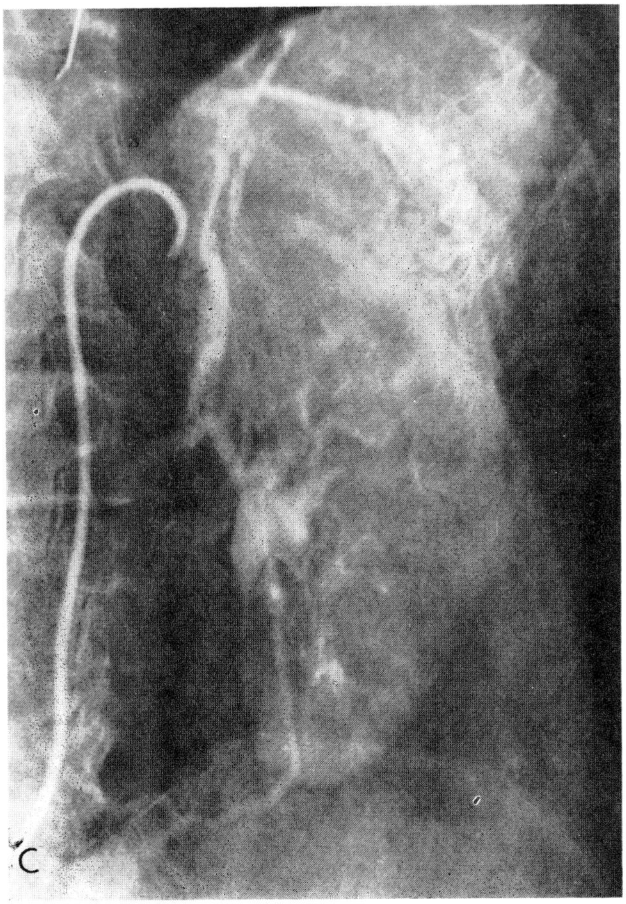

Figure 26.34. Left Gastric Arteriogram. (B) Arterial phase: There is amorphous collection of contrast material from one of the branches of the left gastric artery (Arrow). (A) Repeat left gastric arteriogram: After 0.2 units per cc per minute of vasopressin for fifteen minutes no extravasation is seen. There is constriction of all the branches supplying the stomach. Reflux of the contrast into the aorta suggests intravascular resistance due to vasoconstrictor infusion. (C) Venous phase: No extravasation is noted. *Diagnosis:* Extravasation of blood into the stomach due to an ulcer. Good control after vasopressin infusion occurs.

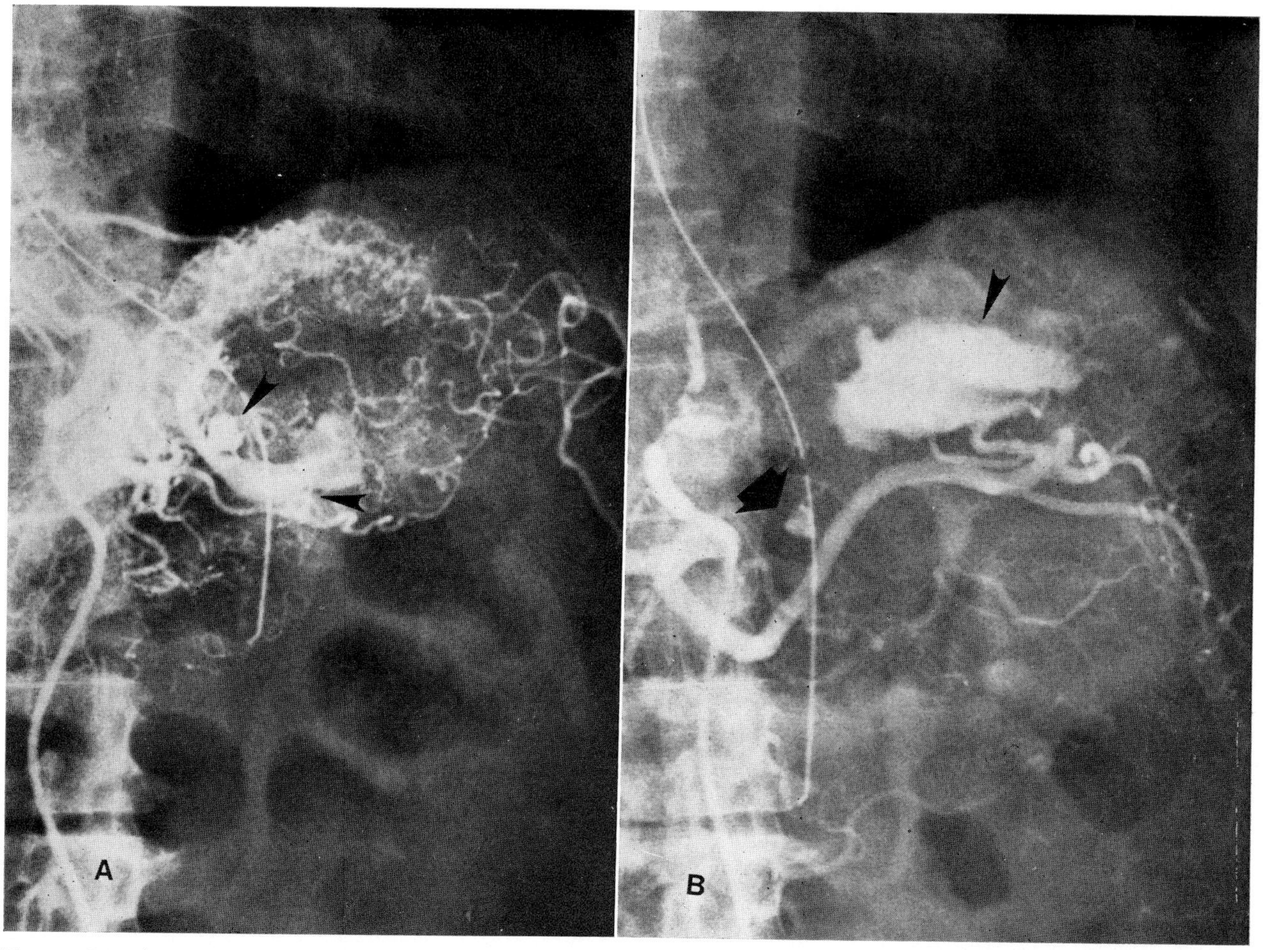

Figure 26.35. Left Gastric Arteriogram. (A) During the routine injection there is discrete collection of contrast in the vicinity of the fundus of the stomach (Arrow). (B) After injection of epinephrine a repeat study again shows the collection of contrast (Arrow). The big puddle of contrast (Arrow Head) is due to previous angiogram. *Diagnosis:* Extravasation into the gastric lumen (A) which was uncontrollable after epinephrine (B). *Surgery:* Penetrating ulcer of the lesser curvature of the stomach. There was periarterial fibrosis of the bleeding artery.

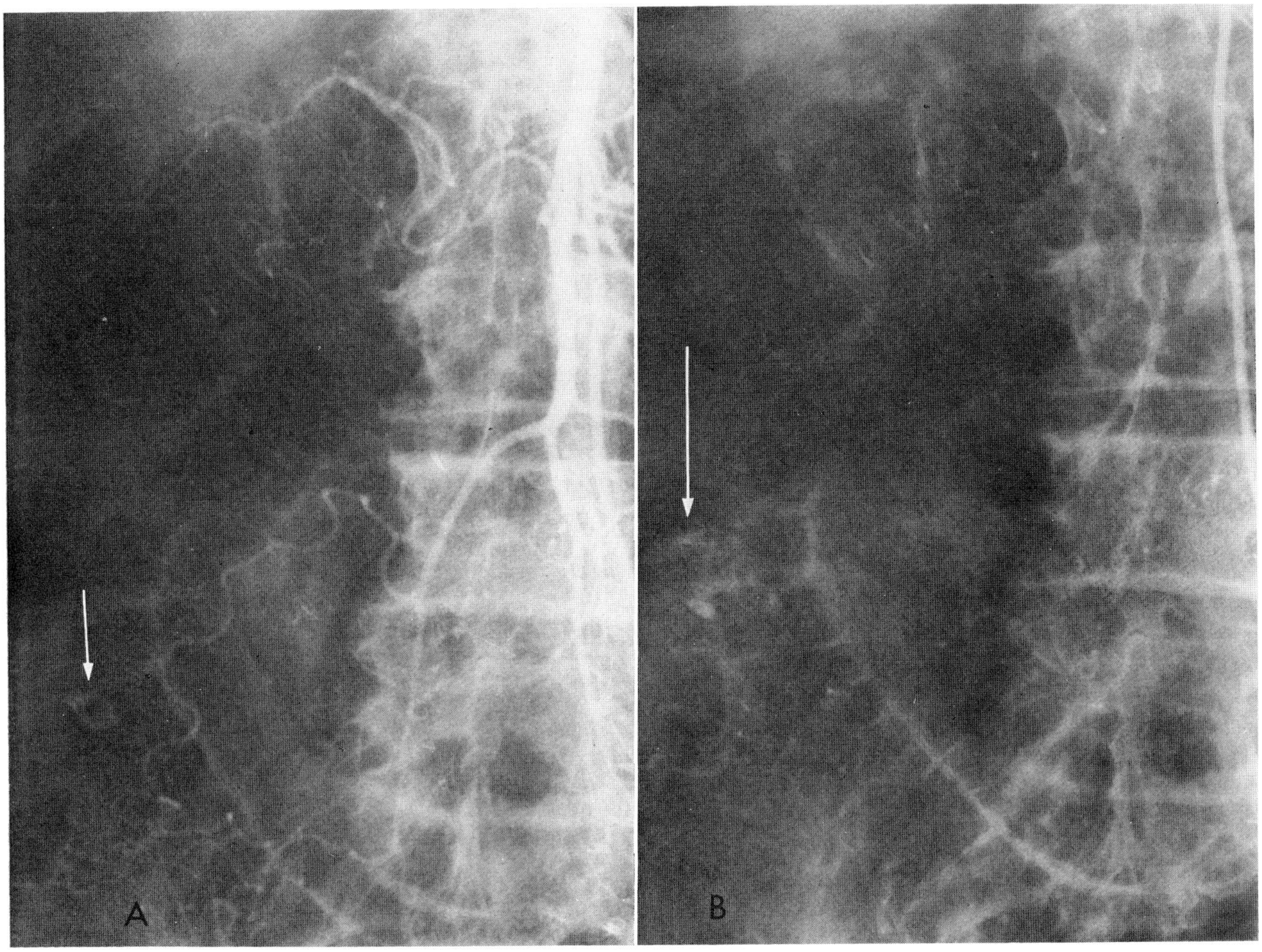

Figure 26.36. Superior Mesenteric Arteriogram. (A) An early abnormal collection of contrast material is seen around translucent area in the vicinity of the ascending colon. (B) Later in the arterial phase a further collection is noted. This patient was bleeding per rectum. *Diagnosis:* Arterial extravasation into the ascending colon probably due to diverticuli. This was confirmed at surgery.

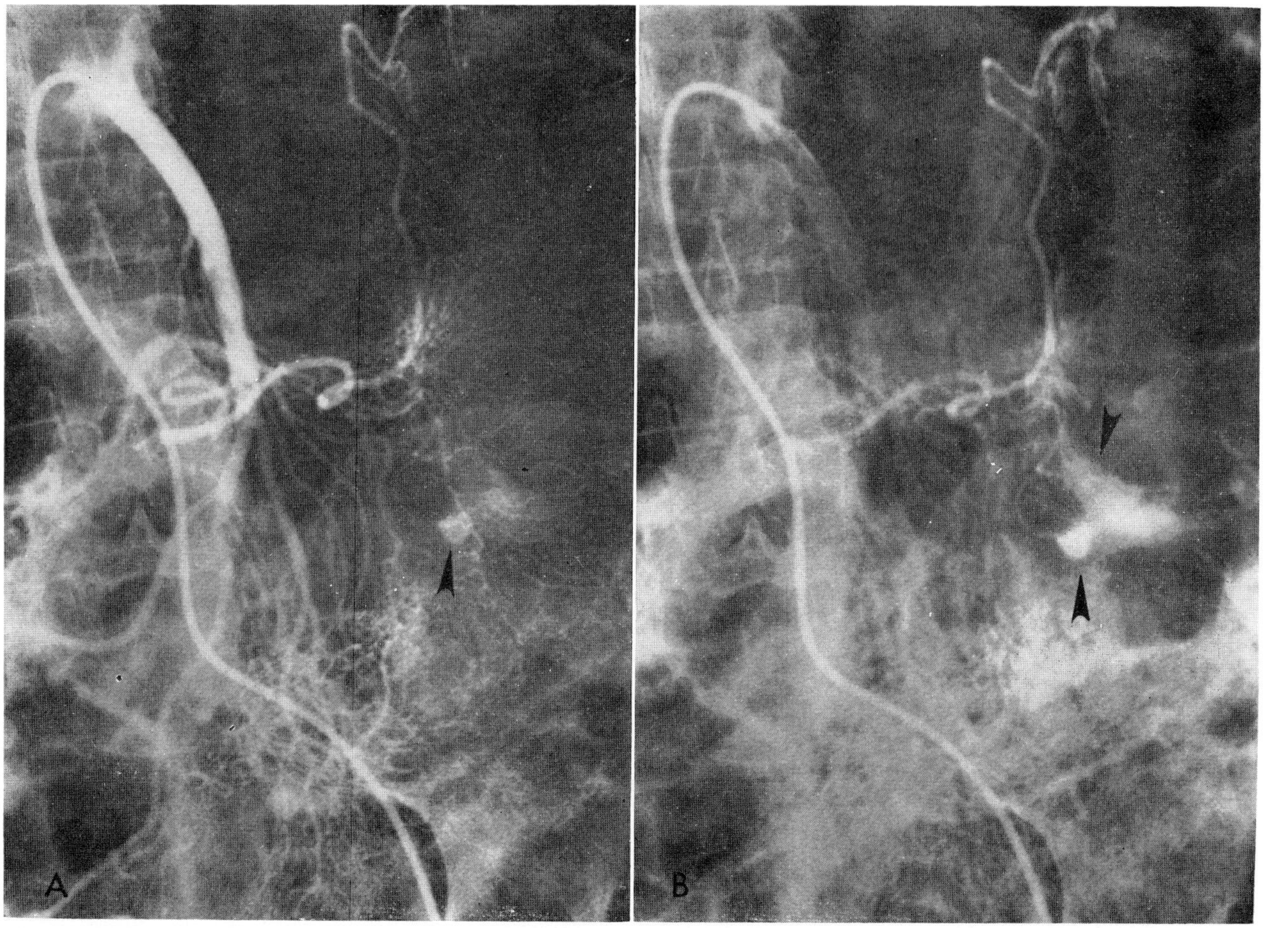

Figure 26.37. Superior Mesenteric Arteriogram. (A) Arterial phase reveals collection of contrast from the middle colic branches in the vicinity of the distal transverse colon. (B) Further increase amorphous collection of contrast is noted. *Diagnosis:* Extravasation of contrast due to arterial bleeding from a diverticulum confirmed at surgery.

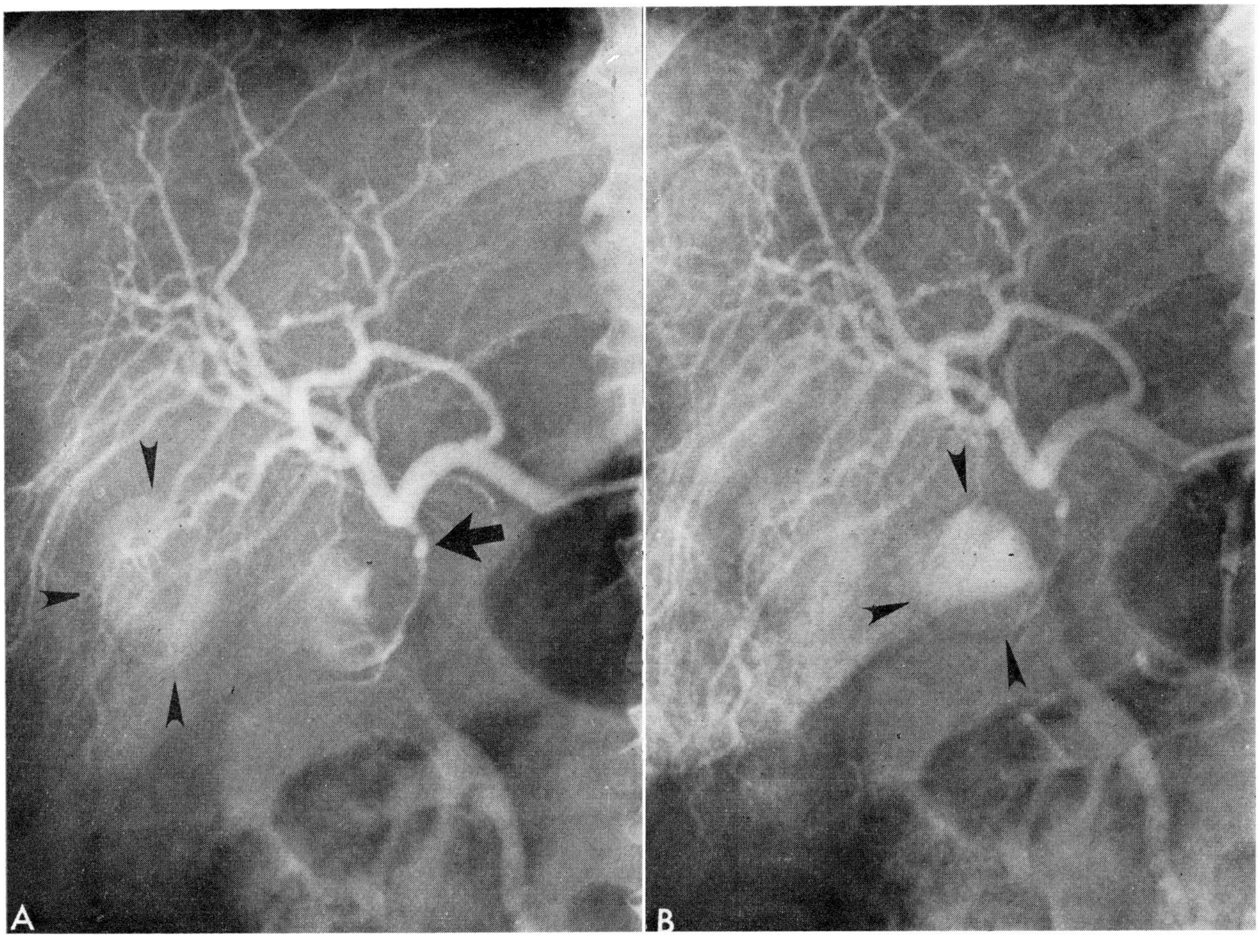

Figure 26.38. Hepatic Arteriogram. (A) Arterial phase: The cystic artery (arrow) is narrowed and bowed. There is a large gallstone (Arrow Head). (B) Mid-arterial phase: There is periarterial collection of contrast. The patient presented with painless jaundice and later in the day developed rectal bleeding. *Diagnosis:* Hematobilia. Bleeding into the lumen of the gallbladder from erosion of the cystic artery by chronic cholecystitis and the gallstone. (Courtesy of Angres, G., Zarnow, H., Swamy, S. S. From *JAMA, 228:*1026, 1974. Courtesy of the authors and the publishers.)

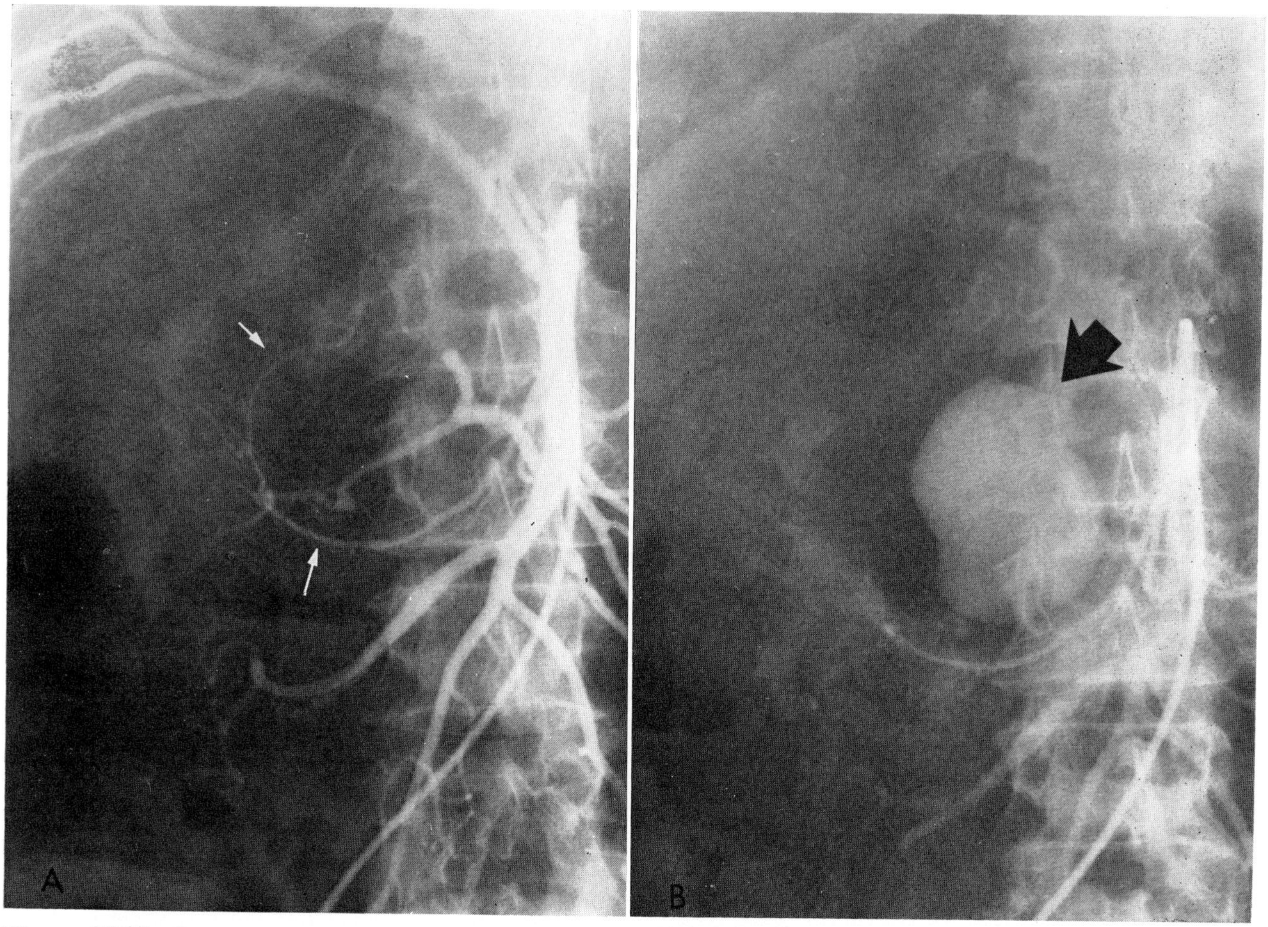

Figure 26.39. Superior Mesenteric Arteriogram. (A) There is stretching and deviation of pancreaticoduodenal arteries around a mass in the vicinity of the head of the pancreas. (B) Later there is an amorphous collection of contrast material. *Diagnosis:* Extravasation of contrast material into a pseudocyst of the pancreas. (Courtesy of Dr. N. Brown, Radiologist, Michael Reese Medical Center, Chicago.)

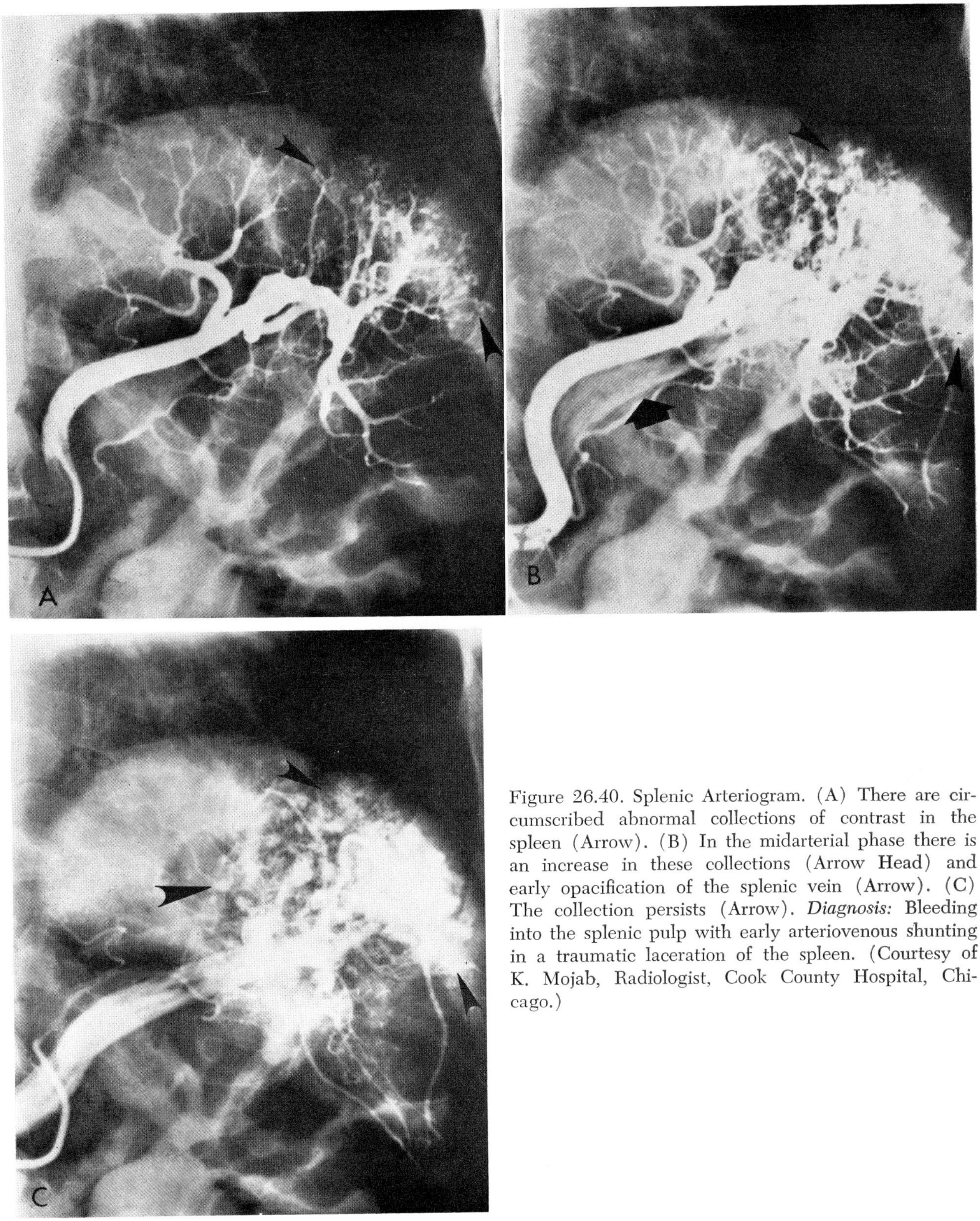

Figure 26.40. Splenic Arteriogram. (A) There are circumscribed abnormal collections of contrast in the spleen (Arrow). (B) In the midarterial phase there is an increase in these collections (Arrow Head) and early opacification of the splenic vein (Arrow). (C) The collection persists (Arrow). *Diagnosis:* Bleeding into the splenic pulp with early arteriovenous shunting in a traumatic laceration of the spleen. (Courtesy of K. Mojab, Radiologist, Cook County Hospital, Chicago.)

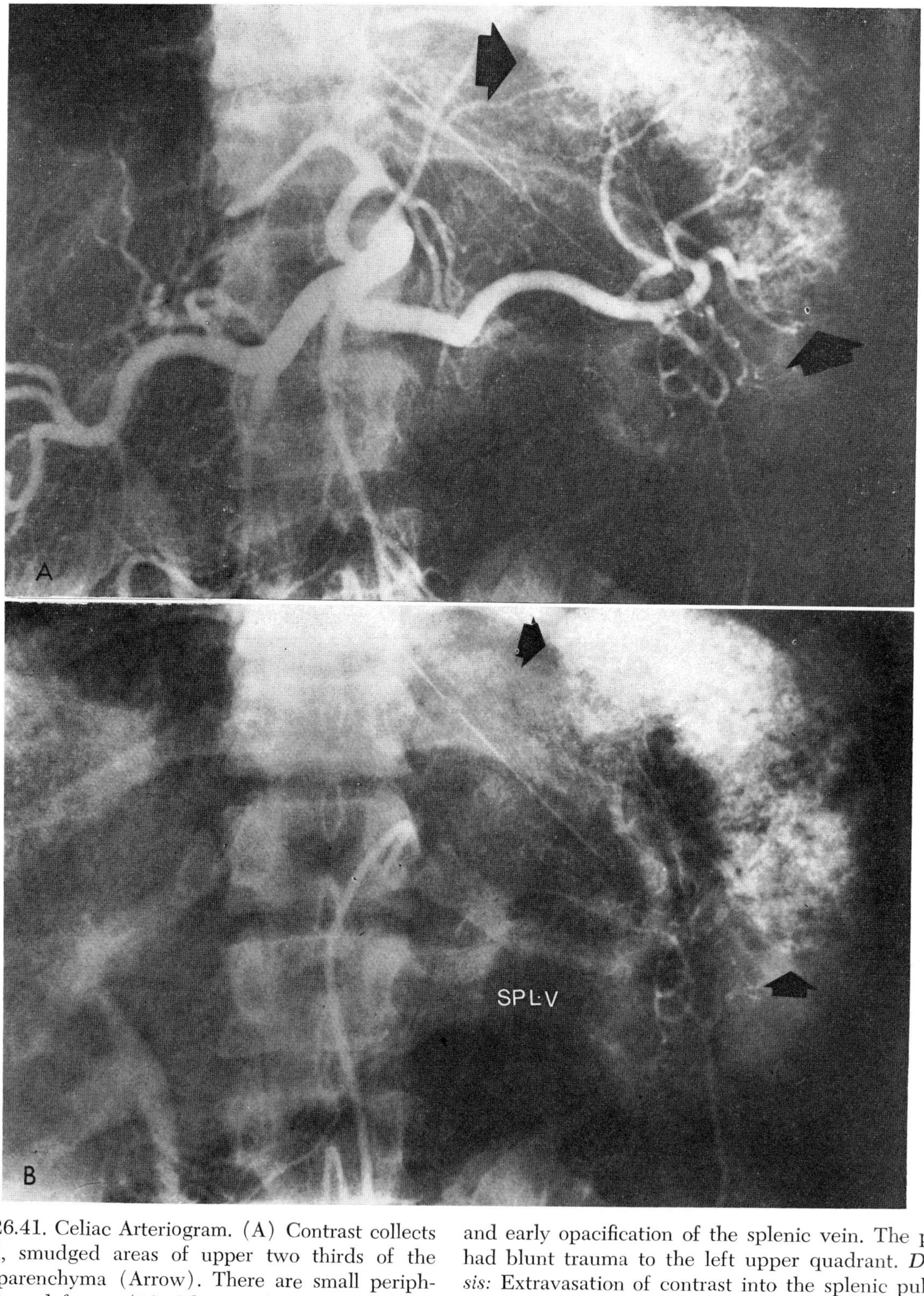

Figure 26.41. Celiac Arteriogram. (A) Contrast collects in small, smudged areas of upper two thirds of the splenic parenchyma (Arrow). There are small peripheral filling defects. (B) These collections (Arrow) persist with better visualization of the filling defects and early opacification of the splenic vein. The patient had blunt trauma to the left upper quadrant. *Diagnosis:* Extravasation of contrast into the splenic pulp due to traumatic laceration of the spleen.

in a heavily diseased vessel. Subintimal extravasation used to be a frequent occurrence when long bevel needles were used, as they prevented the passage of the guide wire into the lumen of the vessel. This can be avoided by using Teflon sleeve needles, those with a short bevel, or those consisting of an inner stylet and outer cannula. Extravasation into the adventitia,[503] though rare, may occur.

Dissecting hematomas of other vessels, usually peripheral, may be due to spontaneous, traumatic, or other predisposing causes, and usually results in obstruction of the lumen. Spontaneous dissections have been described in the splenic;[527] femoral, popliteal;[528] gastroduodenal;[529] and renal arteries.[530, 531] Traumatic dissections occur as a result of blunt trauma or catheterization procedures. *Blunt trauma*[532] may cause contusion of an arterial wall, subsequent weakening, and development of subintimal or medial dissections. Excessive stretching of an artery may also cause dissection. This has been seen in the carotid[533] and popliteal[532] arteries. Undue or excessive manipulation of a guide wire or catheter in a vessel, especially during superselective angiographic procedures, increases the chance of developing dissection. The chances are greater if the vessel happens to have atheromatous change. Predisposing factors, such as *fibromuscular hyperplasia,* have been described as causing dissection of the internal carotid,[534] hepatic,[535] vertebral[536] and renal arteries.[632, 633] These are not necessarily unusual events (Figs. 26-1 to 26-11).

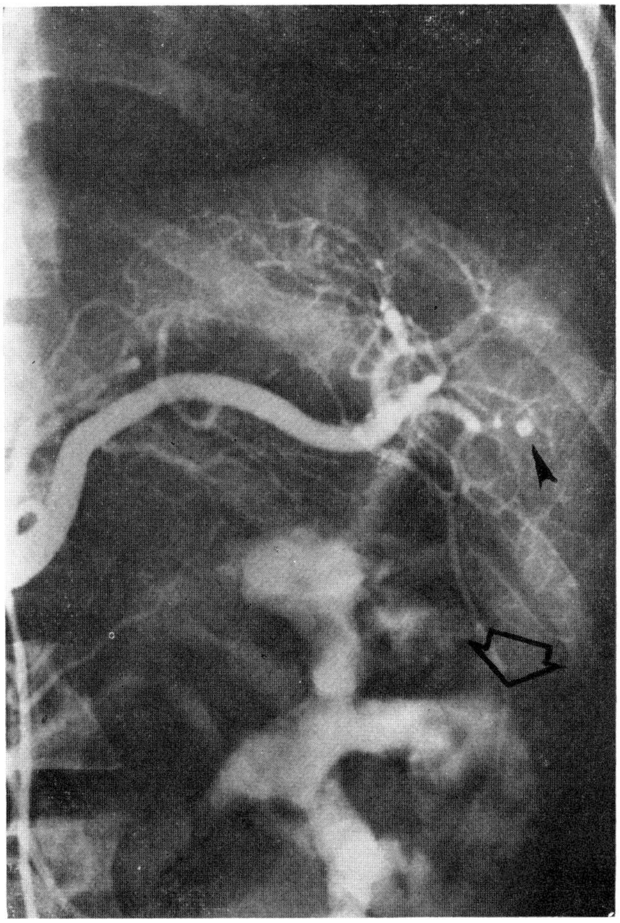

Figure 26.42. Splenic Arteriogram. There is a small, discrete collection of contrast in the spleen (Arrow Head). The patient fell from the second floor of a building. Note also the extravasation of contrast from the renal calyces (Arrow). *Diagnosis:* Posttraumatic extravasation (bleeding) into the spleen and kidney. At surgery the renal bleeding was confirmed. However, the spleen was not explored.

PERIVASCULAR EXTRAVASATIONS

Communicating periarterial hematomas usually are the *result of a defect in the wall of a vessel which was unable to seal itself.* The size and configuration of the hematoma are decided by the nature and resistance of the surrounding tissues, the extent of the trauma, the size of the artery and its hole, the arterial blood pressure, and the efficiency of the coagulation mechanisms. The same factors determine the rapidity with which the aneurysm continues to expand and rupture. In some instances, good defense mechanisms of the body and the slow progression of the bleeding, cause the formation of a fibrous sac. At one end of the spectrum is rupture of the vessel with fatal hemorrhage, and at the other end is a localized, walled-off periarterial hematoma—a *pseudoaneurysm* (Figs. 26-19 to 26-25).

Spontaneous ruptures usually have underlying, predisposing factors such as diseased vessels or congenital malformation of the vessels. Atherosclerotic aneurysms, or aneurysms due to angiitis as seen in polyarteritis nodosa[537] or

(Text continues on page 440)

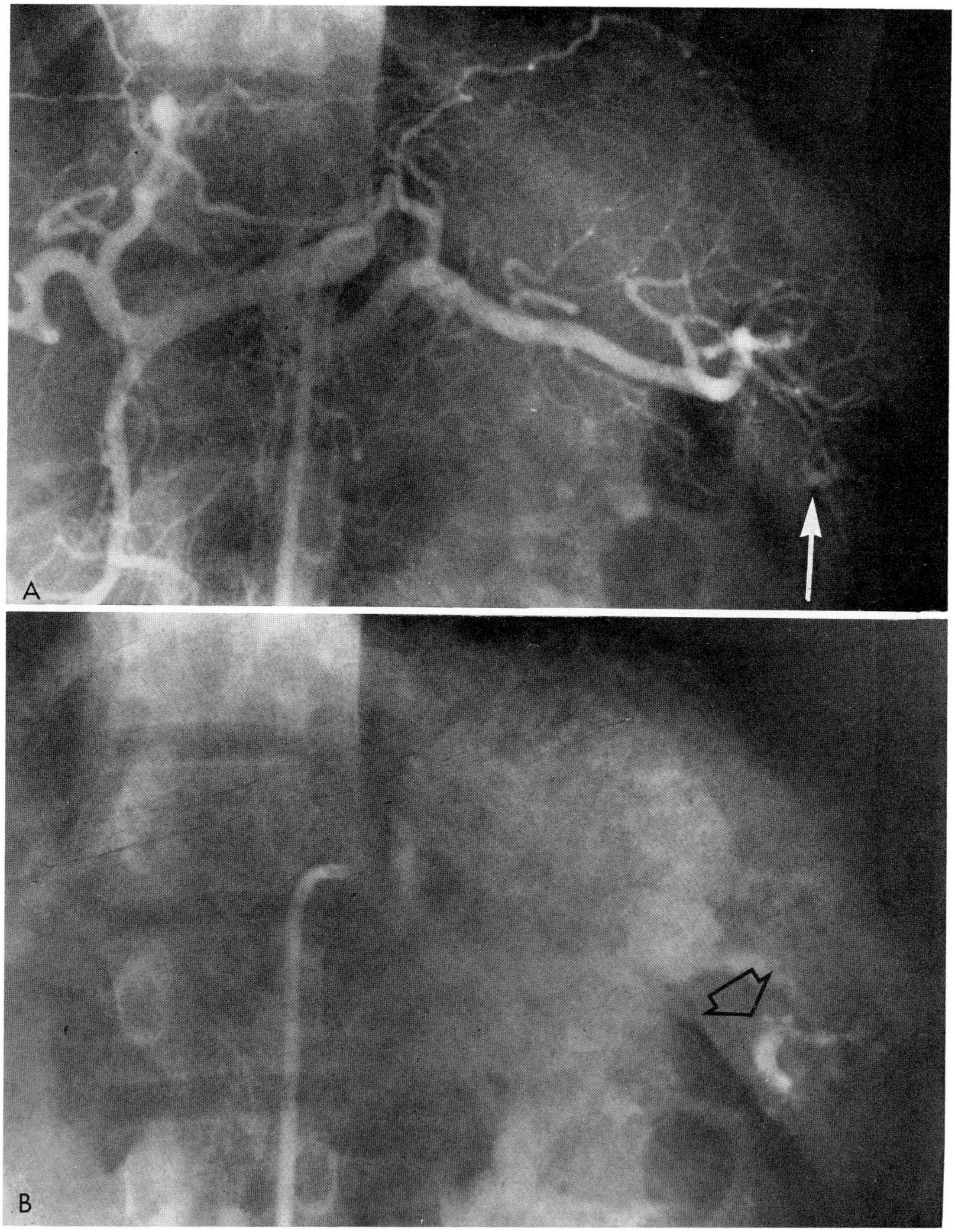

Figure 26.43. Celiac Arteriogram. (A) There is an amorphous collection of contrast in the spleen (Arrow). (B) This persists and increases (Arrow). The patient had left upper quadrant trauma. *Diagnosis:* Posttraumatic extravasation (bleeding) into the splenic parenchyma.

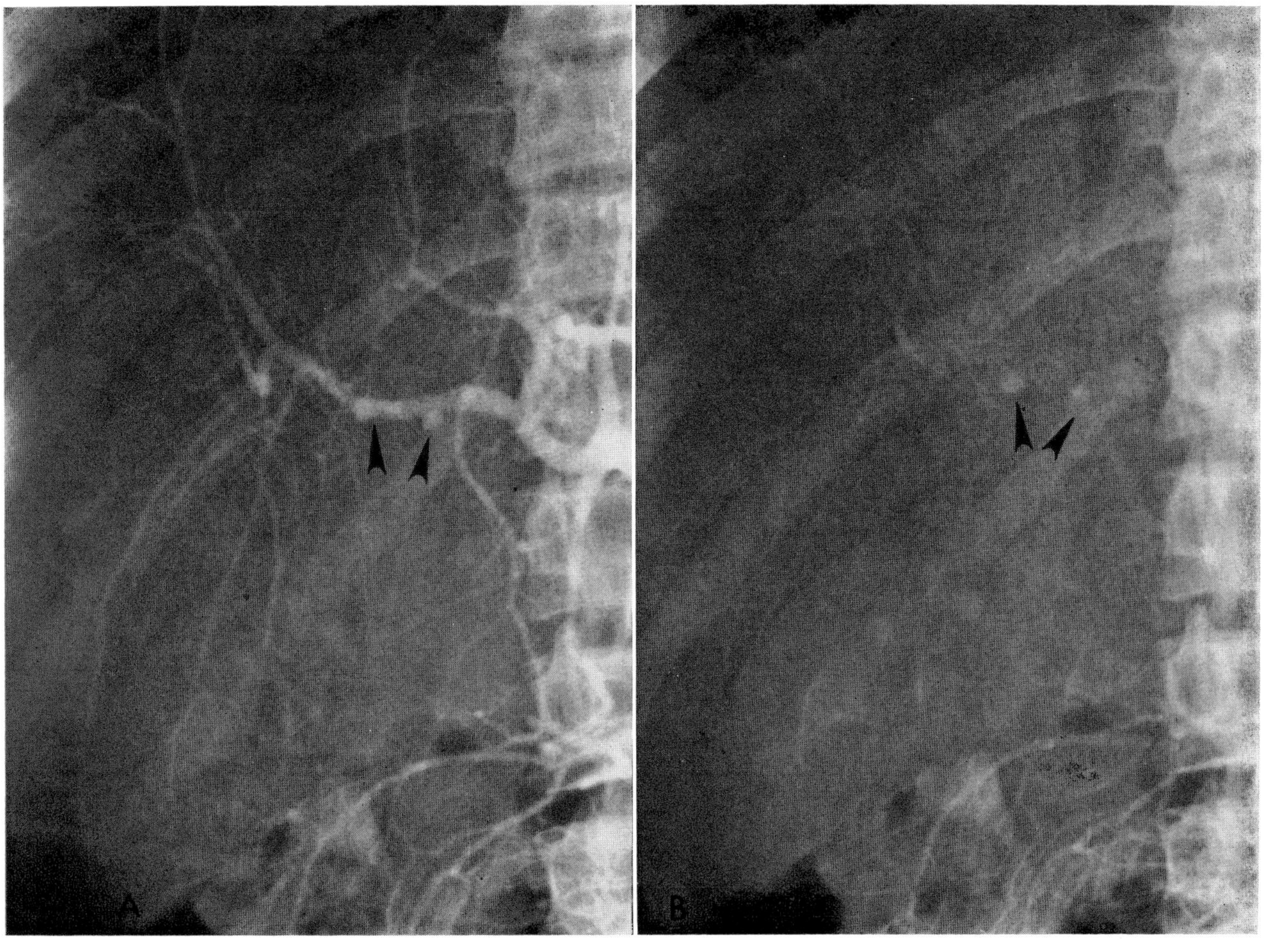

Figure 26.44. Celiac Arteriogram. (A) There are localized periarterial saccular collection of contrast (Arrow) from the intrahepatic artery. (B) The late arterial phase shows persistence of these collections. The patient had blunt trauma to the right upper quadrant. *Diagnosis:* Posttraumatic pseudoaneurysms. (Courtesy of Dr. D. Goldberg, Palos Heights, Illinois.)

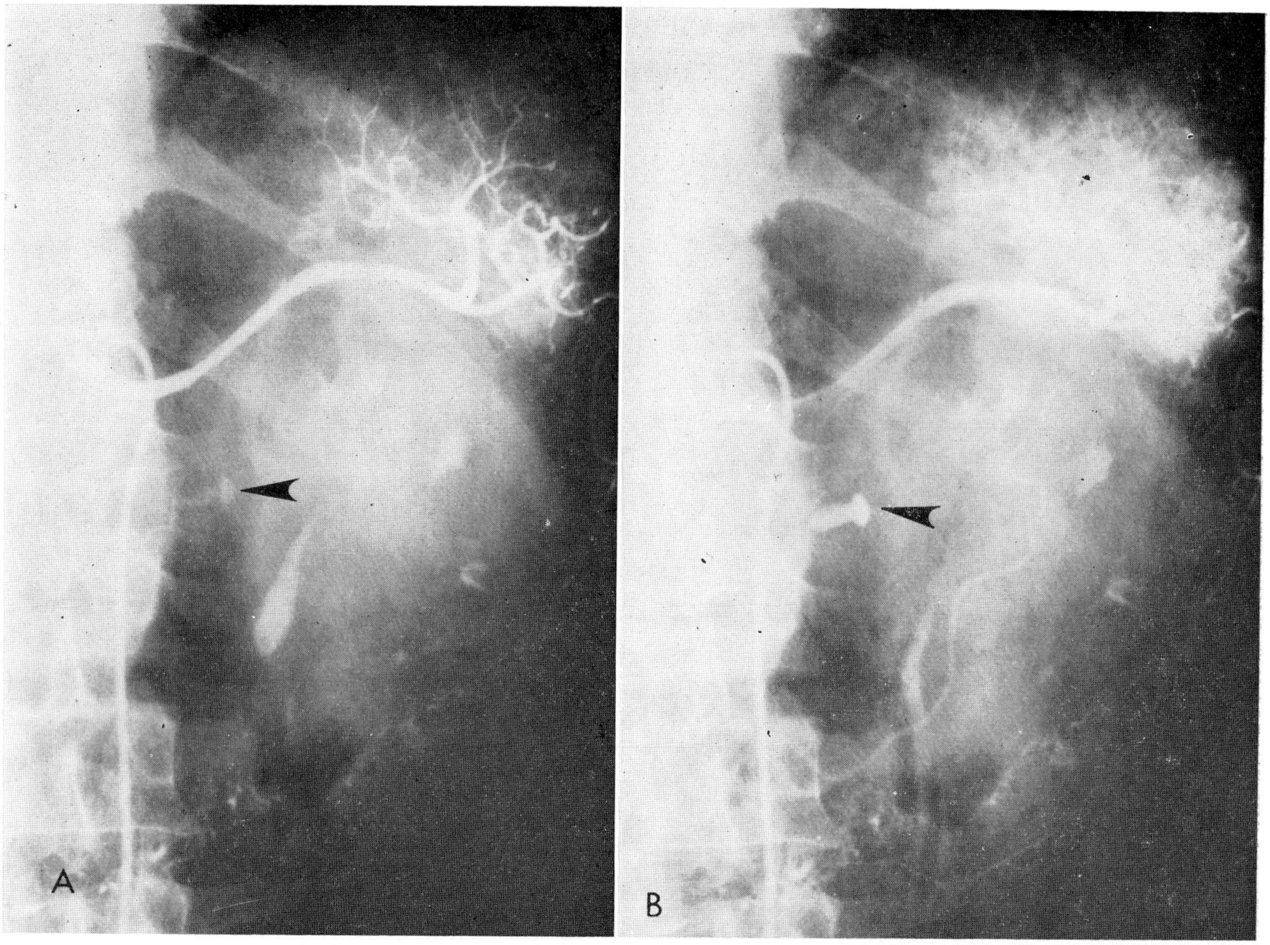

Figure 26.45. Celiac Arteriogram. (A) Early phase reveals a faint collection of contrast inferior to L1 transverse process (Arrow). Please note the elevation of the splenic artery. (B) Midarterial phase reveals more collection of this contrast (Arrow) in a patient who had blunt trauma to the abdomen. *Diagnosis:* Traumatic extravasation into the body of the pancreas with a surrounding hematoma. (Courtesy of Dr. J. Petasnick, Associate Professor, Diagnostic Radiology, Rush Presbyterian-St. Luke Medical Center, Chicago.)

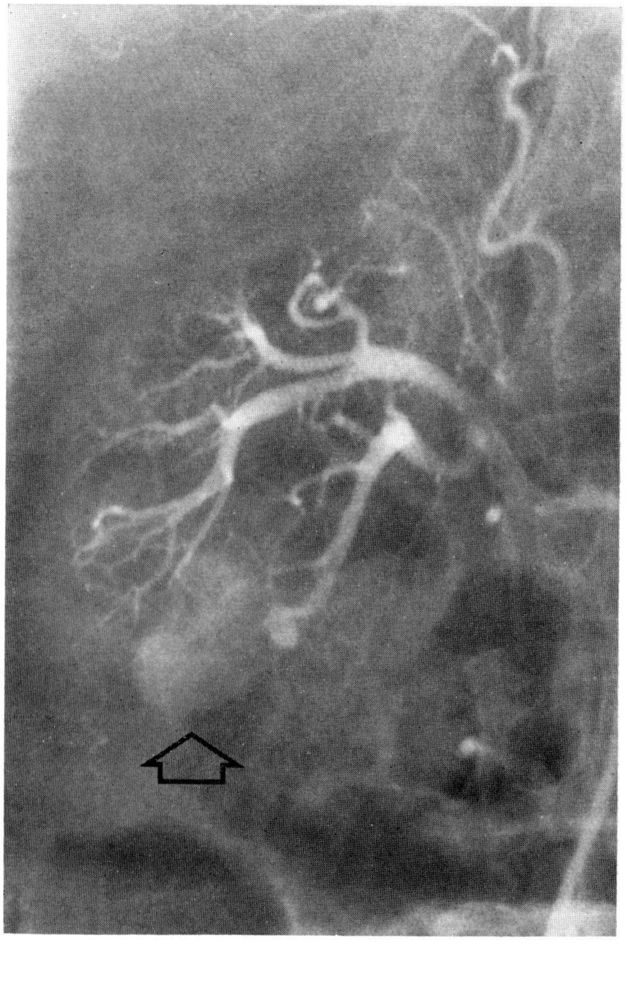

Figure 26.46. Renal Arteriogram. There is an amorphous collection of contrast material in the renal parenchyma. The patient had a recent renal biopsy. *Diagnosis:* Extravasation from the intrarenal arterial branches due to trauma from a recent biopsy.

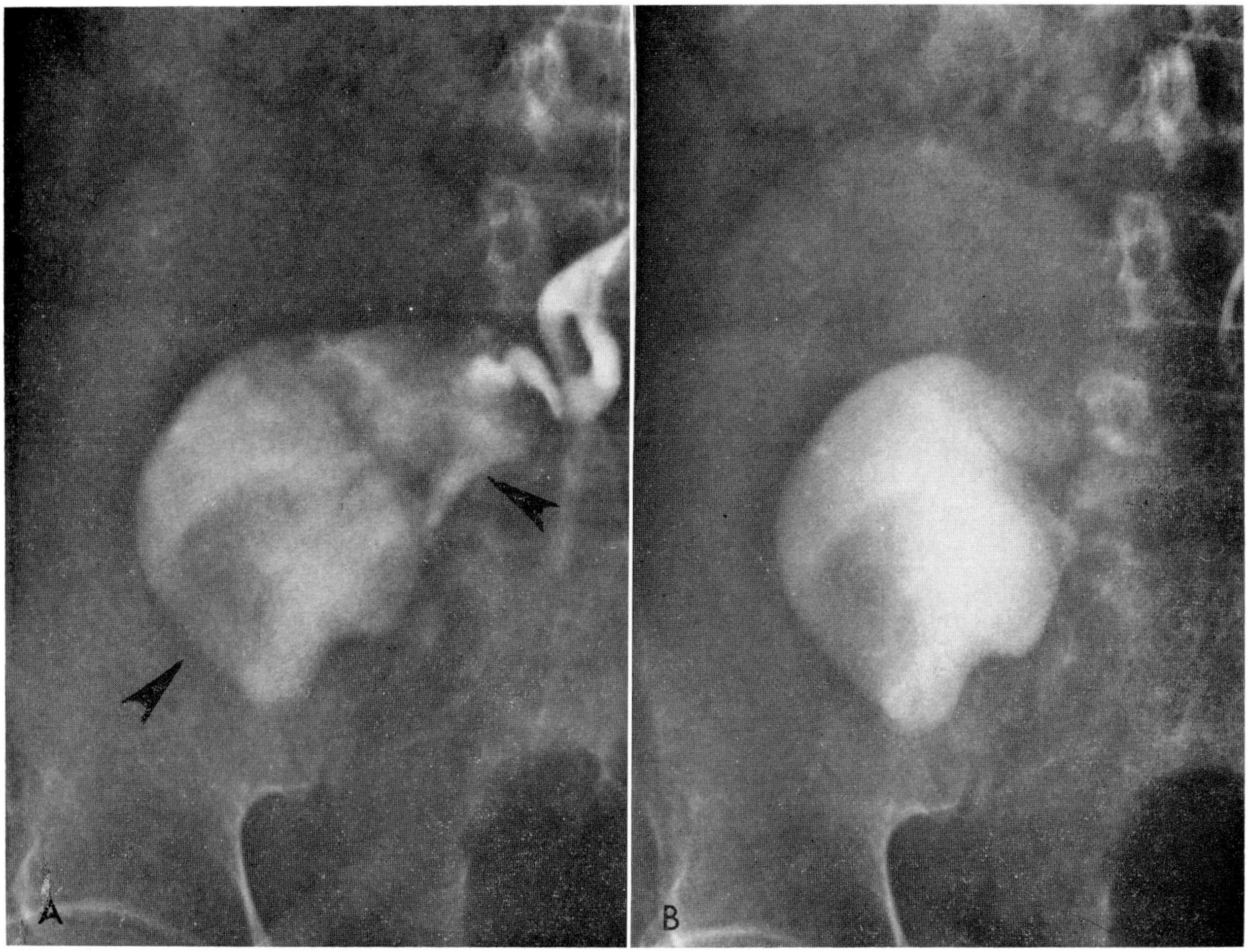

Figure 26.47. Internal Iliac Arteriogram. (A) Early arterial phase: The catheter tip is in the internal iliac artery. A large collection of contrast material is in a soft tissue density. (B) Late arterial phase: The same collection of contrast material is seen with stasis. The patient had a renal transplant with repeated attempts at renal biopsy. *Diagnosis:* Intrarenal pseudoaneurysm with a rind of blood clot around it.

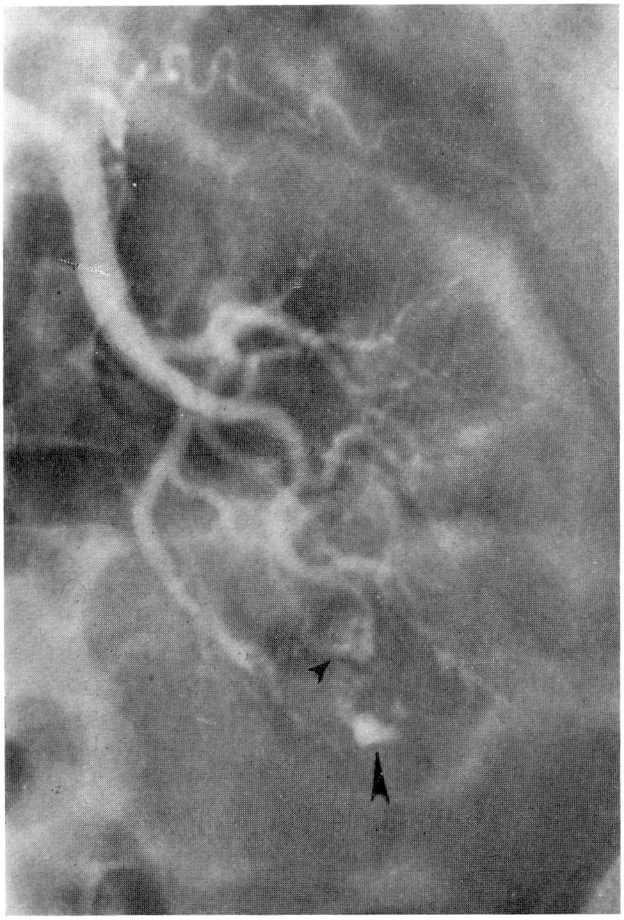

←

Figure 26.48. Renal Arteriogram. There is slight stretching of the lower pole branches and abnormal amorphous collections of the contrast material in the same vicinity (Arrow). The patient had left flank trauma. *Diagnosis:* Laceration of the lower pole of the kidney with extravasation of contrast. *Differential Diagnosis:* Malignant sinusoids of a hypernephroma.

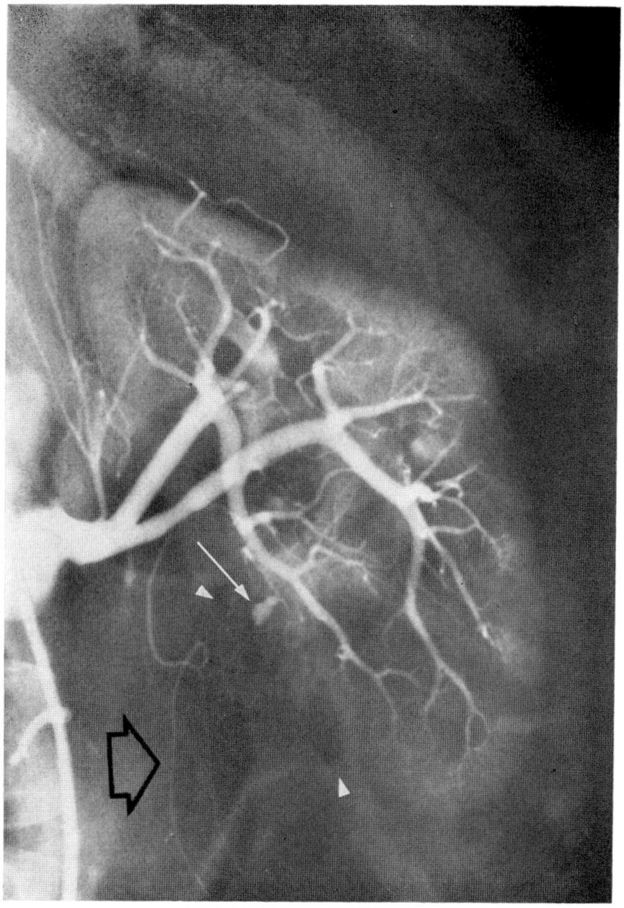

Figure 26.49. Renal Arteriogram. A circumscribed collection of contrast material (Arrow) and poor arterial perfusion to the medial border of the cortex (Arrow Head) and stretching and deviation of the pelviureteral branches (Blank Arrow) are seen in a patient who had blunt trauma to the left flank. *Diagnosis:* Intrarenal as well as perirenal extravasation and an intrarenal blood clot.

Ehler-Danlos syndrome[538] are probably the most common causes. Spontaneous rupture may also occur in a normal vessel and has been described of the splenic vein during pregnancy[539] and of the superior mesenteric artery.[540] Multiple traumatic events may lead to the tearing of an artery with subsequent extravasation. *Blunt trauma* to the aorta, innominate[541] and femoral arteries[542] is another common cause. *Penetrating trauma* is usually related to knife and bullet wounds. Orthopedic devices such as the screws from internal fixation,[543] *osseous trauma* with pelvic fractures,[544] and humeral fractures can cause ruptures. *Following surgery,* ruptures due to vessel erosion from sutures have been described in the abdominal aorta,[545] peripheral arteries,[546] and inferior epigastric artery.[547] Ruptures due to the use of tourniquets have been described involving the ulnar artery.[548] *Catheterization procedures,* unfortunately, are not an infrequent cause of traumatic periarterial extravasation.

Aortic Rupture

Of all the sites previously described, aortic extravasation deserves special mention.[549-553] *The thoracic aorta, heart and renal arteries* are frequent victims of rapid deceleration injuries.

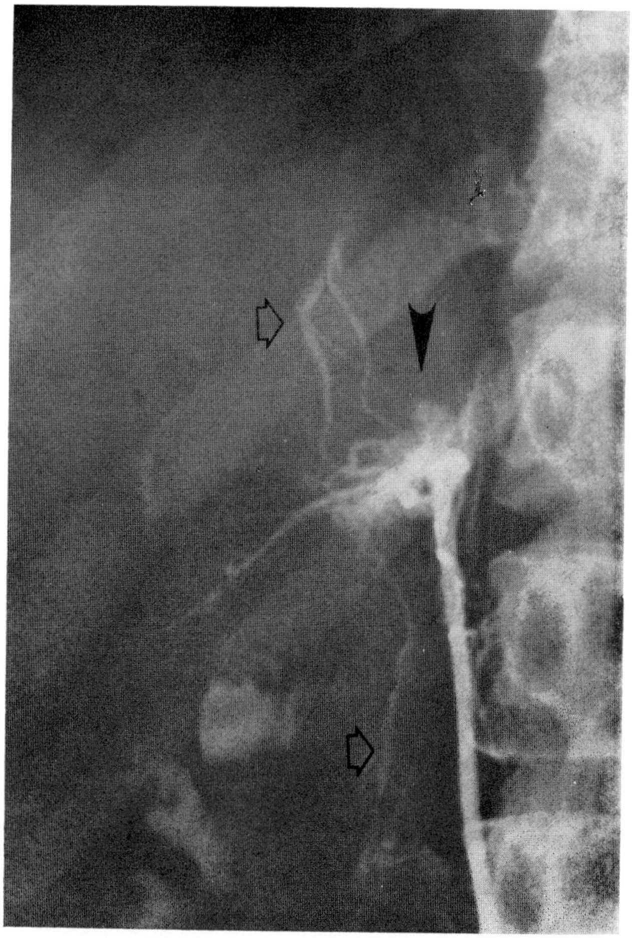

Figure 26.50. Right Adrenal Venogram. There is an amorphous collection of contrast material in the adrenal gland (Arrow Head) and filling of the retroperitoneal veins (Arrow). *Diagnosis:* Extravasation into the adrenal gland.

In the aorta the *greatest strain is at the isthmus* where the relatively mobile thoracic aorta joins the fixed aortic arch. The *other site of great strain* is the ascending aorta which is fixed between the arch and the easily movable heart. Indirect force apparently acts to produce increased intravascular pressure and sudden snapping movements of the relatively mobile segments of the aorta against its fixed segments. This causes intimal hemorrhage, intimal or medial laceration, complete laceration, false aneurysms, or fatal periaortic hemorrhage. The abdominal aorta is not immune either, as it may be compressed against the spine.

The *isthmus of the aorta is the most common site of rupture,* followed in descending order by the descending thoracic aorta, ascending aorta, aortic arch, or abdominal aorta. The rupture may be single or multiple. Immediate death is usual but 10 to 20 percent of patients may live an hour or longer. If the rupture is in the ascending aorta, just above the valve, bleeding into the pericardium develops with subsequent pericardial tamponade. Lucky survivors end up with a pseudo- or true aneurysm. It is difficult to predict which posttraumatic pseudoaneurysms of the aorta will remain quiescent and which will rupture. These pseudoaneurysms are very suceptible to secondary infection (Figs. 26-20, 26-21).

Infectious (Mycotic) Aneurysms

Inflammatory destruction of the elastic wall causes aneurysmal dilatation with rapid growth and even rupture. A damaged intima due to atheromas or thrombus in an aneurysm is fertile soil for infection. These are usually due to staphylococcus, salmonella and enterobacterial infections.[554] There may be direct involvement from an adjacent inflammatory focus as is seen in tuberculous spondylitis involving the aorta.[555]

Extravasation due to *chemical* or *necrotic digestion* involving the splenic or gastroduodenal arteries is seen in pancreatitis. Involvement of the gastroduodenal artery may also be due to penetrating gastric or duodenal ulcers (Figs. 26-12 to 26-27).

EXTRAVASATION INTO A LUMEN

The angiographic extravasation of contrast into a lumen is actually the counterpart of clinical bleeding. This implies that the *artery should be bleeding at a certain optimal rate* in order to demonstrate the extravasation angiographically. To demonstrate active bleeding, the flow of blood into the lumen must be at the rate of 0.5 cc per minute. This is the minimum rate which may be demonstrated by selective catheterization techniques.[594, 595] Of course, *this does not apply to morphologically abnormal vessels* seen in ectasias, angiomas, aneurysms, varices, or arteriovenous fistula. Nor does it apply to other angiographically positive lesions such as Meckel's diverticulum and tumors, which can be demonstrated at any time with proper technical facilities. A flush aortogram may be unable to demonstrate bleeding even if the rate is 3 to 4 cc per minute.

The higher the bleeding rate, the nearer the injection is to the site of bleeding; the more sophisticated the technical facilities, the more rewarding is the end result. Future availability of adhesive contrast material may yield higher positive results in bleeding patients.[596] Discretion in the selection of patients is important when attempting to demonstrate bleeding angiographically. The angiographer should be aware that selection of patients with occult bleeding or suboptimal rates of bleeding may result in a loss of confidence in this valuable procedure. It is not unusual for some arteries to bleed for twenty-three hours, fifty-nine minutes and fifty-five seconds, and then stop immediately prior to the injection of contrast material.

Recognition of extravasation is accomplished by identifying amorphous puddling of contrast which persists for a long time and is easily dispersed within the lumen, smearing the mucosa. Excessive extravasation in respective areas may opacify structures such as the bile ducts or

(Text continues on page 446)

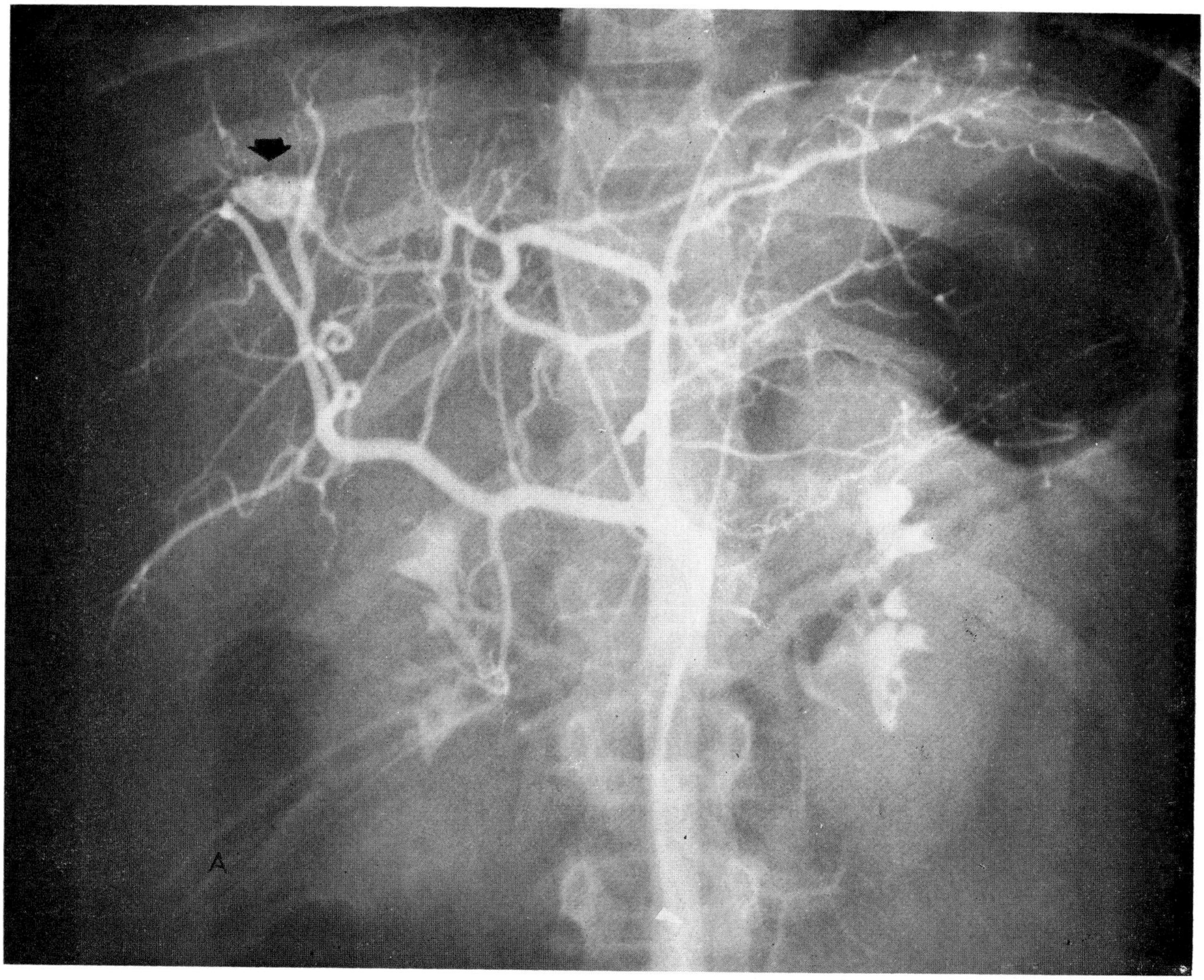

Figure 26.51 A

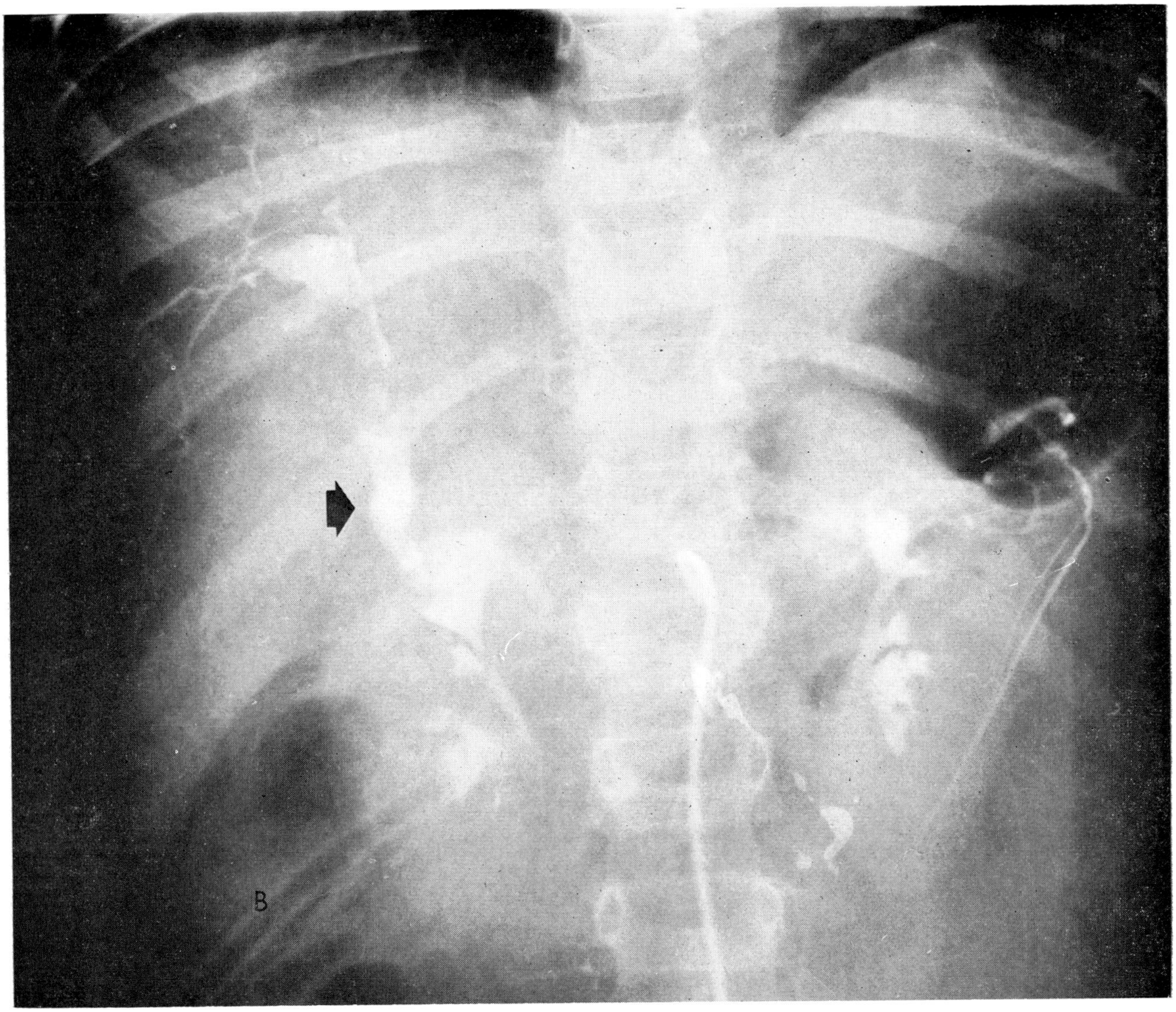

Figure 26.51. Celiac Arteriogram. (A) Arterial phase: Contrast accumulates in the central part of the right lobe of the liver in an irregular manner. (B) Parenchymal phase: Contrast fills the dilated right hepatic duct. *Diagnosis:* Extravasation into the biliary tree (traumatic hemobilia). (From Enge, I., Knutrud, O., and Normann, T. Central rupture of the liver with traumatic hemobilia. *Br J Radiol, 41:*789, 1968. Courtesy of the authors and publishers.)

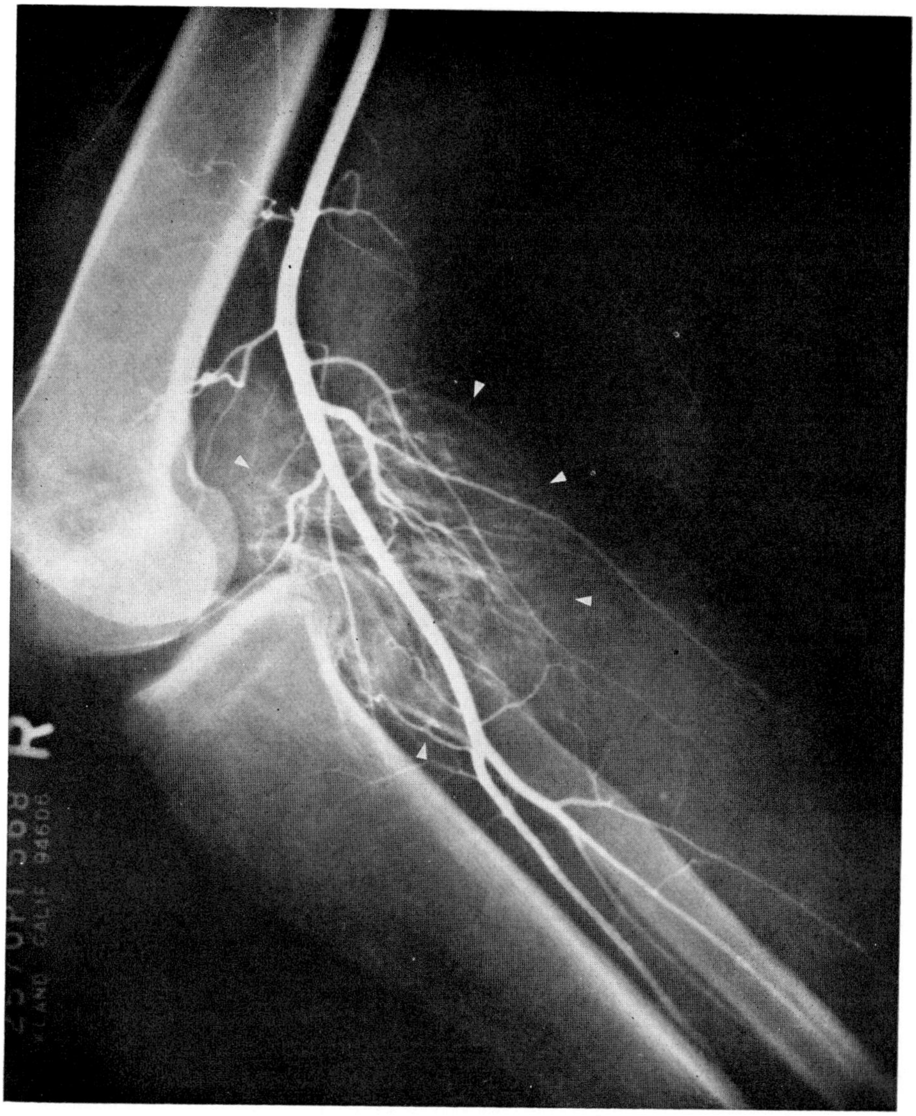

Figure 26.52 A

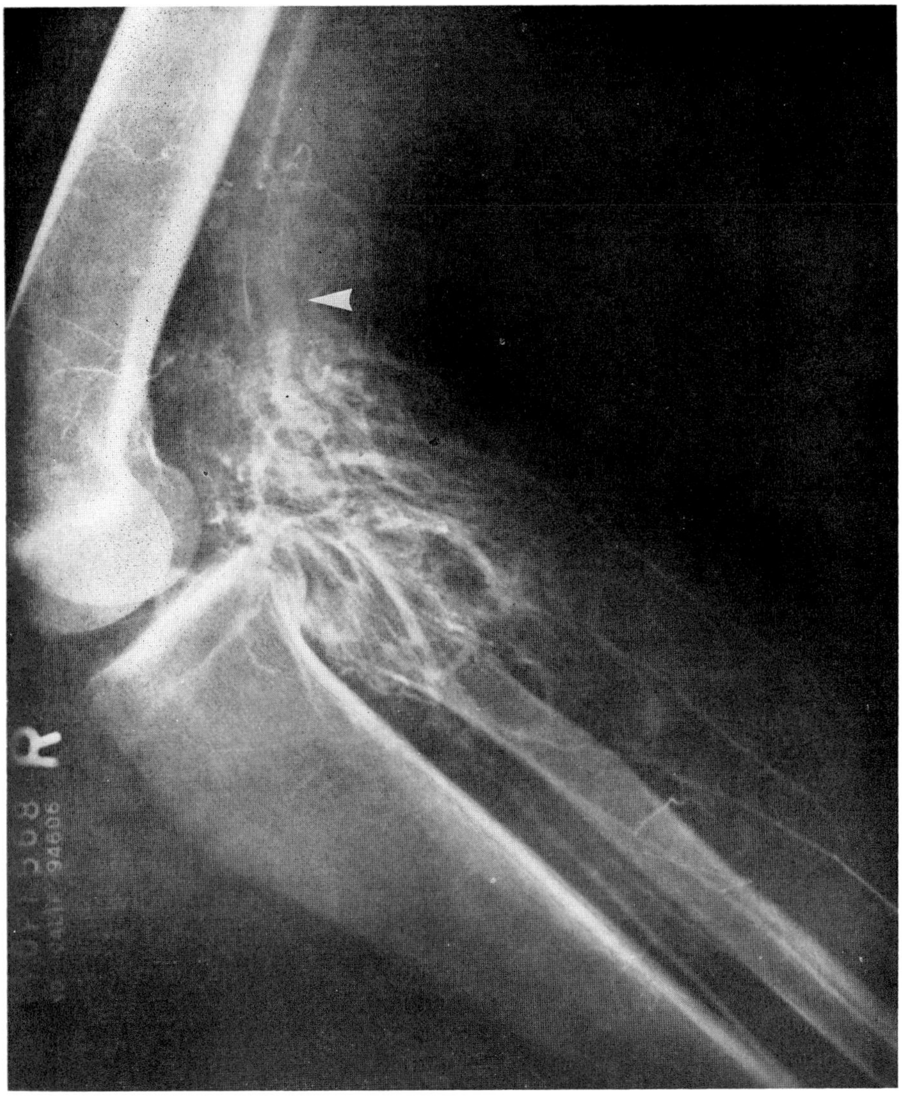

Figure 26.52. Femoral Arteriogram. (A) Arterial phase: There is an appreciable increase in the localized vasculature (Arrow Heads). Also note the early mottled staining of a moderately defined mass. (B) Late phase: Intense staining is seen in the same area as well as early femoral vein opacification (Arrow Head). This patient had taken an overdose of drugs and squatted in an awkward position for thirty hours. *Diagnosis:* Malignant tumor? *Pathology:* Muscle necrosis (ischemic hemorrhagic striated muscle). (From Gronner, A. T. Muscle necrosis simulating a malignant tumor angiographically. *Radiol, 103:*309, 1972. Courtesy of authors and publishers.)

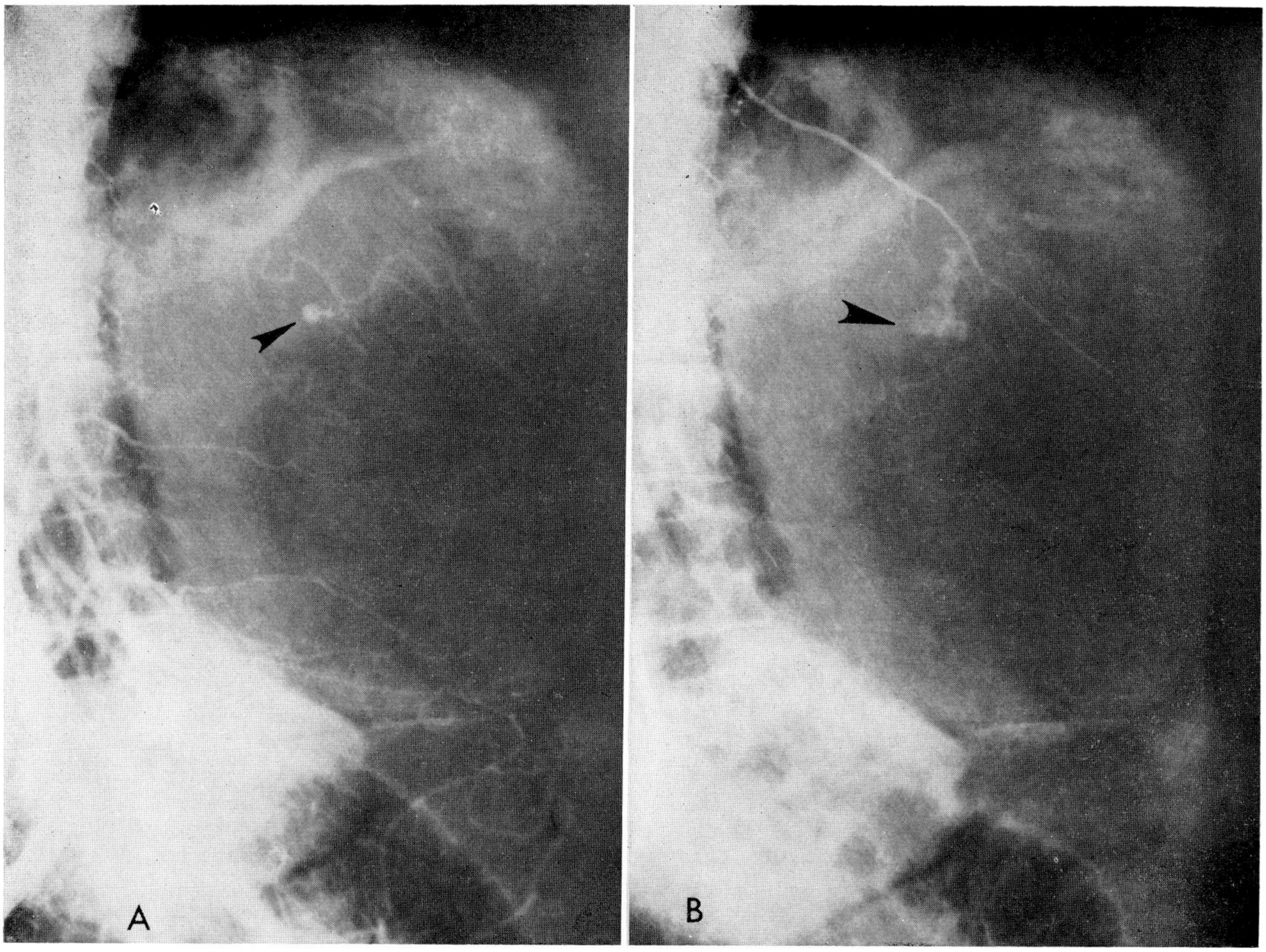

Figure 26.53. (A) Late arterial phase reveals a huge mass in the left hemiabdomen with a central collection of the contrast. (B) The same collection of contrast disperses. Note the inferomedial displacement of the left kidney. *Diagnosis:* Possible left adrenal carcinoma with marked necrosis and extravasation of the contrast. Pathology confirmed the diagnosis.

gallbladder in their entirety. *Locating the anatomic site* of bleeding is accomplished by tracing the extravasation to that particular branch and its parent vessel. Extravasation of contrast into the lumen of the esophagus, stomach, duodenum, small bowel, colon, gallbladder (hemocholecyst), bile duct (hemobilia), pancreatic ducts, and lymphatic ducts (hemochylia) can occur.

Arterial extravasation into the lumen of the *esophagus* usually falls within the arborization of the *left gastric artery*. The usual causes are tears at the cardiac orifice,[562, 563] long-standing nasogastric intubation, or postesophagoscopy. Again, the bleeding may be arterial or venous in nature. Venous extravasation is usually seen in esophageal varices related to portal hypertension (Figs. 26-28 to 26-38).

Extravasation into the lumen of the *stomach* is seen most commonly with ulcers, either peptic or stress, and gastritis. These occur within the arborization of the *left gastric artery*. Extravasation into the *duodenal lumen* is most likely due to benign ulcers in the bulb, or hemorrhagic duodenitis.[564, 565] This bleeding usually involves the branches of the *gastroduodenal artery*. Rare causes of extravasation into the duodenum are related to aortic surgery followed by the development of aortoduodenal fistula.[572]

Extravasation into the lumen of the *small bowel* is seen in Meckel's diverticulum and can be demonstrated either due to extravasation, staining of ectopic gastric mucosa, if any, or by recognition of the embryonic nature of its blood supply (Fig. 34-5). However, this supply may also come from normal ileac vessels.[566–568] Other causes of small bowel extravasation include superior mesenteric venous occlusion,[1014–1016] regional enteritis,[569] intramural aneurysms[570] and diverticulum.[571] Small bowel arterial extravasation falls within the range of the *superior mesenteric artery* branches.

Extravasation into the lumen of the *colon* may fall within the range of the vessels of the *superior and/or inferior mesenteric arteries. Diverticula* are probably the leading causes of massive hemorrhage in the large bowel due to rupture of the vasa recta at the dome of the diverticula.[573, 574] Other causes such as vascular malformations of the appendiceal stump,[575] stress ulcers of the cecum,[576] or granulation tissue of colitis may be demonstrated by extravasation of the contrast providing the study is done at an opportune time. Other lesions such as *submucosal ectasia of the vessels within the right colon* due to aging[108, 577] or associated with aortic stenosis[579] may not show extravasation of contrast but are definitely causes of occult bleeding. These can be demonstrated with the assistance of magnification angiography.[57] Other causes of extravasation into the gastrointestinal tract, though rare, may occur and cause acute hemorrhage. They may be seen following surgery,[581–583] angiitis (polyarteritis nodosa),[584] telangiectasia,[585] pseudoxanthoma elasticum,[586, 587] or bleeding tumors such as leiomyoma[588] (Figs. 26-28 to 26-39).

The Pediatric Patient and Extravasation

In the pediatric age group stress peptic ulcers, portal hypertension, Meckel's diverticulum, duplication of the gastrointestinal tract, ulcerative colitis, and polyps are probably the most common causes of bleeding into the gastrointestinal tract.[589]

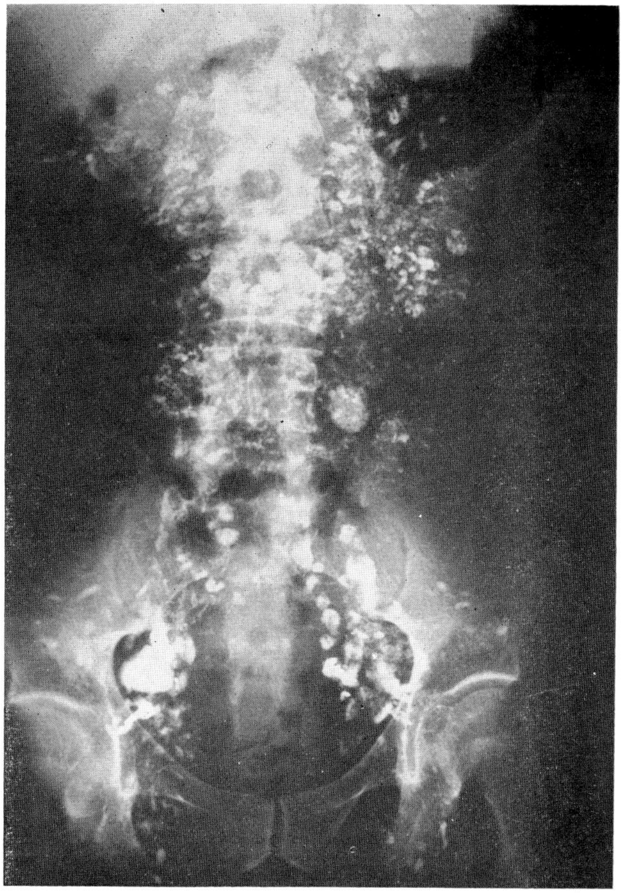

Figure 26.54. Lymphangiogram reveals dilatation of the abdominal lymph vessels with retrograde opacification of dilated mesenteric lymphatics in a patient who developed spontaneous rupture of a congenital splenic artery aneurysm into the portal circulation causing massive flooding of the blood into the dilated abdominal lymphatic system. The same patient happened to have a Lutembacher's syndrome and protein-losing enteropathy. (Courtesy of Stalder, Hans, Joliat, Gerard. Blood in the lymph (hemochylia) and intestinal lymphangiectasia associated with Lutembacher's syndrome. *Am J Med, 55*:99, 1973. Courtesy of the authors and the publishers.)

The Cirrhotic Patient and Extravasation

Patients with cirrhosis and portal hypertension bleed from their esophageal varices the majority of times. However, it is not unusual for them to bleed from gastric ulcers, esophageal ulcers, enteritis, etc.[590, 591]

Catheter Management of Acute Gastrointestinal Bleeding

At the present time *vasopressin* and *epinephrine* are the available vasoconstrictors for the management of acute gastrointestinal hemorrhage,[102–105, 108, 592] When *vasopressin is injected* into the celiac axis, the hepatic artery escapes vasoconstriction unlike the left gastric, splenic and gastroduodenal arteries. The small bowel blood vessels are very responsive to vasopressin. It decreases superior mesenteric arterial flow, thereby decreasing portal flow and pressure. There is a 50 percent reduction of portal pressure in patients with portal hypertension. The most *dramatic effect* in arresting bleeding[108, 593] is seen in patients with esophageal mucosal tears, gastritis, stress ulcers, bleeding due to colitis, diverticula, angioma, vascular ectasias, Curling's ulcer and uremic gastritis.

The vessels which are devoid of contractile elements may not respond to vasoconstricting drugs.[108] Therefore, the management of bleeding may not be satisfactory when there is chemical or necrotic digestion of a bleeding vessel, severe atherosclerosis of the bleeding vessel or parent branch, denudation of the muscle wall of the vessel,[581] or recent inflammatory vasculature. And, of course, a large vessel containing contractile elements may not respond because of the caliber of the vessel. Theoretically, junctional zone areas and hollow viscus with plentiful blood supplies from multiple sources may not respond satisfactorily.

Methods

Vasopressin, 100 units, is mixed with 500 cc of saline or 5% dextrose in water. A continuous perfusion pump such as a sigma motor pump is essential for continuous, monitored infusion. A repeat angiogram is done after the test dose of vasopressin is infused for fifteen to thirty minutes. The final dose of vasopressin depends on the vasoconstrictive response of the branches, arrest of bleeding demonstrated by lack of contrast extravasation, and the reflux of contrast into the aorta. These factors reflect local increased peripheral resistance. *The actual infusion is determined by a trial and error method.* It should be tailored according to the clinical situation. A general dose rate is 0.2 units per cc per minute for the first six to eight hours followed by 0.1 unit per cc per minute for the following twenty-four to thirty hours. Then 5% glucose in water or normal saline is infused at the rate of 0.75 cc to 1.0 cc per minute to avoid clotting of the catheter. If there is no bleeding during the following eighteen to twenty-four hours the catheter may be removed. *An injection rate of more than 0.4 units per cc per minute is neither advisable nor effective.* The closer the tip of the catheter is to the site of arterial bleeding, and the better the selection of a patient who will respond to a vasoconstrictive drug, the higher the rewarding results will be.[102, 105, 108]

Intermittent infusion with periodic *estimations of the serum lactic acid levels* will help in preventing thrombosis of the small veins of the bowel which may result in infarction of the bowel itself.[110] *Fluid overload should be prevented,* as vasopressin is an antidiuretic drug.[59] Elevated systemic vasopressin levels do not appear to have an adverse effect on renal function.[1496] *Careful monitoring of the cardiac response* in elderly individuals and individuals with a history of heart disease is essential.[1497] Blood oozing around the catheter may be a serious problem especially in patients with decreased platelet counts due to repeated transfusion (Figs. 26-34 and 26-35).

Extravasation of Contrast Into the Gall Bladder (Hemocholecyst), Biliary Tree (Hemobilia), Pancreatic Duct and Lymphatic Ducts

Extravasation into the *gallbladder* may occur as a result of chronic cholecystitis and stone formation within the gallbladder. This may cause secondary erosion of the cystic artery.[556–558] Apoplexy of the gallbladder may be seen in patients with essential hypertension due to bleeding from the cystic artery into the gallbladder.[559]

Hemorrhage into or through the *biliary*

tract[560] occurs when injury or disease causes vascular communication with the biliary tree. Thus blood may flow into the intestine with the bile. The origin of this blood is *mostly arterial*, but occasionally may be venous, and while usually massive, can at times be occult. *Etiologies* include trauma, tumors, arteriovenous fistula, aneurysms, or liver biopsy. Bleeding may originate within the liver, biliary ducts, gallbladder, or even in the pancreas. *Trauma* deserves special mention, as it is one of the major causes of hemobilia. Traumatic ruptures of the liver form a cavity which heals poorly. The liver *regenerates quickly and profusely, but heals slowly and badly.* After trauma a certain amount of time is needed before the tissues become necrotic and open communications between the blood vessels and the ducts. *There is no correlation between the size of the cavity or the gravity of the bleeding.* The silent period may be days, weeks, or even years. The diagnosis may be established on the grounds of the past history, laparotomy, or during autopsy, or may never be made.[560]

The clinical triad of gastrointestinal hemorrhage, biliary colic, and jaundice may help establish the diagnosis (Figs. 26-38, 26-39 and 26-51).

Bleeding from the splenic artery into the *pancreatic duct*[560, 561] with transportation of blood into the gastrointestinal tract is not unusual in pancreatic pathologies because of the proximity of the splenic artery to the pancreas. Extravasation of blood into the *lymphatic ducts* has been related to rupture of splenic artery aneurysms into the portal vein. This secondarily floods the blood into the lymphatic ducts.[597] This is an interesting, but rare, occurrence (Fig. 26-54).

Extravasation into Cavities and Spaces

Epistaxis from branches of the *internal maxillary and ethmoidal arteries*[598, 599] is responsible for bleeding into the nasal cavities. *Spinal* subarachnoid bleeding has been shown to occur from the *vertebral artery*.[600] Bleeding into the epidural space is seen with tears of the meningeal vessels (Fig. 27-15). The extravasated contrast may pass into the epidural or subgaleal spaces.[601]

EXTRAVASATION INTO PARENCHYMA

Bleeding may occur into an organ such as the liver, spleen, kidney, pancreas, brain, or into a tumor or into a necrotic area of muscle (Figs. 26-40, 26-44, 26-45 to 26-49).

Parenchymal Extravasation

Unlike bleeding into a hollow cavity or the lumen of a viscus, bleeding into the parenchyma of an organ with an intact capsule tends to arrest the bleeding to a certain extent by providing a tamponade effect. This implies that a certain amount of bleeding into the organ is essential before this tamponade can occur. The balance maintained between the vis-a-tergo of the extravasated blood and the hemostatic forces opposed to it is an exceedingly delicate one. A slight increase in the former or minimal trauma is enough to cause capsular rupture, with fatal exsanguination beyond the confines of the organ.[605] Because of the tamponading effect, the organ, but not the organism, may be in jeopardy. The most common cause of this type of bleeding is *blunt or penetrating trauma.* Occasionally it may be due to rupture of vessels based on predisposing factors[602, 603] such as vasculitis, infarcts, bleeding disorders, and idiopathic reasons.

Because of this tamponade effect, the *bleeding point or extravasation may not be demonstrated at the time the study is conducted.* Thus, indirect signs such as parenchymal filling defects or defects in subcapsular space may be demonstrated. Further effects of these intraparenchymal hematomas are not harmless to the organism as a whole. *Splenic hematomas* may go on to develop delayed rupture.[605] *Renal or perirenal hematomas may* cause loss of function of a kidney[578] or renovascular hypertension.[580, 604] Bleeding into the *liver* or *ducts* may cause a Budd-Chiari syndrome due to pressure on the hepatic veins or hemobilia,[560] respectively (Figs. 26-40 to 26-49).

Extravasation in the Muscle

Posttraumatic necrosis of a muscle with its ruptured small vessels and hemorrhage[111] are faithfully represented as irregular collections of extravasated contrast and increased staining during angiography[607] (Fig. 26-52).

Extravasation into the Parenchyma of a Tumor

Bleeding from vascular tumors, either spontaneously or secondary to minimal trauma, is not an uncommon event.[606] Again, the bleeding may be confined to the tumor parenchyma or extend beyond its capsule or that of the organ (Fig. 26-53). If the organ has a draining apparatus, such as the bile ducts or ureter, or if a connection is established between the bleeding point and the draining ducts continuous bleeding is common (Figs. 26-38 and 26-51).

CHAPTER 27

ARTERIOVENOUS COMMUNICATIONS

VISUALIZATION of a vein before the normally accepted arteriovenous circulation time, signifies shunting of blood from artery to vein at different anatomical levels in that circuit for various reasons. *Flowing blood, like flowing water, has an inherent natural tendency to follow the path of least resistance.*[732] Arteries and veins developing out of a common capillary plexus form the basis for the persistence of direct communication between them. This communication is of varying sizes, either *microscopic* or *macroscopic.*[733, 734]

Arteriovenous communications may be *normal* or *abnormal.* Normal arteriovenous shunts regulate circulation, while abnormal ones disrupt it.[652] The presence of *microscopic arteriovenous shunts* is assumed by the premature visualization of the veins; at macroscopic levels the actual communication can be visualized.

Normal arteriovenous shunts at the microscopic level regulate the circulation in capillary beds. When the capillary network is closed or narrowed, the diversion of blood through these existing shunts occurs. Maximum patency of these normally occurring shunts can cause ischemia of that region by shunting blood away from the area.[742] This shunting at the microscopic precapillary level is present in venous occlusions and stasis, functional or organic ischemia, occlusive disease of the arterial tree,[735, 736] inflammation,[737] regeneration of an organ such as the liver,[738] and distension of a hollow viscus such as the bowel.[739] Normal arteriovenous anastomoses[741] in the stomach[740] are approximately 140 microns in size. In the liver they are 50 to 180 microns, in the spleen 150 to 370 microns, and in the lungs 100 to 400 microns.

Normally during clinical angiography, early visualization of veins may occur when the *tip of the catheter occludes a small vessel because of a spasm or wedging.* This causes precapillary shunting resulting in premature visualization of the contrast in the veins. *A prolonged injection of contrast* beyond the normal arteriovenous circulation time of an organ obviously opacifies both the artery and the vein simultaneously.

ABNORMAL ARTERIOVENOUS ANASTOMOSIS

This, in fact, is a *parasitic short circuit* engrafted upon a normal circulation. It serves no useful purpose and produces deleterious effects. Such a communication, when present, provides an irresistible avenue for shunting of blood from a high pressure, high resistant arterial circuit into a low pressure, low resistant, capacious venous pool.[732] Because of the sudden shunting of blood, an extra burden may be imposed upon the cardiovascular system, causing increase in cardiac output, increased blood volume, and hypertension.[743, 744] *The hemodynamic changes* associated with arteriovenous anastomosis[652, 732] depends on the length and size of the fistula, volume of blood shunted per cardiac cycle, diameter of the feeding artery, presence of collateral vessels, location of the fistula in relation to the heart (either proximal or distal), and interposition of another capillary system between the fistula and the heart as in a portal arteriovenous fistula.

The *clinical signs* of an arteriovenous shunt are observed when the shunt exceeds a certain magnitude.[715] Significant hemodynamic changes occur in only a certain percentage of patients. The farther the fistula is from the heart, the less significant are the hemodynamic changes and vice versa.[652, 745] Thus brachial or popliteal

(Text continues on page 467)

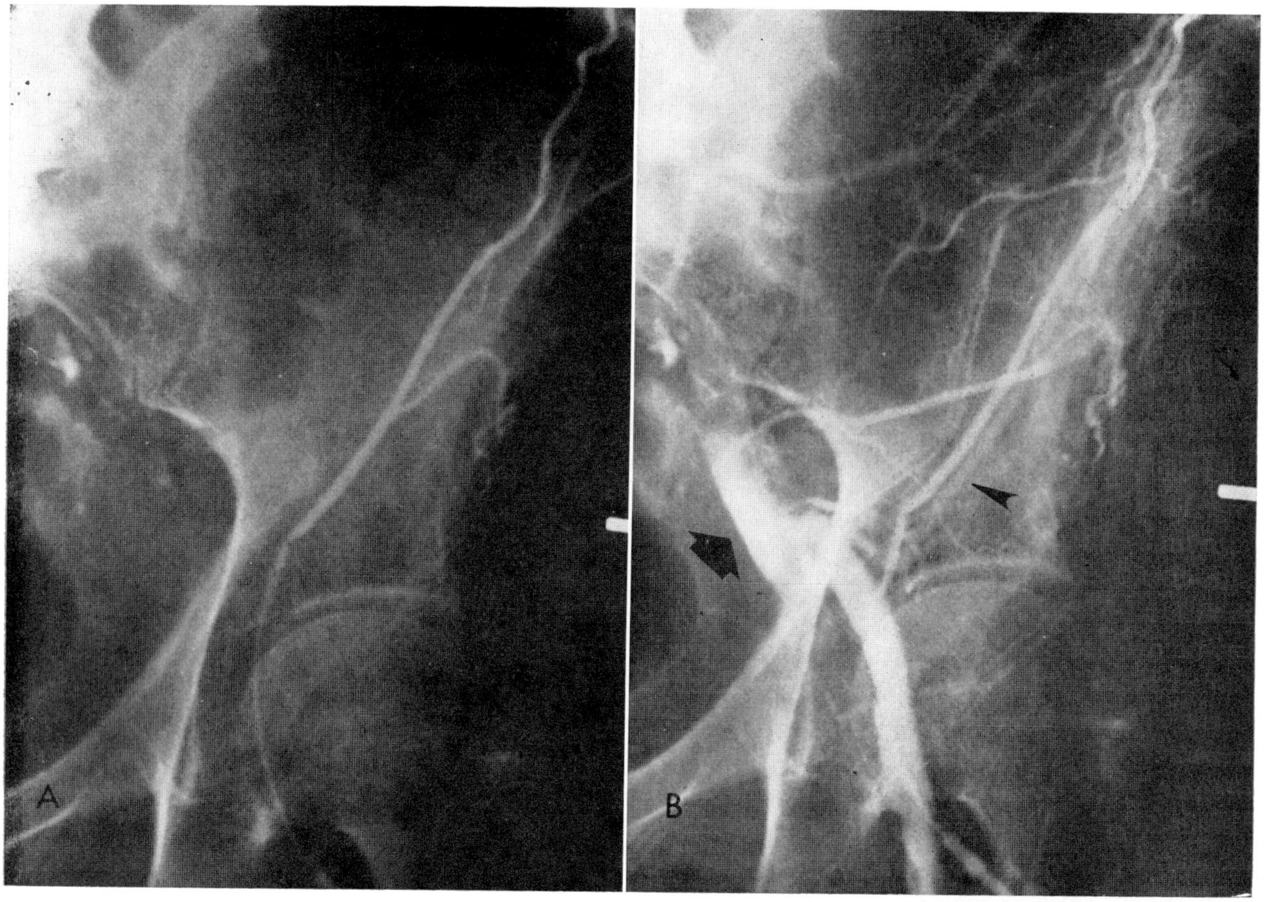

Figure 27.1. Femoral Arteriogram. (A) The plastic cannula is in the superior circumflex iliac artery. (B) Midarterial phase: This reveals premature opacification of the corresponding vein (Arrow) and also of the external iliac vein (Arrow Head). (C) A repeat femoral arteriogram after withdrawing the catheter into the common femoral artery shows no evidence of abnormality. *Diagnosis:* Nonpathological arteriovenous shunting because of injection of a large volume of contrast into a small vessel.

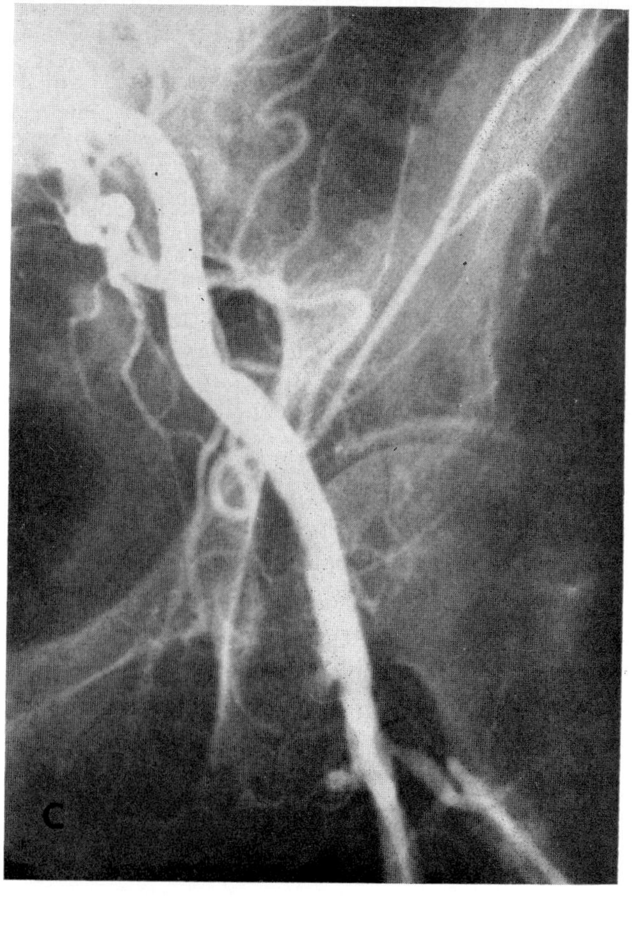

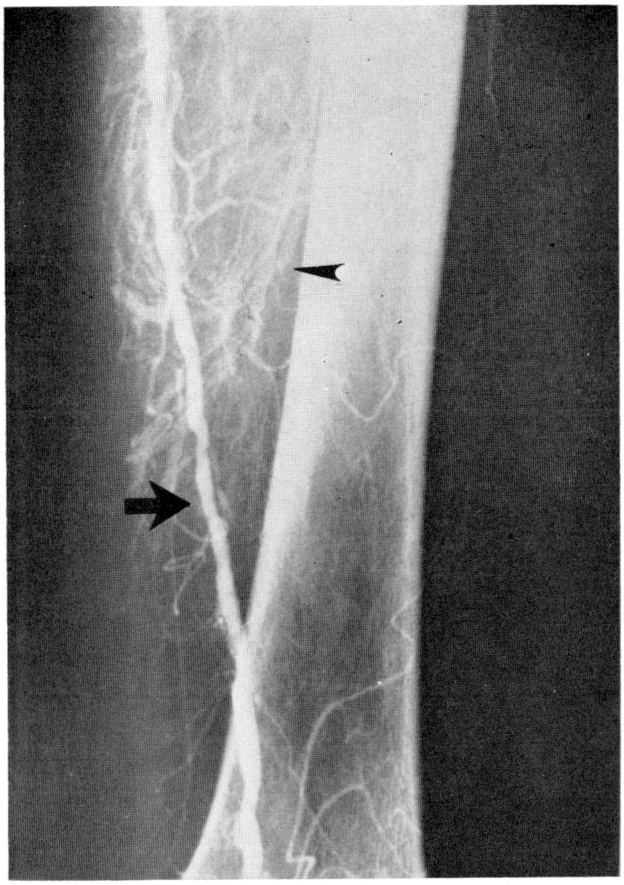

←

Figure 27.2. Femoral Arteriogram. There is arteriovenous (Arrow Head) shunting due to the compromised lumen of an atherosclerotic superficial femoral artery (Arrow).

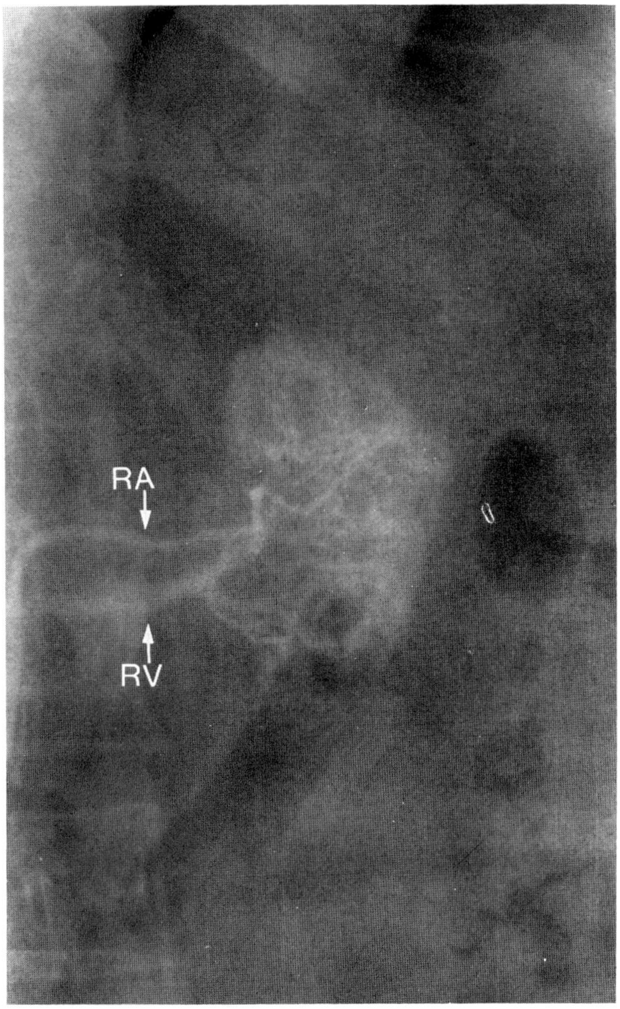

Figure 27.3. Renal Arteriogram. There is a very small kidney with a very small renal artery (R.A.) and simultaneous opacification of the renal vein (R.V.). *Comment:* Hypoplastic small kidney? It is not unusual to demonstrate early venous opacification when the catheter wedges into a small vessel.

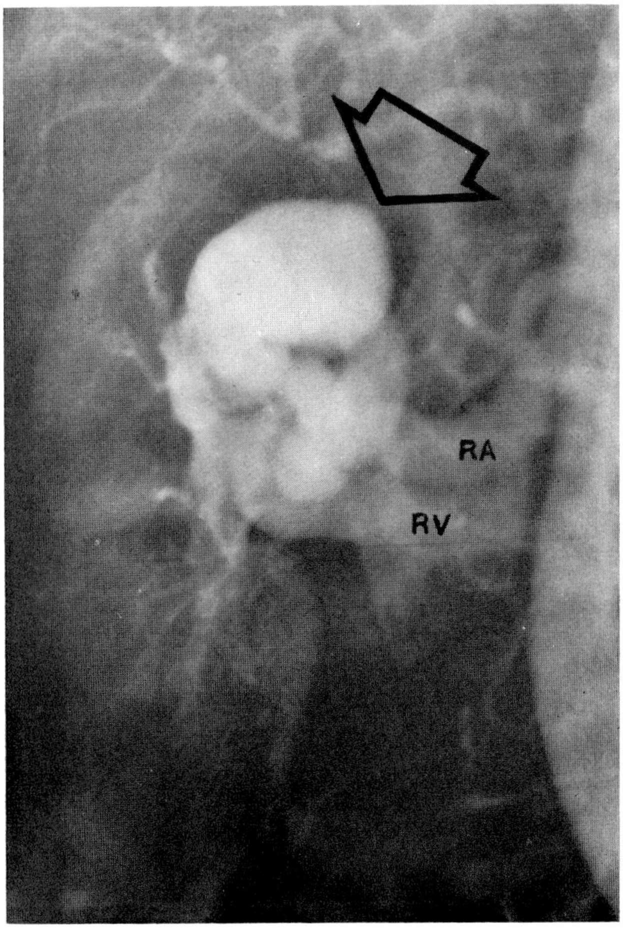

←

Figure 27.4. Flush Aortogram. A dilated right renal artery (R.A.). Circumscribed collection of contrast material (Arrow). Note simultaneous opacification of the renal vein (R.V.). The patient had hypertension without history of previous trauma or any other significant clinical histories. *Diagnosis:* Intrarenal arteriovenous fistula probably congenital in nature.

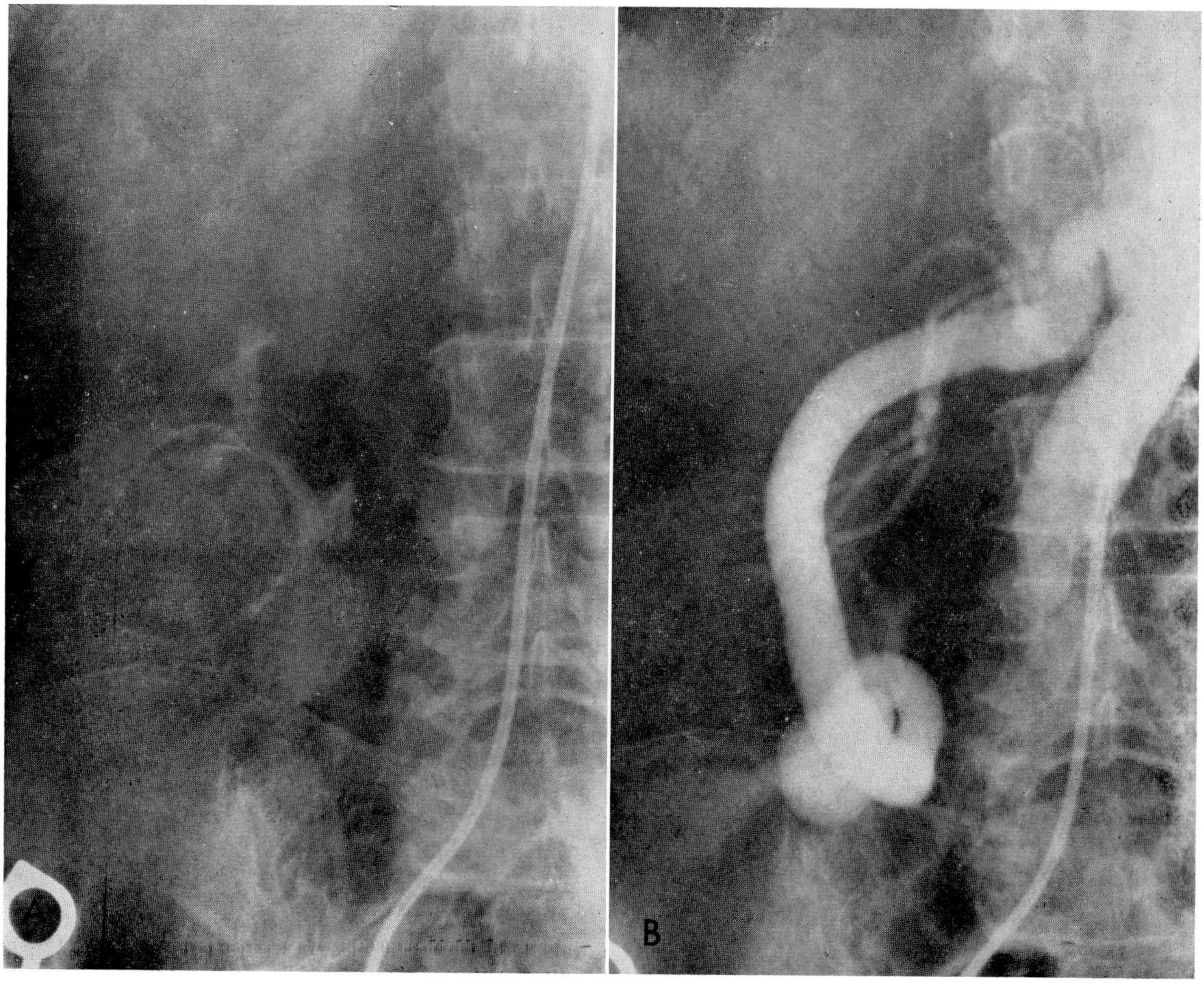

Figure 27.5 A and B

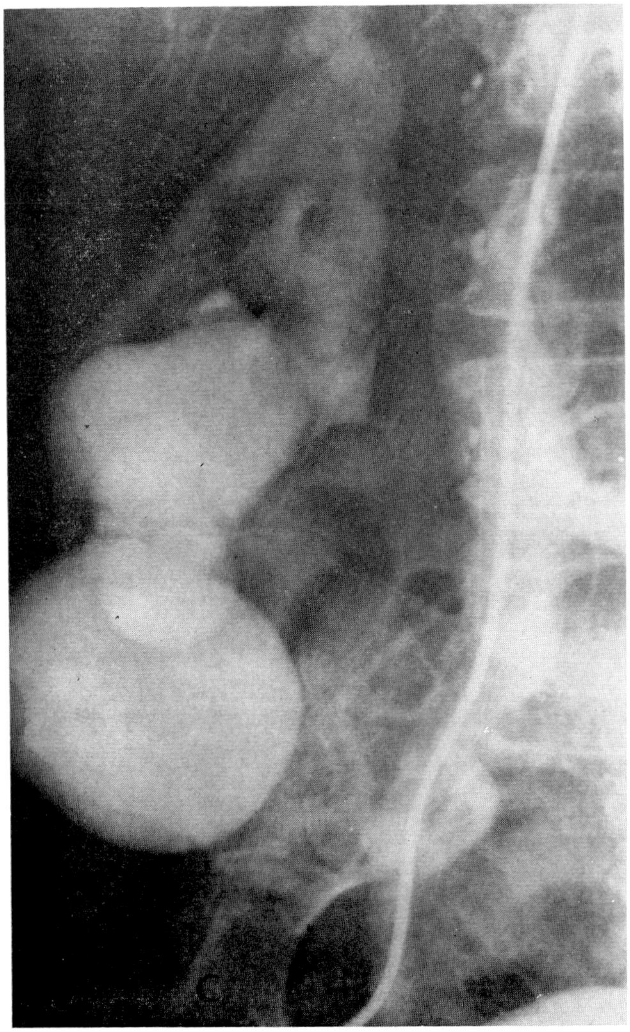

Figure 27.5. Flush Aortogram. (A) Scout film: A mass lesion is seen in the right lower pole of the kidney. (B) Early arterial phase: Note the very prominent right renal artery. (C) Late arterial phase: Saccular collections of contrast material are seen in the same projection with early opacification of a venous sac. *Diagnosis:* Congenital arteriovenous fistula. (Courtesy of Dr. M. Schwartz, St. Theresa Hospital, Waukegan, Illinois.)

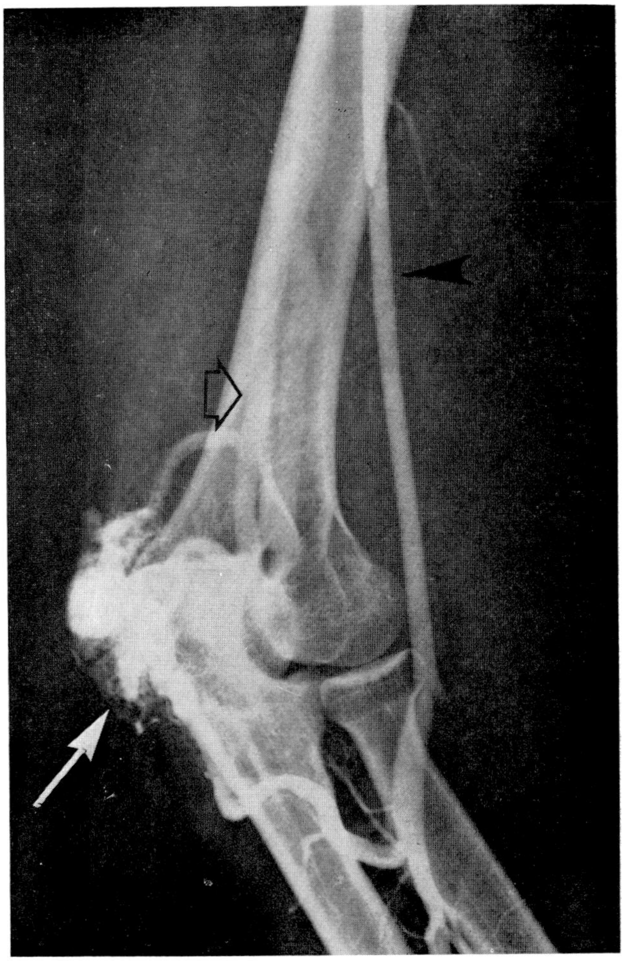

Figure 27.6. Brachial Arteriogram. There are hypertrophied arterial branches (Arrow Head) supplying blood to a vascular pool (White Arrow) with simultaneous venous opacification (Arrow). *Diagnosis:* Arteriovenous malformation—congenital.

Figure 27.7. Brachial Arteriogram. There is an increased number of tortuous vessels with simultaneous opacification of a vein. This patient was a young boy. *Diagnosis:* Congenital arteriovenous malformation.

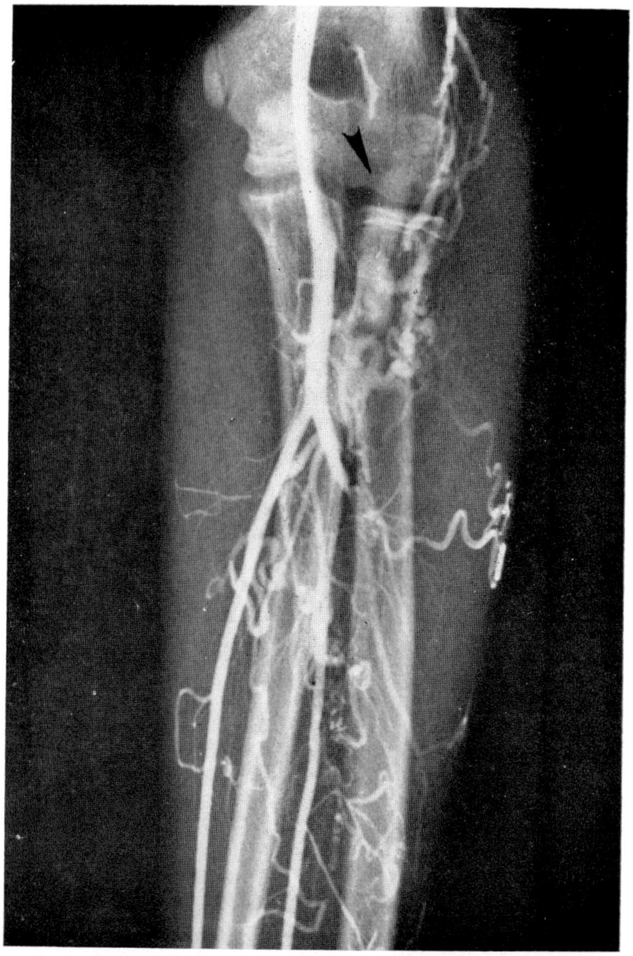

Figure 27.8. Common Carotid Arteriogram. (A) There is a saccular collection of contrast at the level of the internal maxillary artery. (B) Note the early venous filling of the jugular vein (Arrow). The patient was twelve years old. *Diagnosis:* Congenital arteriovenous aneurysm of the internal maxillary artery.

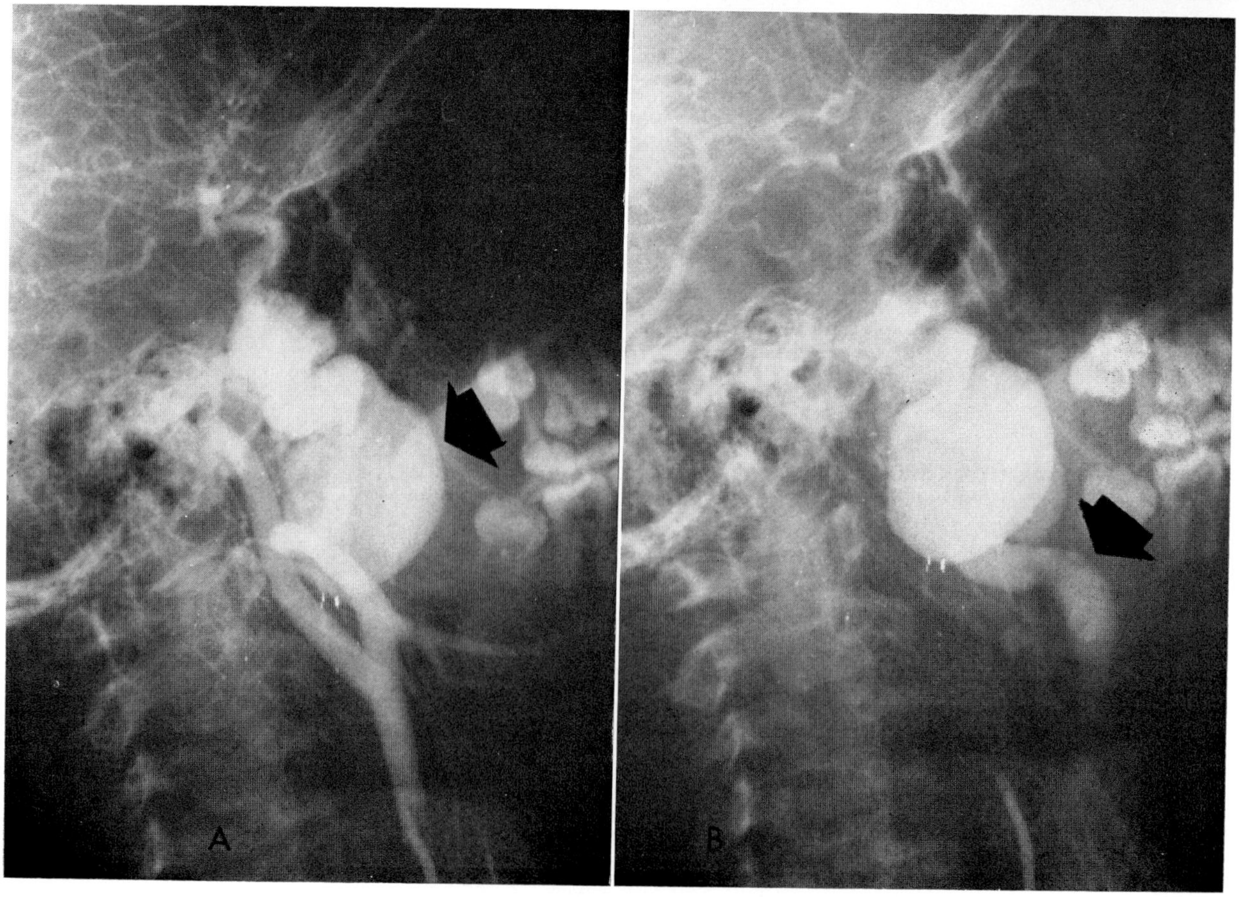

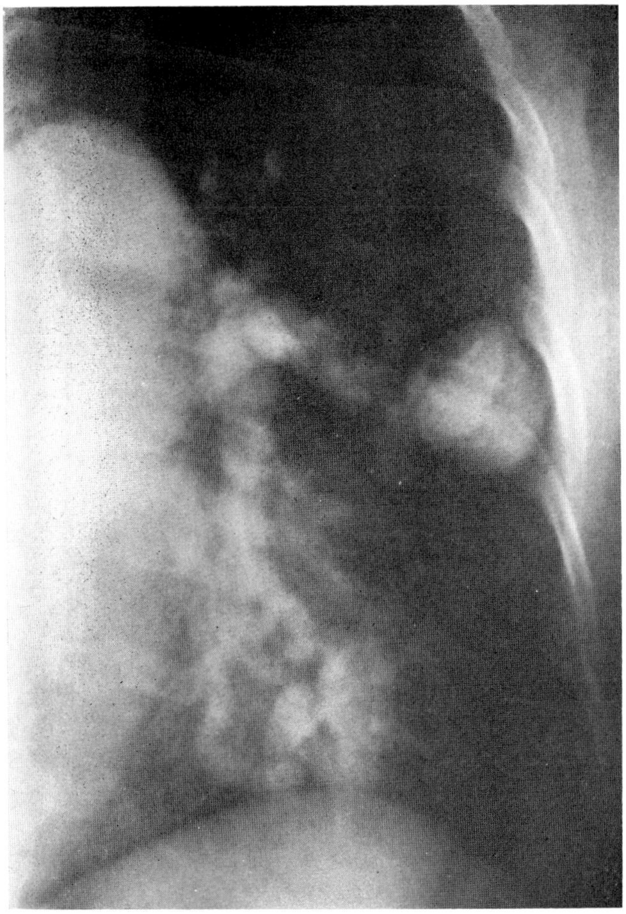

Figure 27.9. Pulmonary Arteriogram. There are very prominent tortuous pulmonary arterial branches, a saccular collection of contrast material and draining veins. *Diagnosis:* Multiple arteriovenous fistulae in a patient who had hereditary hemorrhagic telangiectasia.

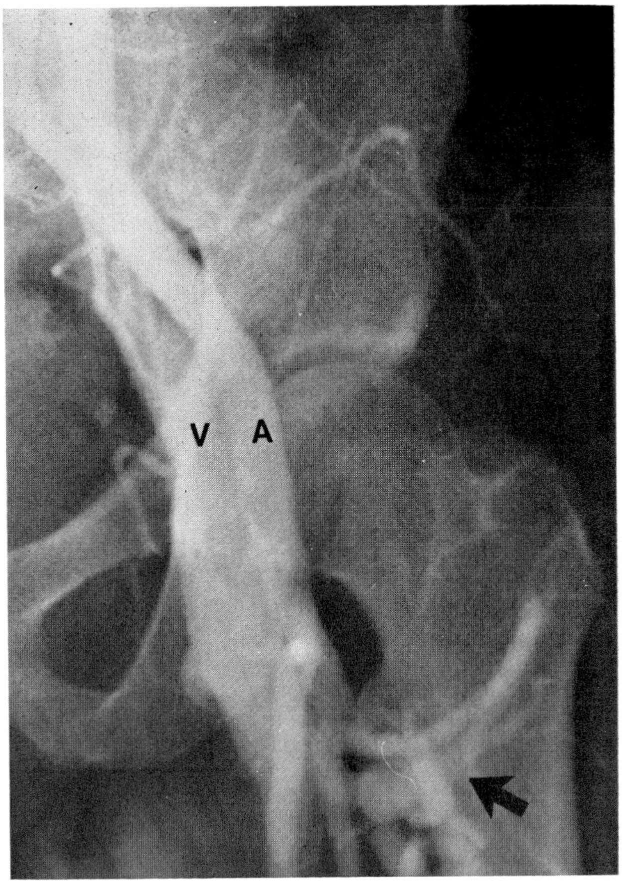

Figure 27.10. Femoral Arteriogram. There is early opacification of the dilated femoral vein due to arteriovenous communication of the circumflex femoral vessel (Arrow). *Diagnosis:* Traumatic arteriovenous fistula.

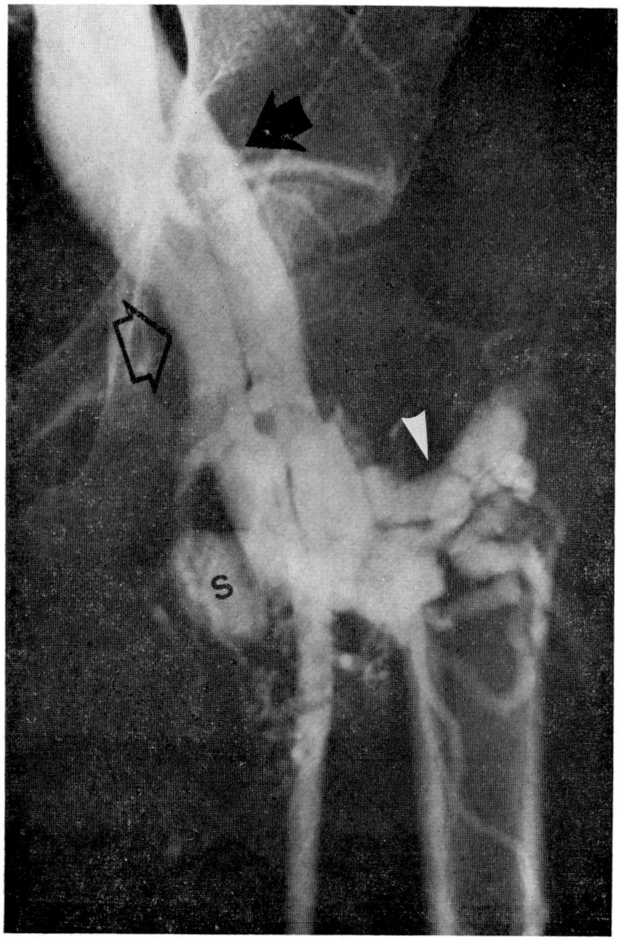

Figure 27.11. External Iliac Arteriogram. There is marked dilatation of the left external iliac artery (Arrow), saccular collection of contrast material (S), marked dilatation of the circumflex femoral branch (Arrow Head), simultaneous opacification of the external iliac vein (Blank Arrow) and tortuous corkscrew branches in the vicinity. *Diagnosis:* Arteriovenous fistula between the circumflex femoral artery and vein with marked collateral vessels.

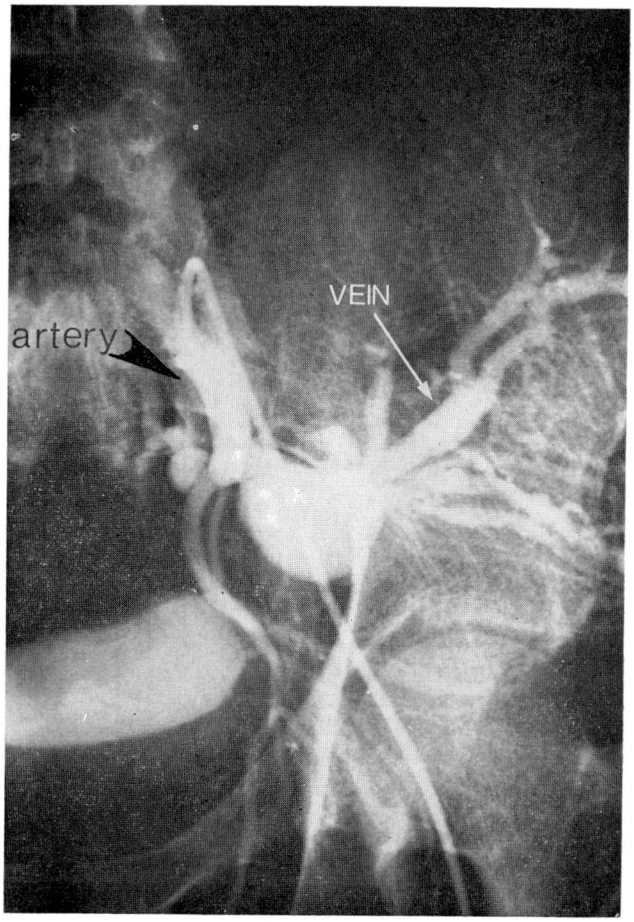

Figure 27.12. Internal Iliac Arteriogram. The internal iliac artery is dilated and there is a periarterial saccular collection of contrast. The venous network at the gluteus maximus is simultaneously opacified. *Diagnosis:* Traumatic arteriovenous fistula between the superior gluteal artery and vein (stab wound).

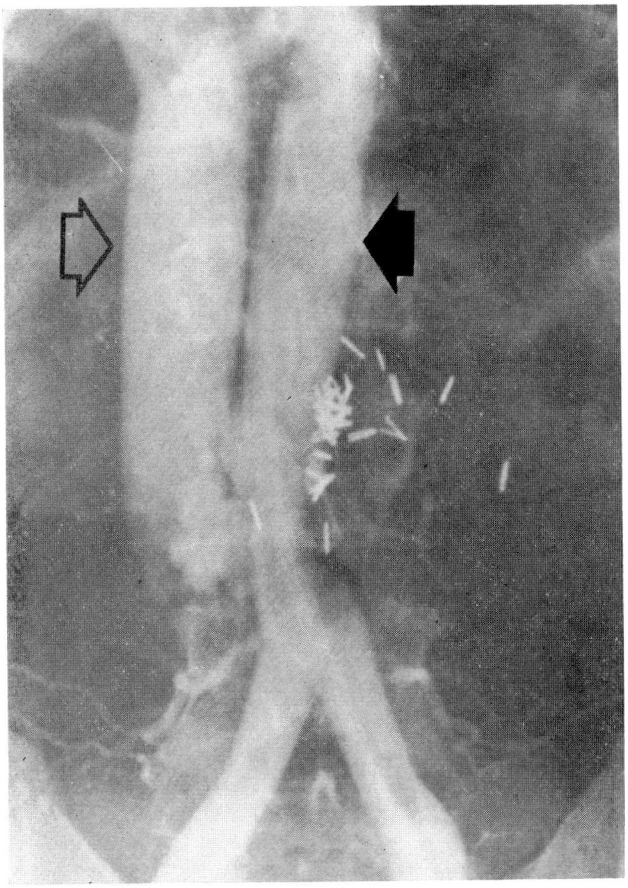

Figure 27.13. Abdominal Angiogram. There is simultaneous opacification of the abdominal aorta (Arrow) and inferior vena cava (Blank Arrow). This patient had been shot. *Diagnosis:* Traumatic aortocaval fistula.

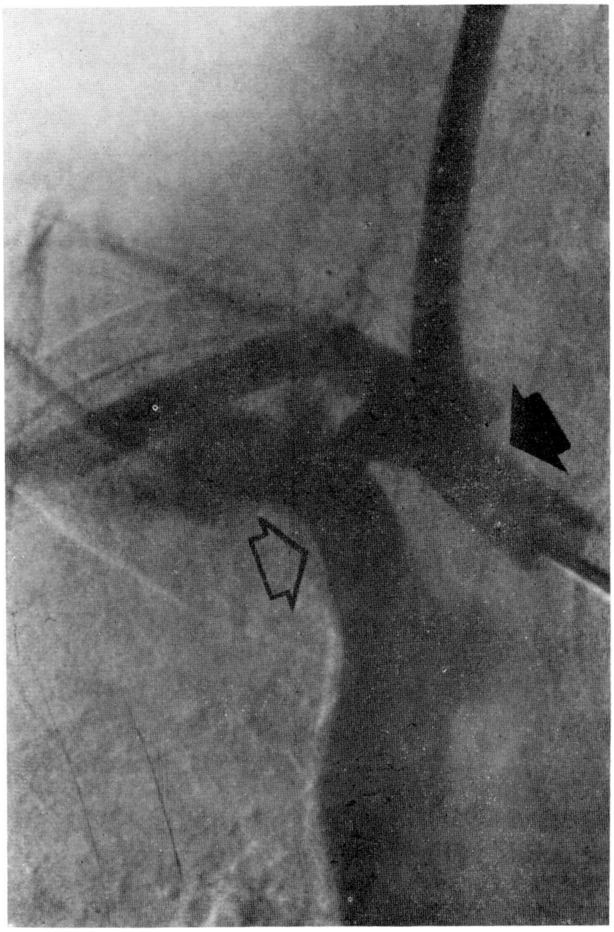

Figure 27.14. Innominate Arteriogram. There is simultaneous opacification of the innominate artery (Arrow) and the innominate vein (Blank Arrow) with a sac-like collection of contrast in between. *Diagnosis:* Traumatic arteriovenous fistula.

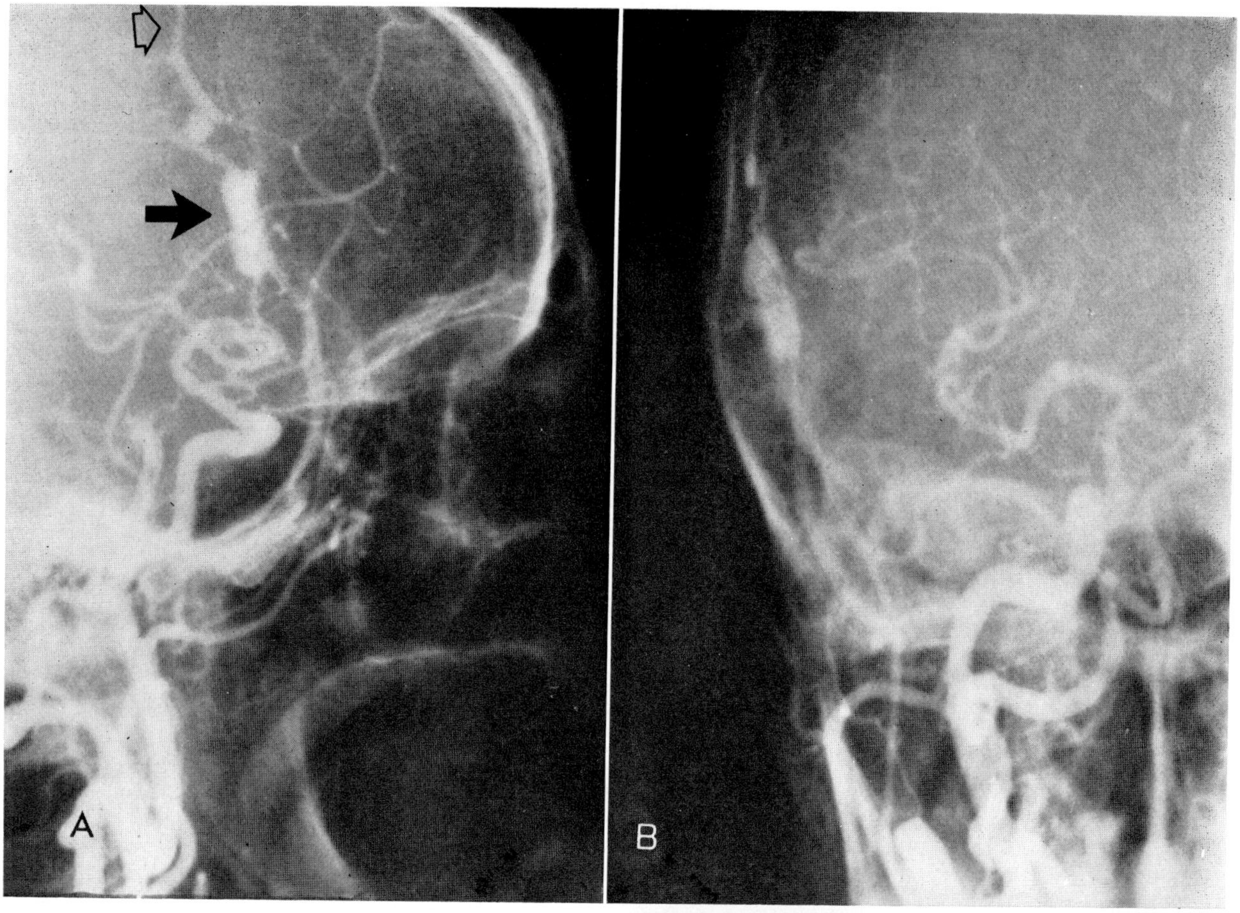

Figure 27.15. Right Brachial Arteriogram. There is periarterial extravasation (Arrow) of contrast with early venous drainage (Blank Arrow) of the middle meningeal vessels. *Diagnosis:* Traumatic arteriovenous fistula with an associated subdural hematoma.

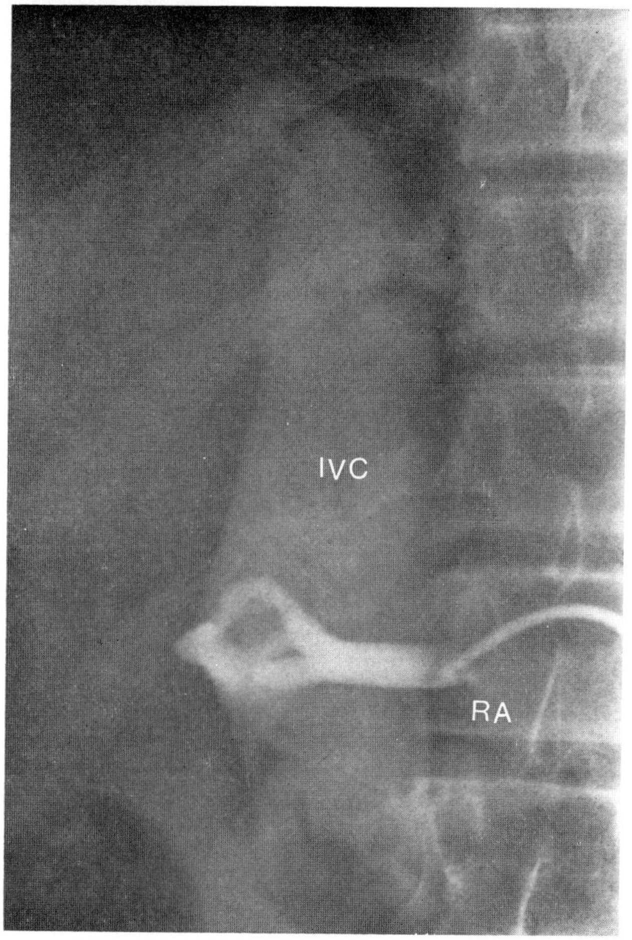

Figure 27.16. Right Renal Arteriogram. There is simultaneous opacification of the inferior vena cava and right renal artery (R.A.) in a patient who had a nephrectomy for an adenocarcinoma of the right kidney. He presented with left flank chronic, gnawing pain since nephrectomy. Left renal arteriogram was within normal limits. The stump of the right renal artery revealed the present finding. *Diagnosis:* Renal artery stump communicating with the vein causing A.V. fistula of the stump. *Comment:* The left flank pain was thought to be due to hemodynamic occlusion of the left renal vein because of arterial blood communicating with the vena cava and increasing the blood pressure of the cava above that of the left renal vein. The A.V.F. was at the same level as the left renal vein and was demonstrated on fluoroscopy. During surgery, after clamping the right renal artery, the left renal vein decreased in size. After surgery, the patient had no more symptoms.

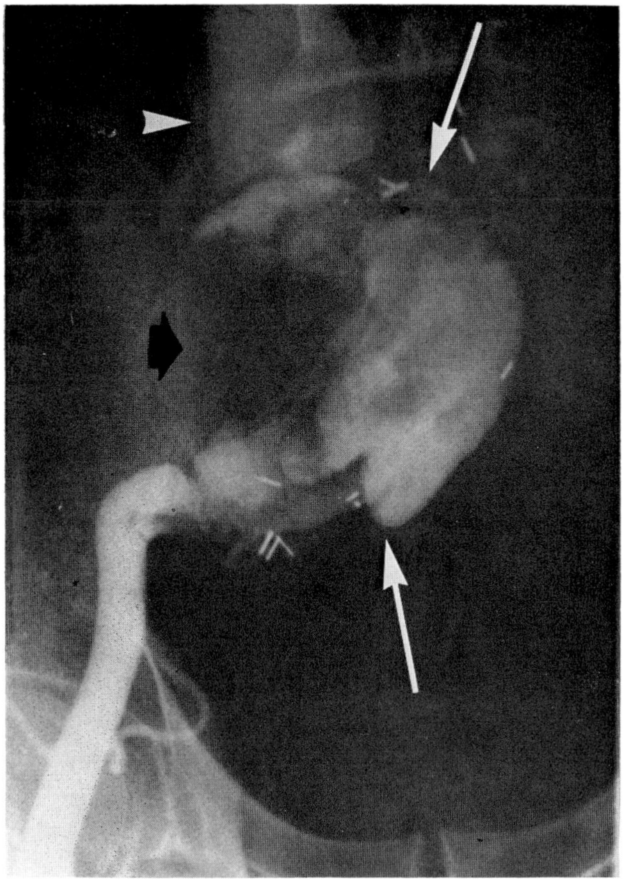

Figure 27.17. Right Femoral Arteriogram. There is a saccular collection of contrast (White Arrow) with a filling defect (Large Arrow) and visualization of the inferior vena cava (Arrow Head). This patient had an abdominal aortic graft and later developed congestive heart failure. *Diagnosis:* Postsurgical arteriovenous fistula at the right common iliac level with a blood clot.

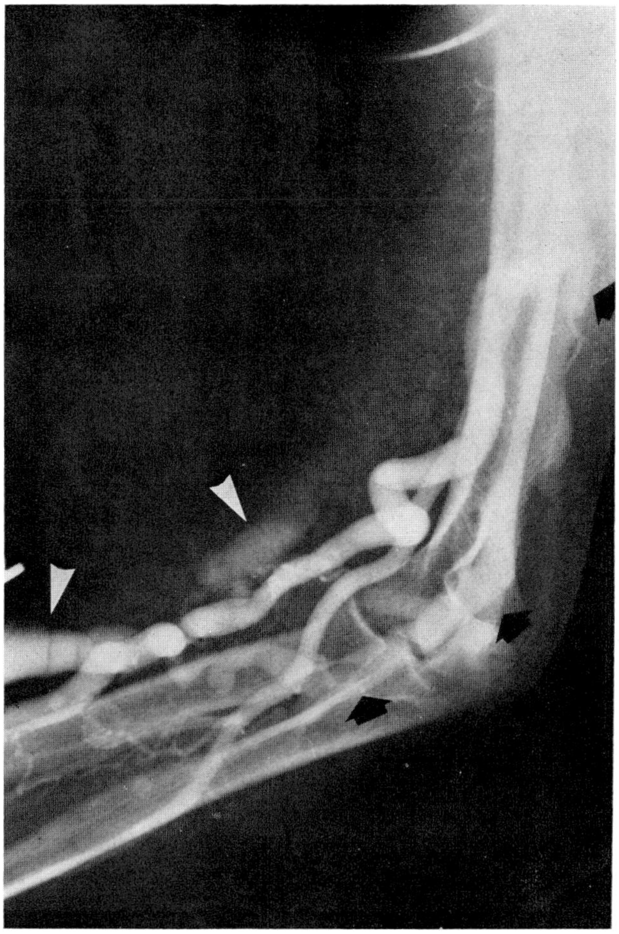

Figure 27.18. Subclavian Arteriogram. The brachial artery is hypertrophied as are its branches. There is simultaneous opacification of the veins (Arrow) and aneurysmal dilatation of the veins (Arrow Head). *Diagnosis:* Arteriovenous fistula in a patient with a shunt for renal dialysis.

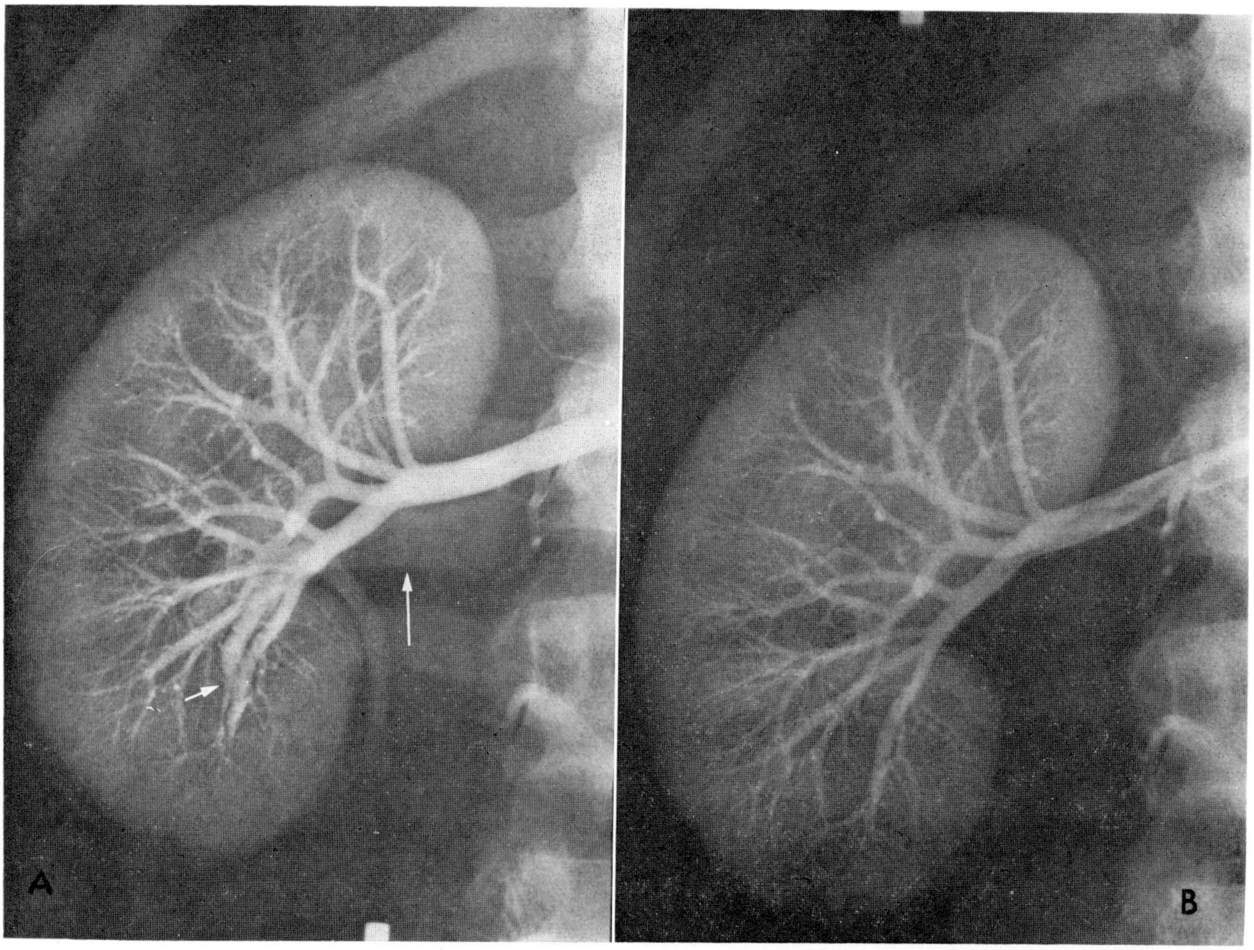

Figure 27.19. Renal Arteriograms. (A) The first injection reveals opacification of a segmental vein in the lower pole of the kidney with faint opacification of the main renal vein. This patient had a recent renal biopsy. (B) A second injection (4 minutes later) does not demonstrate the venous opacification. *Diagnosis:* Post-renal biopsy arteriovenous fistula, which was closed due to accidental embolization?

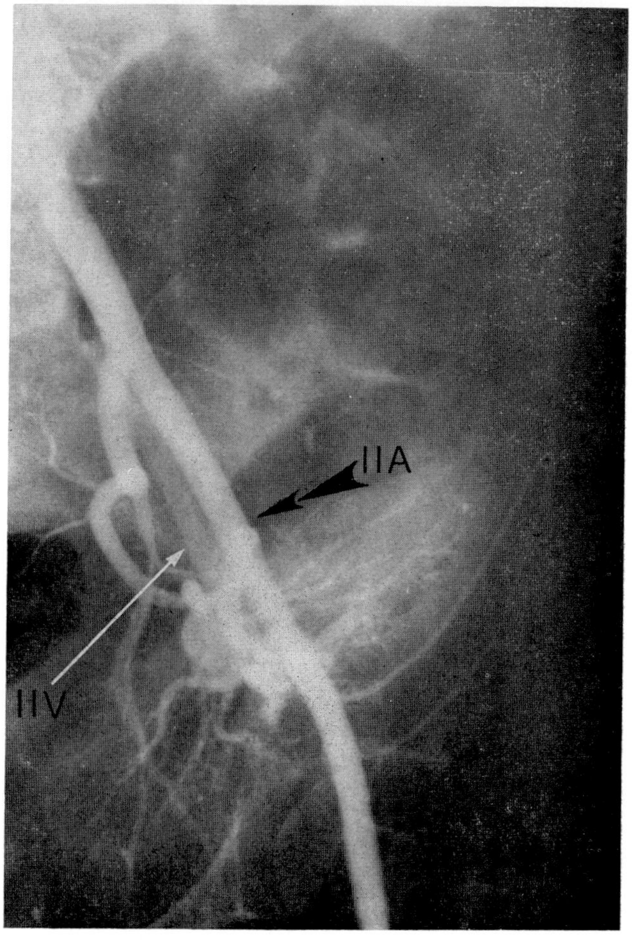

Figure 27.20. Pelvic Arteriogram in a patient who had a transplanted kidney. Left internal iliac artery (I.I.A.) is seen with simultaneous opacification of the vein (I.I.V.). *Diagnosis:* Renal pedicle A.V. fistula.

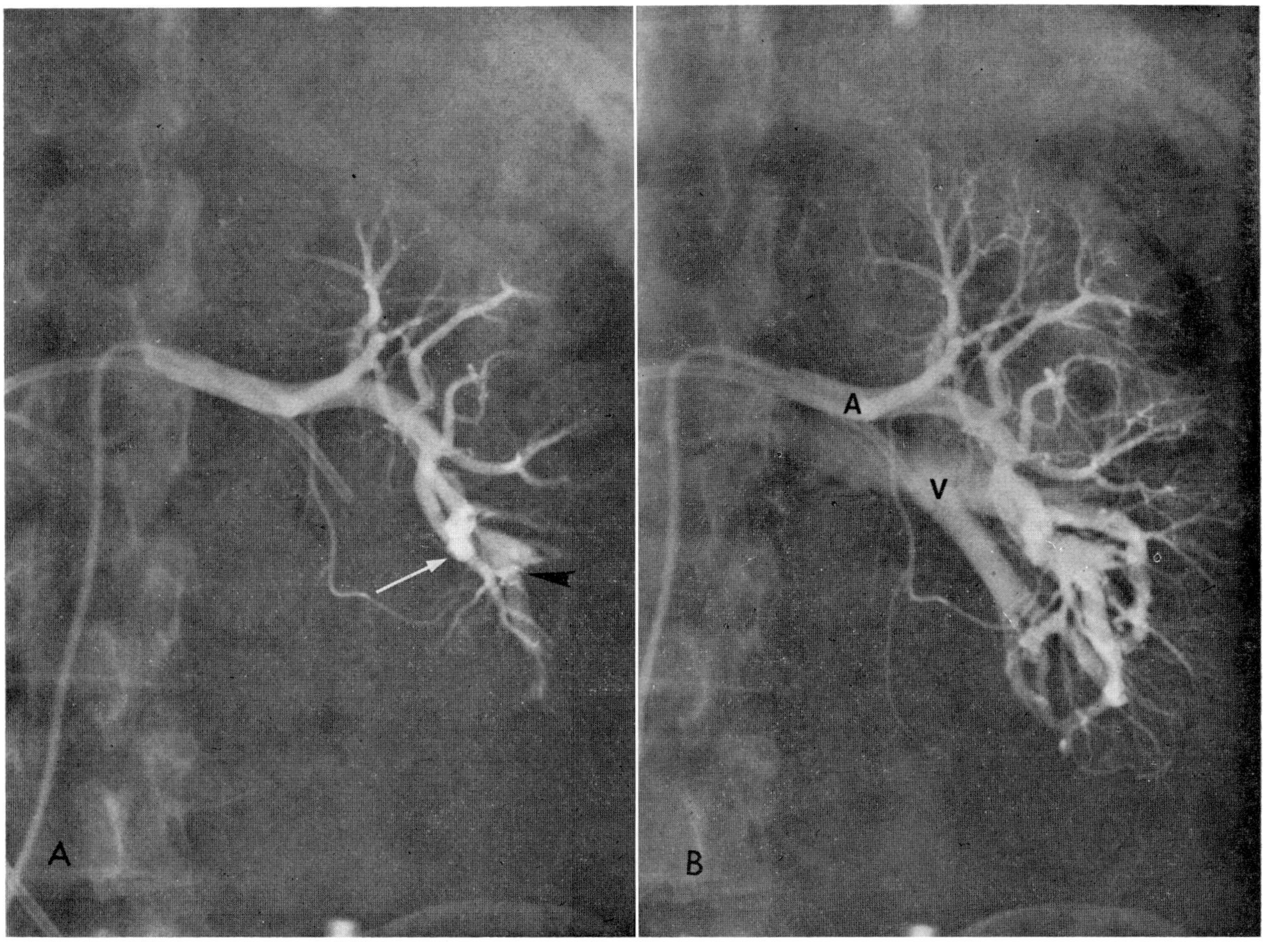

Figure 27.21. Renal Arteriogram. (A) Early arterial phase: A saccular collection of contrast material is adjacent to the intrarenal branches (Arrow) with another tubular collection of the contrast material (Arrow Head). (B) Late arterial phase: Simultaneous opacification of the intrarenal lower pole veins as well as the main renal vein can be seen. This patient had a stab wound to the left flank. *Diagnosis:* Traumatic arteriovenous fistula.

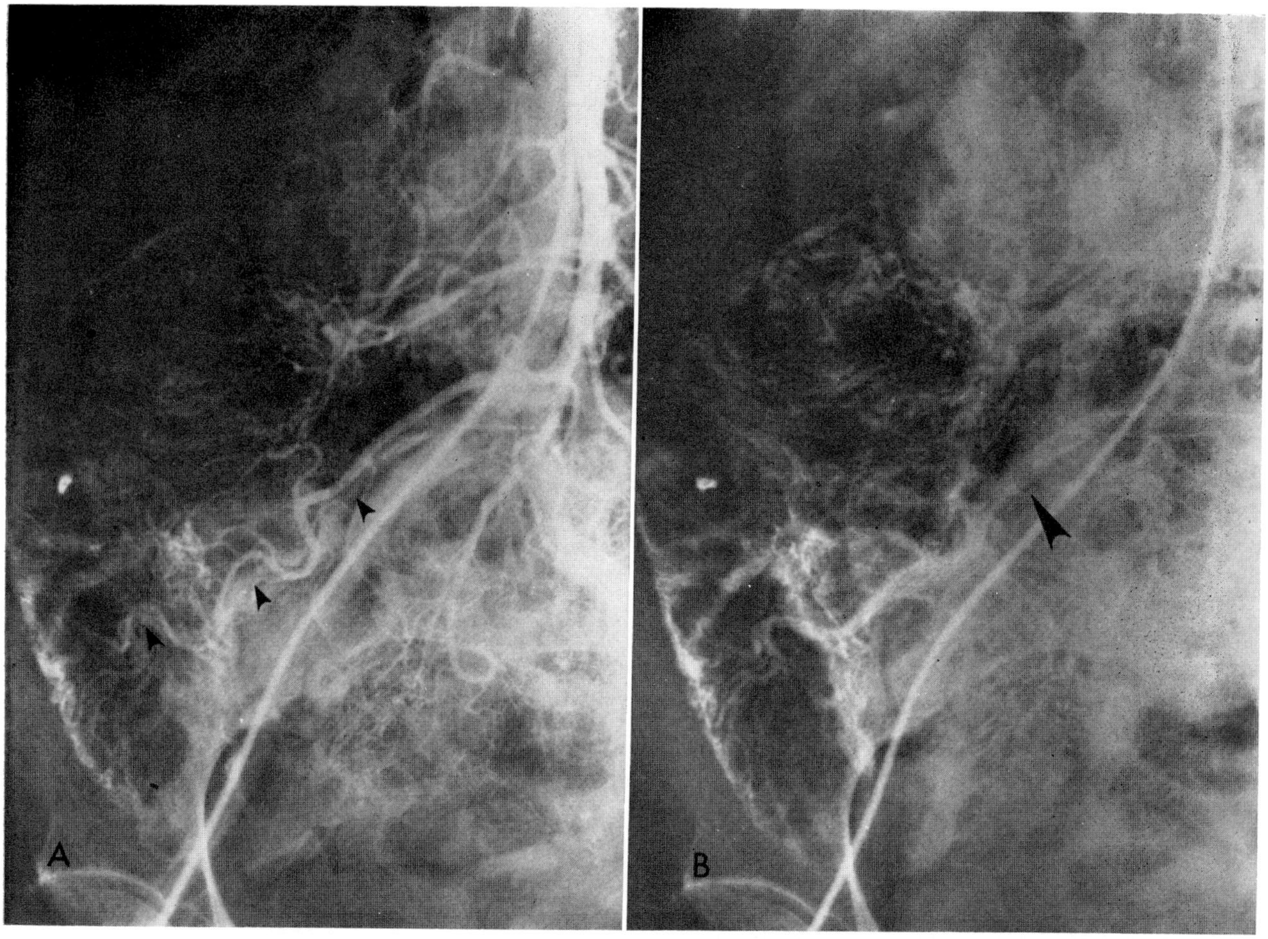

Figure 27.22. Superior Mesenteric Arteriogram. (A) Reveals early opacification of the ileocolic vein. (B) Little later, same is well demonstrated in a chronic lower G.I. bleeder. *Diagnosis:* Angiodysplasia confined to cecum. Surgery confirmed the diagnosis.

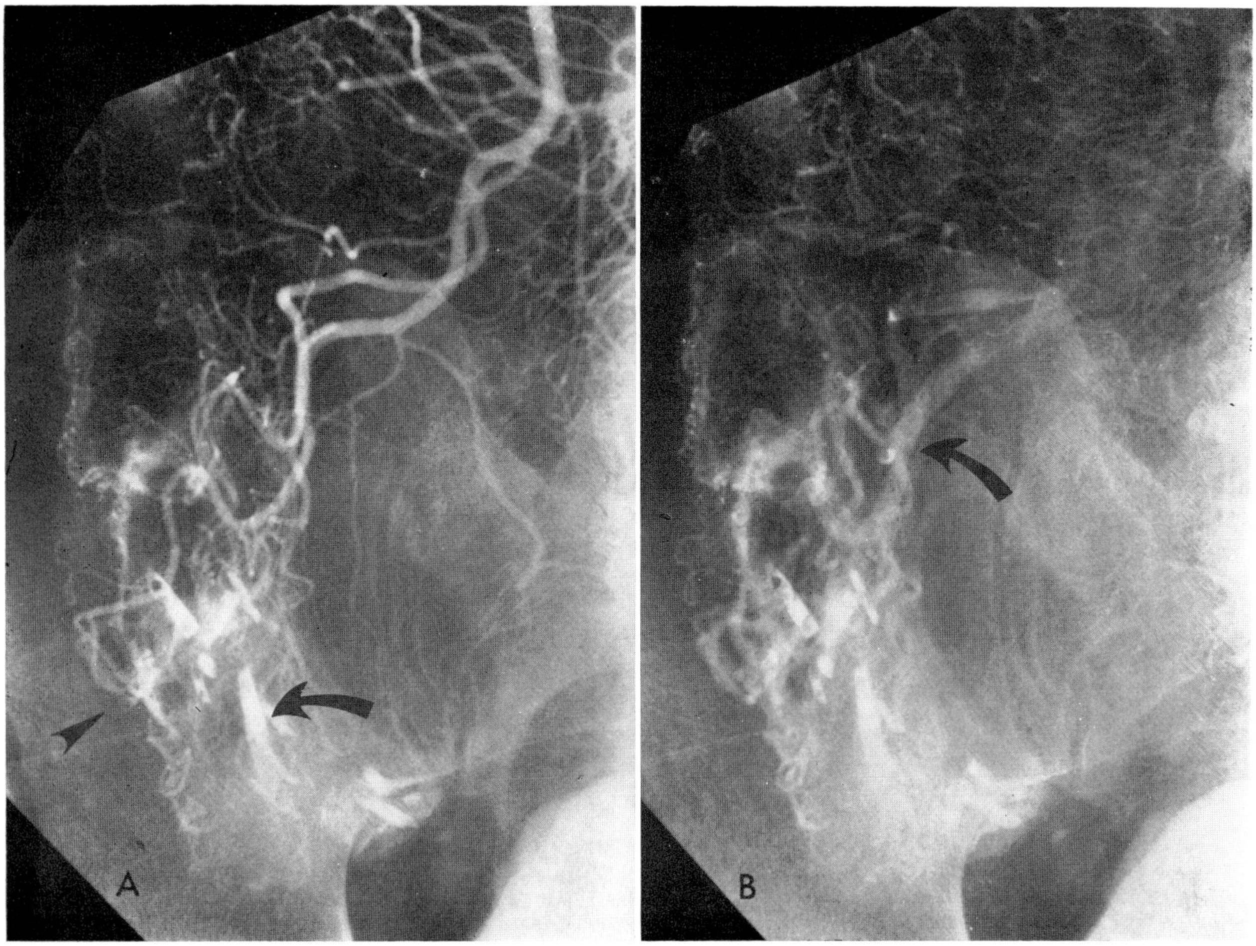

Figure 27.23. Superior Mesenteric Arteriogram. (A) Early phase reveals prominent vessels in the vicinity of cecum (Arrow Head). Retained barium is also noted in the cecum (Arrow). (B) Late arterial phase reveals premature opacification of veins from that segment of the colon (Arrow) in a patient who was a chronic gastrointestinal bleeder. *Diagnosis:* Dysplastic (telangiectatic) vessels. *Pathology:* Angiodysplasia. (Courtesy of Dr. J. Petasnick, Associate Professor, Diagnostic Radiology, Rush Presbyterian-St. Luke Medical Center, Chicago.)

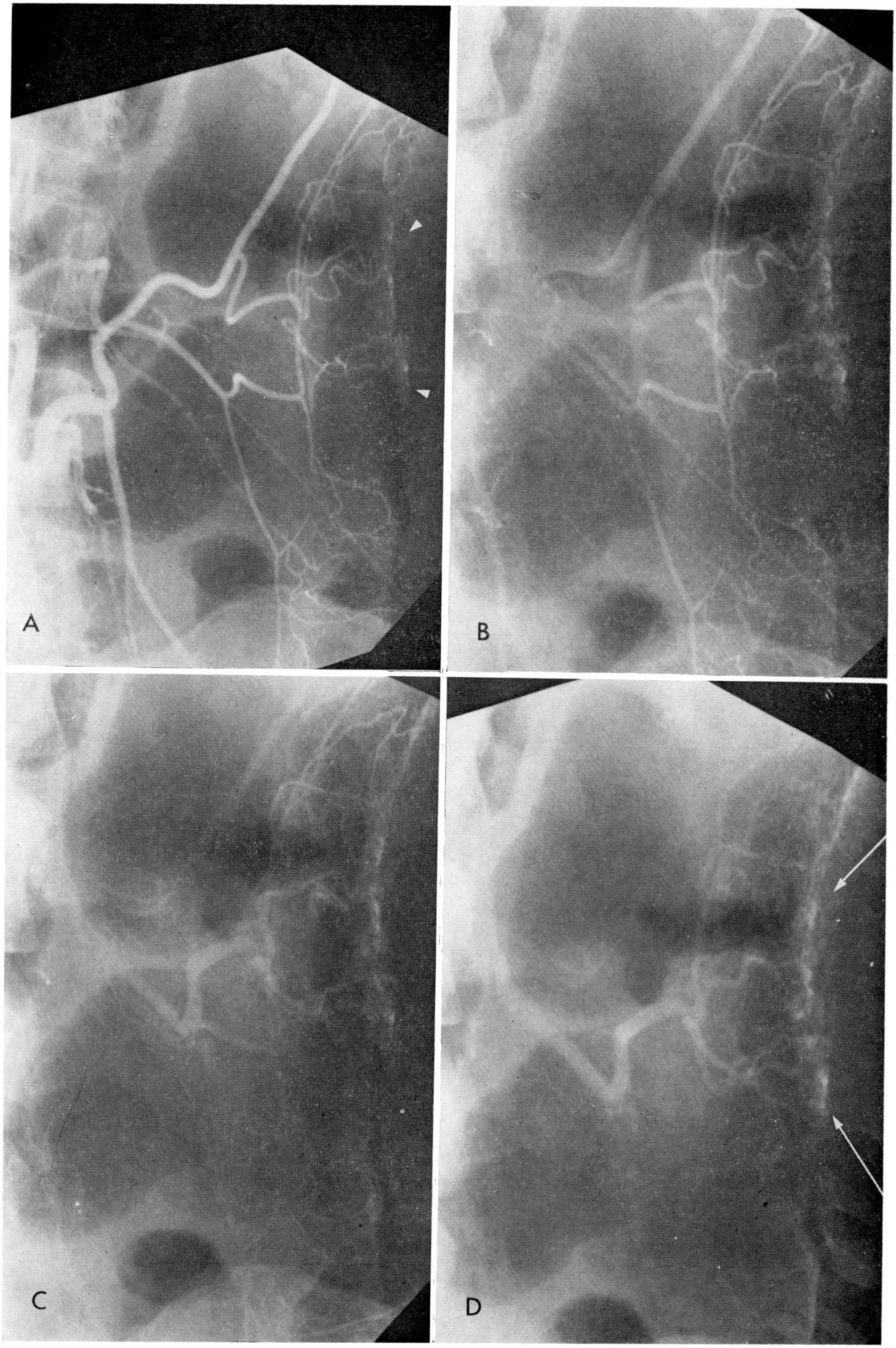
A
B
C
D

arteriovenous fistulae are less significant hemodynamically than aortocaval or aortopulmonary fistulae.

The *anatomical components* of an arteriovenous fistula are the proximal artery and vein and the distal artery and vein. Blood at systemic pressure is shunted totally or partially into the vein. In the distal artery, the blood flow may be away from or toward the fistula depending on its size, adequacy of collaterals, and peripheral resistance. Retrograde flow in the veins occurs after the valves become incompetent due to venous dilatation.[746] Initially, the resistance from venous valves favors segmental dilatation of the veins.[747] The *internal jugular vein* does not dilate in spite of an arteriovenous shunt, as the vein is blessed with a negative pressure.[779] Different names have been given to these arteriovenous communications, depending on the absence or presence of an interposed sac between the communication.[748]

ETIOLOGY OF ABNORMAL ARTERIOVENOUS COMMUNICATION

Congenital arteriovenous communications usually produce little change in the cardiac work because multiple, small, tortuous communications diminish the peripheral resistance[652] minimally. They can occur wherever blood vessels exist. When they are in the extremities, varices of the veins of that extremity[746] and hypertrophy of the soft tissues can occur.

Penetrating or blunt *trauma* is probably the leading cause of arteriovenous fistula. This also includes iatrogenic trauma during surgical or diagnostic procedures, such as biopsy or catheterization.[749] Other causes of arteriovenous fistula include blunt trauma causing hepatic artery and portal vein communication,[750] childbirth causing internal iliac artery and vein communication,[751] following thoracotomy with intercostal artery to pulmonary vein communication,[752] and human bites.[753] They may occur following the use of a Fogerty catheter for thrombectomy,[754] subtotal hysterectomy,[755] and last but not least, priapism may be due to internal

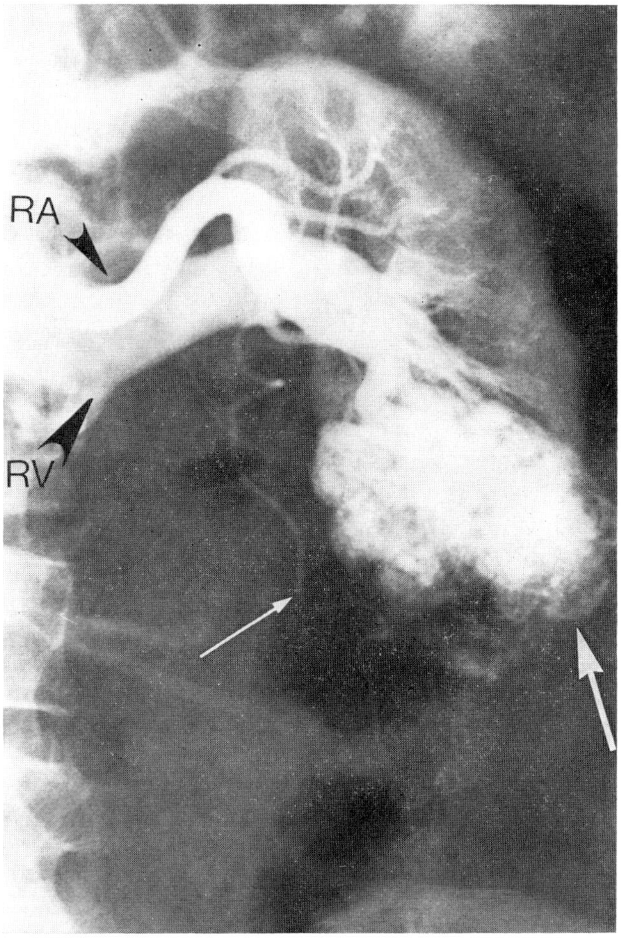

Figure 27.25. Renal Arteriogram. There is a hypertrophied left renal artery with intense staining of an irregular lobulated mass in the lower pole (Large Arrow). A very prominent capsular artery courses toward the inferior aspect of this mass with irregular termination (Small Arrow). Simultaneous opacification of the huge left renal vein occurs (R.V.). *Diagnosis:* Hypernephroma probably rupturing through the renal capsule with parasitic supply from the capsular artery. At the same time marked A.V. shunting is demonstrated.

←

Figure 27.24. Inferior Mesenteric Arteriogram. (A) Early phase reveals a localized area of hypervascularity in the wall of the colon. (B & C) Late arterial phase reveals the increased staining of the wall of the bowel at that level as well as early venous opacification. (D) Venous phase of the same. *Diagnosis:* Early arteriovenous shunting from a diseased segment of the bowel. *Pathology:* Localized area of granulomatous colitis. (Courtesy of Dr. J. Petasnick, Associate Professor, Diagnostic Radiology, Rush Presbyterian-St. Luke Medical Center, Chicago.)

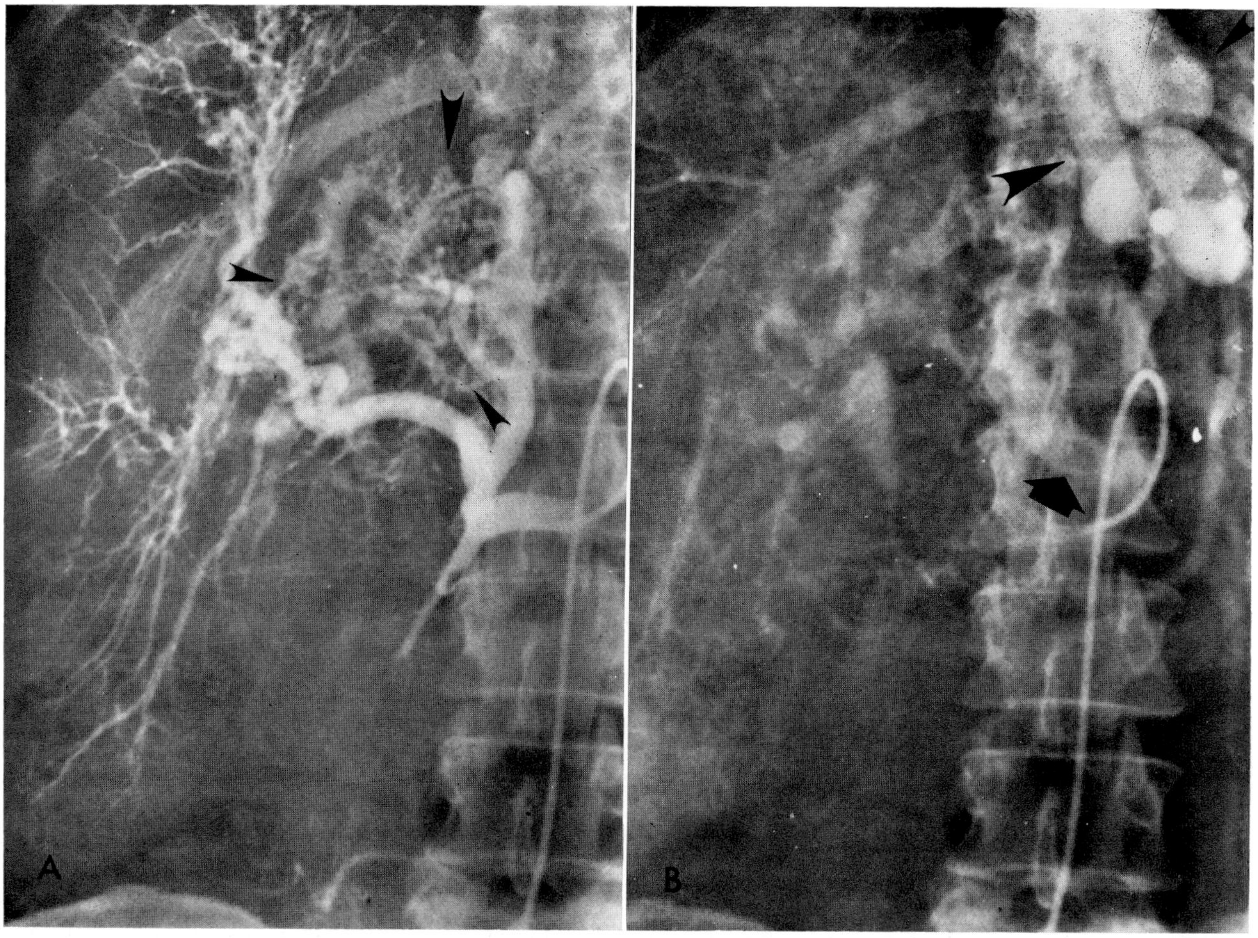

Figure 27.26. Hepatic Arteriogram. (A) Arterial phase: There is hypervascularity with vessels of irregular caliber, which lack tapering (Arrow Head). (B) Late arterial phase: There is early opacification of the dilated tortuous veins which course toward the esophagus (Arrow Head). This fills via abnormal prematurely opacifying portal vein (Arrow). The patient had esophageal varices clinically. *Diagnosis:* Hepatoma with malignant arteriovenous communication causing esophageal varices. *Note:* Normally, during a selective hepatic arteriogram, the portal vein does not visualize.

pudendal artery communication with the corpora cavernosa.[756]

Spontaneous arteriovenous communication may occur if there is a predisposing factor such as aneurysm[759, 760] or a neoplastic process eroding into an adjacent vein. Spontaneous arteriovenous fistula of the great vessels, aorta, and inferior vena cava cause greater hemodynamic change (high output cardiac failure, hypotension) and more severe clinical manifestations (anuria, back pain, shock) compared to traumatic arteriovenous fistula in the same vicinity.[757, 758] Primary or secondary *malignant neoplasms* with their luxurious, chaotic, structureless vessels have all the rights to develop abnormal arteriovenous communications at varying levels in that vascular circuit. Some unusual ones include pulmonary metastatic neoplasms from a thyroid carcinoma,[761] choriocarcinoma[762] causing pulmonary arteriovenous fistula, or malignant mesenchymoma causing an aorta-caval fistula.[763]

Some arteriovenous fistulae are of special clinical interest because of the associated specific manifestations they cause.

Renal arteriovenous fistula[652, 764] may cause both systolic and diastolic hypertension and increased cardiac output. Due to shunting of blood, hematuria as well as incomplete infarction of the renal parenchyma, may develop. Renal pedicle arteriovenous fistula following nephrectomy cannot cause diastolic hypertension by itself. There is a high incidence of renal arteriovenous fistula following biopsy,[765, 766] espe-

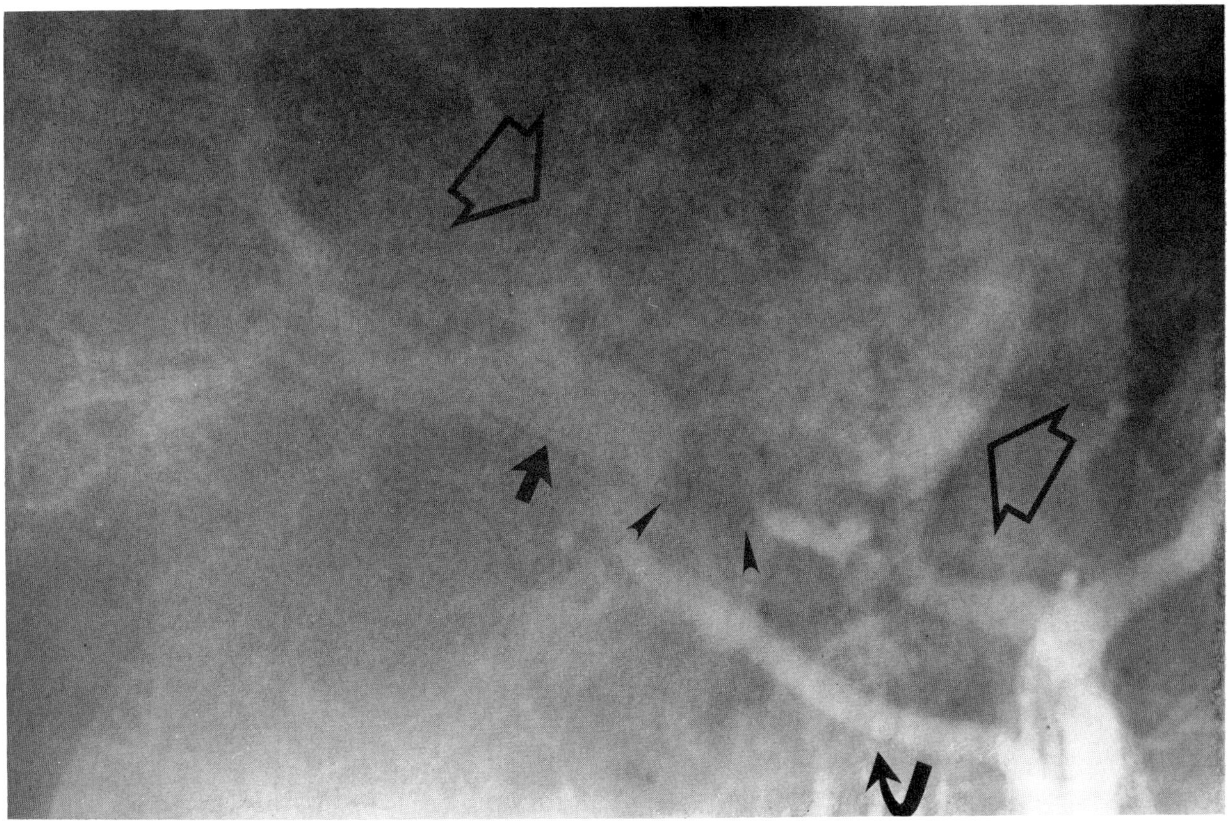

Figure 27.27. Simultaneous Celiac and Superior Mesenteric Angiograms. There is amorphous collection of contrast material and channels of irregular caliber (Blank Arrow). Simultaneous opacification of the portal vein radicals (Arrow) occur. There is a filling defect in the venous trunk (Arrow Head). *Diagnosis:* Hepatoma with malignant arteriovenous communications and a tumor thrombus in the portal vein. *Note:* Replaced hepatic coming from the superior mesenteric artery (Curved Arrow).

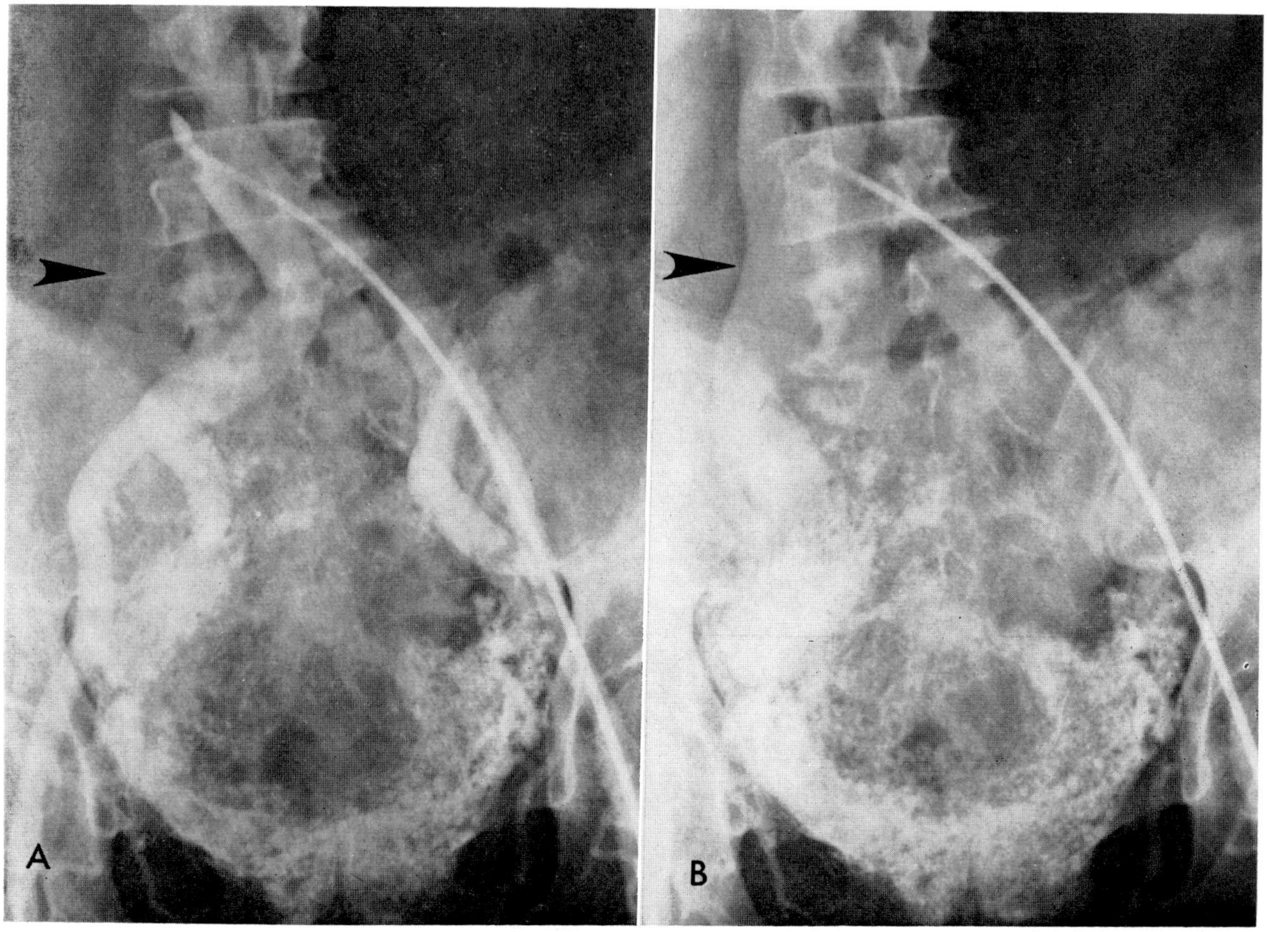

Figure 27.28. Pelvic Arteriogram. (A) Arterial phase: Markedly dilated internal iliac arteries supply sheets of abnormal vasculature in the true pelvis. (B) Late arterial phase: The tremendously hypervascular sheets of abnormal vessels simultaneously opacify the inferior vena cava (Arrow). *Diagnosis:* Malignant tumor of the true pelvis probably arising from the uterus with A.V. shunting. *Pathology:* Hemangioendotheliosarcoma of the uterus.

cially in the presence of nephrosclerosis or hypertension. The chances of arteriovenous communication are higher if the biopsy is taken from the renal medulla, rather than from the renal cortex. Seventy percent of these abnormal communications closes spontaneously.[767]

Arteriovenous Fistula of the Portal Circulation

Because of the interposition of the hepatic venous reservoir between the fistula and the heart, these fistulae[652, 768] rarely lead to cardiac overload.[769, 770] Instead they cause portal hypertension and ascites.[771, 772]

Gastrointestinal Tract Arteriovenous Fistula

These may be the cause of gastrointestinal bleeding either as vascular ectasia with early venous shunting or as large malformations or as only a "blush," or early venous opacification.[773–775] Telangiectasia does not spare the gastrointestinal tract vasculature; one of its representations may be an arteriovenous malformation[683] (Figs. 27-22 to 27-24).

Pulmonary arteriovenous fistula[412] may be associated with hereditary hemorrhagic telangiectasia. They tend to cause cyanosis, because of shunting of blood before it reaches the pul-

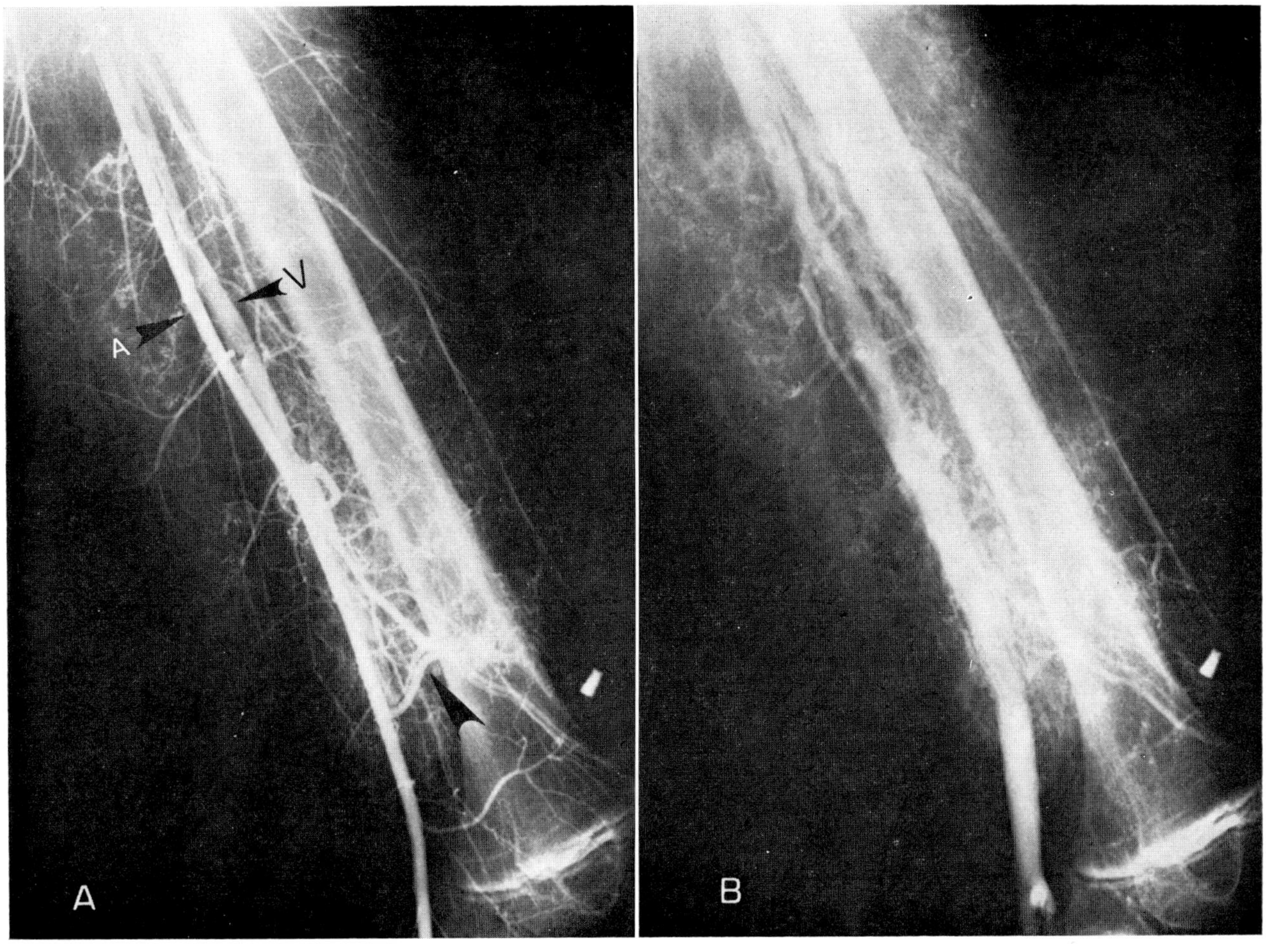

Figure 27.29. Femoral Arteriogram. (A) Arterial phase: Demonstrates diffuse abnormal vessels in the distal thigh with corkscrew appearance. At the same time please note that early dense opacification of the vein (V). (B) Venous phase reveals the extent of this infiltrating process and further opacification of the vein in a 12-year-old girl. *Diagnosis:* Hemangiona. *Pathology:* Diffusely infiltrating skeletal muscle hemangioma.

monary parenchyma.[776, 777] Of particular interest is the association of pulmonary arteriovenous fistula and cirrhosis of the liver.[778] The patient may not be fascinated, but at least the hepatologist, chest physician, and angiographer will find it interesting.

CHAPTER 28
FILLING DEFECTS

FILLING DEFECTS in organs:

1. Cystic masses
   a. Serous cysts
   b. Abscesses
   c. Hematomas
   d. Neoplastic
   e. Parasitic
2. Infarcts
3. Malignant or benign neoplasms
4. Infiltrative disorders
5. Dilatation of normal structures
6. Variation in blood supply
7. Transient

CYSTIC MASSES

The contents of a cystic mass depend on the histologic nature of the lesion. The contents may be serous fluid seen in simple benign cysts, pus as in abscesses, blood found in hematomas or necrotic tumors, exudates seen in cystadenomas, or clear fluid found in parasitic cysts.

The *cyst wall* is actually a reflection of the contents of the cyst. In a *benign cyst* there is a single layer of cells enclosed by a fibrous sac. *Abscesses* have pyogenic membranes with vascular granulation tisse. *Hematomas* have vascular organizing granulation tissue. *Neoplastic* cysts are composed of tumor tissue; and the walls of parasitic cysts have a germinal layer, an elastic layer, and reactive host tissue. The *walls of benign simple cysts* are thin and uniform because the lining cells are not excessively active metabolically. Thus, increased vasculature is not present in this wall. Only in exceptional circumstances, such as an adrenal cyst, the wall may be uniformly thick. The *walls of hematomas* and *abscesses* are of variable thickness depending on the duration and metabolic activity of the wall. This in turn is reflected by the presence of vascular granulation tissue. The *walls* of *neoplastic tissues* are hypervascular, irregular, and of variable thickness due to a metabolically active peripheral rind of viable neoplastic cells. The thickness of the *wall of a parasitic cyst* depends on the biological activity of the cyst and the host's response in that vicinity. The usual angiographic situation in a biologically active parasitic cyst is excellent demonstration of a hyperstaining cyst wall.

A *simple cyst* is usually demarcated against the juxtaposed well-stained parenchyma as a homogeneously lucent mass with a uniform, very thin wall. Because of the expansile nature of the mass, it provides itself with a very sharp interface from the adjacent well-stained parenchyma (Figs. 28-1 to 28-14). If the thin wall of a simple renal cyst acquires any irregularity, thickness, or undue pericystic vascularity, a comparatively higher metabolic rate is suggested. This may be due to infection, hematoma, or a tumor complicating that simple benign cyst (Figs. 28-16, 28-17, and 36-42). *Abscesses,* whether localized *de novo* or an inflamed cyst, develop an active wall composed of granulation tissue. This gives rise to a uniformly thin or thick irregular wall encircling the lucent, tense, expansile mass (Figs. 28-16 and 28-17). The diagnosis of hematoma is made with a history of previous injury. The *hematoma* develops into a tense, expansile, cystic cavity lined by a wall of variable thickness depending on the duration of the hematoma. The wall is hypervascular because of organization of the blood clot and formation of granulation tissue, giving rise to a well-stained regular or irregular wall varying in thickness (Figs. 28-19 and 28-24).

Neoplastic cysts may be due to the original

cystic nature of the tumor with variable proportions of cystic to solid structures (cystadenomas, benign or malignant) or due to central necrosis of a solid tumor or due to a tumor arising in the wall of a simple cyst. The wall of such a cystic mass is obviously irregular, thick and hypervascular due to the presence of metabolically active structures. It is also expansile and tense with a sharp interface with the adjacent parenchyma of a compact organ due to constant bleeding, necrosis or exudation into the cystic cavity with subsequent stretching of the wall (Figs. 28-14, 28-20, 28-21, 28-22, 28-26, 28-27, 36-18, 36-34, 36-35, 36-36, 36-41, 36-42, and 36-63).

Parasitic Cysts (Hydatid)

Tense, expansile, cystic lesions give rise to a well-stained wall of variable thickness.[1105–1108] This wall may represent the reactive tissue of the host varying in thickness from 0.5 mm to 4.0 mm (Fig. 28-18).

Pancreatic Cystic Lesions

These lesions[1092, 1093] include pseudocysts, retention cysts, congenital cysts, traumatic cysts, inflammatory cysts, and neoplastic cysts. The ultimate position and relation[1094] of a *pancreatic pseudocyst* lined by an adventitial wall is influenced by the point of origin of the cyst within the gland, the associated peritoneal reflections, and the arrangement of the underlying viscera (Figs. 28-8, 29-13 and 34-12). They can be located behind the stomach and transverse colon, between the stomach and liver, behind or below the transverse colon, or at the fundus of the stomach. Usually thin walled, they have a great tendency to erode into the adjacent vessels, depending on their location (Fig. 26-39). Thus the splenic, gastroduodenal[1095] arteries, or portal vein[1096] may be involved. On rare occasions these lesions insinuate themselves into the kidney or spleen[1097] mimicking intrarenal or intrasplenic masses. They can cause thrombosis of the veins they come across. *Ten percent of all pancreatic cysts are neoplastic in nature.* Of these, cystadenomas and/or cystadenocarcinomas are the major types seen. Vascularity of these masses depends on the proportion of the cystic and solid (adenomatous) components of the neoplasms (Fig. 36-18).

Adrenal Cysts

Pseudocysts, cystic adenomas, lymphangiomatous cysts, retention cysts, and on rare occasions, parasitic cysts may all involve the adrenal gland.[1089–1091] The thickness of the wall of a pseudocyst may range from 1 mm to 3.0 cm (Fig. 28-7). Others may vary from 1 mm to 5 mm in thickness.

Renal Cysts

Renal cysts may be solitary or multiple simple cysts, peripelvic or in the renal medulla. The medullary cysts may or may not be associated with hepatic fibrosis. Though the etiology is not clear, solitary cysts[1084] are acquired. The mechanism of their production is tubular obstruction followed by anemic degeneration due to circulatory disturbance with or without repeated hemorrhage into the same area. A renal cyst can be multicystic due to dysplasia. Of course, it can be polycystic, either of the infantile or adult type.[202] Polycystic kidneys may be unilateral[1086] or bilateral, and may be associated with cancers and hamartomas.[1087] Arterial rupture due to elastic tissue defects is not uncommon in patients with polycystic kidneys.[1088]

Peritoneal and Retroperitoneal Cysts

Mesenteric cysts[1098, 1099] are more common than omental, and may be unilocular or multilocular. Bleeding into the cysts, malignancies arising within the cysts, or torsion of the cysts are not uncommon events. Other retroperitoneal cysts are embryonic, traumatic, neoplastic, enterogenous, or teratomatous in nature.

Splenic Cysts

Epithelial true cysts are usually dermoids or epidermoids.[1100] Endothelial true cysts include those of lymphangiomatous,[1102] hemangiomatous, polycystic or serous origins. Parasitic cysts, traumatic pseudocysts, postinfarction cysts, and

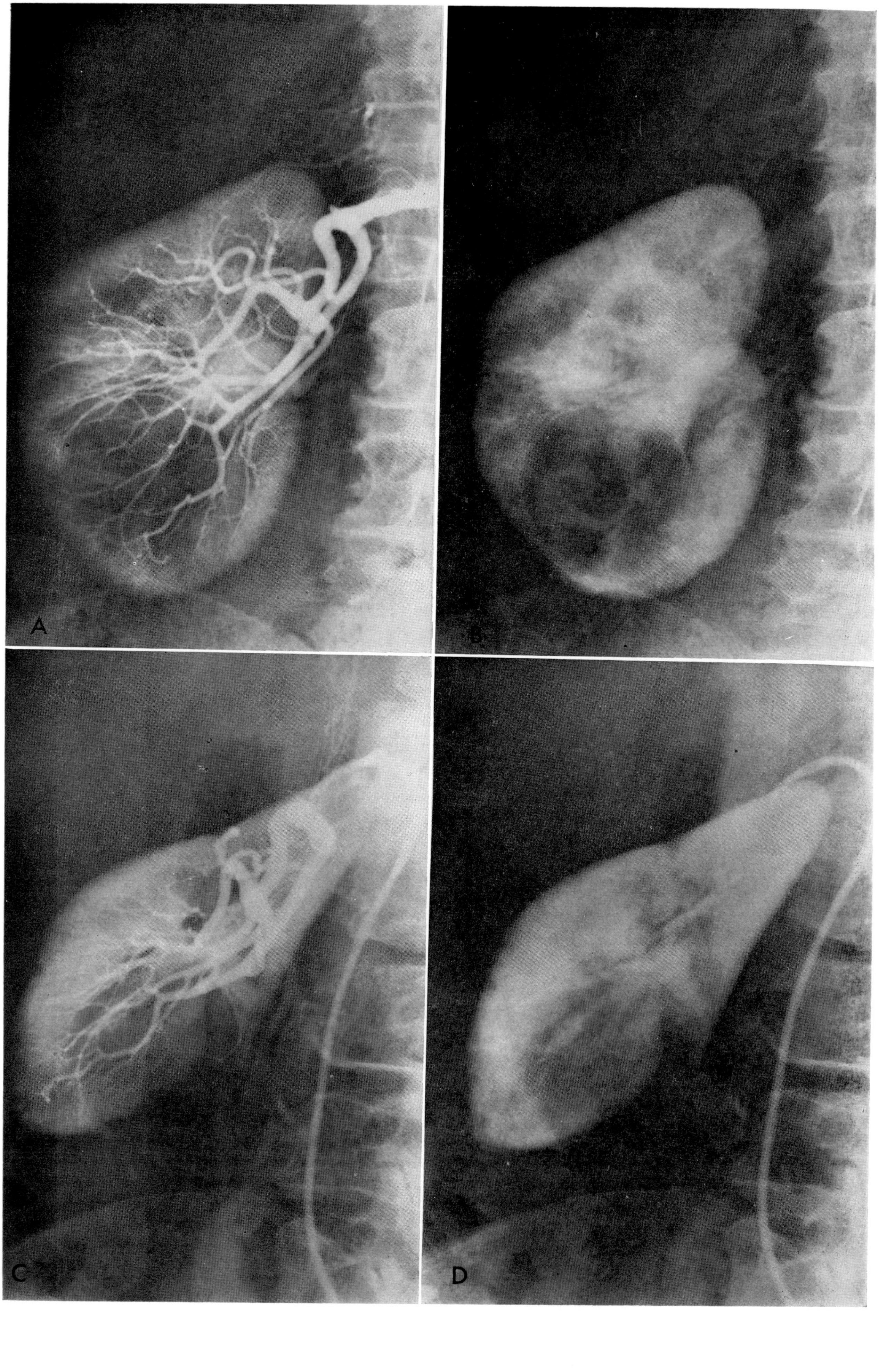
A
B
C
D

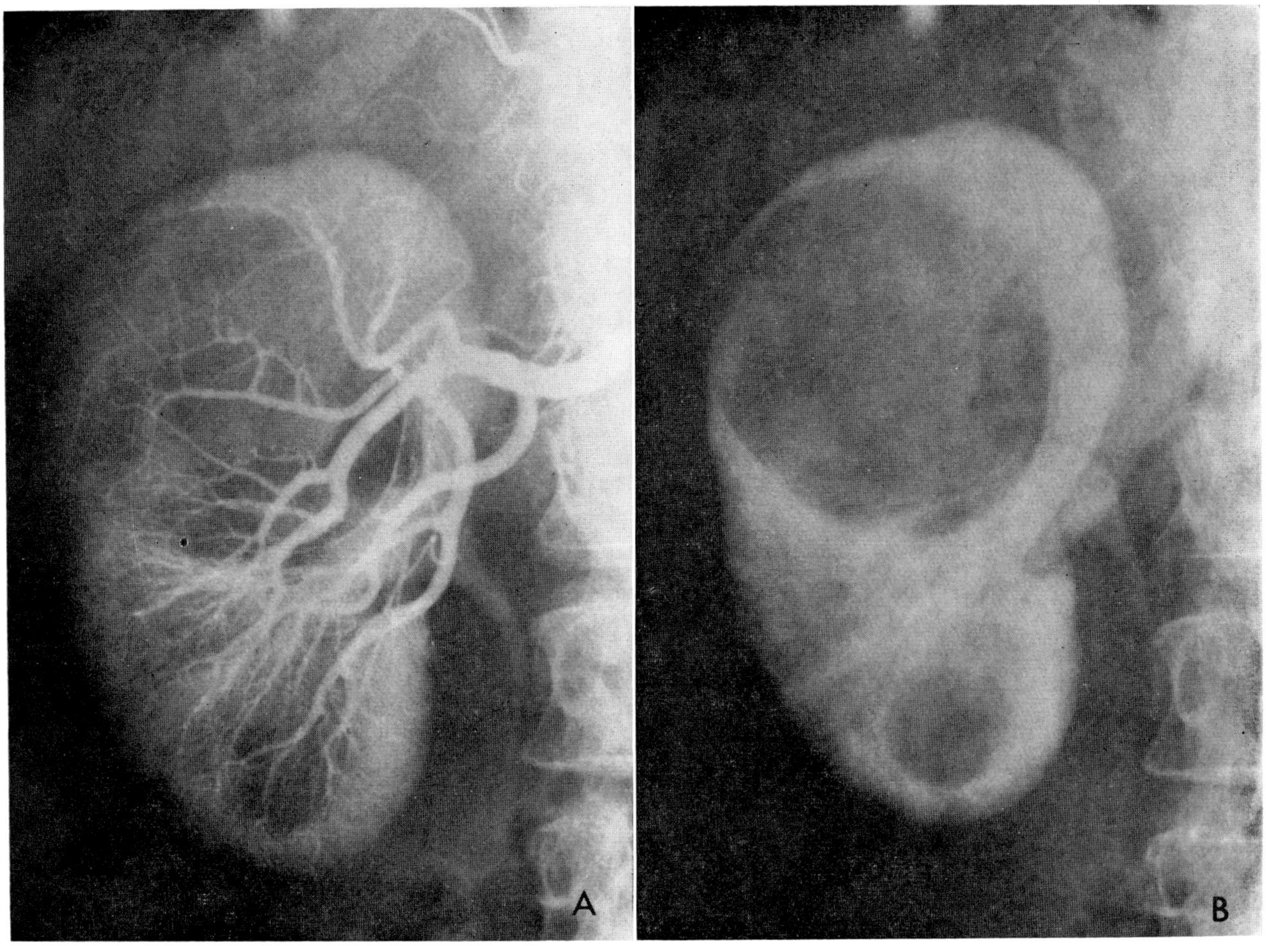

Figure 28.2. Renal Arteriogram. (A) There is stretching and deviation of the intrarenal branches in the proximal portion of the kidney. (B) There are two areas of sharply defined filling defects having a sharp interface with the adjacent parenchyma. *Diagnosis:* Renal cysts.

←

Figure 28.1. Renal Arteriogram. (A) The A.P. projection reveals stretching and deviation of the intrarenal branches around an avascular mass. (B) Reveals a well-defined, circular filling defect outlined by a uniformly thin sharp wall. (C, D) Oblique views of the same. *Diagnosis:* Renal cyst. *Comment:* All the avascular lesions of the kidney should be studied in two projections.

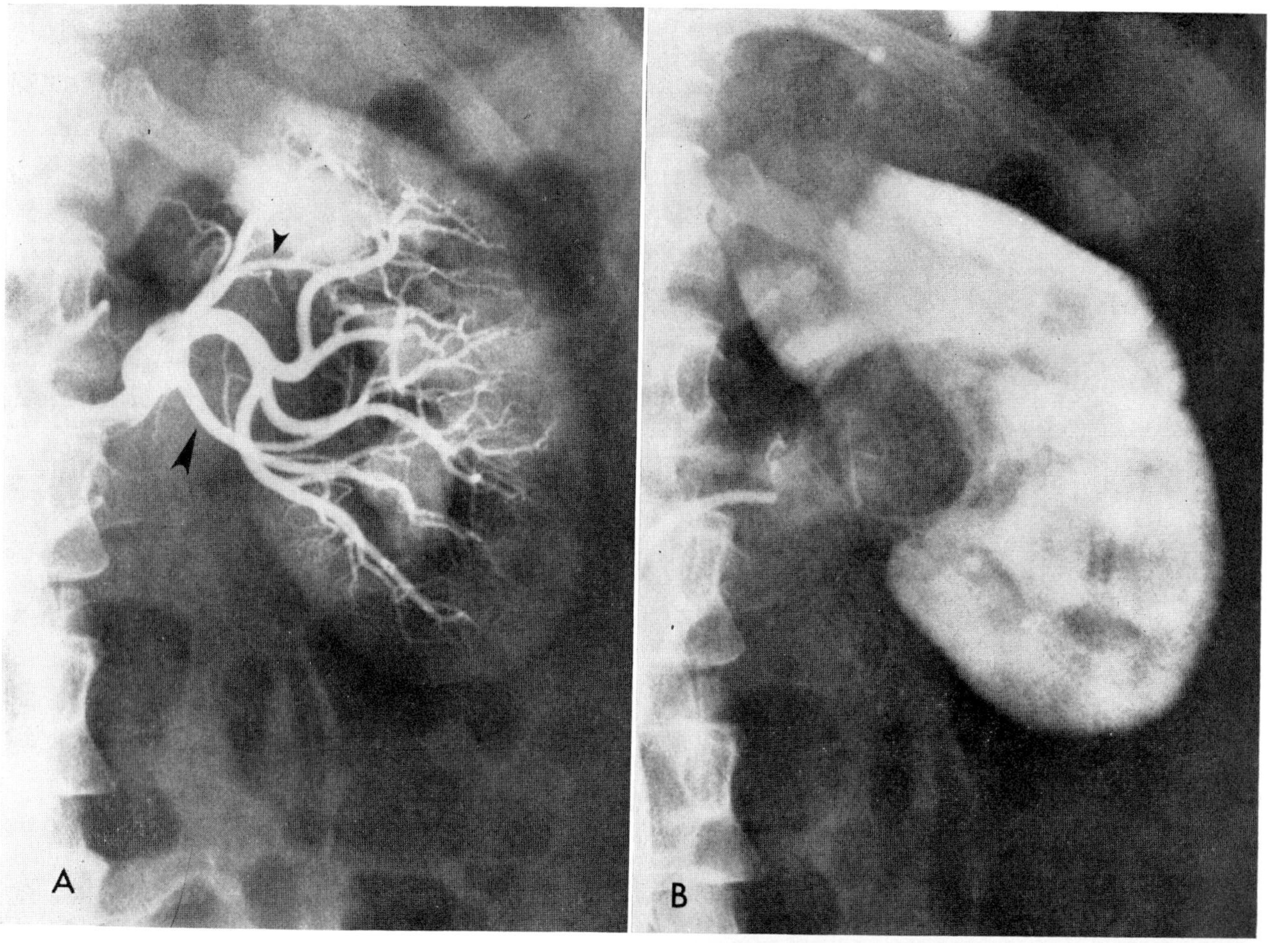

Figure 28.3. Renal Arteriogram. (A) Renal arterial phase: The renal hilar branches are stretched and deviated around an avascular filling defect. The upper pole of the left kidney was perfused by another aberrant artery. (C) An oblique view of the same area reveals the stretching and deviation of the dorsal renal artery better. (B) Renal parenchymal phase: A smooth circular filling defect is in the left renal pelvic area with a sharp interface between the renal parenchyma and the filling defect. *Diagnosis:* Peripelvic cyst.

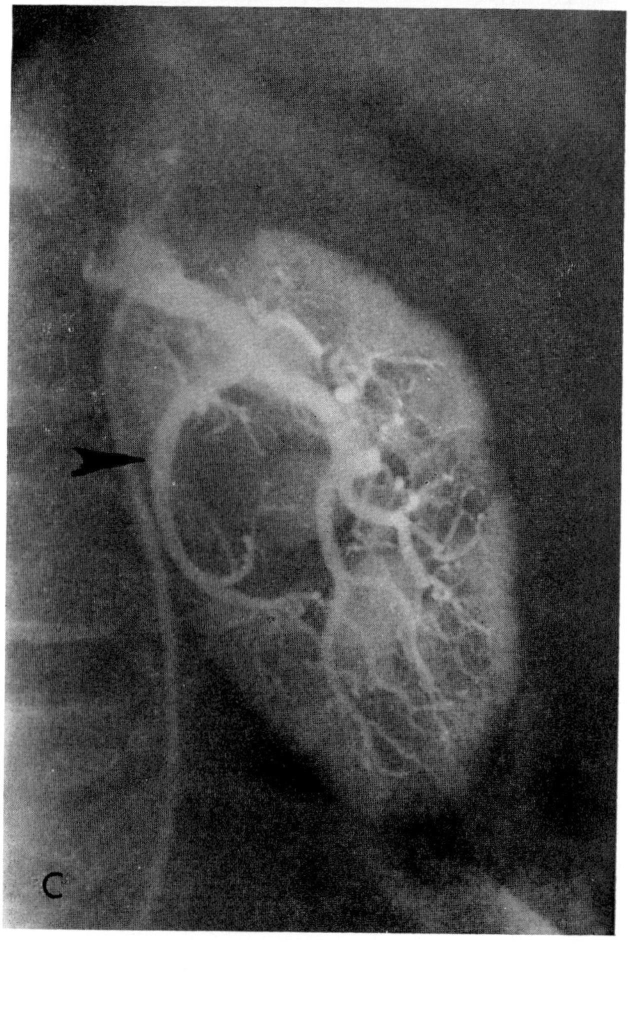

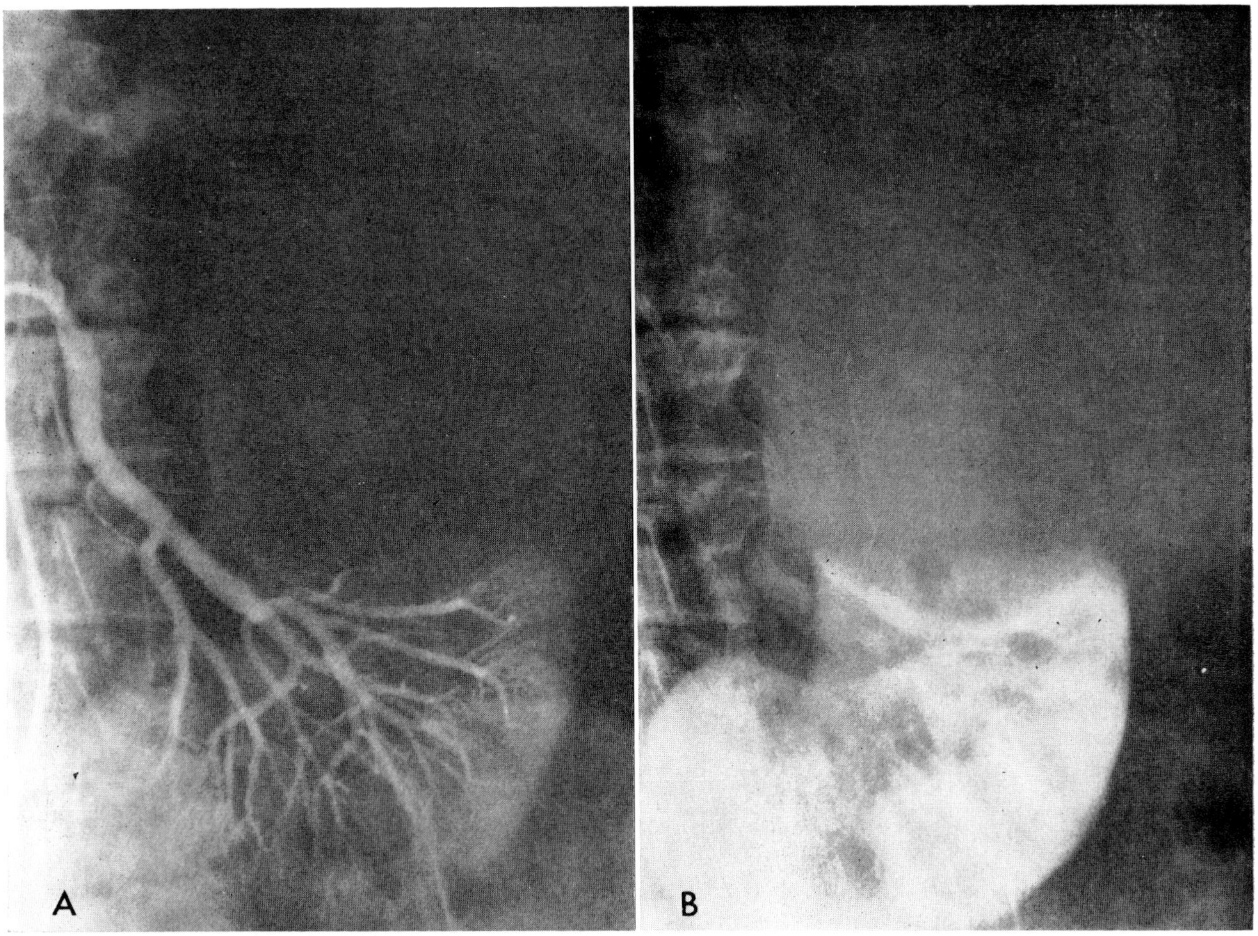

Figure 28.4. (A) Arterial phase: There is marked inferior displacement of the renal parenchyma and pedicle by a huge mass in the left upper pole of the kidney. (B) Parenchymal phase: The same findings are noted with a sharp interface between the mass and the opacified renal parenchyma. *Diagnosis:* A huge avascular mass from the upper pole of the left kidney. *Comment:* It would be very easy to overlook a tumor with such a huge avascular mass as the arterial supply may be from the inaccessible perinephric arteries. Cyst puncture was done and the biochemical findings and cytology pointed towards a benign cyst.

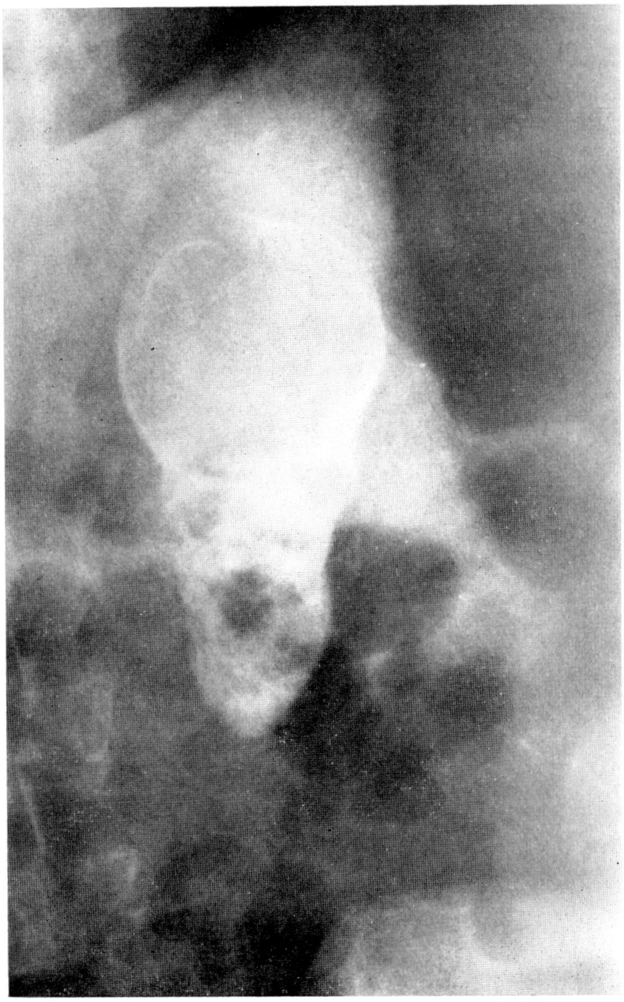

Figure 28.5. Parenchymal Phase of a Renal Arteriogram. A small kidney with multiple, small, circumscribed filling defects is seen with a moderately sized one in the upper pole. It has sharply defined, thinned walls. *Diagnosis:* Dysplastic cystic kidney. No confirmation obtained.

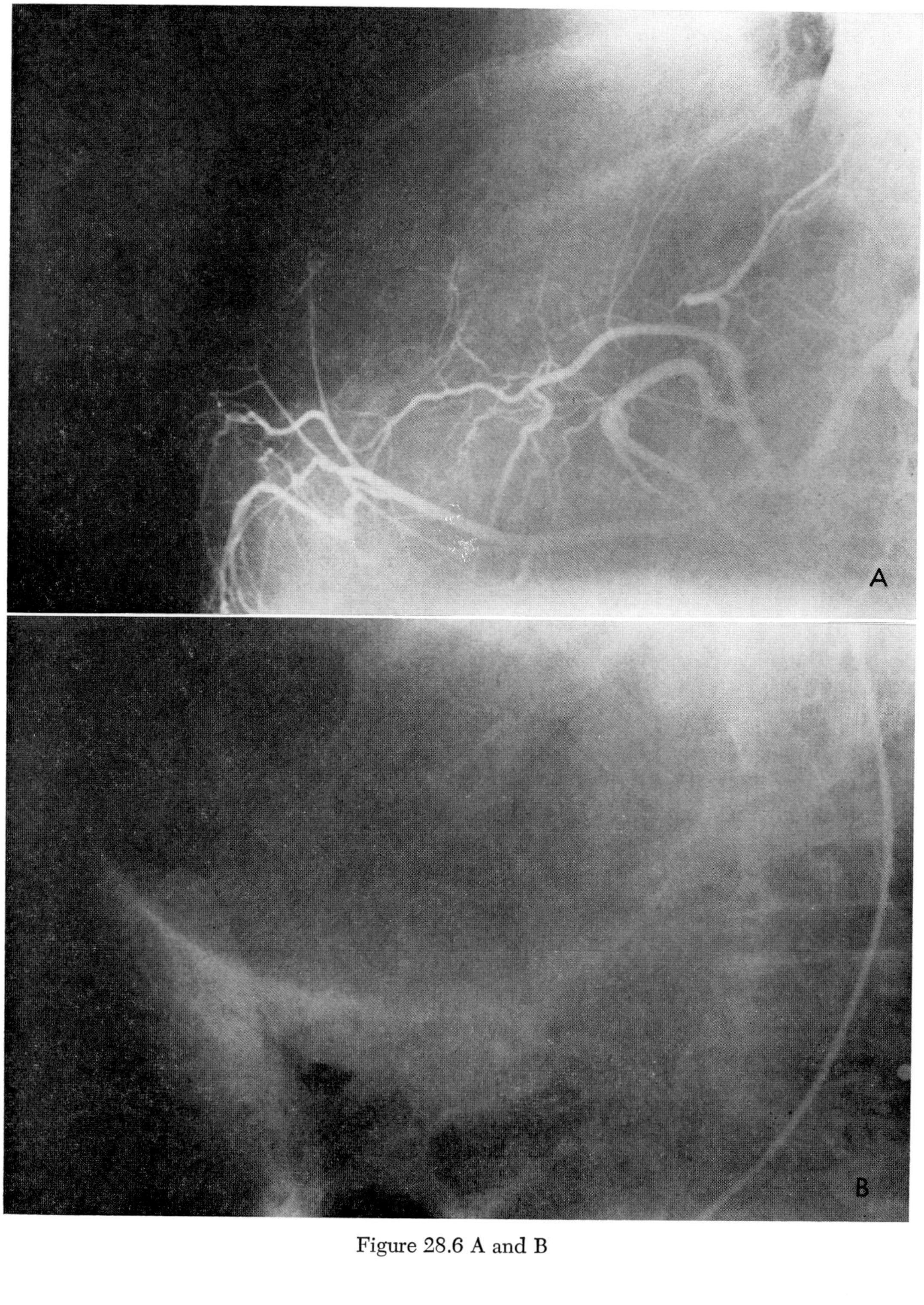

Figure 28.6 A and B

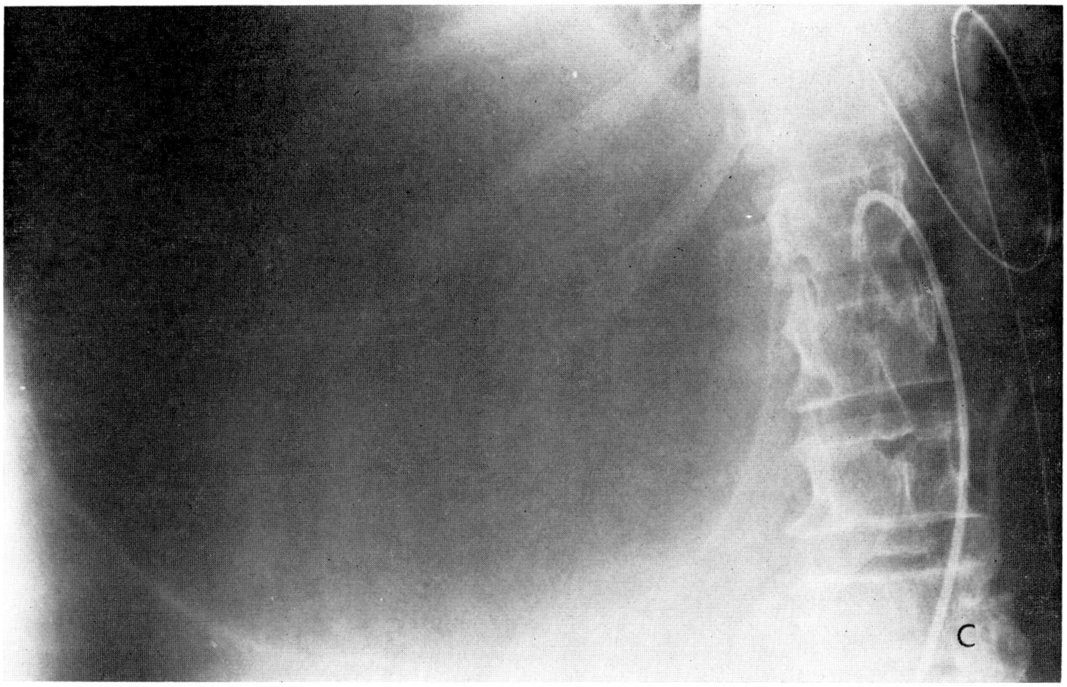

Figure 28.6. Hepatic Arteriogram. (A) Arterial phase: There is caudal displacement of the intrahepatic branches by an avascular mass. (B) and (C) Late phase: A huge avascular mass which has staining of its uniformly thin wall. This fifty-six-year-old patient had mass which was palpable in the right upper quadrant. *Diagnosis:* Congenital hepatic cyst.

neoplastic cysts due to necrotic tumors are also found in the spleen. In any of these, the wall may be either thick or thin.[1101]

Hepatic Cysts

Polycysts,[1103, 1104] either isolated or associated with splenic or renal polycysts, solitary cysts, and retention cysts[1106] are found in the liver. They are usually thin walled. In addition one may find traumatic cysts, biliary cysts,[1072] parasitic cysts, and neoplastic cysts. The last may be cystic hamartomas[1105] and primary or secondary necrotic malignant tumors (Figs. 28-6, 28-20 and 28-22).

INFARCTS

Infarcts[1047] are wedge-shaped zones of ischemic necrosis due to sudden occlusion of an artery or vein. When they are *arterial* infarcts, they are usually *anemic.* Initially, however, they may be hemorrhagic in solid organs due to peripheral anastomotic circulation. In loose tissues such as lung and bowel, they are usually hemorrhagic because of the supply from the bronchial arteries in the lung or anastomotic communications within the bowel vasculature. *Hemorrhagic infarcts* can also occur if emboli fragment and allow blood flow through the large vessels to the infarcted areas. In normal people infarction is uncommon in the lung or liver due to the dual blood supply of these organs. The bronchial and pulmonary arteries supply the lung, while the hepatic artery and portal vein supply the liver. Gradual or partial occlusion of a vein may not cause an infarct. If an organ has a capsule, the subcapsular rim of parenchyma is spared as it receives blood supply from the capsular vessels.[1048] *The angiographically well defined, sharp peripheral filling defect is the clinical counterpart of an anemic infarct. The angiographic intense stain of an ischemic area is the clinical counterpart of a hemorrhagic infarct.*

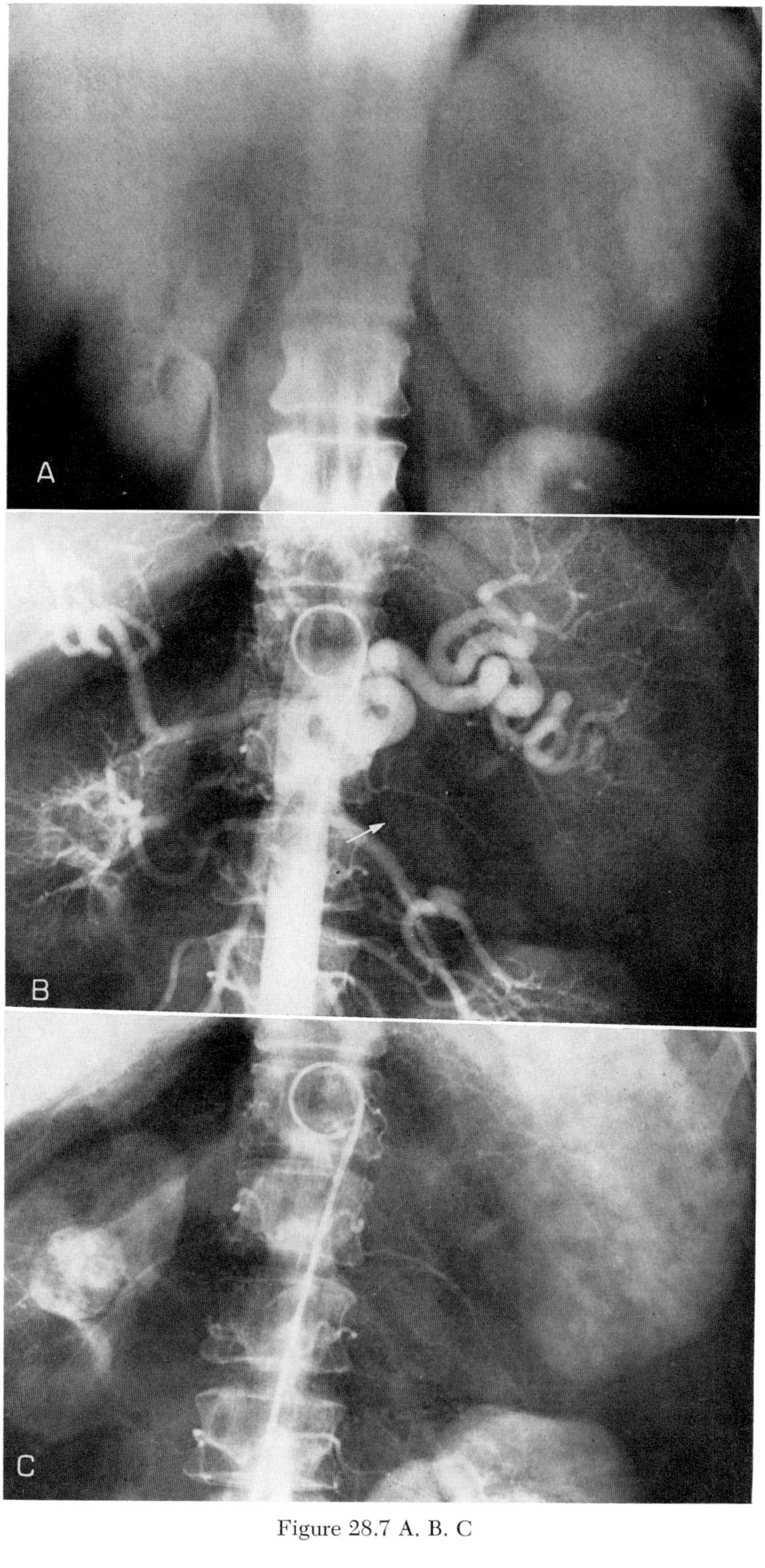

Figure 28.7 A. B. C

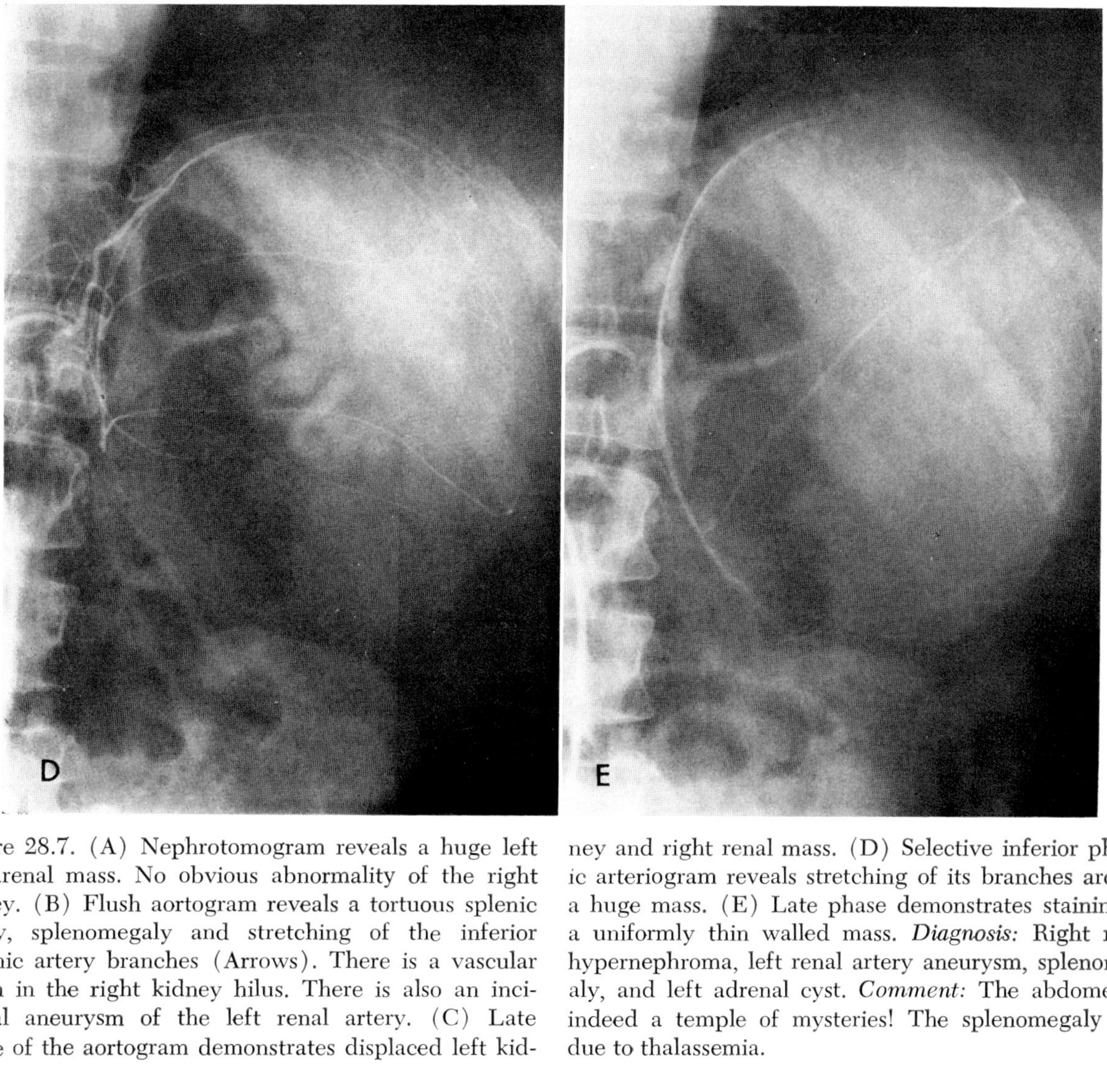

Figure 28.7. (A) Nephrotomogram reveals a huge left suprarenal mass. No obvious abnormality of the right kidney. (B) Flush aortogram reveals a tortuous splenic artery, splenomegaly and stretching of the inferior phrenic artery branches (Arrows). There is a vascular lesion in the right kidney hilus. There is also an incidental aneurysm of the left renal artery. (C) Late phase of the aortogram demonstrates displaced left kidney and right renal mass. (D) Selective inferior phrenic arteriogram reveals stretching of its branches around a huge mass. (E) Late phase demonstrates staining of a uniformly thin walled mass. *Diagnosis:* Right renal hypernephroma, left renal artery aneurysm, splenomegaly, and left adrenal cyst. *Comment:* The abdomen is indeed a temple of mysteries! The splenomegaly was due to thalassemia.

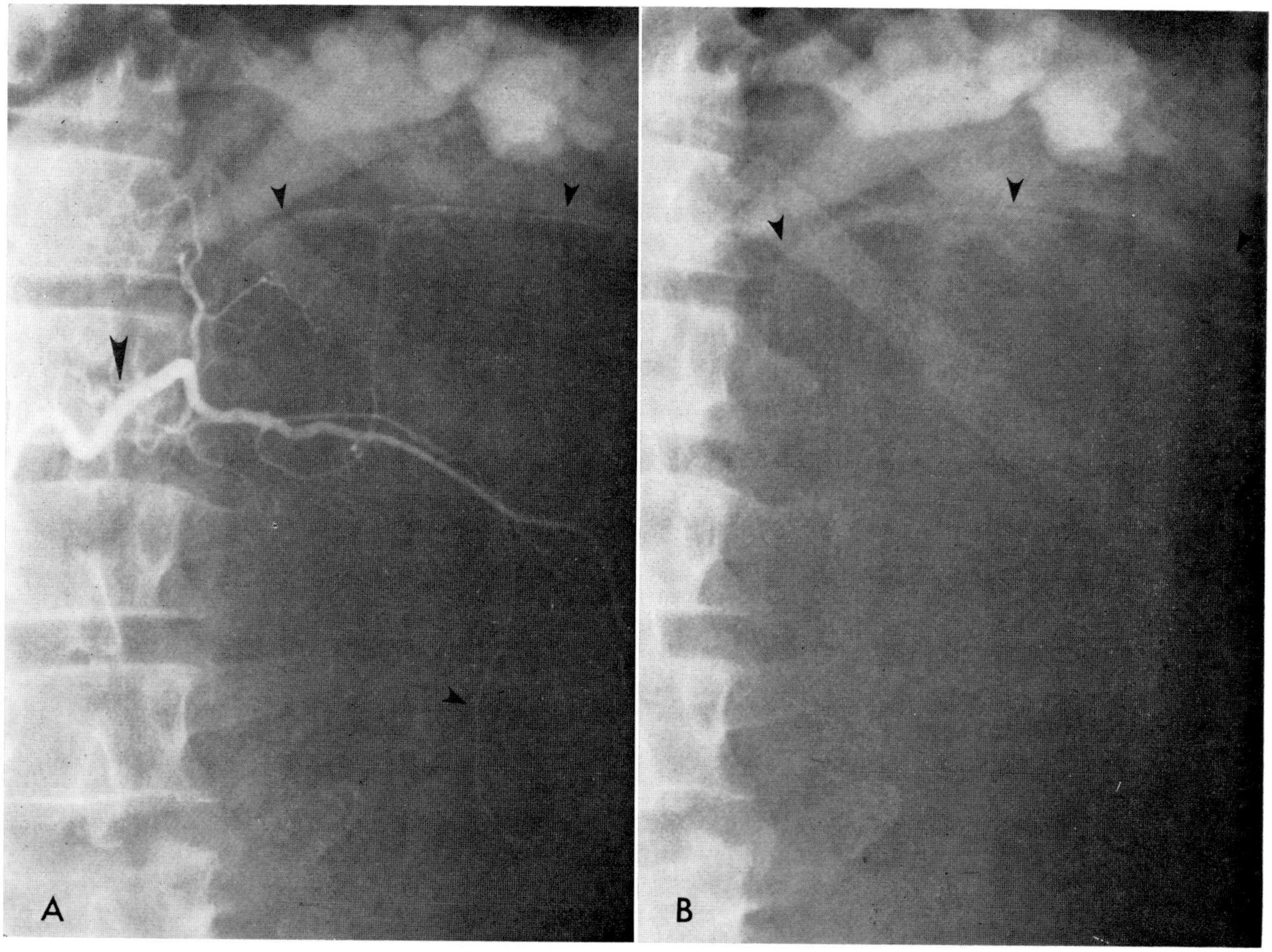

Figure 28.8. Lumbar Arteriogram. (A) Very prominent lumbar artery with normal but prominent branches coursing around a huge mass (Arrow). (B) A lucent mass with uniformly stained thin wall (Arrow) is seen. Notice the cranial displacement of the renal shadow. *Diagnosis:* Retroperitoneal cyst, probably a pancreatic pseudocyst (as the patient was a known alcoholic). *Pathology:* A huge pancreatic pseudocyst with attachment to the psoas muscle.

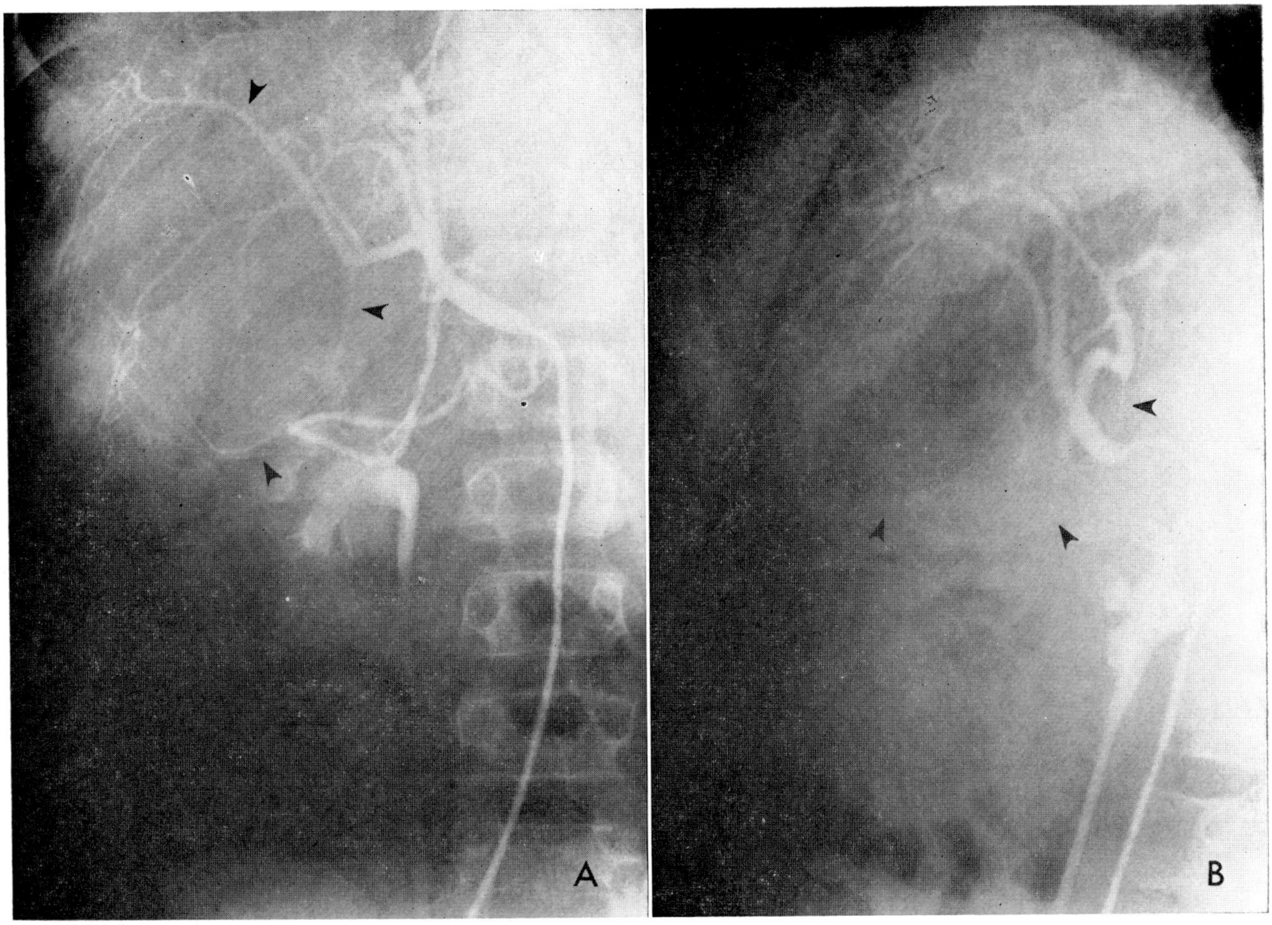

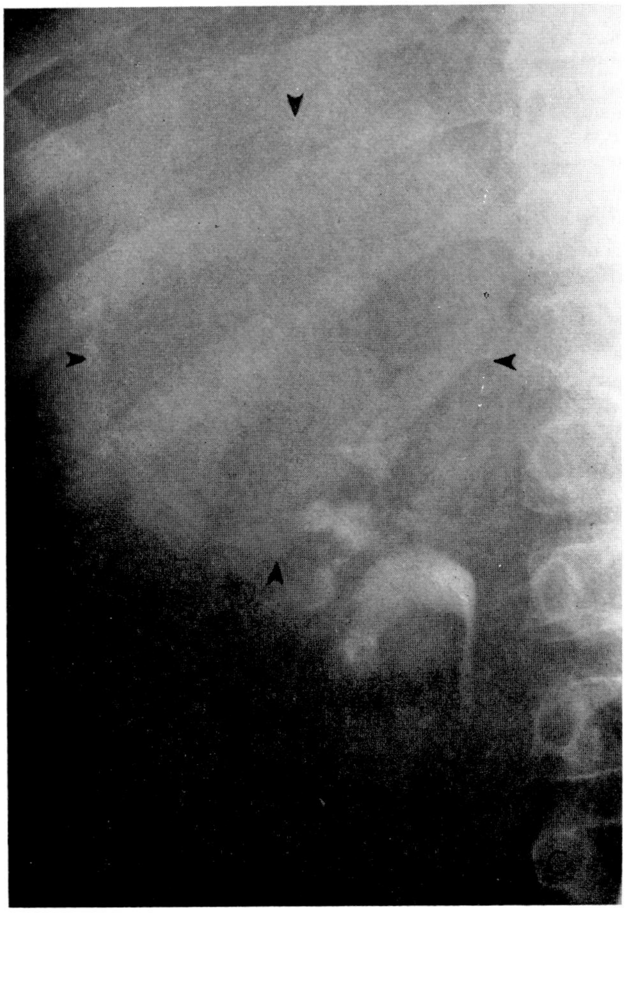

Figure 28.9. (A) Celiac arteriogram reveals stretching and deviation of the intrahepatic branches around a mass in a young individual who had right upper quadrant trauma. (B) Oblique view of the same. (C) A circular filling defect with a very thin wall is seen. *Diagnosis:* Choledochal cyst. *Comment:* This may be mistaken for a hematoma, but the trauma was minimal. *Pathology:* Hepatic duct diverticulum. (Courtesy of Dr. A. Dragomer, Radiologist, Ingalls Memorial Hospital, Harvey, Illinois.)

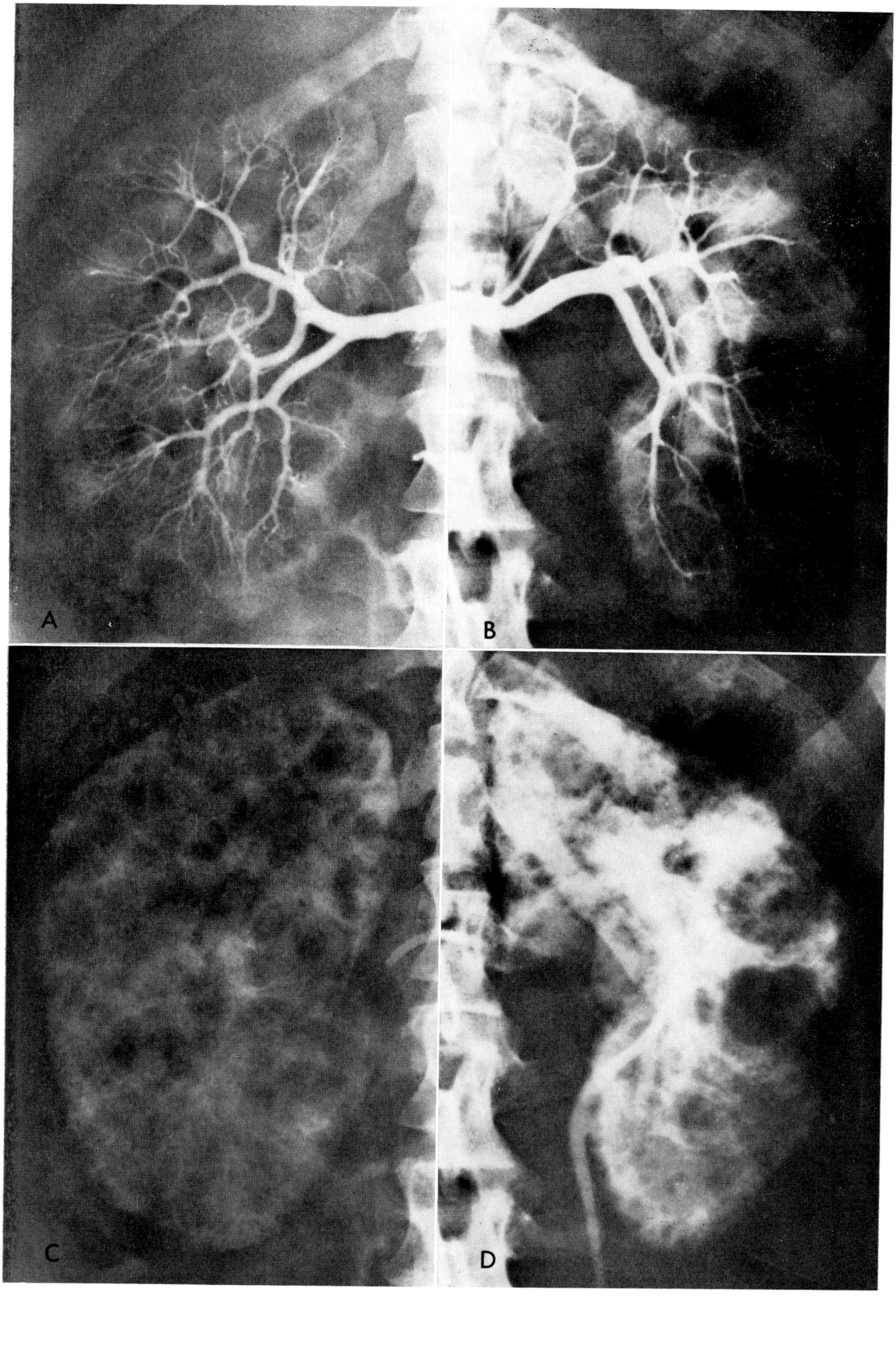
A
B
C
D

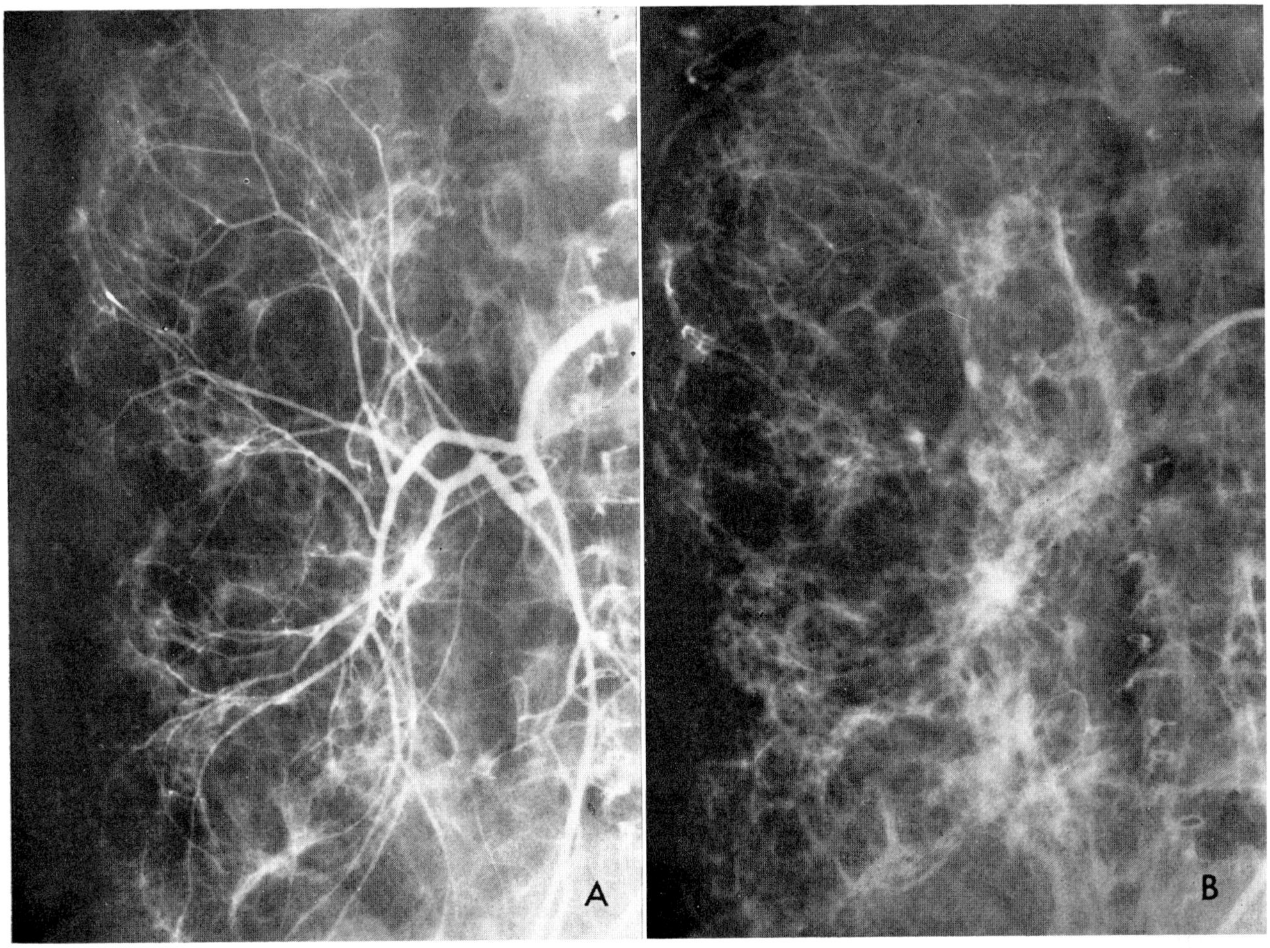

Figure 28.11. Renal Arteriogram. (A) Arterial phase: There is marked increase in the renal size with stretching and deviation of the intrarenal branches. (B) Parenchymal phase: Smooth lucent filling defects with thin walls are seen in the renal parenchyma. No renal parenchyma is discernible. *Diagnosis:* Polycystic kidney with complete compromise of the renal parenchyma by the cysts.

←

Figure 28.10. Renal Arteriogram. (A, B) Arterial phase: Increase in renal size with diffuse stretching and deviation of the intrarenal branches is seen. (C, D) Parenchymal phase: Multiple, well-defined, circular filling defects with thin walls are dispersed irregularly in the renal parenchyma. *Diagnosis:* Polycystic kidneys.

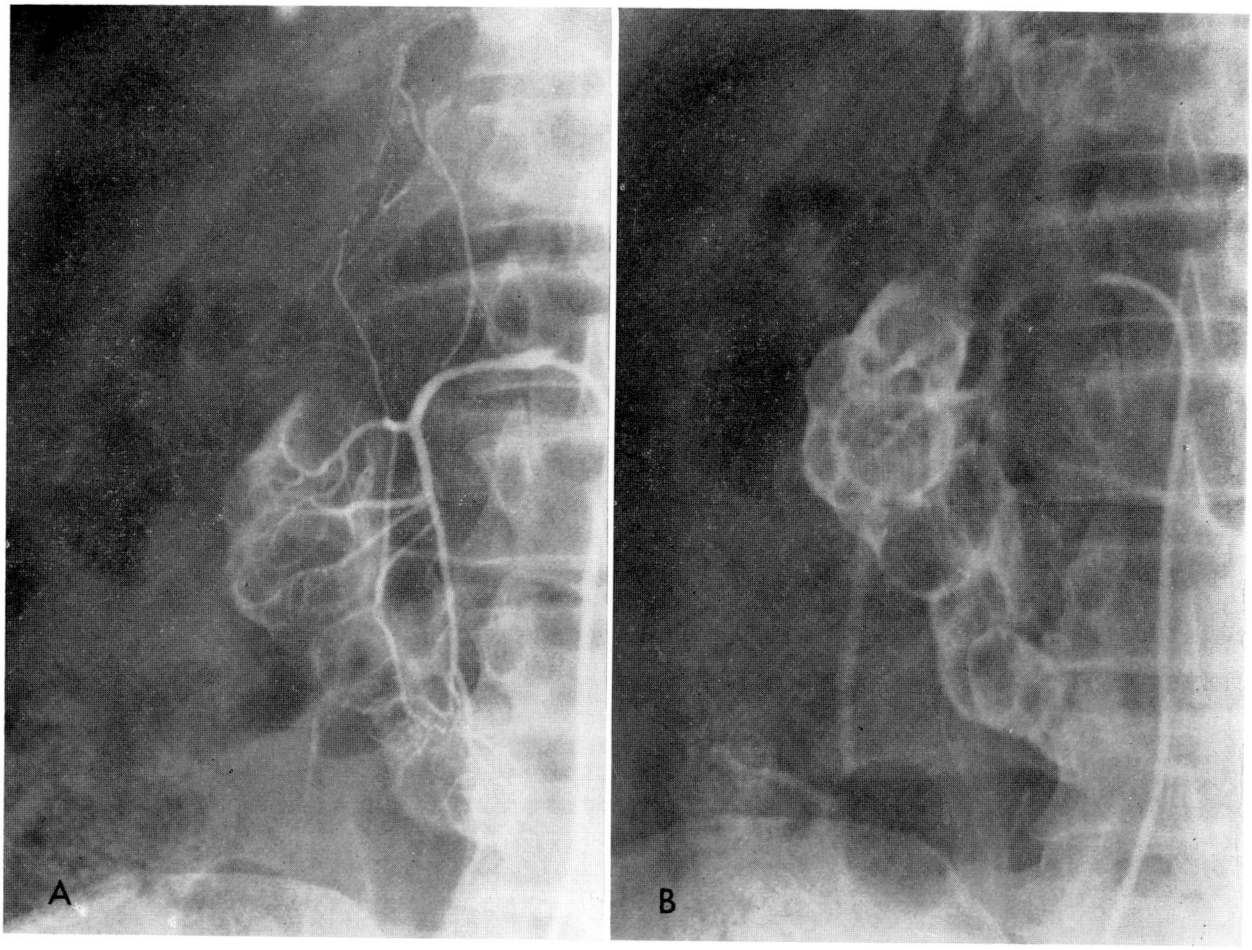

Figure 28.12. Renal Arteriogram. (A) Right renal arteriogram: Thinning of the main renal artery and abnormal arborization of intrarenal vasculature surrounding multiple avascular filling defects is seen in a small kidney. Notice the lower pole of the kidney coursing towards the midline. (B) Parenchymal phase: Multiple, well-circumscribed and sharply delineated avascular filling defects with thin walls replace the entire renal parenchyma. *Diagnosis:* Multicystic kidney. The medial orientation of the lower pole was due to a horseshoe kidney. The other half of the horseshoe was involved with hydronephrosis.

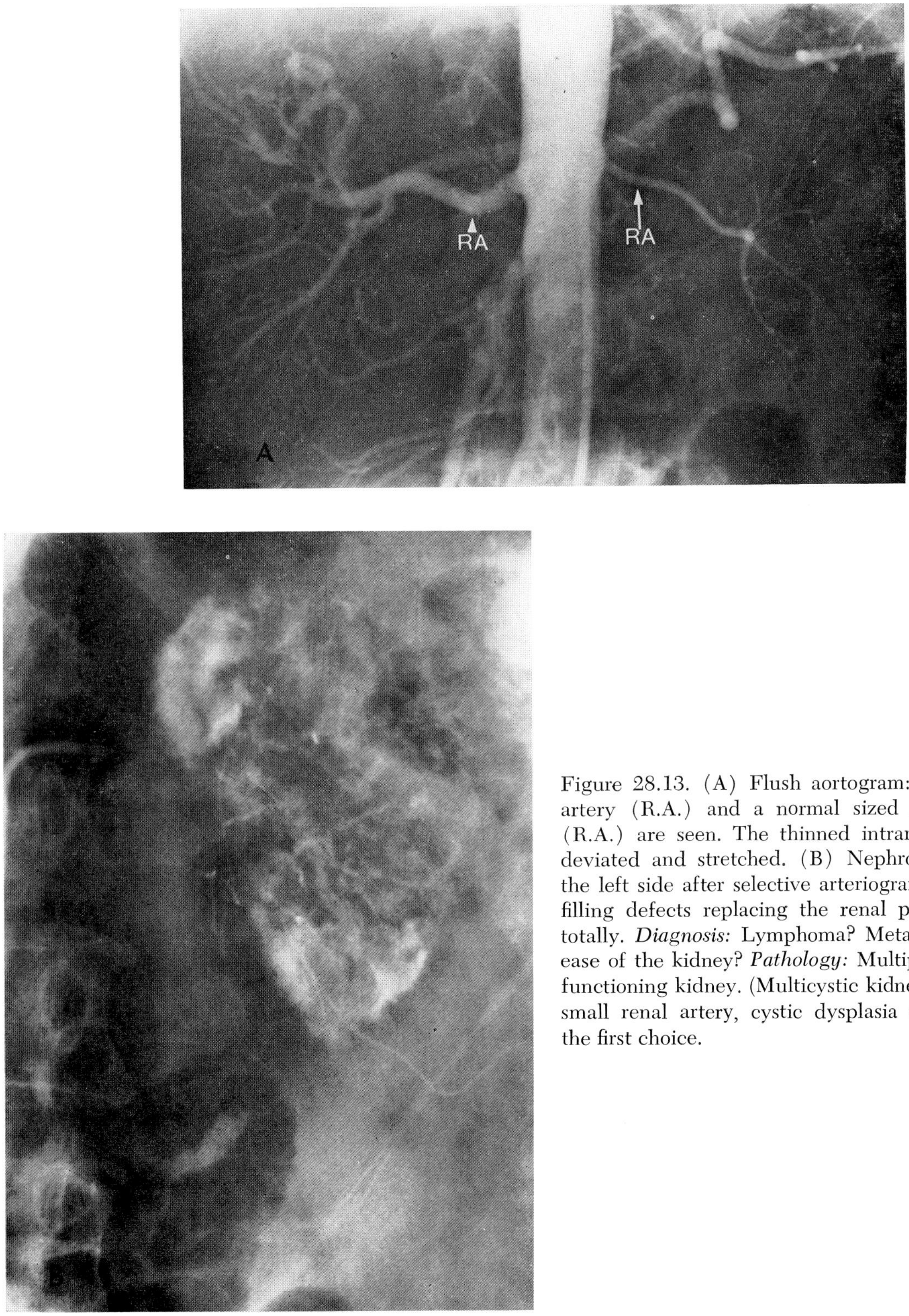

Figure 28.13. (A) Flush aortogram: A thin left renal artery (R.A.) and a normal sized right renal artery (R.A.) are seen. The thinned intrarenal branches are deviated and stretched. (B) Nephrographic phase on the left side after selective arteriogram reveals multiple filling defects replacing the renal parenchyma almost totally. *Diagnosis:* Lymphoma? Metastases? Cystic disease of the kidney? *Pathology:* Multiple cysts in a nonfunctioning kidney. (Multicystic kidney?) In view of the small renal artery, cystic dysplasia should have been the first choice.

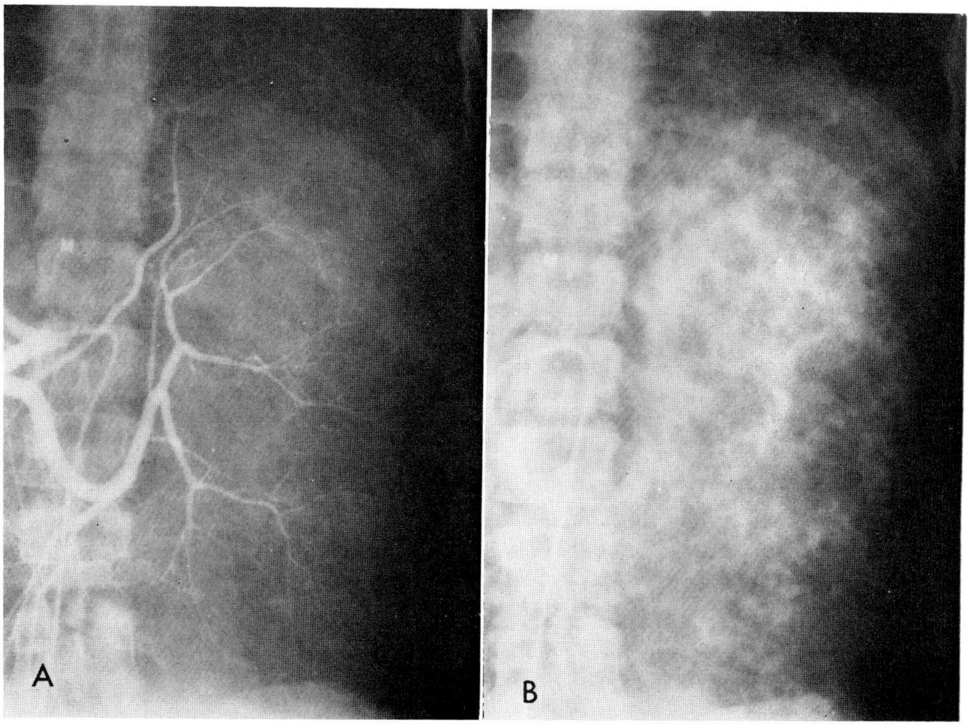

Figure 28.14. Splenic Arteriogram. (A) Arterial phase: The intrasplenic branches are stretched and deviated. (B) Parenchymal phase: Filling defects are revealed in the parenchyma. *Diagnosis:* Cysts? Abscesses? *Pathology:* Lymphangioma of the spleen. (From Shanser, J. D., Moss, A. A., Clark, R. E., and Palubinskas, A. J. Angiographic evaluation of cystic lesions of the spleen, *Am J Roentgenol 119:*166, 1973. Courtesy of the authors and publishers.)

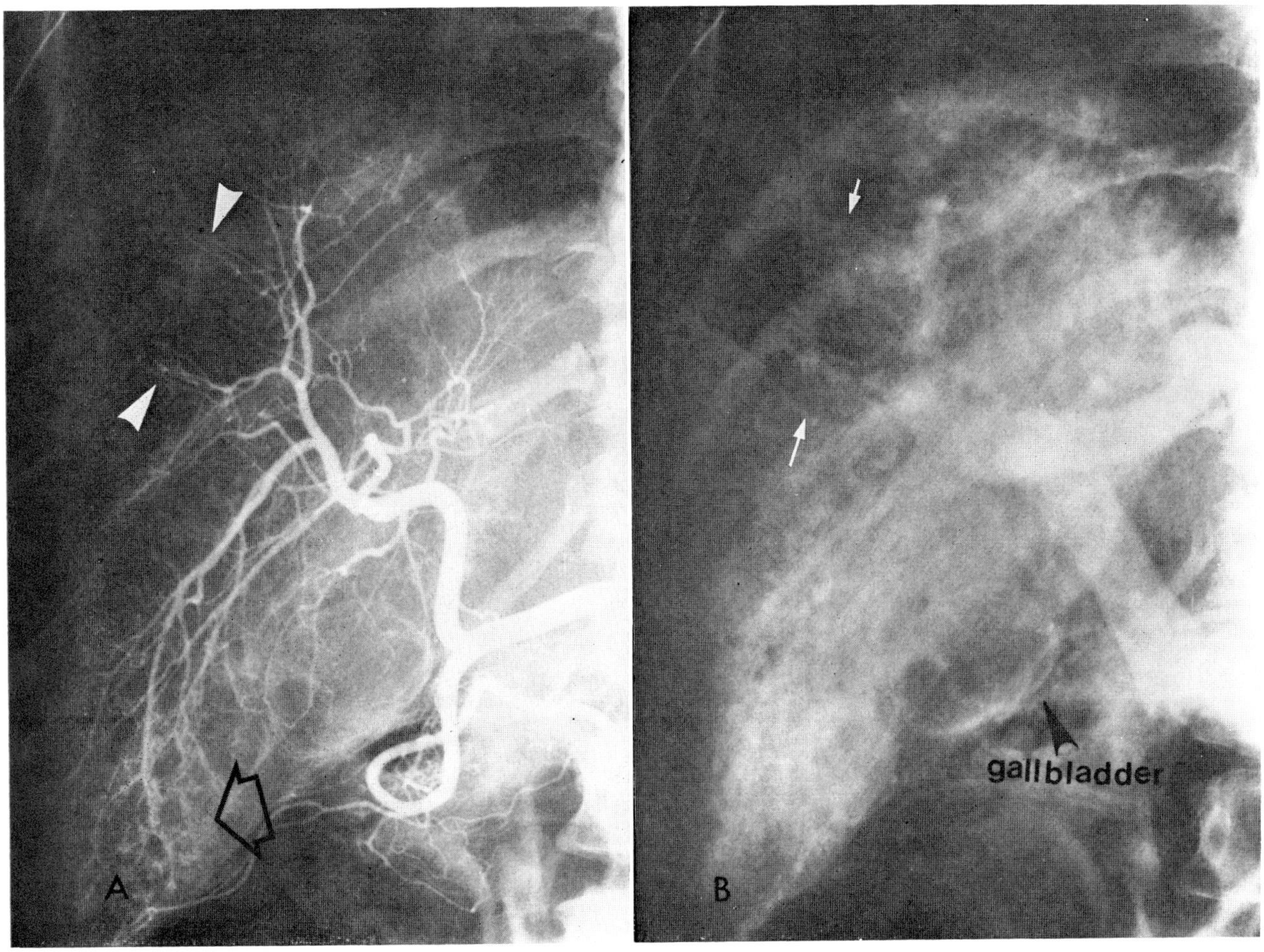

Figure 28.15. Hepatic Arteriogram. (A) There is circumferential stretching of the branches in the upper part of the right lobe of the liver (Arrows) and smudging of contrast material near the inferior portion (Blank Arrow). (B) A lucent filling defect in the upper part of the liver is seen with well-defined margins and irregular filling defect at the inferior angle. There had been a blunt trauma to the right upper quadrant twelve days prior. *Diagnosis:* Acute hematoma of the upper part of the liver with a small laceration at the inferior angle. *Comment:* There is a thin wall around this filling defect because of the short duration of the injury.

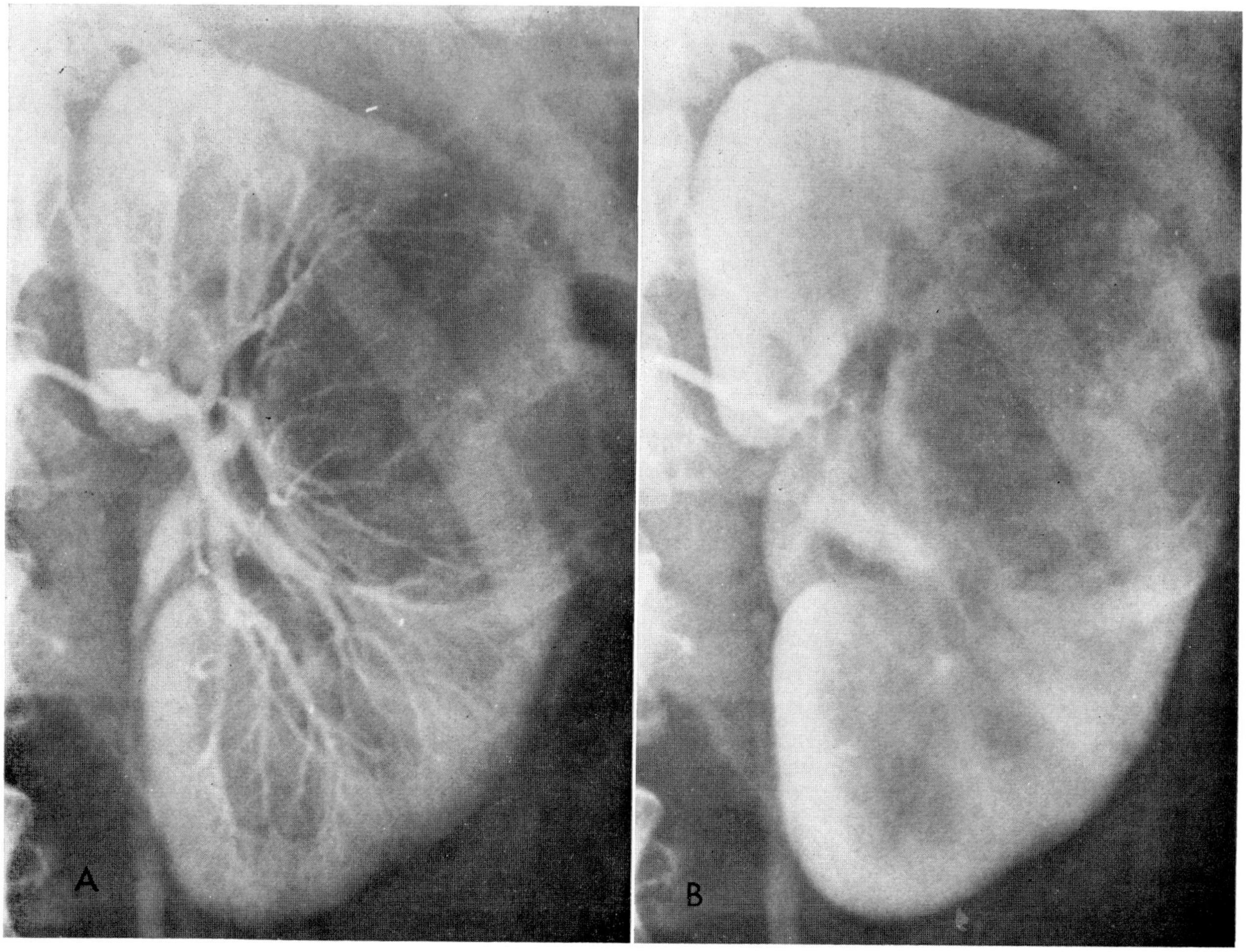

Figure 28.16. Renal Arteriogram. (A) Arterial phase: Stretching and deviation of the intrarenal branches in the midportion of the kidney are seen. (B) Late phase: There is a filling defect with an irregular wall stained with contrast material. *Diagnosis:* Avascular hypernephroma versus abscess. *Surgery:* Abscess of the kidney.

Intestinal Infarction

Occlusion of mesenteric arteries or veins causes infarction of the intestine within eighteen hours.[111] Whether arterial or venous occlusions, they are hemorrhagic infarcts. In *arterial* occlusion there is *stasis of contrast* proximal to the occluded site. In *venous* occlusions, intense and *prolonged opacification of a thickened bowel wall* with or without intraluminal and intramural extravasation of the intraarterially injected contrast is demonstrated.[1014–1016]

Hepatic Infarcts

These infarcts are *relatively uncommon* and are usually due to occlusion of a branch of the portal vein in individuals with underlying predisposing diseases such as hypotension, cardiovascular disorders, gastrointestinal malignancies or splenic diseases. The subcapsular area is frequently spared because of good blood supply from the subcapsular vascular network provided by the inferior phrenic artery.[1048, 1049]

Splenic Infarcts

These are very *common*, usually bland and anemic. They may be due to leukemia, lymphoma, myeloproliferative disorders, sickle cell anemia, polycythemia, polyarteritis nodosa, and splenomegaly due to a variety of other causes[111] (Figs. 28-36, 28-37).

Renal Infarcts

These infarcts are usually anemic since the kidney has an end artery type of blood supply.[1054, 1055] One to two weeks after the episode, the infarcted zone becomes smaller and retracts to become a scar at the end of six to eight weeks.[1050] Depending on the extent of the vascular insult, there may be associated perirenal hematoma. This is especially common with necrotizing angiitis seen in polyarteritis nodosa.[1051] Renal infarcts have gained clinical importance since some are associated with hypertension[1052] (Figs. 28-30 to 28-32).

Cystic degeneration of an infarct is not uncommon. *Venous infarcts* due to venous occlusion are more serious as they are usually septic and may be associated with subcapsular and perirenal hematoma. Unlike arterial infarcts, venous infarcts are swollen, boggy and edematous, giving rise to stretching and deviation of the intrarenal branches. If there is recanalization of the occluded vessel, infarcts may be seen angiographically without an occluded vessel.[465] Thus even a normal angiogram may not exclude the presence of small infarcts.[1495] Microemboli occluding arcuate and interlobar vessels may mimic nephrosclerosis.[1053] Atheromatous emboli occluding small vessels may cause renal failure.[953] Linear infarcts due to needle tracts may be nicely demonstrated angiographically after needle biopsy of the kidney.[1055]

Adrenal infarcts are painful tributes to excessive injection pressure during venography.

DILATATION OF NORMAL STRUCTURES

Tubular Filling Defects

These are usually due to abnormal dilatation of normal tubular structures such as the *hepatic ducts*. Dilatation of bile ducts may be on a congenital basis,[1110] and either solitary or diffuse. If acquired it is usually due to an obstructive etiology. Tubular defects are confined to the distribution of the biliary tree and are of variable dilatation (Figs. 28-81 and 28-82).

Saccular Filling Defects

The most common cause is focal or diffuse dilatation of the collecting system of the kidney most frequently seen with *hydronephrosis*. Each dilated lucent calyx is separated from the other by a thin medullary invagination of the cortex in a rhythmic order. Peripherally, they are lined by a well-stained cortex of variable thickness. This should serve to differentiate hydronephrosis from a polycystic kidney with its masses of different size, diffusely dispersed, which lack the rhythmic arrangement of hydronephrosis. The angiographic findings of focal hydronephrosis in no way differs from that of an intraparenchymal simple cyst (Fig. 28-29).

Traumatic biliary cysts[1066] present as a saccular filling defect within the liver. They are due to posttraumatic pinching of a bile duct with obstruction and secondary dilatation.

(Text continues on page 513)

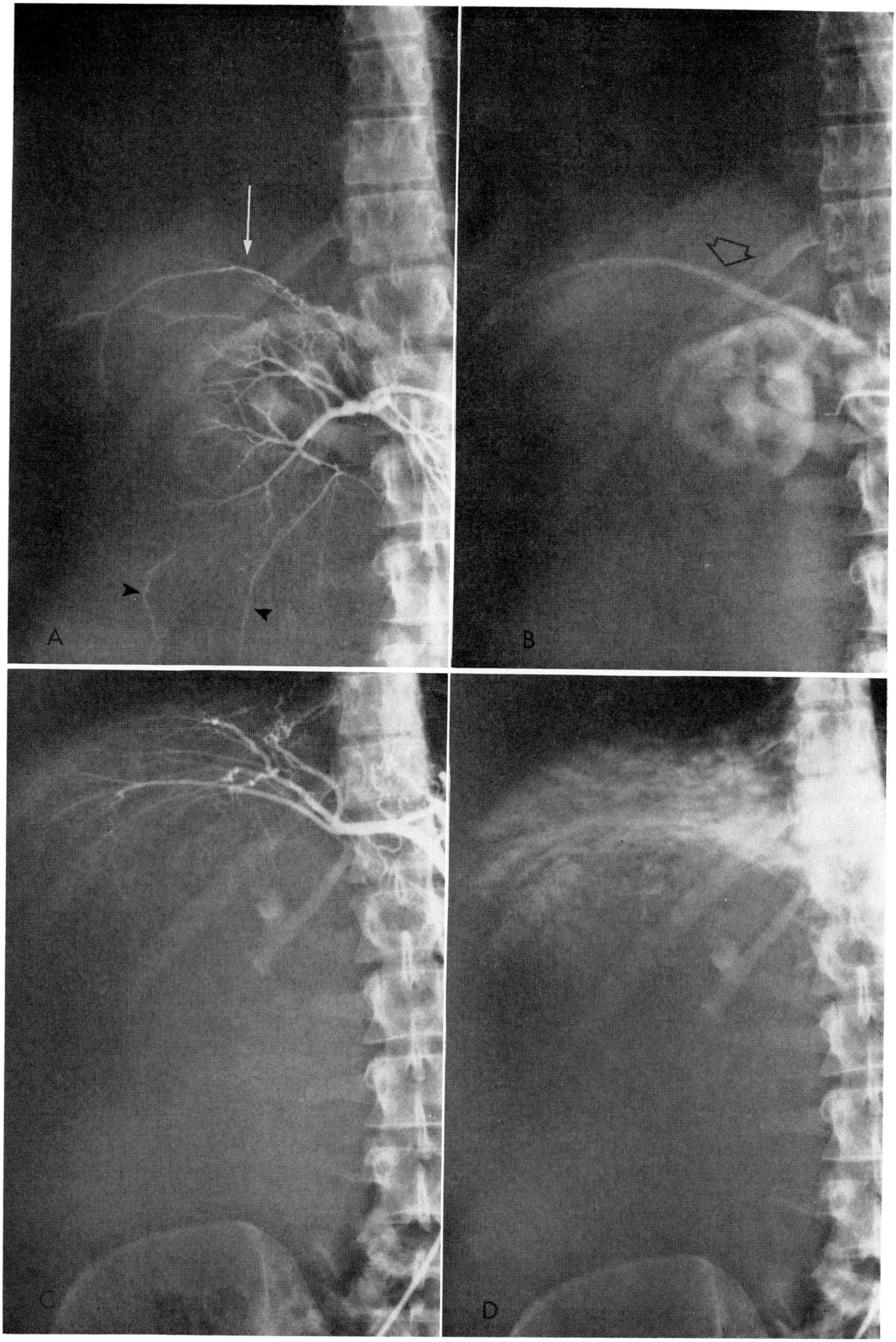
A
B
C
D

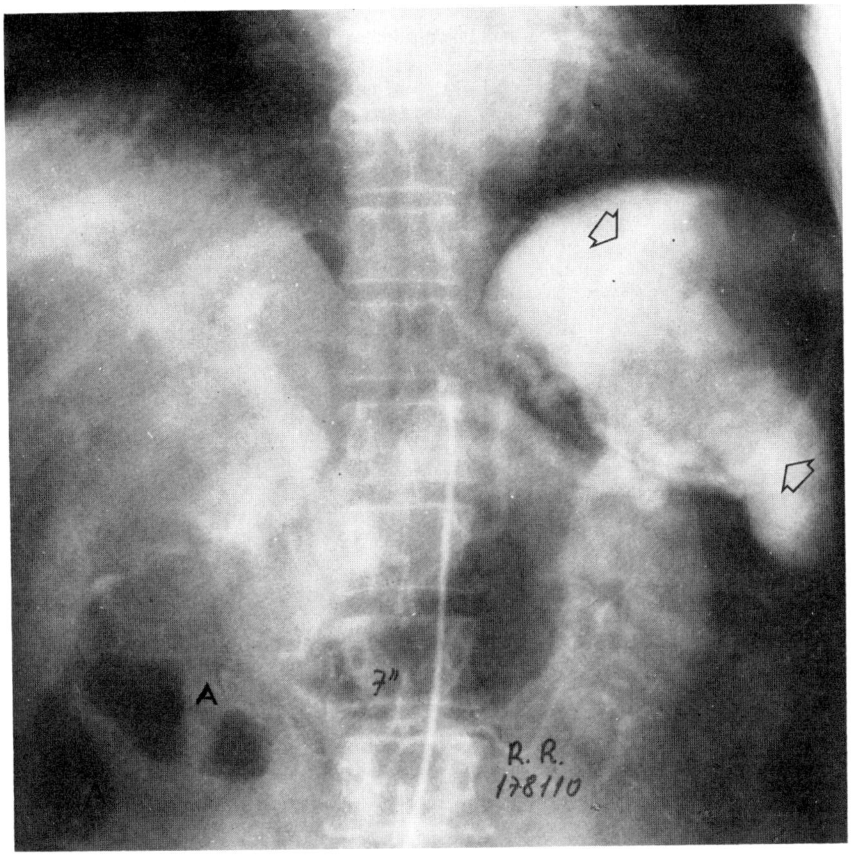

Figure 28.18. Celiac Arteriogram—venous phase. A large filling defect is revealed with a well-defined interface with the opacified splenic parenchyma. A "halo" delineates this filling defect. (B) Close-up of the same. *Differential Diagnosis:* Cyst, abscess, hematoma. *Diagnosis:* Hydatid cyst. (From the angiographic diagnosis of echinococcosis of the liver and spleen. By Dr. I. Garti and V. Deutsch, *Clin Radiol* 22:467, 1971. Courtesy of the authors and publishers.)

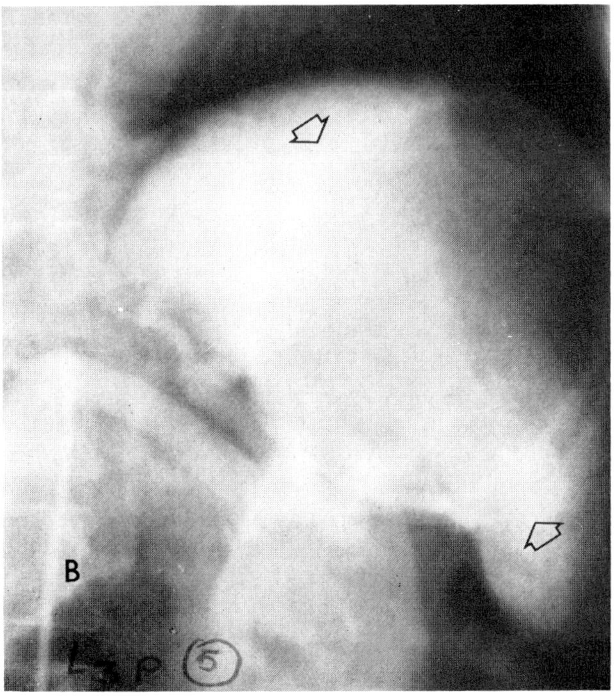

←

Figure 28.17. (A) Selective renal arteriogram: A very prominent renal capsular artery (Arrow) and prominent perforating renal capsular arteries (Arrow Head) are seen. (B) Parenchymal phase: The distal half of the renal parenchyma is not visualized. Marked staining of a thick wall surrounding a huge mass is noted. (C) Celiac arteriogram: There is cranial displacement of the hepatic arteries with compression. (D) Parenchymal phase: There is extrinsic compression of the hepatic parenchyma from this huge mass. The patient was a young female who had recently delivered. *Diagnosis:* Huge intrarenal abscess. (Courtesy of Dr. H. T. Shah, Radiologist, Michael Reese Medical Center, Chicago.)

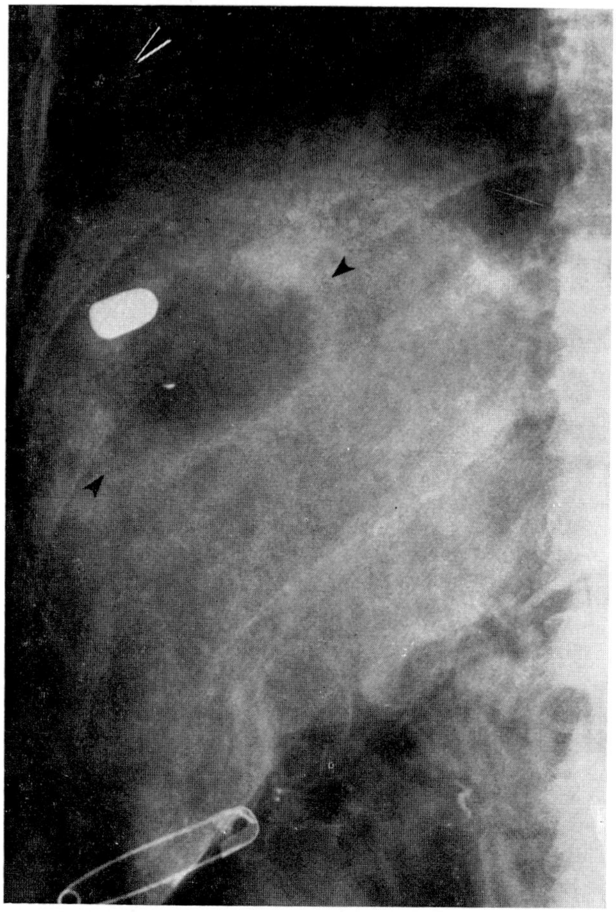

Figure 28.19. Hepatic Arteriogram. There is a circumscribed translucent area with a dense halo about it. The patient had received a gunshot wound three weeks earlier. *Diagnosis:* An organizing intrahepatic hematoma. The halo is due to vascularization of the granulation tissue of the organizing hematoma.

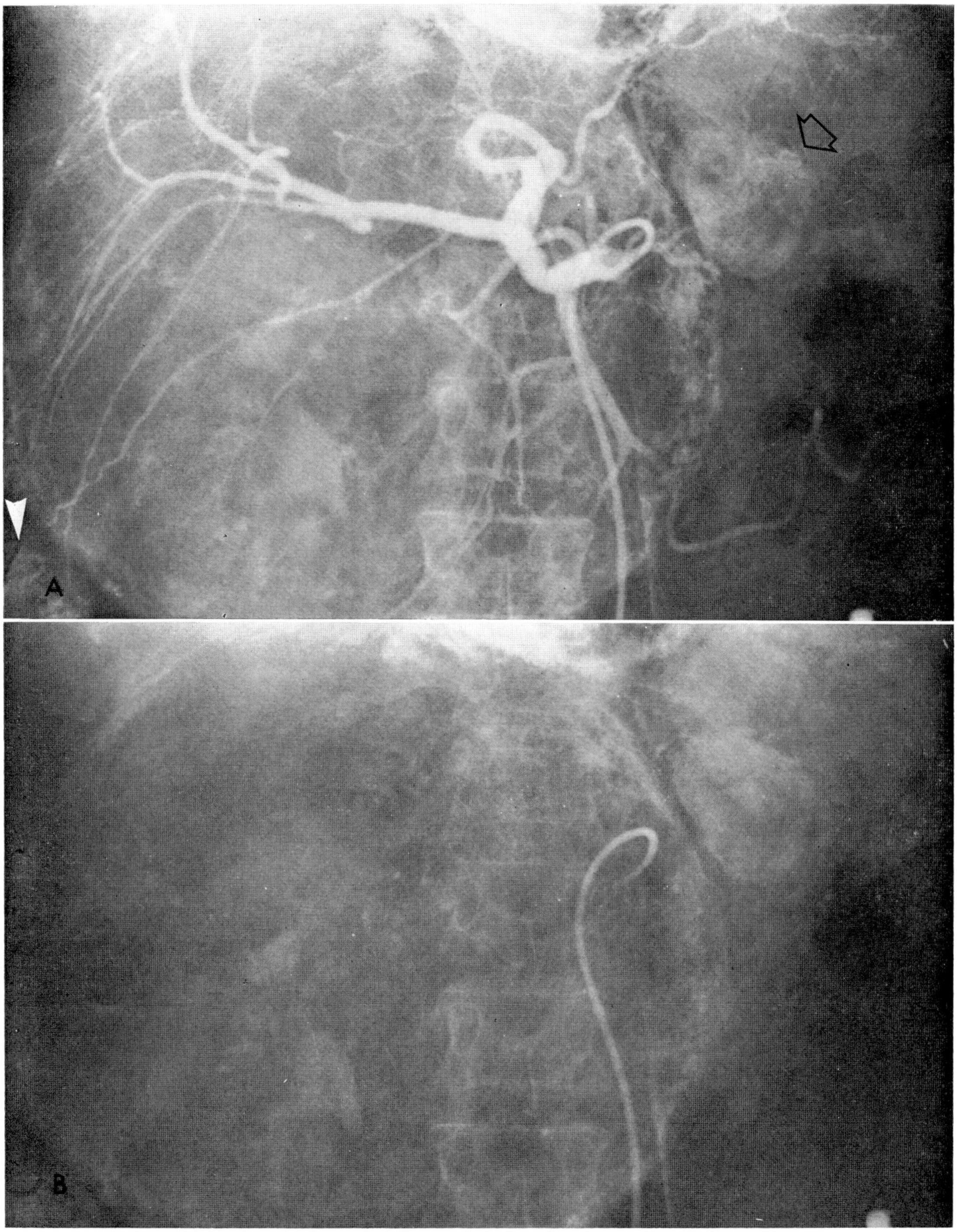

Figure 28.20. Hepatic Arteriogram. (A) Arterial phase: The hepatic artery is prominent with stretching and deviation of the intrahepatic branches around a huge mass occupying the right lobe of the liver. It extends to and crosses the midline. Other masses of smaller sizes are around this huge mass (Arrows). There is an amorphous collection of the contrast material at the periphery of this huge mass and also in the center. (B) Parenchymal phase: There is increased staining of the wall of this huge mass with uneven thickness of the wall and homogeneous staining of the small masses. *Diagnosis:* Necrotic malignant masses of different sizes. This patient had a known leiomyosarcoma of the small bowel. *Comment:* The liver metastases from leiomyosarcomas tend to be very bulky and necrotic in the center.

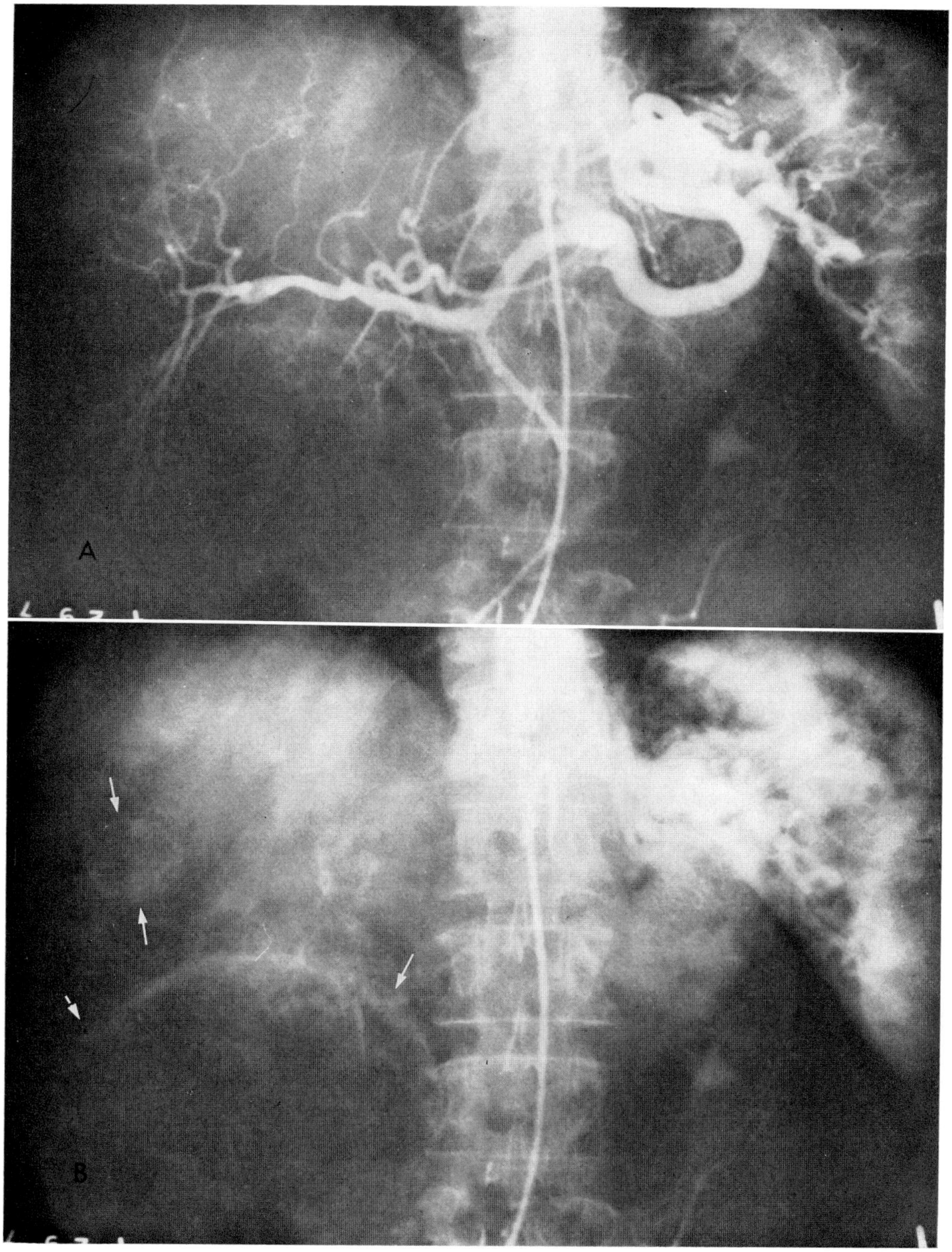

Figure 28.21. Celiac Arteriogram. (A) Arterial phase reveals stretching of the intrahepatic branches in the lower portion. (B) Parenchymal phase reveals two cystic masses with irregular thick walls. *Diagnosis:* Necrotic metastasis versus multiple abscesses. *Pathology:* Metastasis from an adenocarcinoma of the colon.

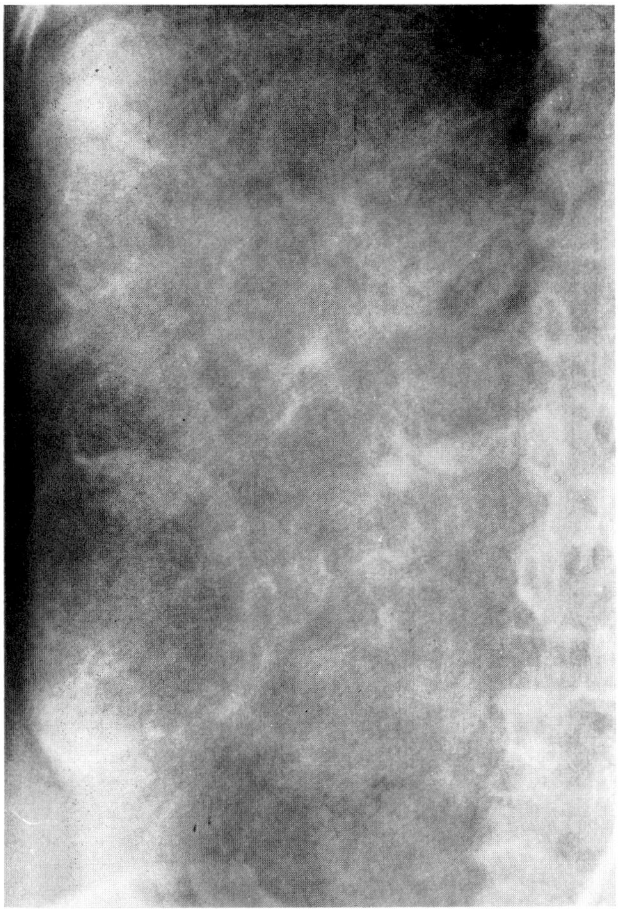

←

Figure 28.22. Celiac Arteriogram—late phase. There are multiple masses with increased staining of their walls. The walls are of irregular thickness, and there are subtle hypervascular areas in the lucent central areas. *Diagnosis:* Multiple necrotic metastases in the liver.

Figure 28.23. Simultaneous Hepatic and Superior Mesenteric Arteriogram. (A) Reveals stretching and deviation of intrahepatic branches around a mass. (B) Late phase reveals a huge filling defect with an irregular wall in the liver. *Diagnosis:* Abscess, hematoma, metastasis. *Pathology:* Amebic abscess. (Courtesy of Dr. J. Petasnick, Associate Professor, Diagnostic Radiology, Rush Presbyterian-St. Luke Medical Center, Chicago.)

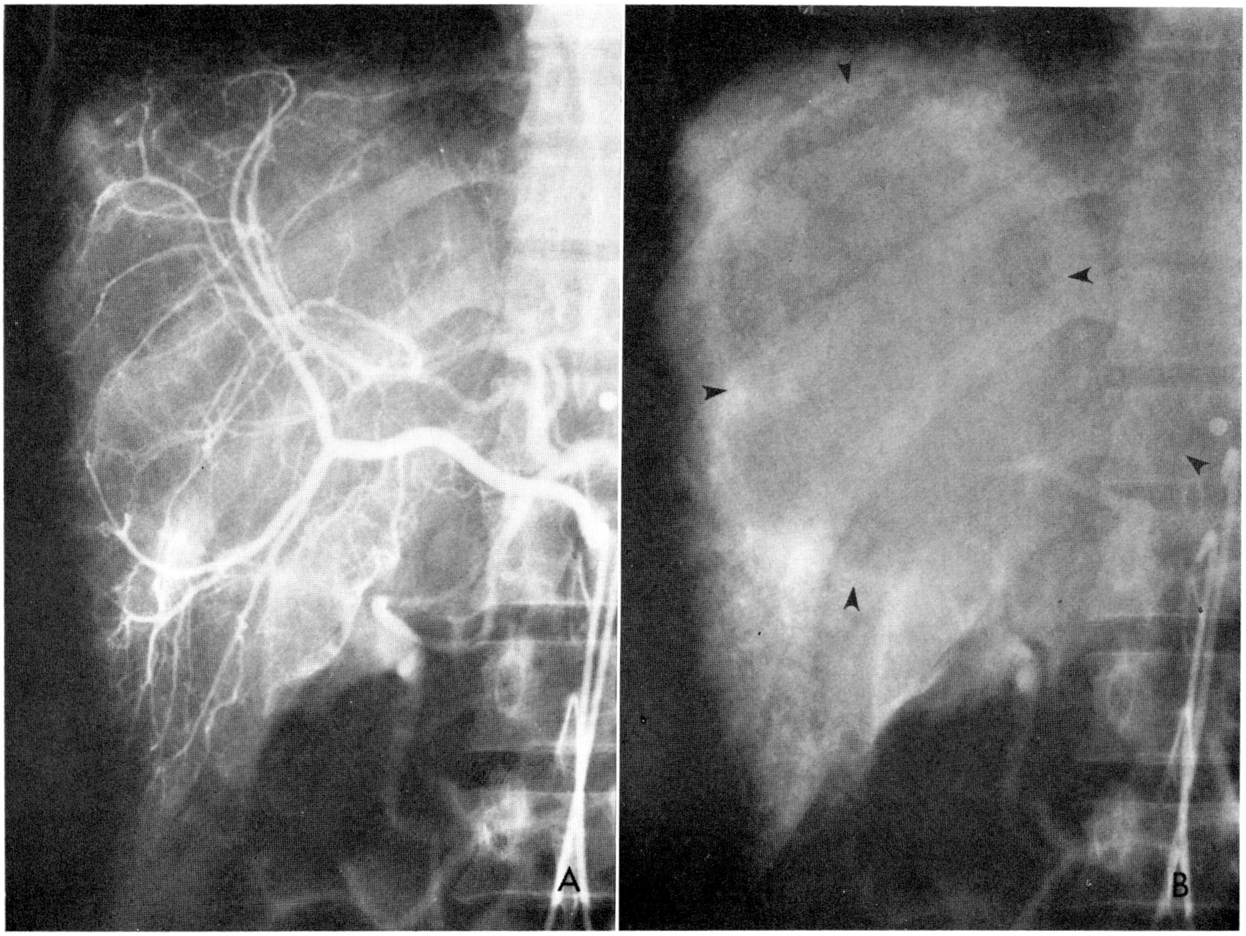

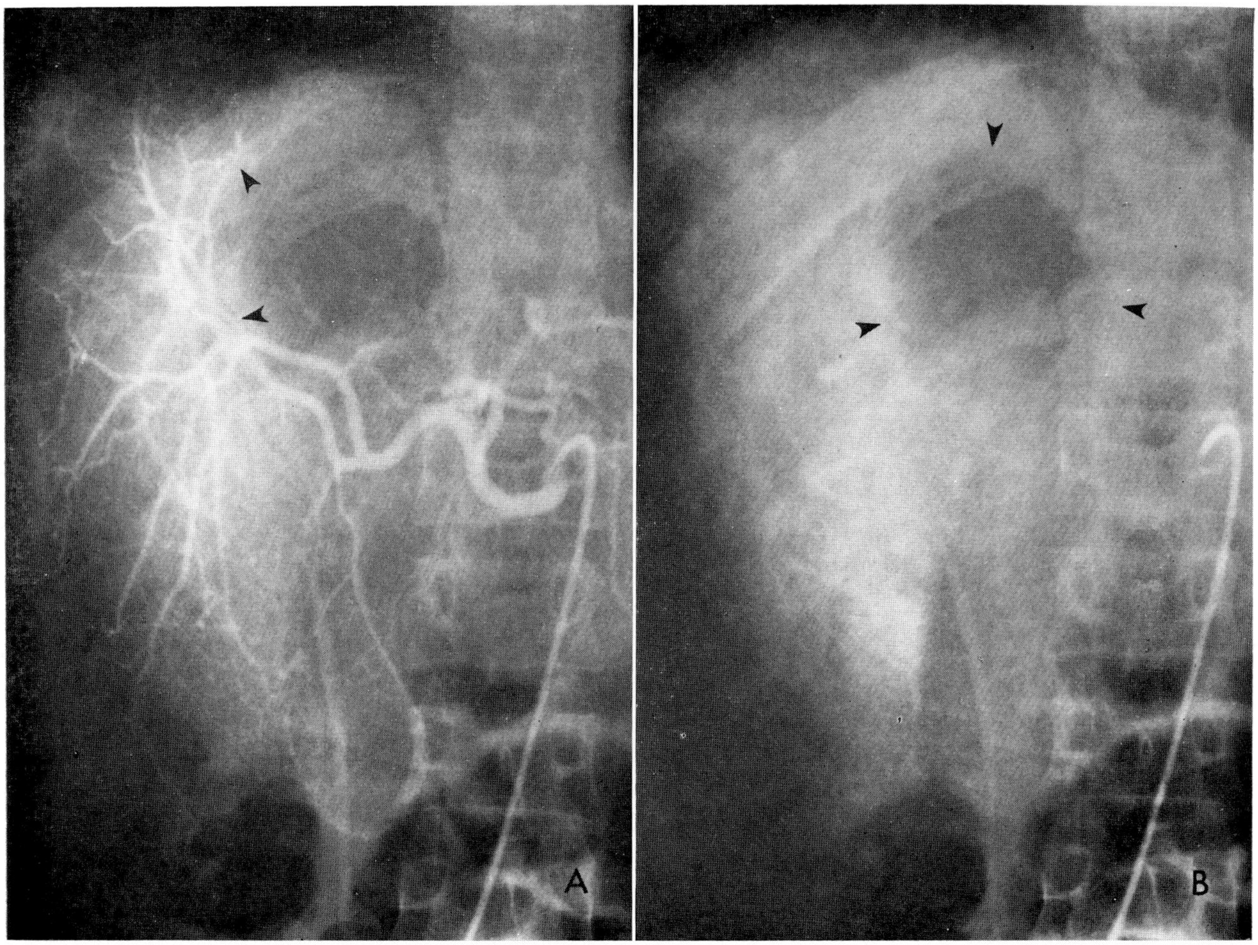

Figure 28.24. Hepatic Arteriogram. (A) Early phase reveals deviation and stretching of the intrahepatic branches (Arrows) around an avascular mass. (B) Late phase reveals a sharply defined filling defect with irregular wall in a patient who had blunt trauma. *Diagnosis:* Hematoma of the liver. (Courtesy of Dr. J. Petasnick, Associate Professor, Diagnostic Radiology, Rush Presbyterian-St. Luke Medical Center, Chicago.)

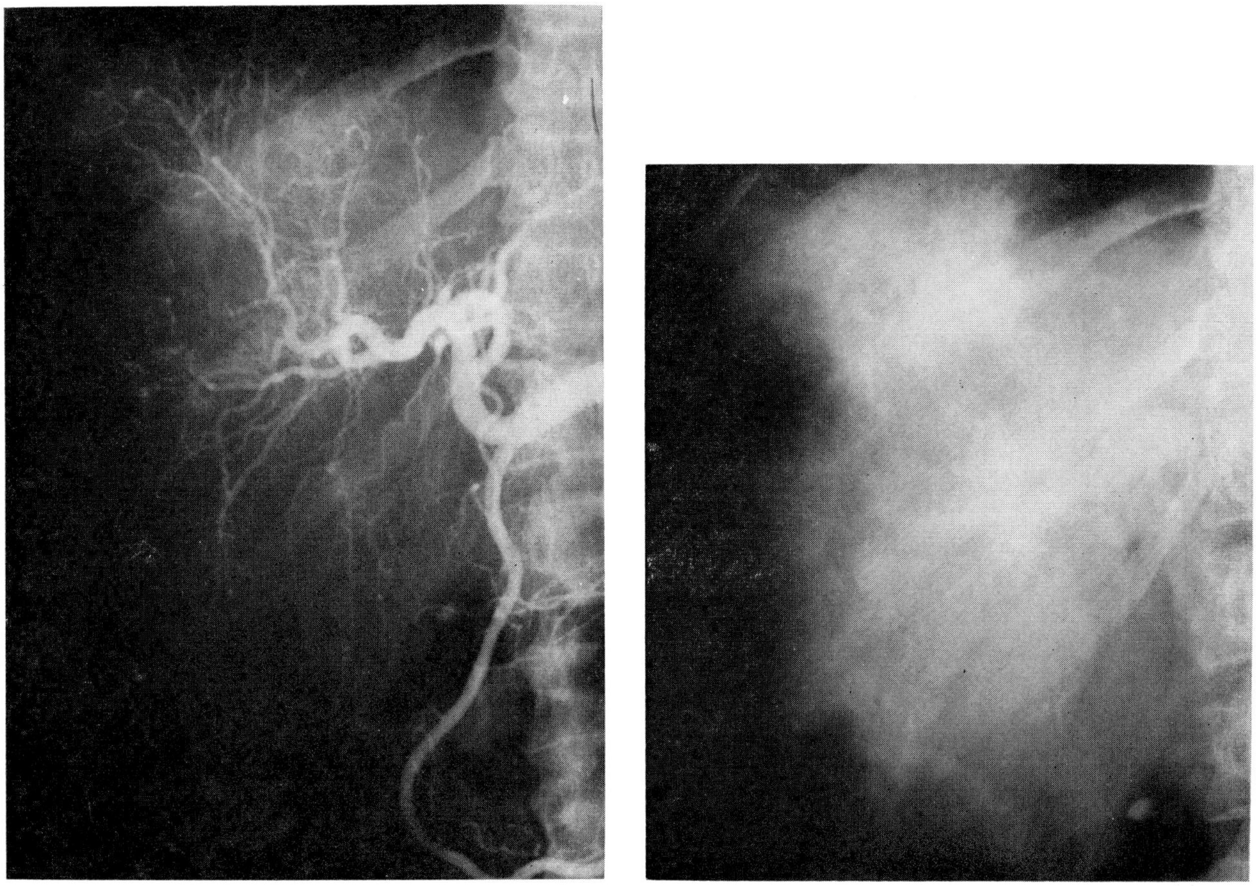

A B

Figure 28.25 A and B. Hepatic Arteriogram. A. Arterial phase: Circumferential displacement of intrahepatic branches around multiple avascular masses. B. Parenchymal: Reveals well defined avascular areas in the liver substance. *Pathology:* Metastasis to the liver from an adenocarcinoma of colon.

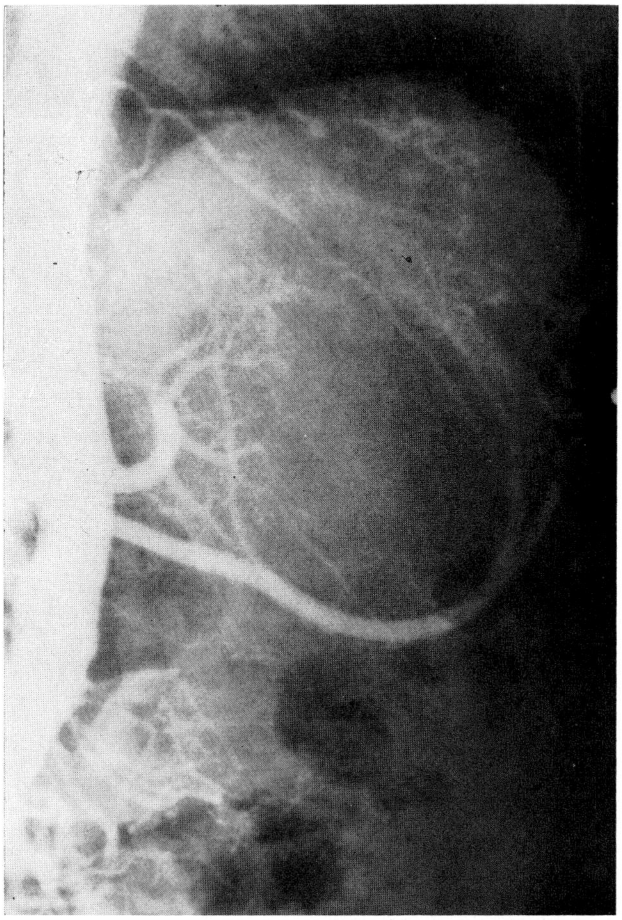

Figure 28.26. Flush Abdominal Aortogram. There is inferior displacement and stretching of the distal portion of the main splenic artery. This occurs around an avascular mass which was palpable in the left upper quadrant. *Diagnosis:* Avascular mass of retroperitoneal origin. Differential diagnosis included pancreatic or splenic masses, etc. *Pathologic diagnosis:* Splenic sarcoma.

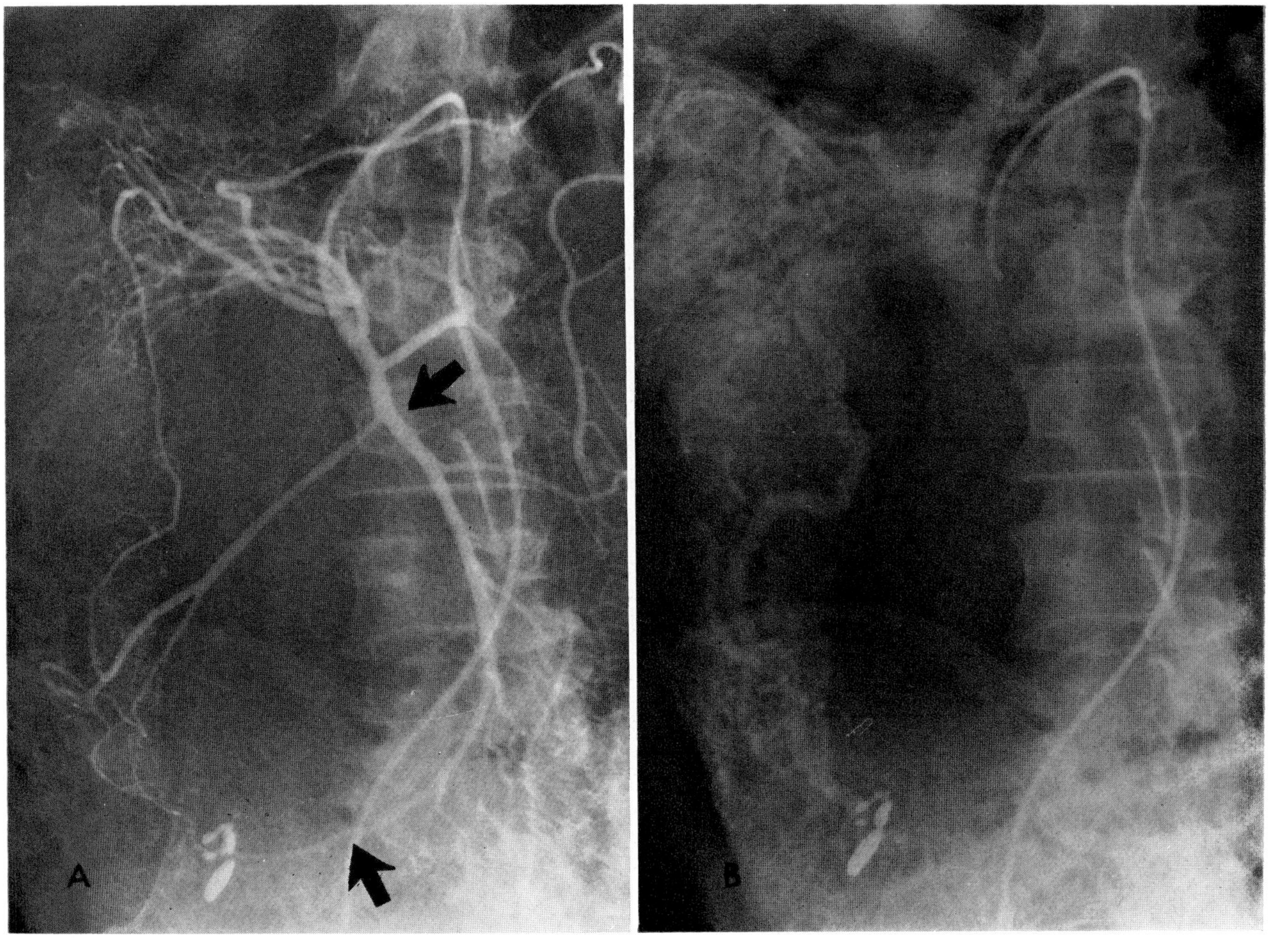

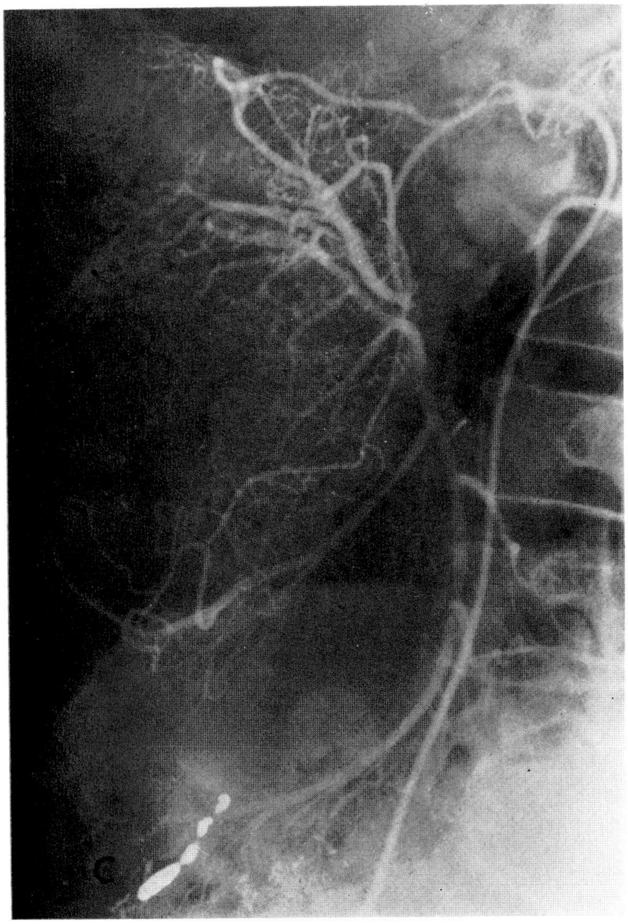

Figure 28.27. Superior Mesenteric Arteriogram. (A) Early phase: Reveals the superior mesenteric artery and its branches splayed around a mass (Arrows) with abnormal vasculature on the surface of this mass (Arrow Heads). (B) Venous phase: Reveals this comparatively avascular mass. (C) An oblique projection reveals the mass to be anterior to the superior mesenteric artery suggesting that the mass is in the peritoneal cavity, probably in the mesentery. *Diagnosis:* Malignant necrotic tumor of the mesentery? Leiomyosarcoma? *Pathology:* Leiomyosarcoma.

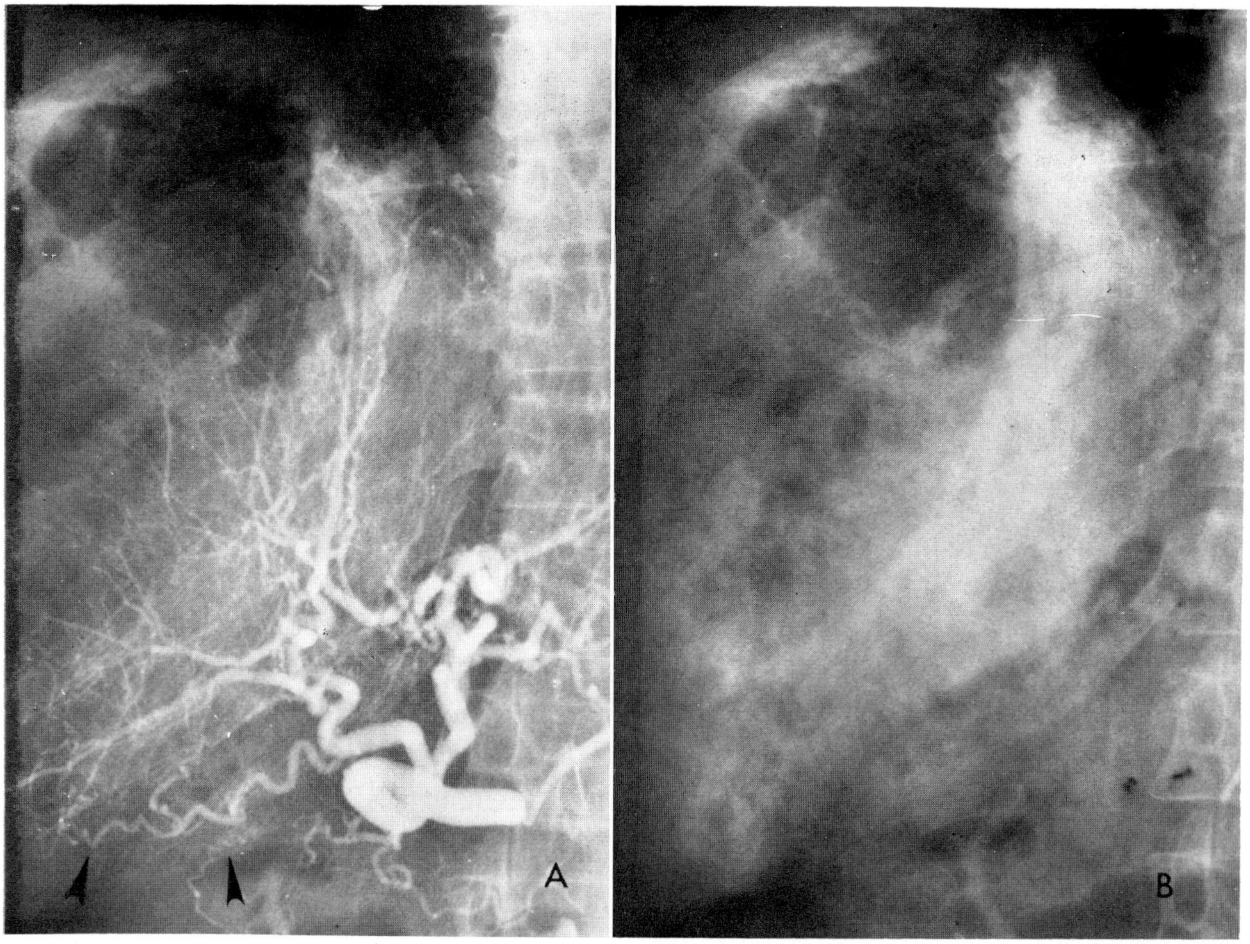

Figure 28.28. Hepatic Arteriogram. There is deviation of distal intrahepatic arteries away from the liver contour. Lucencies in the projection of the liver are seen as well as corkscrew branches (Arrow) from the main hepatic artery near the porta hepatis. The patient was known to have regional enteritis. *Diagnosis:* Intrahepatic abscesses with an inflammatory mass near the porta hepatis.

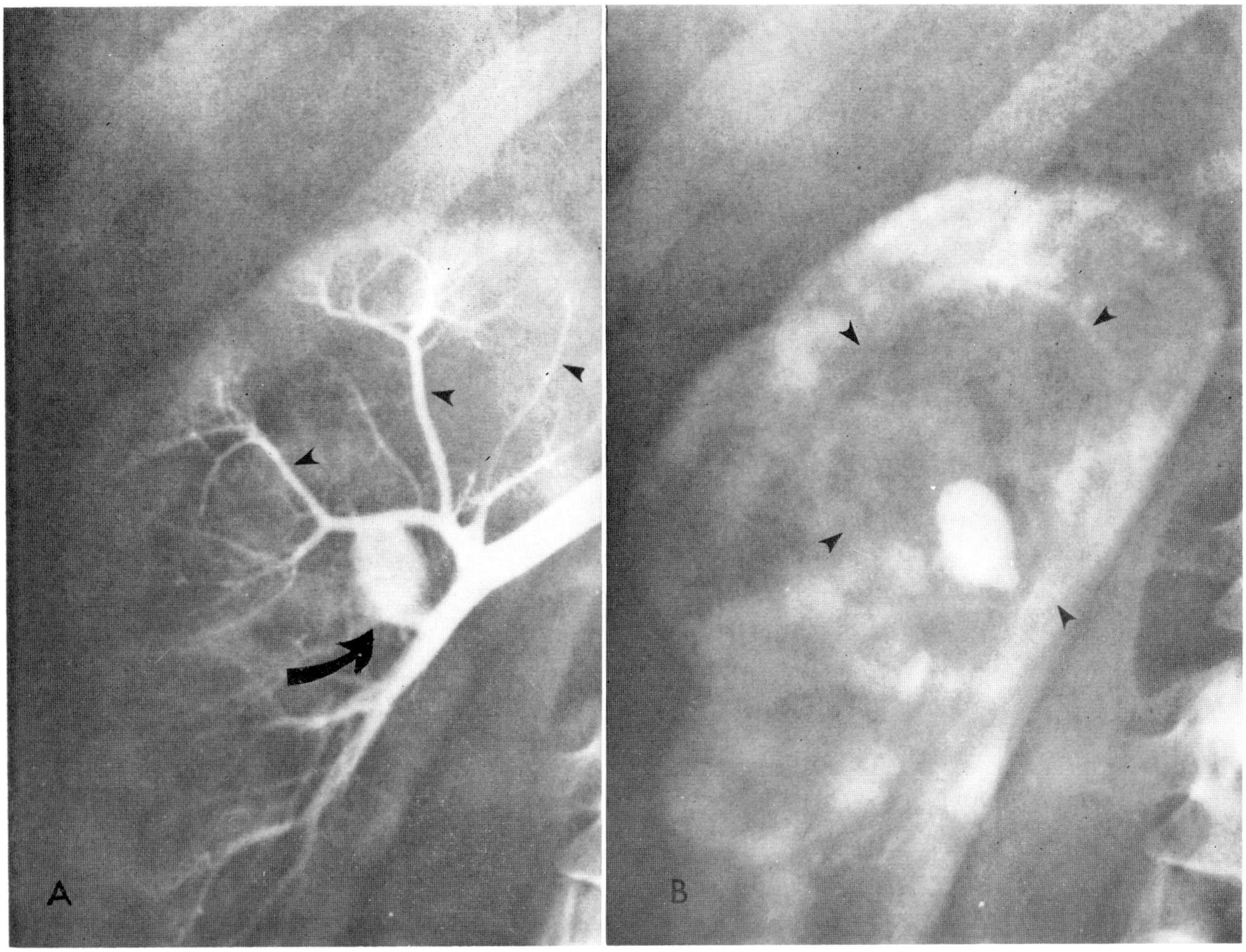

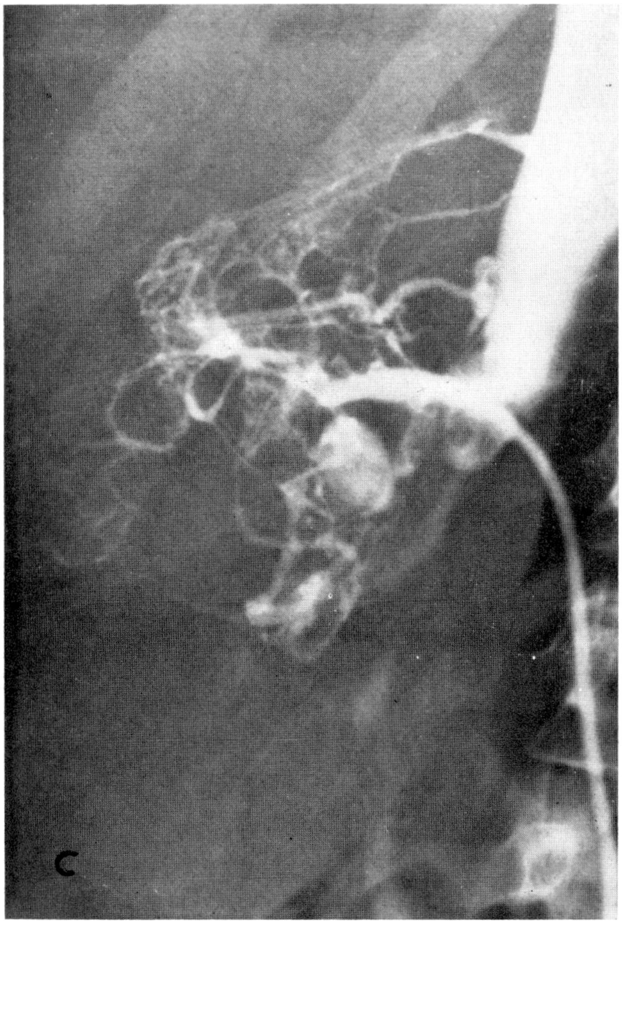

Figure 28.29. Renal Arteriogram. (A) Renal arteriogram: The intrarenal branches in the upper pole of the kidney are stretched and deviated (Arrow Head). Incidental stone in the kidney (Arrow). (B) An intrarenal, well-defined circular filling defect is noted. (C) Renal venogram: There is stretching and deviation of the intrarenal small veins at the same area. *Diagnosis:* Calculus pyonephrosis of the upper calyx of the kidney.

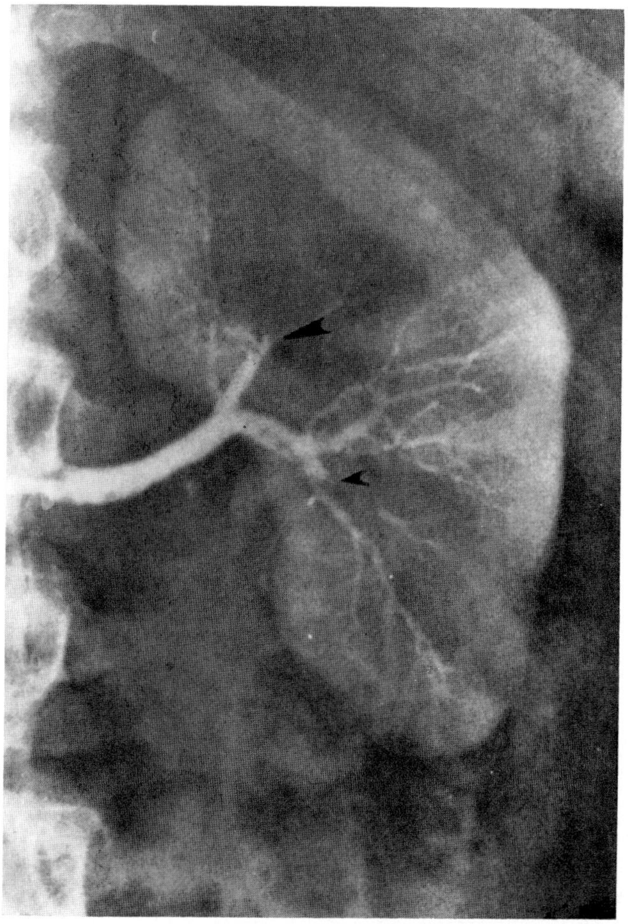

Figure 28.30. Left Renal Arteriogram. Abrupt termination of multiple intrarenal branches exist (Arrow) with wedge-shaped filling defects corresponding to these areas of perfusion. Three minutes prior to this, a flush aortogram was within normal limits. *Diagnosis:* Catheter emboli with infarcts. *Comment:* This would not have happened if the catheter was flushed with saline and heparin solution every few seconds.

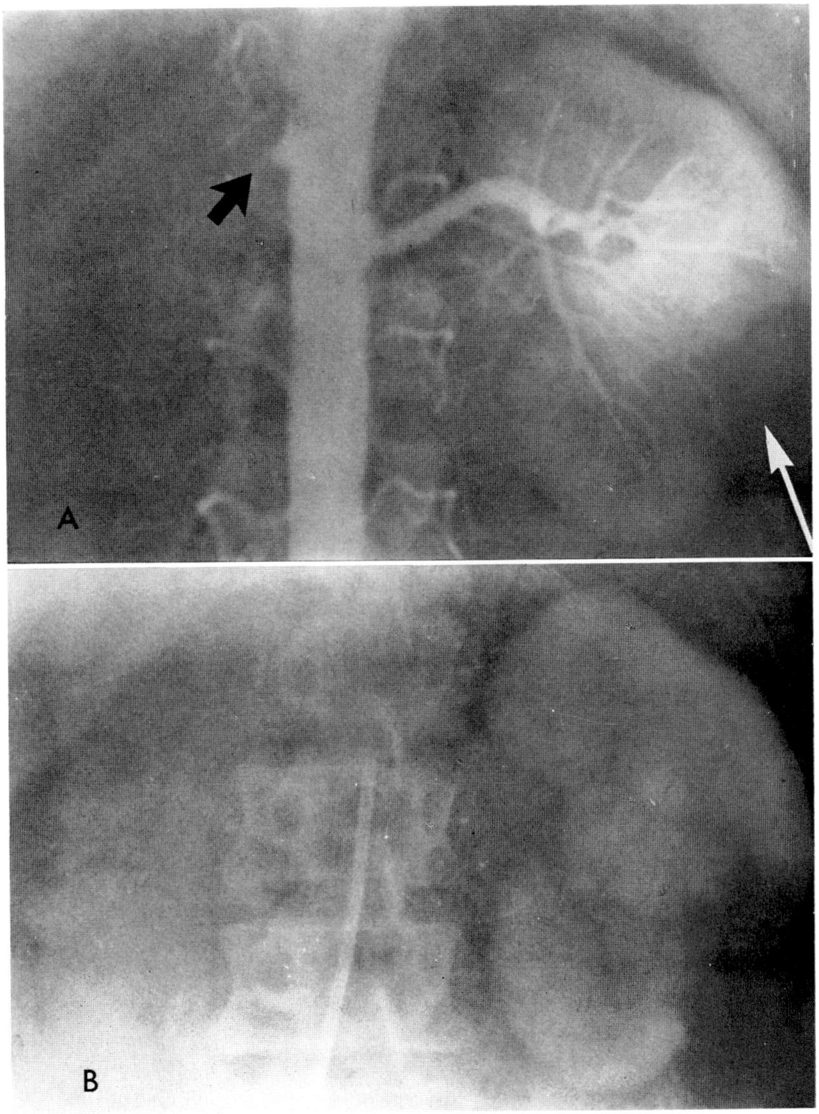

Figure 28.31. Flush Abdominal Aortogram. (A) Early arterial phase: Visualization of only a stump of the renal artery on the right side noted (Arrow). Lack of arterial perfusion of the peripheral portion of the mid-part of the left kidney (White Arrow). (B) Parenchymal phase: No nephrogram on the right side. The same lack of perfusion is well defined in the left kidney. The patient had atrial fibrillation due to mitral stenosis. *Diagnosis:* Embolic occlusion of the right renal artery and occlusions of the smaller intrarenal branches of the left kidney with infarcts.

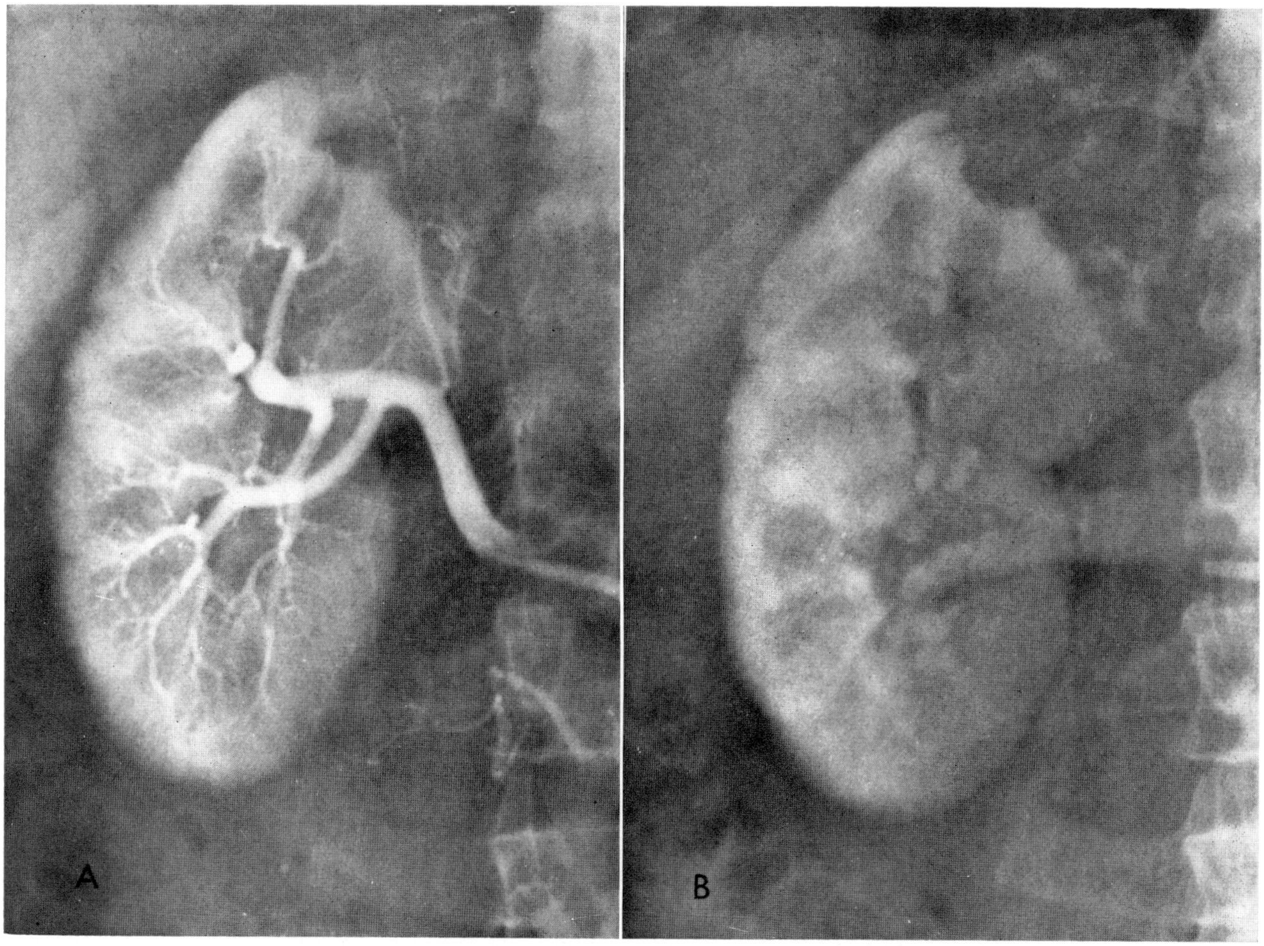

Figure 28.32. Renal Arteriogram. (A) Arterial phase: A sharp avascular area is in the upper pole. (B) Parenchymal phase: Notice the filling defect in the upper pole. A flush aortogram did not reveal any other arteries to that area. *Diagnosis:* Infarct of the upper pole of the kidney. *Surgery:* Confirmed the diagnosis.

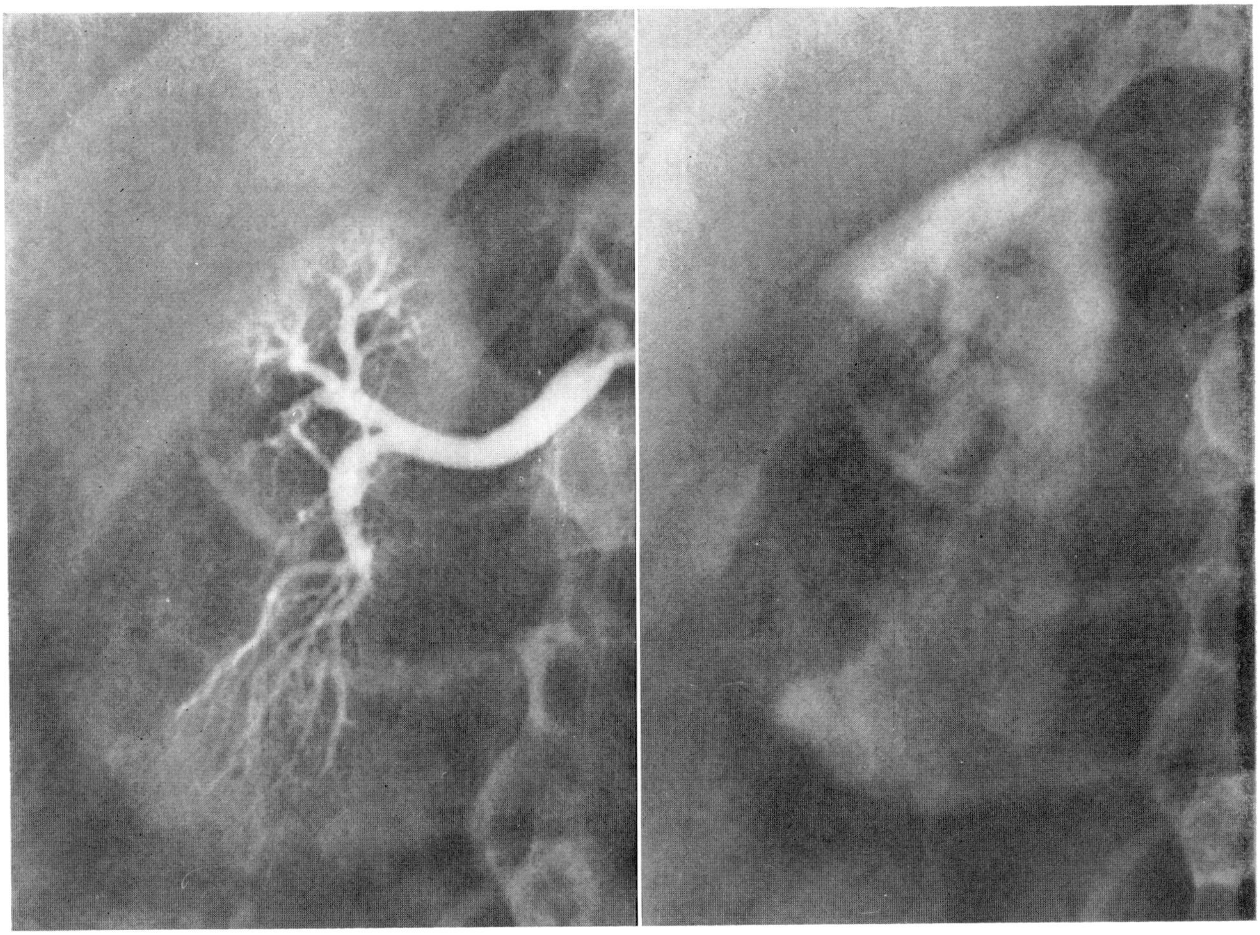

Figure 28.33. Renal Arteriogram. (A) Arterial phase: Lack of arterial perfusion occurs in the midportion of the kidney. (B) Parenchymal phase: An irregular, well-defined filling defect is seen in the same area. The patient had right flank pain, chills and fever. *Diagnosis:* Intrarenal abscess. *Differential Diagnosis:* Intrarenal hematoma or avascular renal malignancies such as renal lymphoma, hypernephroma or metastases.

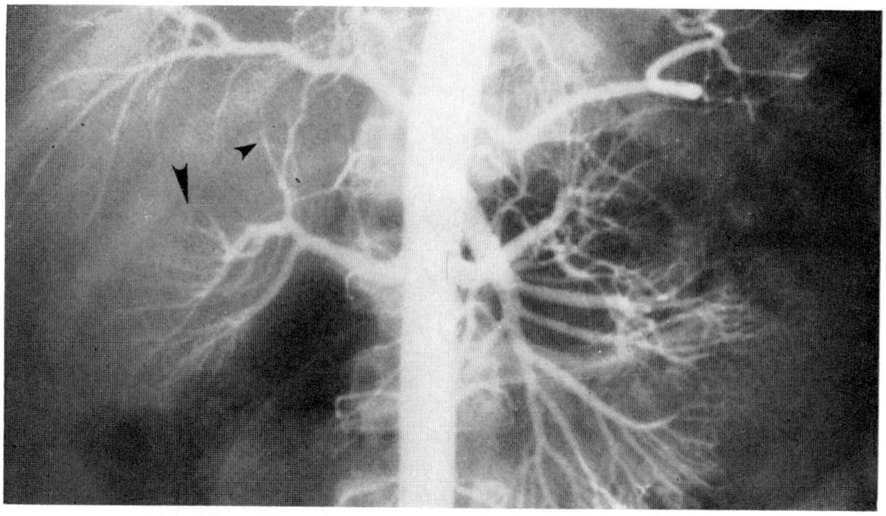

Figure 28.34 A

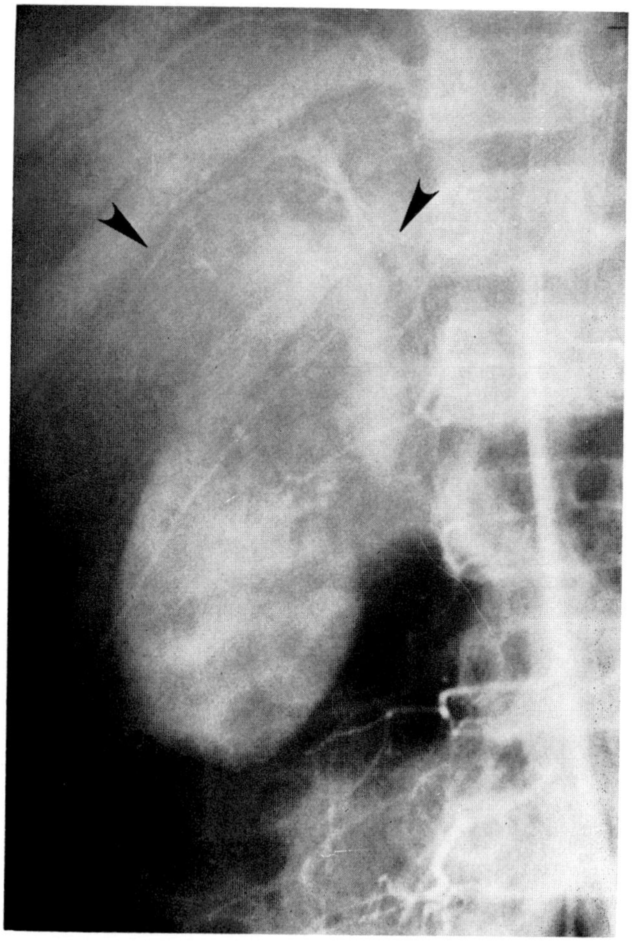

Figure 28.34 B

Figure 28.34. Aortogram. (A) Arterial phase demonstrates nonopacification of arterial supply to the upper part of the kidney. Note the separation of the stretched capsular artery. (B) Parenchymal phase: Sharply defined avascular area in the same location noted. This individual had flank trauma. *Diagnosis:* Posttraumatic laceration with intrarenal and perirenal bleeding.

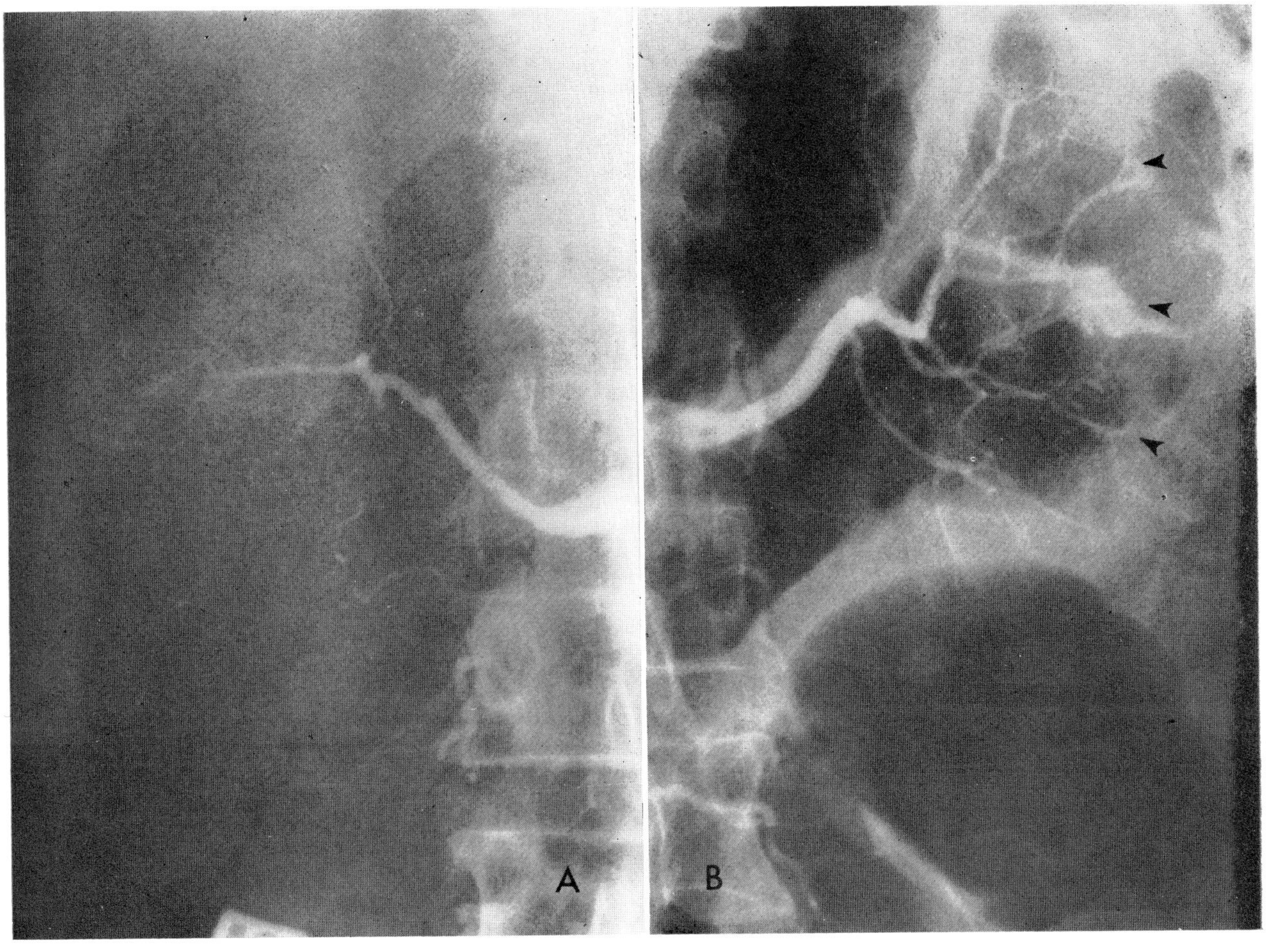

Figure 28.35. (A) Right renal arteriogram: Lack of perfusion of the upper and lower half of the kidney occurs with only one segment perfused by a small renal vessel. (B) Left renal arteriogram: There is abrupt termination of the intrarenal branches. This patient had mitral stenosis with atrial fibrillation. *Diagnosis:* Bilateral massive infarcts of both kidneys due to emboli. (C) An intravenous pyelogram three months later reveals shrunken minimally functioning kidneys bilaterally.

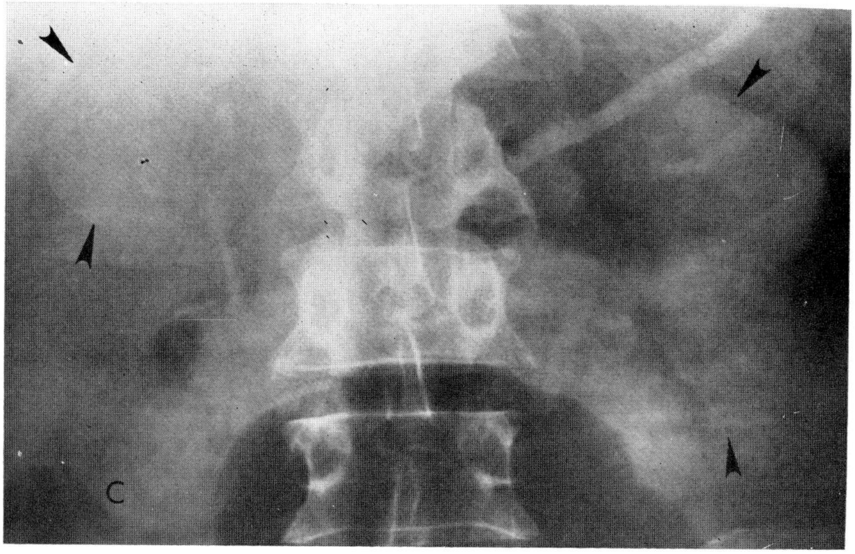

Figure 28.35 C

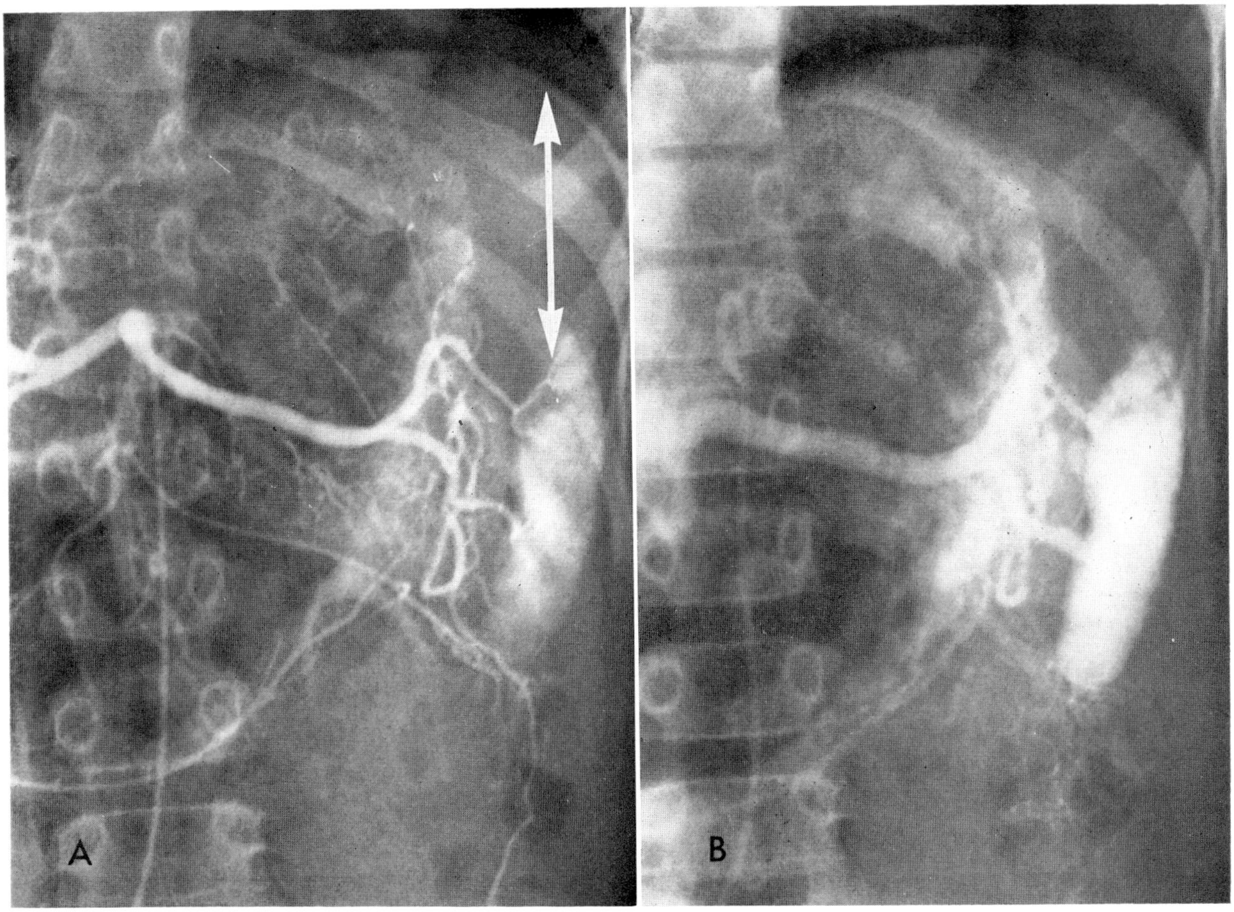

Figure 28.36. Splenic Arteriogram. (A) Arterial phase: There is lack of arterial perfusion of the proximal half of the spleen. (B) Parenchymal phase: The splenogram of the proximal half is absent (Arrow) and the splenic vein is abruptly terminated. This patient had left upper quadrant trauma. *Diagnosis:* Traumatic thrombosis of a branch of the splenic artery with infarction of the spleen.

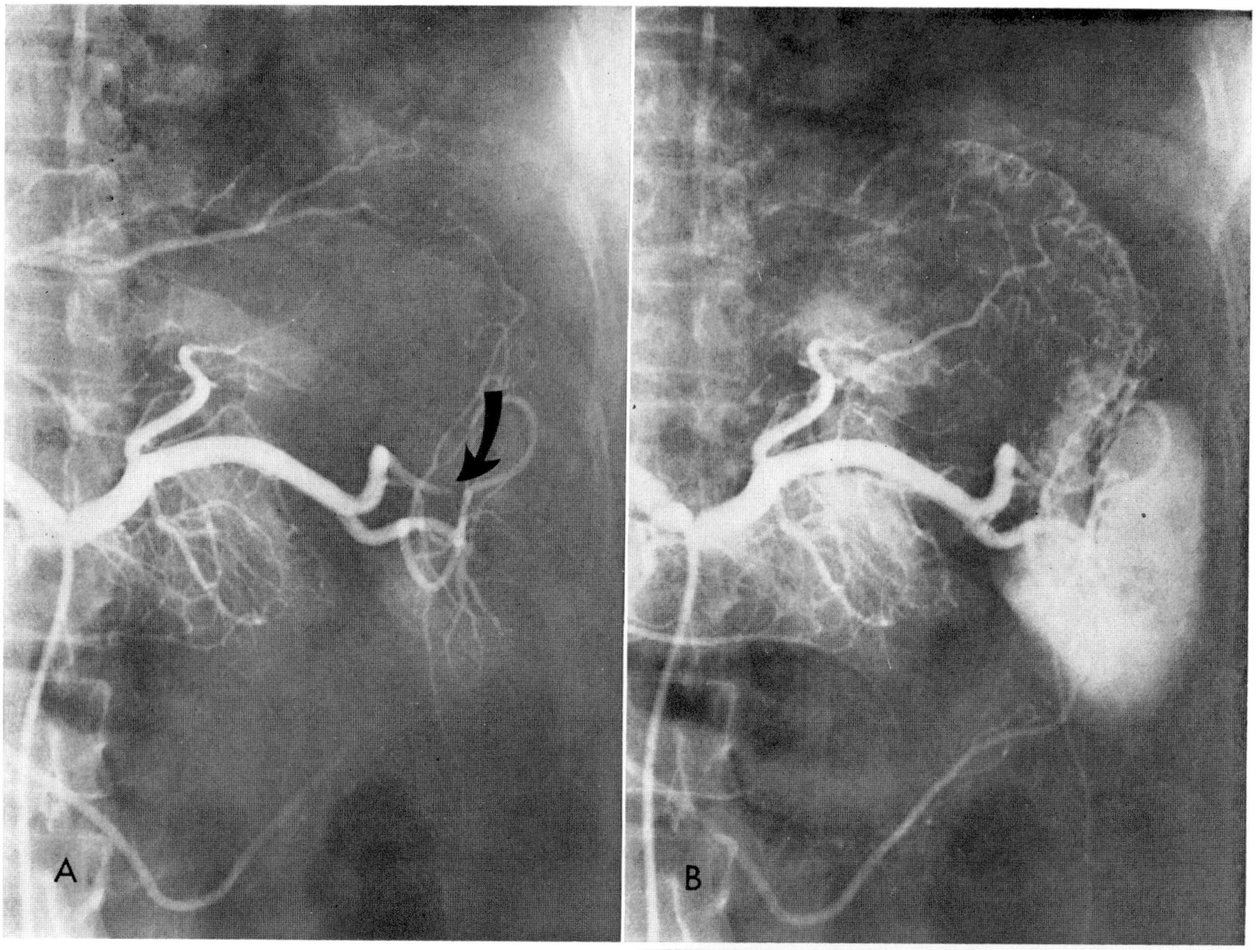

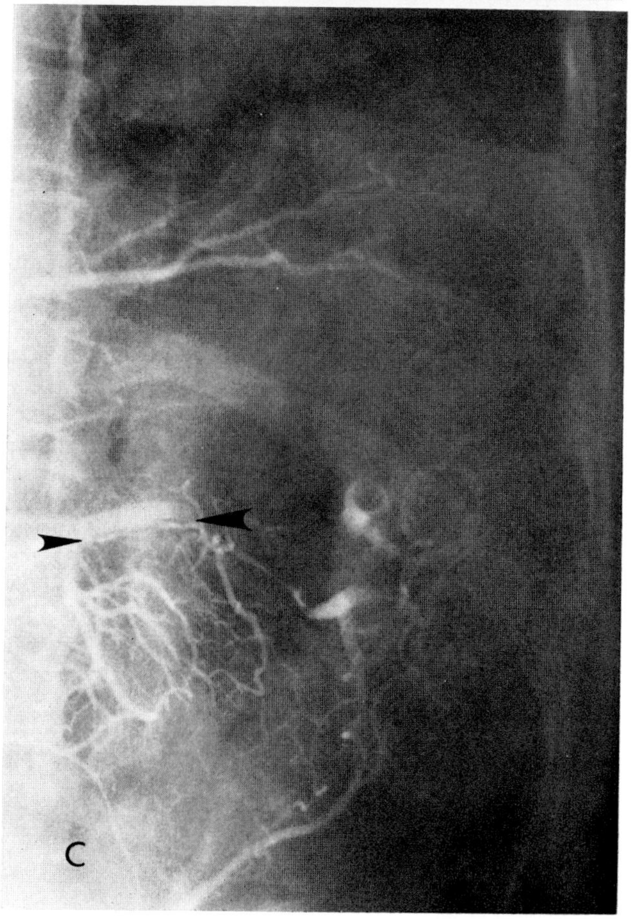

Figure 28.37. Celiac Arteriogram. (A) The proximal half of the spleen is not visualized and there is sudden termination of a major intrasplenic arterial branch (Arrow). (B) Midarterial phase. (C) A repeat injection shows a lucent intimal line (Arrow) in the lumen of the splenic artery. Now the spleen does not opacify. Initially the patient had left upper quadrant trauma. *Diagnosis:* Partial traumatic infarction of the spleen (shown in Figures A and B). The infarction was made complete by intimal dissection due to overzealous manipulation of the catheter in the procedure.

INFILTRATIVE DISORDERS AS FILLING DEFECTS

The angiographic demonstration of infiltrative disorders depend on the nature and extent of involvement of the parenchyma of an organ. They are dependent on whether the infiltration is *discrete* (either focal or multifocal) or *diffuse*. Unlike the expansile cystic masses, infiltrative deposits are incapable of developing a wall around themselves. Therefore, they may acquire discrete, regular, or irregular margins, indistinct margins, or no margins at all if they have a permeative behavior. When there is complete replacement of the normal parenchyma by the infiltrative disorder, a ghost shadow of the organ is seen within its capsular confines on a scaffolding of stretched intrinsic vasculature. Common clinical examples include *lymphoma* infiltrating into the kidney,[1126, 1127] liver[1128] (Figs. 28-38 and 28-52), or spleen[1131] or *fatty infiltration* of the liver seen in alcoholic cirrhosis (Fig. 28-67). *Sarcoidosis* and other granulomatous disease may present as filling defects on an infiltrative basis[1129] (Fig. 28-70). Nonhomogeneous parenchymal defects in large spleens may be seen in any splenomegaly, as well as in those patients with lymphomatous infiltration of the splenic parenchyma. Thus certain reservations should be made when this diagnosis is attempted angiographically.[1130]

MALIGNANT NEOPLASMS

If an infiltrating primary malignant neoplasm totally occludes its own blood supply, it may present as lucent mass with irregular or regular borders and with or without sharp margination from the well-stained adjacent parenchyma (Figs. 28-45, 28-46, 28-58 and 28-69). The same appearance may be given by some metastatic lesions which are incapable of eliciting a neovascular response from the host parenchyma[1438, 1439] (Figs. 28-50 and 28-51). On rare occasions infiltration of an organ by an adjacent extrinsic malignant lesion may give rise to lucent, irregular filling defects of the invaded organ.[913]

Technical errors such as nonopacification of the peripheral tumor vasculature of a necrotic tumor or insufficient amount of contrast injected, or severe tamponade within the tumor parenchyma, may give the existing tumor the appearance of a lucent defect with irregular, nondescript margins (Figs. 28-47 and 28-48).

VASCULAR VARIATIONS

It is a common observation to notice clear-cut filling defects, having sharp interfaces with the adjacent parenchyma during selective catheterization. These are due to variations in the origin of the vessels perfusing that particular segment of the parenchyma. The realization of this fact will aid in avoiding an incorrect diagnosis. The classic example is during *renal angiography* when the kidney has two separate arterial supplies. If one is injected, the area of parenchyma supplied by the second artery will have a relatively lucent appearance and present as a filling defect. A similar occurrence may take place within the *liver* where a dual arterial supply is not uncommon. Because of its large volume, however, this finding is less readily recognized in the liver.

TRANSIENT FILLING DEFECTS—FUNCTIONAL

These small, patchy filling defects of variable size and number are usually seen in the renal cortical area. They may be due to transient ischemia from the induced catheter stress (catheter bitten kidney?). Recognition of this possible cause suggests a second study which usually reveals partial or complete disappearance of these lesions, further delineating their transient nature. An extreme condition of such a situation may be seen when there is functional intrarenal redistribution of blood, causing complete cessation of perfusion of the outer two thirds of the renal cortex. This may be the result of regional or general stressful clinical situations[265, 1133] (Figs. 28-62 to 28-63).

FILLING DEFECTS—SUMMARY

1. Thin-walled, well-defined defects with sharp interface against adjacent parenchy-

(*Text continues on page 545*)

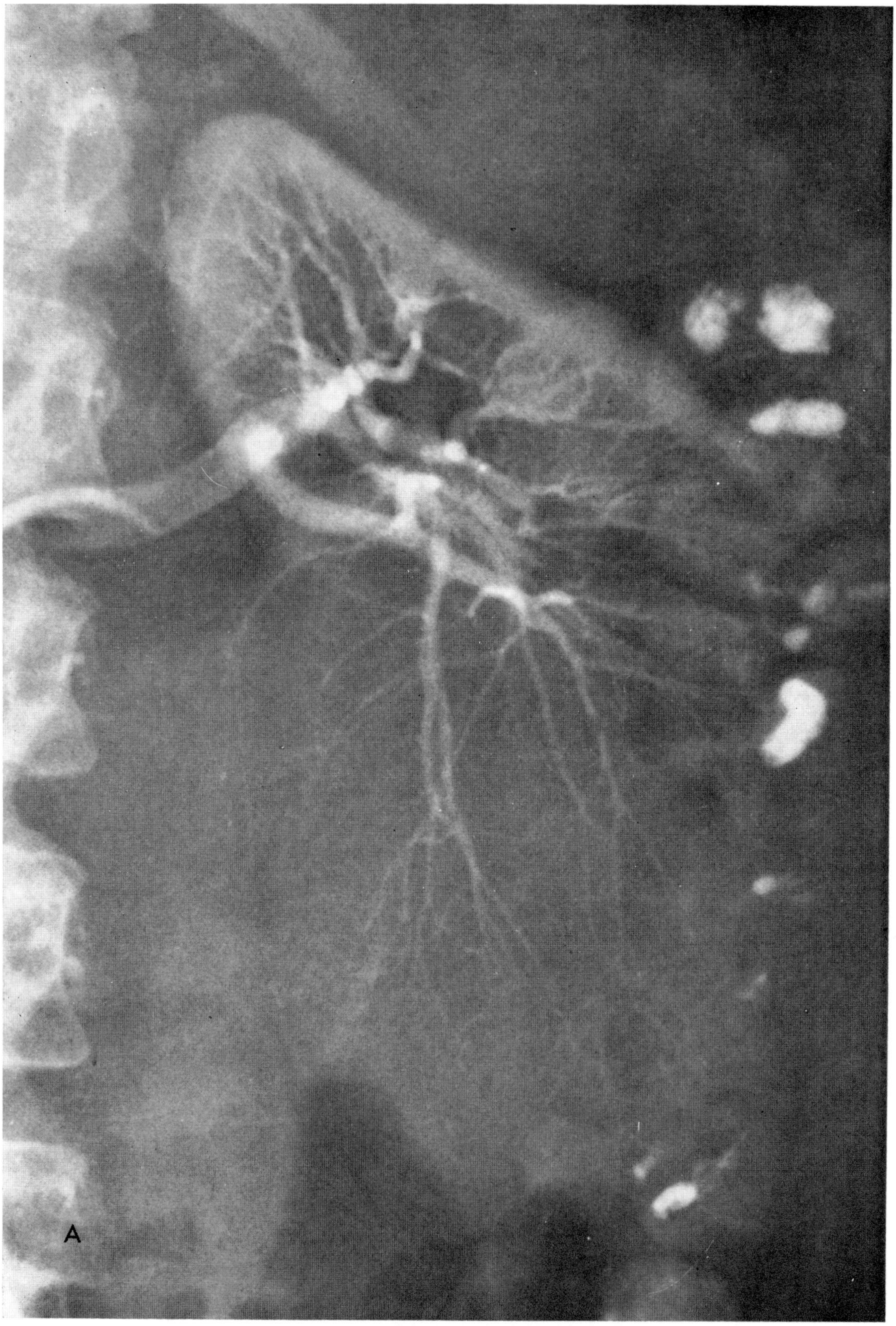

Figure 28.38 A

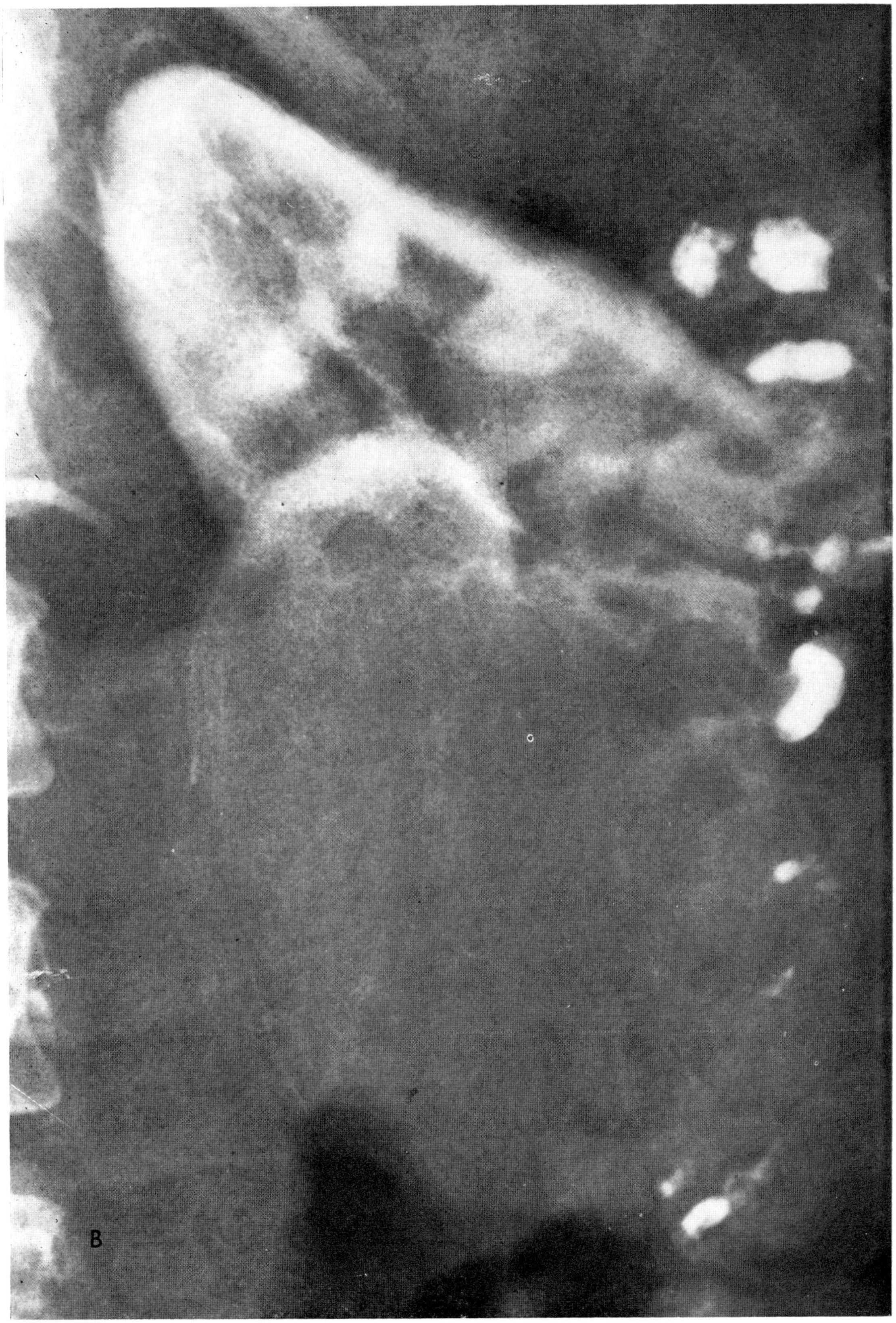

Figure 28.38. Renal Arteriogram. (A) Arterial phase: Stretched and thinned intrarenal branches are in the lower half of the kidney. Barium in the colon is noted. (B) Nephrographic phase: There is a lack of nephrogram in the lower half of the kidney. *Diagnosis:* Infiltrative disorder of the kidney, such as lymphoma, metastases or infiltrating primary tumor of the kidney. *Pathology:* Lymphoma.

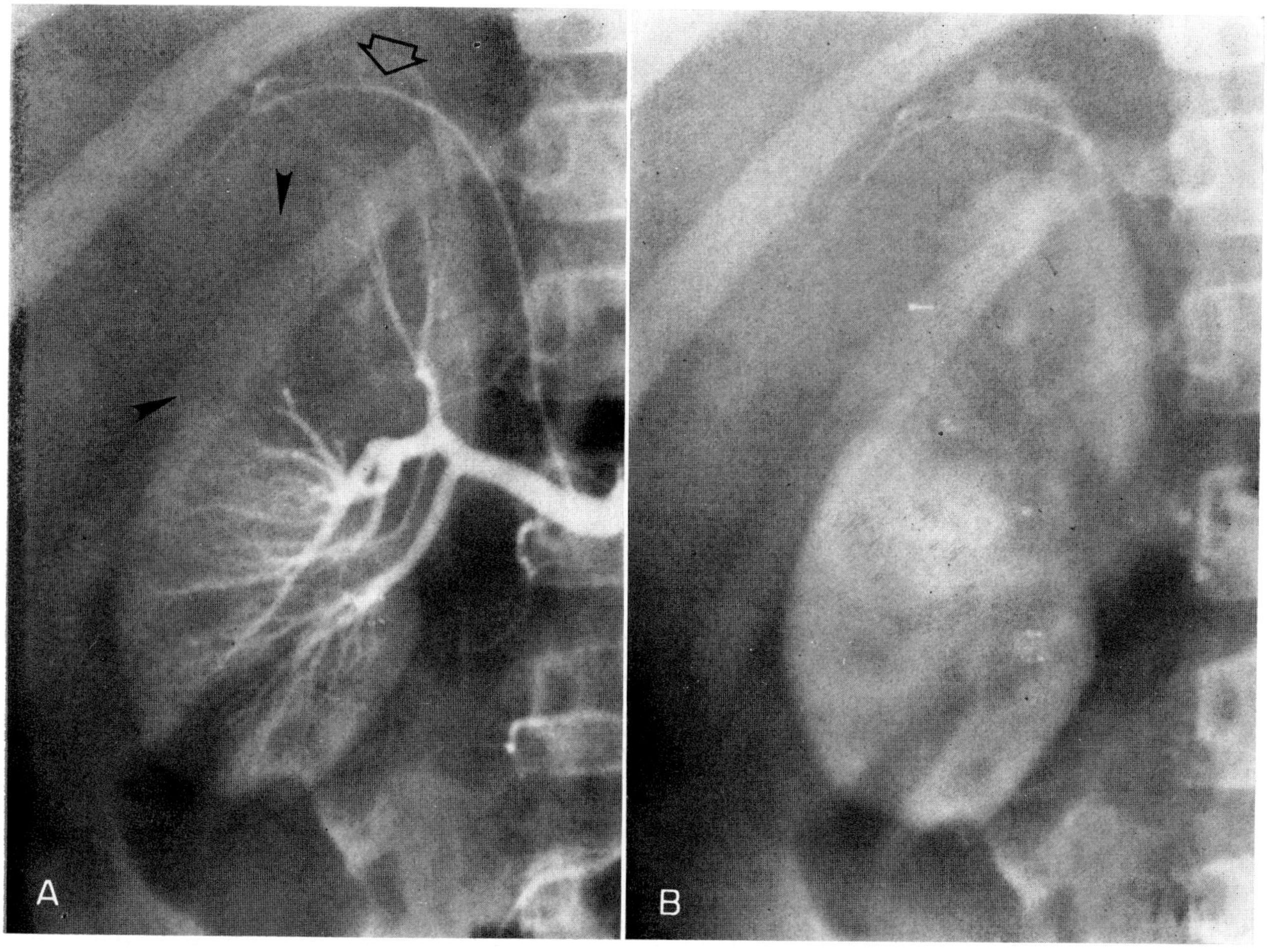

Figure 28.39. Renal Arteriogram. (A) Arterial phase: A filling defect is in the midportion of the kidney (Arrow Head). A stretched and deviated renal capsular artery (Arrow). (B) Parenchymal phase: The same filling defect is well shown extending from the medial to the lateral border at the same location in the kidney. The patient had left flank trauma. *Diagnosis:* Renal laceration with intrarenal and perirenal hematoma.

Figure 28.40. Renal Arteriogram. (A) Early arterial phase: There is lack of arterial perfusion in the midportion of the kidney (Arrow) and abrupt termination of an intrarenal branch (Arrow Head). (B) Parenchymal phase: A well-defined filling defect is seen (Arrow). This patient had penetrating trauma to the left flank. (C) A repeat arteriogram after six months again reveals slight stretching of intrarenal branches with lack of arterial perfusion in the same area. (D) The filling defect is not very obvious. There is a depression in the renal parenchymal contour. *Diagnosis:* Posttraumatic laceration of the intrarenal branch with intrarenal hematoma and infarct. Follow-up films reveals gradual shrinkage and fibrosis.

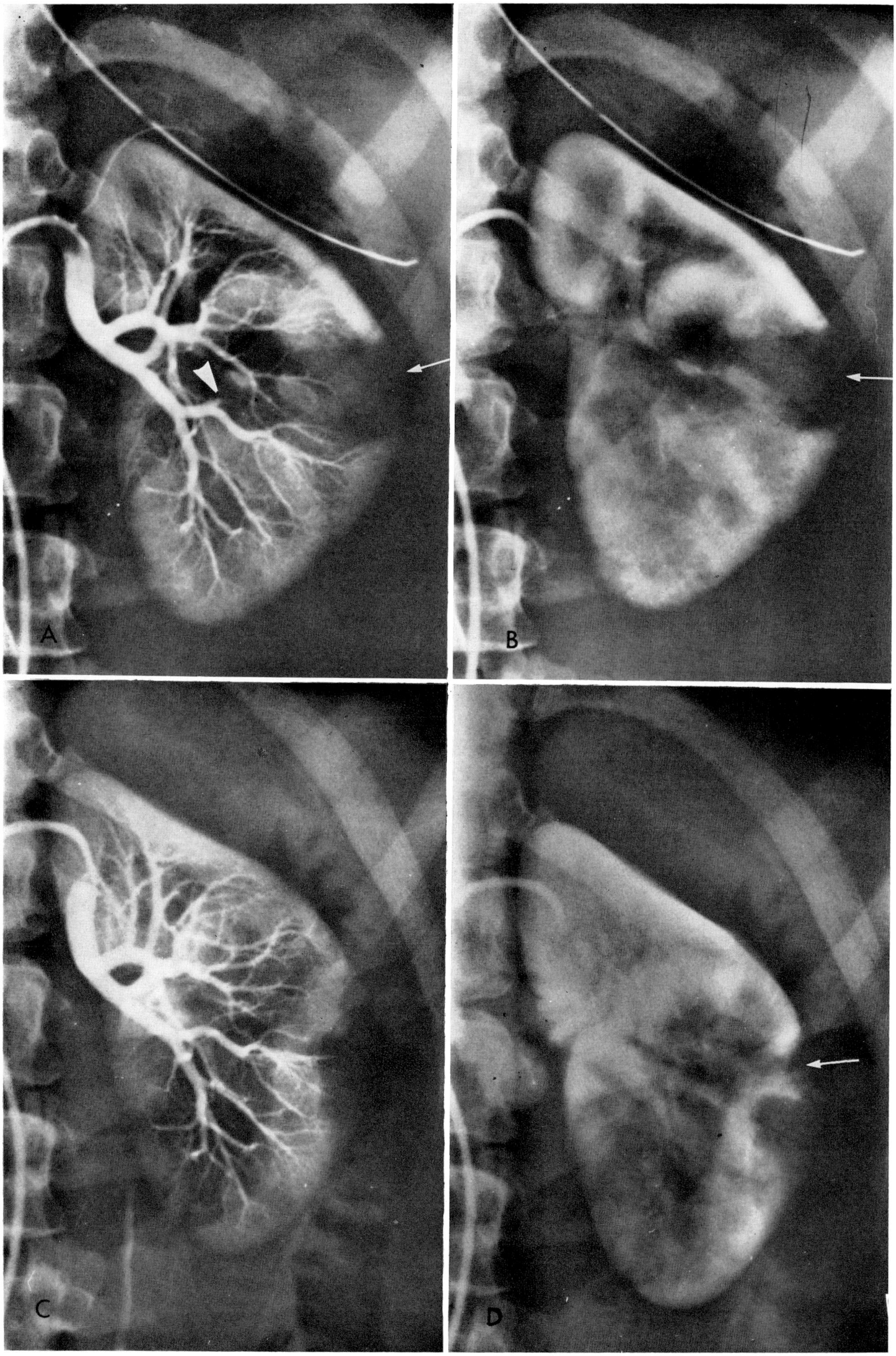
A
B
C
D

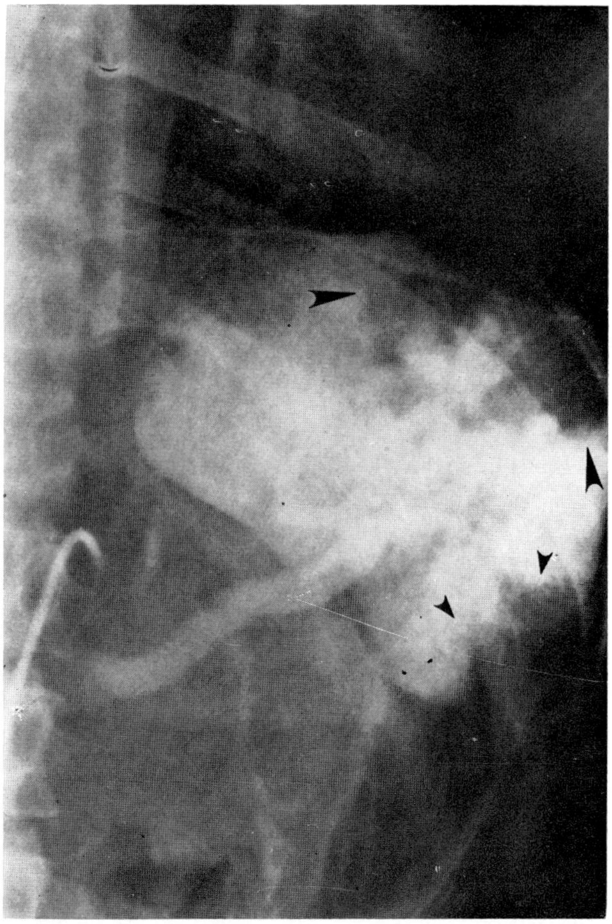

Figure 28.41. Celiac Arteriogram—venous phase. Wedge-shaped filling defects (Arrow) are seen in the spleen. The patient had an automobile accident. *Differential Diagnosis:* Splenic laceration (most likely) or splenic infarcts. *Pathology:* Splenic lacerations with hematomas.

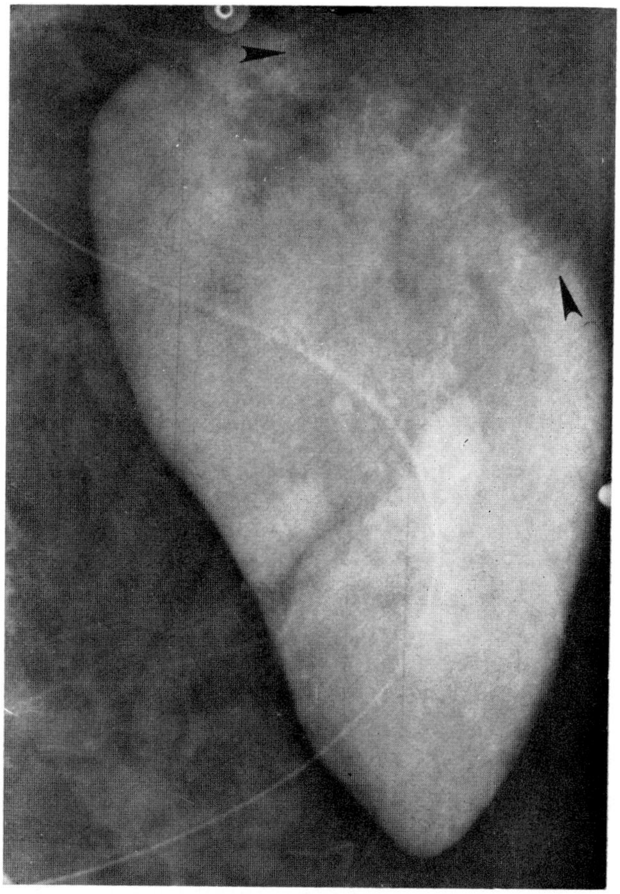

Figure 28.42. Splenic Arteriogram—venous phase. Peripheral irregularities and filling defects are seen in this enlarged spleen. The patient had portal hypertension. *Diagnosis:* Splenic infarcts.

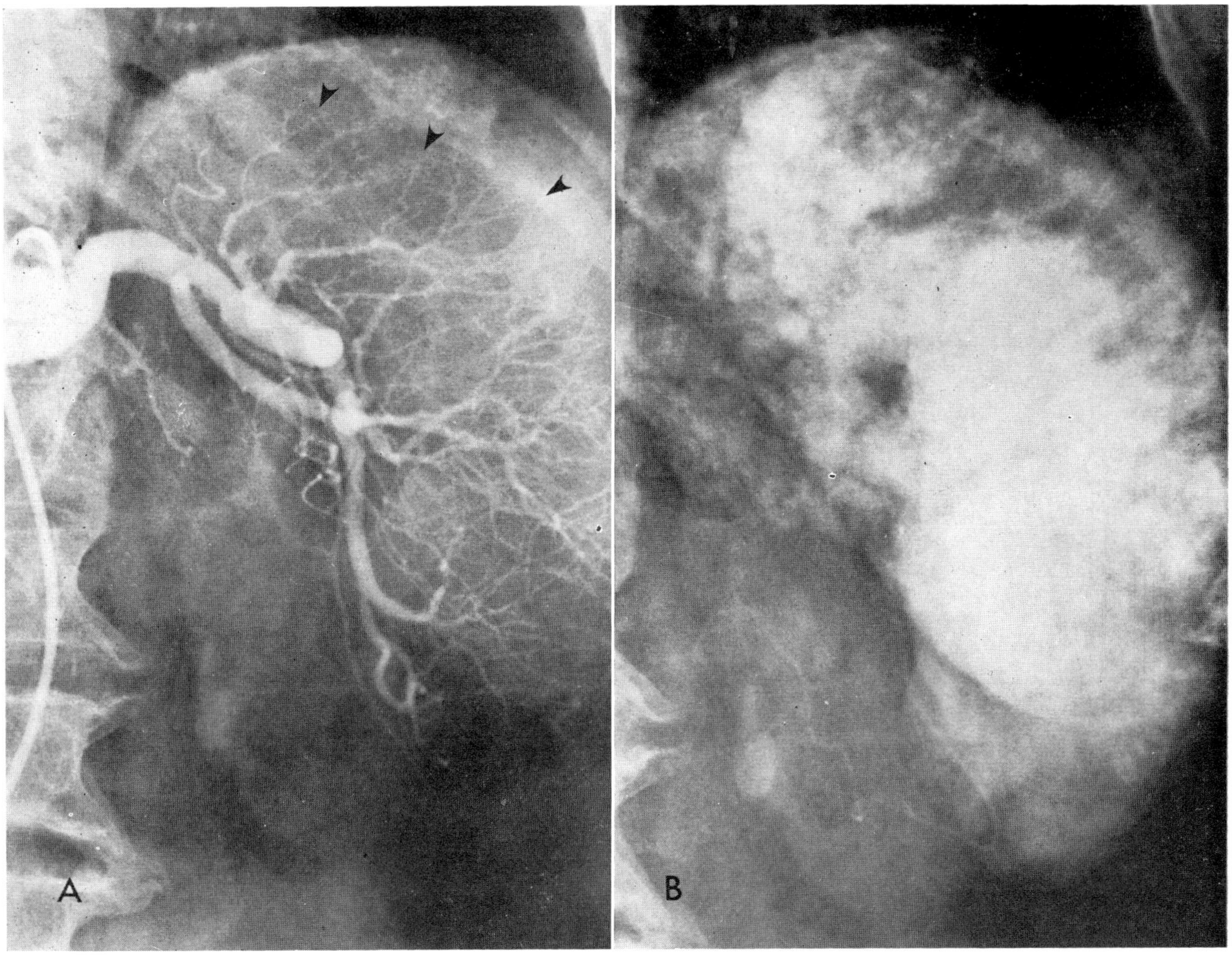

Figure 28.43. Splenic Arteriogram. (A) There is stretching of the intrasplenic branches, and abrupt termination of the stretched vessels (Arrow). (B) There are irregular peripheral filling defects. The patient had portal hypertension. *Diagnosis:* Splenomegaly with multiple infarcts.

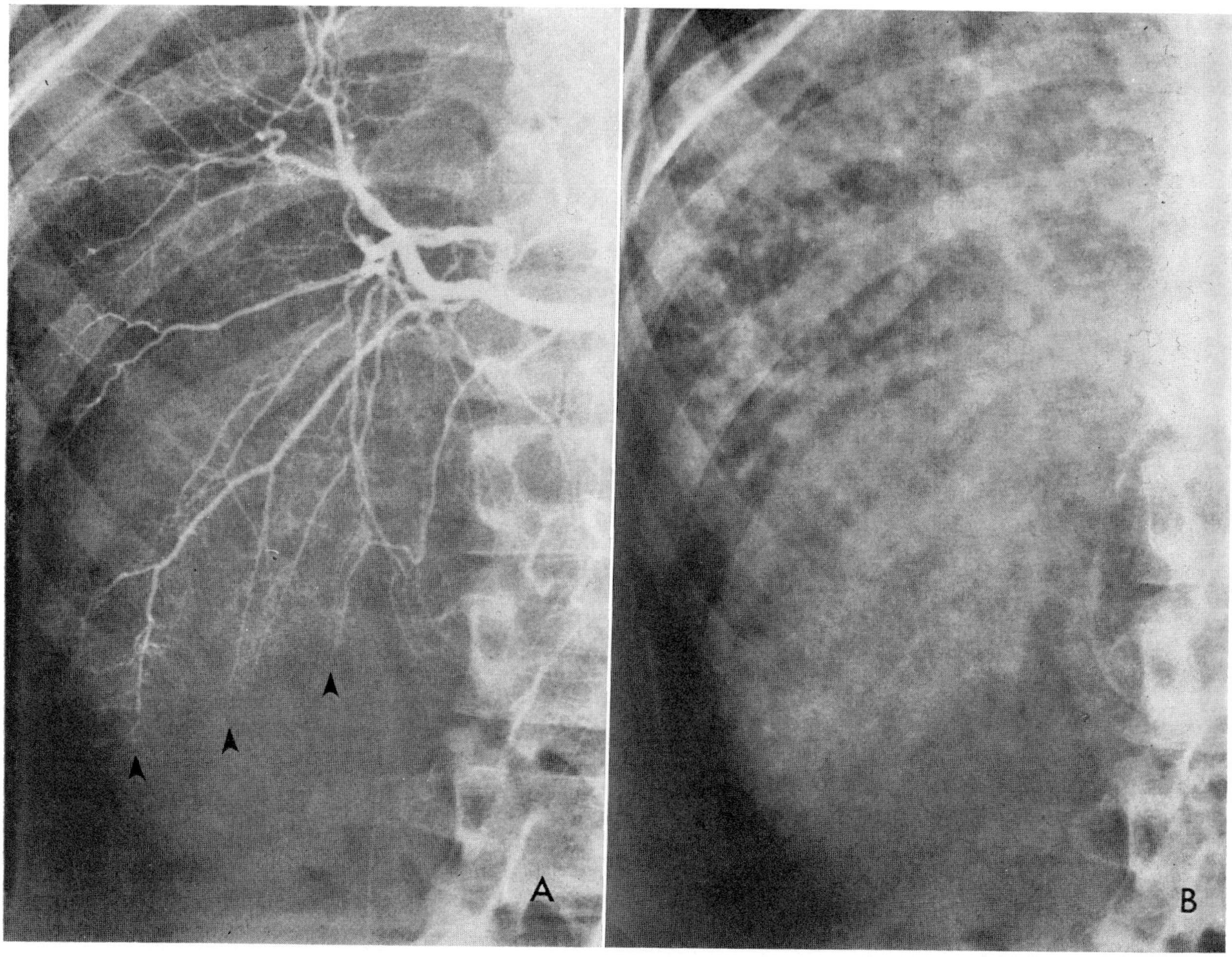

Figure 28.44. Hepatic Arteriogram. (A) There is stretching and abrupt termination of the intrahepatic branches (Arrow). (B) The lower edge of the right lobe of the liver is poorly defined with absent hepatogram. Note the irregular filling defects in the upper portion of the liver. The patient fell from the second story of a building. *Diagnosis:* Contusion of the lower portion of the liver. This was confirmed at autopsy. In addition, fatty infiltration of the liver was found.

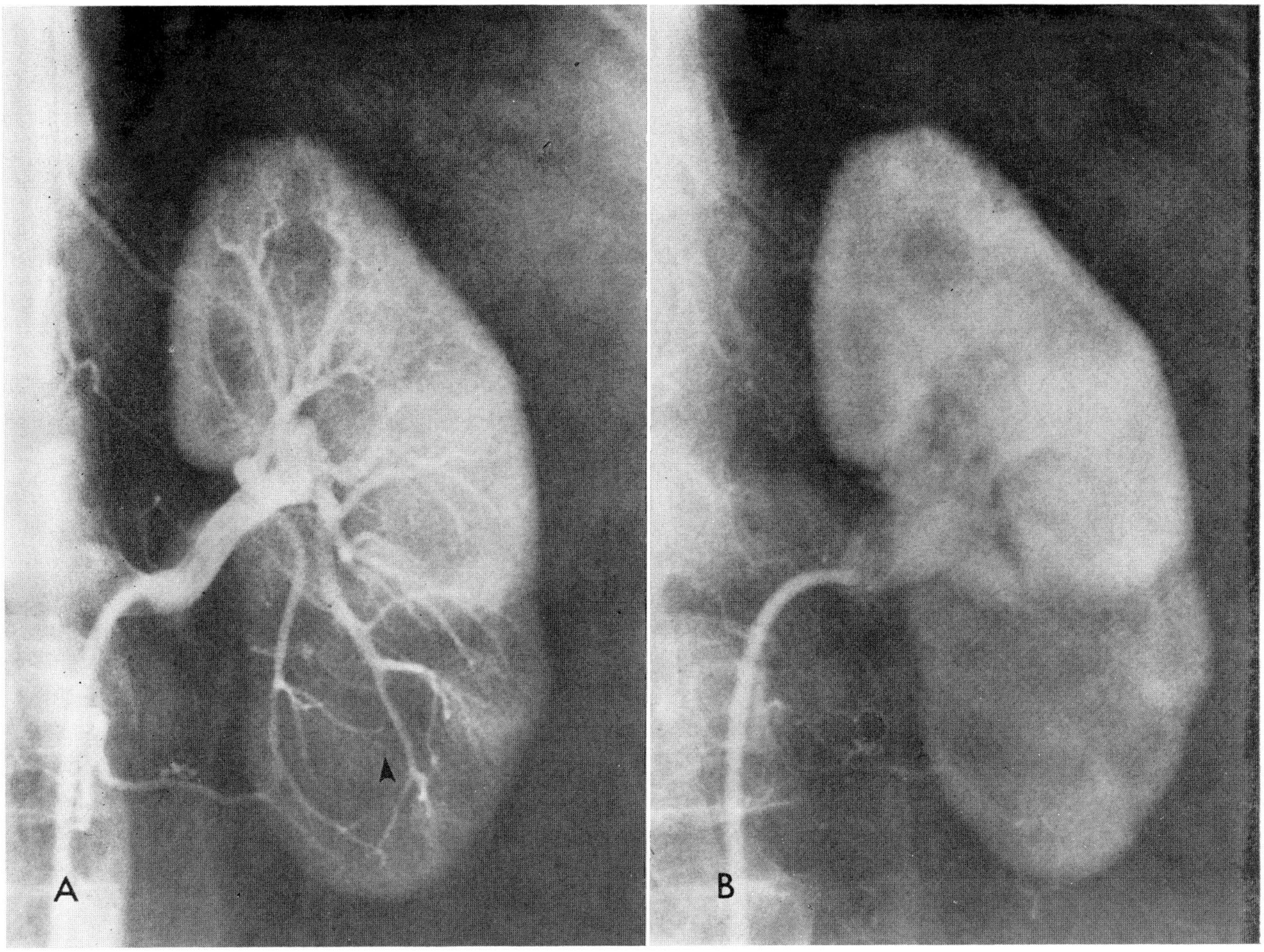

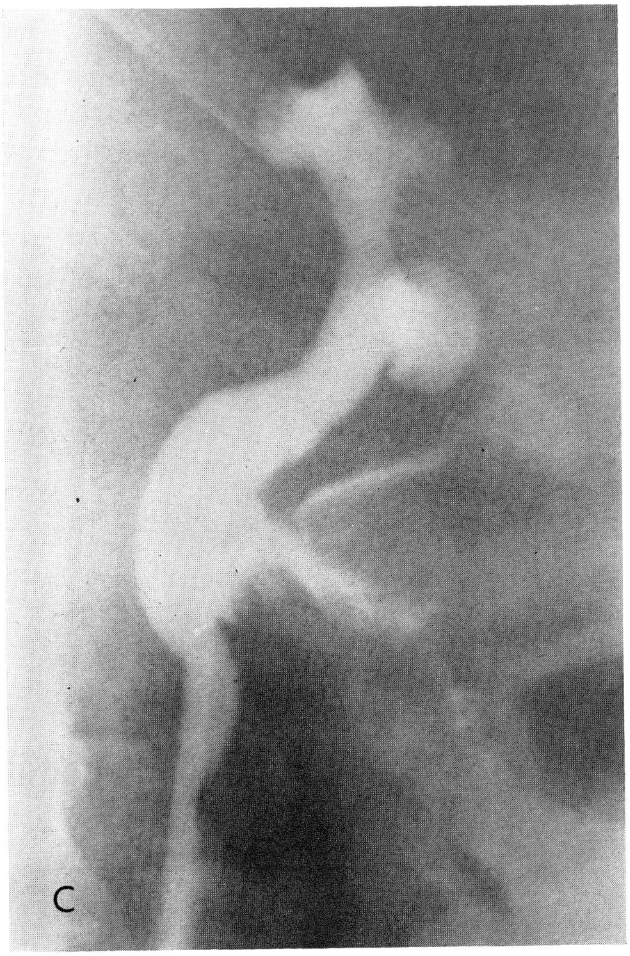

Figure 28.45. (A) Arterial phase reveals stretching and deviation of the intrarenal vessels in its lower half. There are occlusions of some of the small branches seen (Arrow). (B) Parenchymal phase reveals a well-defined filling defect in the same portion with irregular borders. (C) Retrograde pyelogram reveals destruction of the lower half of the calyces. *Diagnosis:* Transitional cell carcinoma. Differential diagnosis on the basis of angiography only: metastasis, lymphoma, abscess, granuloma. (Courtesy of Dr. Himmat T. Shah, Radiologist, Michael Reese Medical Center, Chicago.)

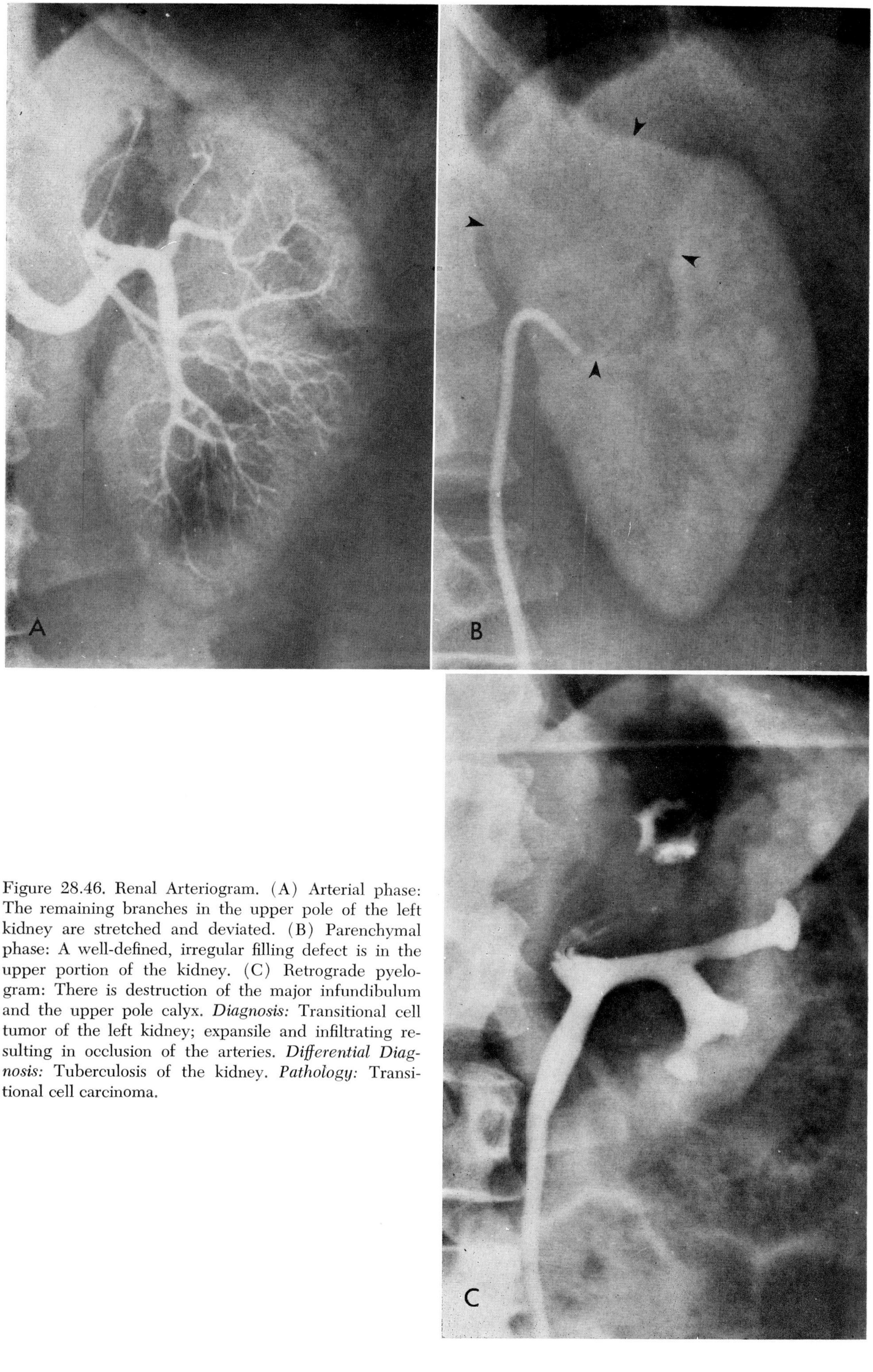

Figure 28.46. Renal Arteriogram. (A) Arterial phase: The remaining branches in the upper pole of the left kidney are stretched and deviated. (B) Parenchymal phase: A well-defined, irregular filling defect is in the upper portion of the kidney. (C) Retrograde pyelogram: There is destruction of the major infundibulum and the upper pole calyx. *Diagnosis:* Transitional cell tumor of the left kidney; expansile and infiltrating resulting in occlusion of the arteries. *Differential Diagnosis:* Tuberculosis of the kidney. *Pathology:* Transitional cell carcinoma.

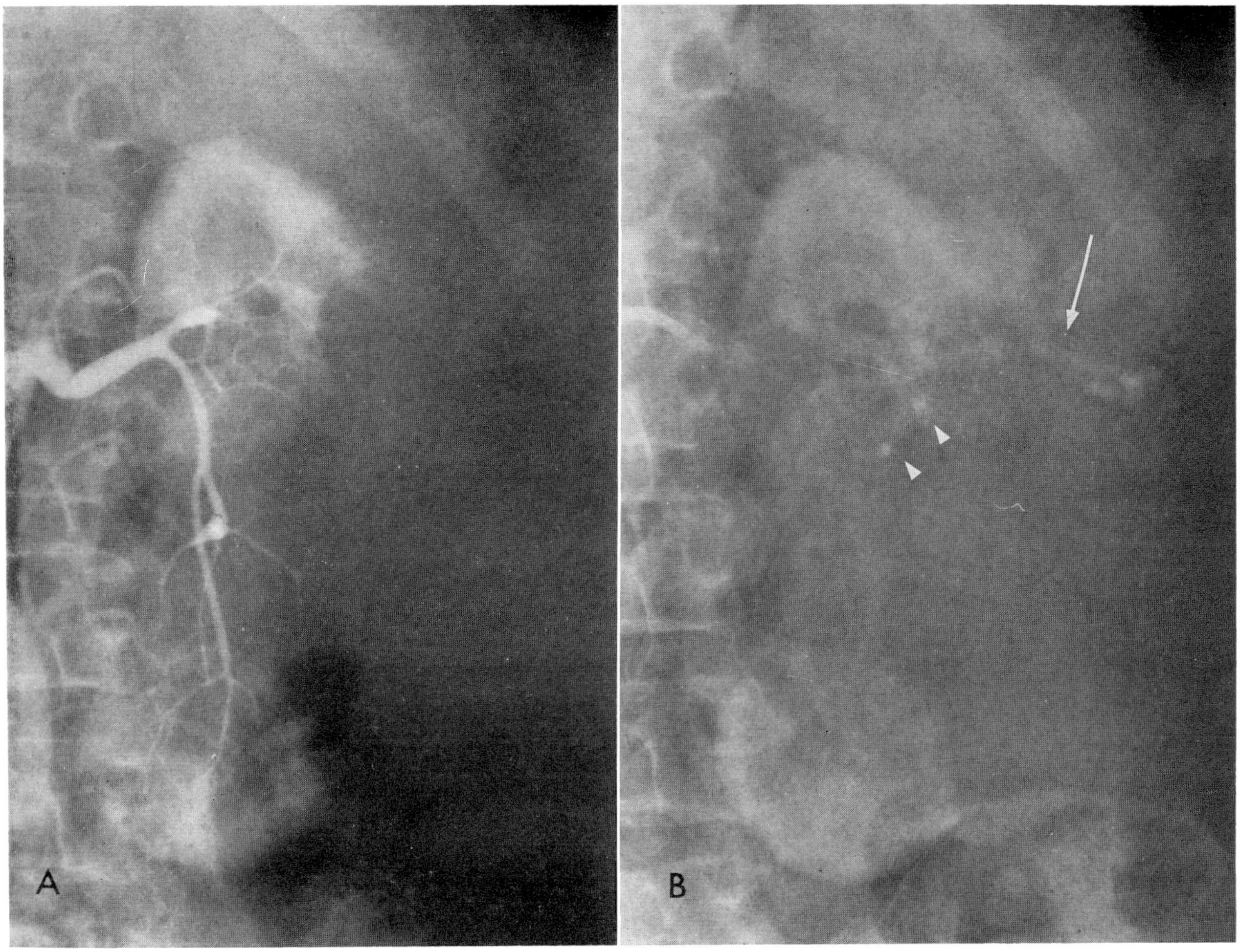

Figure 28.47. Renal Arteriogram. (A) Arterial phase: Note the stretching and deviation of the sparse intrarenal branches in the midportion of the kidney with lack of perfusion of the parenchyma. (B) Parenchymal phase: An irregular filling defect with no sharp interface with the renal parenchyma is seen. Abnormally dilated veins course from the periphery of the mass towards the renal hilus (Arrow). Two small areas of abnormal collection of contrast material can be seen (Arrow Head). *Diagnosis:* Necrotic hypernephroma with tumor sinusoids. *Differential Diagnosis:* Intrarenal hematoma with perinephric extension and extravasation of contrast material. *Pathology:* Necrotic hypernephroma.

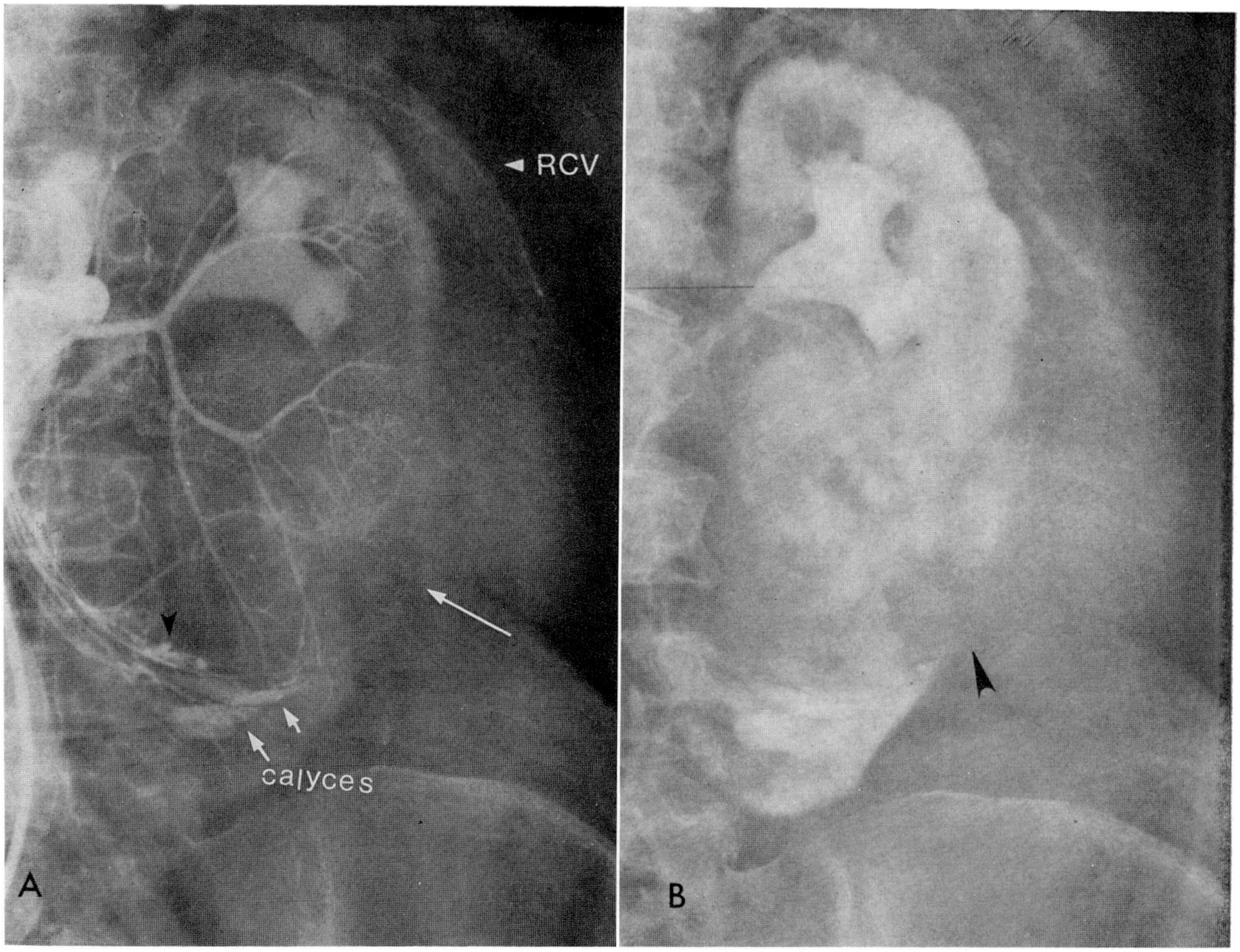

Figure 28.48. Renal Arteriogram. (A) Early arterial phase: Stretching and deviation of the renal hilar as well as intrarenal branches is seen with an abnormal amorphous collection of contrast material (Arrow Head). The left midrenal border is not clearly visualized (Arrow). The renal capsular vessel (R.C.V.) is stretched. (B) Parenchymal phase: A huge filling defect is in the midportion of the kidney splitting the kidney with perinephric extension. An irregular filling defect is noted at the lower portion of the renal contour with no cortex (Arrow). This patient developed a left flank mass of recent origin. *Diagnosis:* Hypernephroma with intrarenal as well as perirenal bleeding. *Differential Diagnosis:* Traumatic intrarenal hematoma and perirenal hematoma with extravasation of the contrast material.

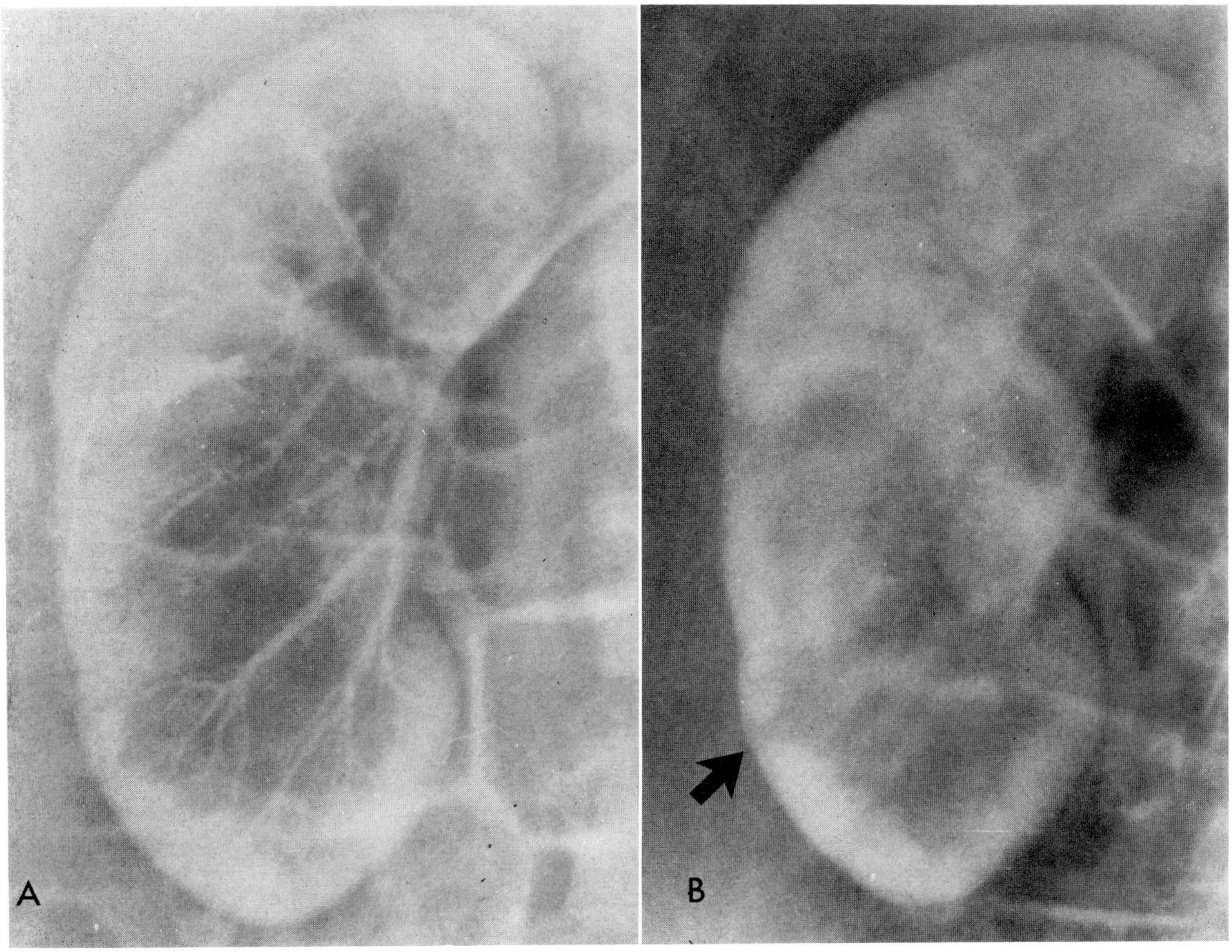

Figure 28.49. Renal Arteriogram. (A) Arterial phase: Slight sparsity of the vessels in the lower pole of the kidney is noted. (B) Late phase: A filling defect is seen in the intramedullary portion of the lower pole of the kidney. Notice the absence of cortical invagination into the medulla and absence of the cortex in the same area. A patient with flank pain and fever. *Diagnosis:* Filling defect due to intrarenal abscess.

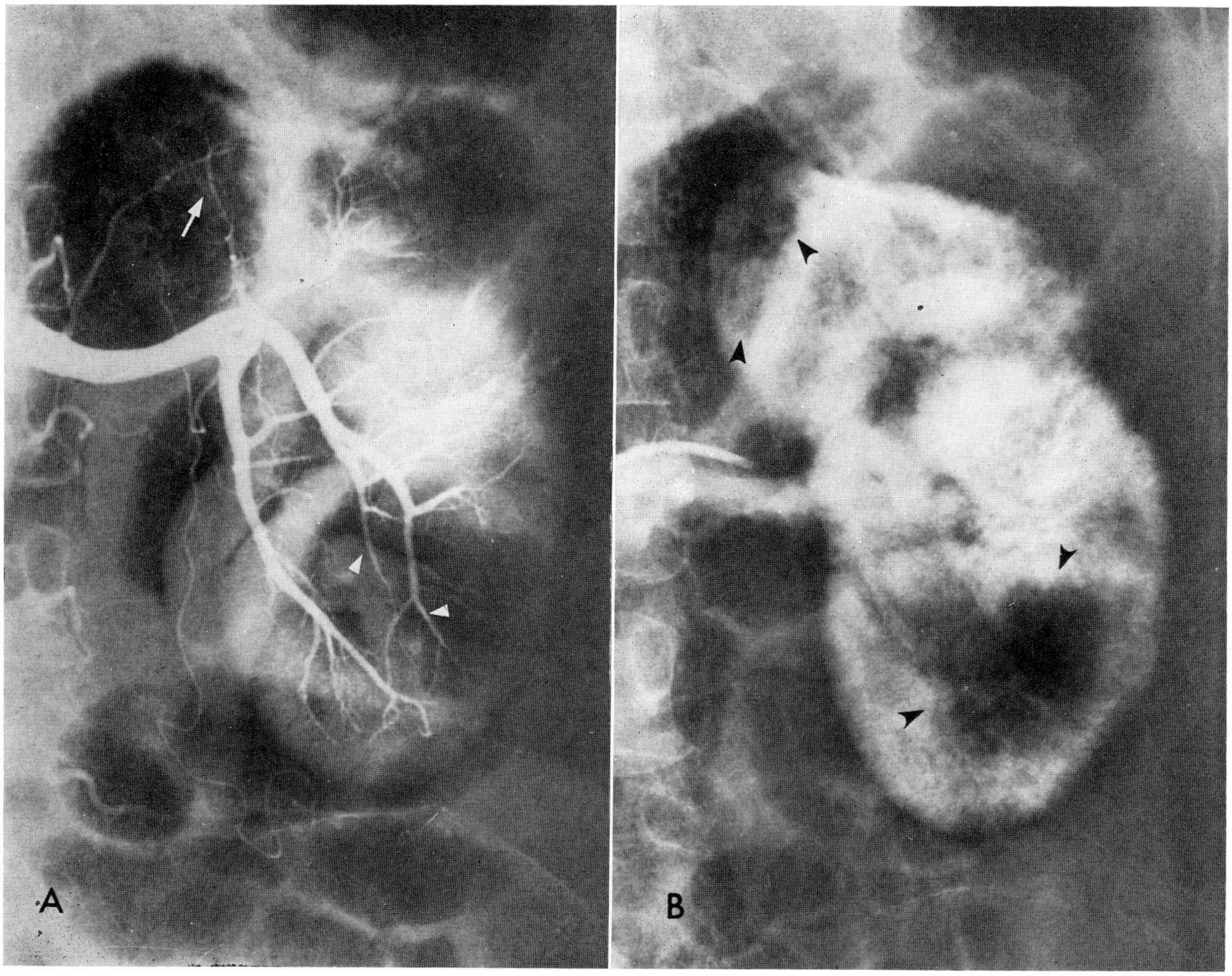

Figure 28.50. Renal Arteriogram. (A) Increased renal size, stretching of the intrarenal arterial branches and smooth narrowing of some of the intrarenal arterial branches with abrupt tapering can be seen. (B) Parenchymal phase: There are multiple irregular filling defects without sharp interface with renal parenchyma. *Differential Diagnosis:* Multiple metastatic lesions to the kidney, or infiltrative diseases such as lymphoma, or multiple abscesses. *Pathology:* Metastatic lesions to the kidney from anaplastic carcinoma from an unknown primary site.

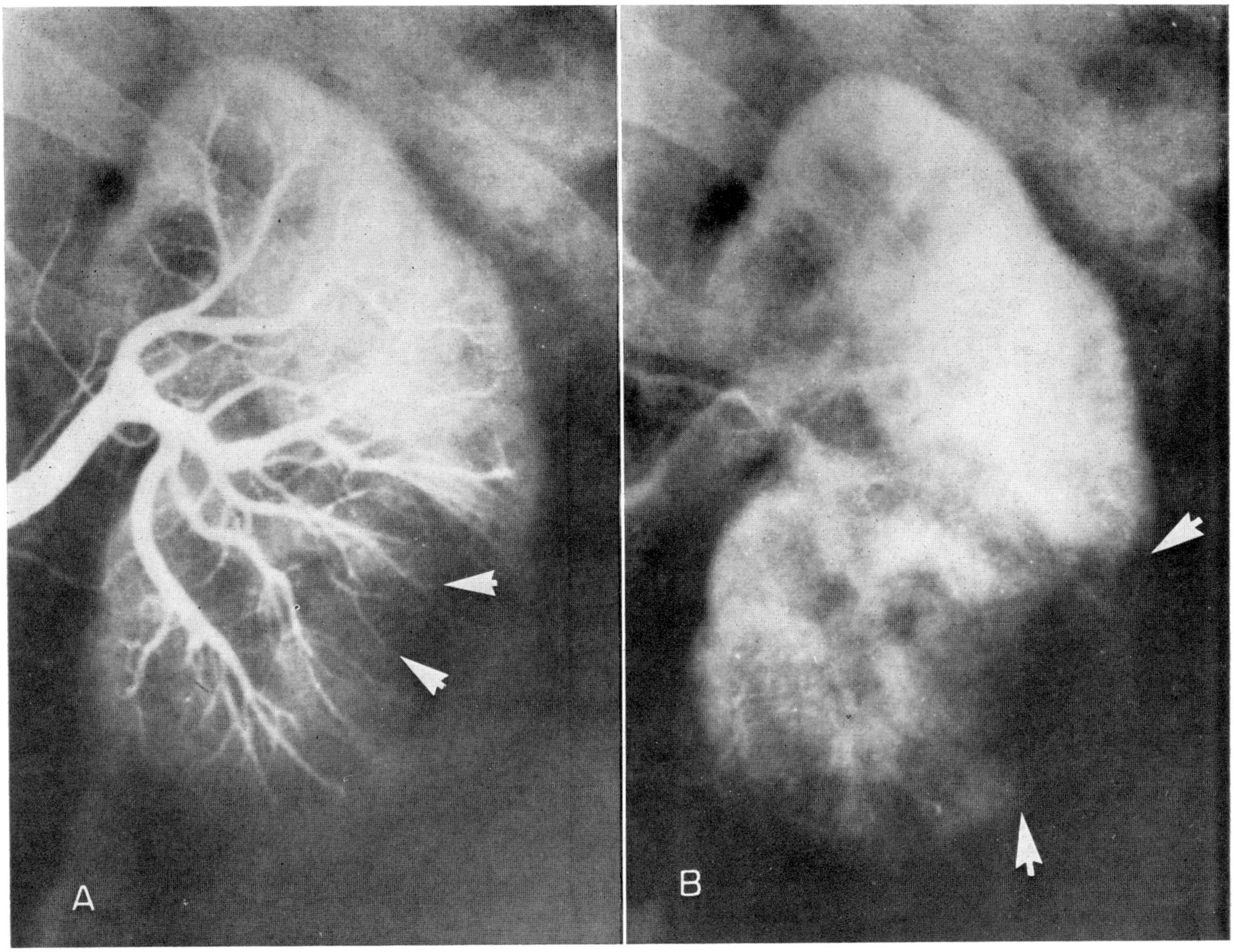

Figure 28.51. Renal Arteriogram. (A) The early phase reveals sparsity of peripheral small vessels in the mid-portion of the kidney. There is occlusion of some of these branches (Arrow Heads). (B) The late phase reveals a nondescript filling defect without sharp margination (Arrow Heads) in a patient who had a squamous cell carcinoma. *Diagnosis:* Metastasis. *Pathology:* Metastasis.

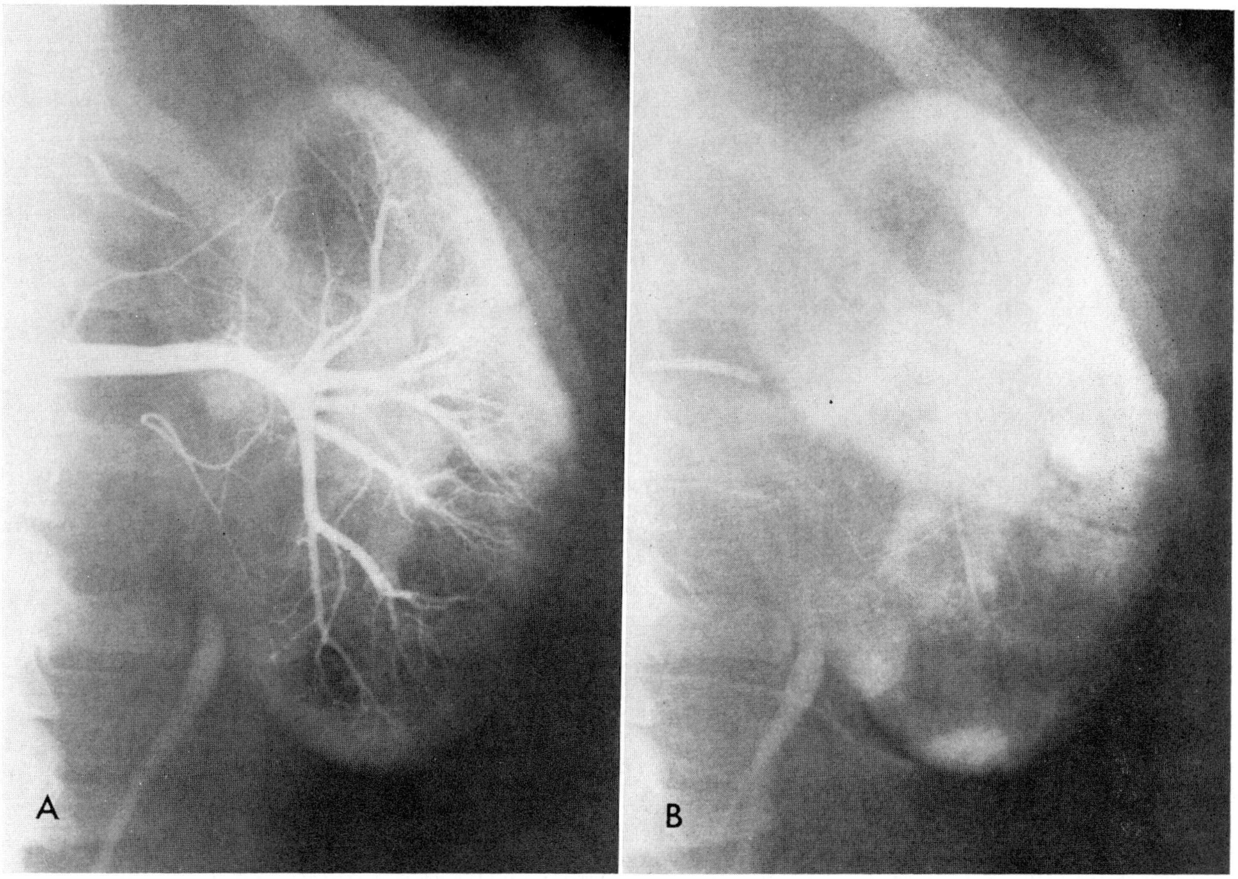

Figure 28.52. Renal Arteriogram. (A) Arterial phase reveals stretching of the sparse intrarenal branches. (B) Parenchymal phase reveals filling defects with irregular borders. *Diagnosis:* Metastasis, lymphoma. *Pathology:* Metastasis from an anaplastic carcinoma.

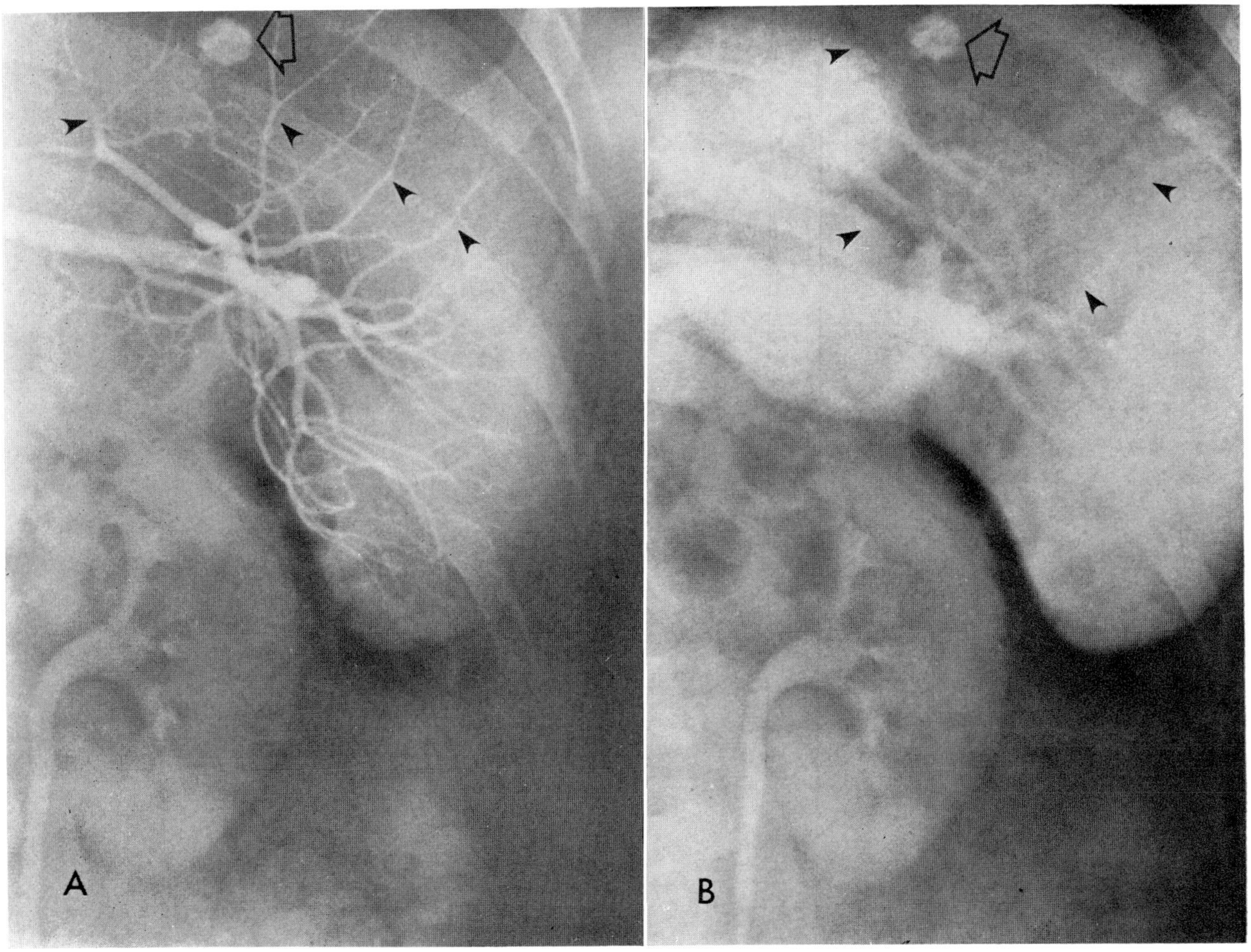

Figure 28.53. Splenic Arteriogram. (A) The intrasplenic arteries (Arrow Head) are stretched. Note an incidental calcification (Arrow). (B) There is relative lucency in the same area. The patient had a history of left upper quadrant trauma. *Radiographic Diagnosis:* Intrasplenic hematoma. *Surgical Diagnosis:* Normal spleen. *Pathologic Diagnosis:* Histiocytic granuloma of the spleen.

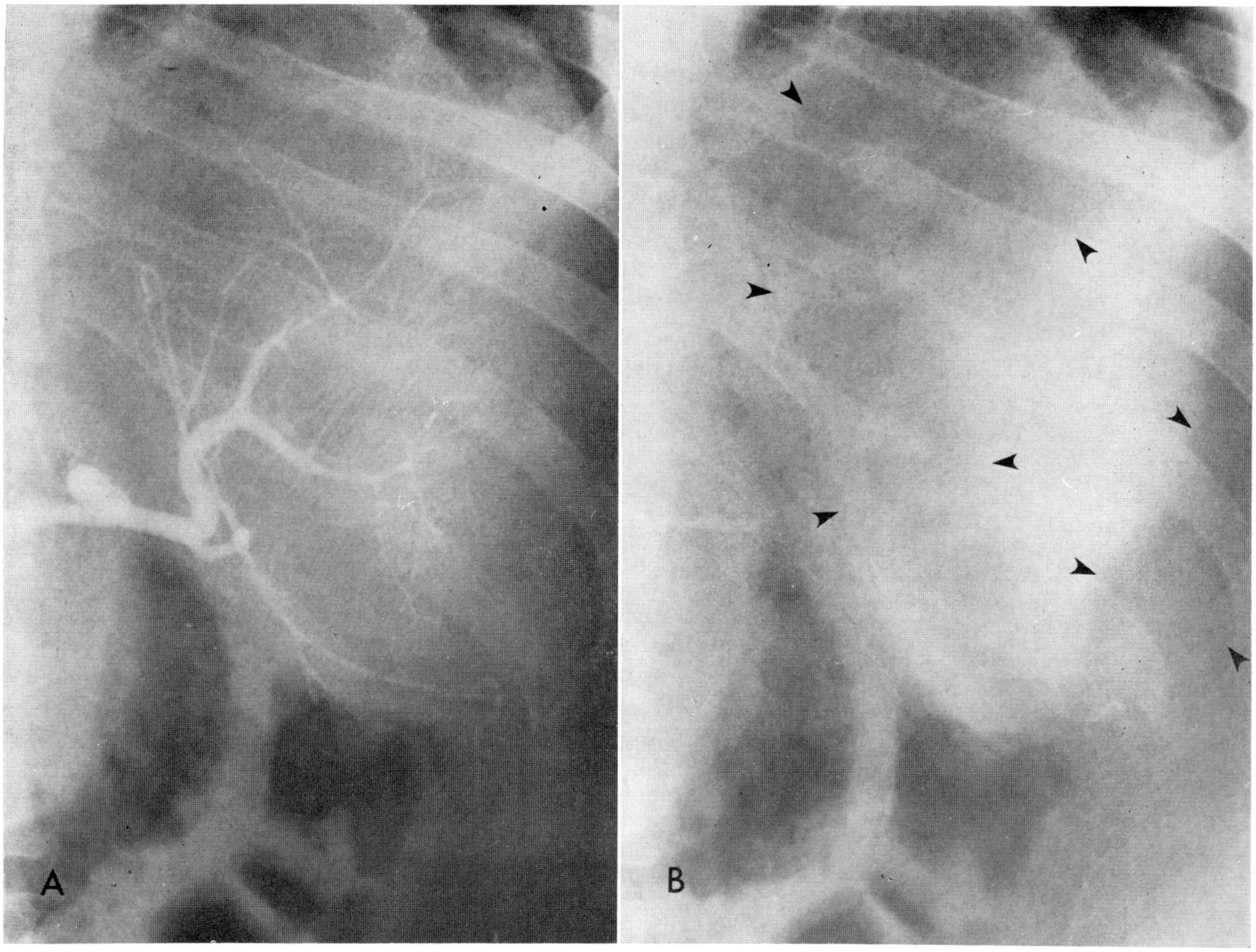

Figure 28.54. Splenic Arteriogram. (A) Arterial phase: Stretching and deviation of the intrasplenic branches in an enlarged spleen is seen. (B) Parenchymal phase: There are multiple, irregular filling defects (Arrow). This patient had trauma two weeks prior to the study. *Diagnosis:* Multiple intrasplenic hematomas.

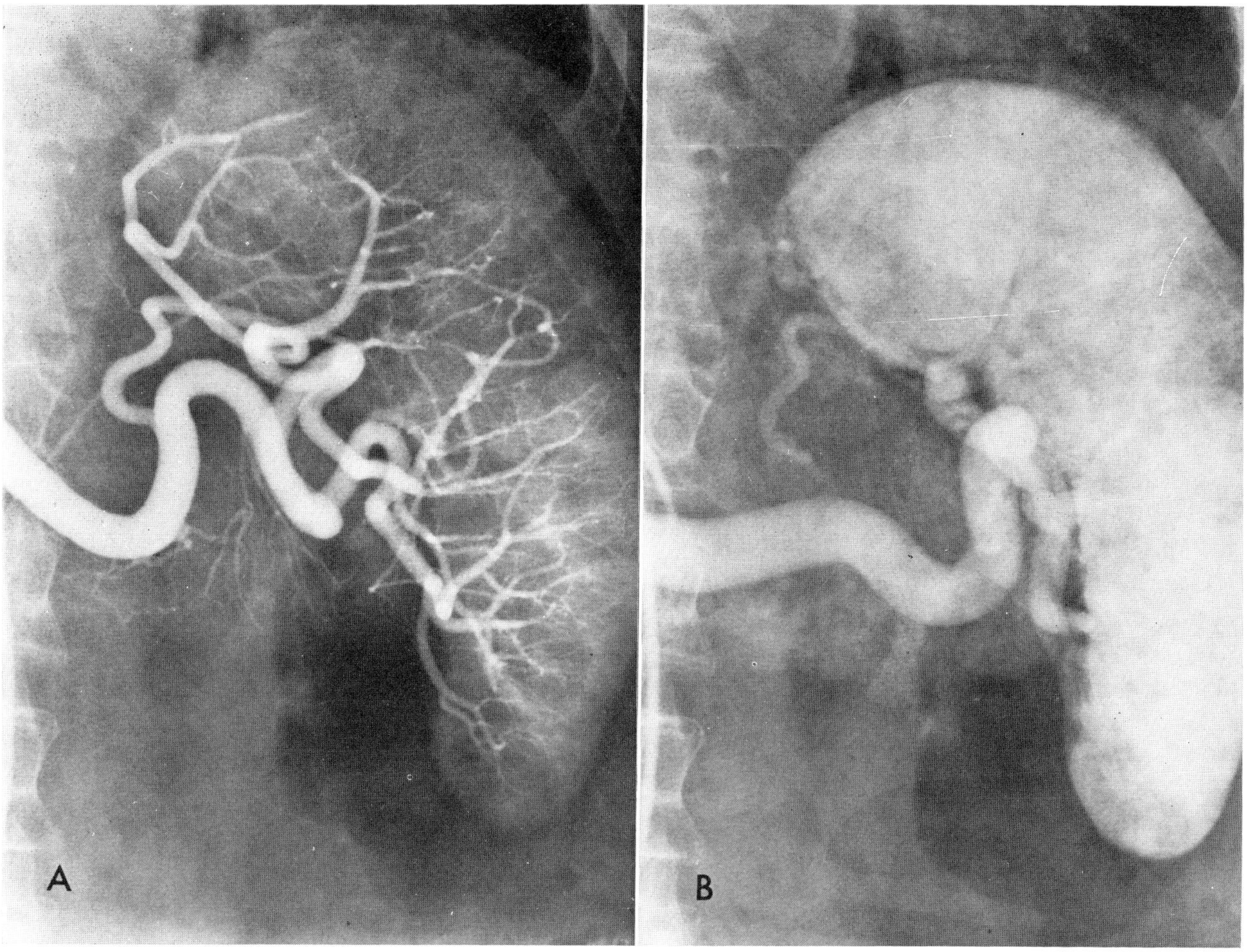

Figure 28.55. Splenic Arteriogram. (A) Arterial phase: The intrasplenic branches of this enlarged spleen are stretched. (B) Venous phase: There is nonhomogeneous opacification of the splenic parenchyma. The patient had lymphoma. *Diagnosis:* Splenomegaly with either small lymphomatous infiltrates or small infarcts. *Surgery:* Lymphoma infiltrating into the splenic parenchyma.

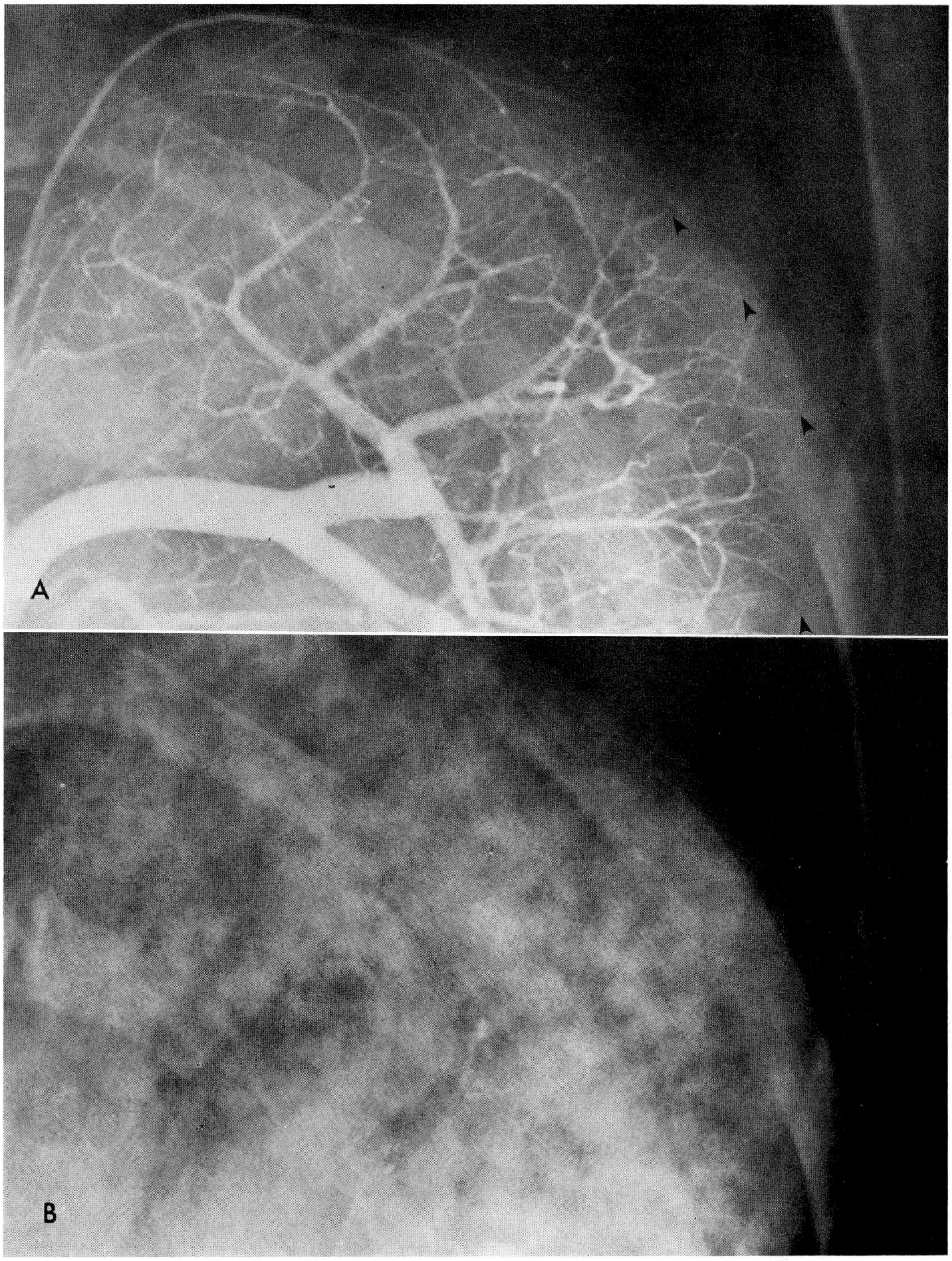

Figure 28.56. Splenic Arteriogram. (A) There is abrupt termination of the intrasplenic distal branches. (B) The parenchymal phase shows multiple, small filling defects, causing a mottled appearance. The patient had sickle-cell hemoglobinopathy. *Diagnosis:* Multiple small infarcts.

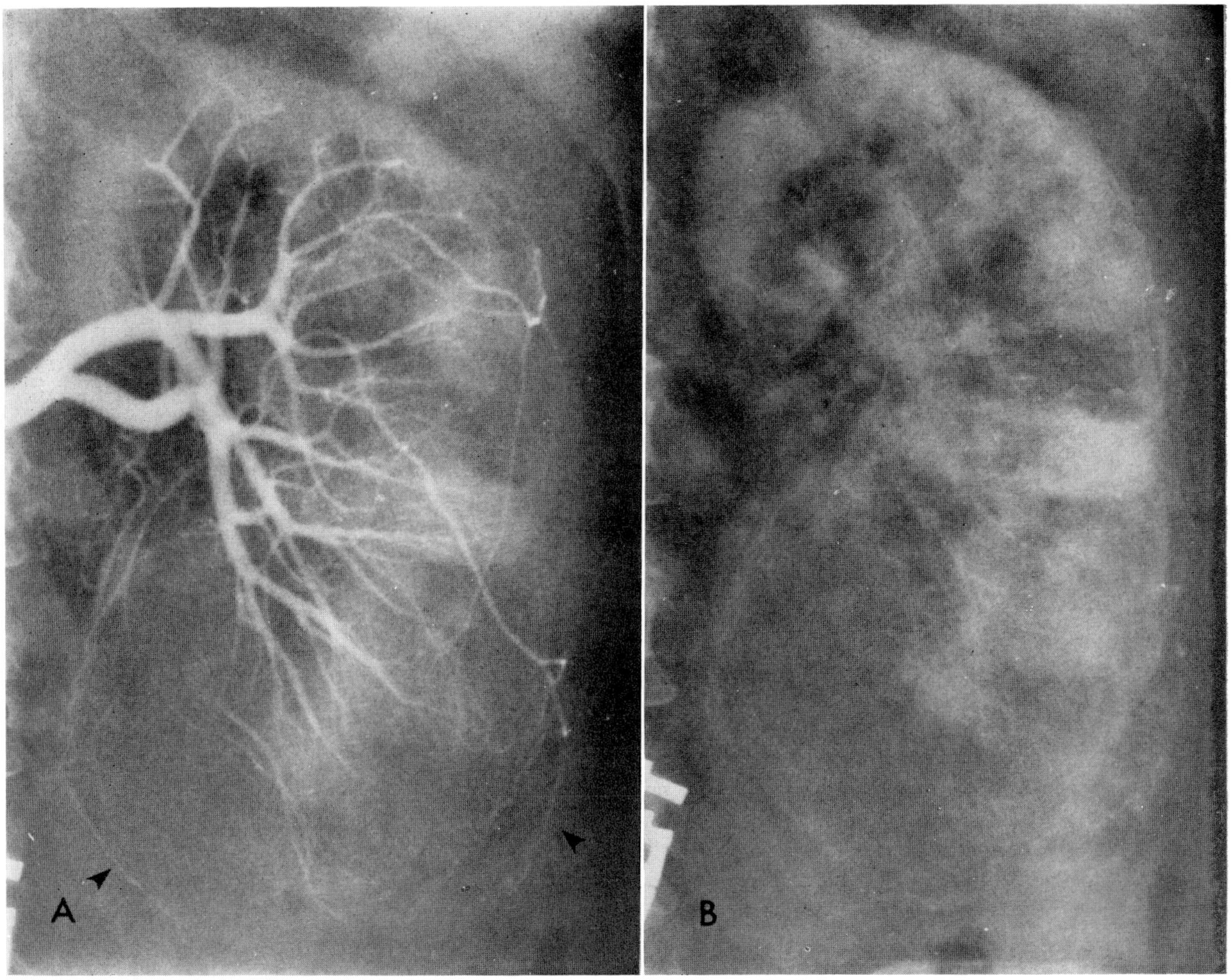

Figure 28.57. Renal Arteriogram. (A) Arterial phase: The intrarenal branches are stretched and deviated. Some of them are amputated. The perinephric circulation is increased (Arrows). (B) Parenchymal phase: Multiple, irregular filling defects of different sizes. *Diagnosis:* Multiple intrarenal abscesses.

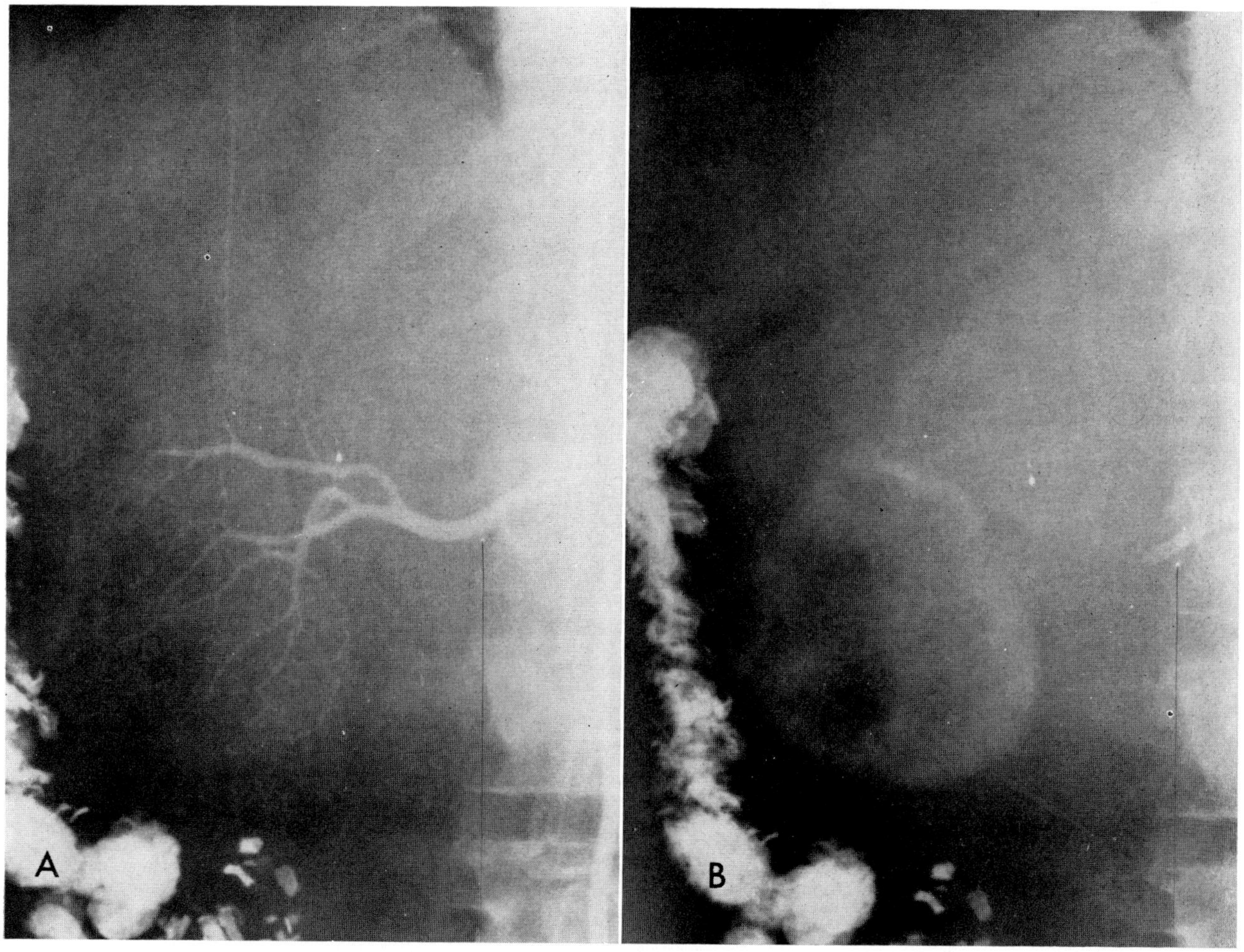

Figure 28.58. Renal Arteriogram. (A) Arterial phase: A small renal artery with stretching and thinning of the intrarenal branches is seen. Lack of perfusion of the proximal portion of the same kidney occurs. Incidental barium in the colon. (B) Parenchymal phase: Note the very poor perfusion in the proximal portion of the kidney with irregular geographic filling defect occupying almost the entire volume of the kidney. *Differential Diagnosis:* Infiltrating disorders of the kidney, lymphoma, metastases, or squamous cell carcinoma, infiltrating adenocarcinoma of the kidney, or tuberculosis. *Pathology:* Infiltrating adenocarcinoma of the kidney.

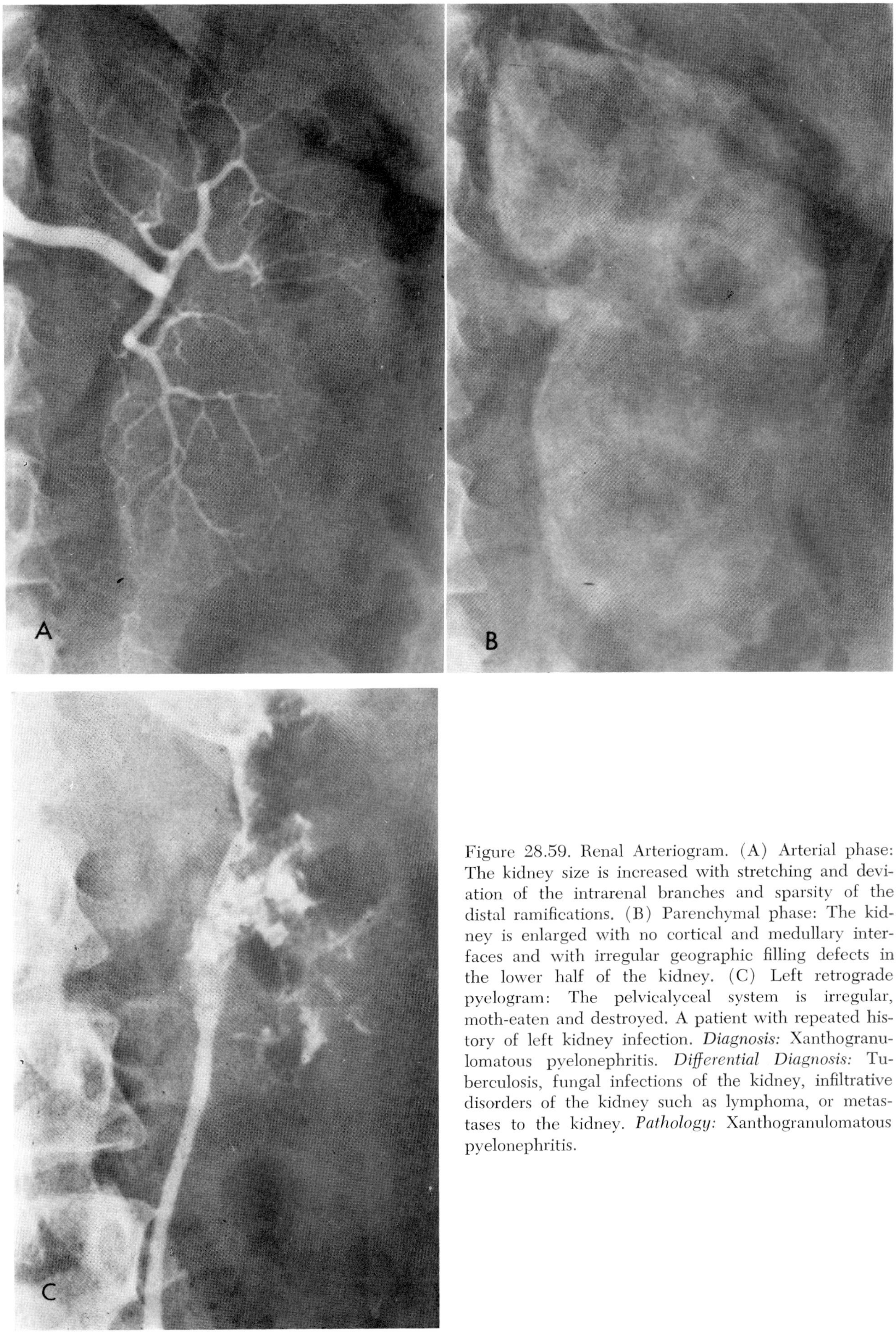

Figure 28.59. Renal Arteriogram. (A) Arterial phase: The kidney size is increased with stretching and deviation of the intrarenal branches and sparsity of the distal ramifications. (B) Parenchymal phase: The kidney is enlarged with no cortical and medullary interfaces and with irregular geographic filling defects in the lower half of the kidney. (C) Left retrograde pyelogram: The pelvicalyceal system is irregular, moth-eaten and destroyed. A patient with repeated history of left kidney infection. *Diagnosis:* Xanthogranulomatous pyelonephritis. *Differential Diagnosis:* Tuberculosis, fungal infections of the kidney, infiltrative disorders of the kidney such as lymphoma, or metastases to the kidney. *Pathology:* Xanthogranulomatous pyelonephritis.

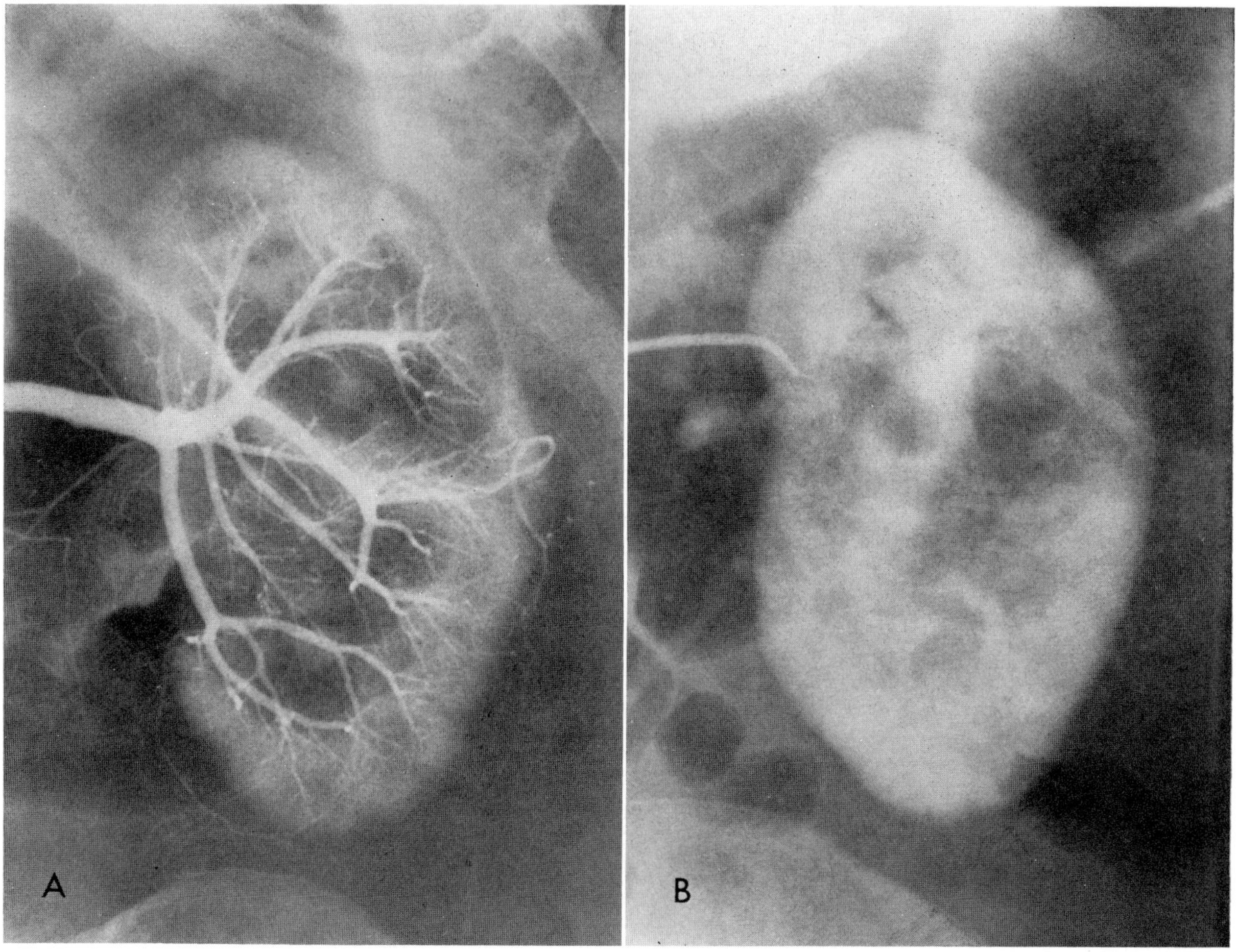

Figure 28.60. Renal Arteriogram. (A) Arterial phase: Stretching and deviation of the intrarenal branches occurs with deviation and prominence of the pelviureteric branches. (B) Nephrogram: There is effacement of the corticomedullary borders and destruction of the cortical invaginations into the medullary spaces. A patient who had repeated chronic infections. *Diagnosis:* Xanthogranulomatous pyelonephritis.

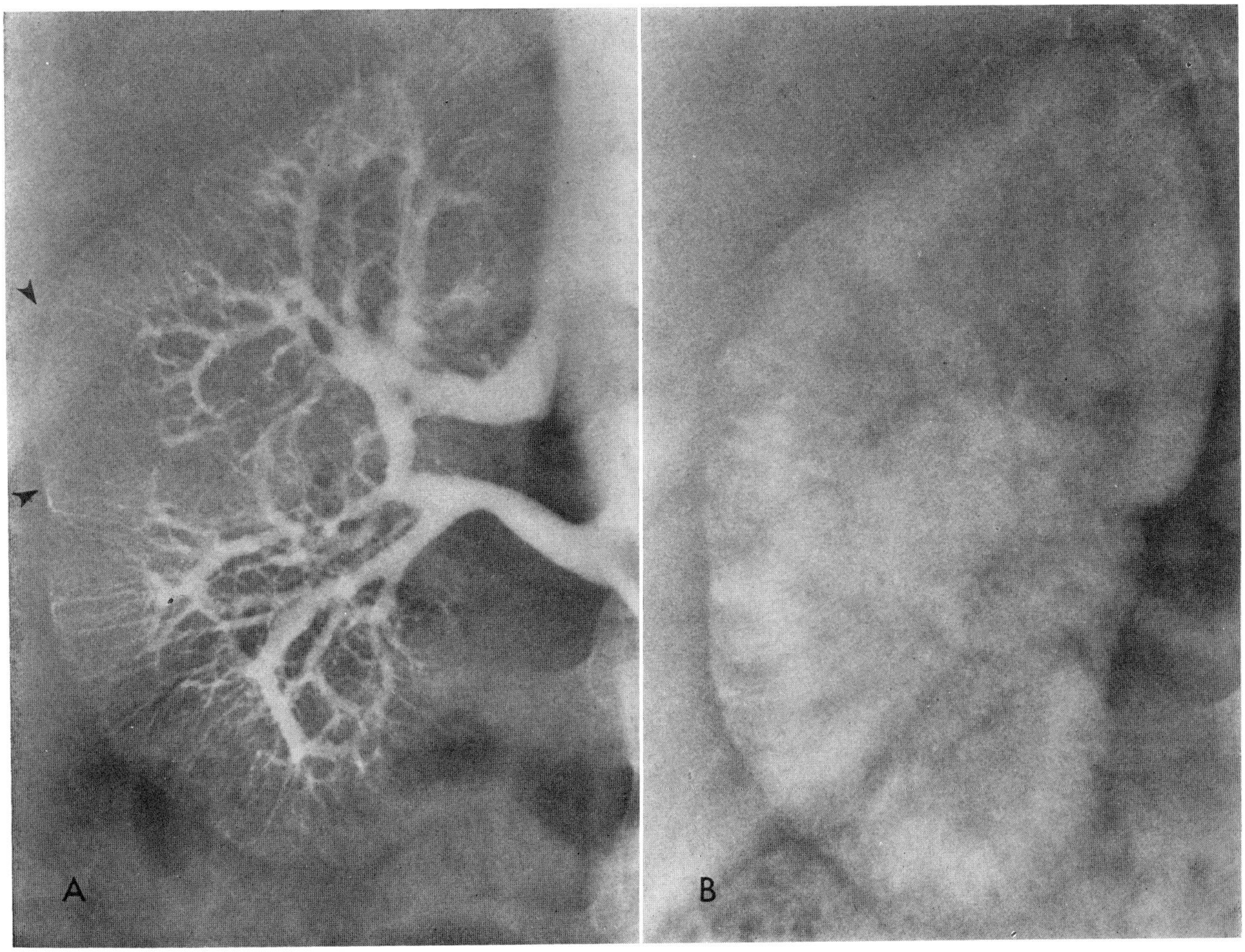

Figure 28.61. Renal Venogram. (A) There is no filling of the interlobular veins in a segment. (B) Renal arteriogram—late phase: Multiple, small peripheral filling defects are in a patient with sickle-cell hemoglobinopathy. *Diagnosis:* Multiple infarcts.

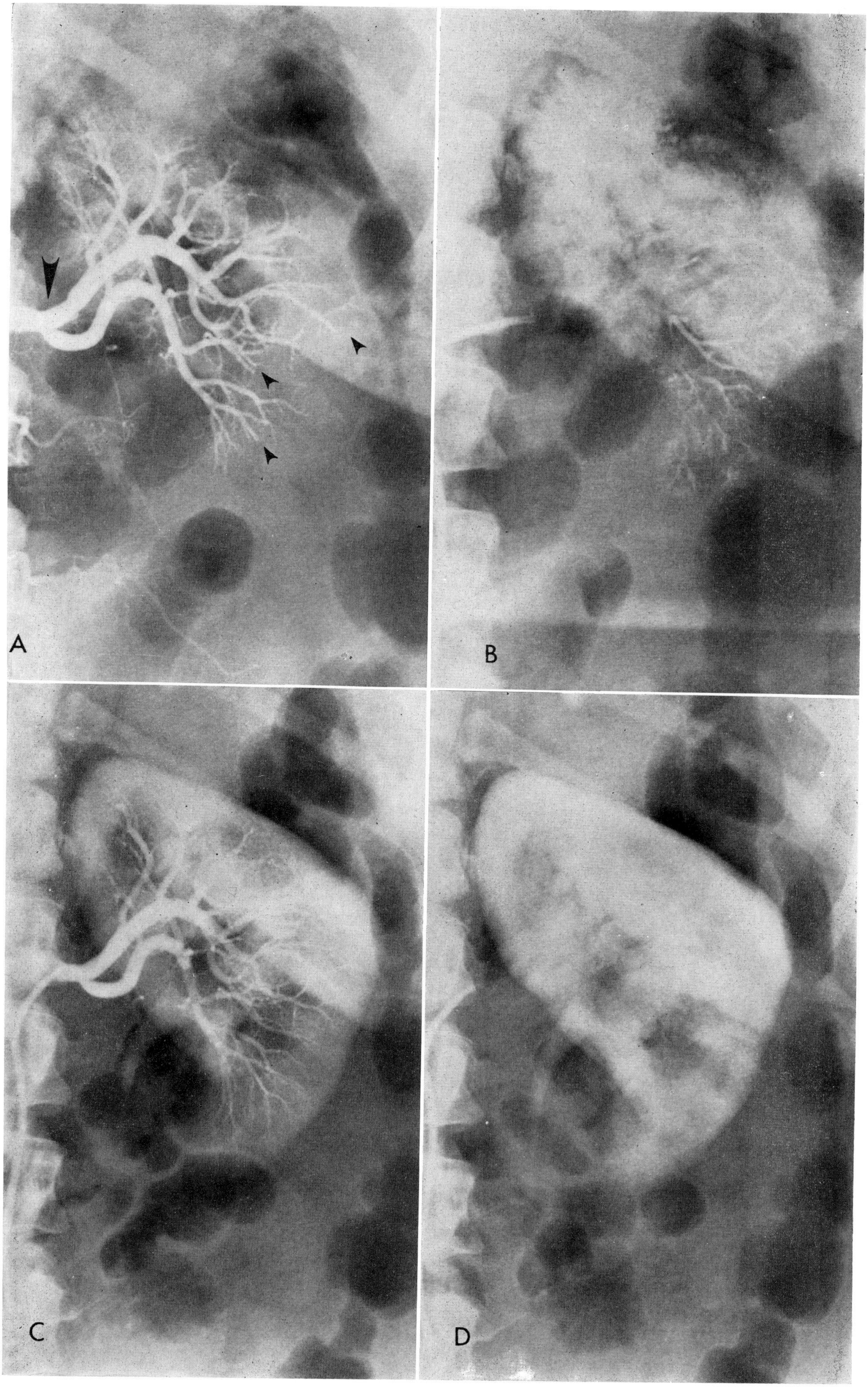
A
B
C
D

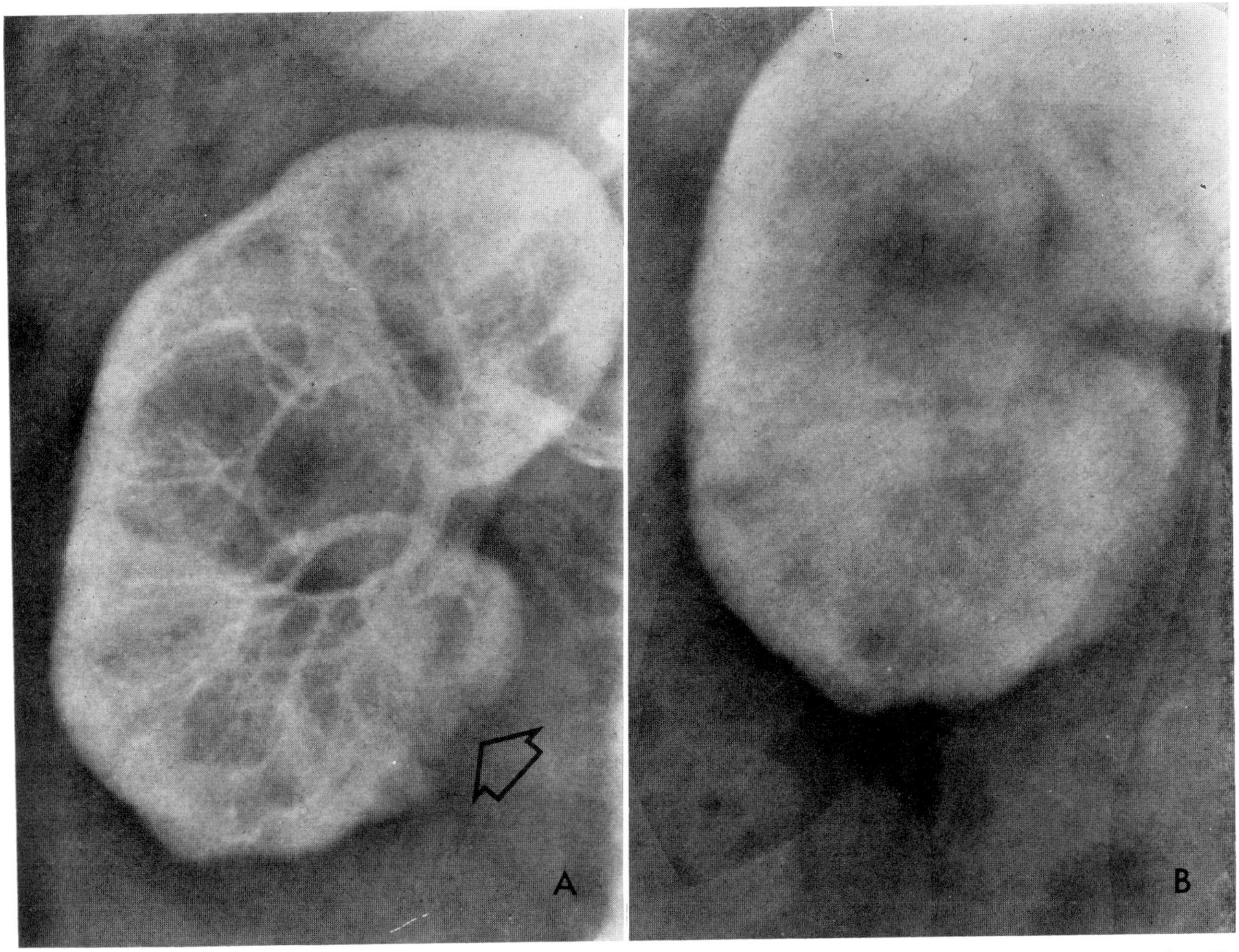

Figure 28.63. Renal Arteriogram. (A) Renal arteriogram: An irregular peripheral filling defect is in the medial border of the renal parenchyma. Incidental stretching of the intrarenal arterial branches around an avascular mass can be seen. (B) Repeat arteriogram—late phase: The renal parenchyma is smooth and well stained. *Diagnosis:* Functional ischemic changes causing filling defect due to under perfusion. Incidental cyst in the midportion of the kidney.

←

Figure 28.62. Renal Arteriogram. (A) Renal arterial phase: There is minimal narrowing of the proximal renal artery (Large Arrow Head) and sudden termination of the intrarenal arterial branches (Small Arrow Head). (B) Parenchymal phase: Small, diffuse irregular filling defects are seen throughout the kidney with some stasis in the small intrarenal arterial branches. (C) A repeat arteriogram two minutes later on the same side shows good filling of the entire renal vasculature. (D) Parenchymal phase: A good nephrogram and an incidental aberrant artery perfusing the lower pole can be seen. *Comment:* The dramatic appearance in the first study is probably due to functional intrarenal redistribution of blood. Trueta phenomena or due to spasm of the vessels?

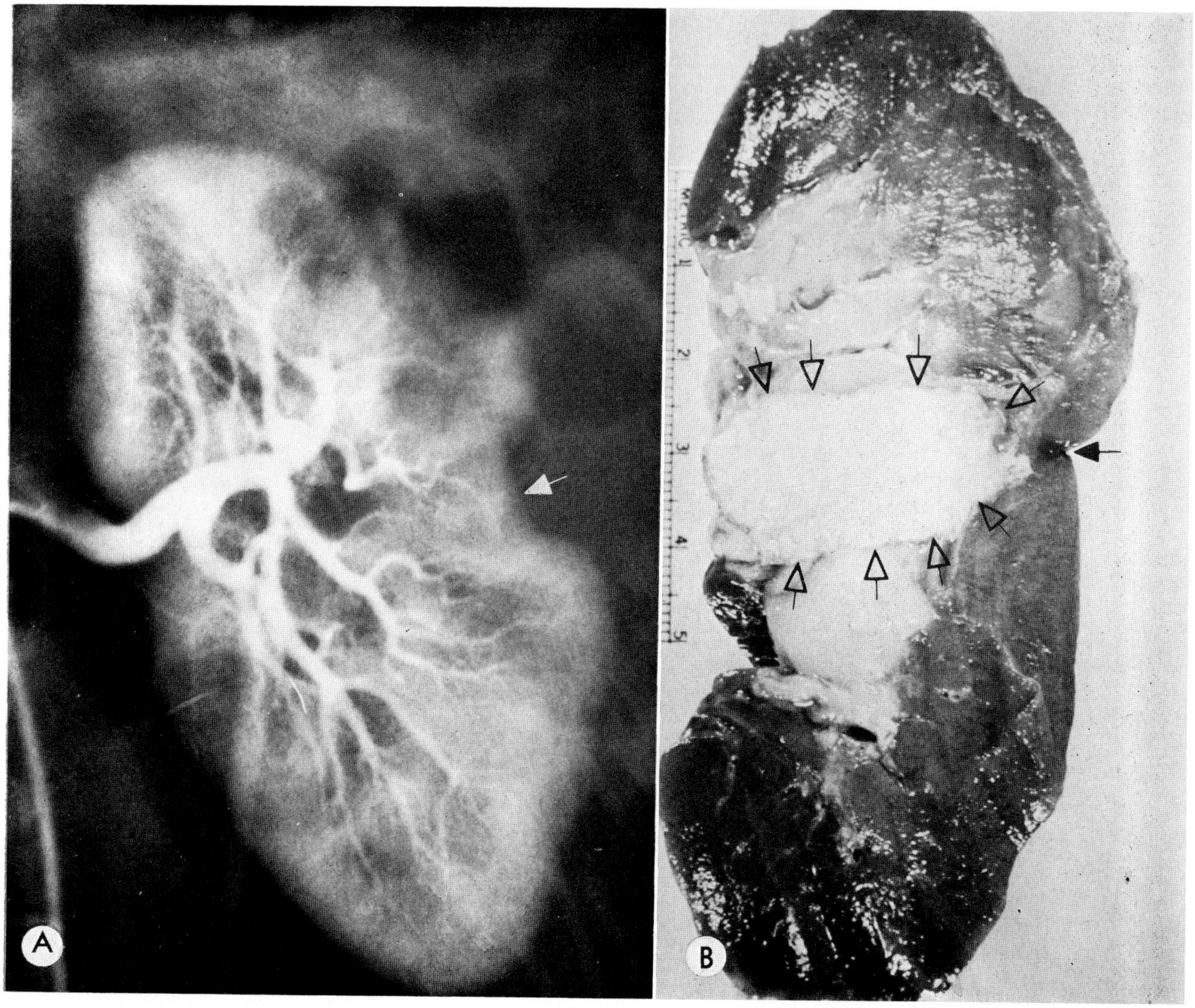

Figure 28.64. (A) A renal arteriogram shows a comparatively avascular area with a large cortical retraction (the dimple—White Arrow). (B) Pathological specimen: Note the large tumor (Blank Arrows) and the cortical dimple (Black Arrow). (From Baltaxe, H. A., Sos, T. A., and Gray, G. F., Jr. Malignant renal tumors producing cortical retraction—"the dimple sign." *Am J Roentgenol, 120:*648, 1974. Courtesy of the authors and publishers.)

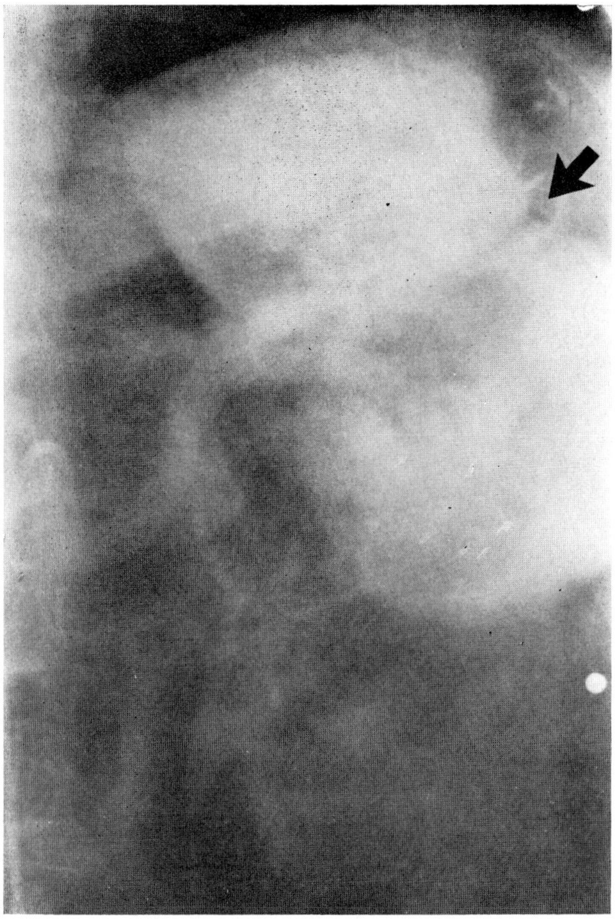

Figure 28.65. Celiac Arteriogram—venous phase. Note the splenic lobulation (Arrow).

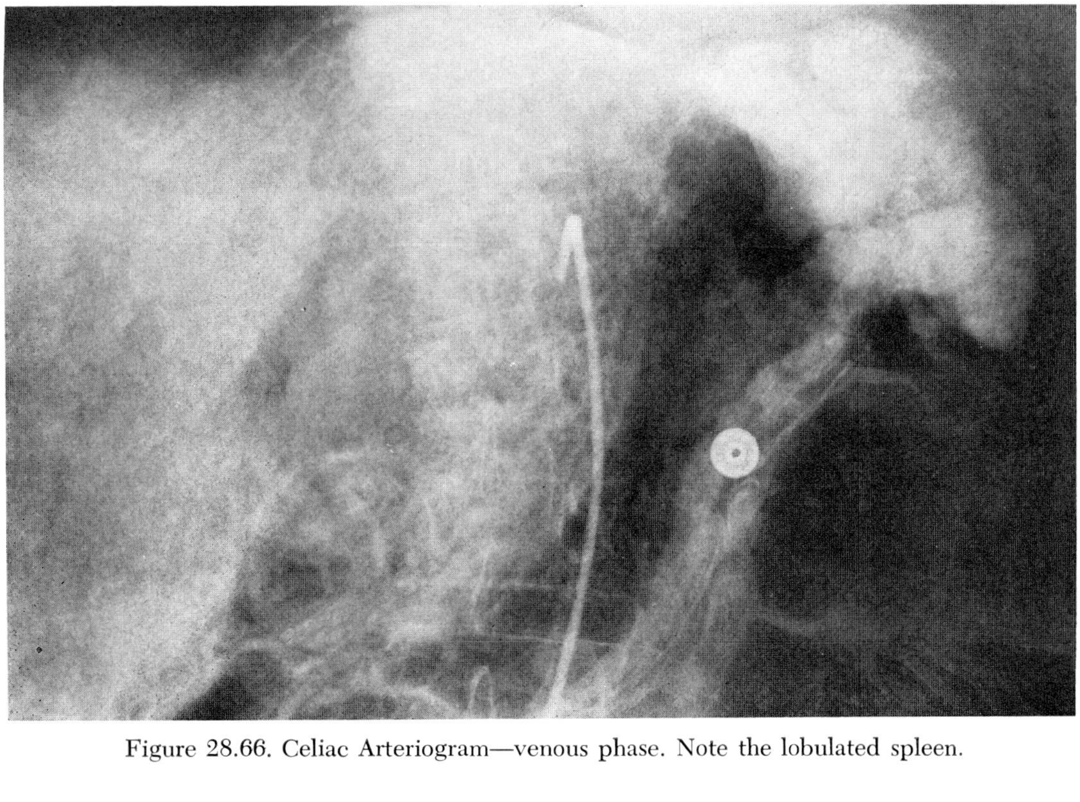

Figure 28.66. Celiac Arteriogram—venous phase. Note the lobulated spleen.

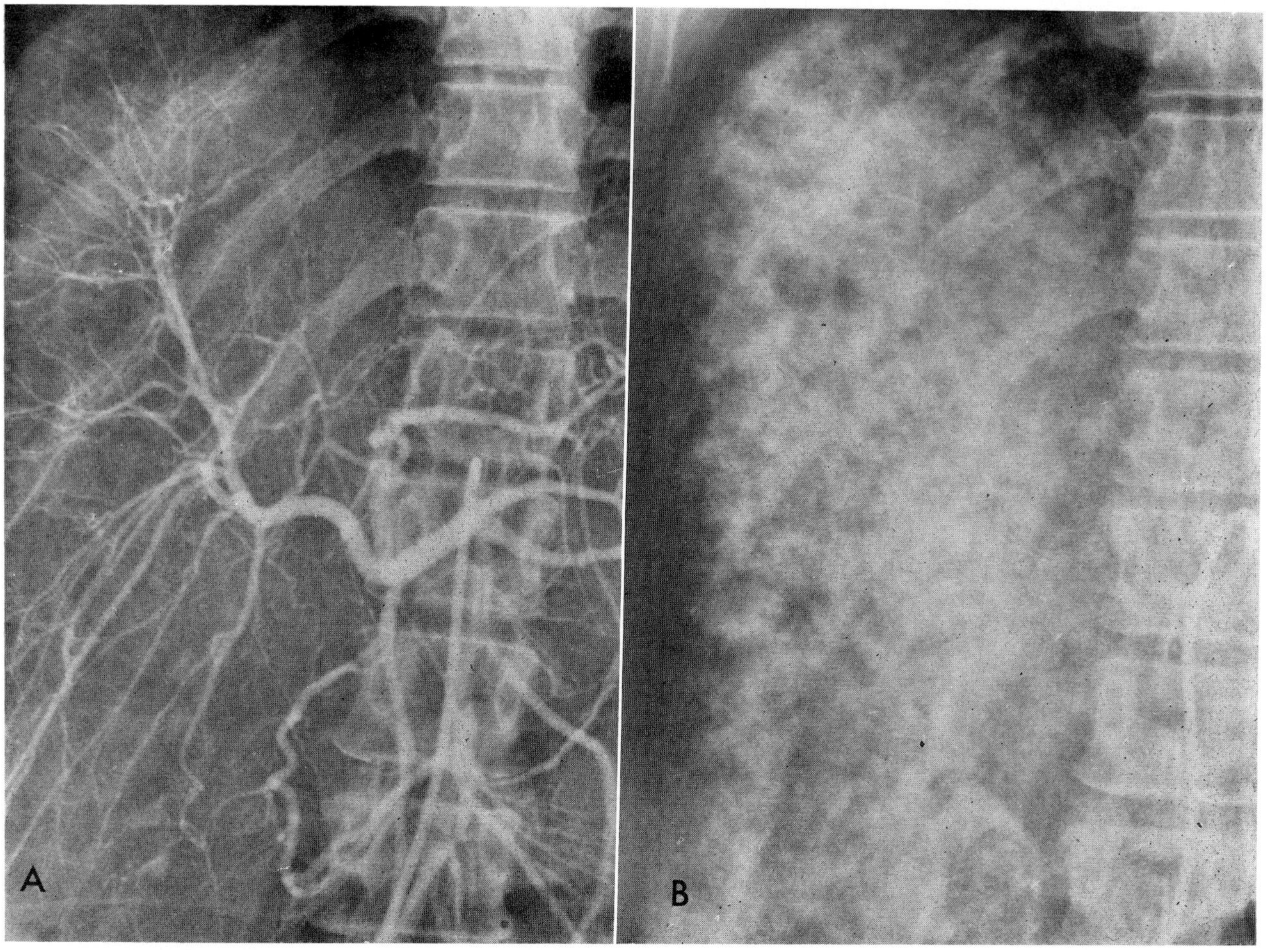

Figure 28.67. Celiac Arteriogram. (A) There is stretching of the intrahepatic branches and reduplication of the distal hepatic branches. (B) There are multiple tiny filling defects in the parenchyma giving mottled appearance. The patient was an alcoholic. *Diagnosis:* Advanced alcoholic cirrhosis with fatty infiltration of the liver.

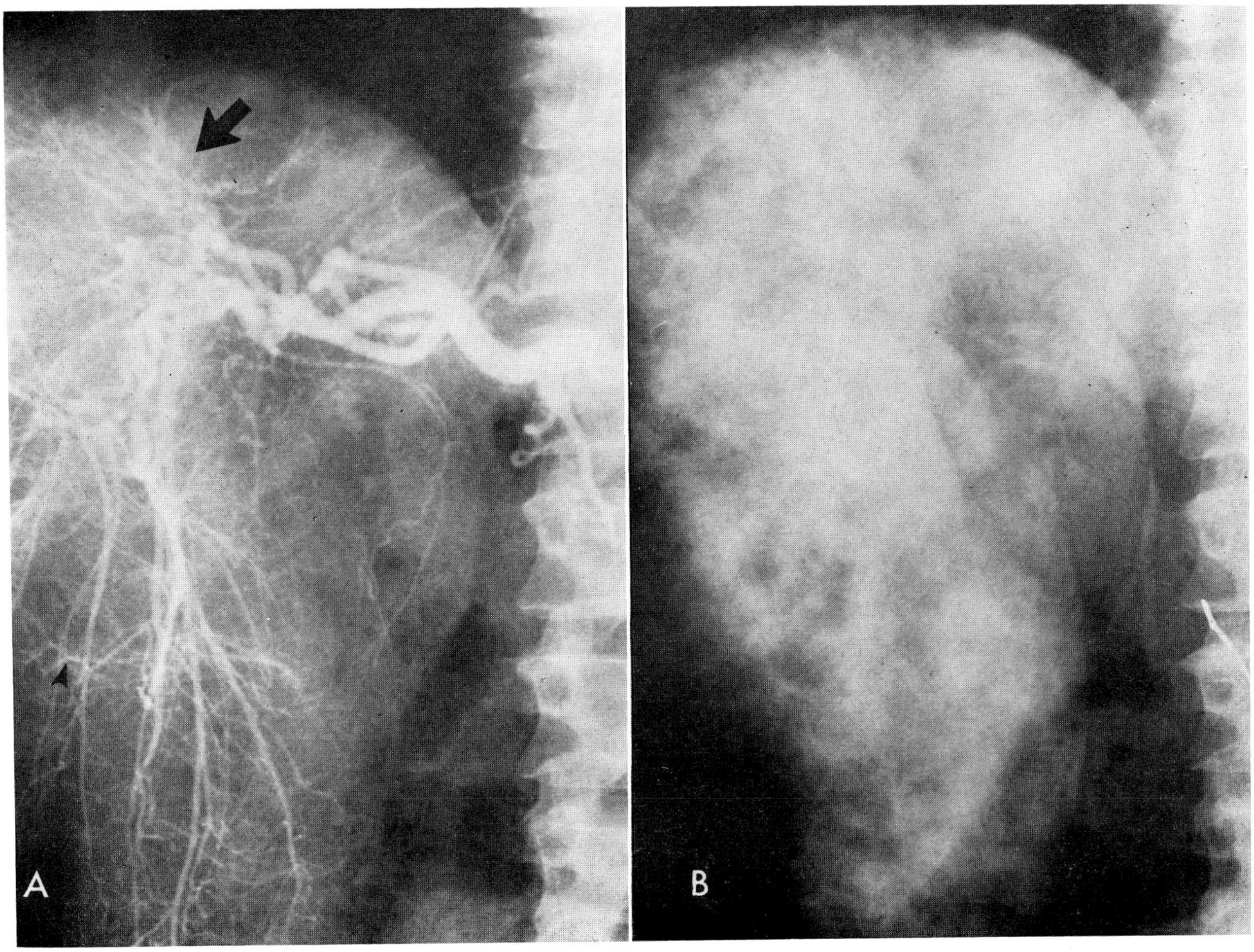

Figure 28.68. Hepatic Arteriogram. (A) Arterial phase reveals stretching and deviation of the intrahepatic branches in certain areas (Arrow Heads), crowding and corkscrew appearance in certain areas (Arrow). (B) Parenchymal phase: Demonstrates multiple filling defects in an enlarged liver. *Diagnosis:* Metastasis to a cirrhotic liver. *Pathology:* Metastasis from an adenocarcinoma of the pancreas to the cirrhotic liver.

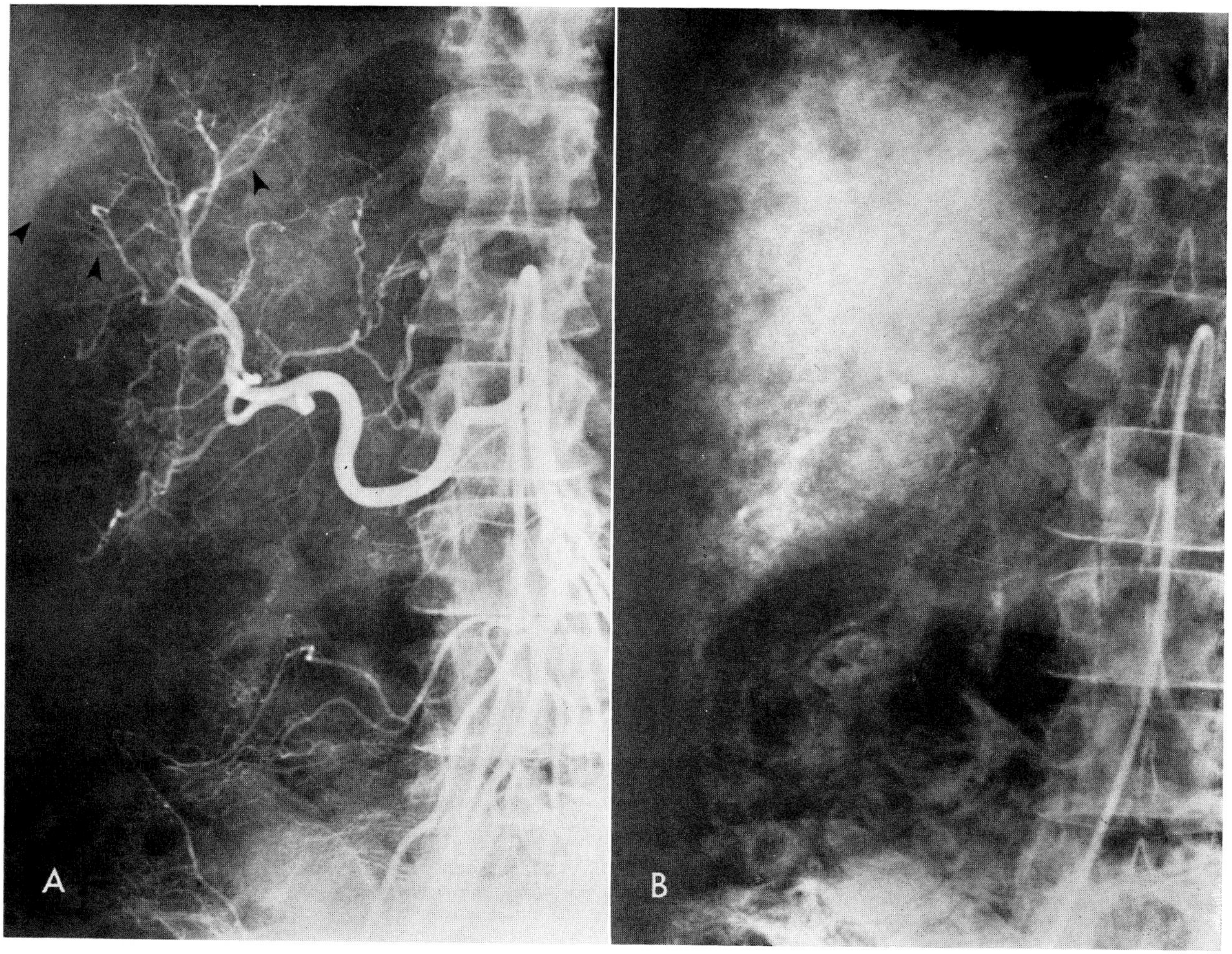

Figure 28.69. Superior Mesenteric Arteriogram. (A) Arterial phase: There is deviation and stretching of the distal small branches of the intrahepatic vasculature (Arrow). Note the replaced right hepatic artery from the superior mesenteric artery. (B) Parenchymal phase: There are multiple filling defects. *Differential Diagnosis:* (1) avascular metastasis, (2) fatty infiltration, (3) other infiltrative disorders. *Biopsy Diagnosis:* Cholangioadenoma.

ma are (a) single, multiple, or polycystic benign cysts; (b) hematomas or abscesses of recent duration; (c) inactive parasitic cysts.

2. Thick-walled, regular or irregular, well-defined defects with sharp interfaces against the adjacent parenchyma are (a) subacute and chronic abscesses; (b) subacute and chronic hematomas; (c) biologically active parasitic cysts; (d) benign[1132] or malignant neoplastic cysts; (e) infarcts, after degenerative liquification; (f) simple adrenal cysts.
3. Well defined defects with a sharp interface, regular borders, but no walls, single or multiple, are (a) infarcts; (b) acute or subacute abscesses or hematomas; (c) malignant, primary or secondary neoplastic lesions; (d) focal infiltrative disorders; (e) vascular variations seen during selective catheterization.
4. Ill defined filling defects with irregular borders and no walls—single, multiple or diffuse—are (a) very acute abscesses or hematomas, (b) neoplastic processes, (c) infiltrative processes, (d) occasional adenomas.[1129]
5. Tubular filling defects in the liver are dilatation of the biliary tree.
6. Saccular filling defects are hydronephrosis, traumatic biliary cysts, and saccular dilatation of the biliary ducts.

FILLING DEFECTS IN THE LUMEN OF VESSELS

Arteries

Emboli, whether bland, atherosclerotic plaques, or tumoral, are the causes of intra-arterial filling defects. Usually there is a *meniscus* sign at the interface of contrast material and embolus. Huge atheromatous plaques can also be demonstrated as irregular filling defects of variable sizes within arterial lumens. Although rare, malignant tumors of the aorta[1122, 1123] (Fig. 28-86), or pulmonary arteries,[1124] and intraluminal metastasis from melanoma[1125] also produce intraluminal filling defects.

Venous

The most common cause of venous filling defects are *bland* thrombi or emboli. *Tumor thrombus* is an expression of an aggressive tumor extending into the draining vein of an organ and drawing an abnormal arterial supply from the artery of that organ. The common examples are hypernephroma and adrenal carcinomas growing into the inferior vena cava toward the right atrium. Hepatomas may grow into the portal and/or hepatic veins. Other rare tumor thrombi are caused by lymphosarcoma growing into the femoral vein,[1111] undifferentiated malignant tumors into the popliteal vein,[1112] and, rarely, continuous columns of leiomyomatosis extending from uterine leiomyomas[1113] into the vena cava. Tumors arising from the wall of the vessel can also be demonstrated as filling defects after contrast injection. This includes leiomyosarcomas and other tumors of the inferior vena cava[1114] and hemangioma of the external jugular vein[1115] (Figs. 28-110 and 28-111).

Other venous filling defects are caused by membranes[1116–1118] (Fig. 28-112), webs,[1119] persistent Eustachian valve of the inferior vena cava,[1120] hypertrophied valves,[1008] and diaphragms of the subclavian vein[1007] and bands of the common iliac vein[1121] (Fig. 28-109). Transverse webs, longitudinal channels, and eccentric webs may be demonstrated in organized emboli.[868]

TRAUMA AND THE ORGAN

Whether because of their easy accessibility, location or size, certain compact organs such as the liver, spleen and kidney are more prone to external blunt trauma than are other structures.[1056–1059] Most of the early, delayed, or fatal posttraumatic complications are due to the extent and magnitude of the applied traumatic force, secondarily injuring the vasculature of that organ. The nature of the injuries includes *thrombosis, laceration or avulsion of the vessel.* Associated shattering splits or vertical or horizontal tears of the parenchyma determine the extent of bleeding. In turn, this determines

(Text continues on page 573)

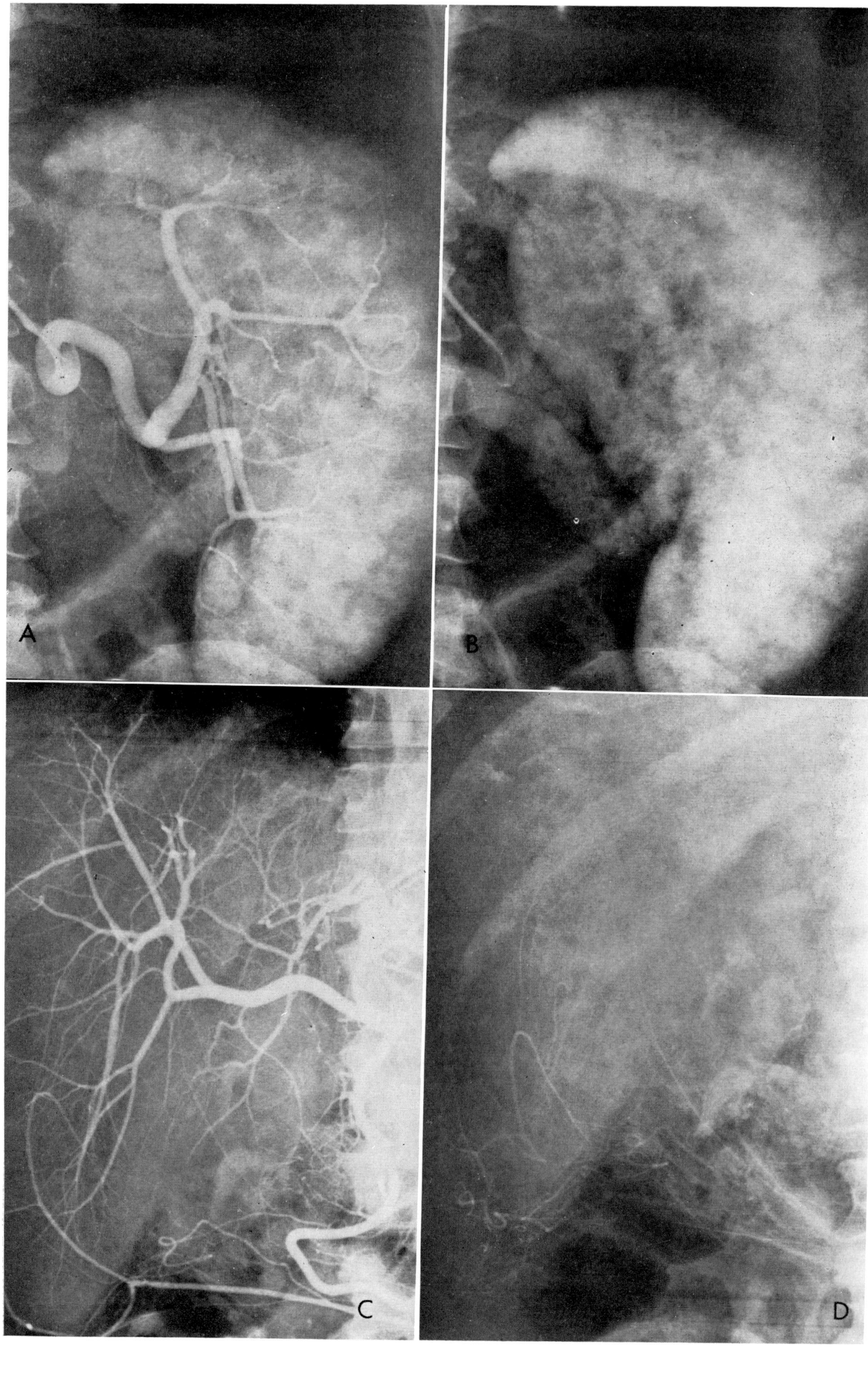
A
B
C
D

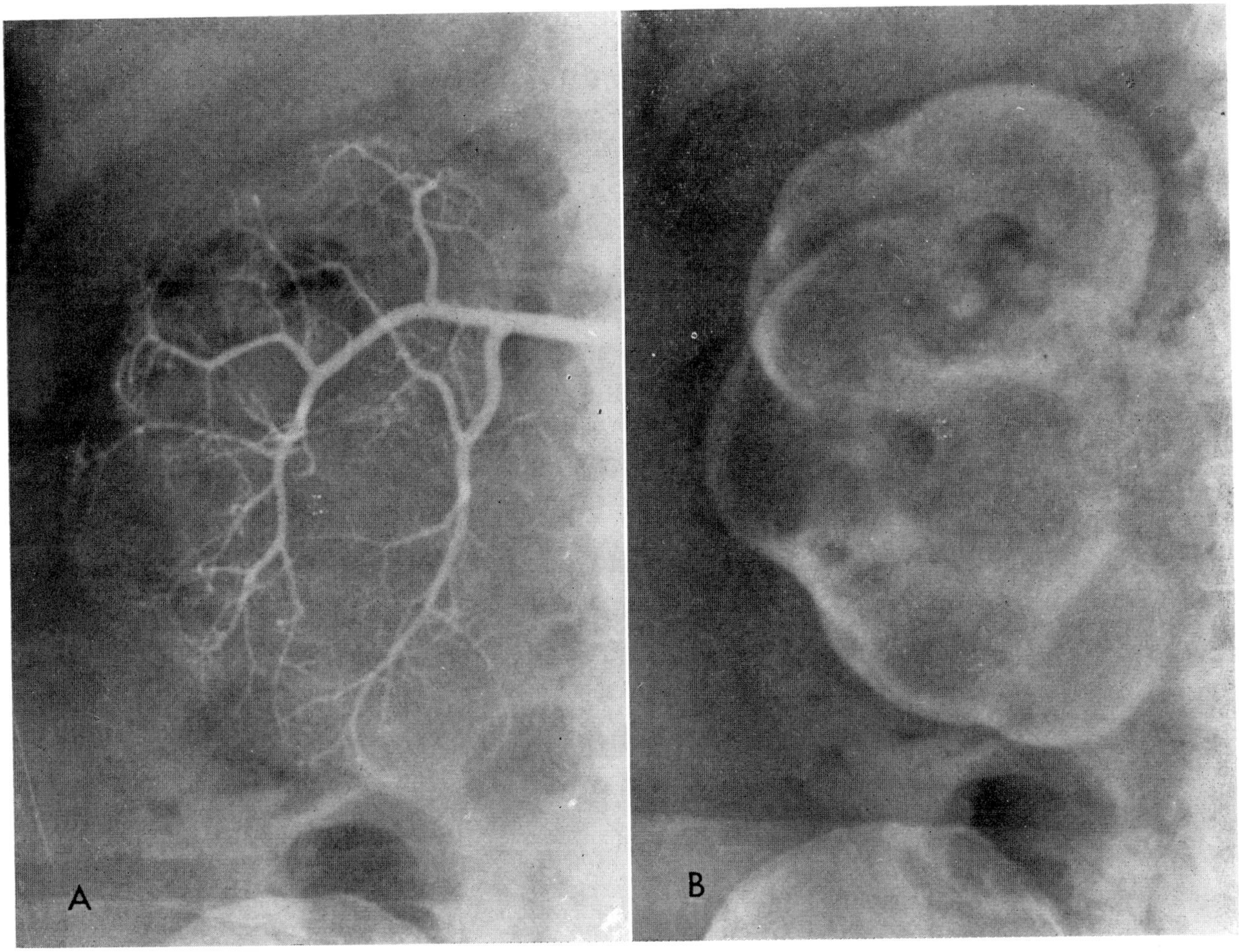

Figure 28.71. Renal Arteriogram. (A) Arterial phase: There is narrowing of the main renal artery and intrarenal diffuse stretching and deviation of the arterial branches. Notice the increase in the size of the kidney. (B) Parenchymal phase: Extreme thinning of the cortex is seen with smooth circular symmetrical filling defects throughout the kidney. *Diagnosis:* Hydronephrosis.

←

Fgure 28.70. Selective Splenic Arteriogram. (A) There is an enlarged spleen with stretching of the intrasplenic vessels. Notice the sparsity of the intrasplenic vessels. (B) The spleen is enlarged with multiple, small filling defects. (C) Celiac arteriogram: Stretching and deviation of the intrahepatic branches in an enlarged liver is seen. (D) There is very poor staining of the liver. *Conclusions:* Hepatosplenomegaly. The stretching of the intrahepatic and intrasplenic branches is due to an infiltrative disorder. *Biopsy of the liver:* Sarcoidosis.

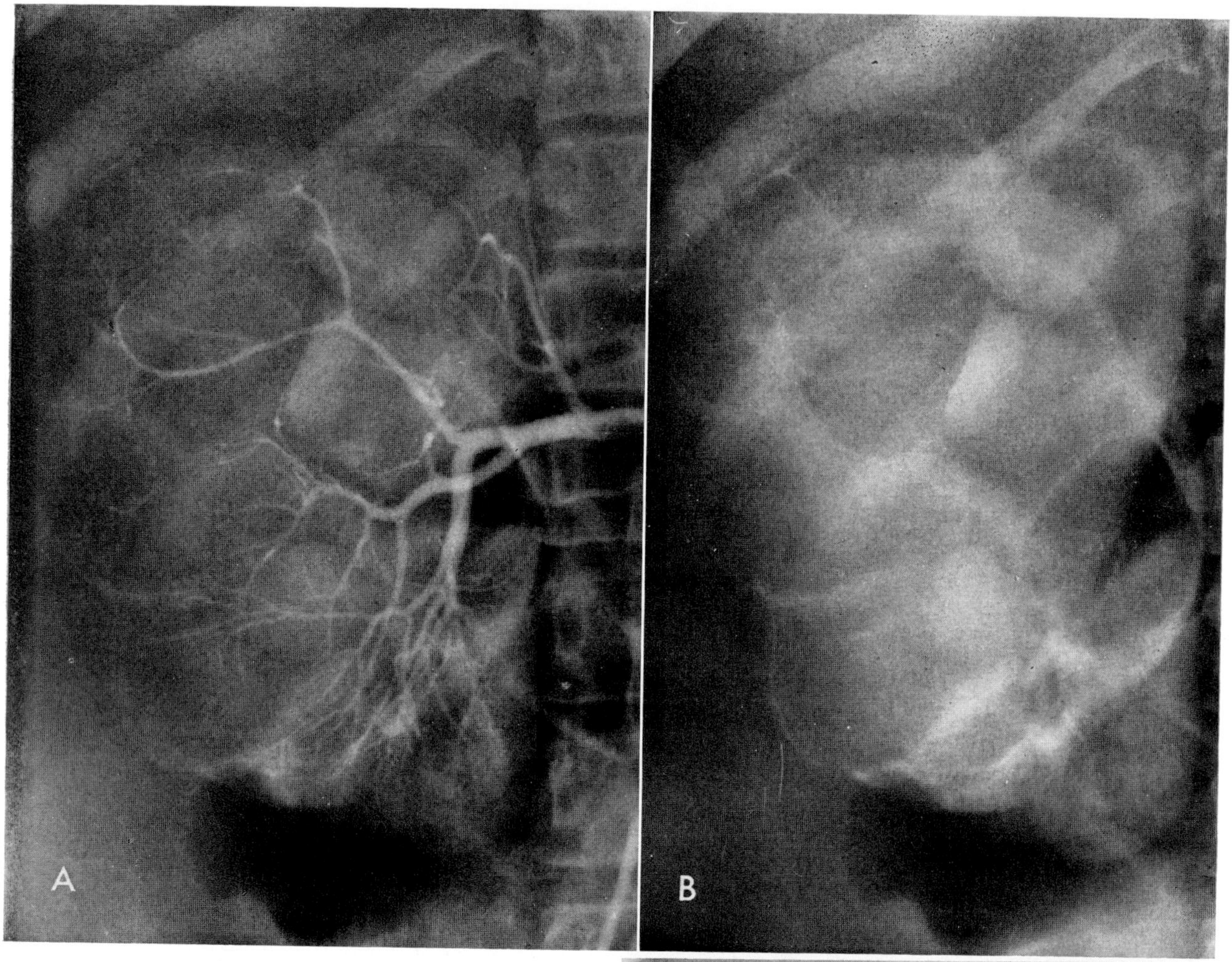

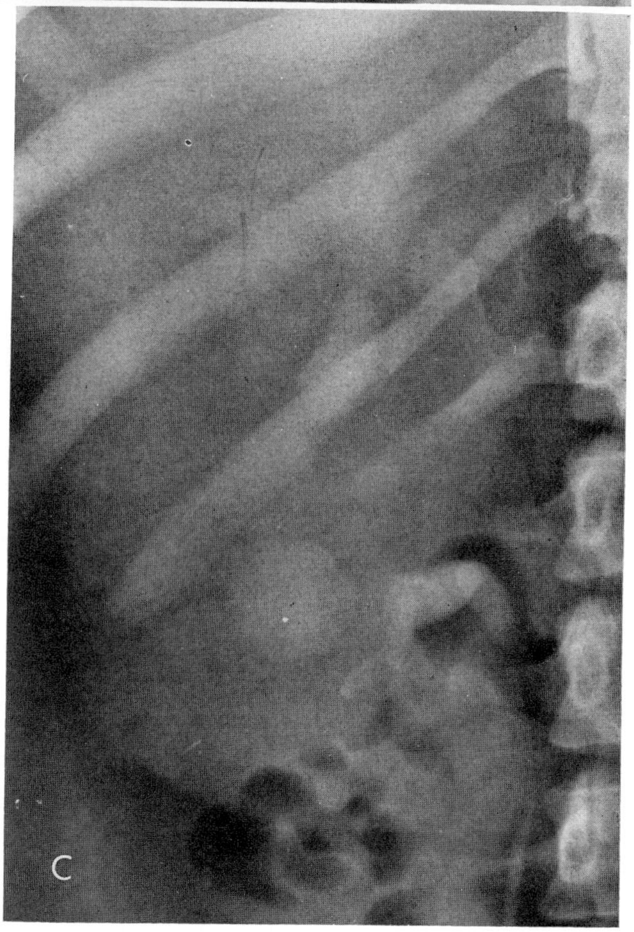

Figure 28.72. Renal Arteriogram. (A) Arterial phase: Stretching and deviation of the intrarenal vessels is seen in the upper two-thirds. (B) Parenchymal phase: Well-stained, thin walls with symmetrical filling defects are separated by cortical invaginations. (C) Intravenous pyelogram: Dilation of the upper collecting systems and normal lower pole collecting systems are seen. *Diagnosis:* Hydronephrosis in a duplicated kidney. The filling defects are due to dilated calyces and the stain is due to compressed cortex.

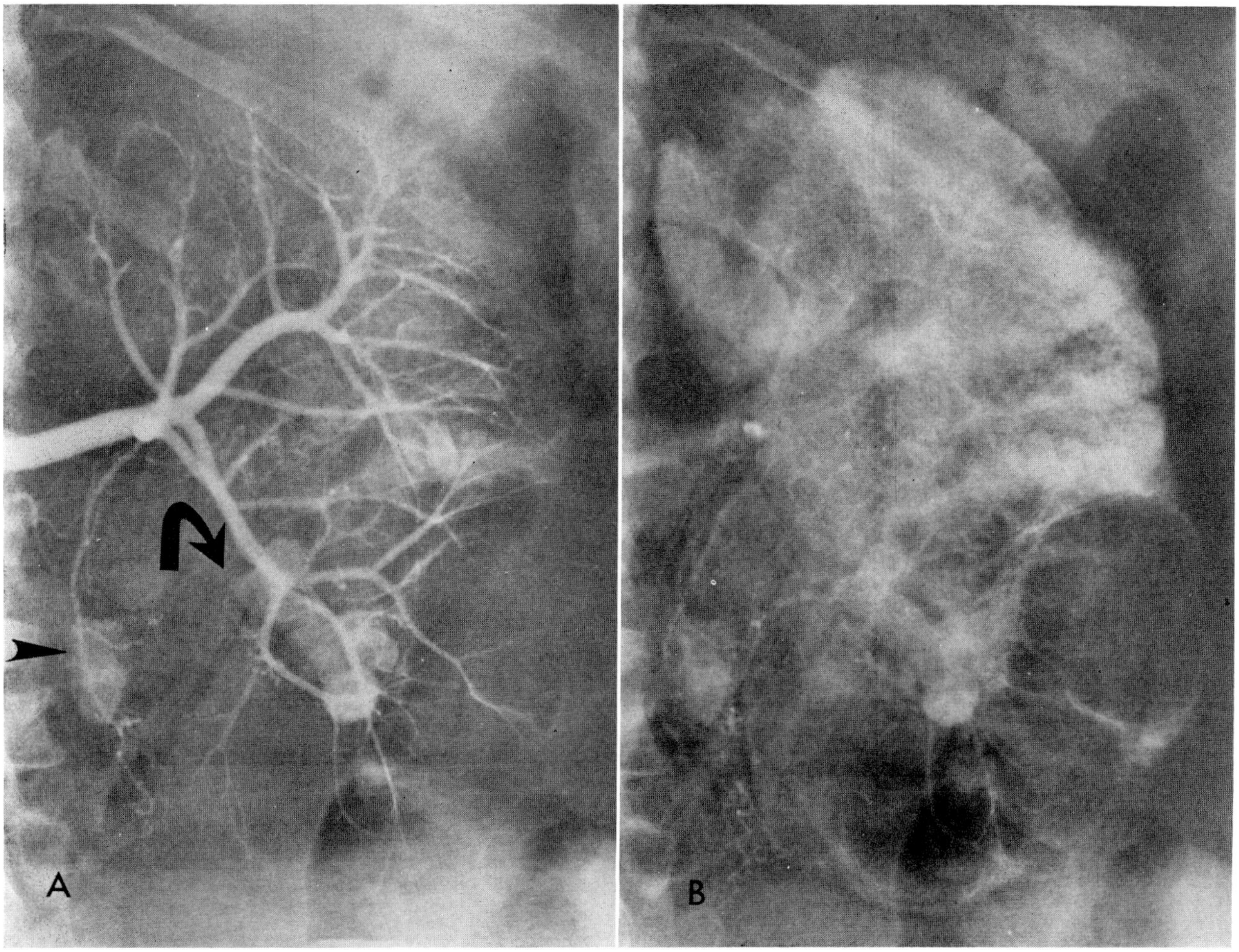

Figure 28.73. Renal Arteriogram. (A) The size of the kidney is increased. Stretching and deviation of intrarenal branches is more pronounced in the lower half with comparatively diminished arterial perfusion. Note the very prominent pelviureteric branch (Arrow Head). The density seen (Arrow) is a segment of a staghorn calculus. (B) Parenchymal phase: Smooth, well-defined, regularly placed, circumscribed filling defects are separated by thin cortical invaginations of the renal cortex. Thinned out peripheral renal cortices are seen. A smooth interface exists between the filling defects and the renal parenchyma. *Diagnosis:* Calculus pyonephrosis in the lower half of the kidney.

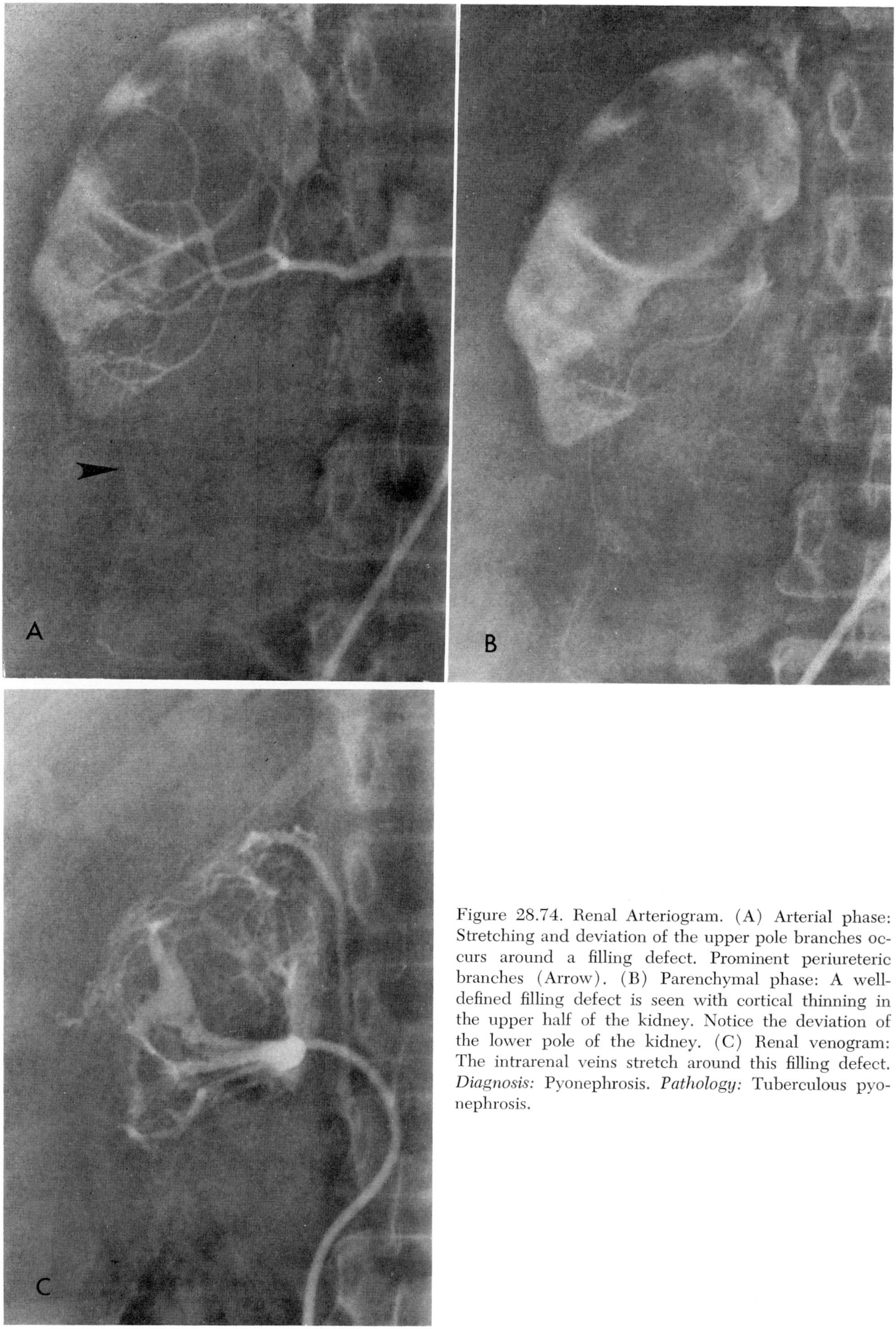

Figure 28.74. Renal Arteriogram. (A) Arterial phase: Stretching and deviation of the upper pole branches occurs around a filling defect. Prominent periureteric branches (Arrow). (B) Parenchymal phase: A well-defined filling defect is seen with cortical thinning in the upper half of the kidney. Notice the deviation of the lower pole of the kidney. (C) Renal venogram: The intrarenal veins stretch around this filling defect. *Diagnosis:* Pyonephrosis. *Pathology:* Tuberculous pyonephrosis.

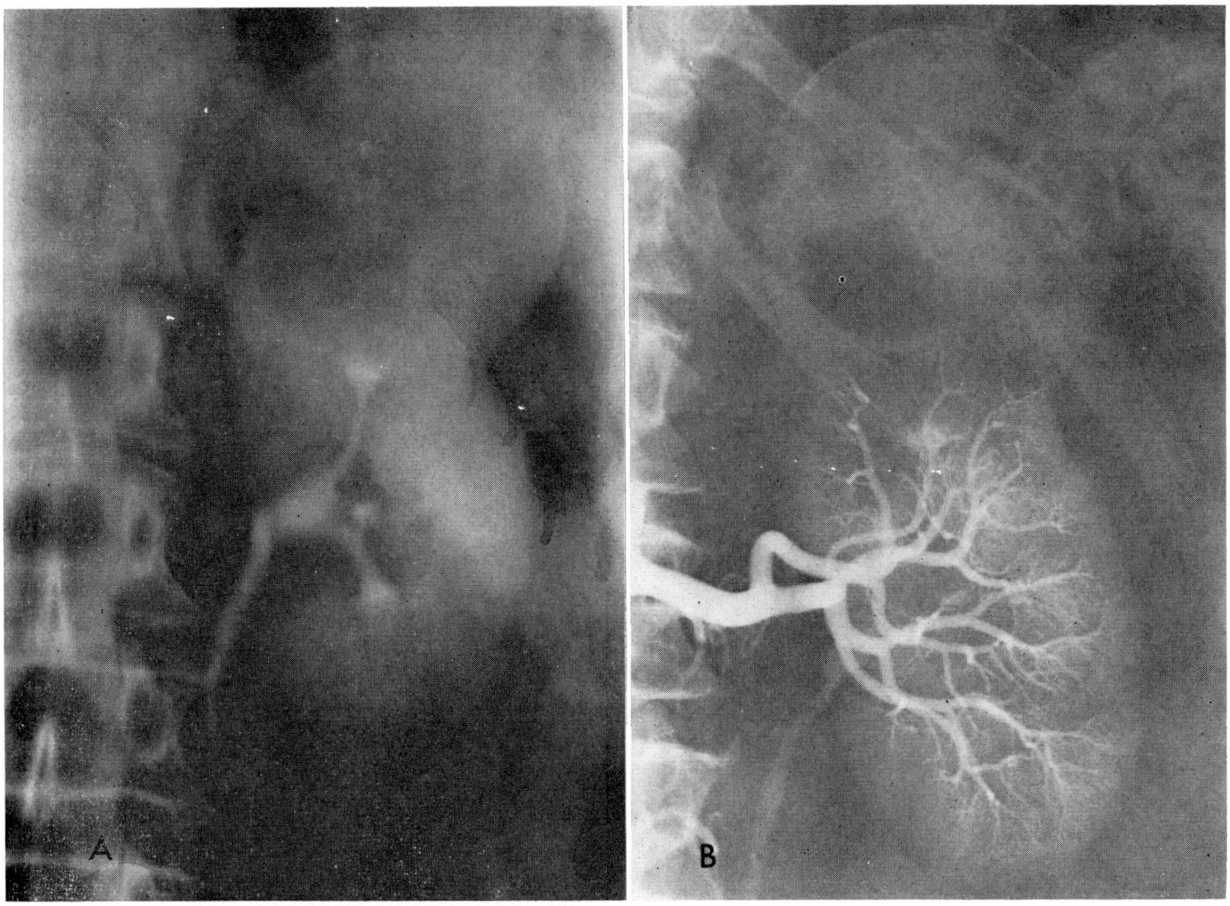

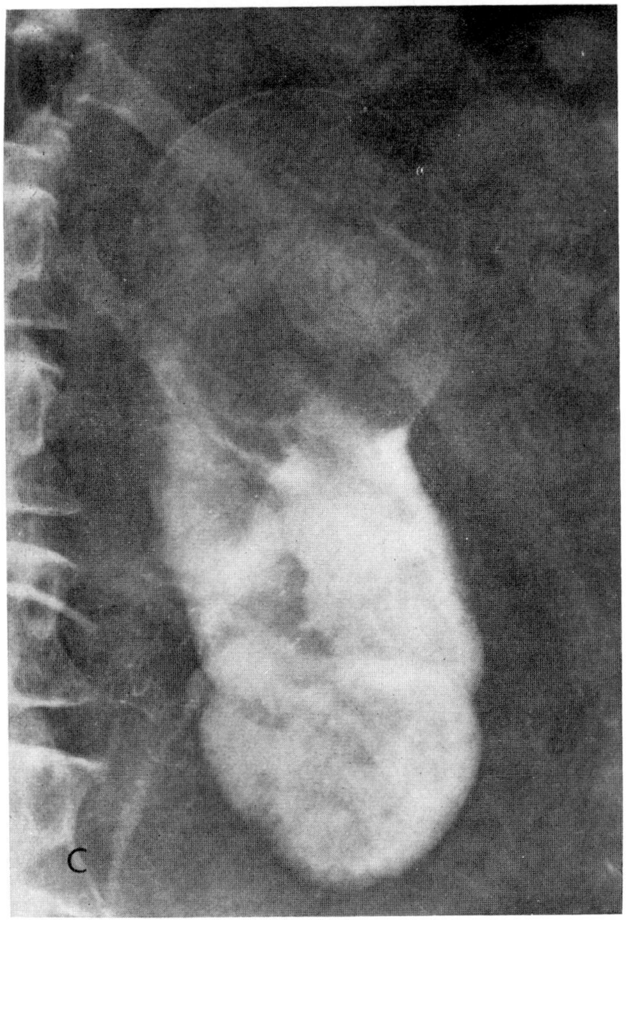

Figure 28.75. Renal Angiogram. (A) A nephrotomogram reveals a mass with a peripheral rim of calcification. (B) Arterial phase: Distortion of the upper pole vessels is revealed. (C) Parenchymal phase: A parenchymal defect at the area of the mass without other abnormalities is observed. *Diagnosis:* Angiography noncontributory. *Pathology:* Necrotic hypernephroma. *Comment:* In masses with peripheral, rim-like calcification a noncontributory angiogram is not a surprise.

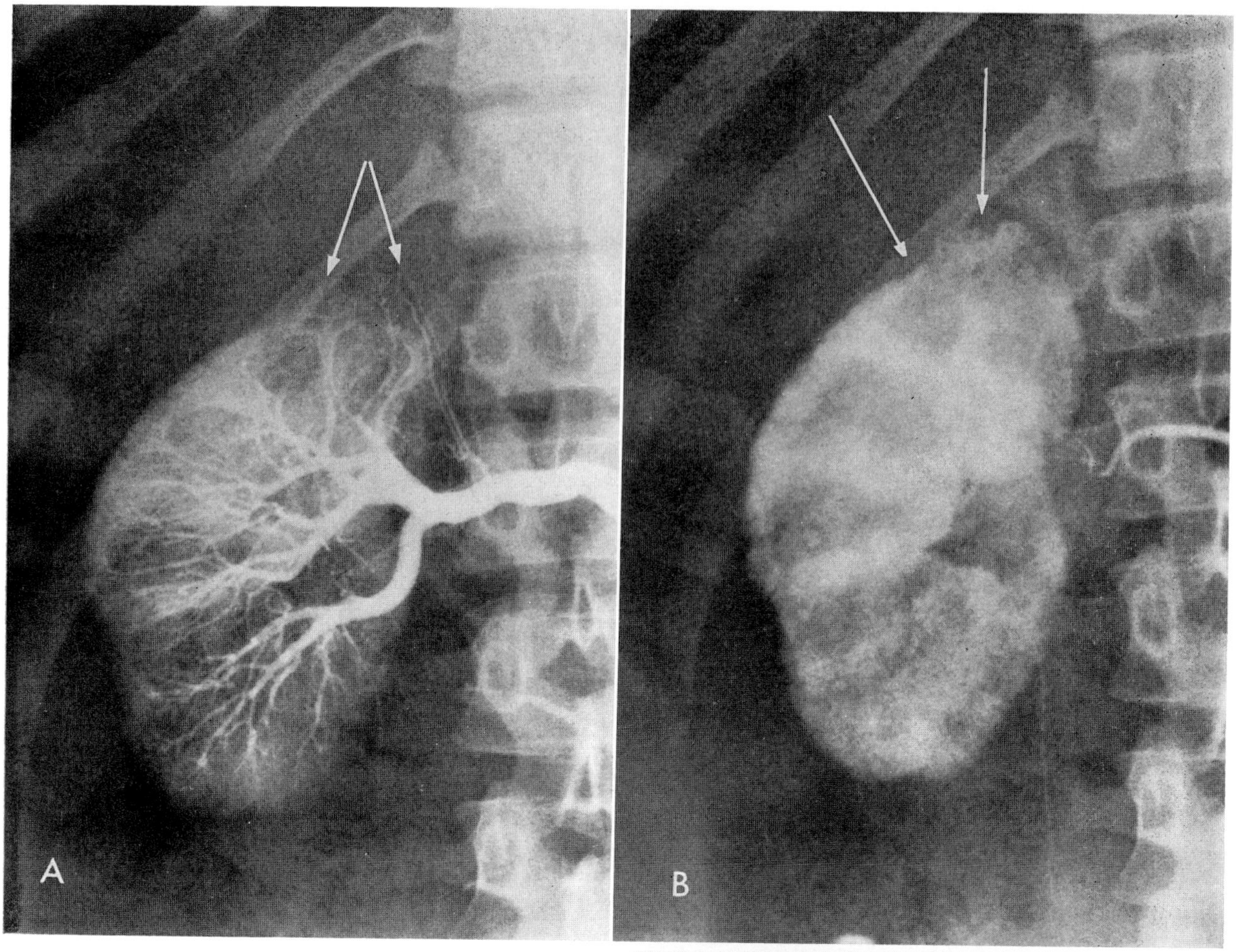

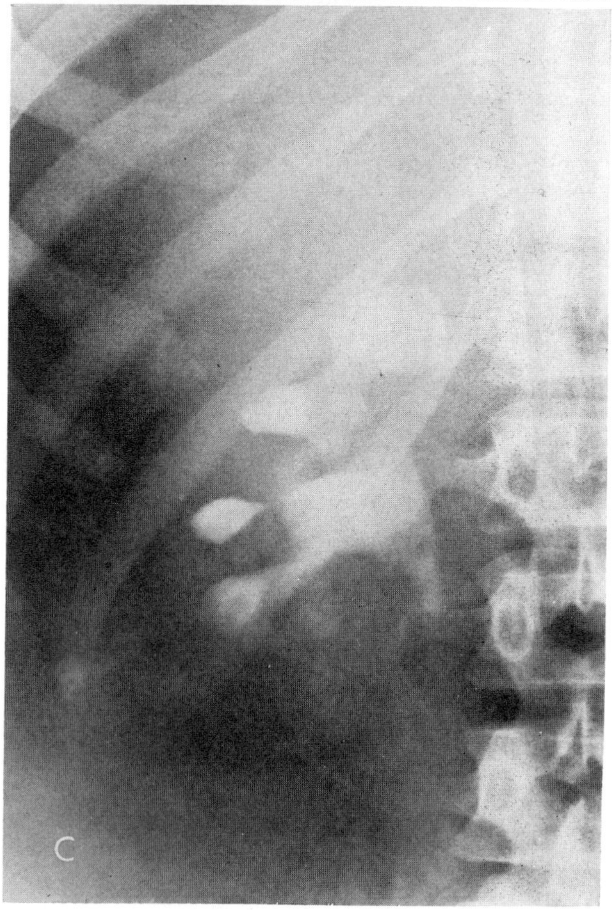

Figure 28.76. (A) Renal arteriogram: Slight stretching and deviation of the upper pole intrarenal branches is seen (Arrow) without cortical perfusion in the same area. A depression on the renal cortical surface. (B) Parenchymal phase: The renal cortex is thinned in two areas (Arrow). (C) Intravenous pyelogram reveals focal dilatation of the upper pole calyx with thinning of the cortex in the same area. *Diagnosis:* Pyelonephritic scars with secondary changes in the adjacent branches.

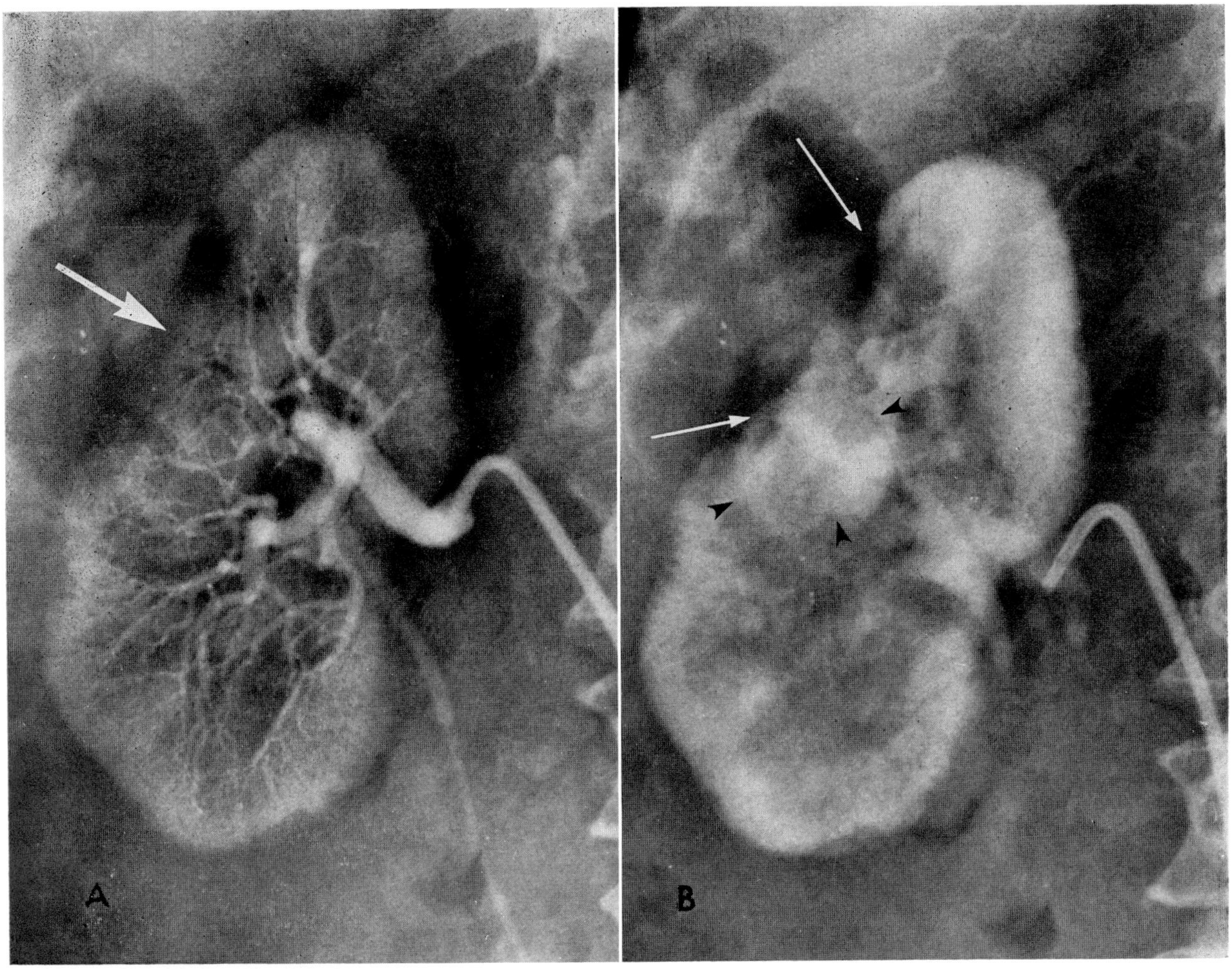

Figure 28.77. Renal Arteriogram. (A) Arterial phase: Crowding of the branches in a segmental area (Arrow). No filling of the arcuate and interlobular arteries. (B) Parenchymal phase: There is flattening and thinning of the cortex (Arrow Head) and increased localized staining of the renal parenchyma (Arrow). *Diagnosis:* Pyelonephric scar with adjacent hypertrophy.

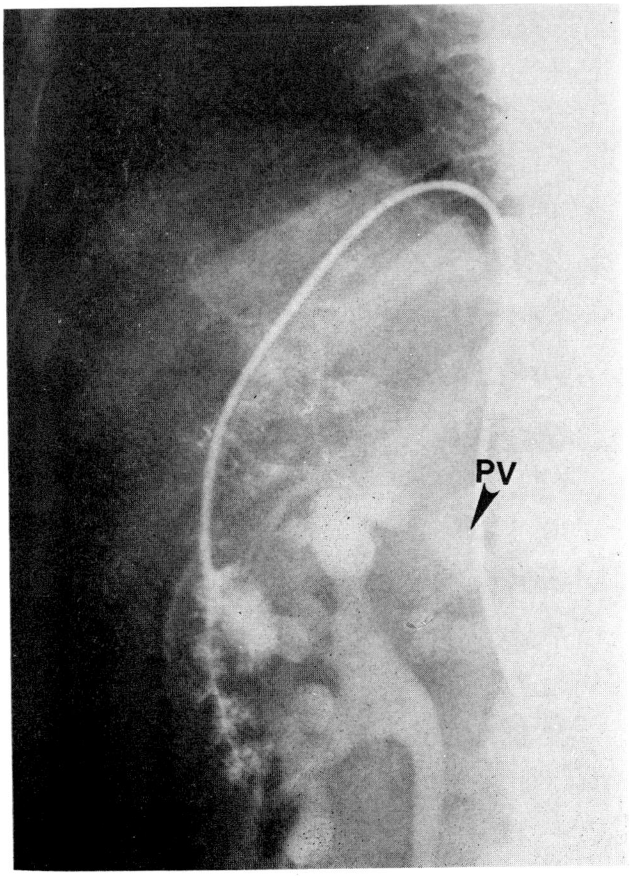

Figure 28.78. Wedge Hepatic Venogram. Dilated liver sinusoids and coarse nonhomogenous pattern in a known alcoholic with cirrhosis. At the same time, please note the retrograde filling of the portal vein (P.V.).

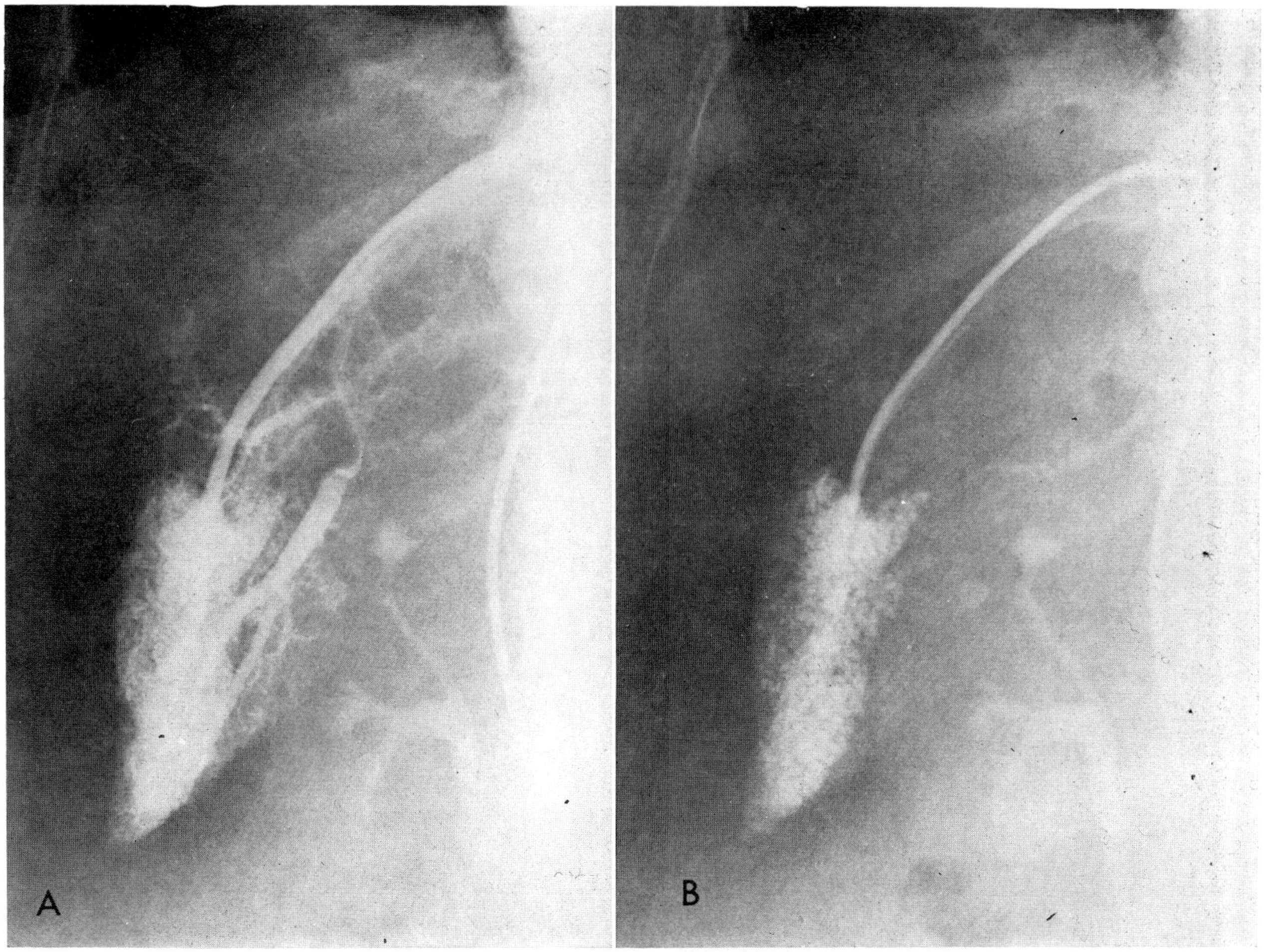

Figure 28.79. Hepatic Venogram. (A) There is hepatic venous opacification with cross-filling of the other branches. (B) There is a nonhomogeneous sinusoidal phase with filling defects causing nodularity. The patient was an alcoholic. *Diagnosis:* Distortion of the normal sinusoidal pattern due to cirrhosis.

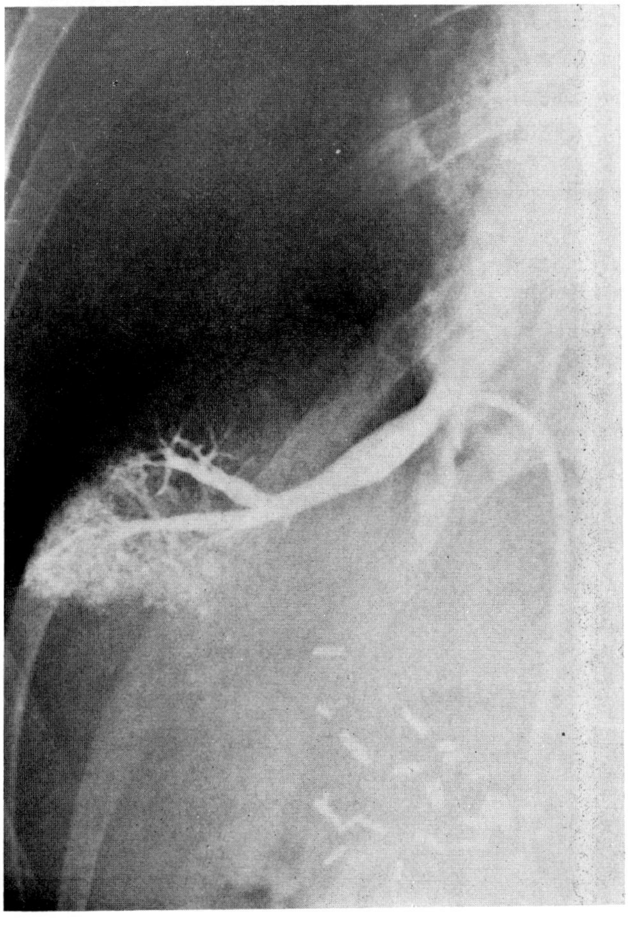

→

Figure 28.80. Hepatic Venogram. There is nonhomogeneous filling of the sinusoids in a patient with cirrhosis.

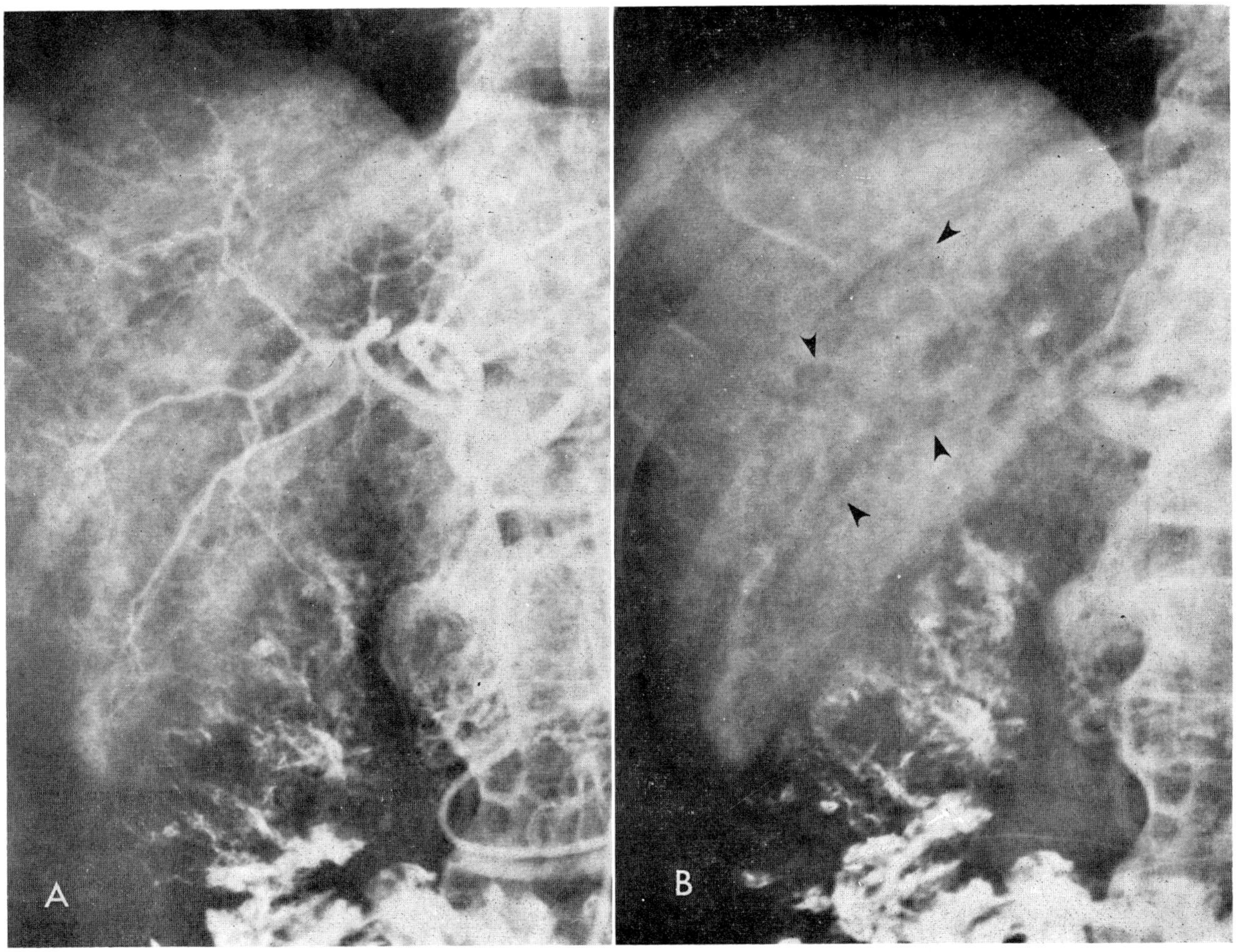

Figure 28.81. Hepatic Arteriogram. This patient had painless jaundice. A late venous film shows tubular defects (Arrow) in the hepatic parenchyma. *Diagnosis:* Pancreatic carcinoma with obstruction and dilatation of the biliary tree.

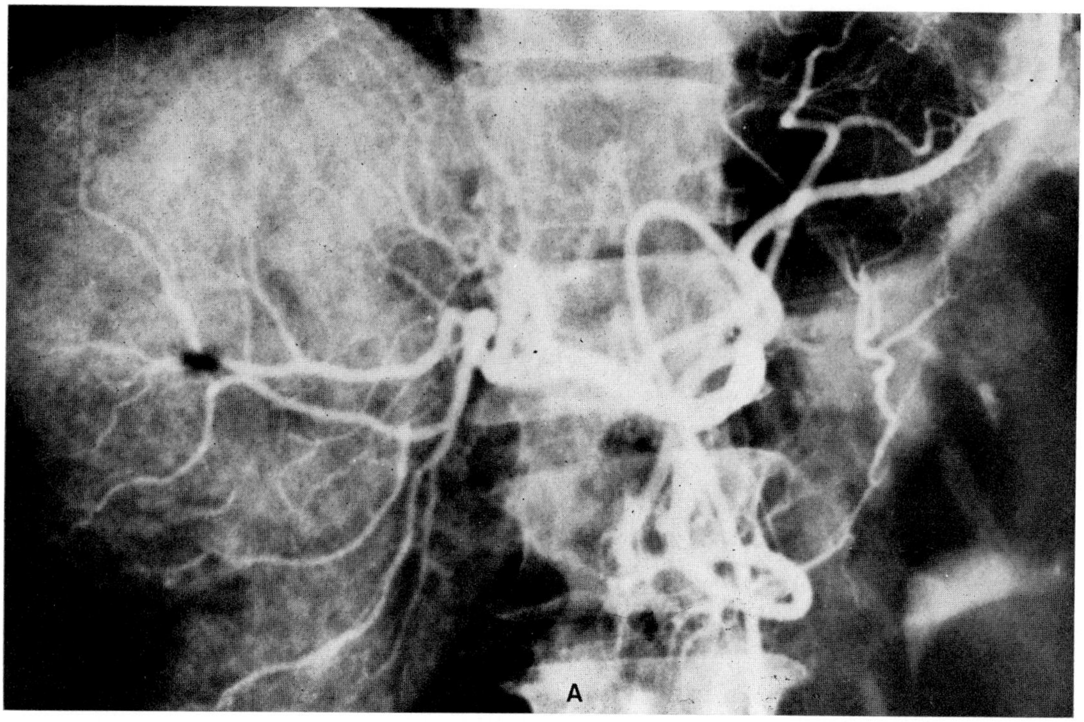

Figure 28-82 A

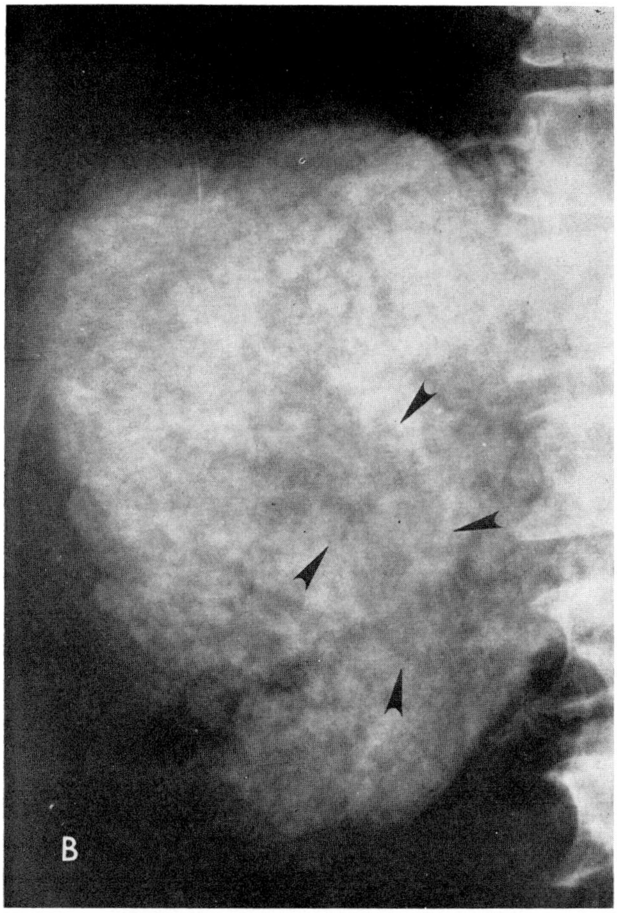

Figure 28.82. Celiac Arteriogram. (A) The intrahepatic branches are stretched and deviated. (B) Parenchymal phase: Filling defects extend toward the porta hepatis. (C) The percutaneous transhepatic cholangiogram reveals dilated bile ducts with distal obstruction. The patient had painless jaundice. *Diagnosis:* Carcinoma of the head of the pancreas with the filling defects in the liver parenchyma caused by a dilated biliary tree.

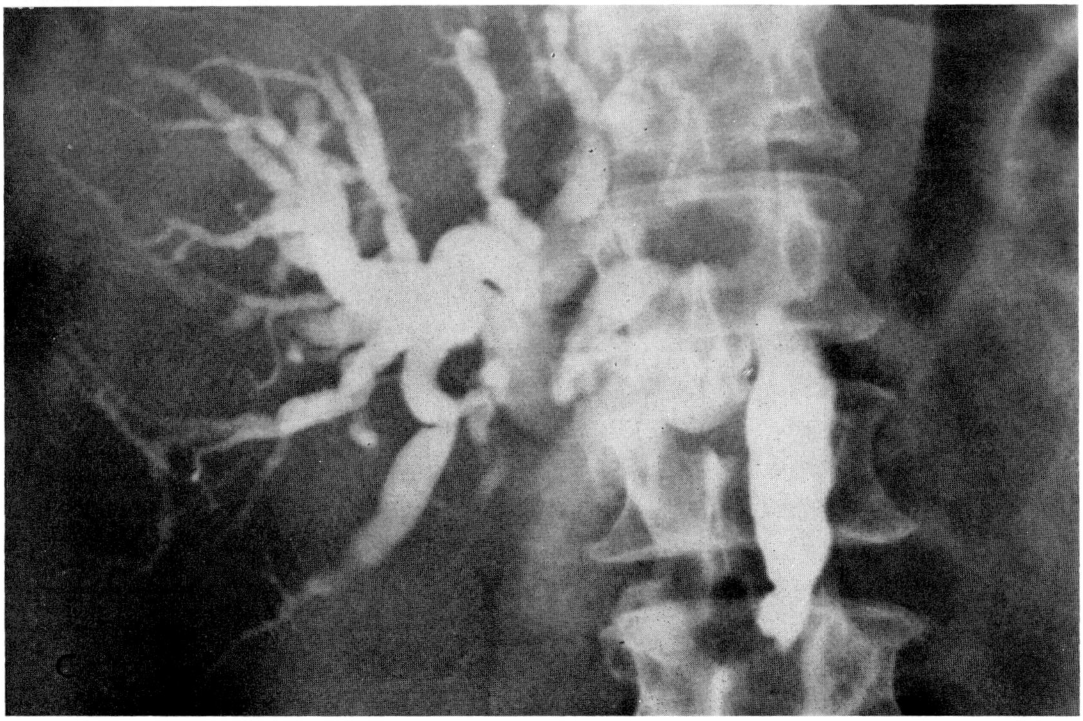

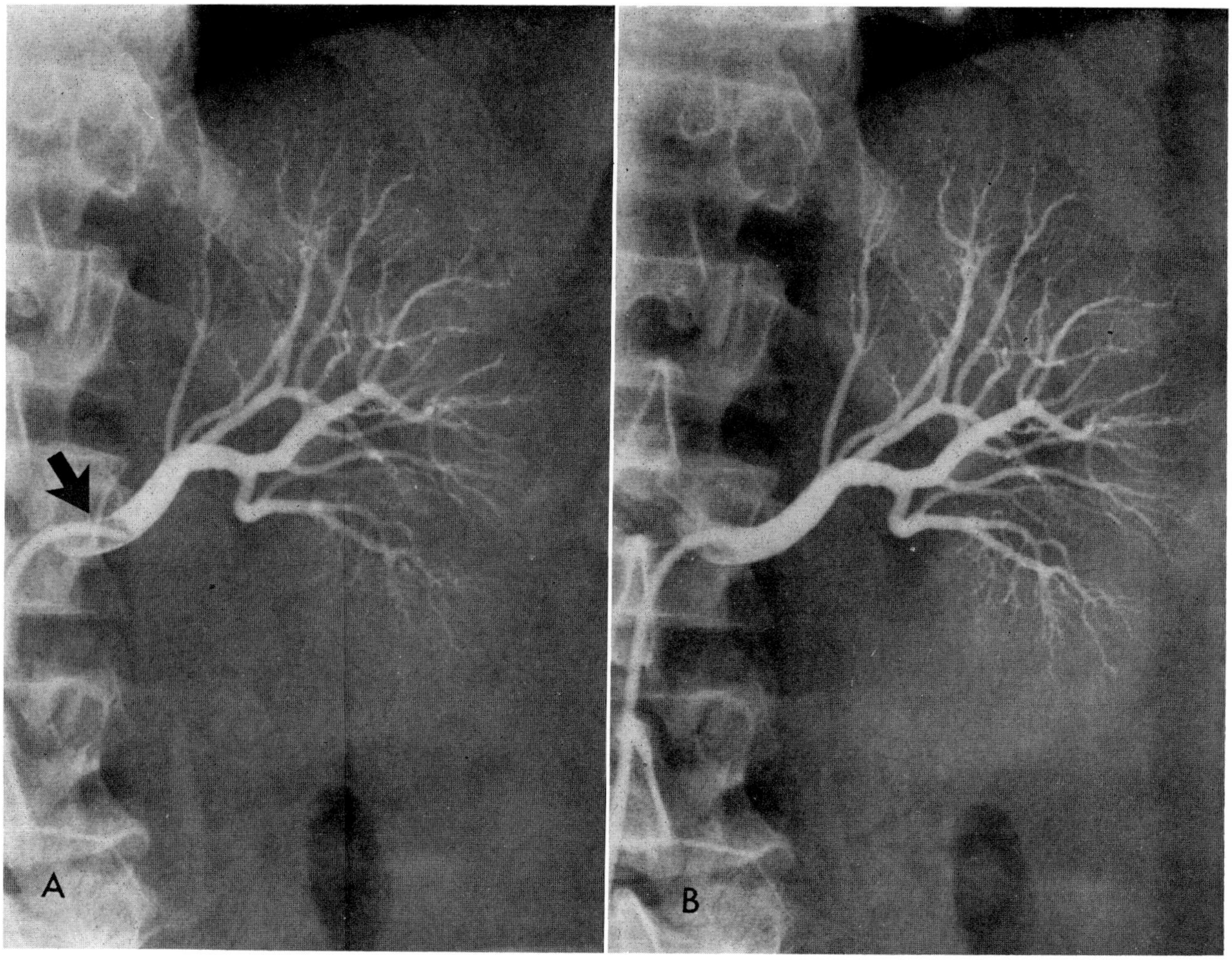

Figure 28.83. Renal Arteriogram. (A) Renal arteriogram: A filling defect is seen at the very proximal renal artery. (B) The filling defect is no more seen. *Comment:* Blood flow during systolic phase causing this filling defect.

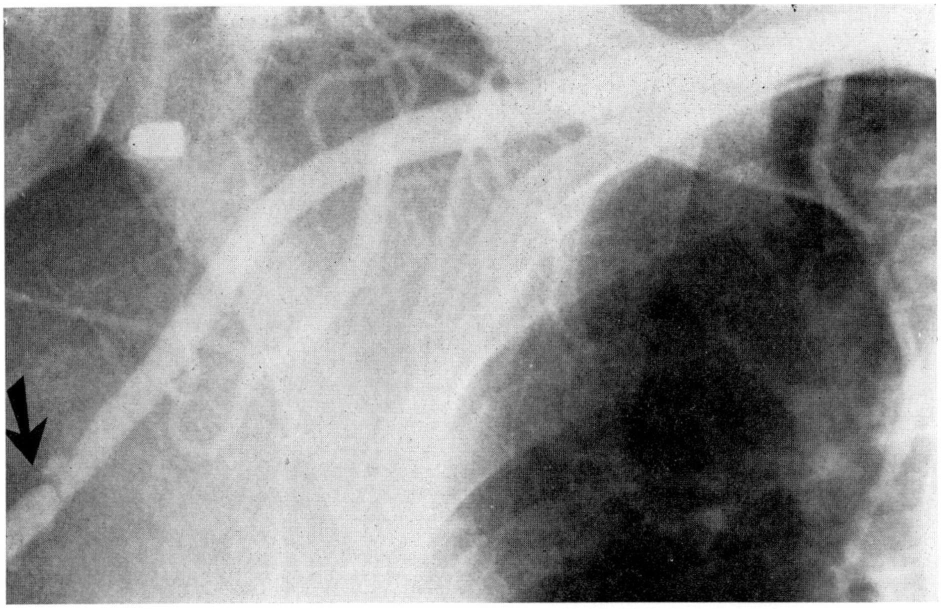

Figure 28.84. Subclavian Arteriogram. There is a linear lucent defect in the brachial artery (Arrow). *Diagnosis:* Traumatic intimal tear due to bullet passing adjacent to but not through the artery.

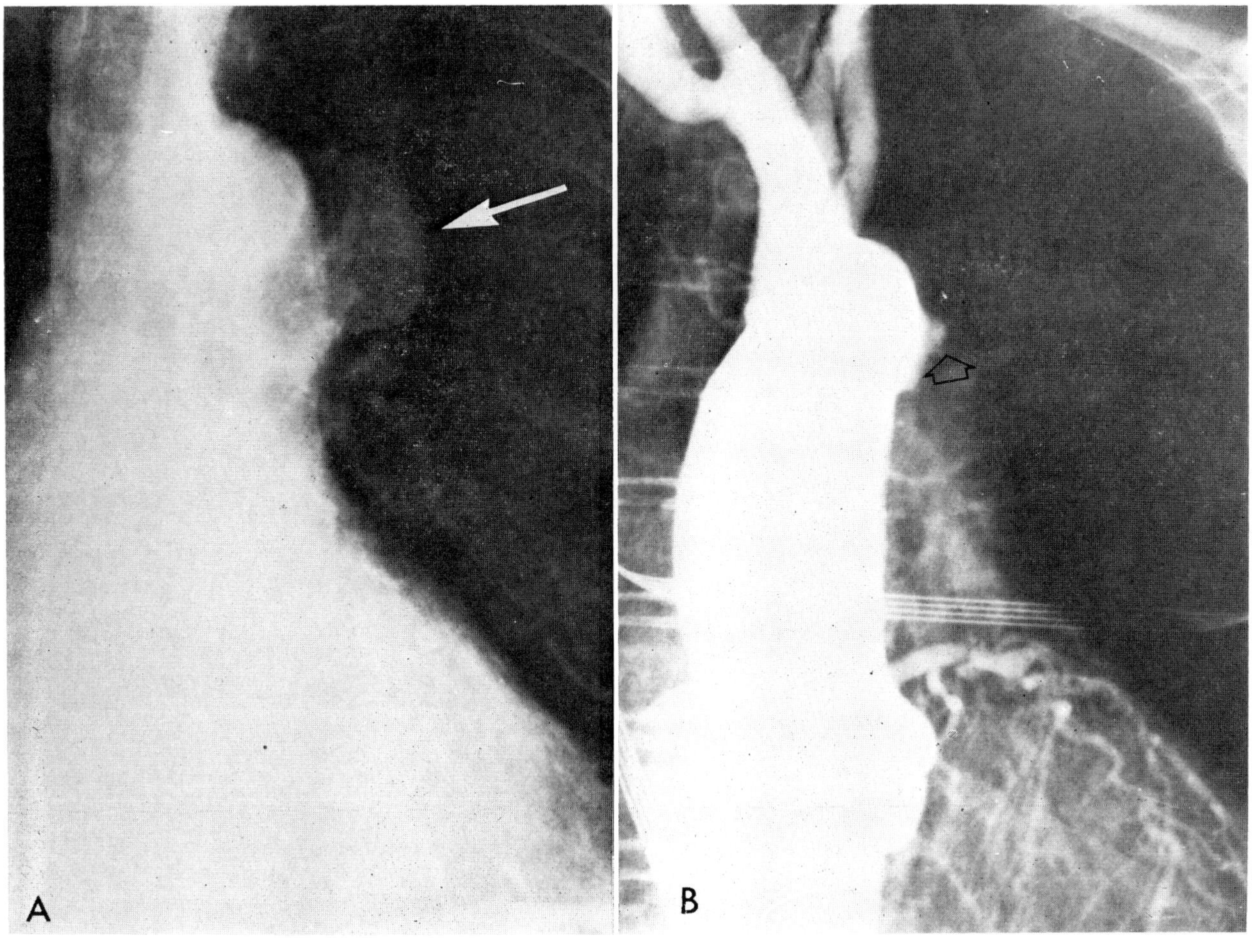

Figure 28.85. Arch Angiogram. (A) The plain chest film shows a mass next to the aortic arch. (B) In the A.P. projection, a small collection of contrast extends beyond the contour of the aorta toward the mass. This seventy-year-old patient was asymptomatic. *Diagnosis:* Clotted aortic aneurysm.

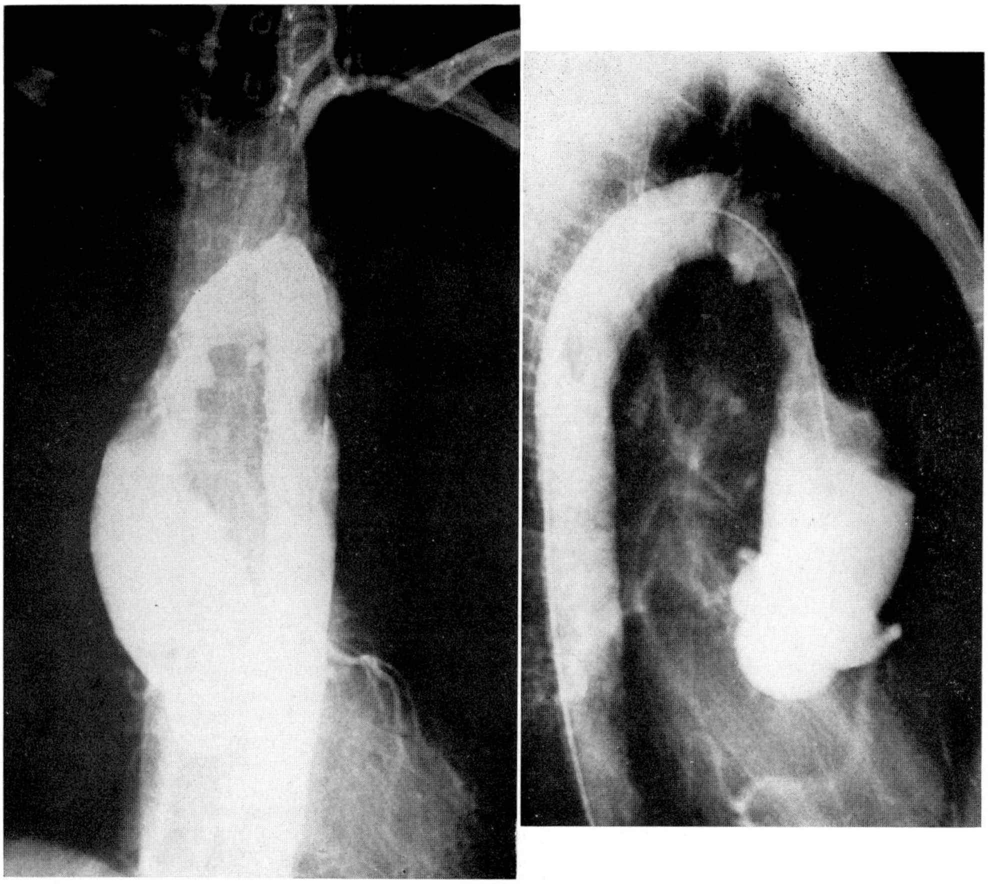

Figure 28.86. Aortogram. (A) Frontal view. (B) Lateral view: Irregular intraluminal filling defects are seen in the opacified aorta. The brachiocephalic vessels do not visualize and the left subclavian fills via collaterals. The patient had episodes of headache, dizzy spells and recent onset of hypertension and gradual loss of radial pulses. *Diagnosis:* Primary intraluminal tumor of the aorta. *Pathology:* Aortic myxoma. (From Silverman, J. F., and Wexler, L. Primary intraluminal tumor of the aorta. *Radiol, 102:*581, 1972. Courtesy of the authors and publishers.)

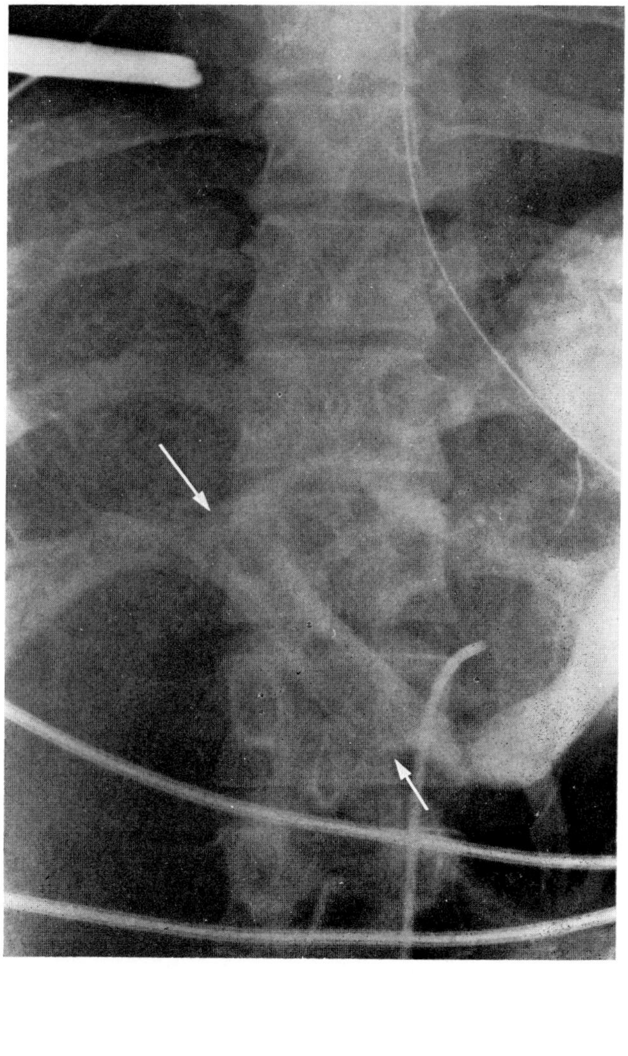

Figure 28.87. Celiac Arteriogram. Venous phase: There is a longitudinal filling defect in the main trunk of the portal vein. *Comment:* Unopacified blood from superior mesenteric vein draining into the portal vein.

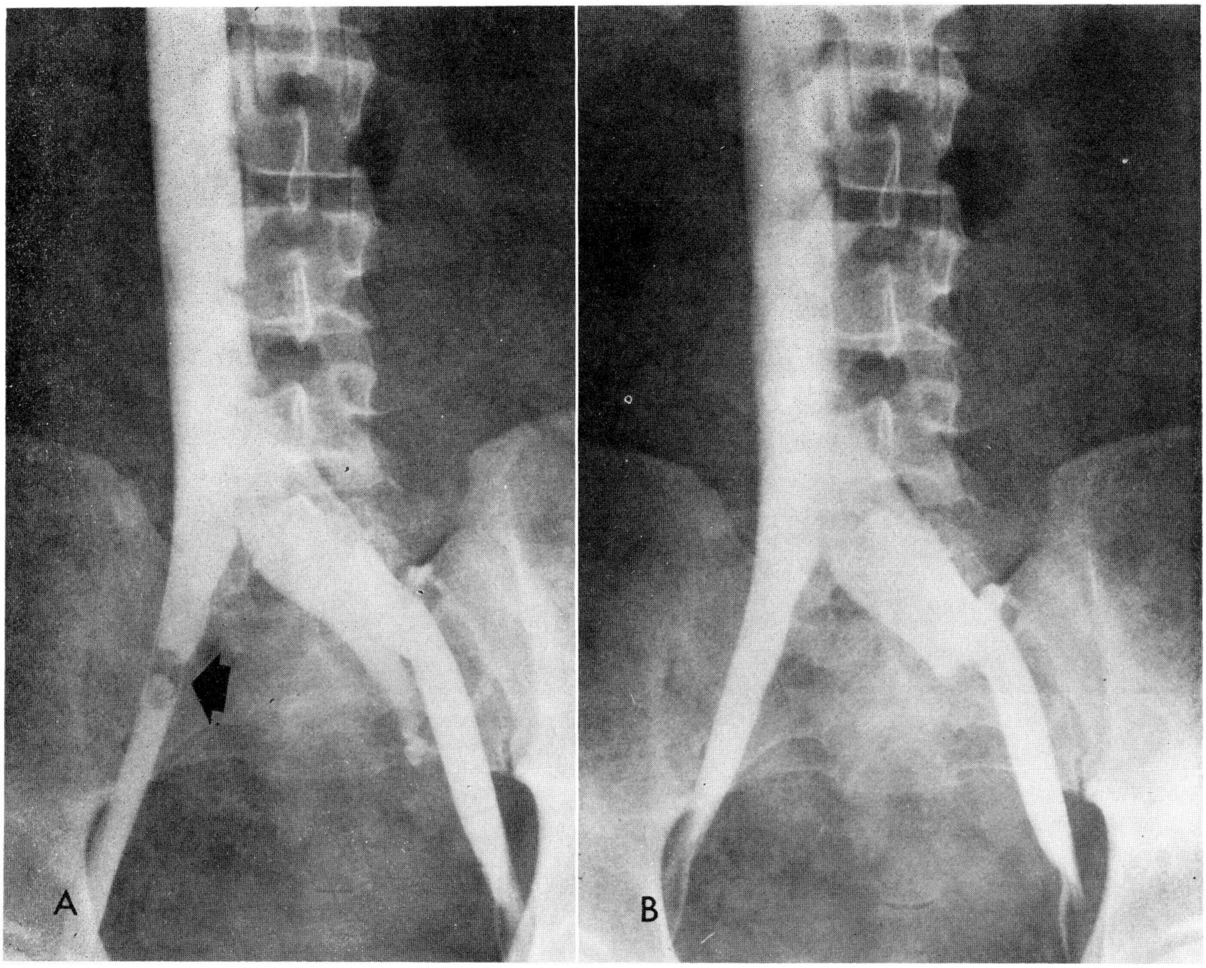

Figure 28.88. Inferior Vena Cavogram. (A) There is a filling defect (Arrow) at the junction of the right external and internal iliac veins. (B) The filling defect is gone. *Comment:* Intermittent venous drainage into the common iliac vein via the internal iliac causes a flow defect.

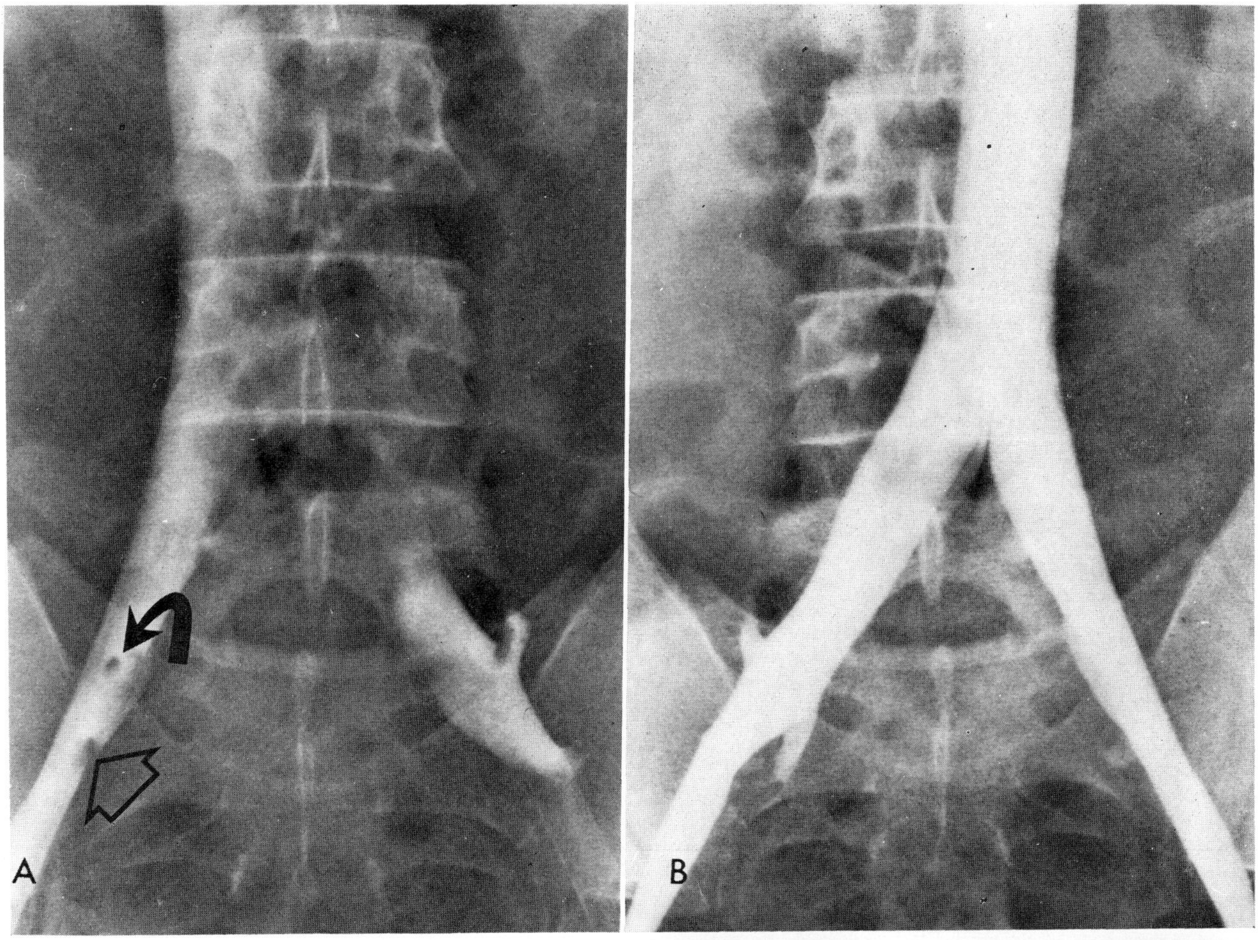

Figure 28.89. Inferior Vena Cavagram. (A) Well-defined, circumscribed filling defects are in the right common iliac vein. The left common iliac vein does not fill. (B) Good filling of both the common iliac veins occurs after a large bolus of contrast is injected. *Comment:* The circumscribed filling defects are due to blood flow from the pelvic veins.

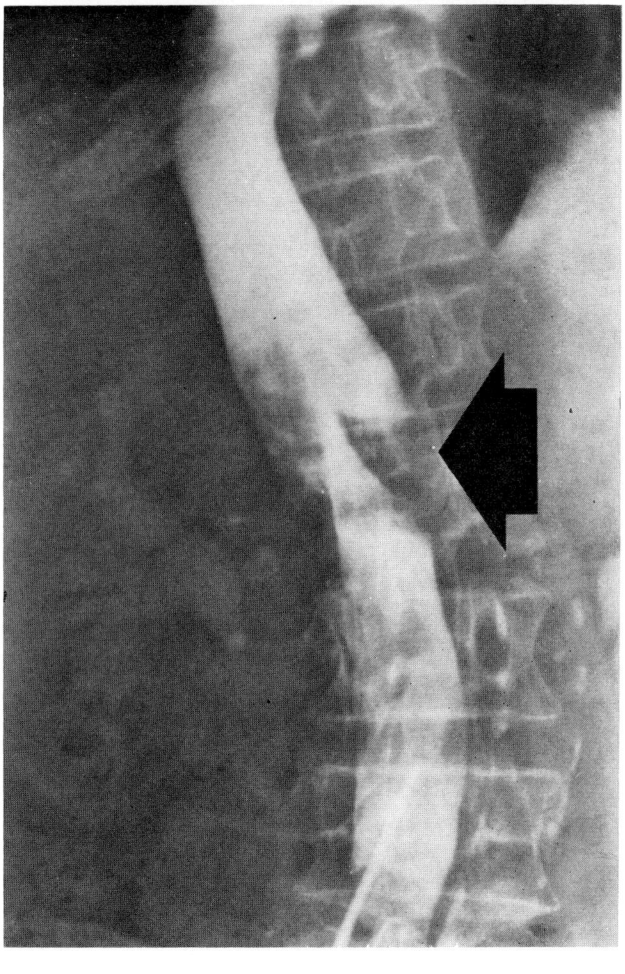

Figure 28.90. Inferior Vena Cavagram. A bizarre filling defect is seen at the level of the renal vein (Arrow). *Comment:* Incomplete mixing of the renal vein blood with the contrast.

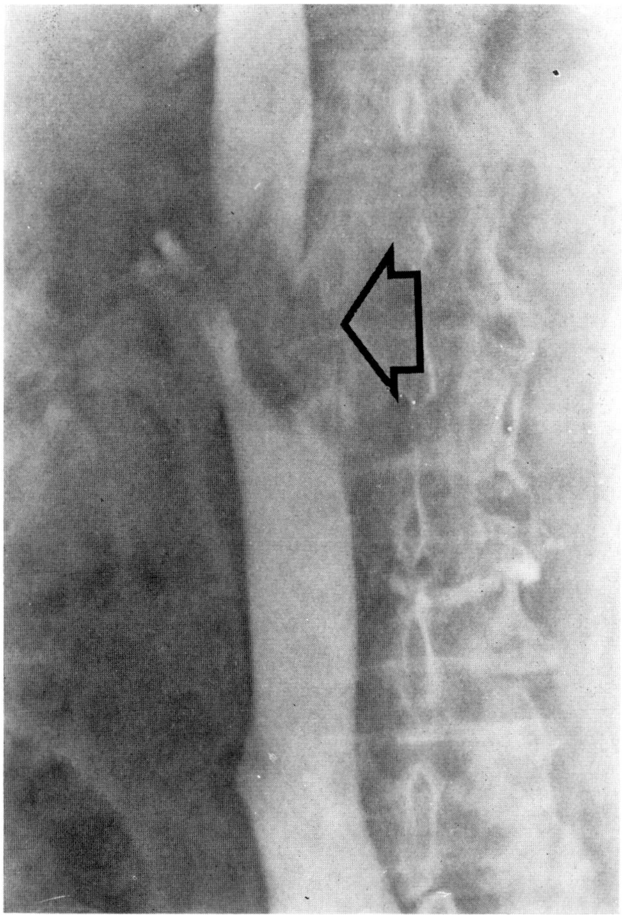

Figure 28.91. Inferior Vena Cavagram. A filling defect is seen at the level of the renal veins. *Comment:* Filling defect due to the blood flow from the renal veins and incomplete mixing of the contrast with the blood.

Figure 28.92. Inferior Vena Cavagram. There is a filling defect in the superior aspect of the left common iliac vein. A repeat injection with a higher injection rate and repositioning of the patient with that side dependent shows the filling defect is seen no more. *Comment:* Incomplete mixing of contrast material with blood.

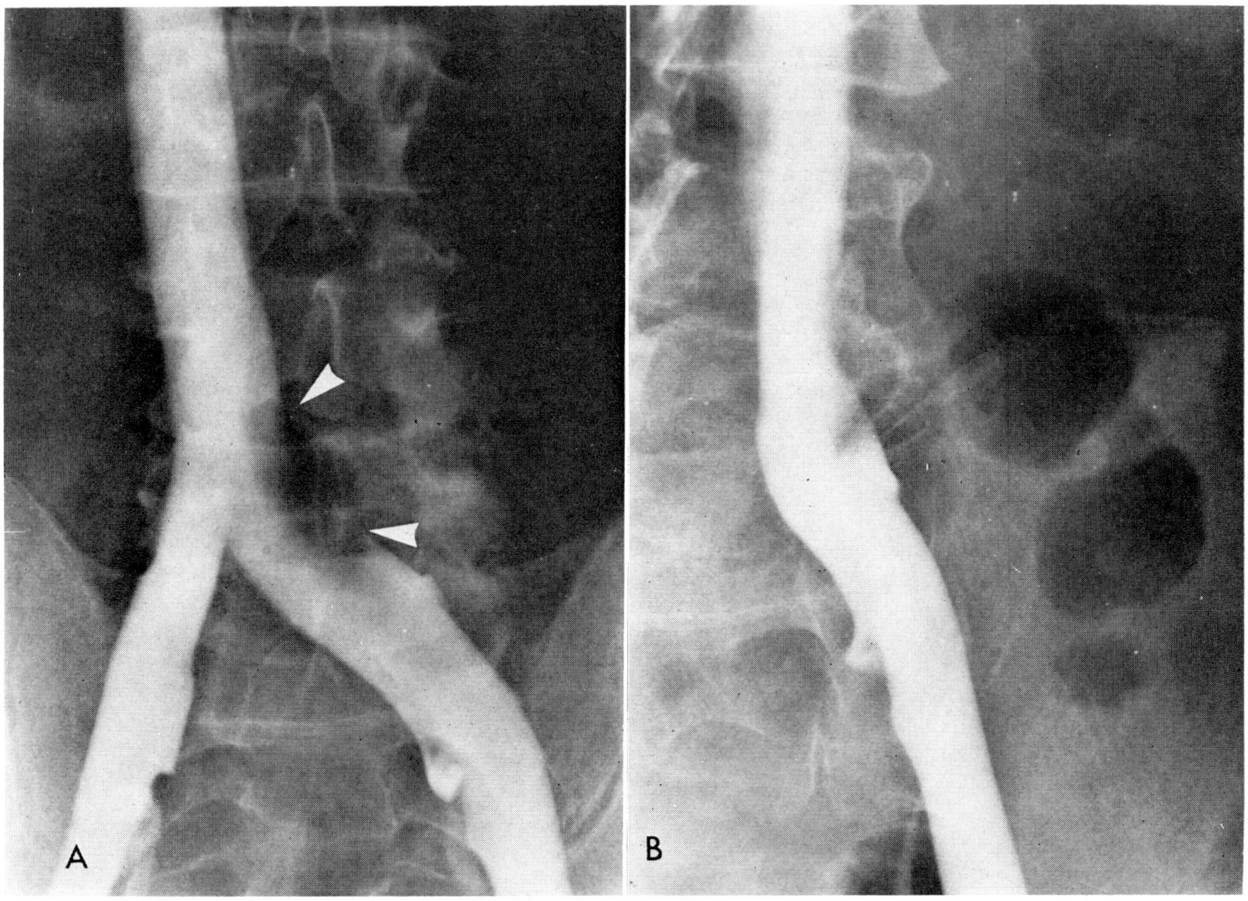

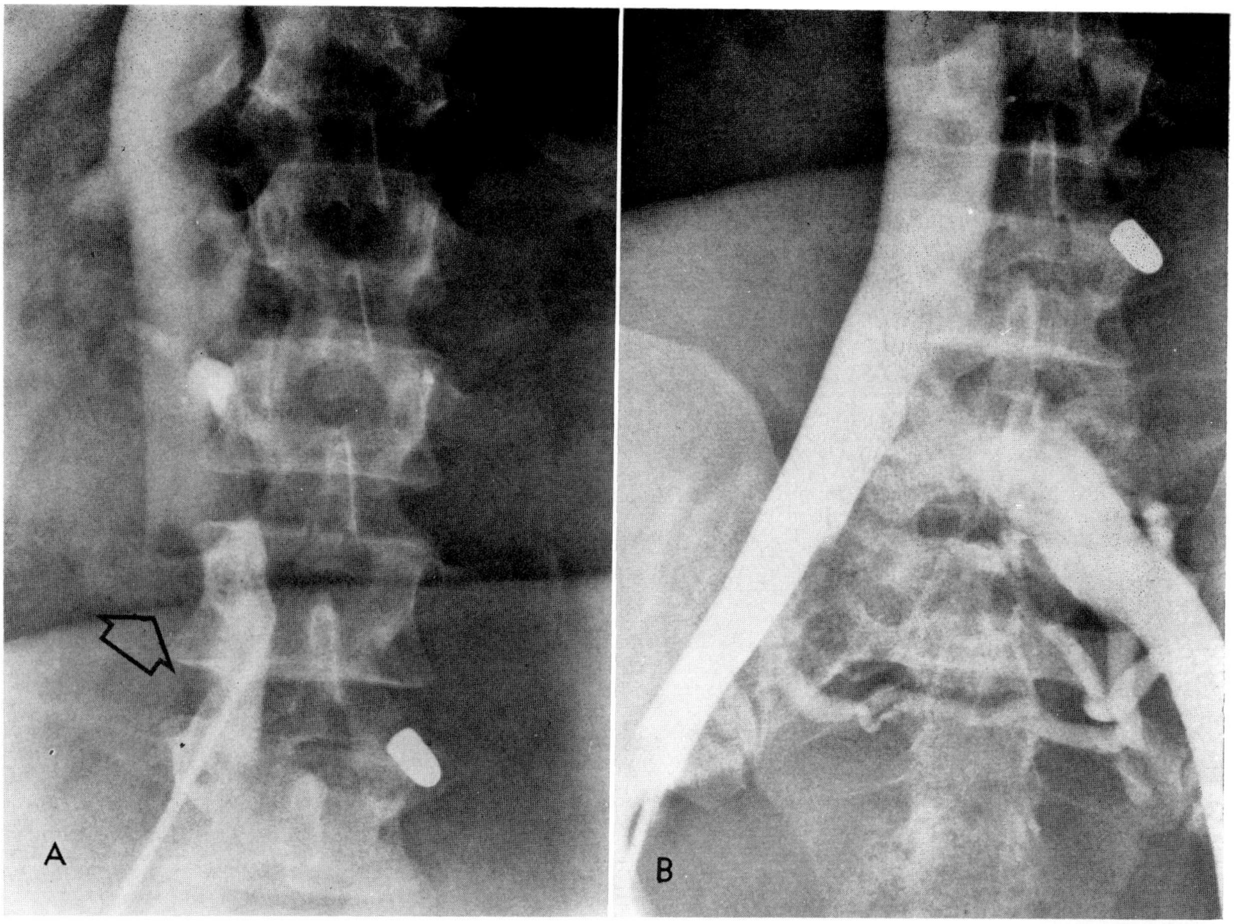

Figure 28.93. Inferior Vena Cavagram. (A) A well-defined, lucent area with a meniscus is in the distal inferior vena cava (Arrow). (B) After withdrawing the catheter to the common iliac vein, a repeat injection does not show the filling defect. *Comment:* Artifact due to incomplete mixing of the blood from the right common iliac vein and the contrast material.

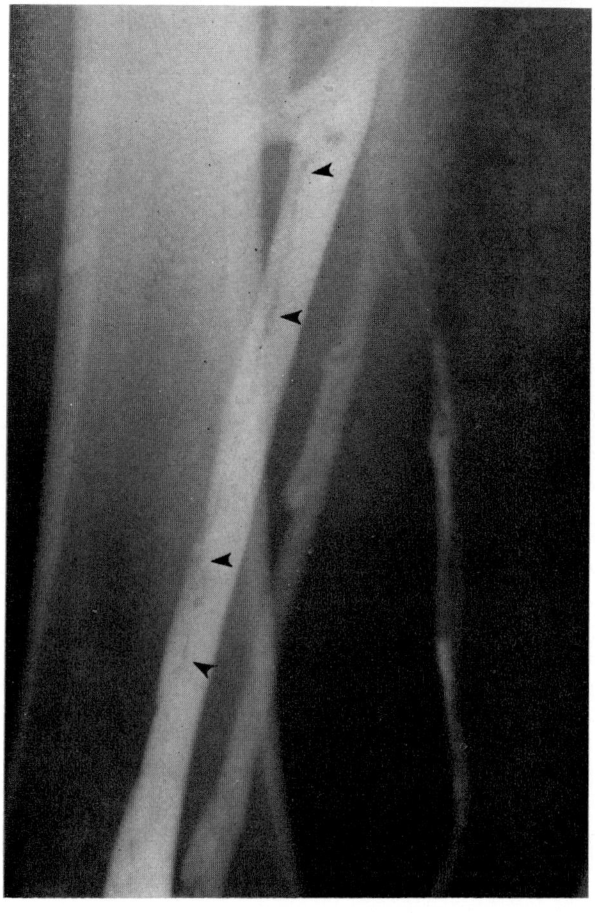

→

Figure 28.94. Lower extremity venogram reveals linear filling defects in the lumen of the femoral vein, in a patient who had repeated attacks of deep venous thrombosis of the entire lower extremity veins. *Diagnosis:* Recanalization of the thrombus.

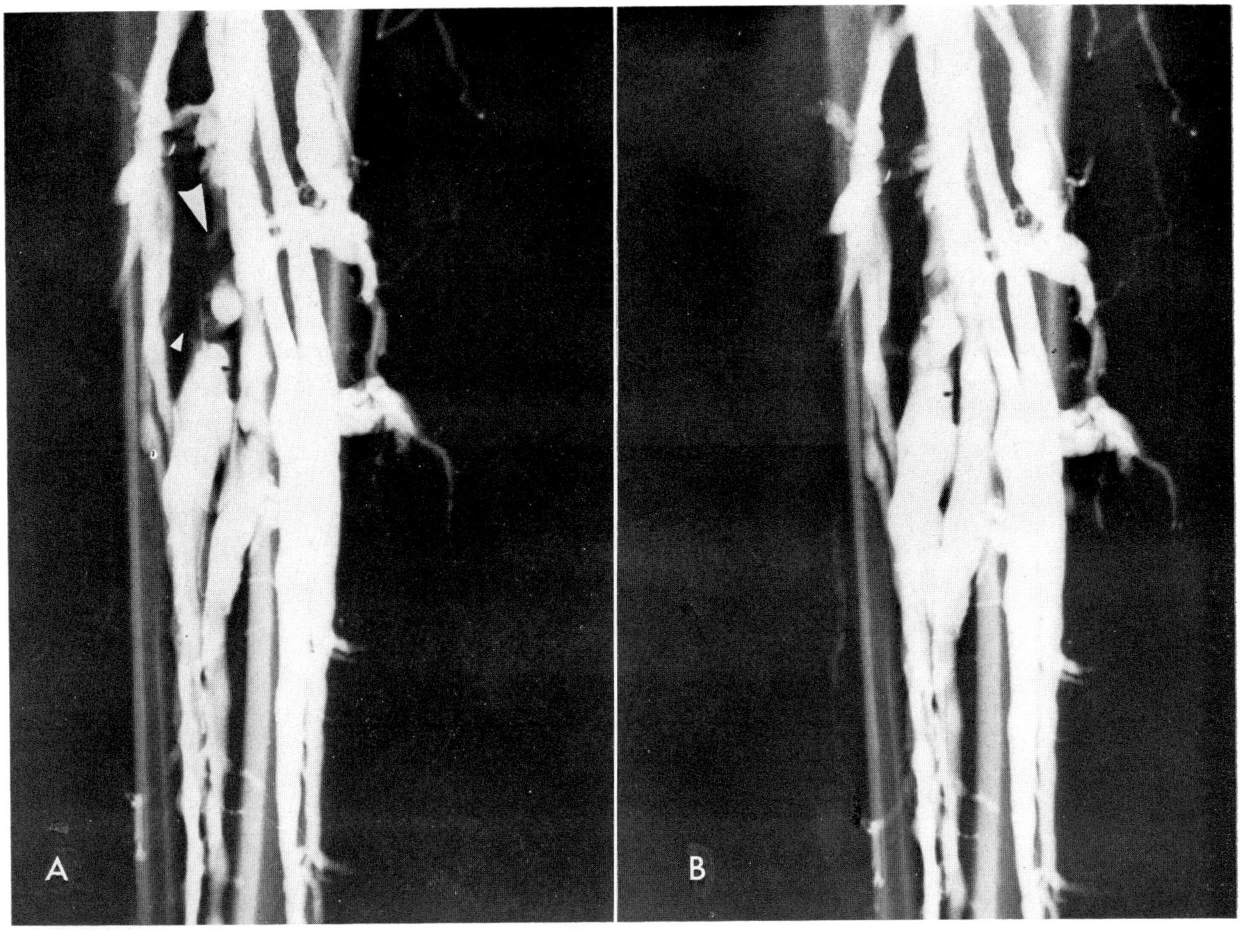

Figure 28.95. Lower Extremity Phlebogram. (A) The deep veins of the calf opacify and a segment of the deep vein (Arrow) does not visualize. (B) A repeat injection after relaxing the calf muscles shows the same segment well opacified. *Comment:* The artifactual non-opacification of a segment is due to contraction of the calf muscles during injection of the contrast material.

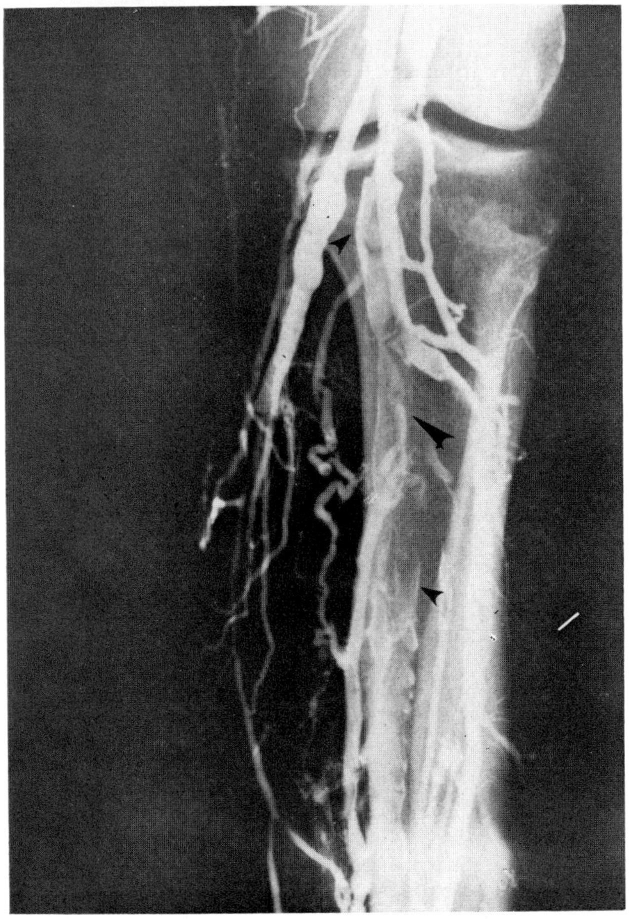

←

Figure 28.96. Lower Extremity Venogram. A long, sausage-shaped filling defect is in the deep venous system. *Diagnosis:* Thrombosis of the deep venous systems of the calf.

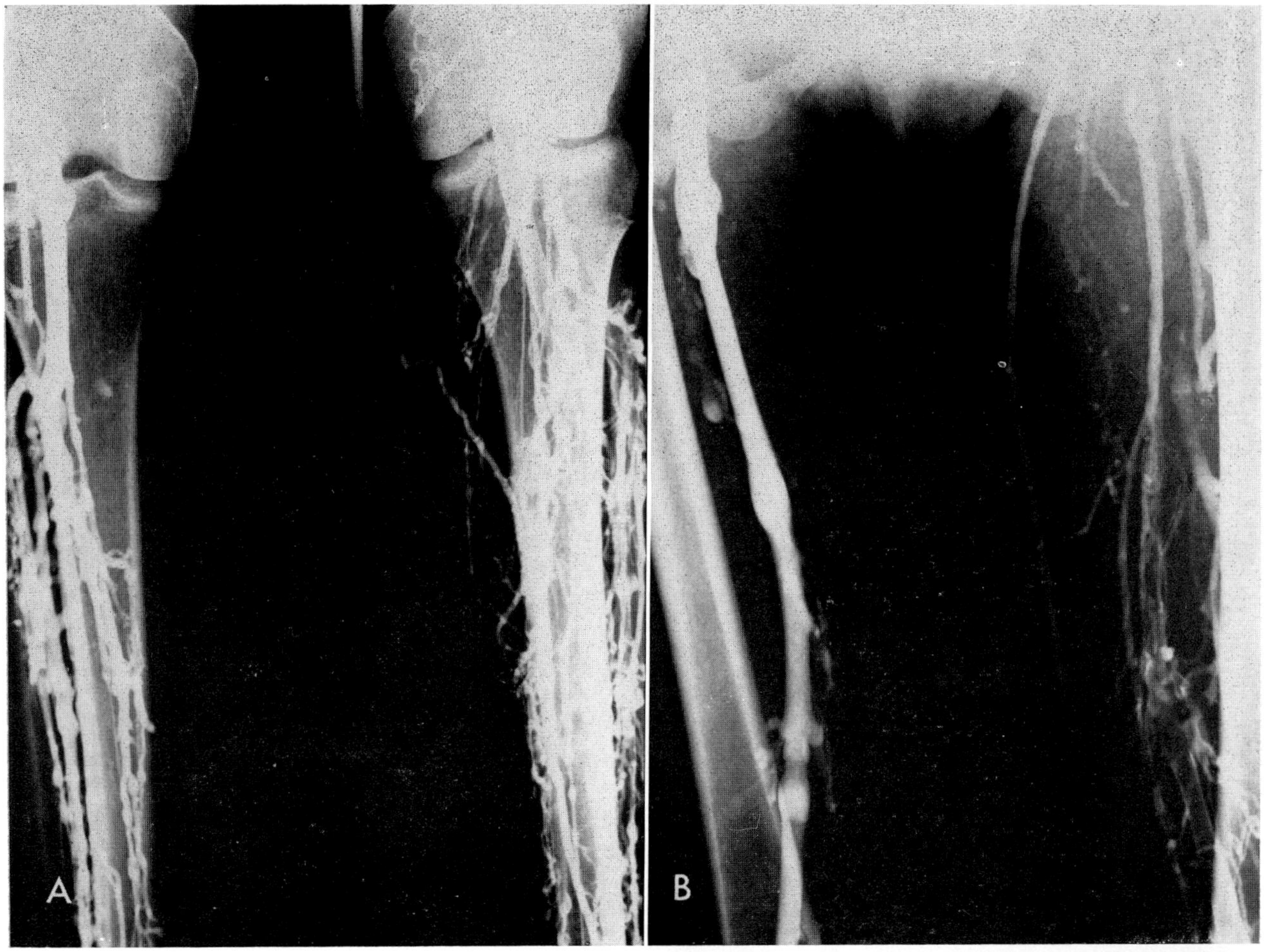

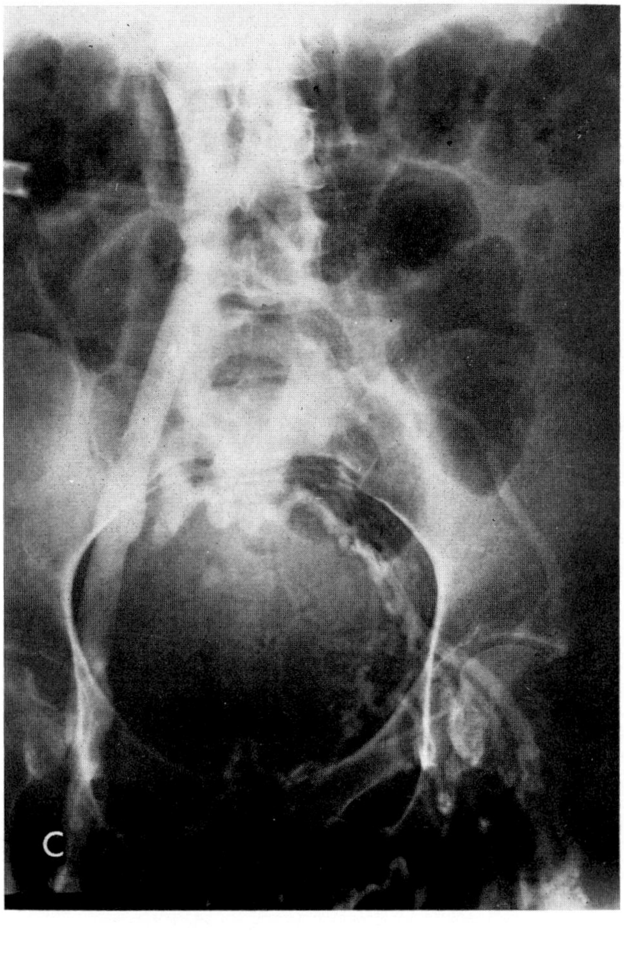

Figure 28.97. Phlebogram—both lower extremities. (A) Lower leg reveals numerous superficial veins in the left calf and a translucent filling defect in the left popliteal vein (Arrow). Compare these findings with the normal right side. (B) Veins of the thighs: The deep veins of the left thigh are not seen. Notice the filling defect in the femoral vein. (C) Veins of the pelvis: Nonvisualization of the common iliac vein on the left, but numerous collateral veins (Arrow) are trying to bridge the occlusion. *Diagnosis:* Thrombosis of deep veins of the left lower extremity.

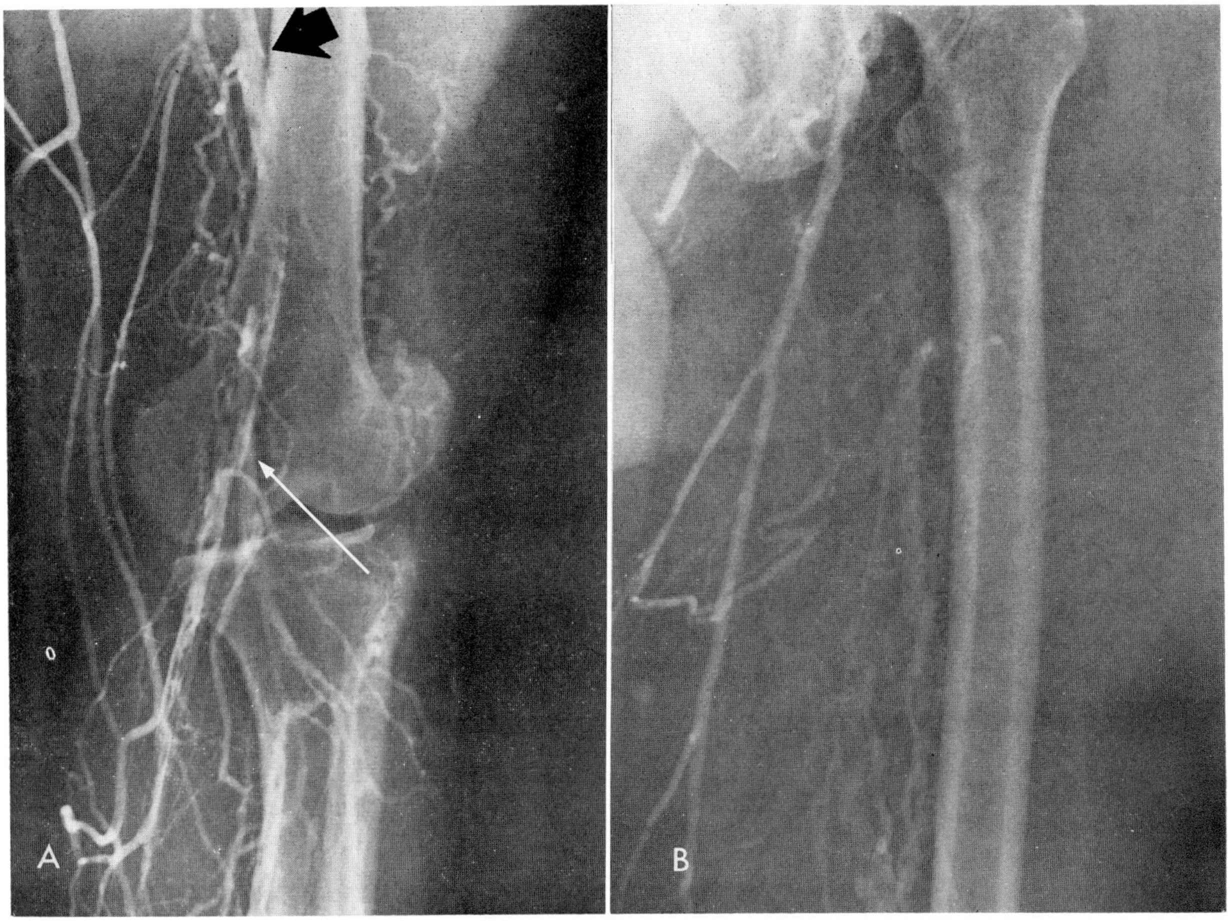

Figure 28.98. Lower Extremity Phlebogram. (A) Filling defects are seen in the deep veins. (B) Nonfilling of the deep veins of the thigh. Note the dilated tortuous veins. *Diagnosis:* Extensive deep venous thrombosis of the lower extremity.

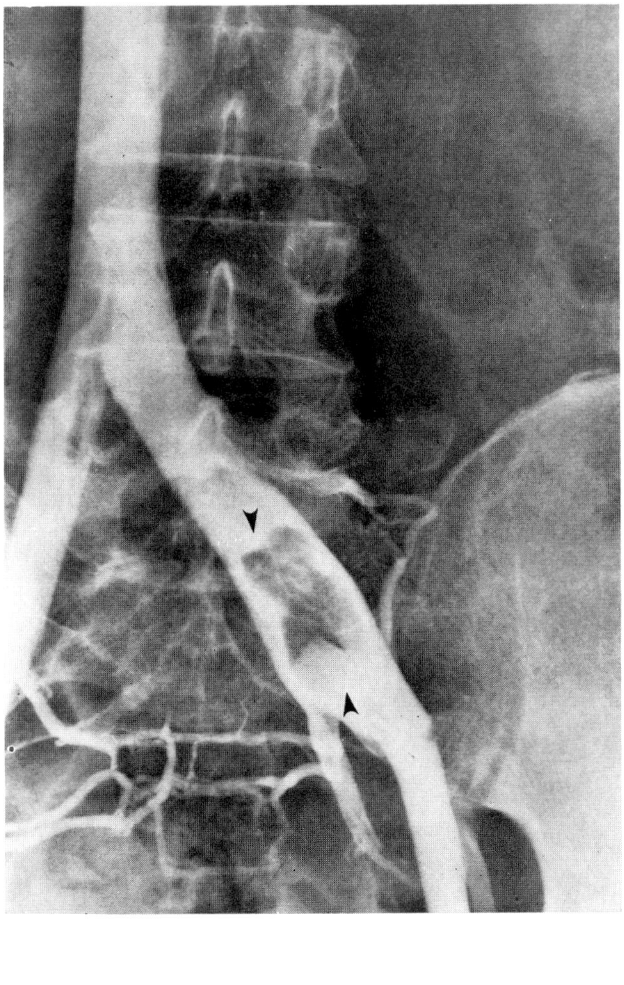

←

Figure 28.99. Inferior Vena Cavagram. An irregular, well-defined filling defect is in the left common iliac vein. *Diagnosis:* Thromboembolic disease.

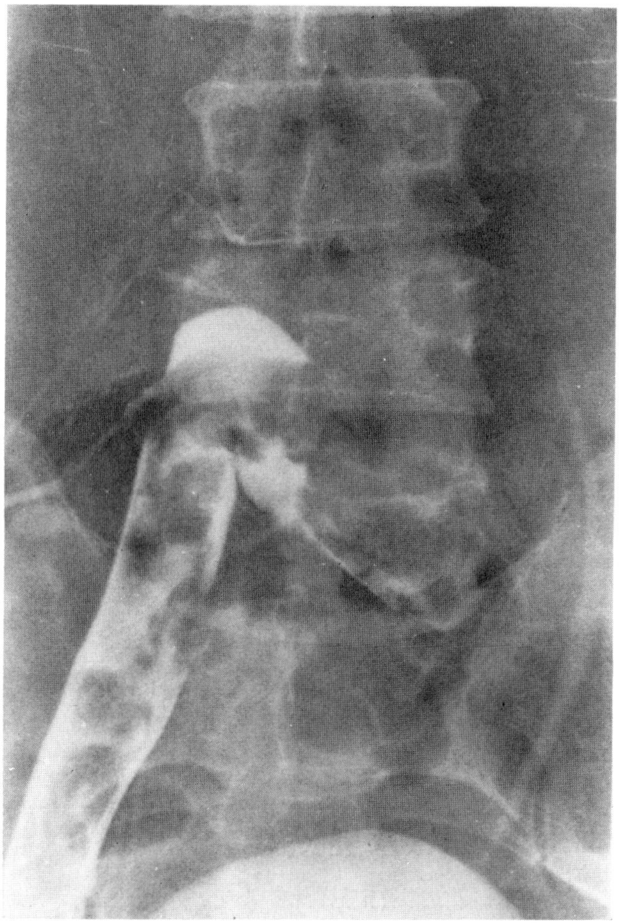

Figure 28.100. Inferior Vena Cavagram. This patient had an umbrella placed into the vena cava. Multiple numerous filling defects occupy both common iliac veins with complete occlusion of the left common iliac vein lumen. *Diagnosis:* Multiple thromboemboli in the common iliac veins.

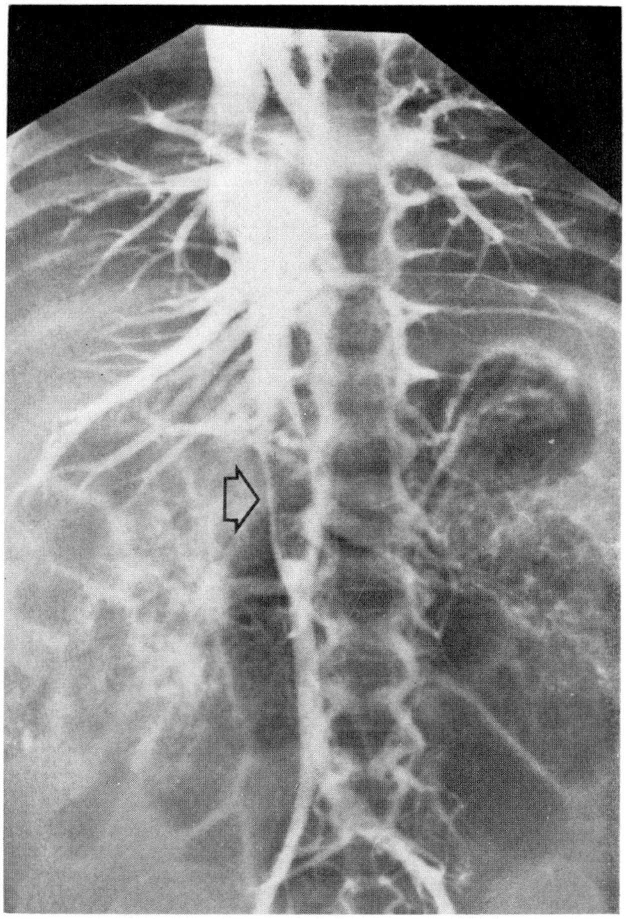

Figure 28.101. Inferior Vena Cavagram. A moderately sized filling defect is in the suprarenal segment of inferior vena cava. *Diagnosis:* Thromboembolus.

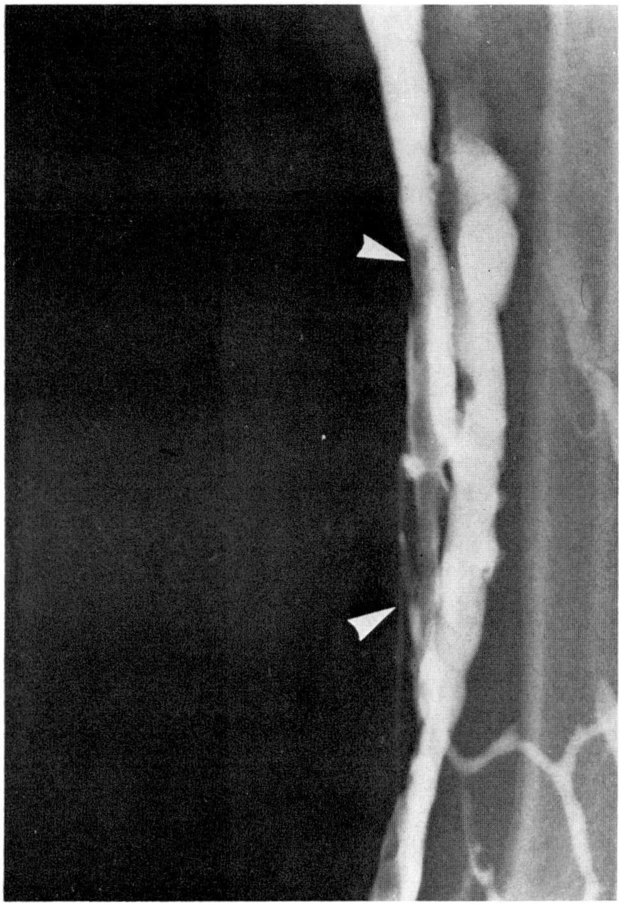

Figure 28.102. Upper Extremity Venogram. An elongated filling defect is in the deep venous system of the arm. *Diagnosis:* A floating thrombus.

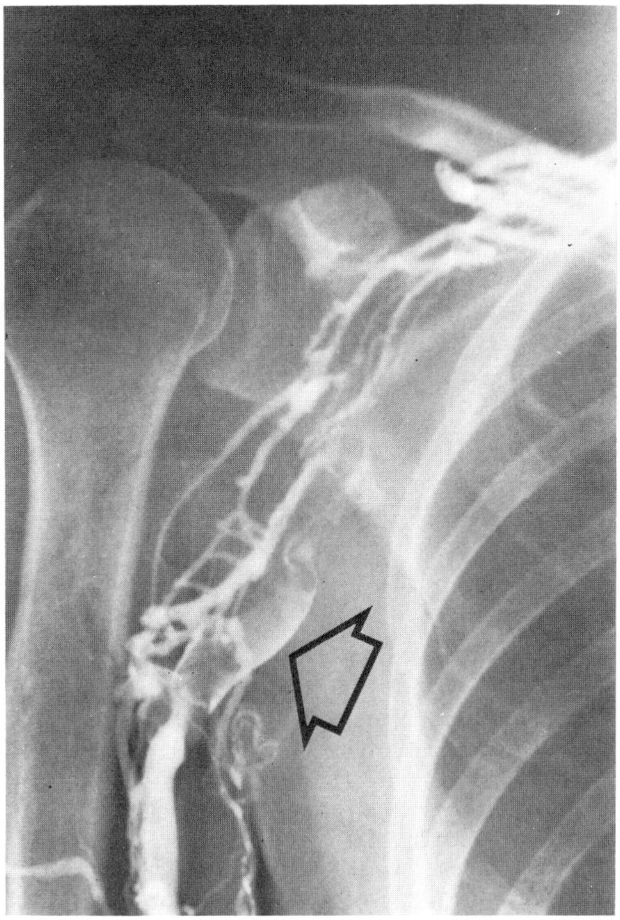

Figure 28.103. Right Upper Extremity Venogram. A filling defect is in the brachial vein at its junction with the axillary vein with expansion of that segment of the vein (Arrow). The patient used the arm excessively the previous night. *Diagnosis:* Effort thrombosis of the brachial vein extending into the axillary vein.

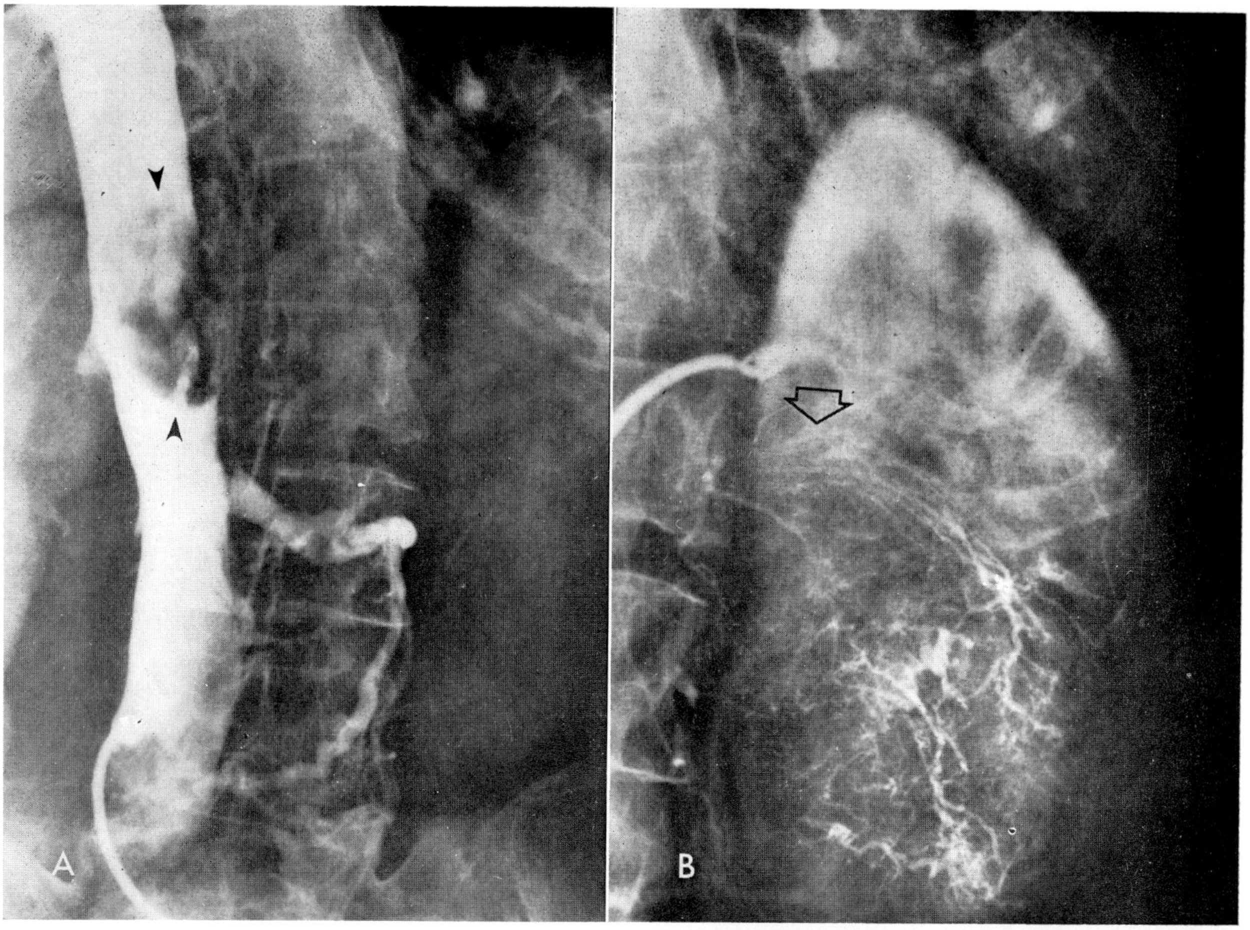

Figure 28.104. (A) Inferior vena cavagram: A smooth, oval filling defect is in the midinferior vena cava at the level of the renal vein. (B) Renal arteriogram—arterial phase: Irregularly dilated vessels with abnormal arborization in the lower half of the kidney and linear vessels traversing along the course of the left renal vein are seen (Arrow). *Diagnosis:* Hypernephroma with tumor thrombus growing into the inferior vena cava via the left renal vein.

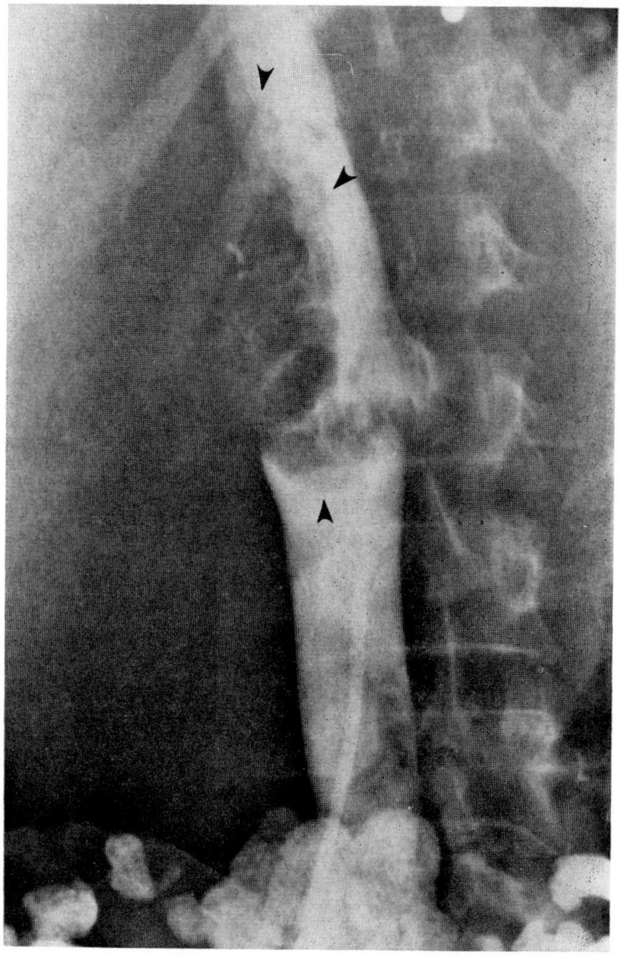

Figure 28.105. Inferior Vena Cavagram. A big filling defect with an inferior meniscus and proximal loculations in the inferior vena cava is noted in a patient who had a nonvisualized kidney and hematuria. *Diagnosis:* Hypernephroma with tumor thrombus extending into the inferior vena cava.

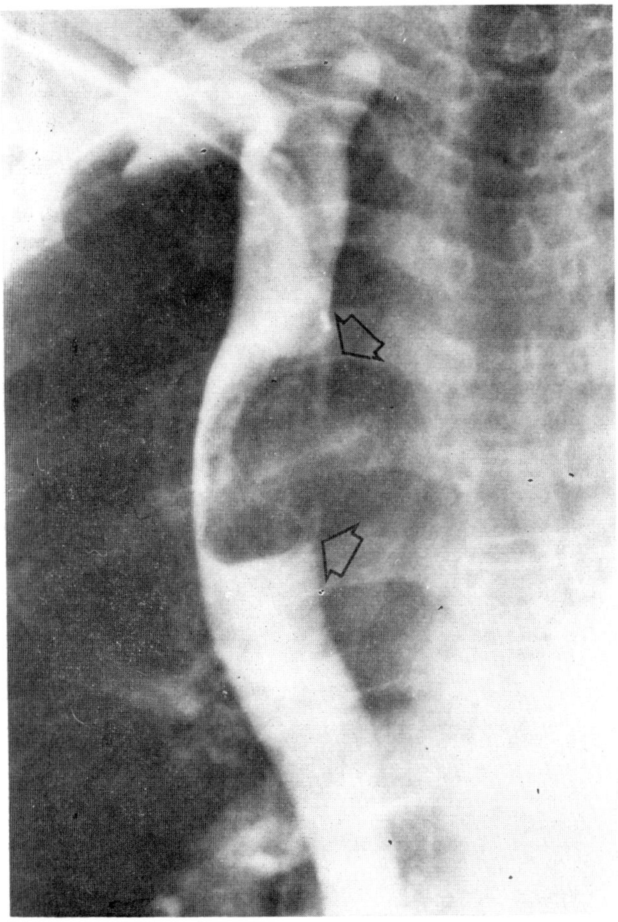

Figure 28.106. Superior Vena Cavagram. A moderately sized filling defect is seen in the superior vena cava with no visualization of the medial wall. This patient had a right paratracheal mass. *Diagnosis:* Bronchogenic cancer growing into the lumen of the superior vena cava.

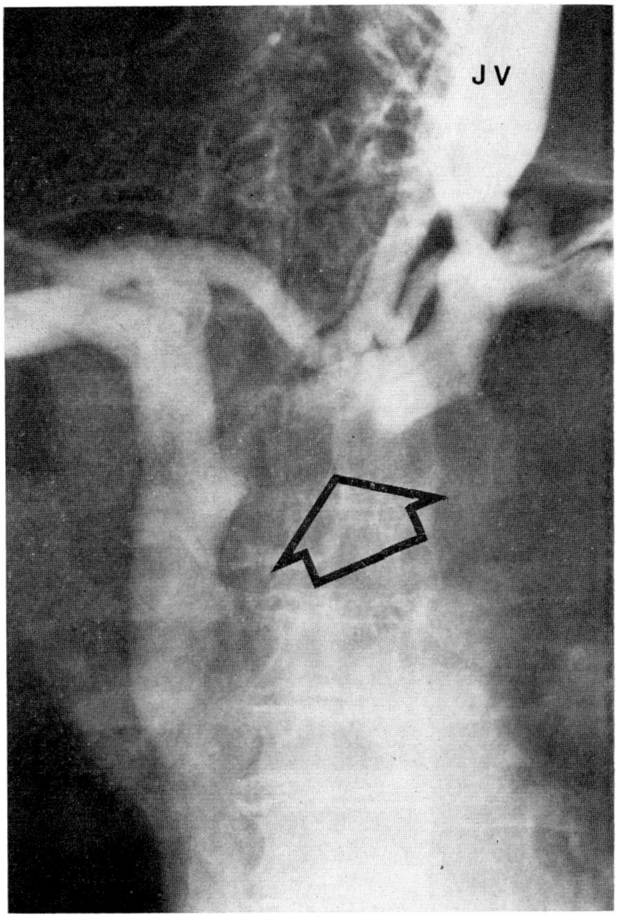

Figure 28.107. Superior Vena Cavagram. A filling defect is in the left innominate vein (Arrow). Contrast refluxes into the jugular vein (J.V.). *Diagnosis:* Malignant tumor infiltrating into the left innominate vein. *Comment:* The advantage of doing venography through both upper extremities is obvious.

Figure 28.108. Superior Vena Cava. A filling defect is in the superior vena cava. Notice the mass adjacent to the filling defect. There is diffuse interstitial fibrosis. *Diagnosis:* Bronchogenic carcinoma. Bronchogenic carcinoma in a patient who had sarcoidosis. Benign lymph nodes by themselves do not infiltrate the veins, but they will deviate and compress the veins.

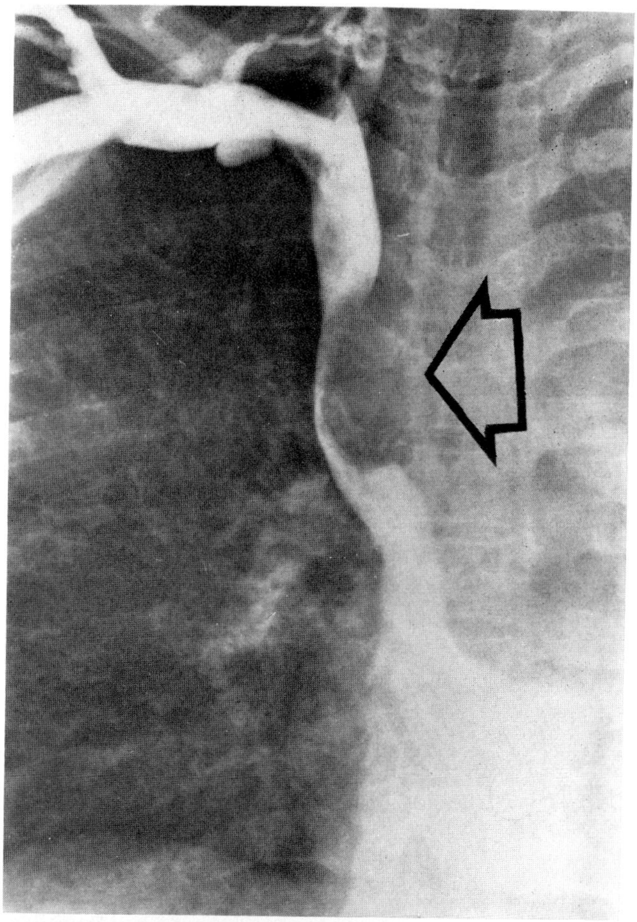

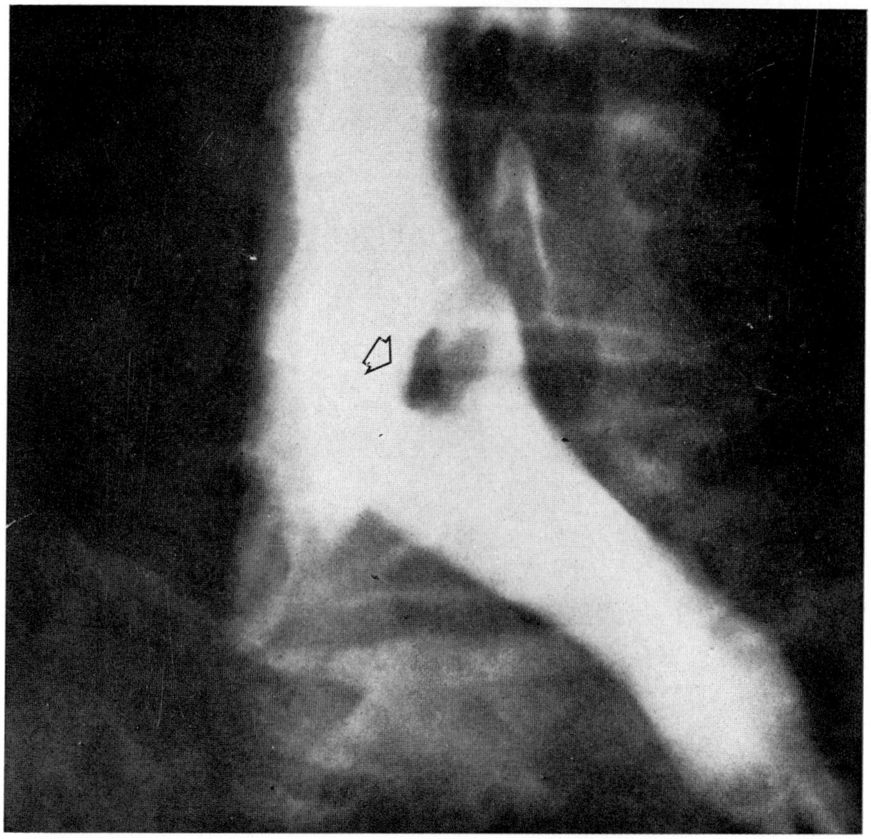

Figure 28.109. Common Iliac Venogram. A filling defect is seen in the mouth of the left common iliac vein. *Diagnosis:* Thrombus? Tumor? *Pathology:* A band joining the anterior wall of the vein to the posterior. (From Negus, D., Fletcher, E. W. L., Cockett, F. B., and Thomas, M. Lea. Compression and band formation at the mouth of the left common iliac vein. *Br J Surg*, 55:369, 1968. Courtesy of the authors and publishers.)

whether there is intraparenchymal, subcapsular or pericapsular fatal exsanguination into the peritoneal or retroperitoneal spaces. *Delayed effects* can range from hypertension related to renal trauma, hemobilia due to hepatic trauma, or even death due to delayed rupture of the spleen. In decreasing order, the *kidney, spleen, liver and pancreas* are the most frequently involved organs when there is a history of blunt trauma. The *vulnerability of these organs increases if they are enlarged.*

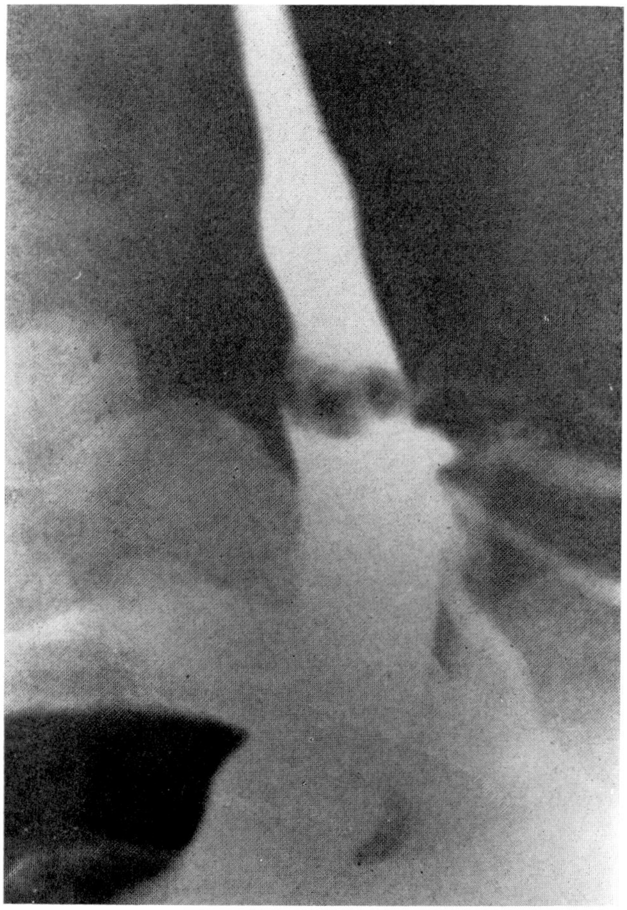

Figure 28.110. External Jugular Venogram. A sharply outlined polypoid filling defect is located between the valves. No thrombus tail is seen. There is associated incomplete obstruction. The filling defect reveals a reticulated pattern. The patient had nodular swelling in the neck. *Diagnosis:* Tumor arising from the wall of the vein. *Pathology:* Hemangioma of the external jugular vein. (From Meyers, M. A. Hemangioma of the external jugular vein. *Radiol,* 89:483, 1967. Courtesy of the authors and publishers.)

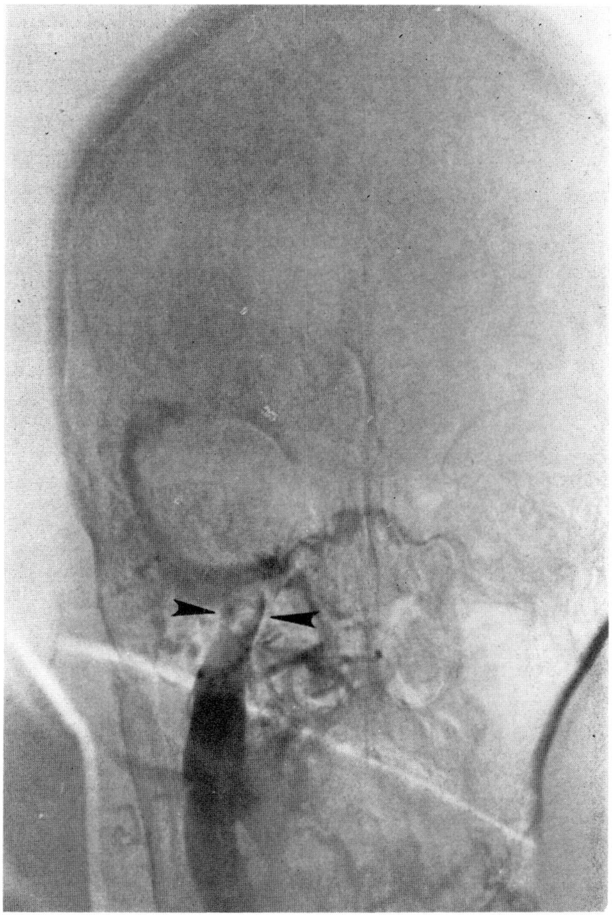

Figure 28.111. Jugular Venogram. A substraction film reveals a filling defect with a meniscus in the internal jugular vein at the level of jugular fossa in a patient with known glomus jugulare tumor. *Diagnosis:* Tumor thrombus in the jugular vein.

Radiographic findings include stasis or irregular accumulation of contrast and increased vascularity in focal or multifocal areas. This would suggest contusion of an organ. Occlusion of a vessel or vessels of varying caliber with lack of perfusion in that portion of the parenchyma suggests thrombosis, laceration or avulsion of the vessels depending on the anatomic extent of the traumatic lesions. Extravasation of the contrast indicates a ruptured vessel. Premature opacification represents an arteriovenous communication at that level of injury. Circumferential deviation of the intraparenchymal branches of an organ reflects either early or delayed intraparenchymal bleed-

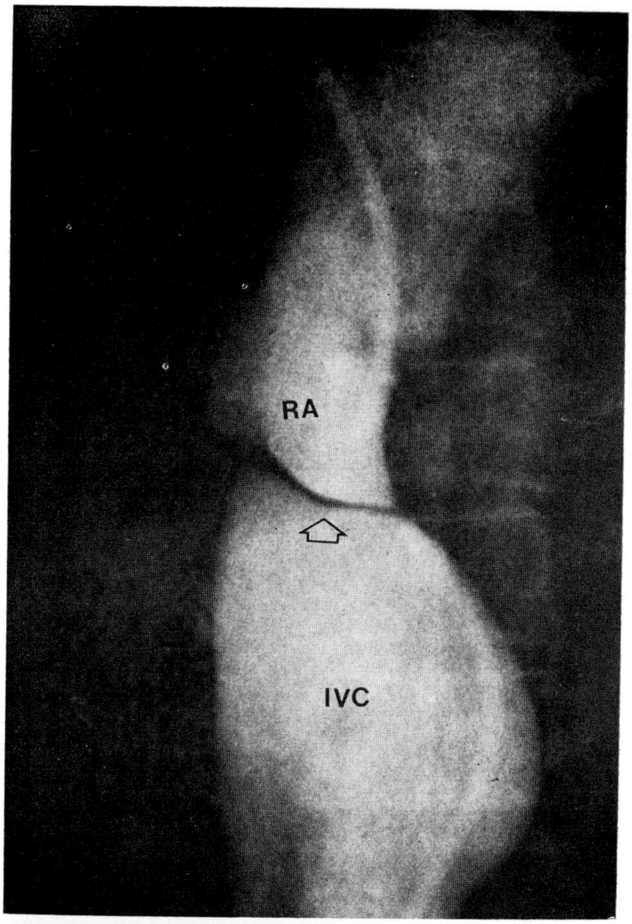

Figure 28.112. Simultaneous opacification of the inferior vena cava and the right atrium (R.A.) reveals a linear filling defect consistent with membranous obstruction of the inferior vena cava (I.V.C.). (From Kimura, C., Matsuda, S., Koie, H., and Hirooka, M. Membranous obstruction of the hepatic portion of the inferior vena cava. *Surgery, 72*:551, 1972. Courtesy of the authors and publishers.)

Figure 28.113. (A) Renal arteriogram: A bullet is in the projection of the right kidney. (B) Lateral view: The filling effect is due to the bullet in the renal vein.

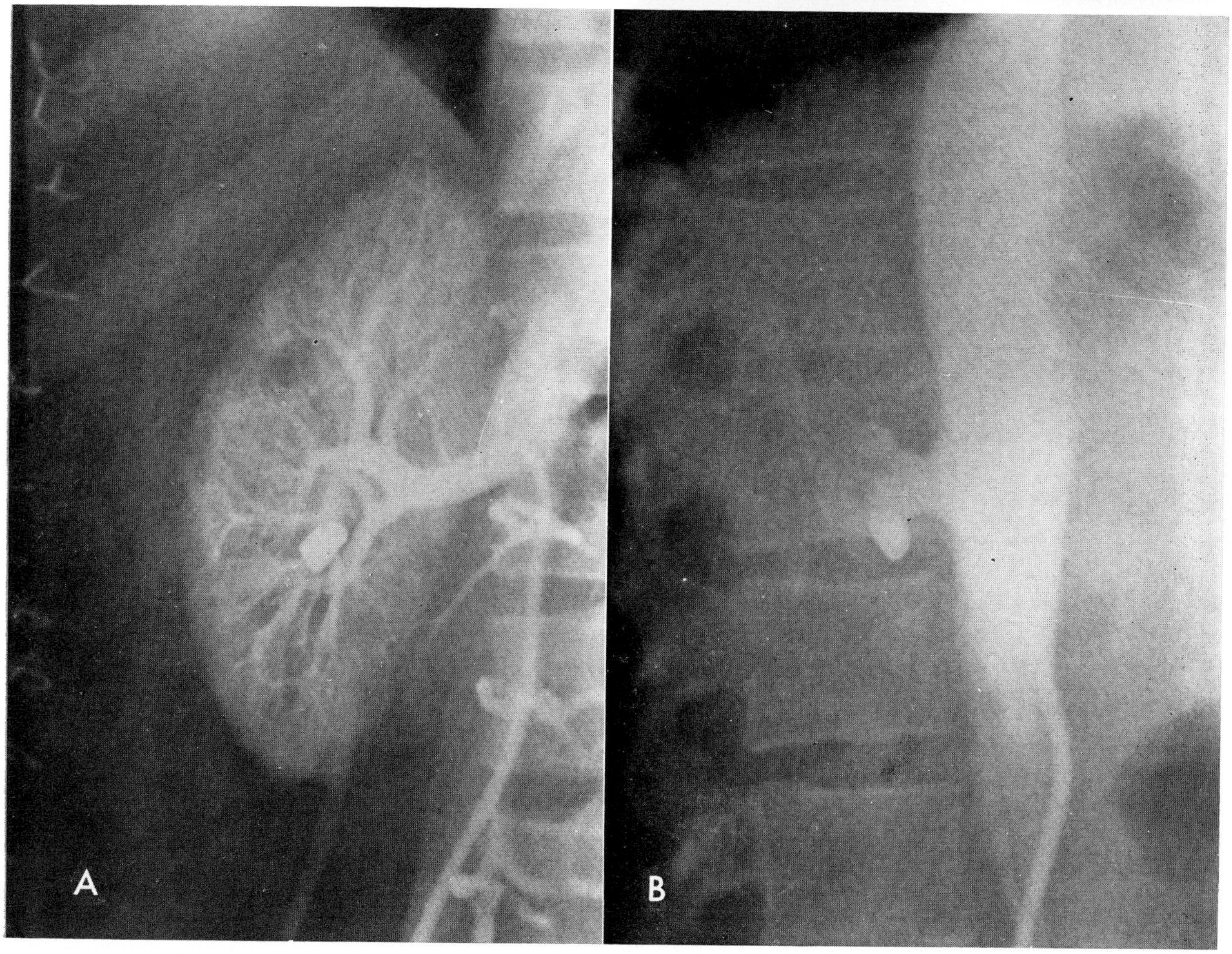

ing, abscess formation, or hemorrhagic cysts. The last two are delayed phenomena. Separation of the subcapsular branches from the capsular boundary indicates a subcapsular hematoma.

Splenic Trauma

The spleen is unusually susceptible to rupture from blunt trauma because of its friability, engorgement, or prior enlargement.[605, 1063, 1065] Retention of the spleen in the left upper quadrant of the abdomen[1060, 1061] makes it relatively immobile. This is due to filaments of the greater omentum with its vasa brevia inserting into the splenic capsule and hilum. During trauma the filaments may peel away the splenic capsule. This may also occur if there are adhesions between the spleen and diaphragm. The long tortuous splenic vessels are susceptible to avulsion, while the soft parenchyma may develop single or multiple lacerations or transverse parenchymal tears which may be either partial or complete. They usually tend to be complete in children[1062] (Figs. 28-36, 28-37, 28-41, 28-54, 26-40, 26-41 and 29-46).

The extravasated blood may collect in the parenchyma, extend into the subcapsular space (Fig. 26-46), or extend beyond the capsule if it is also torn. The initial intraparenchymal bleeding always holds the threat of fatal rupture of the spleen,[605] because the balance maintained between the vis-a-tergo of the extravasated blood and the opposing hemostatic force of the splenic parenchyma is an exceedingly delicate one. A slight increase in the former or initiation of minimal secondary trauma is enough to cause delayed secondary rupture. The delayed rupture can occur from forty-eight hours to many months following trauma. One should be aware of *pitfalls*[1064] such as fetal lobulations which may resemble a parenchymal tear, gastric fundal stains, avascular incidental masses in the spleen, or mesentery adherent to the spleen. All may cause misinterpreting a normal spleen as a torn one.

Hepatic Trauma

Because of its relation to many important structures and its draining ducts, trauma to the liver can cause a spectrum of clinical and angiographic manifestations.[1070–1072] Apart from arteriovenous fistula, periarterial hematomas, and traumatic bile cysts,[1066] hematomas of the liver have a great potential for mimicking many different clinical findings[1066] (Figs. 26-44, 28-15, 28-19, 28-24 and 28-44) (Structure 1).

Structure 1

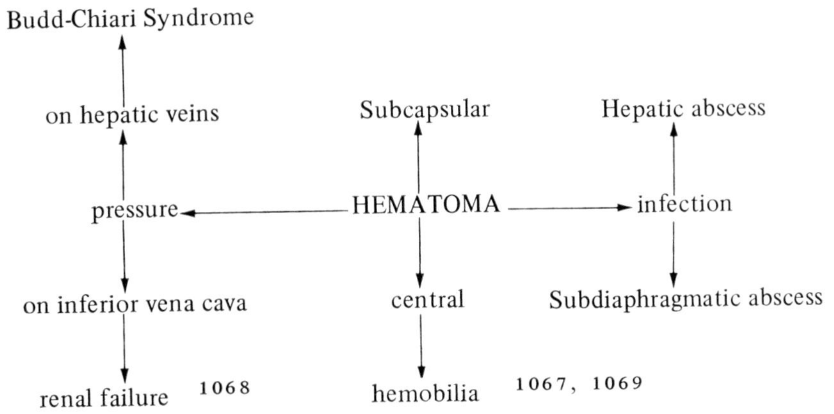

Renal Trauma

The morphological changes that can occur in the vessel and parenchyma of the kidney due to trauma[1074, 1075] in no way differ from changes in other compact organs.[1076] Hematuria after trauma may be minimal or absent if the rupture happens to be intraperitoneal. Delayed renovascular hypertension due to perinephric hematoma and organization causing a *page* kidney is one of the sequelae of renal trauma[1073,

[1077, 1078] (Figs. 26-42, 26-46 to 26-49, 27-19, 27-20, 27-21, 28-34, 28-39 and 28-40).

Pancreatic Trauma

Arterial occlusions due to vascular lacerations and displacement of the adjacent arteries due to edema and hematoma are the usual findings in pancreatic trauma.[1080–1082] Extravasation due to ruptured arteries may not be an infrequent finding[1083] (Fig. 28-45). Traumatic lesions of the pancreas are usually due to massive abdominal trauma associated with other organ injuries. The head and body of the pancreas are the most frequently involved segments because of their proximity to the unyielding, rigid vertebral bodies.[1079]

CHAPTER 29
DEVIATION

DEVIATION OF A CONTRAST POOL

THE BEST EXAMPLE of deviation of a contrast pool is in the cardiac chamber due to pericardial processes. Thus *pericardial effusions, pericardial thickening,* and pericardial effusion with *cardiac tamponade* may all cause deviation of the contrast pool in the right atrium.

Simple pericardial effusions are demonstrated angiographically as a contrast-filled right atrium with a *border* that is *convex* and almost parallel to the separated soft tissue shadow of the right cardiac border. The displacement seen is variable depending on the degree of effusion. The normal distance between the right cardiac shadow and contrast-filled right atrium should be 3 to 4 mm[1134] (Fig. 29-1). The most important factor influencing the *distribution of pericardial fluid* is the fixation of the posterior surface of the heart to the soft tissues of the posterior mediastinum by the six pulmonary veins that enter the left atrium posteriorly. Factors which influence the accumulation of fluid, either inferiorly, laterally or posteriorly, include the phase of the cardiac cycle, individual or generalized chamber enlargement, the phase of inspiration, and the presence of cardiac tamponade.[1135] Because of these influencing factors, a biplane study may be mandatory in some cases. Masses adjacent to the right atrial border or thrombus in the right atrium may be misleading[1138] (Figs. 29-2 and 29-3).

A *thick pericardium* tends to *flatten* the contrast-filled right atrial border (Fig. 29-4), while a *tamponade,* because of its increased pressure, tends to indent the contrast pool of the right atrium, causing a *concave* right atrial border (Fig. 29-5). The presence and degree of indentation depends on the degree of pressure in the pericardial cavity.[1136, 1137]

DEVIATION OF THE CONTRAST COLUMN

Deviation of the contrast column in a vessel is best demonstrated by the discrepancy between the contrast border and the soft tissue border of the artery. This is due either to the presence of a nonfilled false lumen seen in a *dissecting hematoma* or variable layers of clot which are seen in *aneurysms* of the aorta (Figs. 29-6, 29-7).

DEVIATION OF A VESSEL

Though *diagnostically nonspecific,* deviation and stretching of a vessel, either artery or vein, may give a clue as to the presence of a mass in the vicinity. Although this may not aid in establishing the histologic diagnosis of the mass, it is nonetheless of great diagnostic help in establishing the presence of a *mass in certain inaccessible areas.* It serves as further clinical assistance in arriving at the functional or pathologic significance of a detected mass.

Veins

Deviation of the *inferior vena cava* by masses such as lymph nodes above the right renal pedicle or deviation of the azygos vein by mediastinal lymph nodes assist in proper evaluation (Figs. 29-8, 29-9 and 29-10). Stretching of multiple *veins* in the *adrenal* gland is seen in hyperplasia, or deviation and stretching of the adrenal intrinsic venous system may help to establish the diagnosis of multinodular hyperplasia or masses of different histologies (Figs. 29-30 to 29-32, 29-36 and 29-37).

Arteries

Cephalad deviation and stretching of the *splenic vessels* is noted in left upper quadrant masses primarily related to the pancreas. Distortion of a normal configuration of the *in-*

(Text continues on page 619)

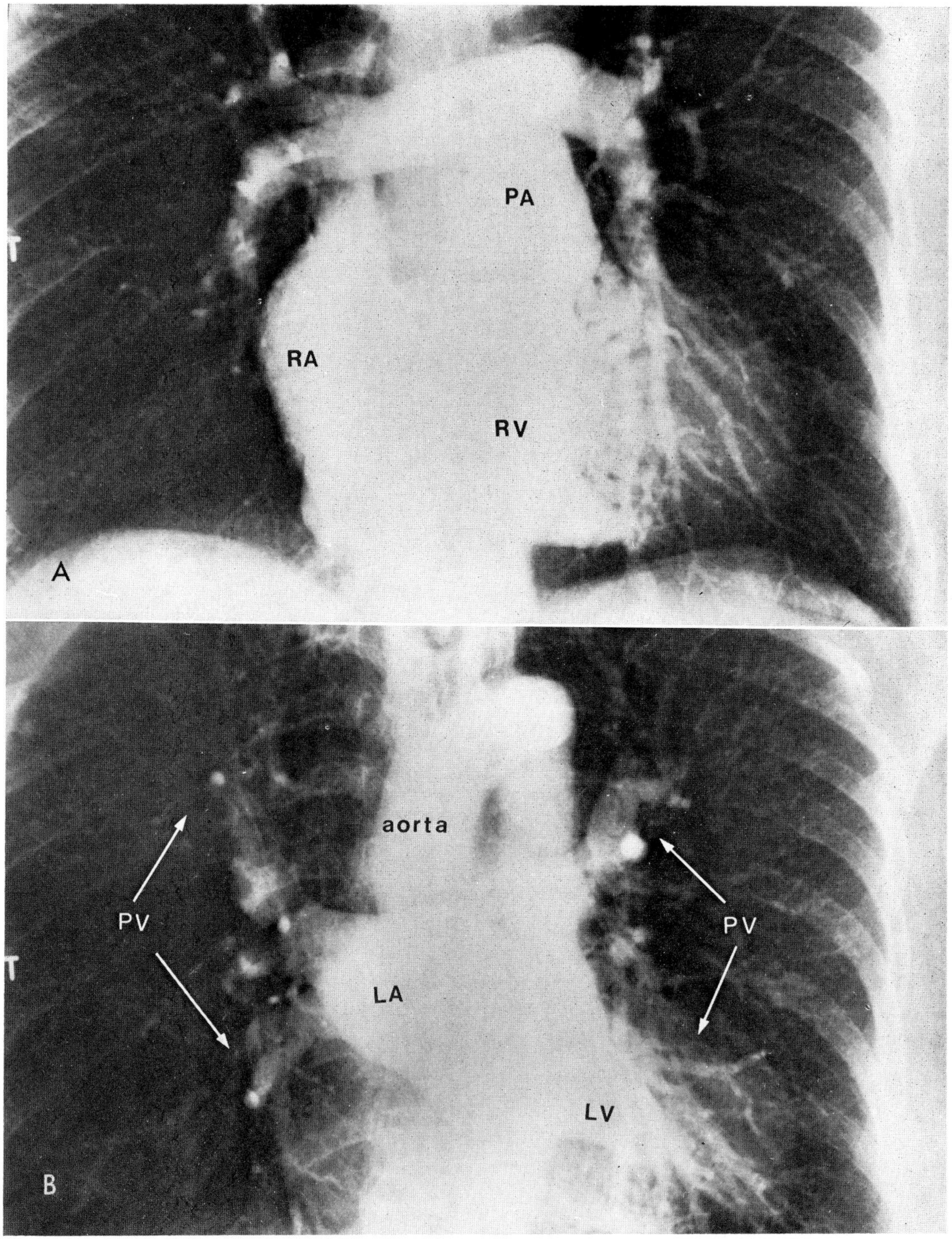

Figure 29.1. Venous Angiocardiogram. (A) Opacification of the right side of the heart. Right atrium (R.A.), right ventricle (R.V.) and pulmonary artery (P.A.). Notice the approximation of the right atrial contrast pool and the right cardiac border. (B) Opacification of the left-sided cardiac structures are shown. Pulmonary veins (P.V.), left atrium (L.A.), left ventricle (L.V.) and aorta. *Comment:* Normal dextro and levo phases of the heart.

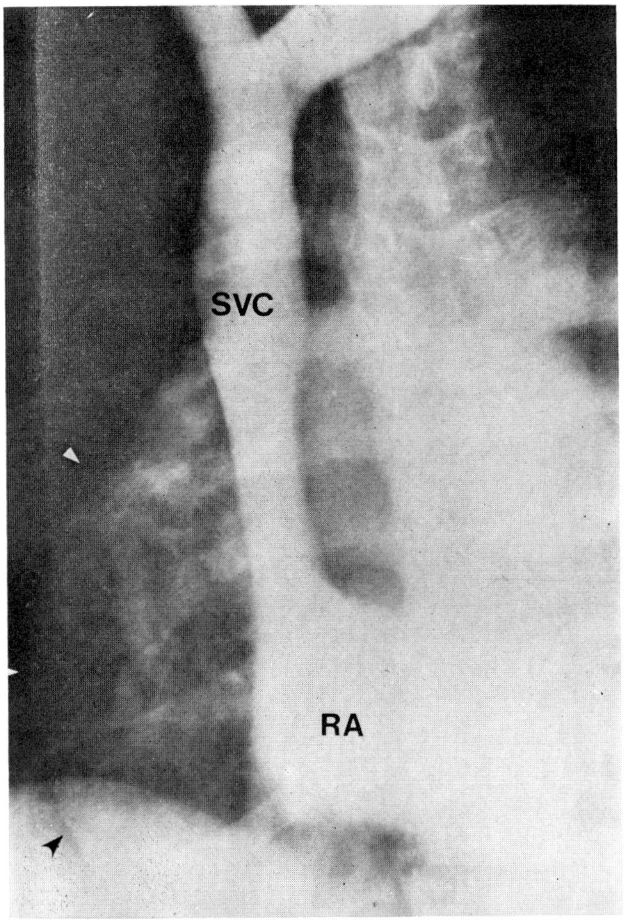

Figure 29.2. Intravenous Angiocardiogram. A marked increase in the distance between the cardiac contour and the contrast pool in the right atrium is seen. *Diagnosis:* Marked pericardial effusion displacing the contrast pool away from the cardiac margin.

Figure 29.3. Intravenous Angiocardiogram. (A) The distance between the cardiac contour and the contrast pool in the right atrium is increased. (B) A little later there is further increase in the distance between the contrast in the right atrial pool and the cardiac contour. *Comment:* Pericardial effusion giving an exaggerated appearance during different phases of cardiac cycle.

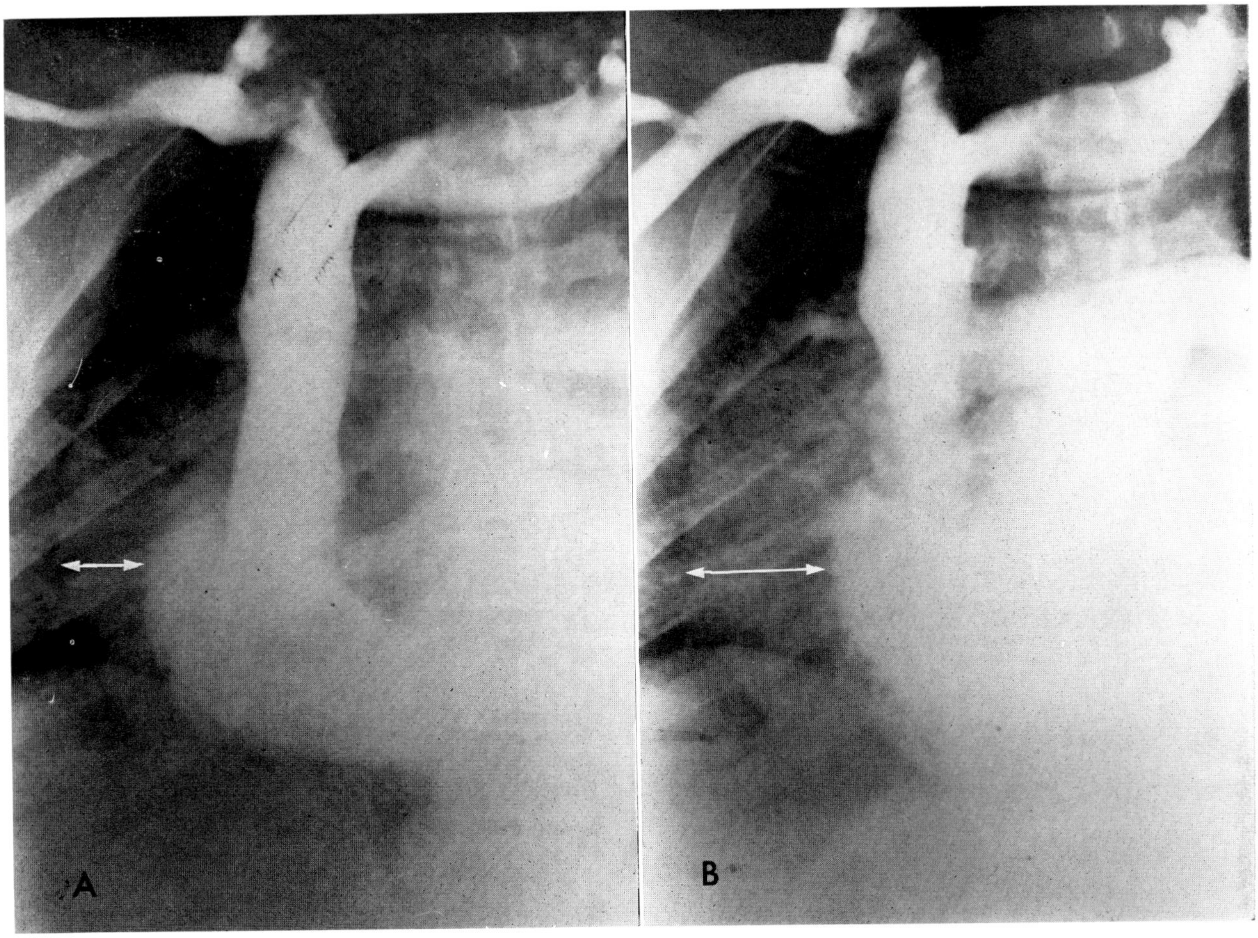

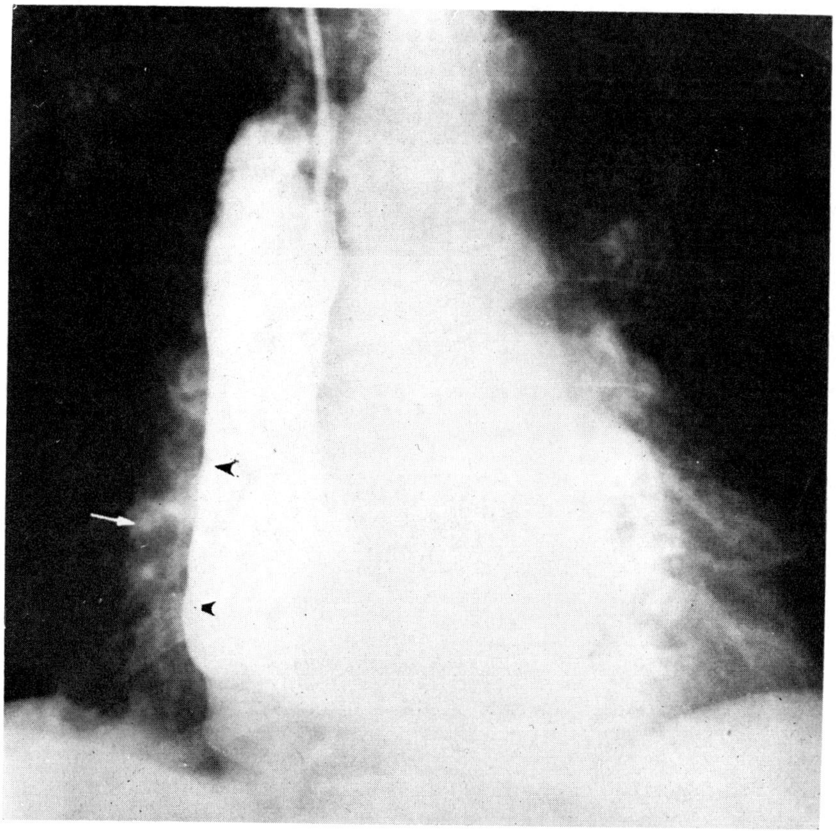

Figure 29.4. Intravenous Angiocardiogram. The contrast pool in the right atrium is deviated from the pericardial stripe (White Arrow) causing an abnormal increased distance between the right atrial contour and the cardiac silhouette. Notice the straight margin of the right atrium (Black Arrow Heads). The patient had constrictive pericarditis due to tuberculosis. *Diagnosis:* Constrictive pericarditis. (From Spitz, H. B., and Holmes, J. C. Right atrial contour in cardiac tamponade. *Radiol, 103:*69, 1972. Courtesy of the authors and publishers.)

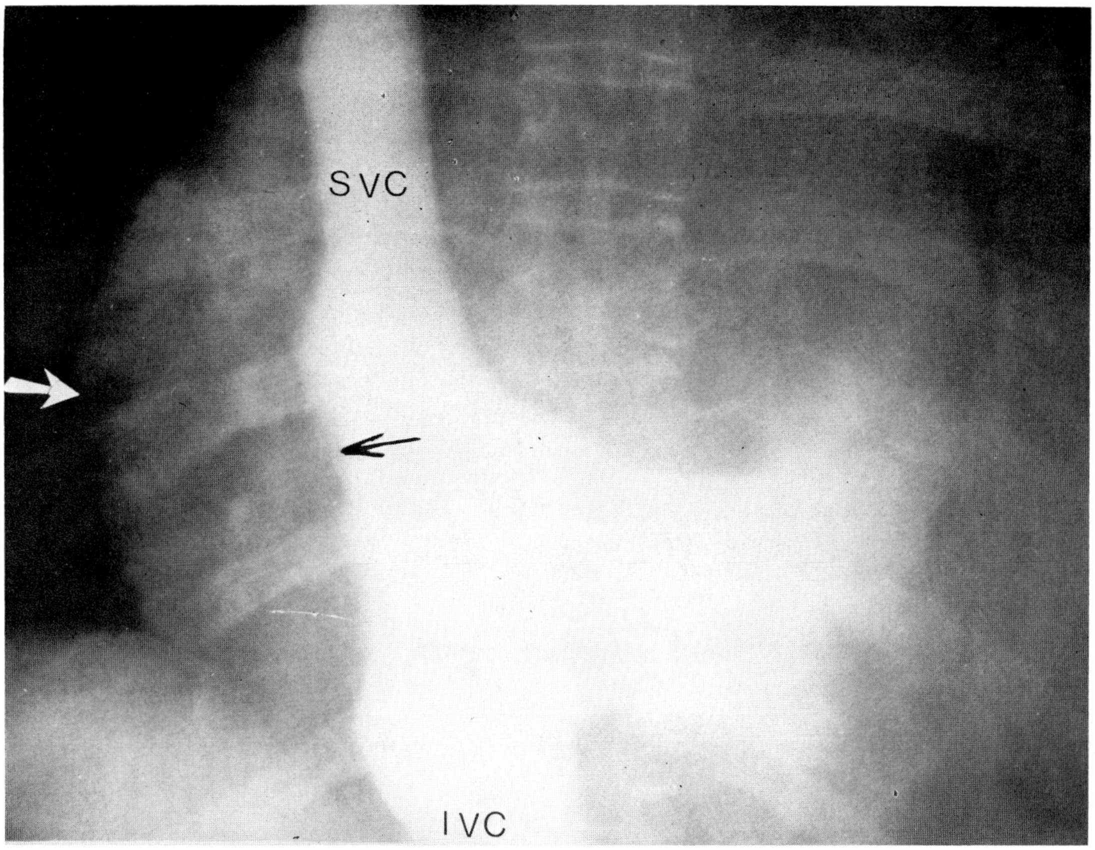

Figure 29.5. Injection into the right atrium reveals marked separation of the contrast pool in the right atrium (Black Arrow) from the pericardial contour (White Arrow). Please note the concave inner border of the right atrial margin, marked reflux into the superior vena cava and a wide inferior vena cava. The patient had tuberculosis and pericardial tamponade. *Diagnosis:* Pericardial tamponade. (From Spitz, H., and Holmes, J. C. Right atrial contour in cardiac tamponade. *Radiol, 103:*69, 1972. Courtesy of the authors and publishers.)

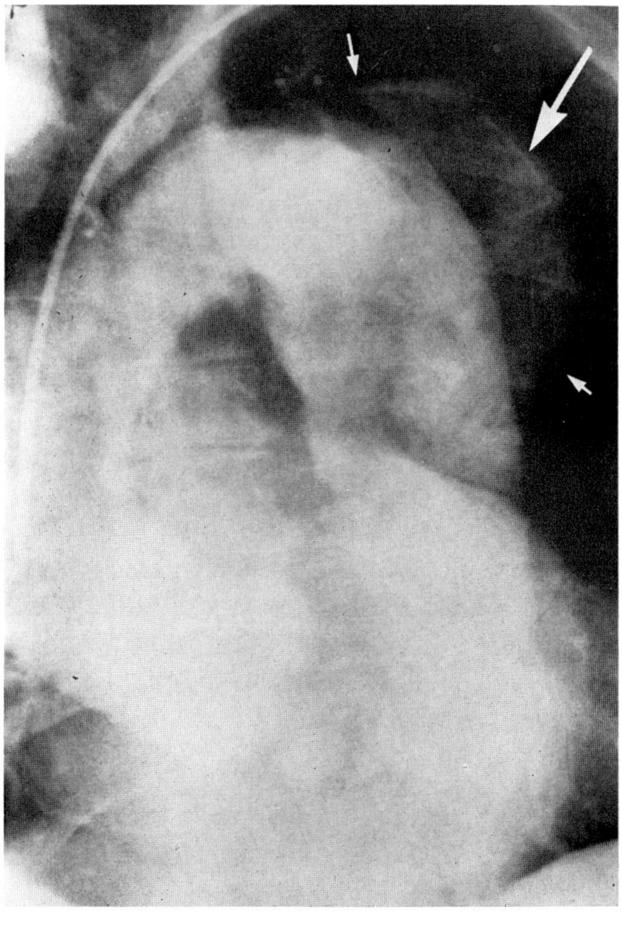

Figure 29.6. Aortic Arch Angiogram. The wall of the aorta (Small Arrow) is separated from the column of contrast. Note the position of the intimal calcification (Large Arrow). *Diagnosis:* Partial thrombosis of an aortic aneurysm.

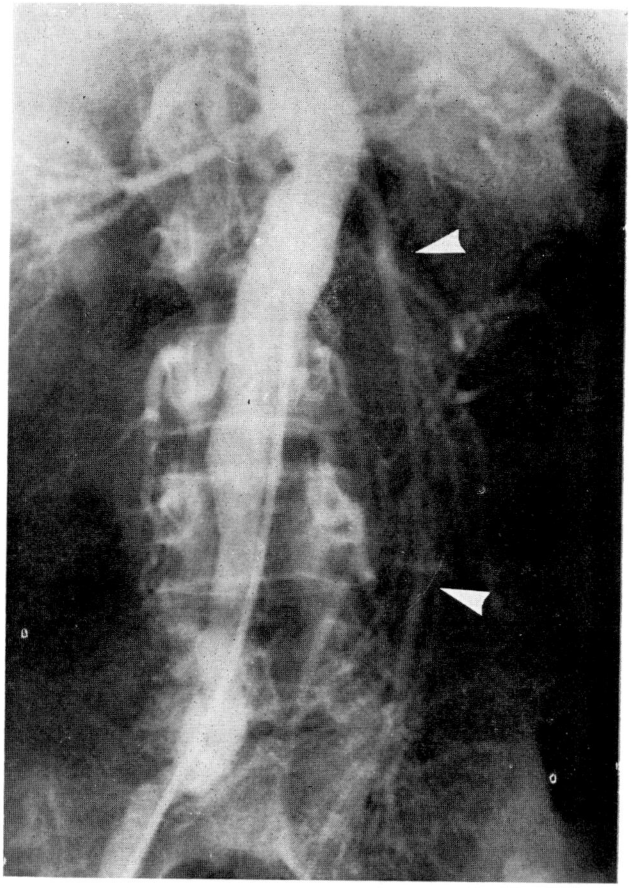

Figure 29.7. Abdominal Aortogram. There is lateral displacement of the superior mesenteric artery (Arrow Head). An appearance of extraluminal course of the catheter. *Diagnosis:* Thrombosed fusiform arteriosclerotic aneurysm of the infrarenal portion of the abdominal aorta. The catheter is passing through the thrombus, confirmed at surgery.

Figure 29.8. (A) There is questionable infiltration of the lymph nodes at the level of the renal pedicle on the right side. (B) Inferior vena cavagram: Note the marked compression with deviation of the inferior vena cava at this level. *Diagnosis:* Lymph node mass probably due to metastases deviating the inferior vena cava. *Comment:* One of the advantages of the inferior vena cavagram is the demonstration of masses above the renal pedicular level if the lymphangiogram is not contributory especially on the right side. Left renal vein and left gonadal vein may behave identically for left paravertebral masses.

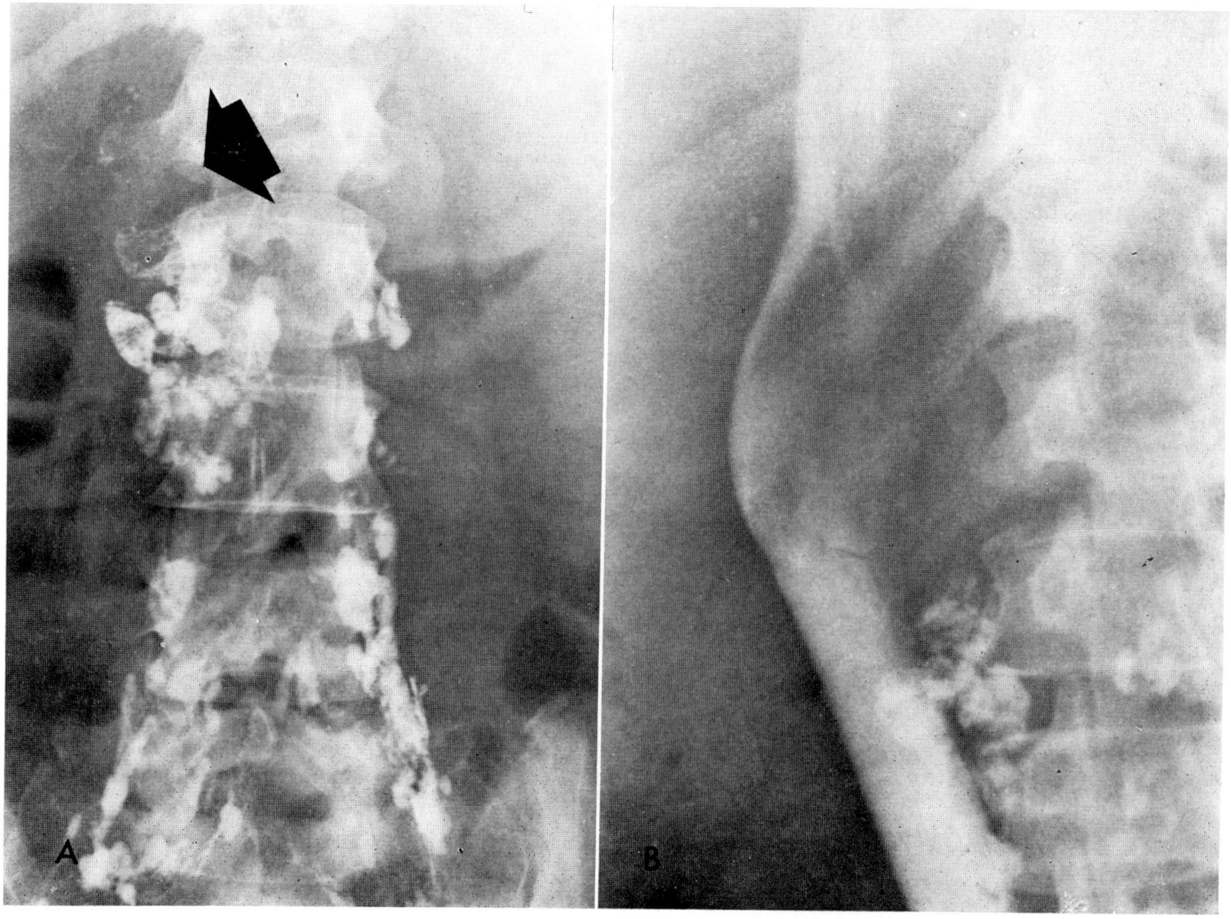

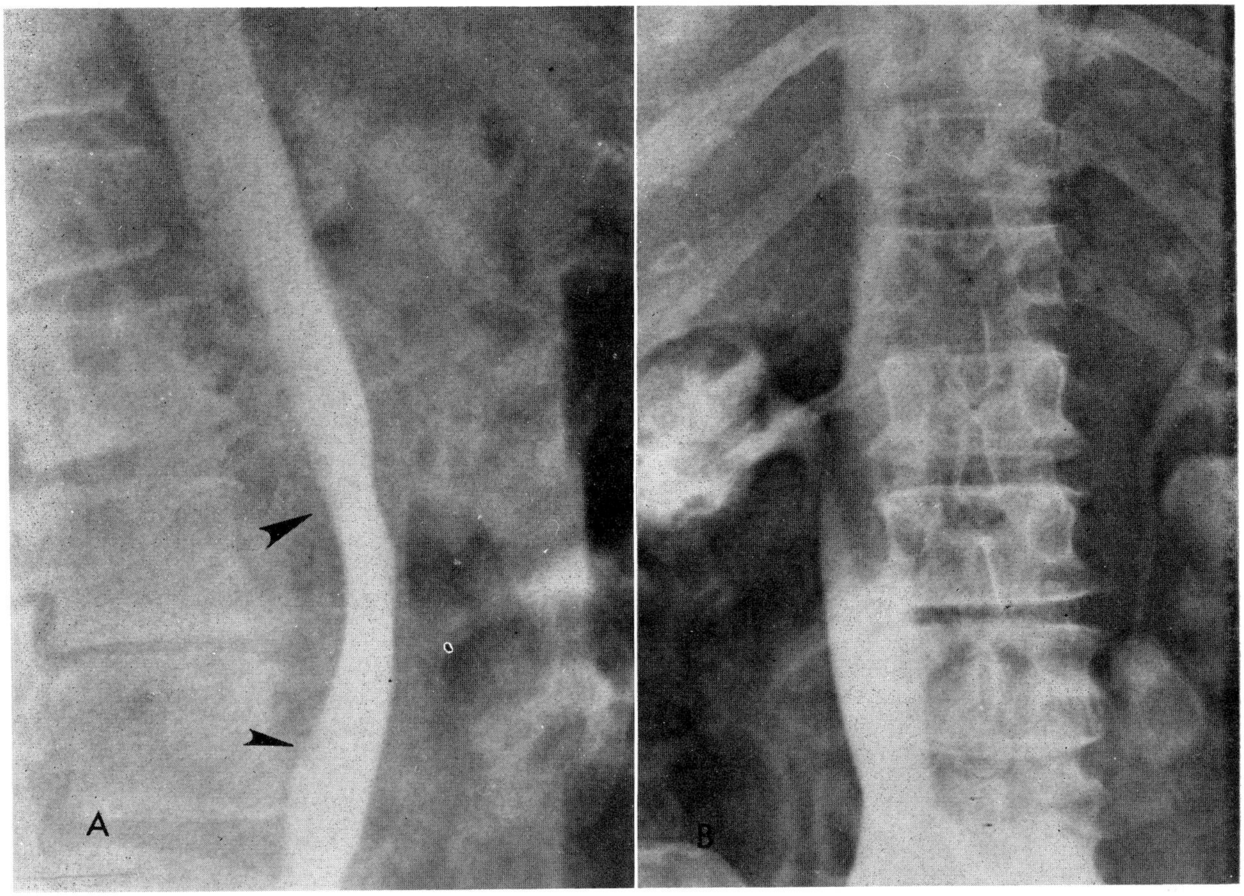

Figure 29.9. Inferior Vena Cavagram—lateral projection. (A) There is localized anterior deviation of the inferior vena cava. (B) A.P. projection: No apparent abnormalities are seen. *Diagnosis:* Retrocaval mass causing deviation of the inferior vena cava probably due to lymph nodes. *Pathology:* Lymph node metastases from ovarian carcinoma. *Comment:* The advantage of the lateral projection is obvious.

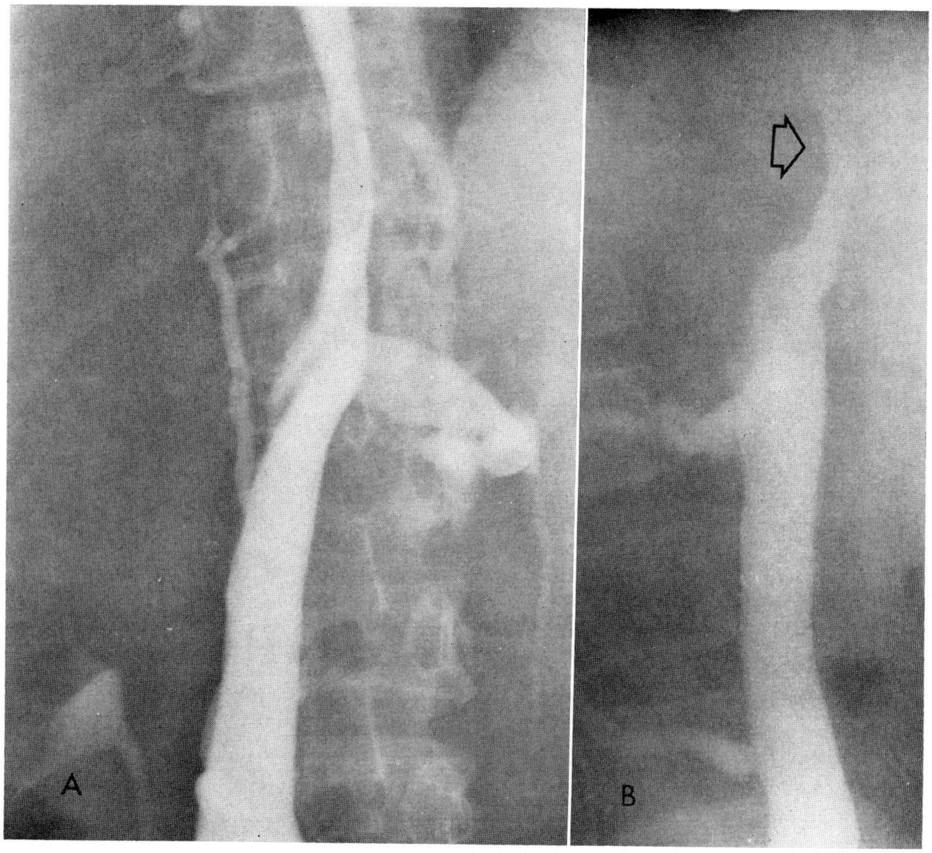

Figure 29.10. Inferior Vena Cavagram. (A) A.P. projection: There is smooth narrowing of the suprarenal segment of the inferior vena cava and deviation to the left. (B) Lateral projection: There is anterior deviation with extrinsic compression on the same segment of inferior vena cava. *Diagnosis:* Masses are probably lymph nodes deviating the inferior vena cava. *Pathology:* Metastases from a bronchogenic carcinoma.

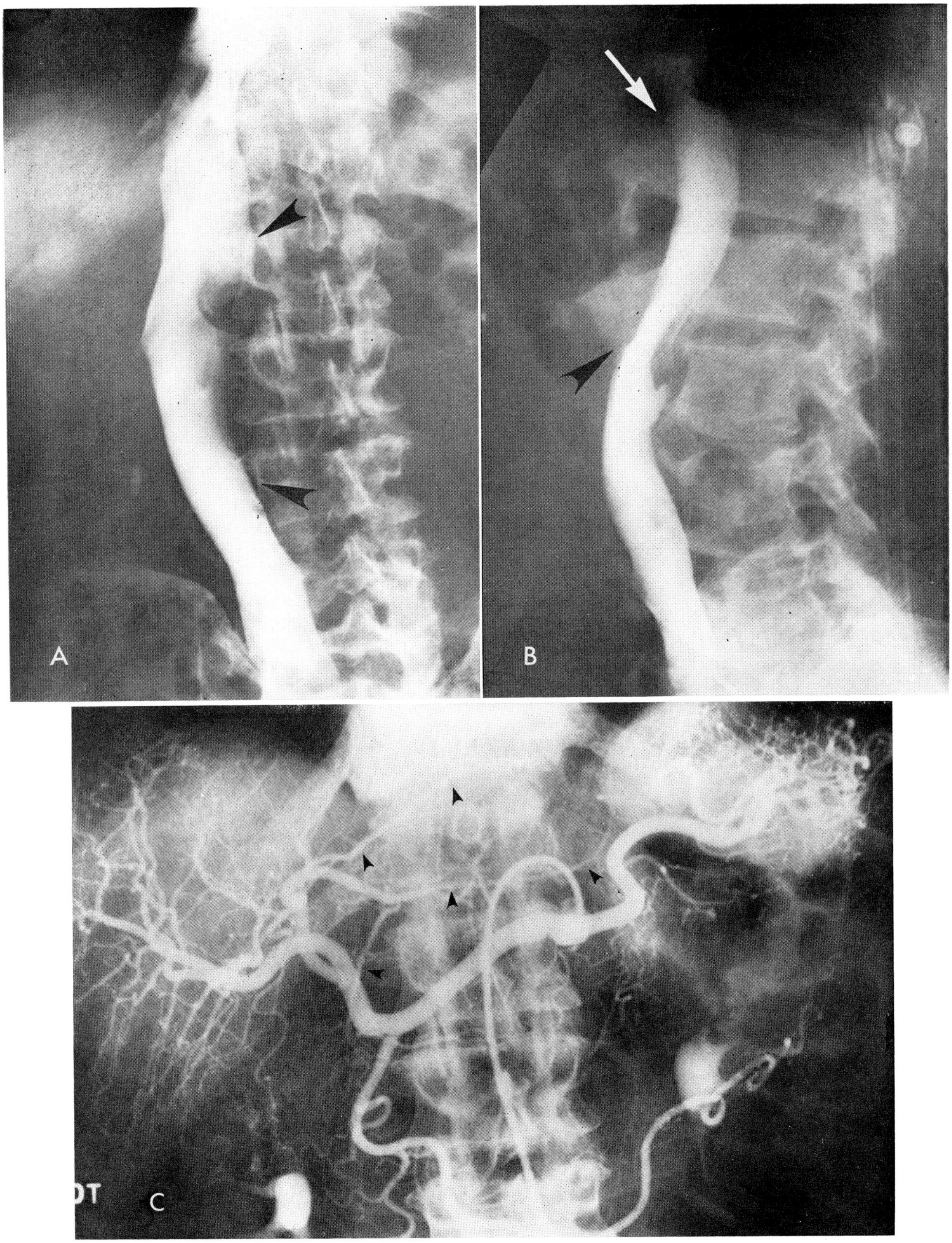

Figure 29.11. Inferior Vena Cavagram. (A) A.P. projection reveals mild deviation of the upper half of the cava to the right side. (B) Lateral view of the same demonstrating gentle posterior deviation of the cava. (C) Celiac arteriogram reveals a small right lobe of the liver and stretching and deviation of the left hepatic branches. *Radiographic Diagnosis:* Regeneration of the left lobe of the liver versus metastasis. A colloidal isotope scan revealed normal concentration in the left lobe suggesting "regeneration of the left lobe of the liver."

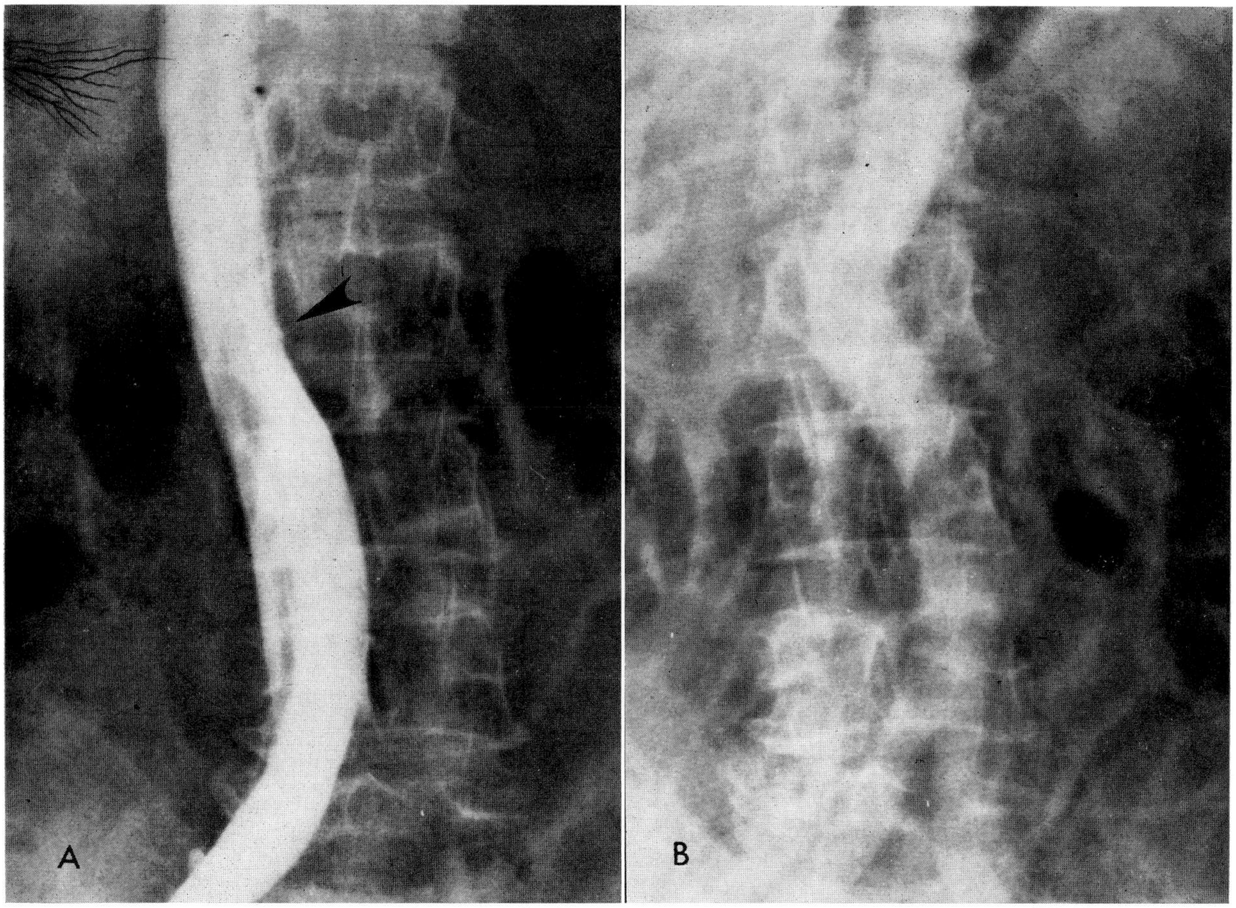

Figure 29.12. (A) Inferior vena cavagram: Note the gentle deviation of the proximal portion of the inferior vena cava. (B) Intravenous aortogram: The aorta is very tortuous. *Comment:* The change in the course of the inferior vena cava is due to the change in the aortic course.

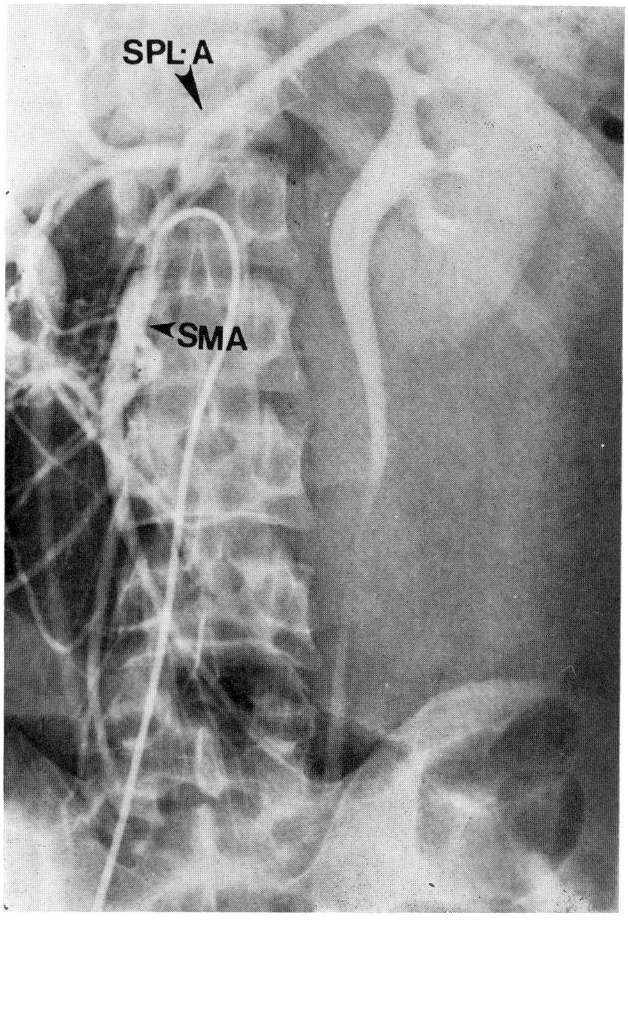

Figure 29.13. Superior Mesenteric Arteriogram. Deviation of the superior mesenteric artery occurs towards the right (S.M.A.) with elevation of the splenic artery (Spl. A.) around a huge avascular mass. There is good filling of the celiac axis via the pancreatic arcade. The patient is a known alcoholic. *Diagnosis:* Huge pancreatic cyst with secondary extrinsic compression of the celiac axis with the celiac axis drawing its blood supply from the superior mesenteric artery via the pancreaticoduodenal arcade.

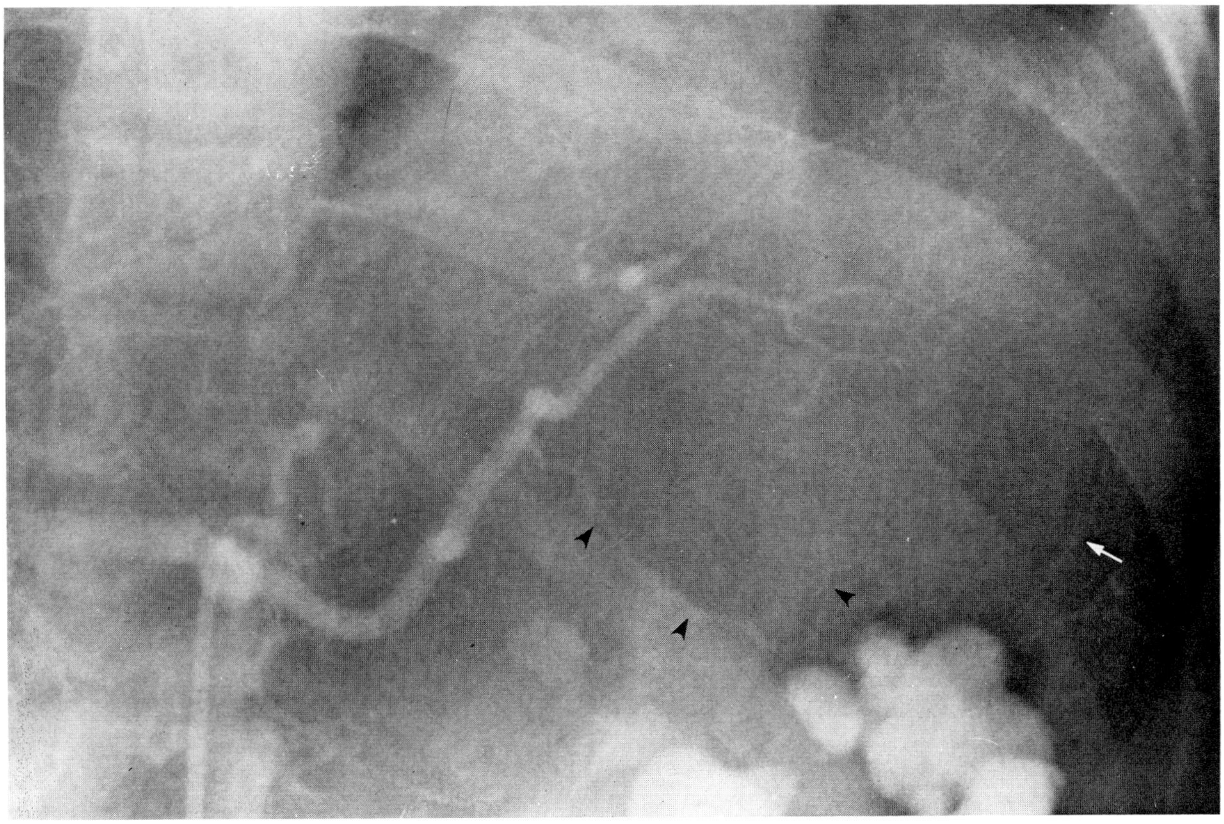

Figure 29.14. Celiac Arteriogram. The pancreatic branches which originate from the splenic artery are stretched and deviated. This young patient presented with fever and left upper quadrant pain ten weeks after a history of left upper quadrant trauma. *Radiographic Diagnosis:* Pancreatic mass near the tail. *Surgical Diagnosis:* Infected hematoma in the tail of the pancreas.

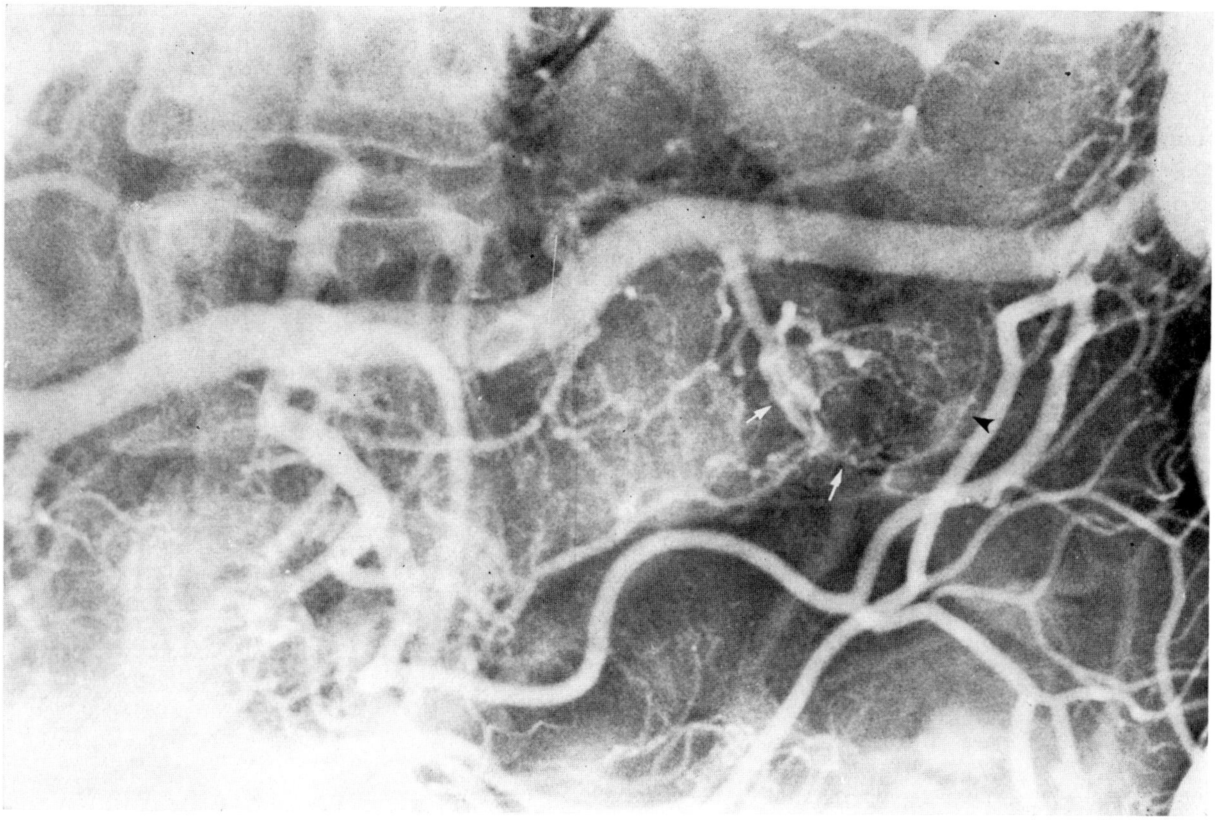

Figure 29.15. Celiac Arteriogram. The pancreatic vessels arising from the splenic artery (Arrow) are deviated. The patient was an alcoholic. *Diagnosis:* Pancreatic pseudocyst. *Surgery:* Island of fibrosis acting like a mass in the pancreas.

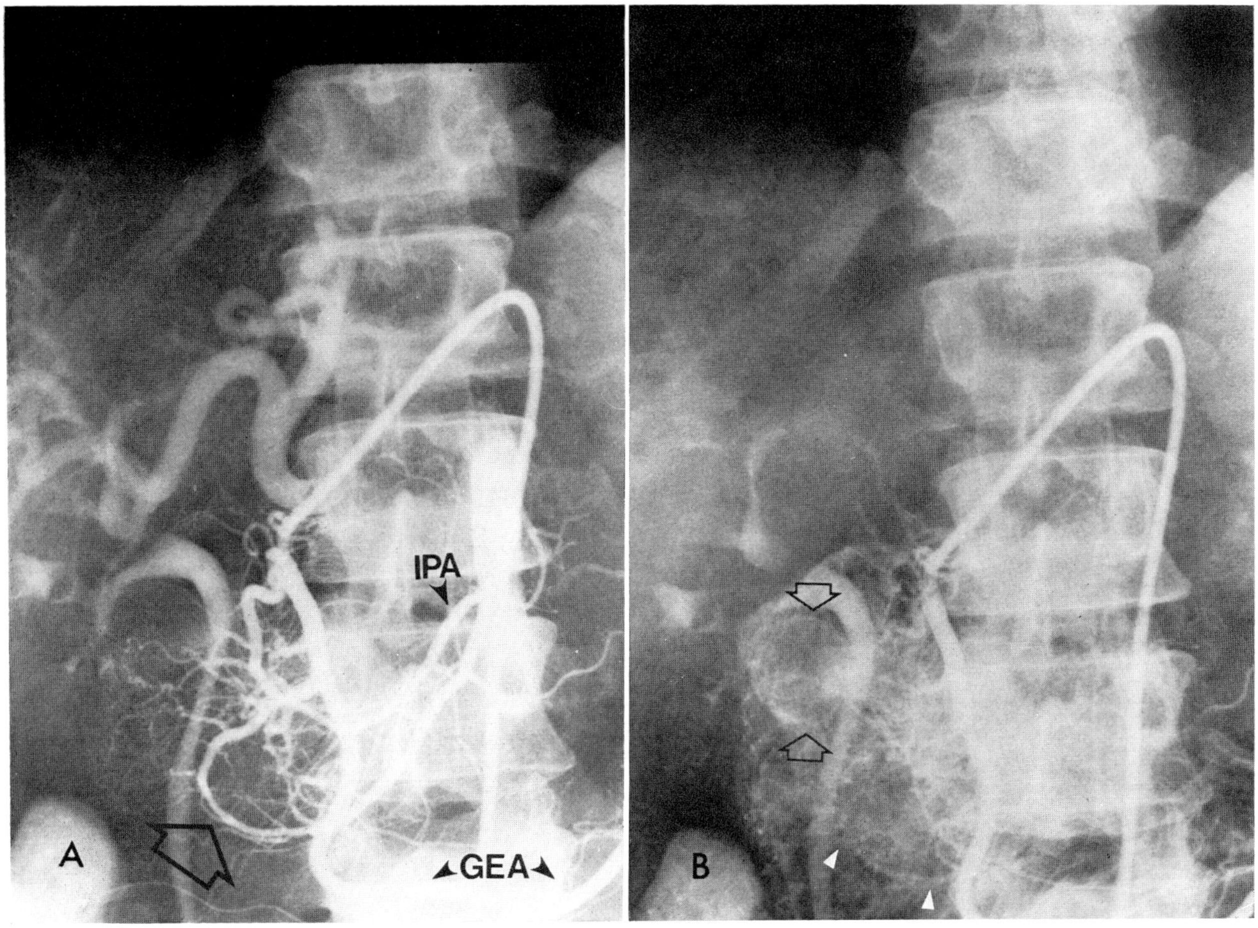

Figure 29.16. Gastroduodenal Arteriogram. (A) Arterial phase: There is deviation of the inferior pancreatic arcade (Arrow) and visualization of the inferior pancreaticoduodenal artery and its branches (I.P.A.). Note gastroepiploic artery (G.E.A.). (B) Late arterial phase: There is extrinsic compression on the medial portion of the duodenal sweep (Arrow Head) and visualization of bowel on end with staining of its mucosa (Arrow). *Diagnosis:* Pancreatic cyst in the head of the pancreas. *Surgical Diagnosis:* Edema of the head of the pancreas without evidence of a cyst.

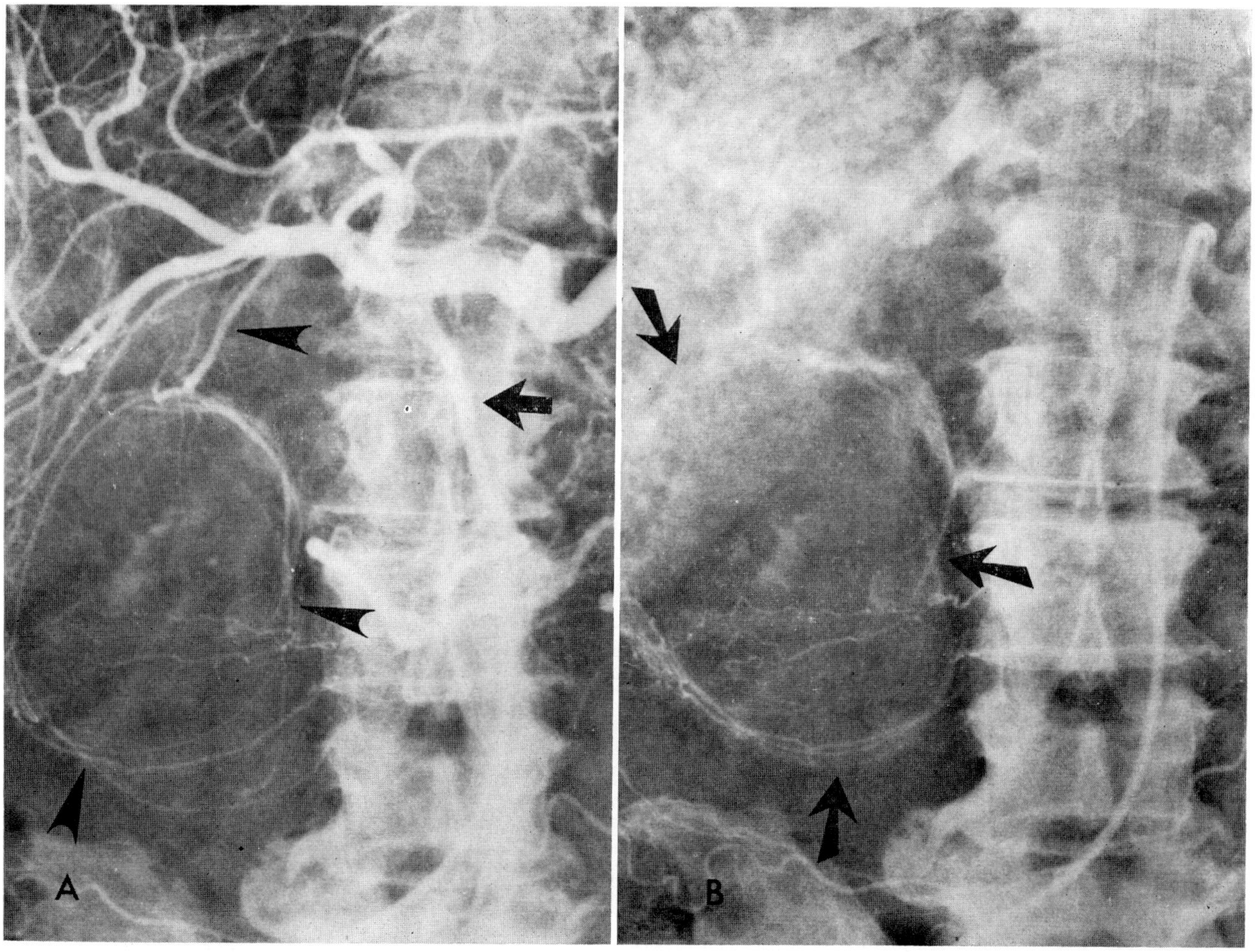

Figure 29.17. Celiac Arteriogram. (A) The gastroduodenal artery (Arrow) is straightened and deviated. There is a prominent cystic artery (Arrow Head) and its branches encircle an enlarged gallbladder. (B) The gallbladder is enlarged. The patient had painless jaundice. *Diagnosis:* Mass in the vicinity of the head of the pancreas with obstructive jaundice. *Pathologic Diagnosis:* Carcinoma of the head of the pancreas.

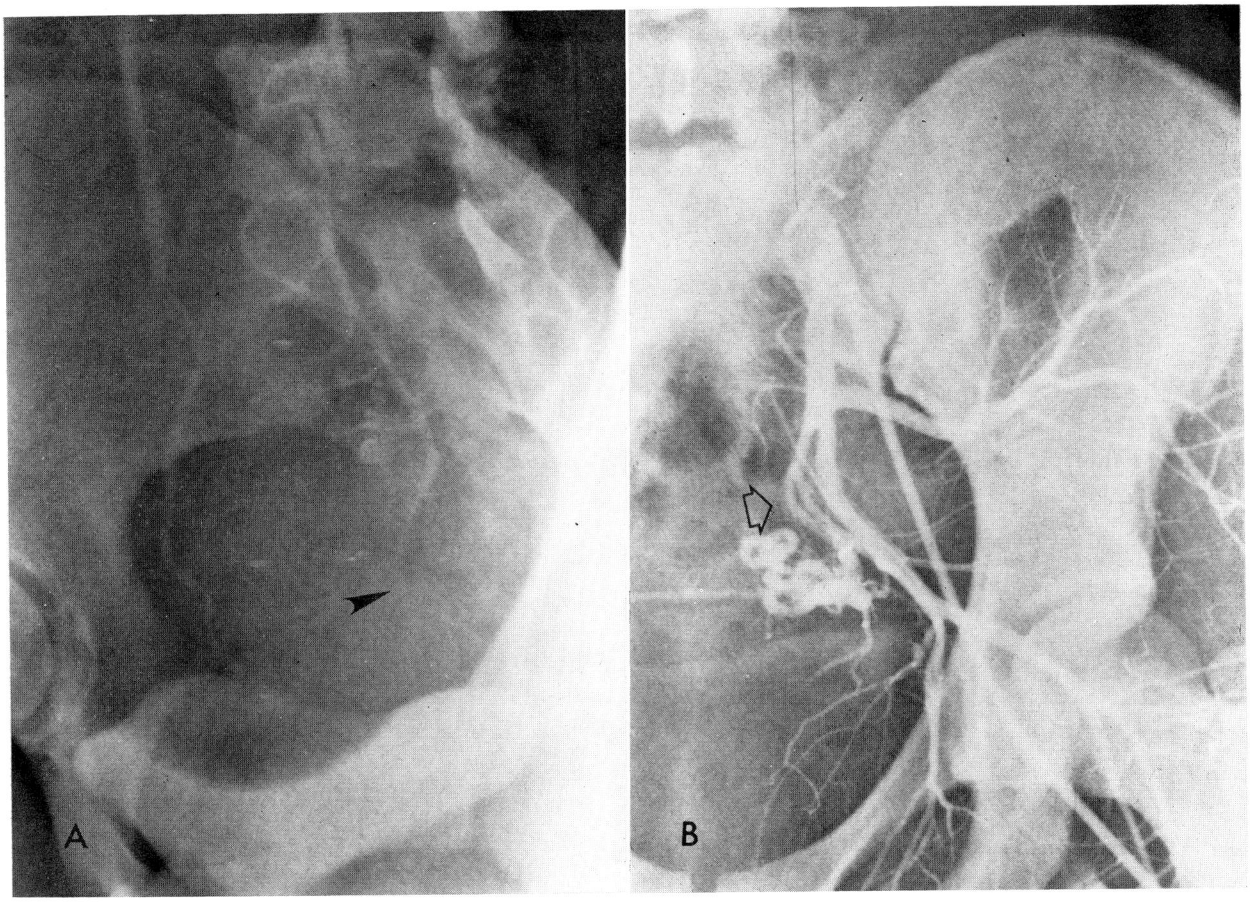

Figure 29.18. Internal Iliac Arteriogram. (A) A right posterior oblique film of an intravenous pyelogram examination revealed anterior deviation of the left ureter. (B) The arteriogram revealed separation of the internal iliac artery branches at the level of the sciatic notch (Arrow). No other obvious abnormalities are seen. This young lady had pain radiating along the distribution of the sciatic nerve. *Diagnosis:* Avascular mass at the sciatic notch. *Pathologic Diagnosis:* Sciatic nerve neurofibroma.

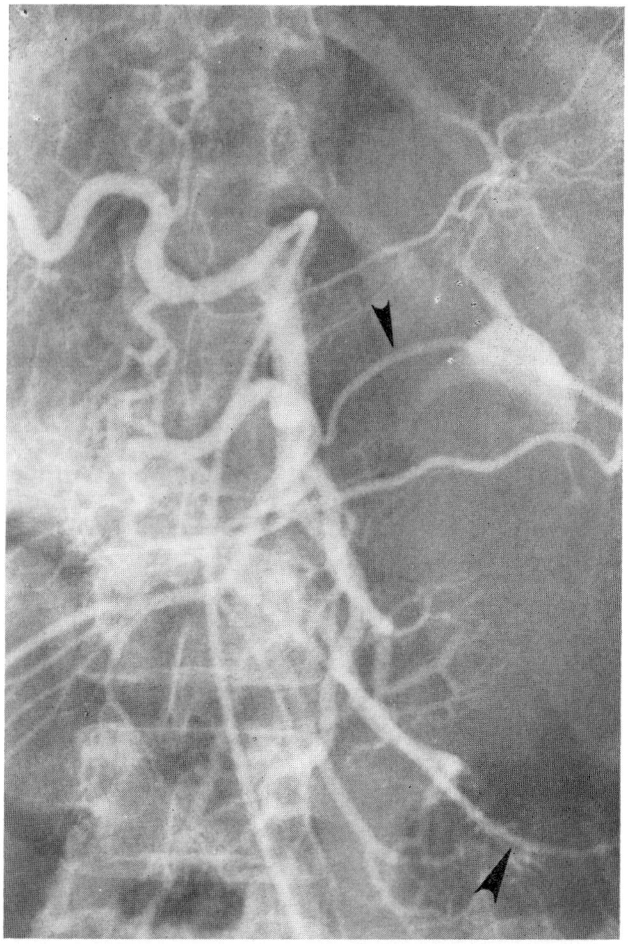

Figure 29.19. Superior Mesenteric Arteriogram. There is stretching and deviation of the proximal branches of the superior mesenteric artery. *Diagnosis:* Masses in the mesentery such as lymphoma. *Pathology:* Lymphoma in the mesenteric lymph nodes and in the kidney.

Figure 29.20. Hepatic Arteriogram. Gastroduodenal (Arrow) and pancreatic (Arrow Head) branches are stretched. The dorsal pancreatic artery arises from the hepatic artery (Blank Arrow). The patient had paravertebral abdominal masses. *Pathologic Diagnosis:* Lymphoma.

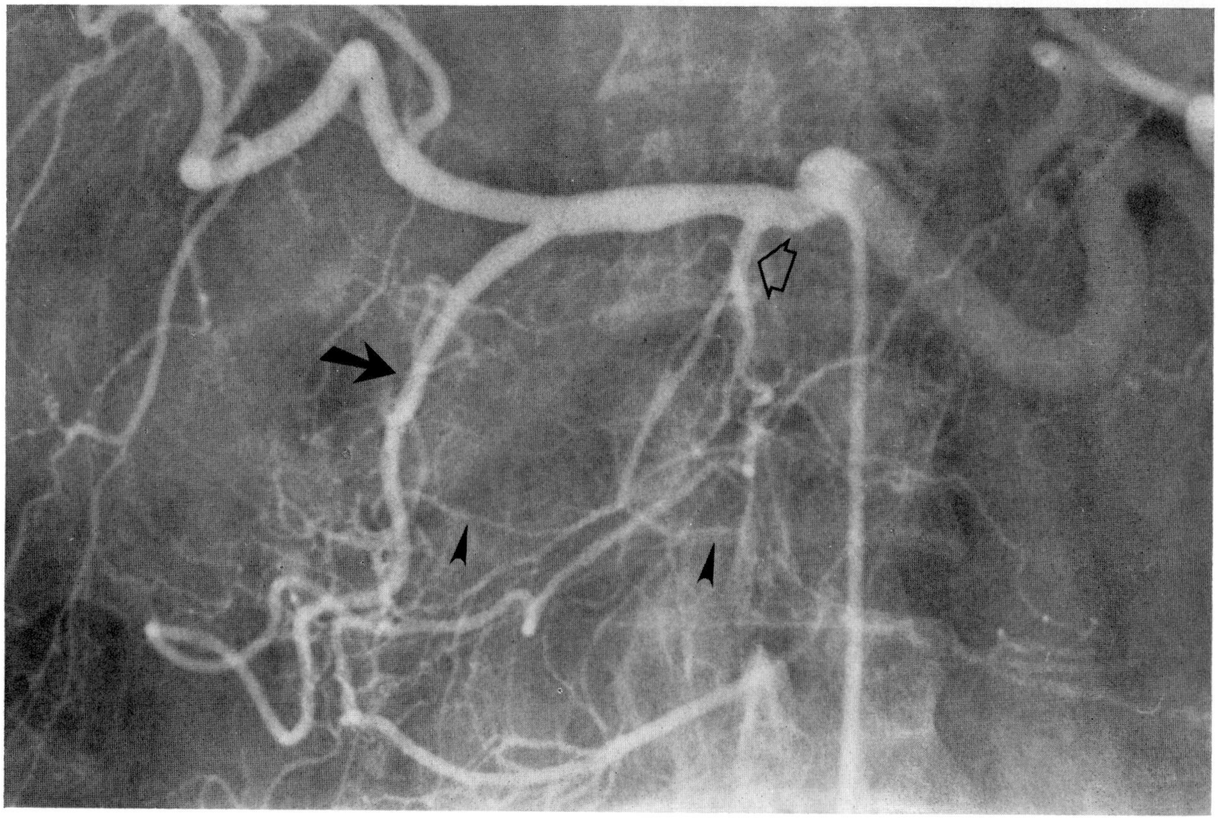

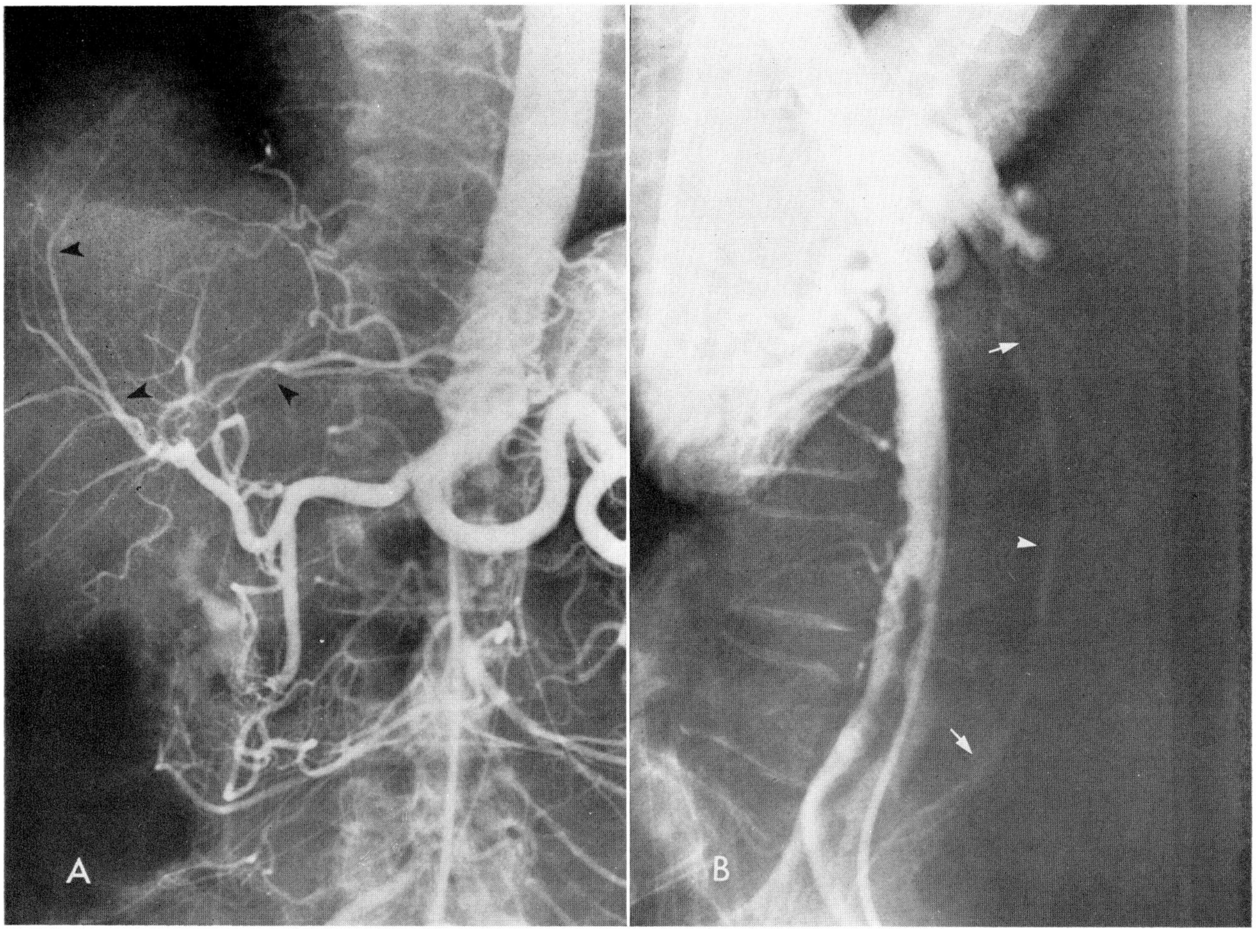

Figure 29.21. Celiac Arteriogram. (A) The intrahepatic branches are stretched and deviated. (B) Cross-table lateral aortogram: Stretching and deviation of the main stem of the superior mesenteric artery are seen. *Conclusion:* Multiple paravertebral masses deviating the superior mesenteric artery, and multiple masses in the liver deviating and stretching the intrahepatic arteries. *Radiographic Diagnosis:* Probable lymphoma. *Surgical Diagnosis:* Reticulum cell sarcoma.

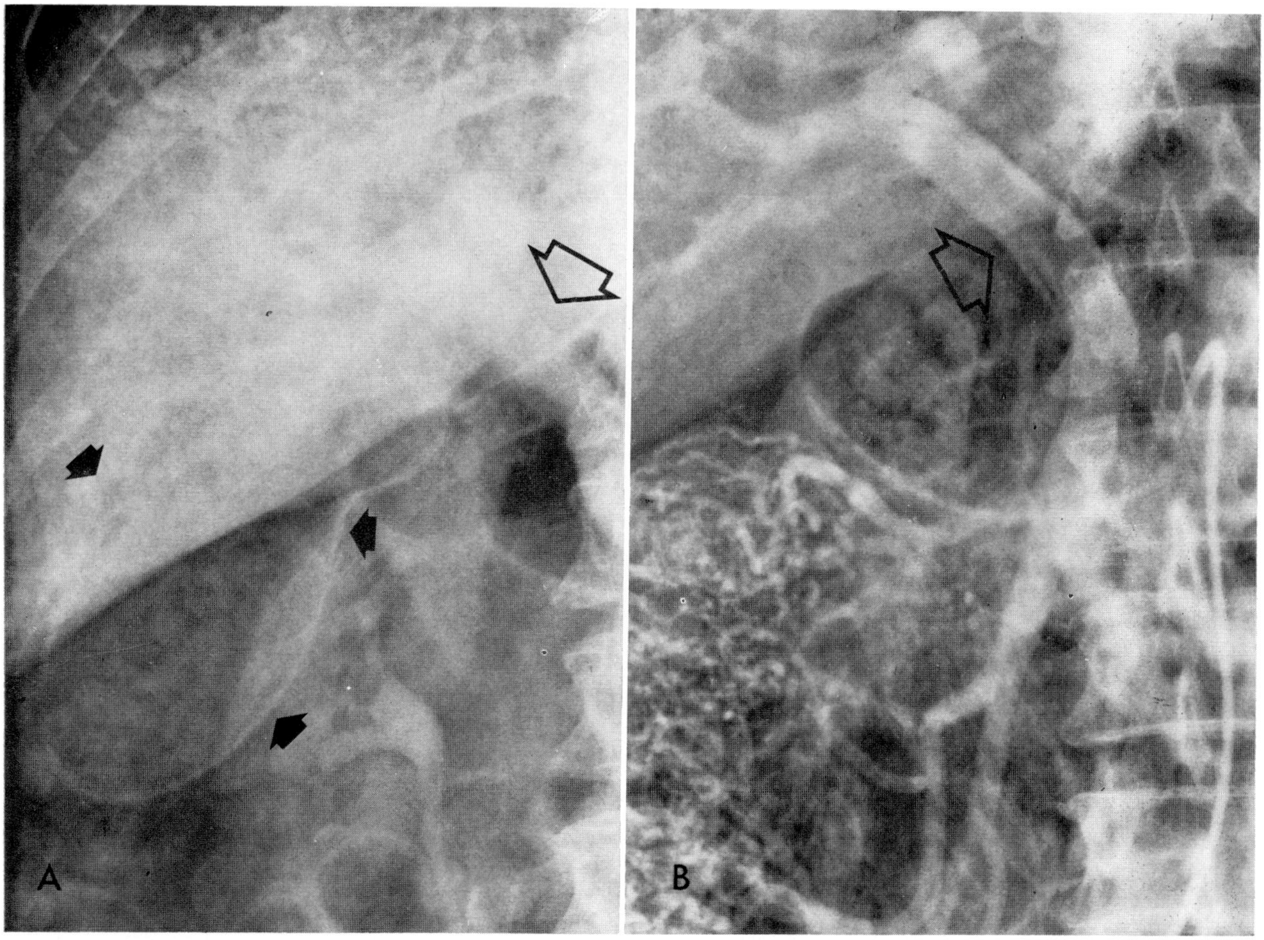

Figure 29.22. Celiac Arteriogram. (A) Venous phase: The gallbladder is dilated (Arrow) and the portal vein (Arrow Head) is elevated. (B) Superior mesenteric arteriogram—venous phase: The superior mesenteric vein (Arrow Head) is bowed. *Diagnosis:* Obstructive jaundice due to a mass adjacent to the porta hepatis. *Pathology:* Lymphoma with lymph nodes at the porta hepatis.

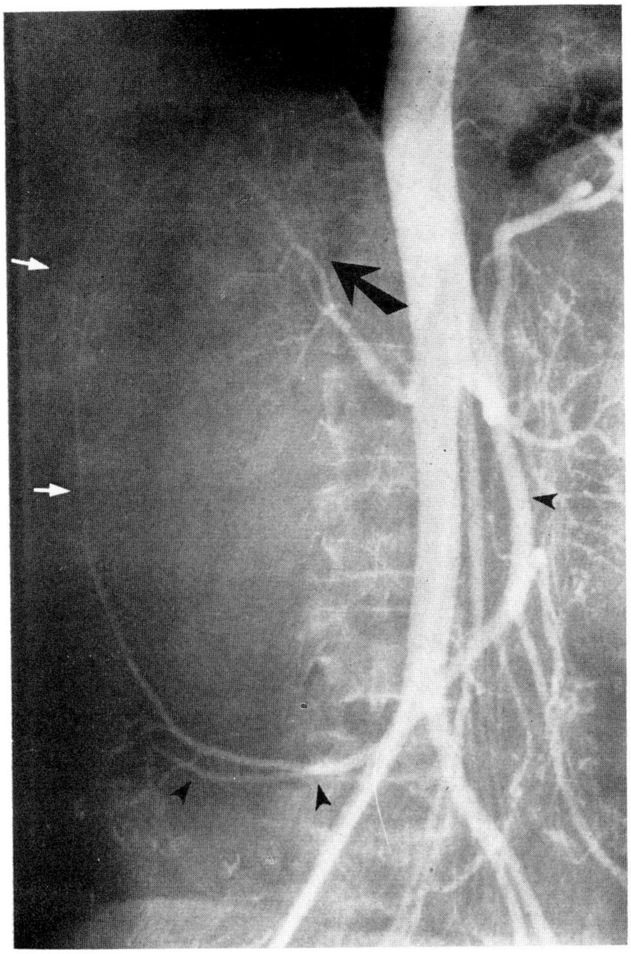

Figure 29.23. Flush Aortogram. Please note the inferior displacement of the right hepatic artery around a huge intrahepatic mass (Arrow Heads) and cranial displacement of the right kidney (Arrow). This was due to a hemangioendothelioma of the liver.

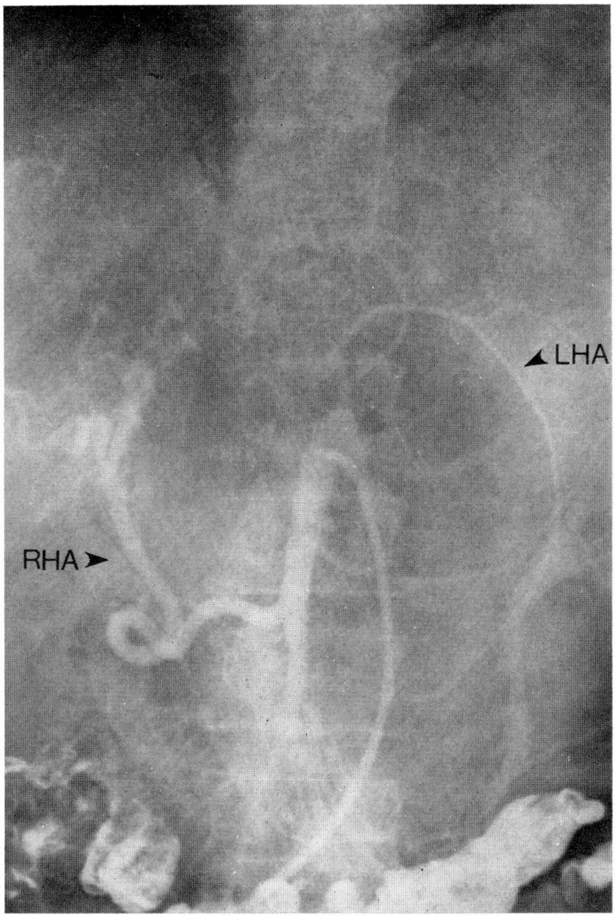

Figure 29.24. Superior Mesenteric Arteriogram. Replaced hepatic arteries from the superior mesenteric artery. Right hepatic (R.H.A.) and left hepatic (L.H.A.). This patient had metastases to the left lobe of the liver, causing stretching and deviation of the replaced left hepatic artery.

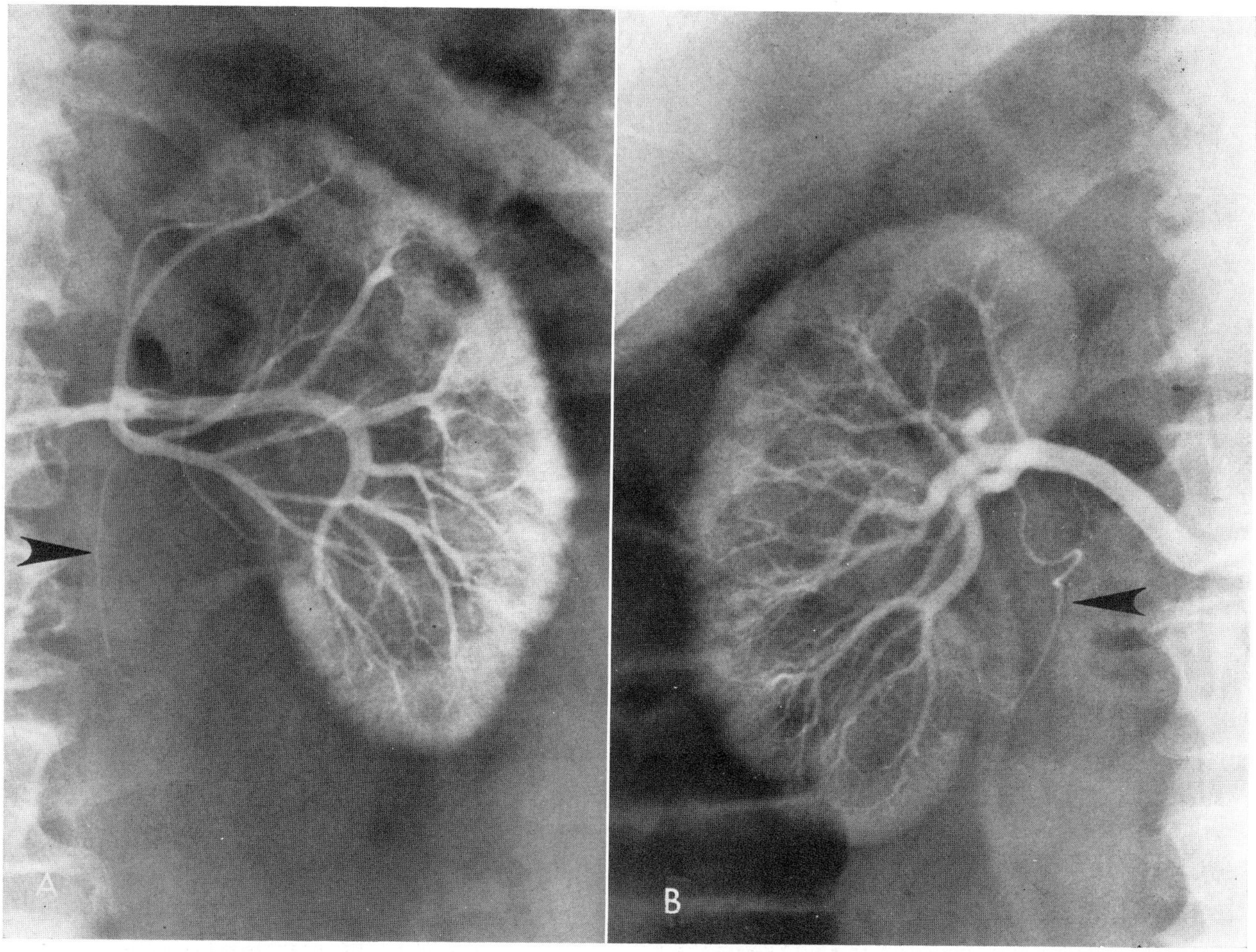

Figure 29.25. Renal Arteriogram. (A) Left renal arteriogram reveals stretching and deviation of the intrarenal branches around an avascular filling defect and deviation of the peripelvic vessels (Arrow). (B) Same patient—right renal arteriogram: Notice the normal course of the peripelvic vessel. *Comment:* Deviation of the peripelvic vessel on the left side due to a huge intrarenal cyst protruding through the left renal hilus.

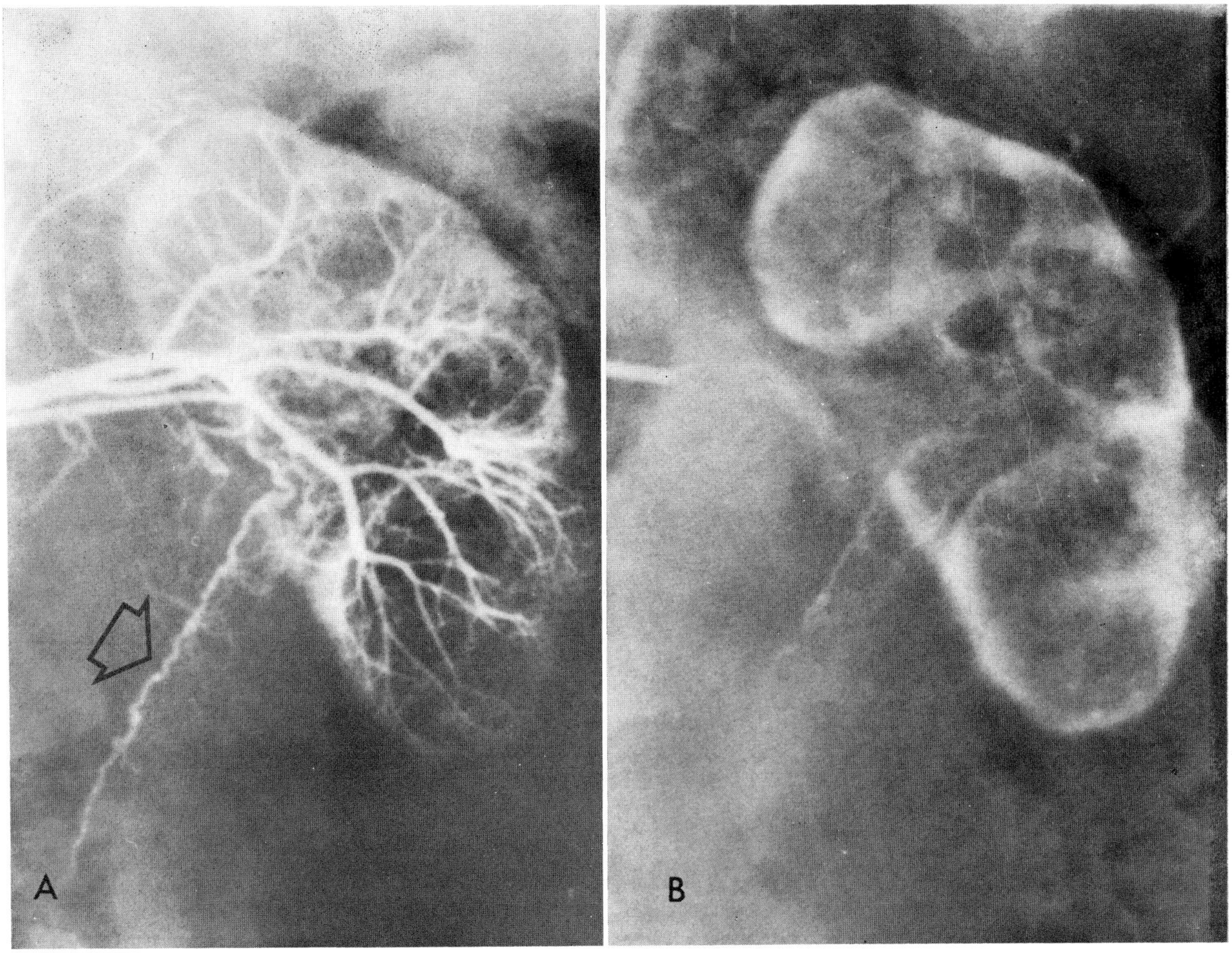

Figure 29.26. Renal Arteriogram. (A) Renal arteriogram reveals stretching of the left main renal branch with prominent peripelvic branch (Arrow). Uniform stretching and deviation of the intrarenal branches occurs. (B) Parenchymal phase: Multiple, well-defined, lucent filling defects are symmetrically arranged and separated by white columns of renal cortex. *Diagnosis:* Hydronephrosis with possible pyonephrosis, with secondary hypertrophy of the renal pelvic and ureteral branches. *Pathology:* Pyonephrosis.

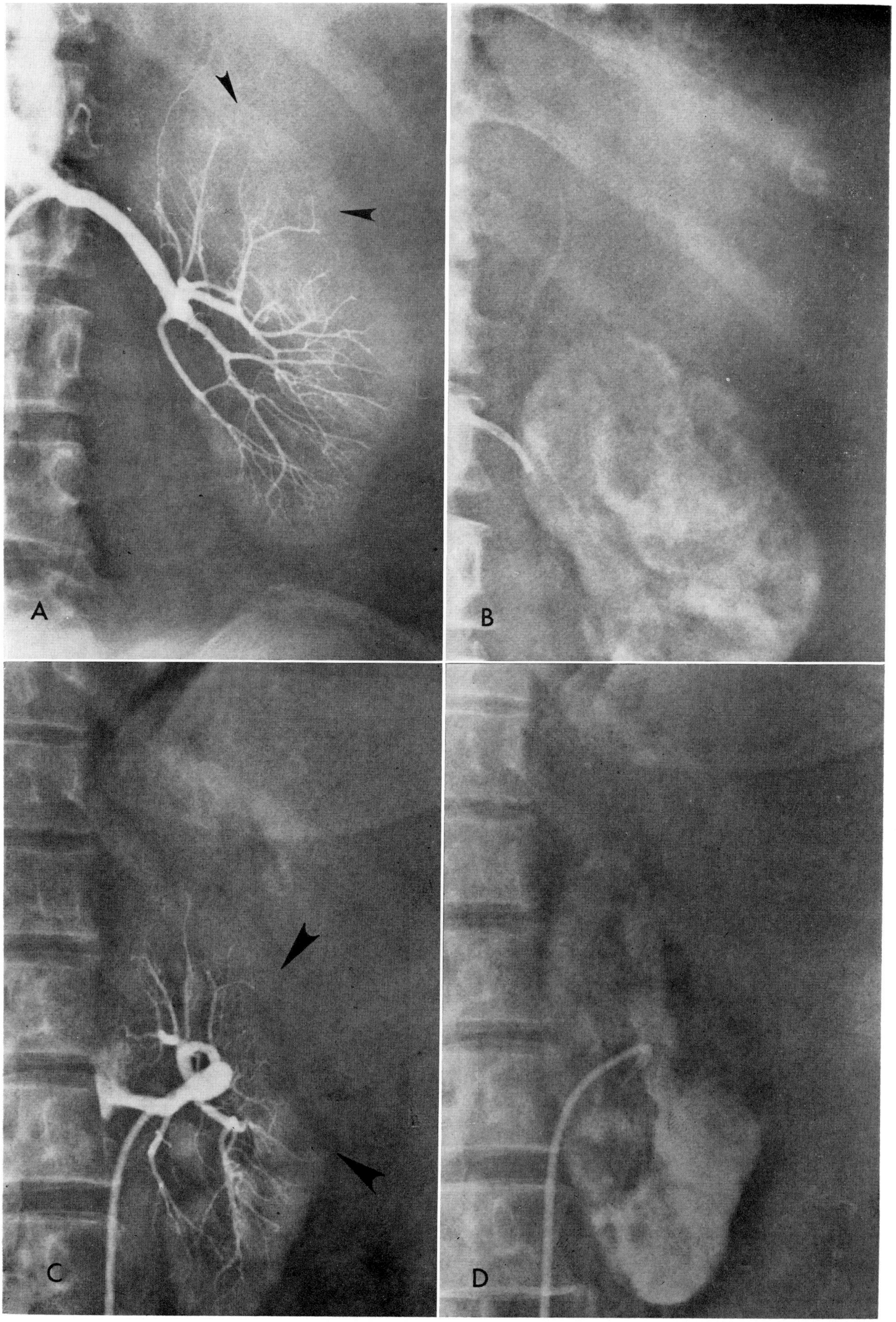
A
B
C
D

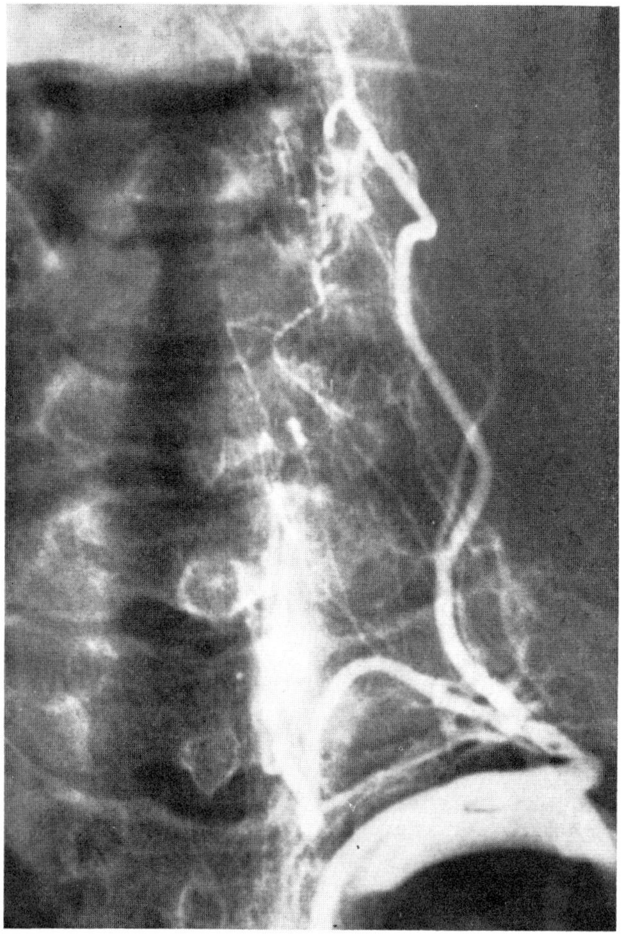

Figure 29.28. Thyrocervical Arteriogram. Reveals distortion of the "S" loop of the inferior thyroid artery in a patient who had hyperparathyroidism. *Diagnosis:* Parathyroid mass versus thyroid mass. *Pathology:* Adenoma of the parathyroid.

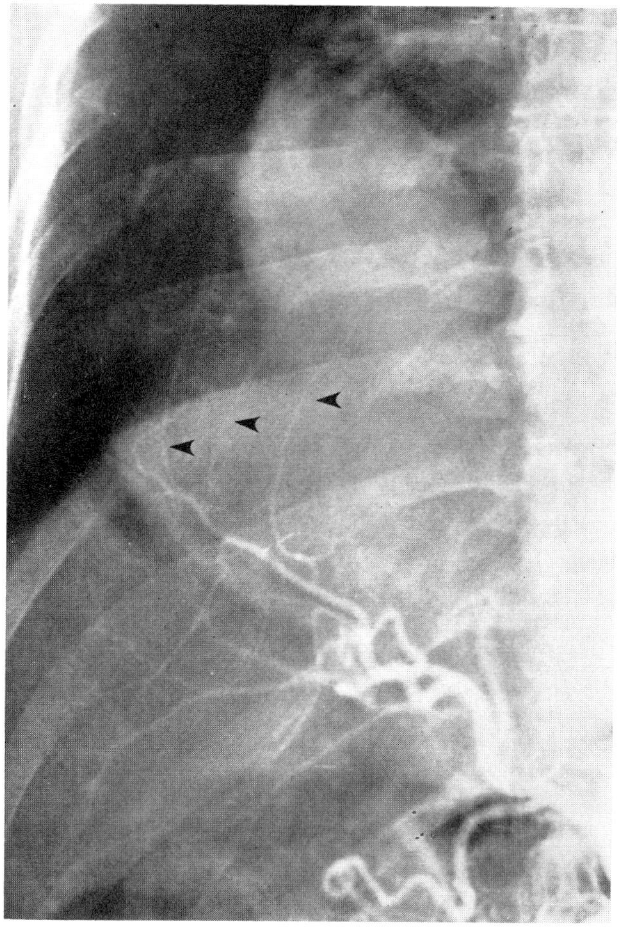

Figure 29.29. Hepatic Arteriogram. Abnormal course of the segmental intrahepatic vasculature above the contour of the diaphragm (Arrow) is seen. *Diagnosis:* Intrathoracic herniation of part of the right lobe of the liver. An isotope scan confirmed the diagnosis.

←

Figure 29.27. Renal Arteriogram. (A) Left renal arteriogram: The upper pole intrarenal arterial branches are stretched and splayed. (B) There is slight splaying of the renal parenchyma with minimal corticular irregularity. (C) Left posterior oblique renal arteriogram: There is poor filling of the renal cortex with compressed intrarenal peripheral branches. (D) Same projection—parenchymal phase: This reveals differential concentration of the contrast in the renal cortex compared to the proximal half. The patient had left flank pain and fever and marked splenomegaly. *Diagnosis:* Possible intrarenal abscess with perinephric extension. *Surgery:* The kidney was intact. *Comment:* Extreme compression by the spleen caused stretching and splaying of the intrarenal branches and led to the false diagnosis because of the clinical information.

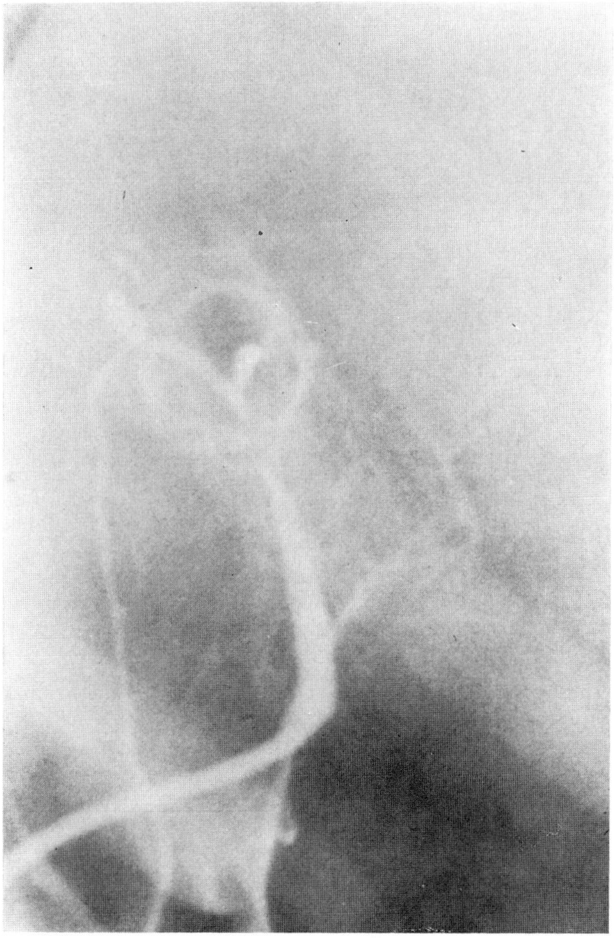

Figure 29.30. Adrenal Venogram. Reveals deviation of intraadrenal veins circumferentially around a mass. In a patient who was thought to have an aldosteronoma. *Diagnosis:* Adrenal mass probably adenoma. *Pathology:* Aldosteronoma. (Courtesy of Dr. Suresh A. Patel, Associate Professor, Rush Medical College, Senior Attending Physician, Presbyterian-St. Lukes Hospital, Chicago.)

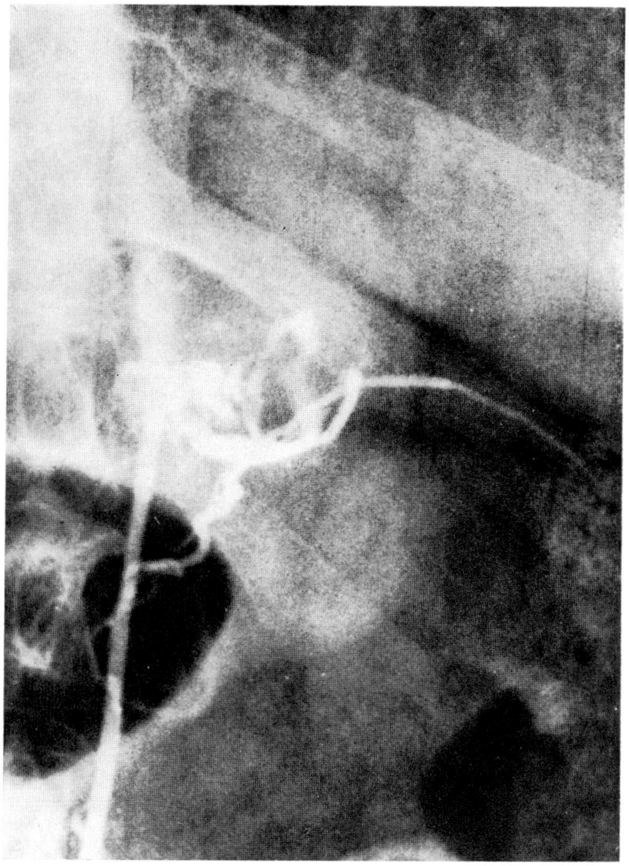

Figure 29.31. Adrenal Venogram. Reveals deviation of the intraadrenal vein around a mass. *Diagnosis:* Adrenal mass. Clinical and laboratory studies suggested an aldosteronoma. *Pathology:* Aldosteronoma.

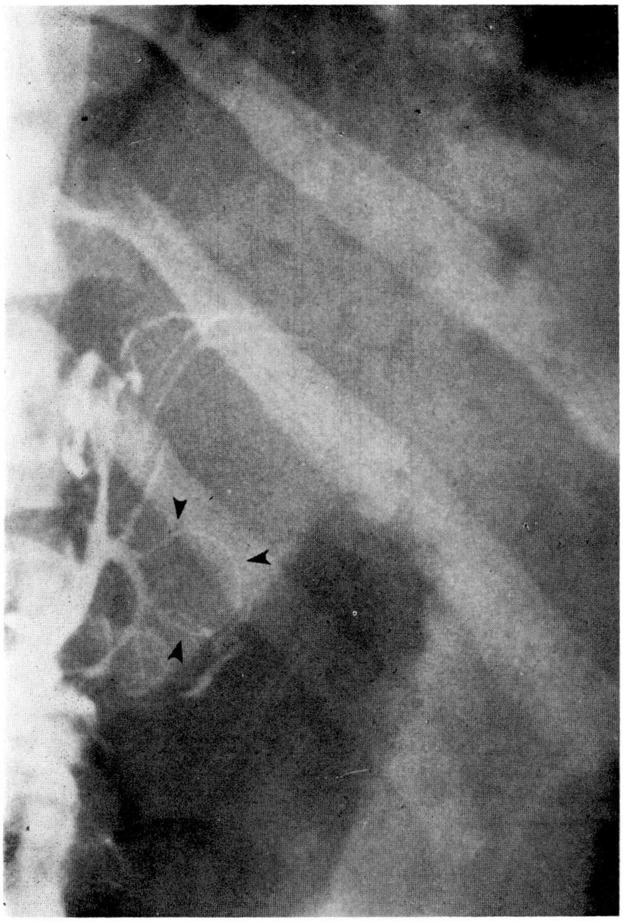

Figure 29.32. Adrenal Venogram. Reveals deviation of the intraadrenal vein around a mass. *Diagnosis:* Adrenal mass. Clinical and laboratory studies suggested an aldosteronoma. *Pathology:* Aldosteronoma. (Courtesy of Dr. K. Mojab, Radiologist, Cook County Hospital, Chicago.)

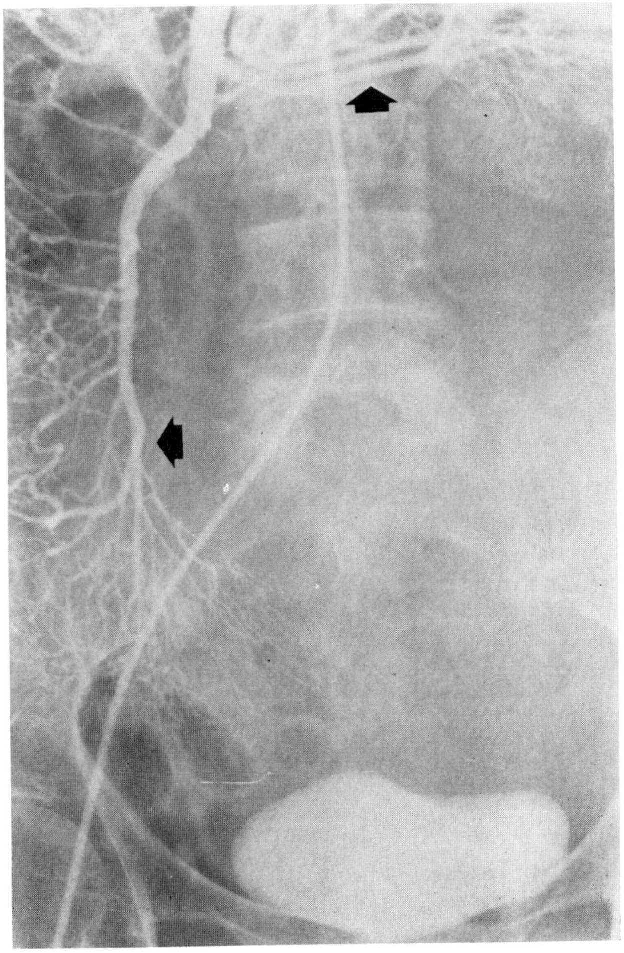

Figure 29.33. Superior Mesenteric Arteriogram. There is splitting, stretching and deviation of the superior mesenteric artery branches by a huge mass arising from the pelvis. *Surgery:* Ovarian carcinoma.

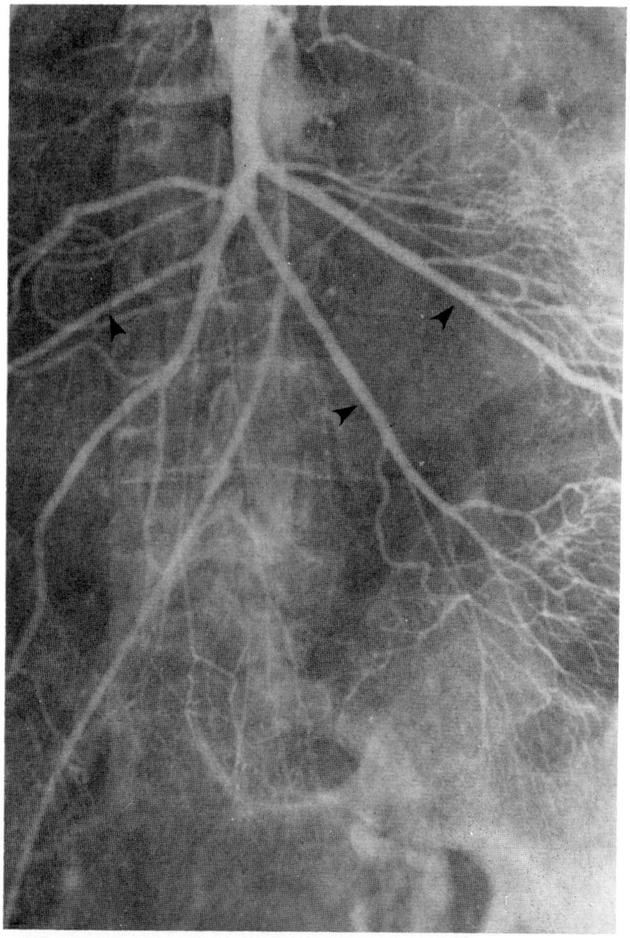

Figure 29.34. Superior Mesenteric Arteriogram. Diffuse stretching of all the main branches of the superior mesenteric artery can be seen. *Diagnosis:* Diffuse masses stretching and separating the mesenteric arterial branches. *Pathology:* Lymphoma in the paravertebral areas as well as in the mesenteric lymph nodes.

Figure 29.35. Celiac Angiogram. (A) Plain abdominal film: A mandible and tooth are seen in a right upper quadrant mass. (B) The vascular arcade arising from the gastroduodenal artery is stretched (Arrow). *Diagnosis:* Teratoma. *Pathologic Diagnosis:* Benign teratoma. (Courtesy of H. Katzen, Chairman, Department of Radiology, Chicago Osteopathic Hospital, Chicago.)

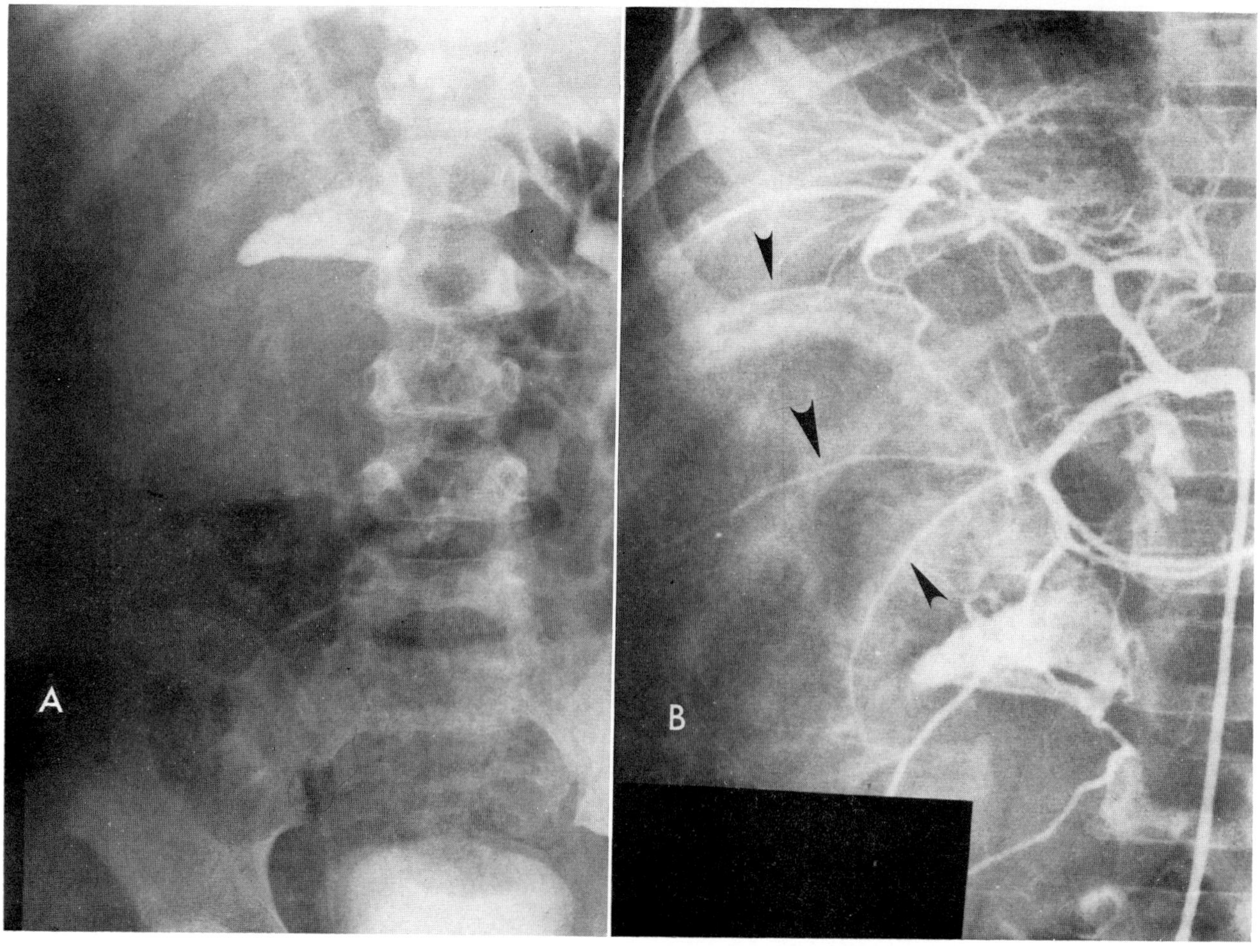

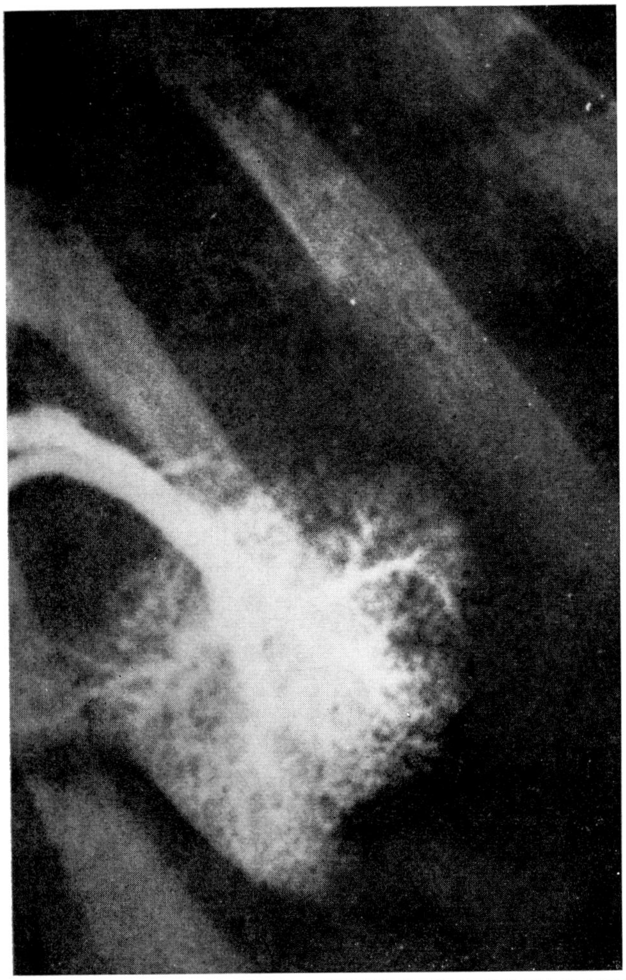

Figure 29.36. Adrenal Venogram. Demonstrates an enlarged adrenal gland with stretching of its intrinsic venous arcade. The same was shown on the opposite side in a patient who had a Cushing's syndrome. *Diagnosis:* Adrenal hyperplasia.

Figure 29.37. Left Adrenal Venogram. (A) The early phase reveals diffuse stretching and deviation of the intraadrenal veins in an enlarged gland. (B) Late phase reveals an avascular mass. The same findings were seen in the right adrenal also in a patient who had long standing essential hypertension. *Diagnosis:* Nodular hyperplasia of the adrenal glands.

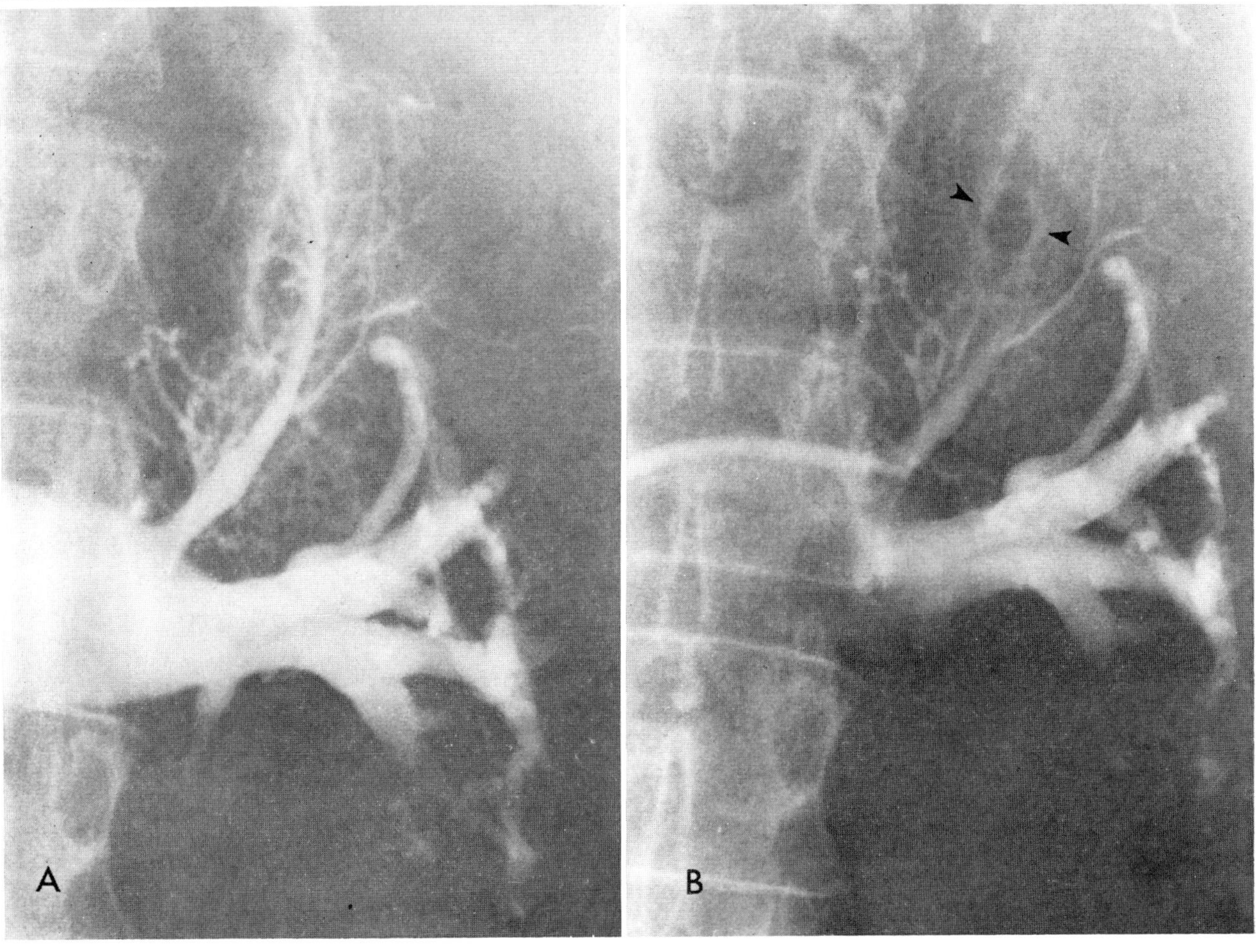

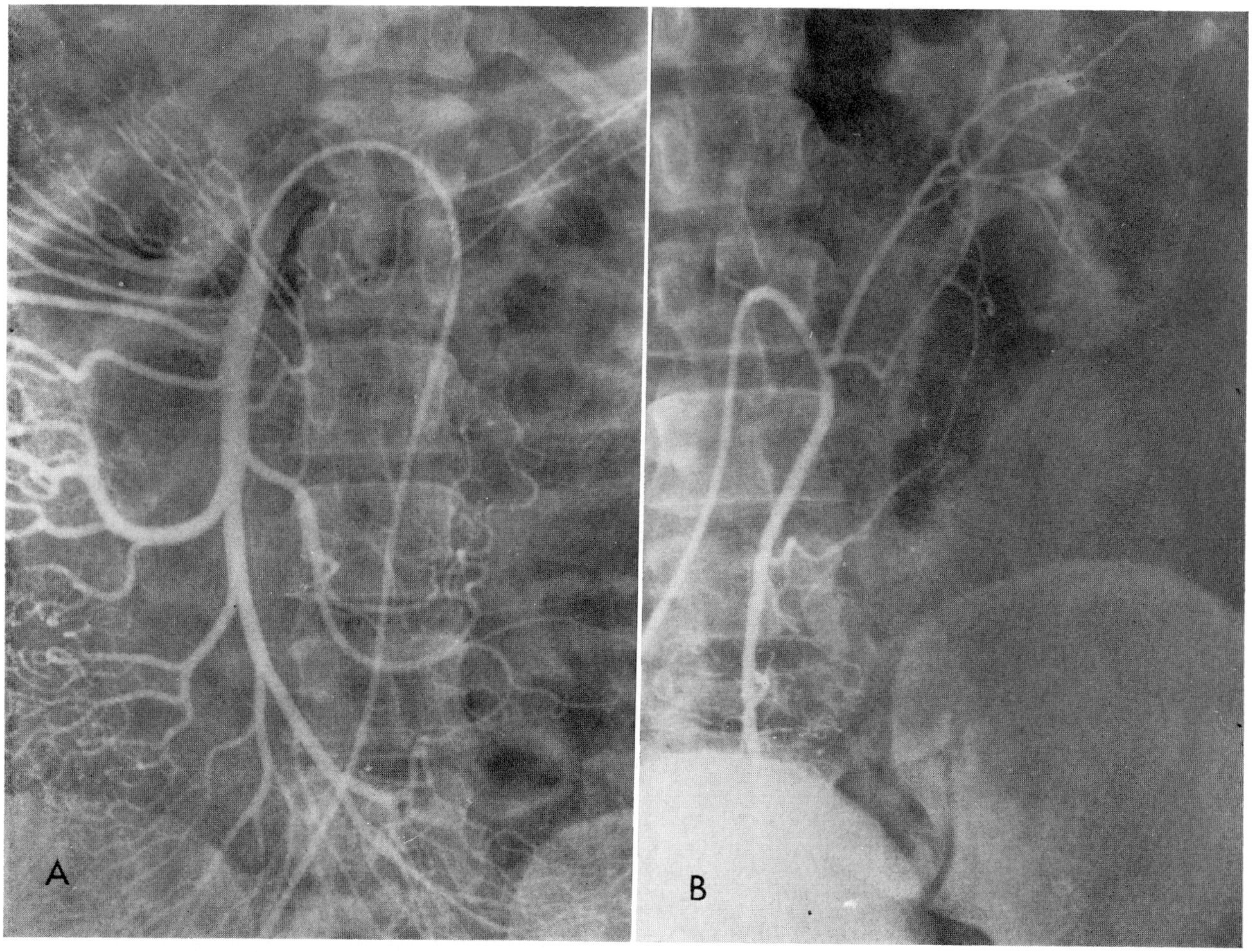

Figure 29.38. (A) Superior mesenteric arteriogram: The main trunk of the superior mesenteric artery and its branches course toward the right. (B) Inferior mesenteric arteriogram: An abnormal medial position of the descending colon branches is seen. This patient had total malrotation of the small and large bowel.

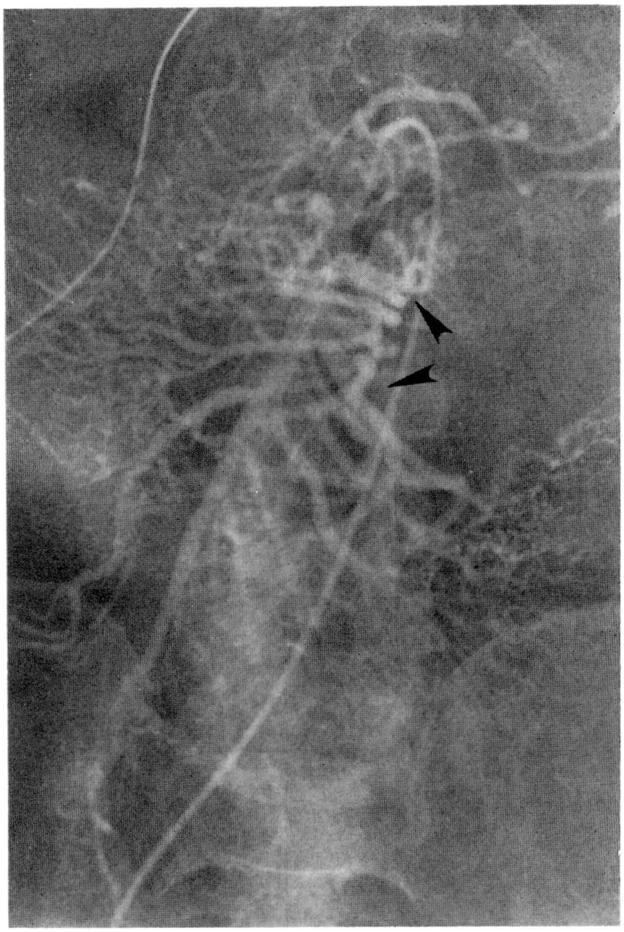

Figure 29.39. Superior Mesenteric Arteriogram. There is abrupt hairpin angulation of the proximal jejunal branches towards the right upper quadrant in a patient who had a known malrotation of the proximal small bowel loops.

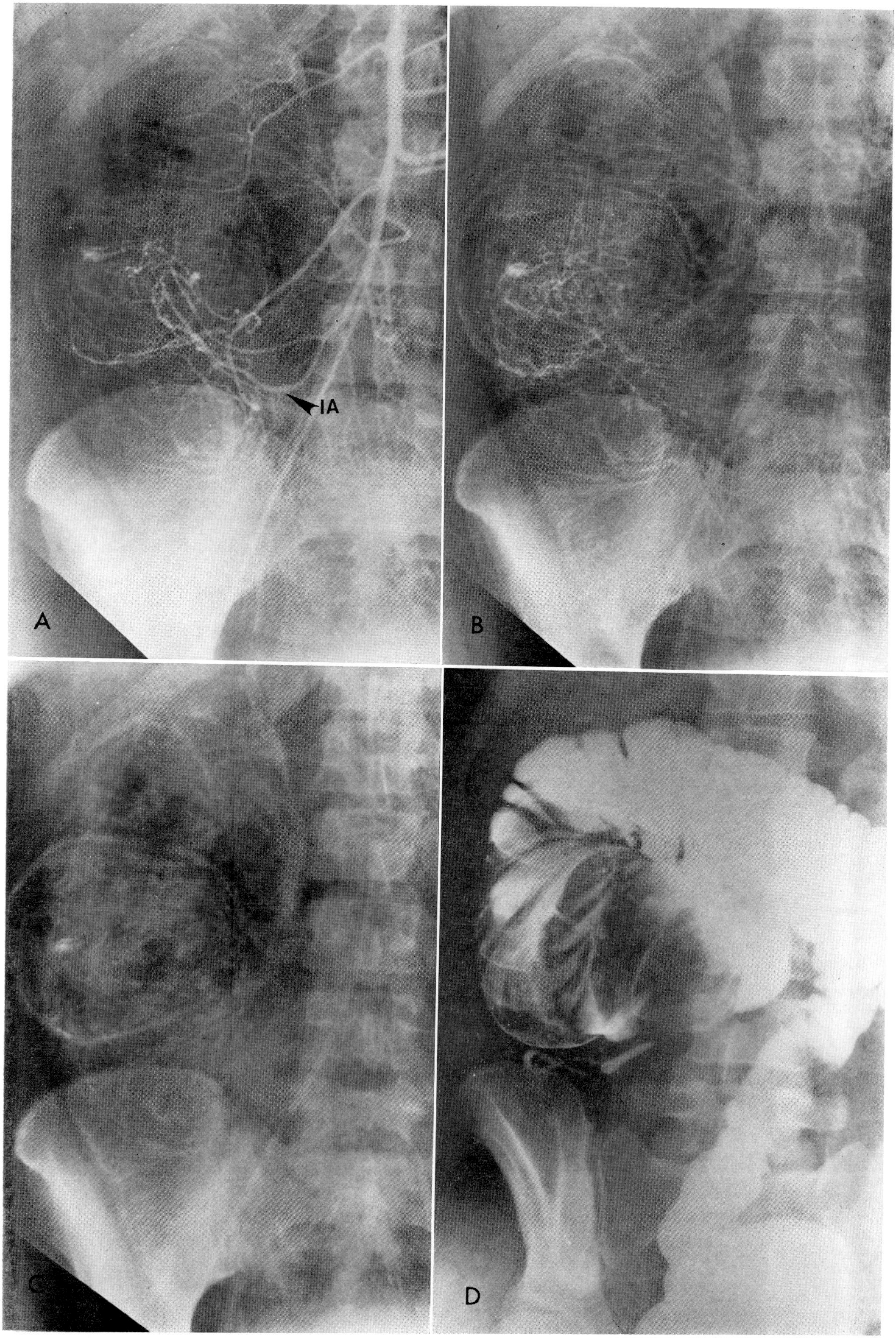
IA
A
B
C
D

←

Figure 29.40. (A) Superior mesenteric arteriogram reveals whorl-like arrangement of ileocolic vessels and with ileac vessels coursing centrally. (B, C) Mid- and late arterial phases reveal the same in a patient who had a palpable mass. (D) Barium enema done next morning reveals an ileocolic intussusception. (Courtesy of Dr. J. Petasnick, Associate Professor, Diagnostic Radiology, Rush Presbyterian-St. Luke Medical Center, Chicago.)

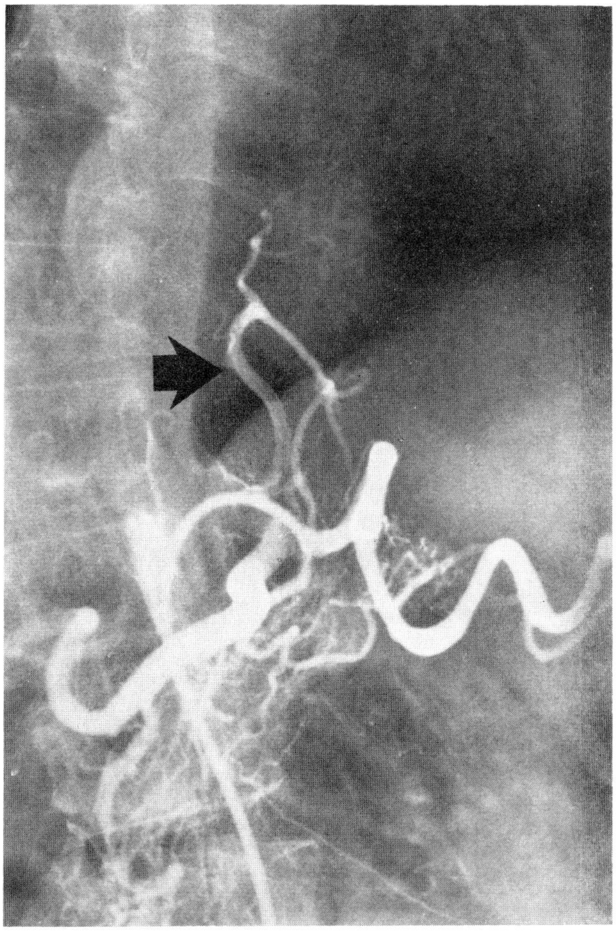

→

Figure 29.41. Celiac Arteriogram. The left gastric artery has an abnormal course toward the hemithorax. The patient had a hiatal hernia.

Figure 29.42. Hepatic Angiogram. The intrahepatic vessels have a corkscrew appearance. Some have a stretched and splayed appearance primarily of the left intrahepatic vessels (Arrow). A colloidal isotope scan revealed normal concentration in the left lobe of the liver. *Diagnosis:* Cirrhosis with enlargement of the left lobe due to regeneration. The loss of volume in the right lobe is due to fibrosis.

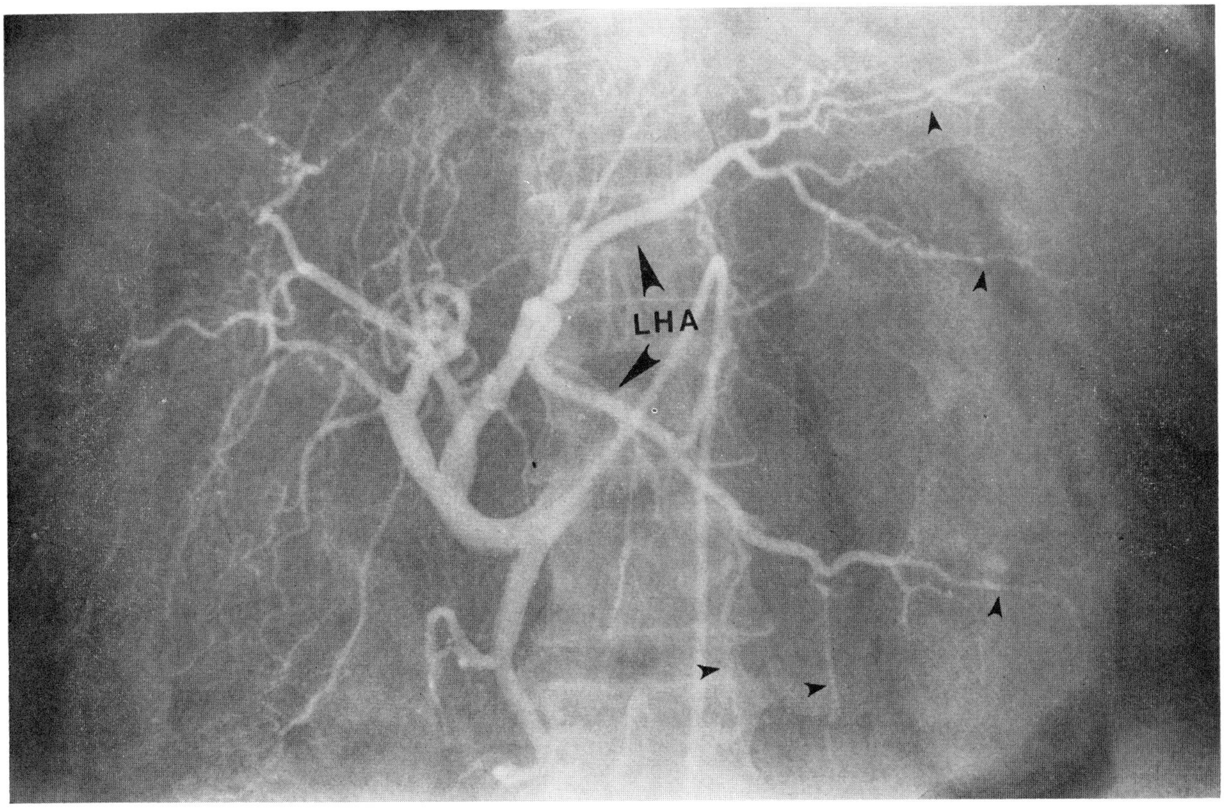

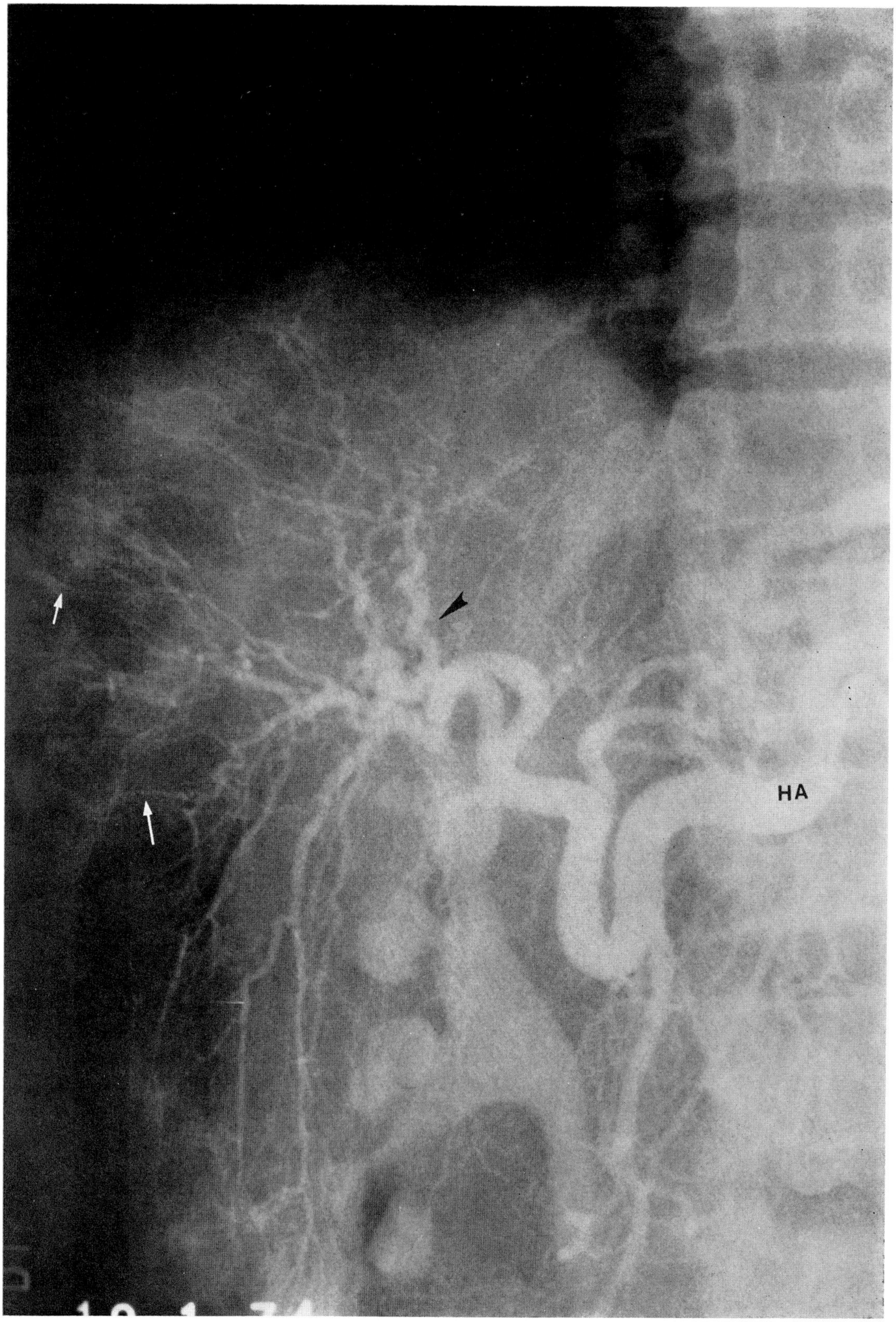

Figure 29.43. Hepatic Arteriogram. The main hepatic artery and its branches (H.A.) are dilated and the intrahepatic branches (Arrow) are tortuous with stretching of the small peripheral branches (White Arrow). This young man was a known chronic alcoholic. *Diagnosis:* Alcoholic cirrhosis causing corkscrew vessels because of fibrosis and stretching of other vessels due to fatty infiltration.

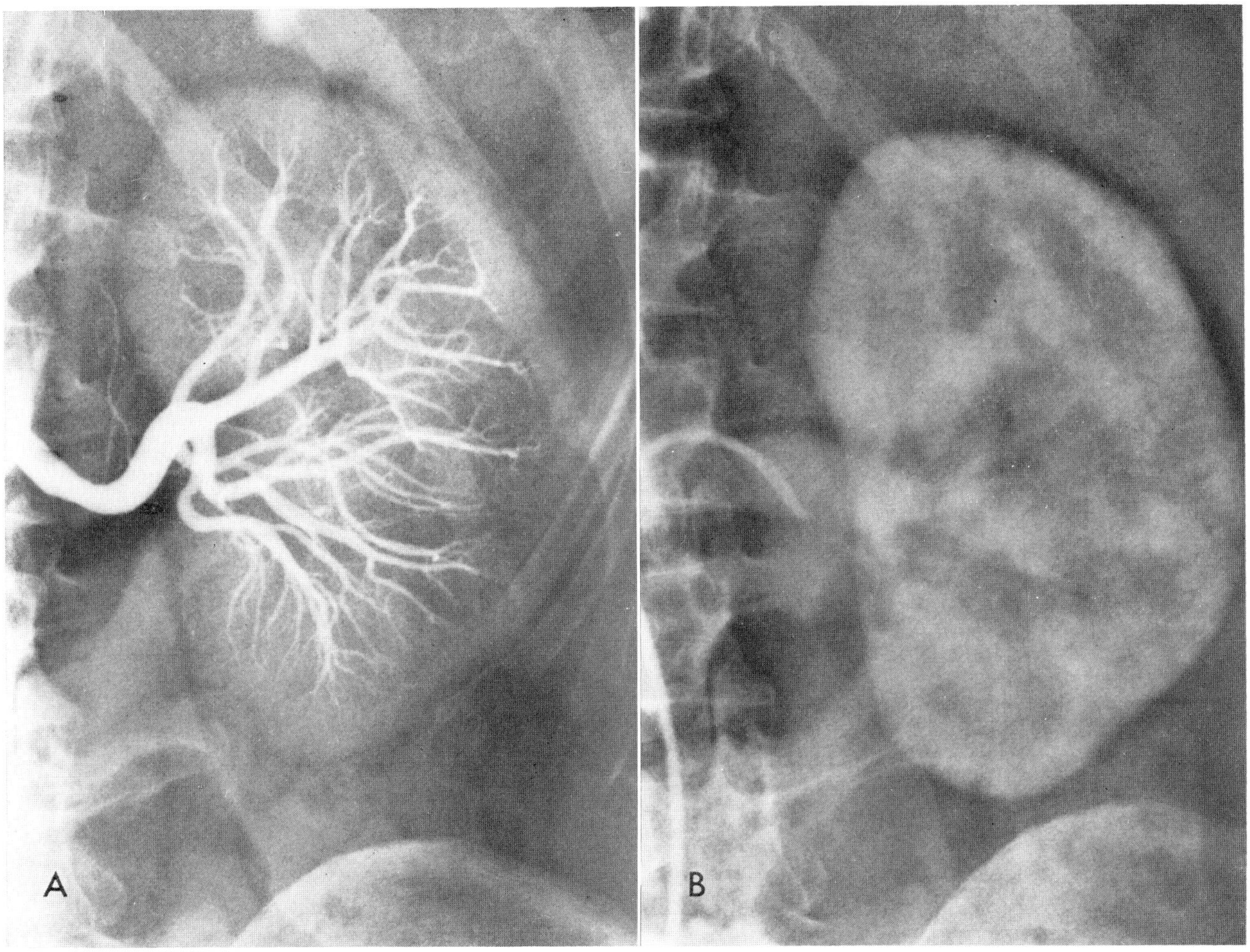

Figure 29.44. Renal Arteriogram. (A) Early arterial phase: Note the slight diffuse stretching of the intrarenal arteries. (B) Parenchymal phase: The renal size is slightly increased and the cortical medullary junction slightly blurred. This young patient had acute glomerulonephritis. *Comment:* Diffuse intrarenal swelling due to edema.

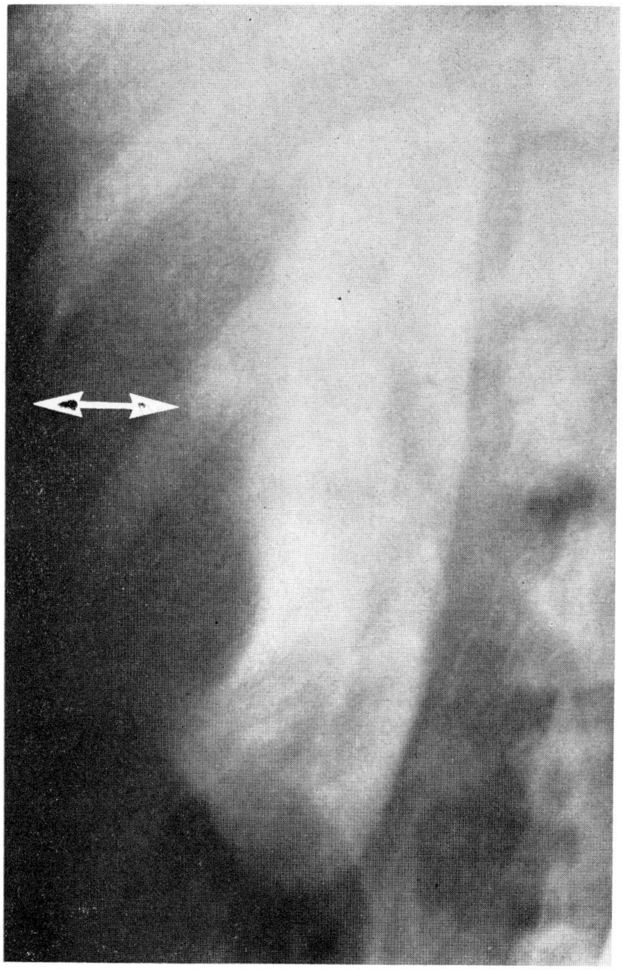

Figure 29.45A

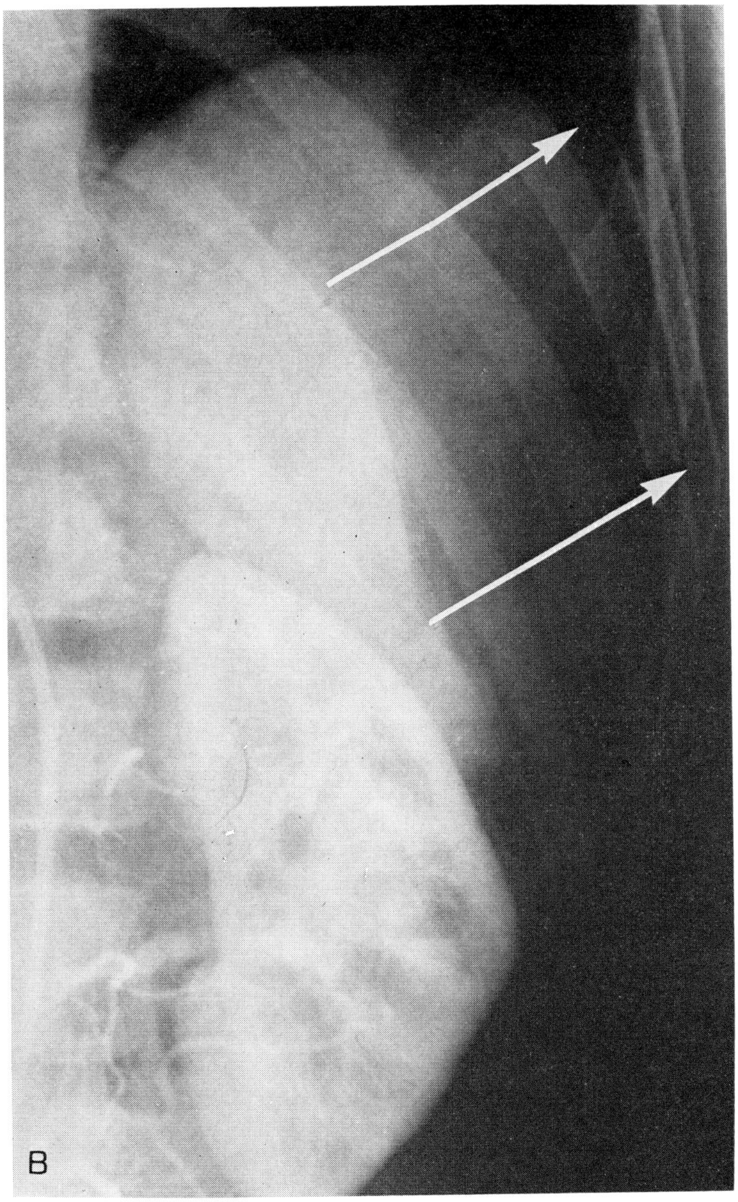

Figure 29.45. (A) Late phase renal arteriogram demonstrates compression and deviation of the opacified renal parenchyma from its capsule in a patient who had flank trauma a week prior to the study. (B) Late phase splenic arteriogram reveals compression and deviation of the opacified splenic parenchyma from its capsule in a patient who had left upper quadrant trauma 2 weeks prior to the study. *Diagnosis:* Subcapsular hematomas of the kidney and spleen. *Comment:* The same finding may be given by accumulation of pus in the subcapsular area.

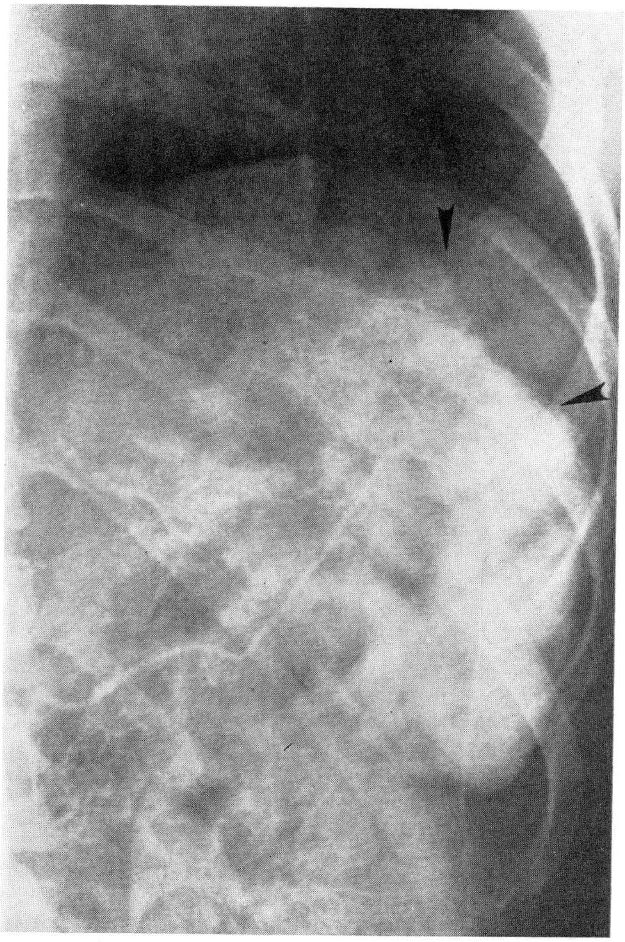

Figure 29.46. Splenic Arteriogram—parenchymal phase: There is smooth, localized deviation of the splenic parenchyma away from its normal contour. This young patient had left upper quadrant trauma. *Diagnosis:* Subcapsular splenic hematoma.

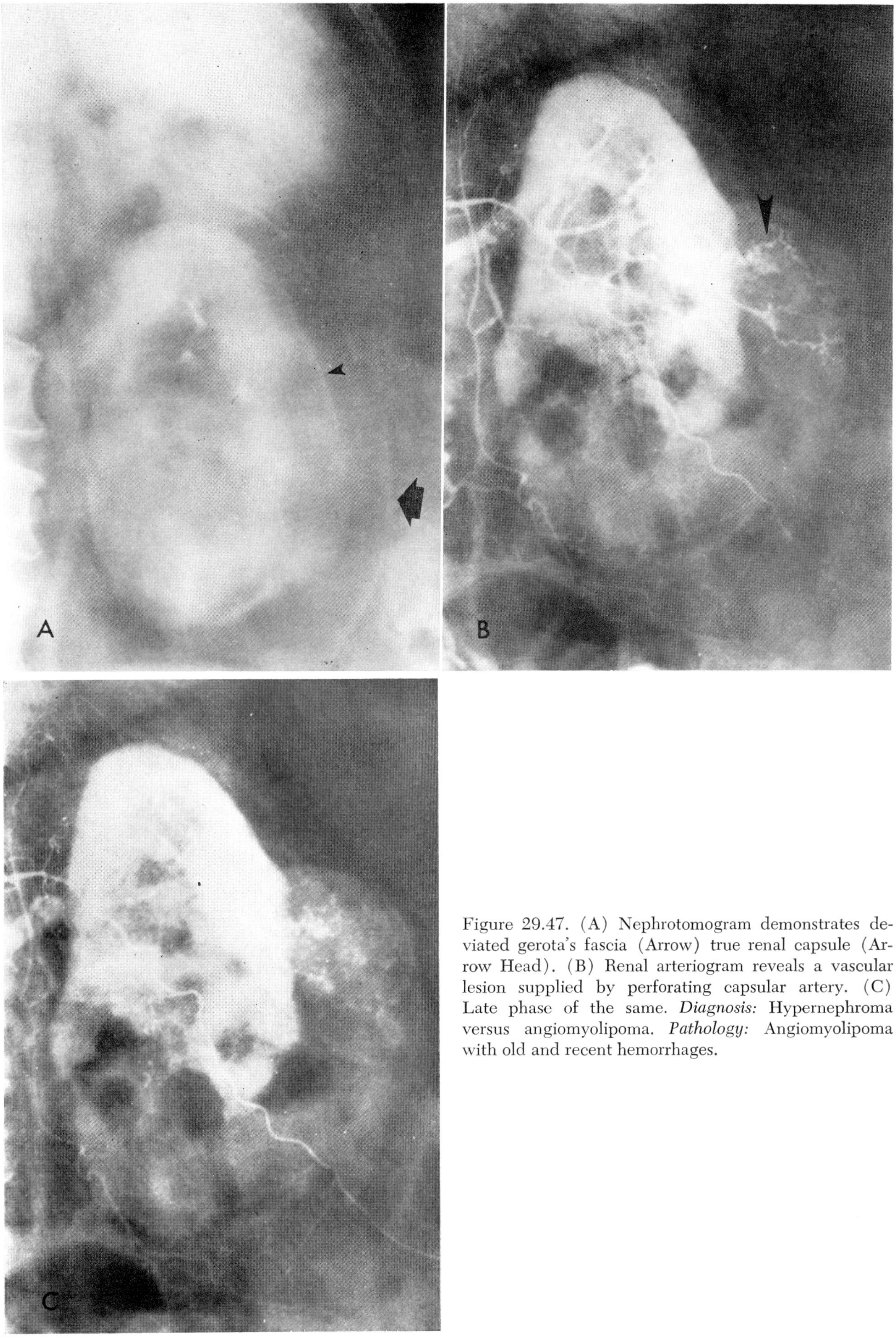

Figure 29.47. (A) Nephrotomogram demonstrates deviated gerota's fascia (Arrow) true renal capsule (Arrow Head). (B) Renal arteriogram reveals a vascular lesion supplied by perforating capsular artery. (C) Late phase of the same. *Diagnosis:* Hypernephroma versus angiomyolipoma. *Pathology:* Angiomyolipoma with old and recent hemorrhages.

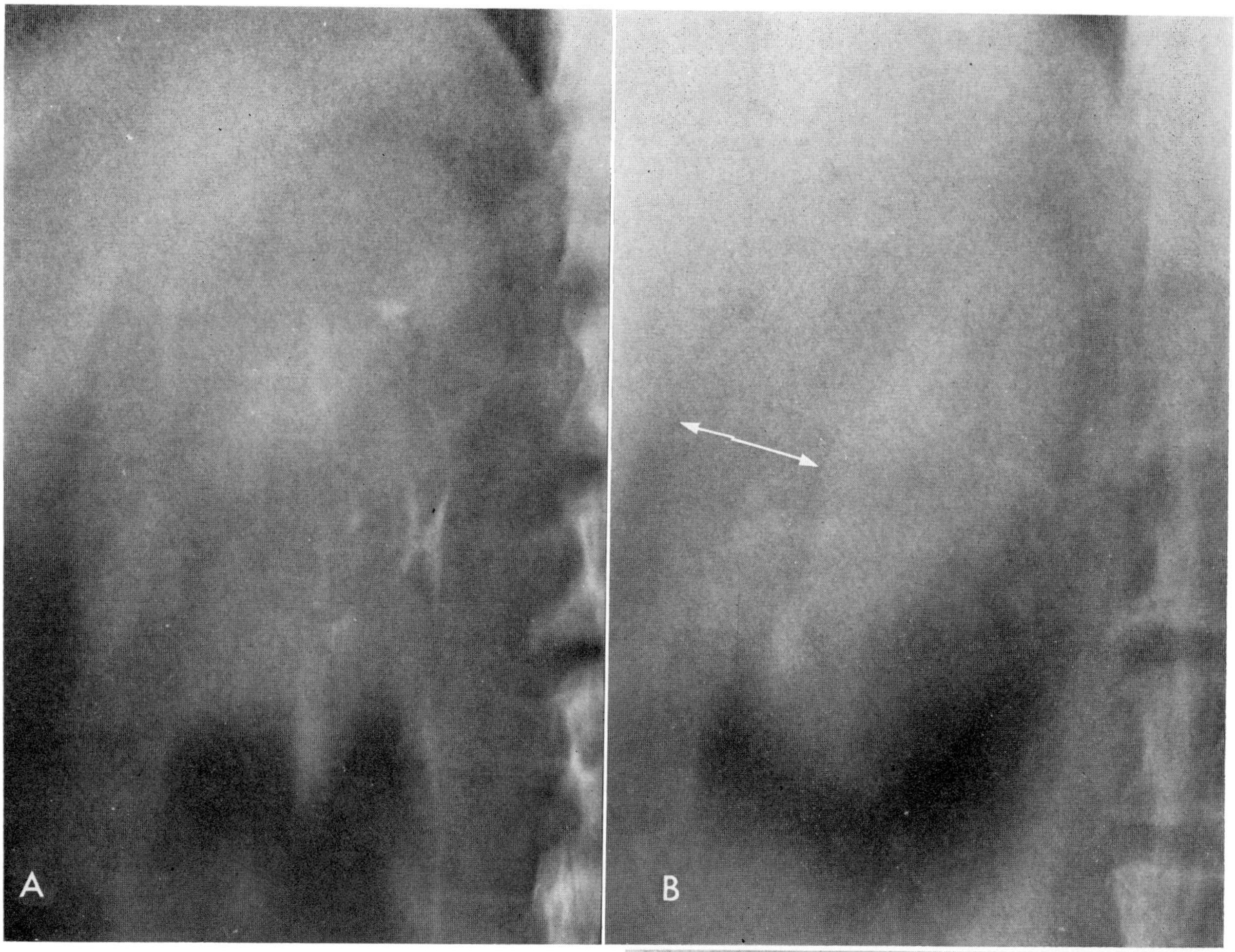

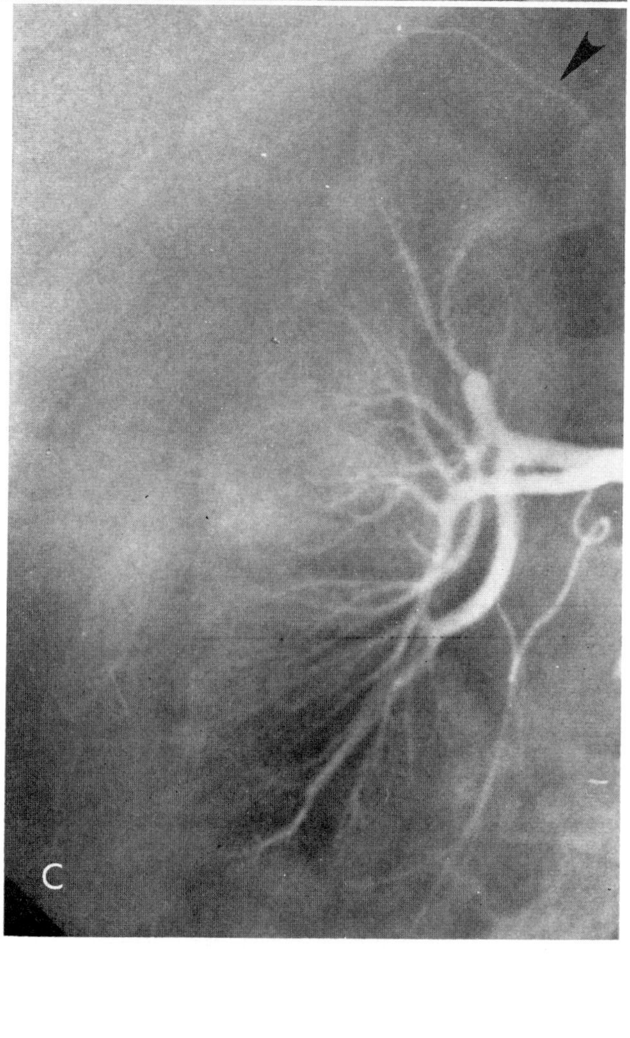

Figure 29.48. (A) Intravenous pyelogram: There is increased contour of the right kidney with undue separation of the calyces from the renal contour. (B) Staining of the renal parenchyma occurs with an irregular lateral contour. There is no correspondence with the renal contour of the intravenous pyelogram. (C) Renal arteriogram: The normal renal cortical border does not reach the renal contour. Separation of the renal capsular artery (Arrow). This patient is receiving anticoagulants. *Diagnosis:* Subcapsular hematoma.

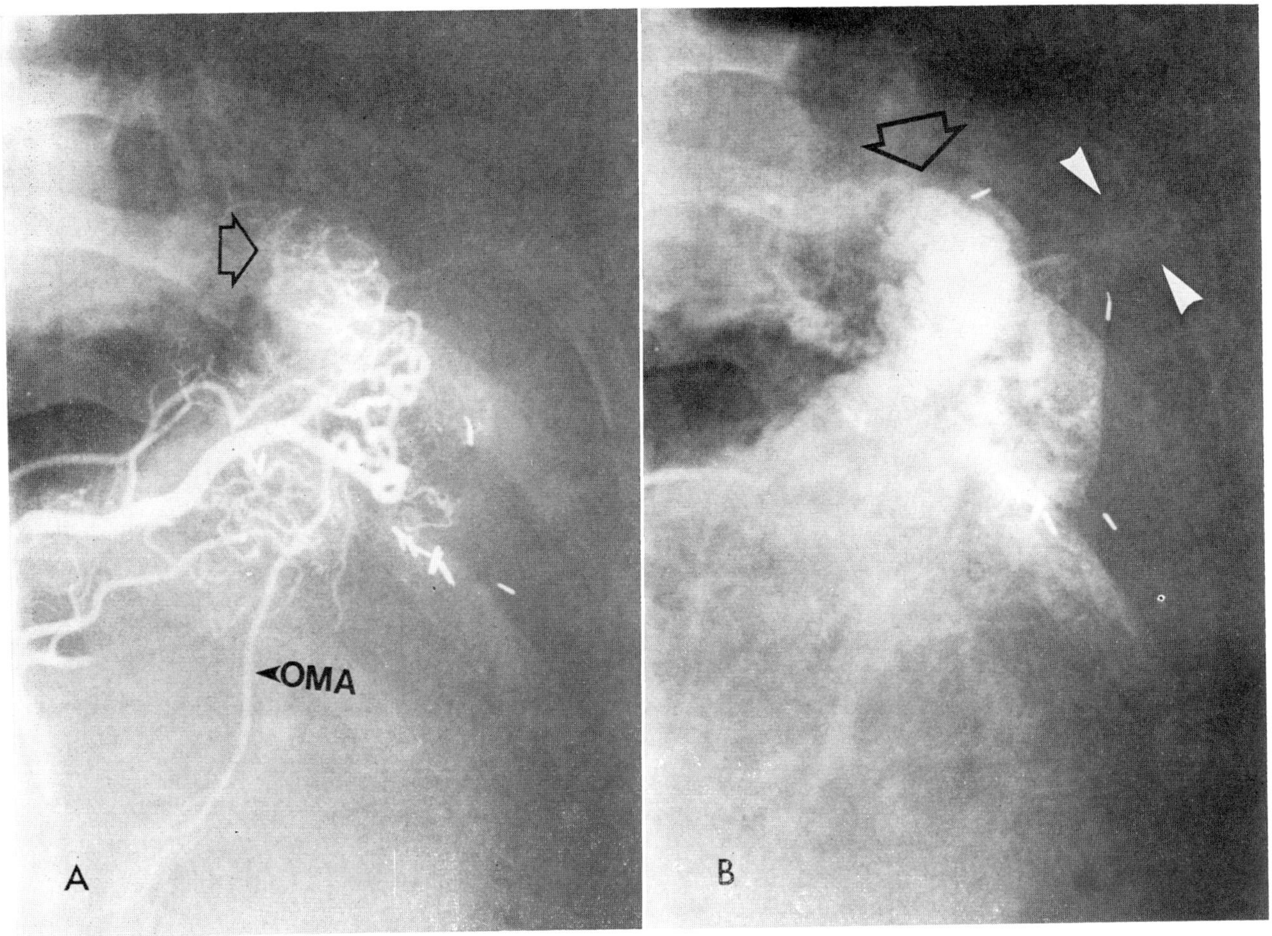

Figure 29.49. Splenic Arteriogram. (A) Arterial phase: There is filling of the branches of the gastric fundus and visualization of the pancreatic branches. There are prominent omental branches (O.M.A.). (B) Late phase: The fundic stain (Arrow) is seen as well as staining of thickened omentum adherent to the diaphragm (White Arrow Head) an avascular space between the omentum and lateral peritoneal surface. The patient had ascites following a recent splenectomy and clinically there was suspicion of a left upper quadrant subphrenic abscess. *Diagnosis:* Possible loculated left subphrenic abscess. At surgery no evidence of an abscess was noted. The omentum was adherent to the diaphragm.

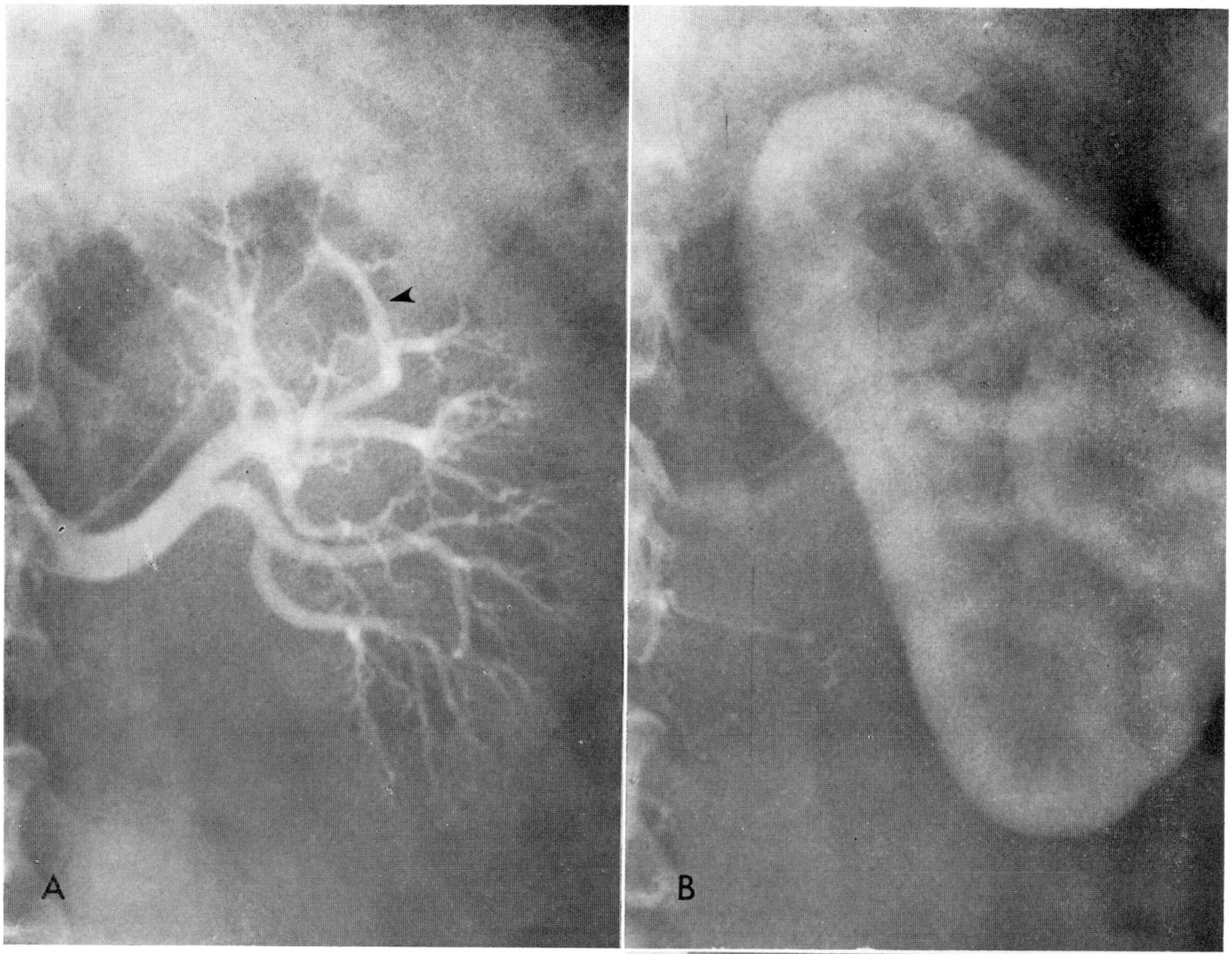

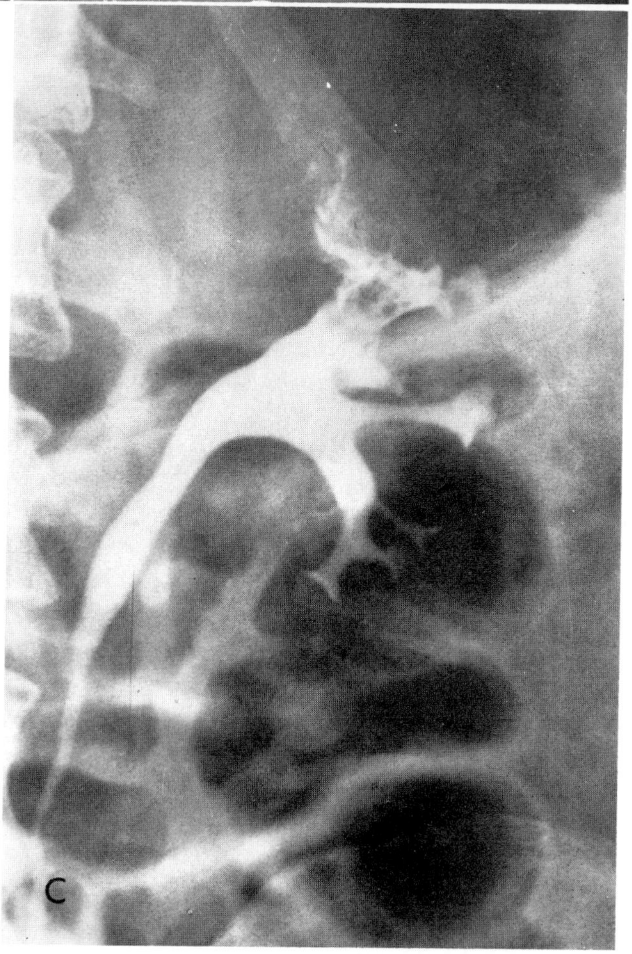

Figure 29.50. Renal Arteriogram. (A) Arterial phase: There is slight deviation and stretching of one of the intrarenal branches. (B) Nephrogram. No apparent abnormalities. (C) Retrograde pyelogram reveals destruction of the upper pole calyx. *Diagnosis:* Transitional cell tumor. *Comment:* Angiography in this case is noncontributory toward the diagnosis of this transitional cell tumor as it may be in some.

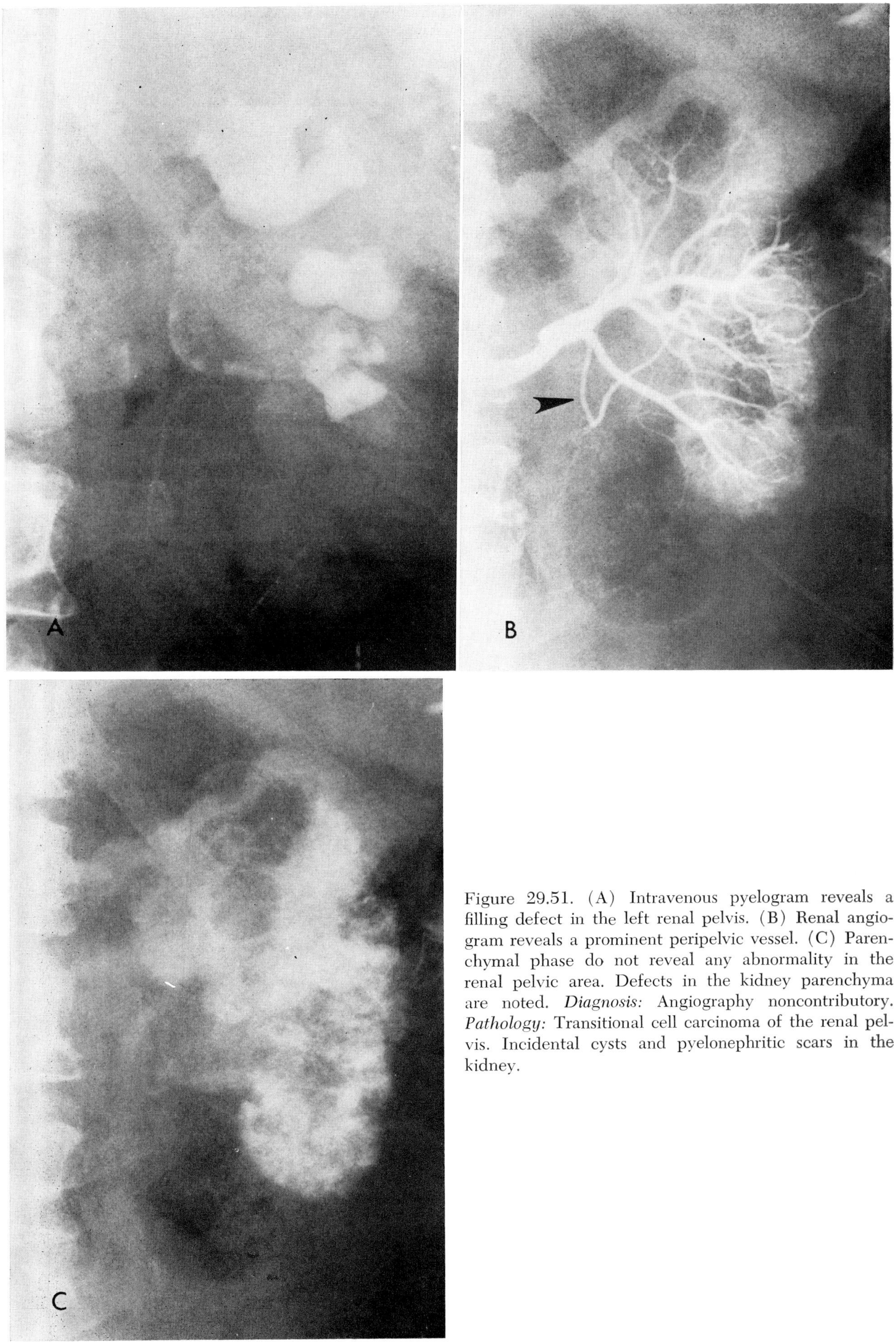

Figure 29.51. (A) Intravenous pyelogram reveals a filling defect in the left renal pelvis. (B) Renal angiogram reveals a prominent peripelvic vessel. (C) Parenchymal phase do not reveal any abnormality in the renal pelvic area. Defects in the kidney parenchyma are noted. *Diagnosis:* Angiography noncontributory. *Pathology:* Transitional cell carcinoma of the renal pelvis. Incidental cysts and pyelonephritic scars in the kidney.

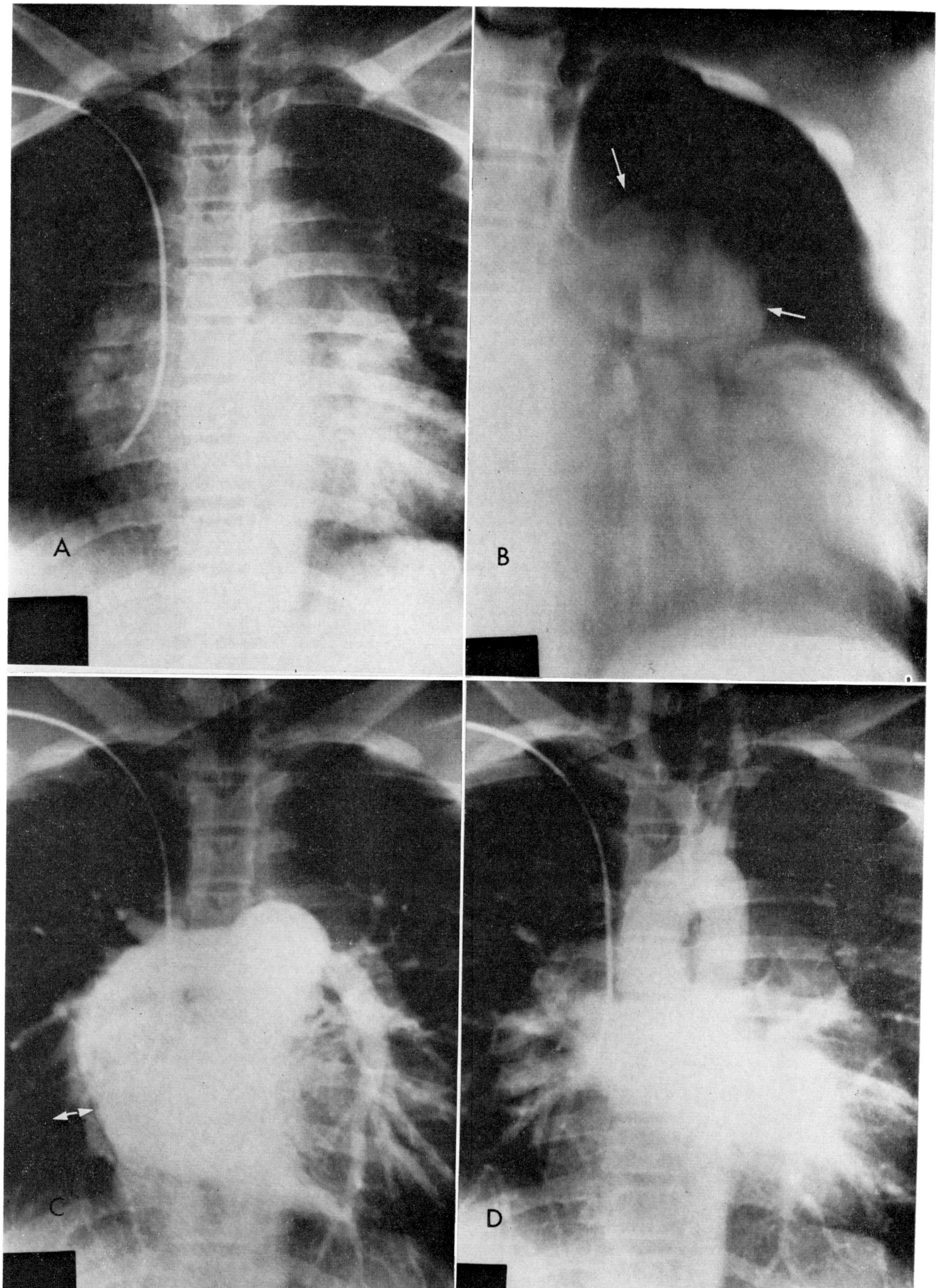
A
B
C
D

ferior thyroid artery often indicates the presence of thyroid or parathyroid masses (Fig. 29-28). Masses in the vicinity of the sciatic notch cause deviation of *gluteal arteries* (Fig. 29-18). Deviation and stretching of the *renal capsular arteries* are clues to perinephric lesions due to tumor, trauma or inflammation. Medial deviation of the *popliteal artery* at the knee causing intermittent claudication in young individuals can be the result of popliteal artery entrapment.[660, 835] Acute hairpin curves of the *intestinal arteries* beyond their origin with redirection medially and posteriorly to the superior mesenteric artery is a clue to internal hernias.[1138] This is best demonstrated in a lateral projection. Furthermore, crowding and abnormal hairpin curves of intestinal branches may suggest adhesions.[1139] A vertical course of the ileocolic artery amidst the branches of the right colic artery signifies an ileocolic intussusception[1140] (Fig. 29-40). Twisting of the mesenteric vessels upon themselves with dilatation of the superior mesenteric artery resembling a *barber pole* helps detect the cause for patient's obscure abdominal problems as malrotation of the gut with volvulus.[1141]

DEVIATION OF THE PARENCHYMA OF AN ORGAN

Deviation or compression of the stained parenchyma usually occurs in the *subcapsular region* of an organ with an intact capsule. These deviations are usually caused by accumulations of *blood or pus.* Extrinsic masses may cause compression of an organ and even cause stretching of the intrinsic vessels of that compressed organ. This can usually be established by obtaining additional studies in oblique or lateral projections, depending on the situation.

Stretching

Stretching of vascular arborization and ironing out of the inherent curves of vessels during their course through an organ has several etiologies. Stretching of the vessels may be seen in *organ enlargement.* It is also seen with infiltrating pathologies such as *edema; lymphoma; leukemia, or sarcoidosis; primary and secondary malignant neoplasms; or multiple masses surrounding the vessel in a circumferential manner. Hyperplasia* of an entire organ such as the kidney, or localized hyperplasia such as regenerating nodules of a lobe of the liver (Figs. 29-42 and 29-43), postpyelonephritic hypertrophy of the kidney, or diffuse enlargement of the endocrinal glands may all stretch the intrinsic vessels.

Hyperplasias of Endocrinal Glands

The affected gland may be normal or enlarged in size.[1279] The hyperplastic cells are in no way different from the adjacent normal cells. As hyperplasia is usually diffuse in nature, the vessels are also *diffusely* and *uniformly stretched.* Prolonged hyperplasias may produce nodular lesions which deviate the already stretched vessel (Figs. 29-36 and 29-37). As the metabolic needs of these hyperplastic cells are not significantly greater than normal cells, the vasculature is usually not increased. *Angiographically* diffuse stretching of the vessels with or without deviation may be seen. From the angiographic point of view it may be difficult, or even impossible, to recognize hyperplasias in organs such as the parathyroid glands or pancreas (islet cell hyperplasia).

←

Figure 29.52. (A) The left hilum is prominent in a young and otherwise asymptomatic individual. (B) Tomograms of the same. (C, D) Intravenous angiocardiogram reveals that this mass is extravascular at the same time please notice the pericardial effusion. *Diagnosis:* Lymphoma or thymoma with pericardial involvement. *Surgery:* Tuberculous lymphadenitis and pericarditis with effusion.

CHAPTER 30
TORTUOSITIES AND KINKS

TORTUOSITY

Tortuosity of a vessel is usually associated with arteriosclerosis or loss of elastic tissue. It is a *normal* finding in some vessels such as the inferior phrenic, splenic, occipital in general, and in ovarian arteries in a multiparous individual. Dilatation of preexisting vessels can cause extreme tortuosity seen with collateral vessels and those with granulation tissue. Apart from these, tortuosity of the intrinsic vessels may be due to *loss of volume of a compact organ. Periarterial and arterial fibrosis* can also cause tortuosity.

Tortuosity Due to Loss of Elastic Tissue

This is seen in arteriosclerosis, hyperelastosis, and congenital defects of the elastic tissues. Generalized lengthening and tortuosity of all elastic arteries and the proximal portions of muscular arteries may be seen.[1146, 1147] An extreme expression of such is *arteria dolicho et magna*, revealing tortuous, dilated vessels with

(*Text continues on page 624*)

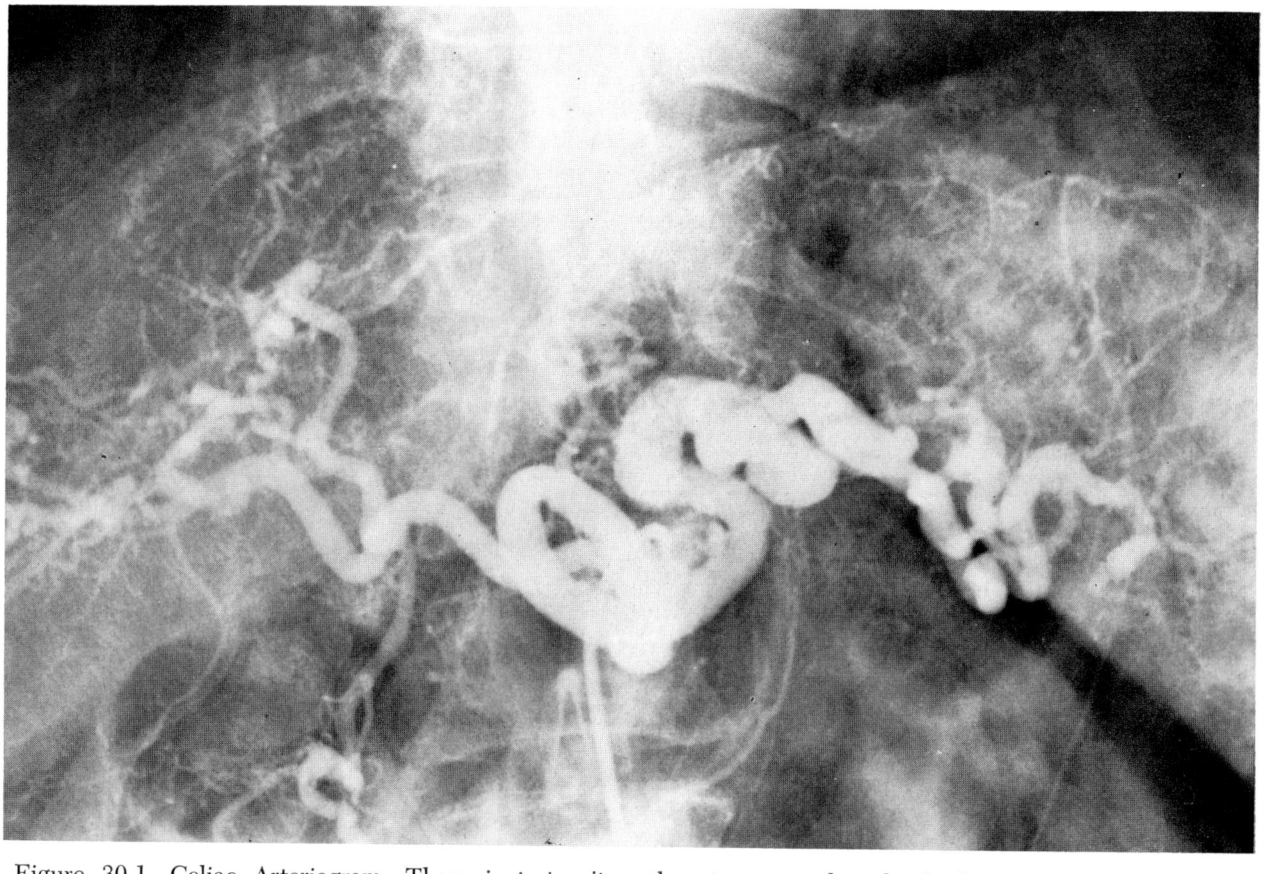

Figure 30.1. Celiac Arteriogram. There is tortuosity and coiling of the splenic artery in a fifty-year-old individual. *Comment:* Tortuosity of the splenic artery in otherwise normal individuals is not an uncommon event.

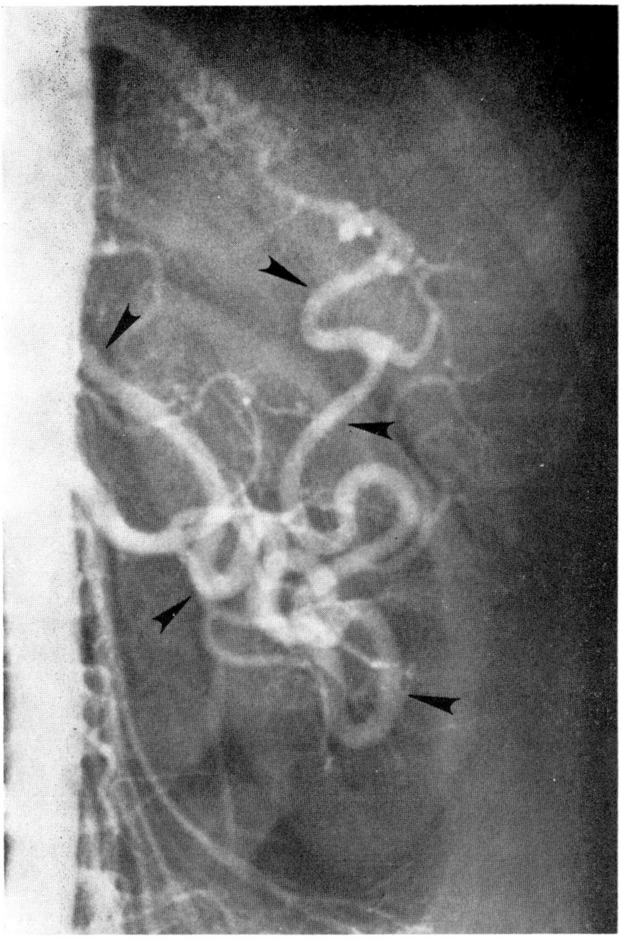

← Figure 30.2. Abdominal Aortogram. There is a long, tortuous splenic artery (Arrow) in a young woman who is otherwise normal.

Figure 30.3. Renal Arteriogram—right and left kidneys. Very tortuous renal hilar branches are present in a young patient with long-standing hypertension.

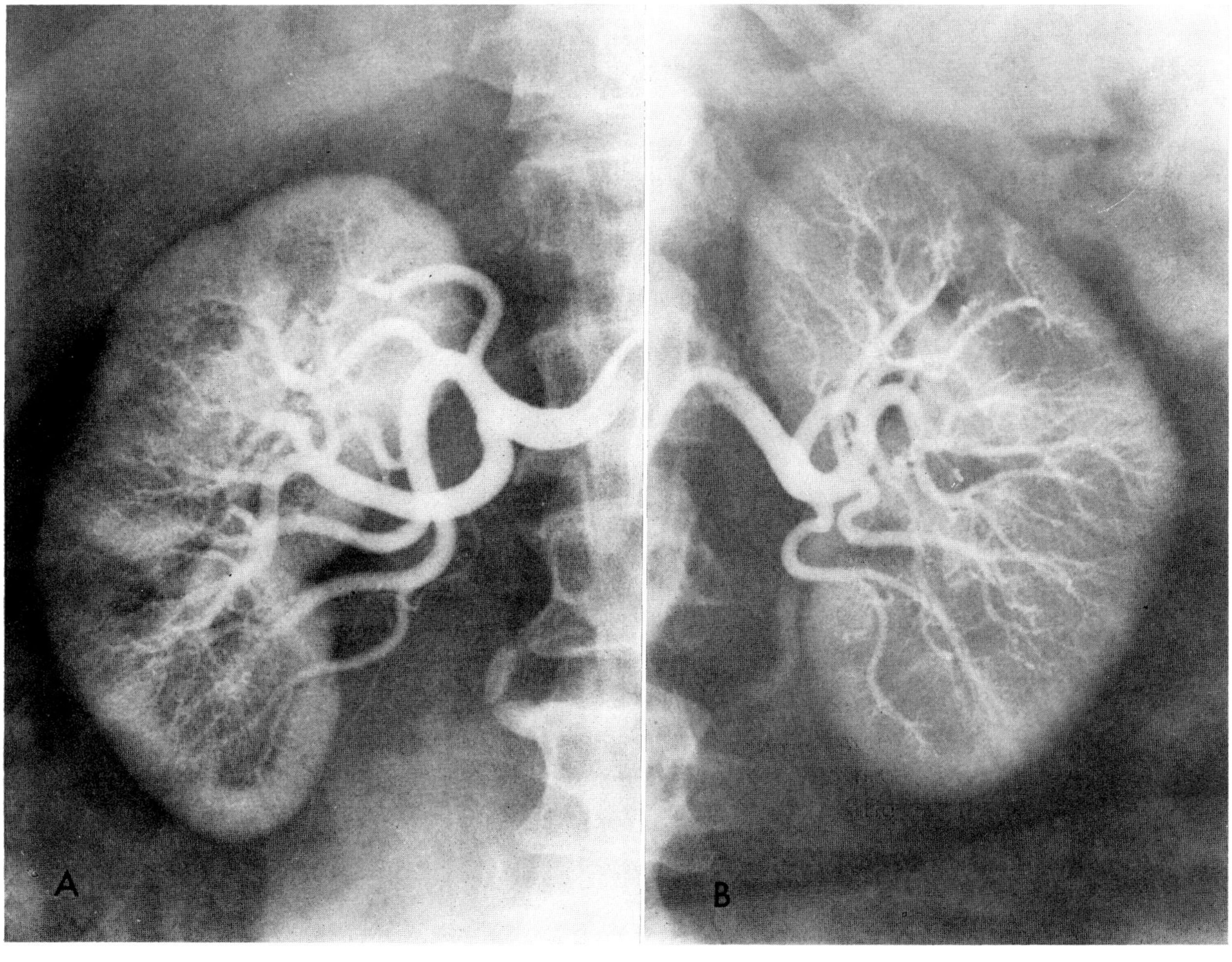

Figure 30.4. Aortic Arch Arteriogram. The innominate artery is ectatic (Arrow), and the subclavian artery is tortuous (Arrow Head). *Comment:* Kinking of the ectatic innominate.

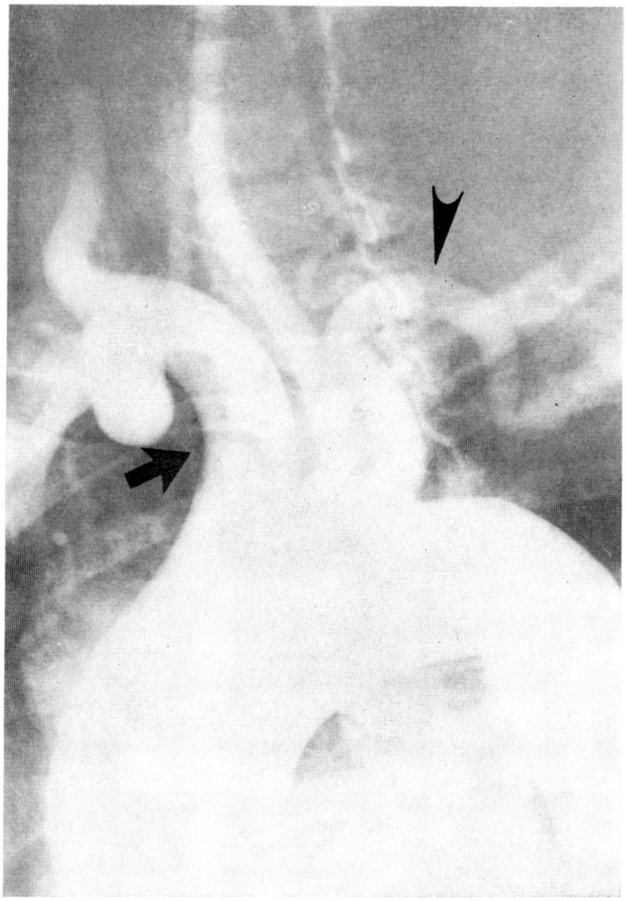

Figure 30.5. Thoracic Aortogram. There is eccentric narrowing (Arrow) of the aortic arch distal to the origin of the left subclavian artery. The patient was asymptomatic. *Diagnosis:* Pseudocoarctation of the aorta.

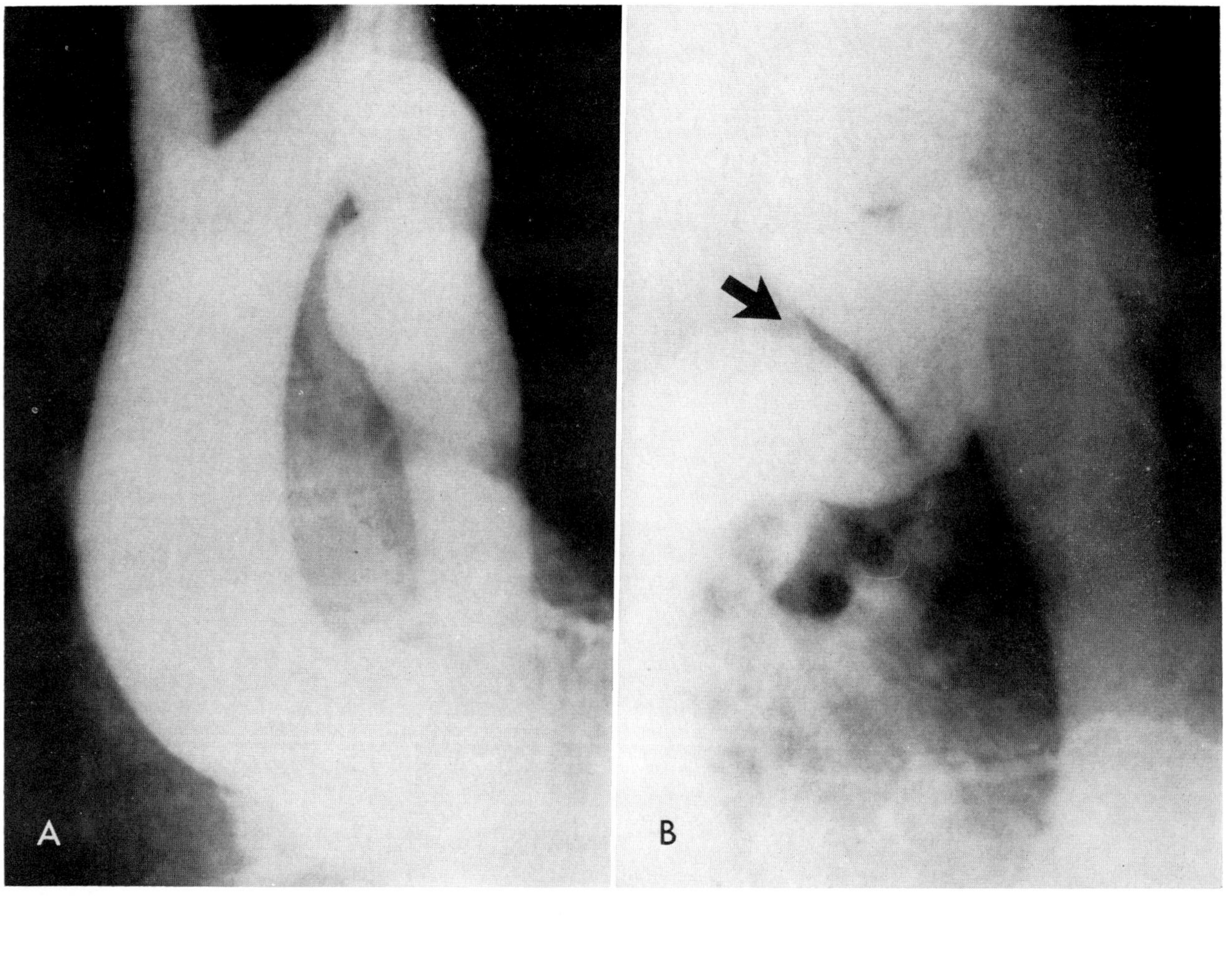

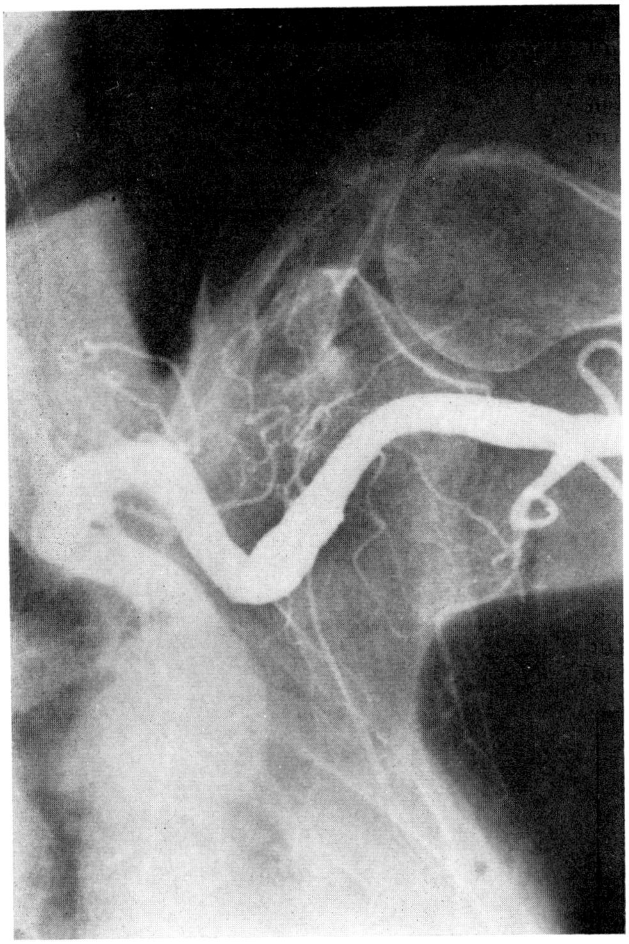

Figure 30.6. Left Subclavian Arteriogram. This type of tortuous, kinked left subclavian artery may cause technical difficulties when attempting to catheterize the descending aorta via left axillary artery.

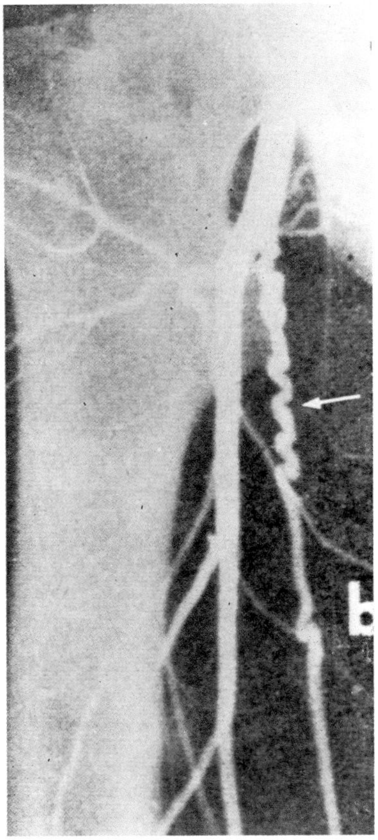

Figure 30.7. Femoral Arteriogram. The superficial femoral artery has a corkscrew appearance which suggests recanalization. The patient had Buerger's disease. (From McKusick, V. A., Harris, W. S., Ottesen, O. E., Goodman, R. M., Shelley, W. M., and Blookwell, R. D. Buerger's disease: A distinct clinical and pathological entity. *JAMA, 181:5*, 1962. Courtesy of the authors and publishers.)

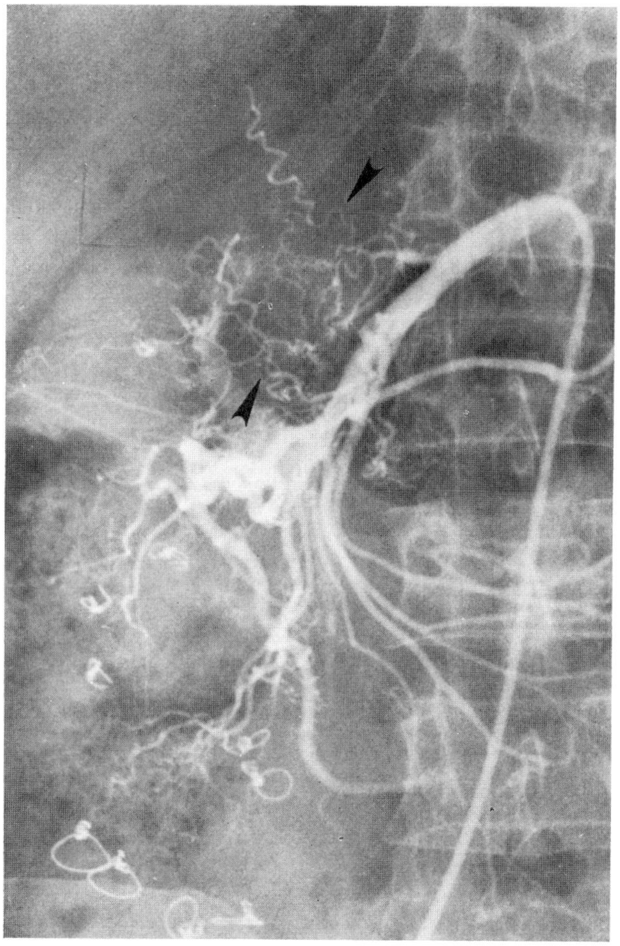

Figure 30.8. Superior Mesenteric Arteriogram. Numerous corkscrew vessels from the proximal superior mesenteric artery travel toward the porta hepatis. In a patient who had an inflammatory mass due to regional enteritis.

slow blood flow causing claudication, thrombosis, embolization and even rupture[1148, 1149] (Fig. 21-17).

Tortuosity Due to Loss of Volume of a Compact Organ

When a normal-sized solid organ loses volume either because of aging or fibrosis, its intrinsic vessels curl upon themselves and have a *corkscrew* appearance. This is due to the associated loss of supporting tissue elements. This is well exemplified in the *liver and the kidney.* Therefore, diseases which can cause loss of parenchymal volume may present angiographically with tortuosity of the intrinsic vasculature. At the same time a confusing second pattern may be superimposed upon the organ, depending on the stage of the particular disease.

The *renal arterial bed* per se is capable of only limited responses to a wide variety of disease states. As a result, the arterial bed alone cannot provide a basis for accurate differentiation of the many disease processes of the renal parenchyma.[1150] Distal small vessel tortuosity, sharp angulation and abrupt termination of arcuate arteries, a thin renal cortex, small defects due to tiny infarcts, beading and small aneurysms of the small vessels, slow flow, poor venous filling, and effacement of the corticomedullary injunction, in combination or alone, may be seen in many nonsurgical diseases of the kidney.[1151–1160] Thus, the above findings may be seen in arterial nephrosclerosis in association with arteriosclerosis elsewhere, arteriolar nephrosclerosis in association with essential hypertension, in malignant nephrosclerosis, and as a manifestation of old age, particularly in those patients over eighty years old. Pyelonephritis,[1161, 1164, 1165] radiation nephritis,[1162] scleroderma,[1163] and other diseases can also cause spiralling of the small vessels (Figs. 30-17 to 30-20).

Hepatic

Tortuous distorted vessels are not uncommon in the liver because of *loss of volume and fibrosis* related to cirrhosis, aging, and radiation hepatitis.[1166] In cirrhosis[111] diffuse fibrous scarring preceded by fatty changes and accompanied by regenerating nodules produces a spectrum of changes including corkscrew vessels, stretched vessels, and hypo- or hypervascularity. All the findings may be present at the same or at different times in the liver.[479, 1167–1169] It is interesting to note that childhood postnecrotic cirrhosis may not cause significant tortuosity of the vessels since the liver never has had a chance to grow to a normal size[1170] (Figs. 30-11 to 30-15).

Periarterial and Arterial Fibrosis

Periarterial and arterial fibrosis can be a cause of tortuosity or kinks in different vascular beds. The common examples are pancreatic lesions, including pancreatitis and pancreatic

(Text continues on page 632)

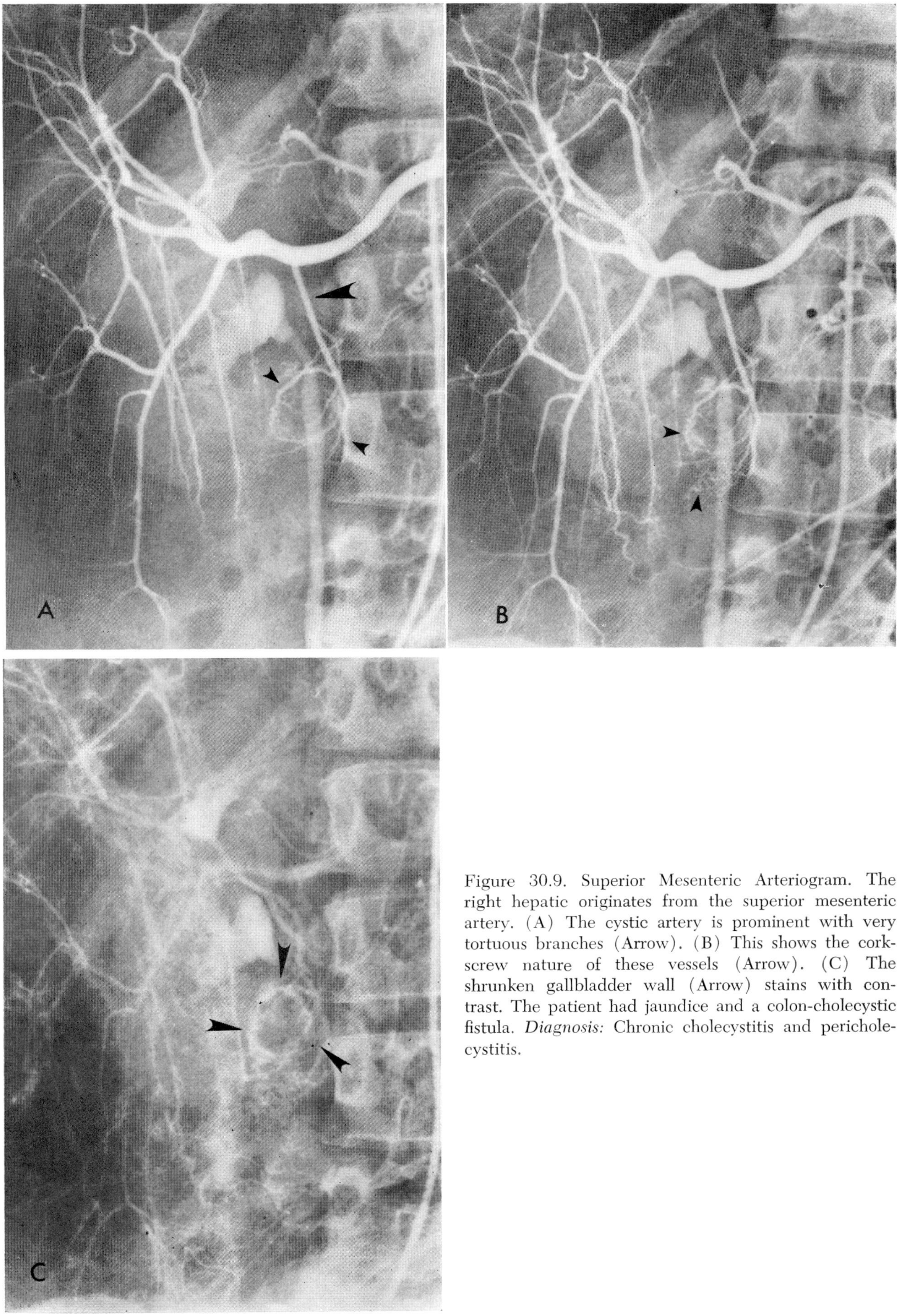

Figure 30.9. Superior Mesenteric Arteriogram. The right hepatic originates from the superior mesenteric artery. (A) The cystic artery is prominent with very tortuous branches (Arrow). (B) This shows the cork-screw nature of these vessels (Arrow). (C) The shrunken gallbladder wall (Arrow) stains with contrast. The patient had jaundice and a colon-cholecystic fistula. *Diagnosis:* Chronic cholecystitis and pericholecystitis.

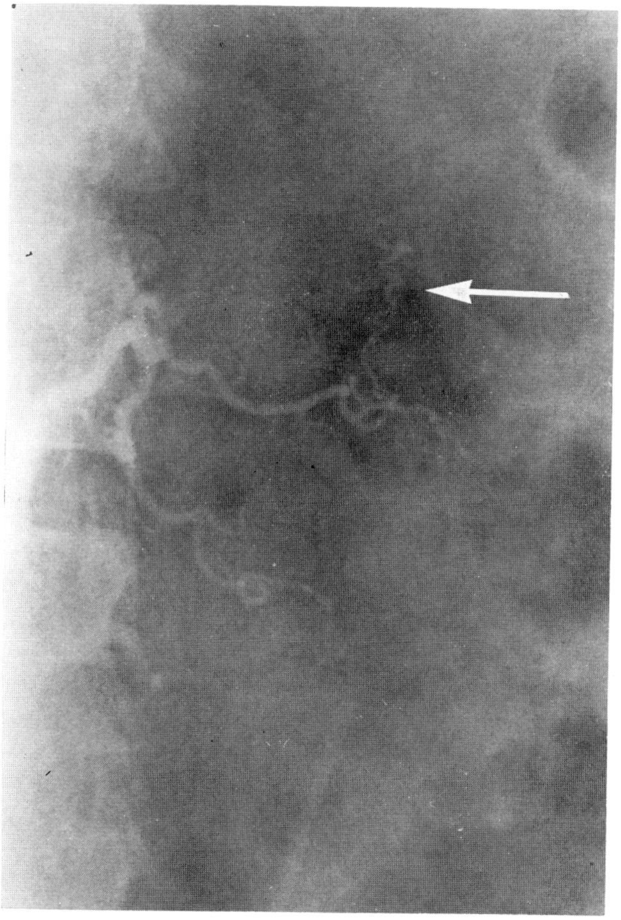

Figure 30.10. Lumbar Arteriogram. A prominent retroperitoneal branch is present with a markedly corkscrew course (Arrow). This patient had left flank pain and fever. *Diagnosis:* Abscess in the retroperitoneal area. Surgery confirmed the diagnosis.

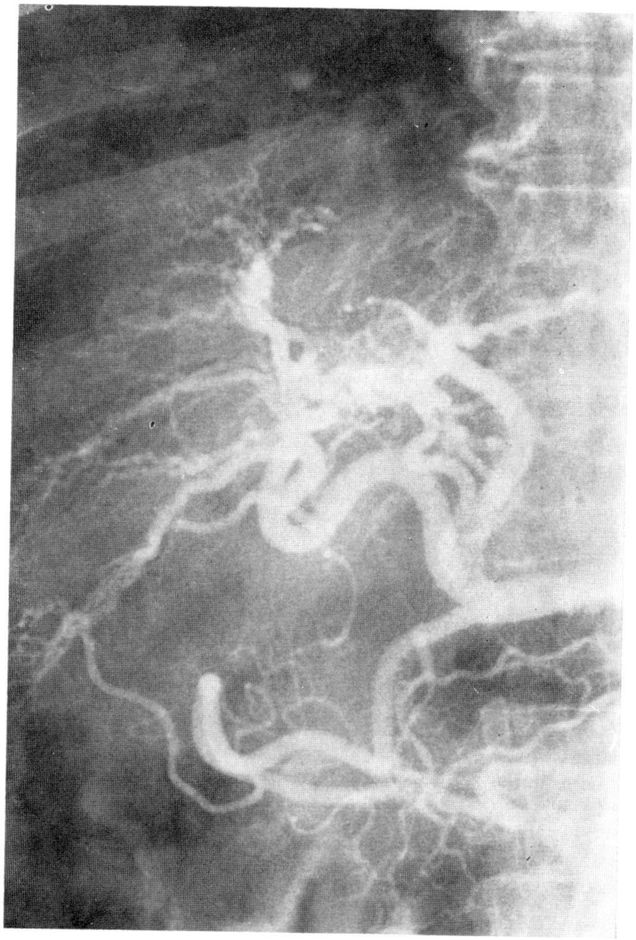

Figure 30.11. Hepatic Arteriogram. The main hepatic artery and its branches are dilated. The intrahepatic branches are crowded with a marked corkscrew configuration. The patient was a known alcoholic with portal hypertension. *Diagnosis:* Loss of volume of liver parenchyma due to fibrosis. There is compensatory increased blood flow from the hepatic artery. The diagnosis of cirrhosis was confirmed by biopsy.

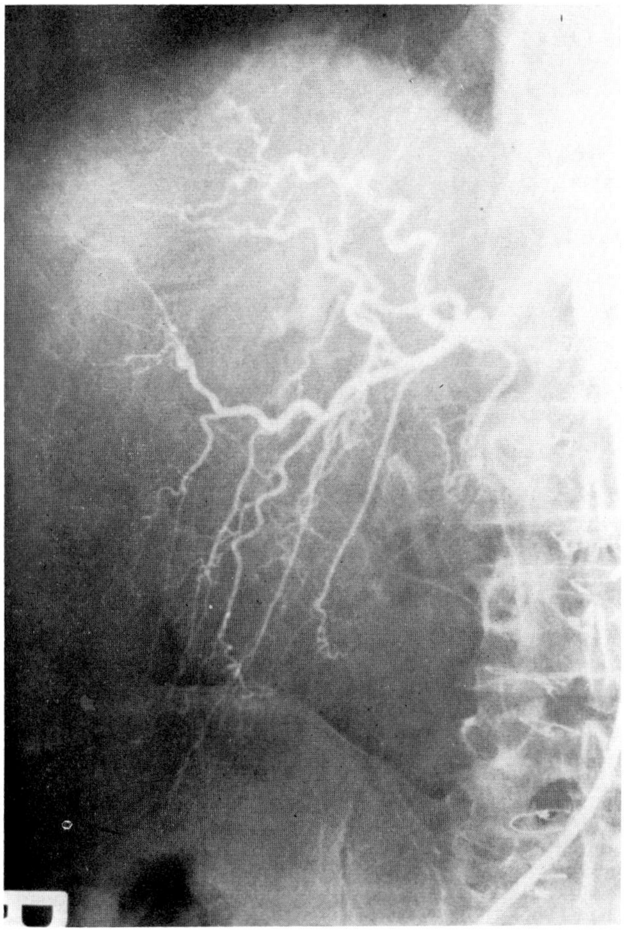

Figure 30.12. Hepatic arteriogram reveals corkscrew intrahepatic branches. This patient is a young alcoholic. *Diagnosis:* Loss of hepatic parenchyma due to fibrosis. Liver biopsy confirmed the diagnosis.

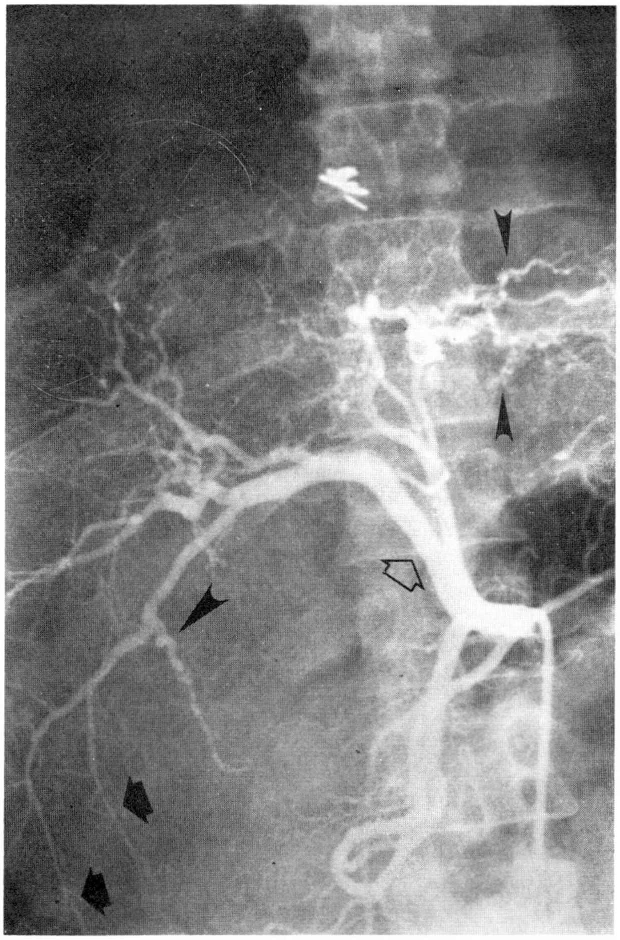

Figure 30.13. Hepatic Arteriogram. The main hepatic artery (Blank Arrow) is dilated and there are corkscrew intrahepatic branches (Arrow Head). The peripheral vessels are stretched. The patient was known to be an alcoholic with portal hypertension. *Diagnosis:* Loss of liver volume with fibrosis in the area of corkscrew vessels. There is regeneration of the liver in the areas of stretched vessels.

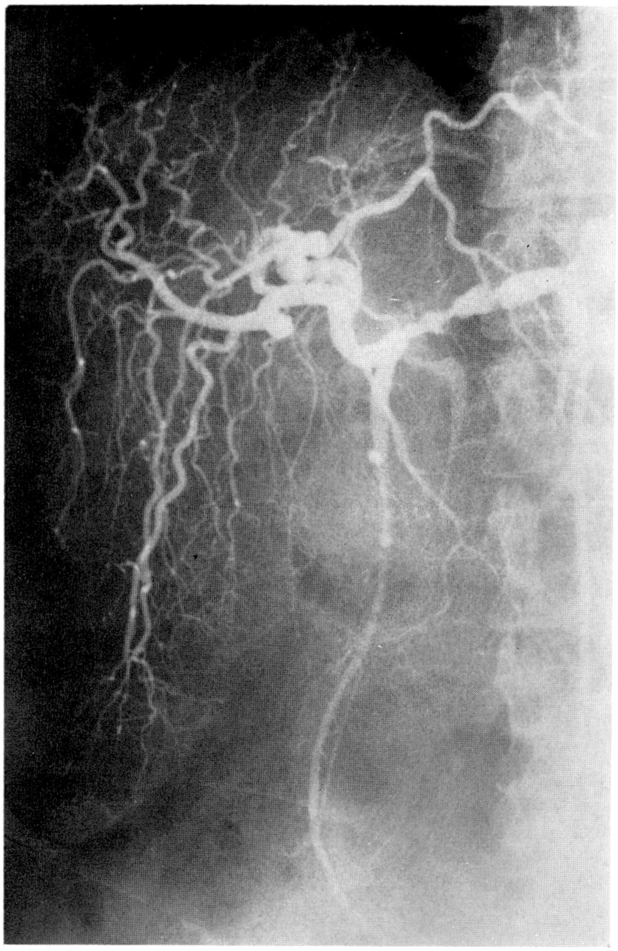

Figure 30.14. Celiac Arteriogram. Tortuous intrahepatic branches with a corkscrew appearance are seen in a patient who had known biliary cirrhosis. At the same time notice the alternating areas of dilatation and narrowing in the main hepatic artery (Arrows) due to catheter induced spasm.

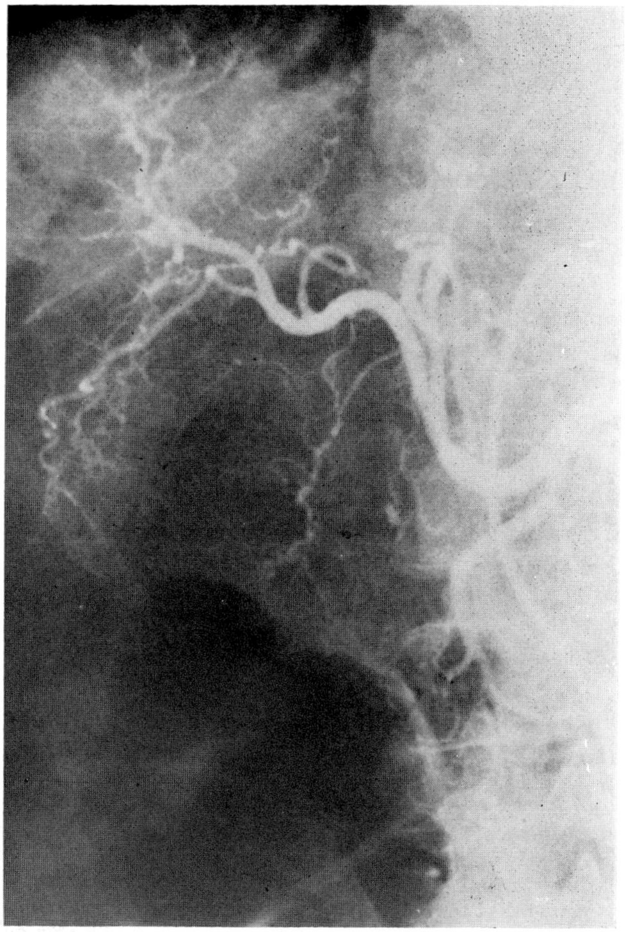

Figure 30.15. Celiac Arteriogram. Please note the corkscrew hepatic branches in a small liver. This patient was an eighty-five-year-old female (nonalcoholic). *Comment:* Fibrosis of the liver due to aging.

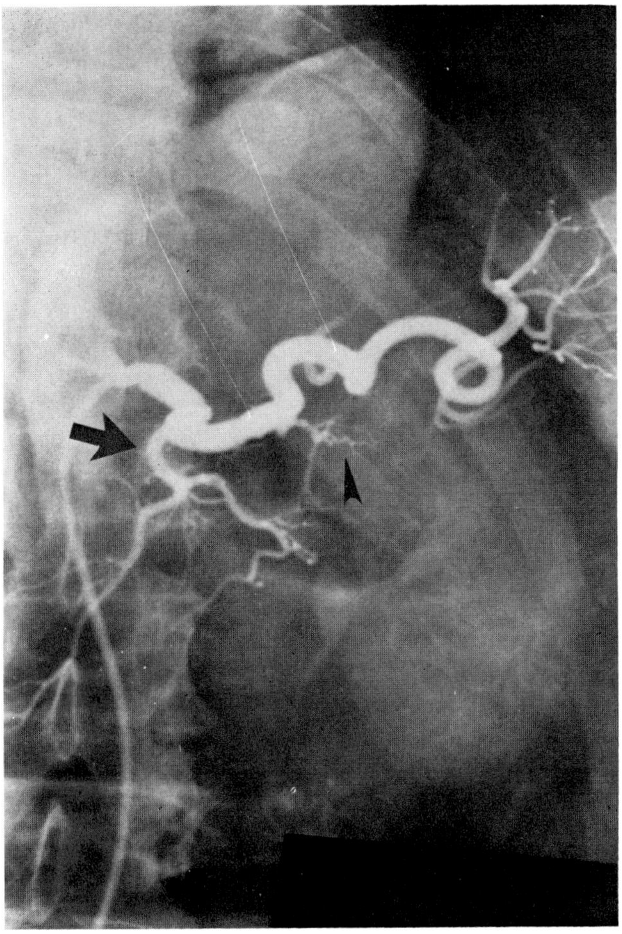

Figure 30.16. Splenic Arteriogram. Deviated, corkscrew branches arise from the splenic artery (Arrow Head). The patient was an alcoholic with repeated attacks of pancreatitis. *Diagnosis:* Chronic pancreatitis. *Note:* The dorsal pancreatic artery arising from the splenic is prominent (Arrow).

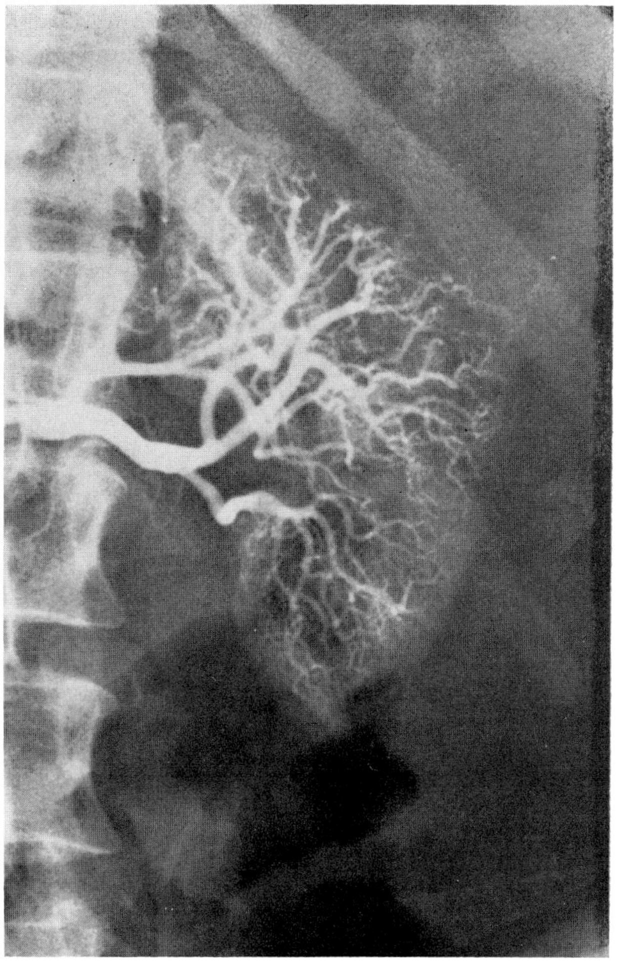

Figure 30.17. Renal Arteriogram. Diffuse crowding of the intrarenal arterial branches, marked tortuosity of the vasculature and thinning of the cortex is seen with a small kidney. This twenty-seven-year-old patient had malignant hypertension. *Comment:* Malignant nephrosclerosis.

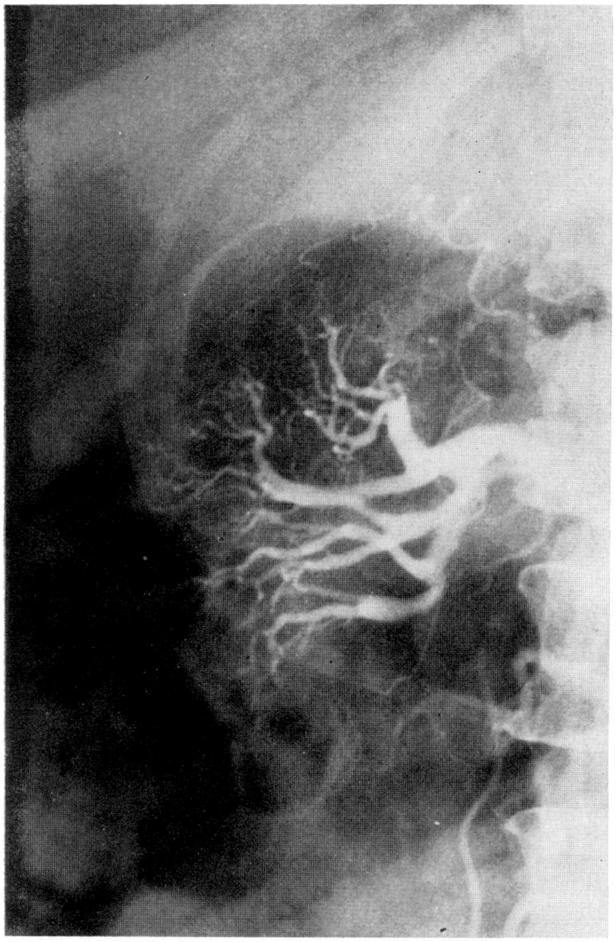

Figure 30.18. Renal Arteriogram. A renal arteriogram reveals dilatation and tortuosity of the hilar branches and intrarenal small vessels with a corkscrew appearance. Crowding of the intrarenal branches and slow circulation. This patient was forty years old with malignant hypertension. *Comment:* Malignant nephrosclerosis.

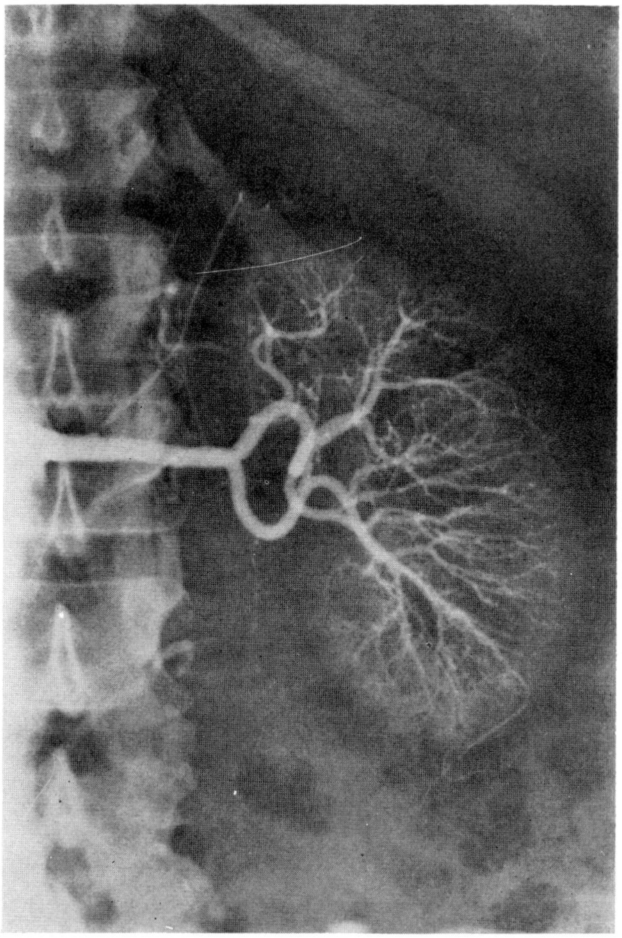

Figure 30.19. Renal Arteriogram. Slight tortuosity of intrarenal branches and crowding of the intrarenal branches is seen in a patient who has been moderately hypertensive for the last eight years. *Comment:* Nephrosclerosis.

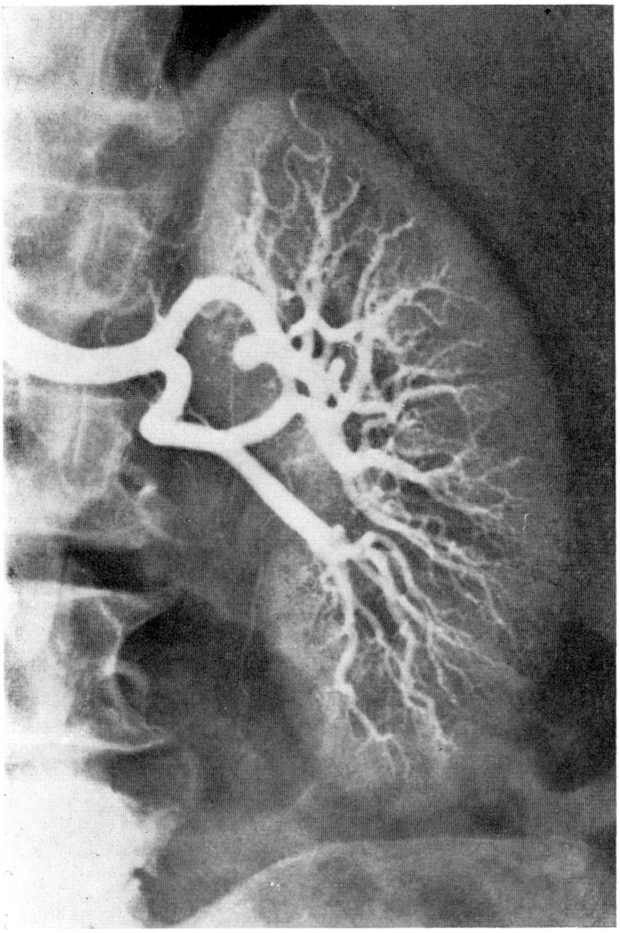

Figure 30.20. Renal Arteriogram. The arterial phase reveals tortuosity and minimal corkscrewing of the peripheral branches of the kidney in a nonhypertensive seventy-two-year-old individual. *Comment:* Aging phenomenon.

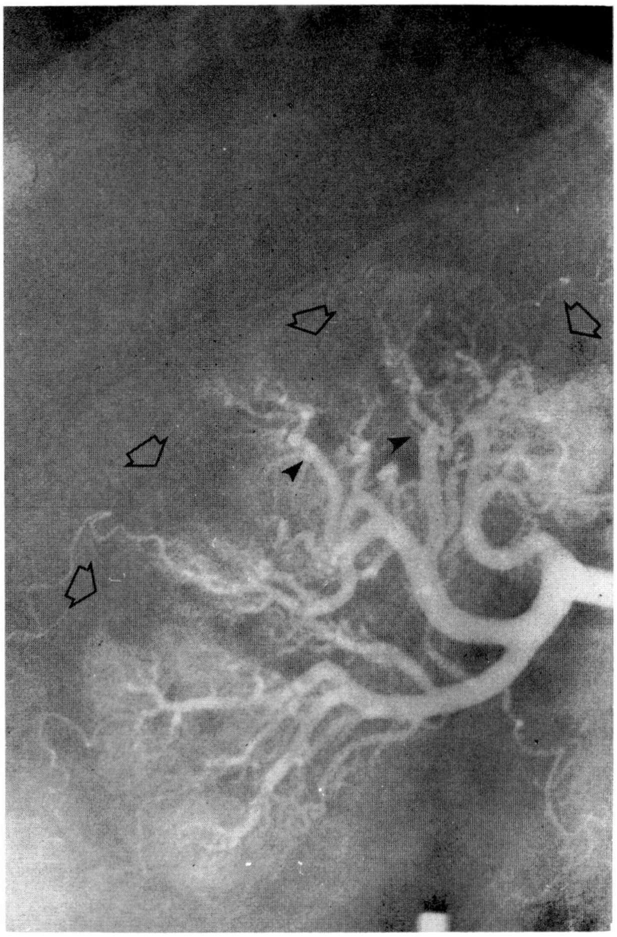

Figure 30.21. Renal Arteriogram—renal arterial phase: Corkscrew branches with slight dilatation of the intrarenal branches are seen (Arrow Head) with multiple filling defects (Arrow). A patient with chronic urinary tract infection. *Diagnosis:* Chronic pyelonephritis with scars.

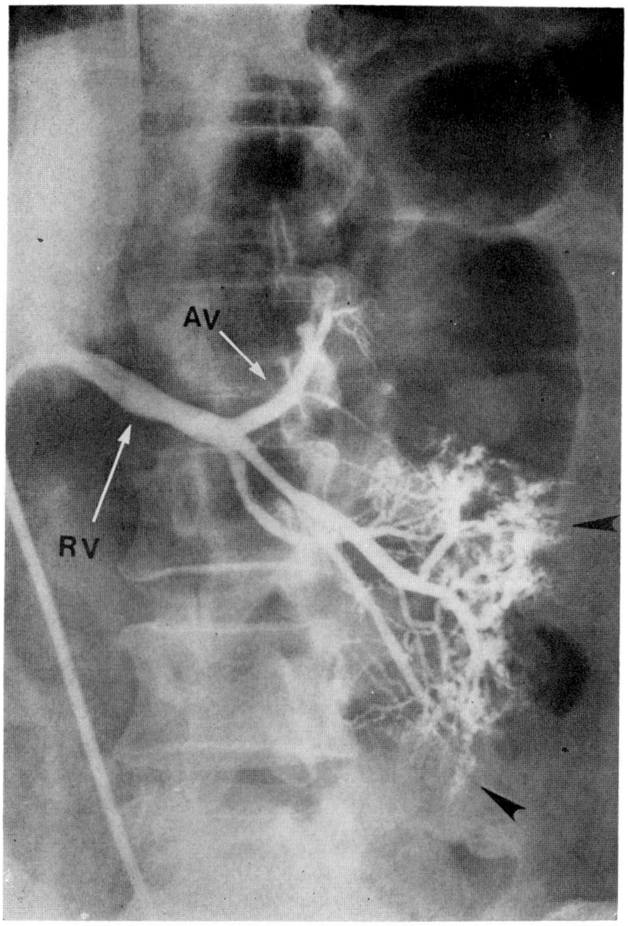

Figure 30.22. Left Renal Venogram. There is crowding of intrarenal branches with marked narrowing of the left main renal vein (R.V.), corkscrewing of the intrarenal small venous branches (Arrow) and prominent filling of the adrenal vein (A.V.). This patient had a nonvisualized kidney on the left side with absence of the left hemitrigone and the left ureteric orifice. *Comment:* Dysplastic kidney?

carcinoma, radiation,[1172, 1173] and carcinoid with mesenteric fibrosis.

KINKING

Kinking of an artery is another expression of localized elongation causing tortuosity due to loss of elastic tissue or traction by juxta-arterial fibrous tissue.

Kinking of the Innominate Artery

This entity would not be so popular if it were not for enthusiastic diagnoses of superior mediastinal mass lesions, most likely aneurysms, by new house staff members. This finding is seasonal, peaking in the beginning months of each academic year.

Kinking of the Aorta

In the thoracic aorta distal to the origin of the left subclavian artery, kinking occurs as the aorta swings forward and downward near the attachment of the ligamentum arteriosum, and then abruptly swings backwards and laterally.[1174] This may or may not be associated with cardiac or other valvular abnormalities.[1175–1177] Aortic kinking is also popular as it can be diagnosed on plain chest films under the label of *pseudocoarctation* (Fig. 30-5).

Kinking of the Internal Carotid Artery

These kinks are not uncommon and may often have decreased blood flow and blood pressure across the kinked area.[1178–1180] They appear to have a predisposition to thrombosis or even intrinsic occlusion at the site of the kink.

CHAPTER 31

FLOW

THE NORMAL VOLUME and/or velocity of flow may be increased, decreased, or even reversed within a vessel.

INCREASED FLOW

Reactive hyperemia is noticeable in extremities after exercise and helps provide good filling of the collateral vessels. It decreases the transit time of contrast and demonstrates the distal ends of occlusion in a better manner.[289, 290] Increase in hepatic arterial flow has been noted during acute alcoholic hepatitis[1142] or in advanced cirrhosis. Of interest is the decrease in the total hepatic blood flow in cirrhosis.[1171] There may be an obvious increase in regional

(Text continues on page 641)

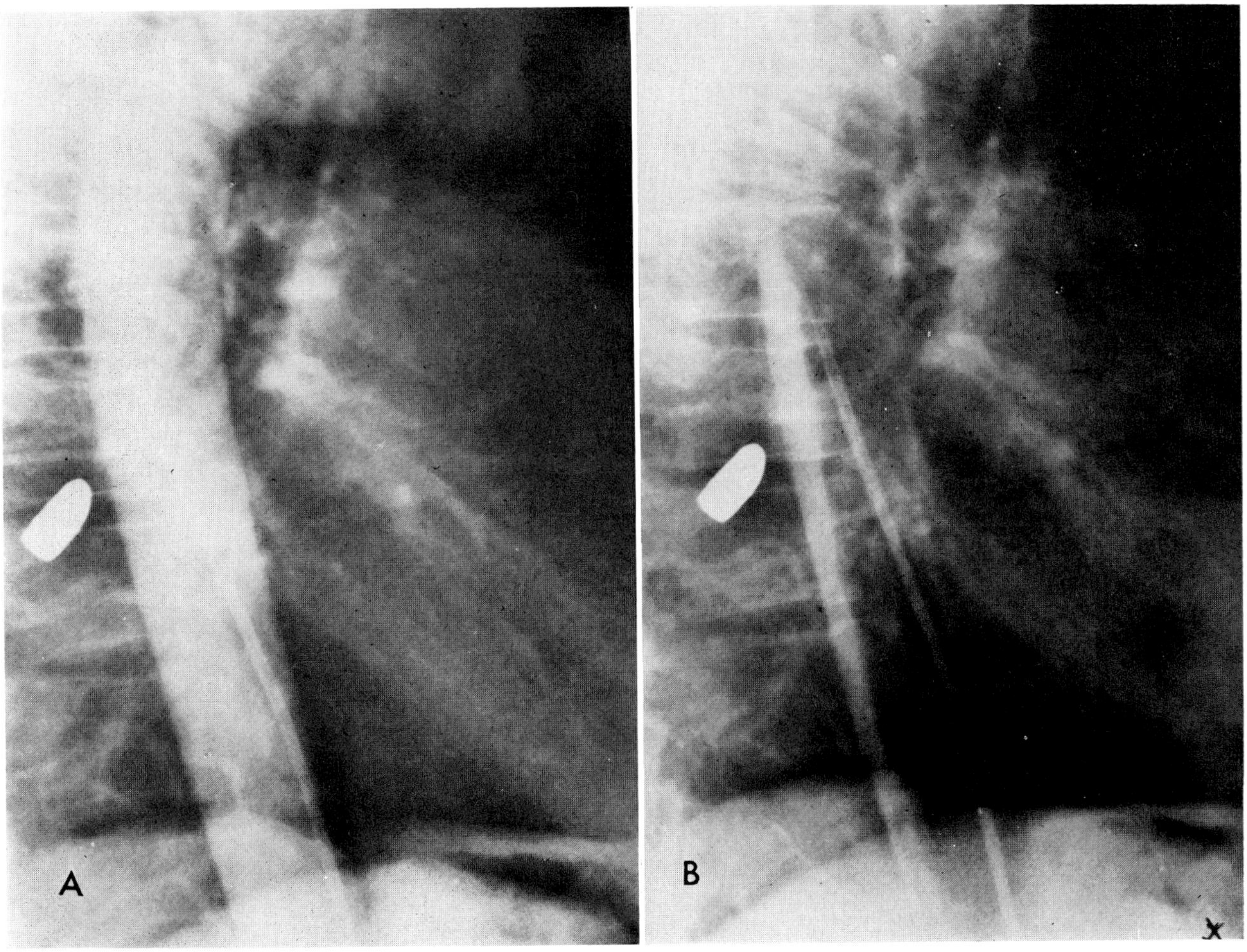

Figure 31.1. Thoracic Aortogram. (A) Early arterial phase (cross-table) lateral. (B) Late arterial phase (cross-table) lateral. The contrast collects in a linear manner along the posterior aortic wall. *Comment:* The relative heavy contrast material lingers along the dependent portion of a vessel.

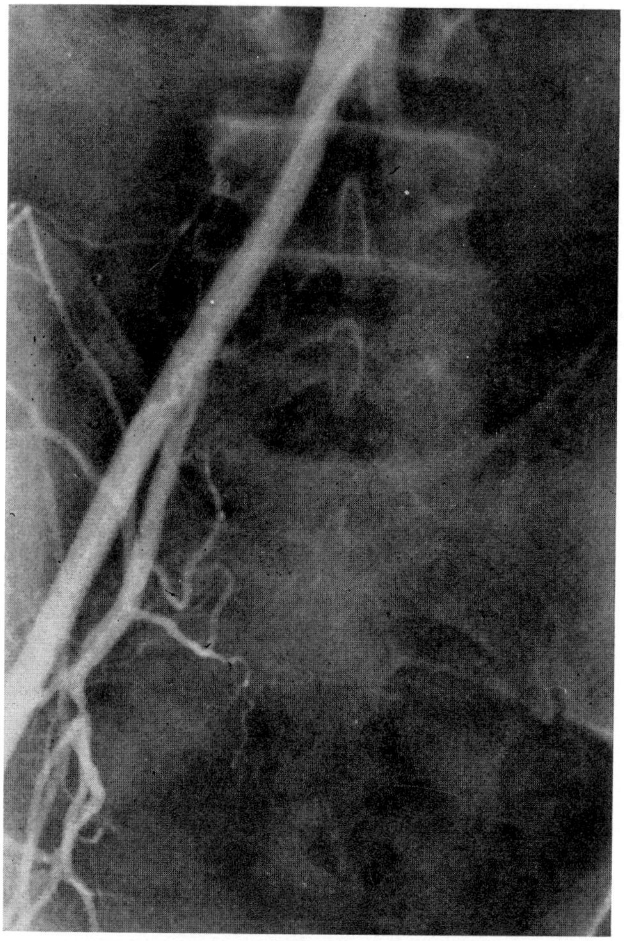

Figure 31.2. Pelvic Arteriogram. The catheter tip is just above the bifurcation of the aorta, filling the ipsilateral vessels and not filling the contralateral iliac vessel. *Comment:* Without enough room for turbulent mixing of contrast and blood, this streamline flow phenomena occurs.

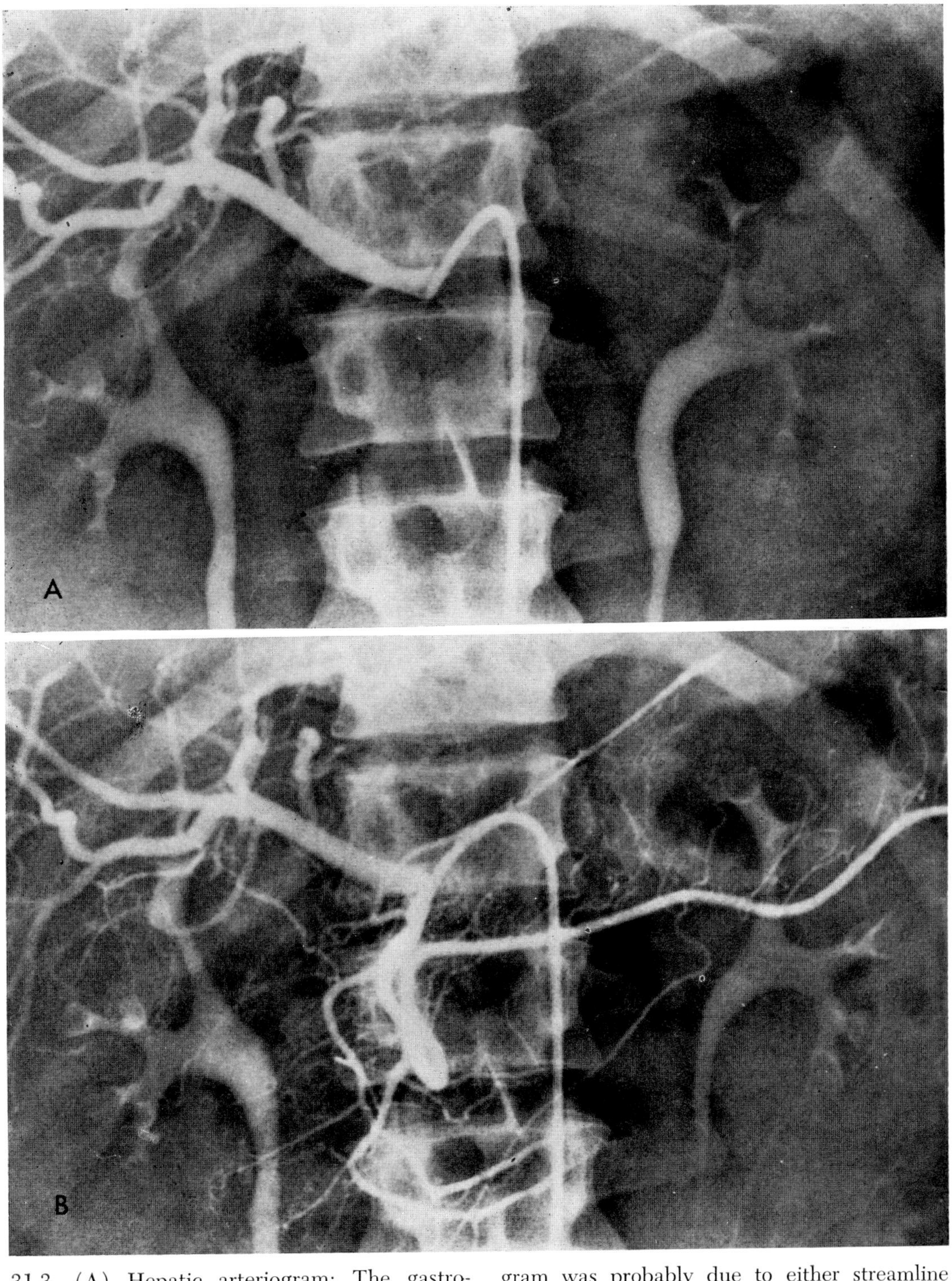

Figure 31.3. (A) Hepatic arteriogram: The gastroduodenal artery does not fill. (B) Selective gastroduodenal injection: There is excellent filling. *Comment:* In this case the lack of filling during the hepatic arteriogram was probably due to either streamline flow or perfusion of the gastroduodenal artery from superior mesenteric artery flow.

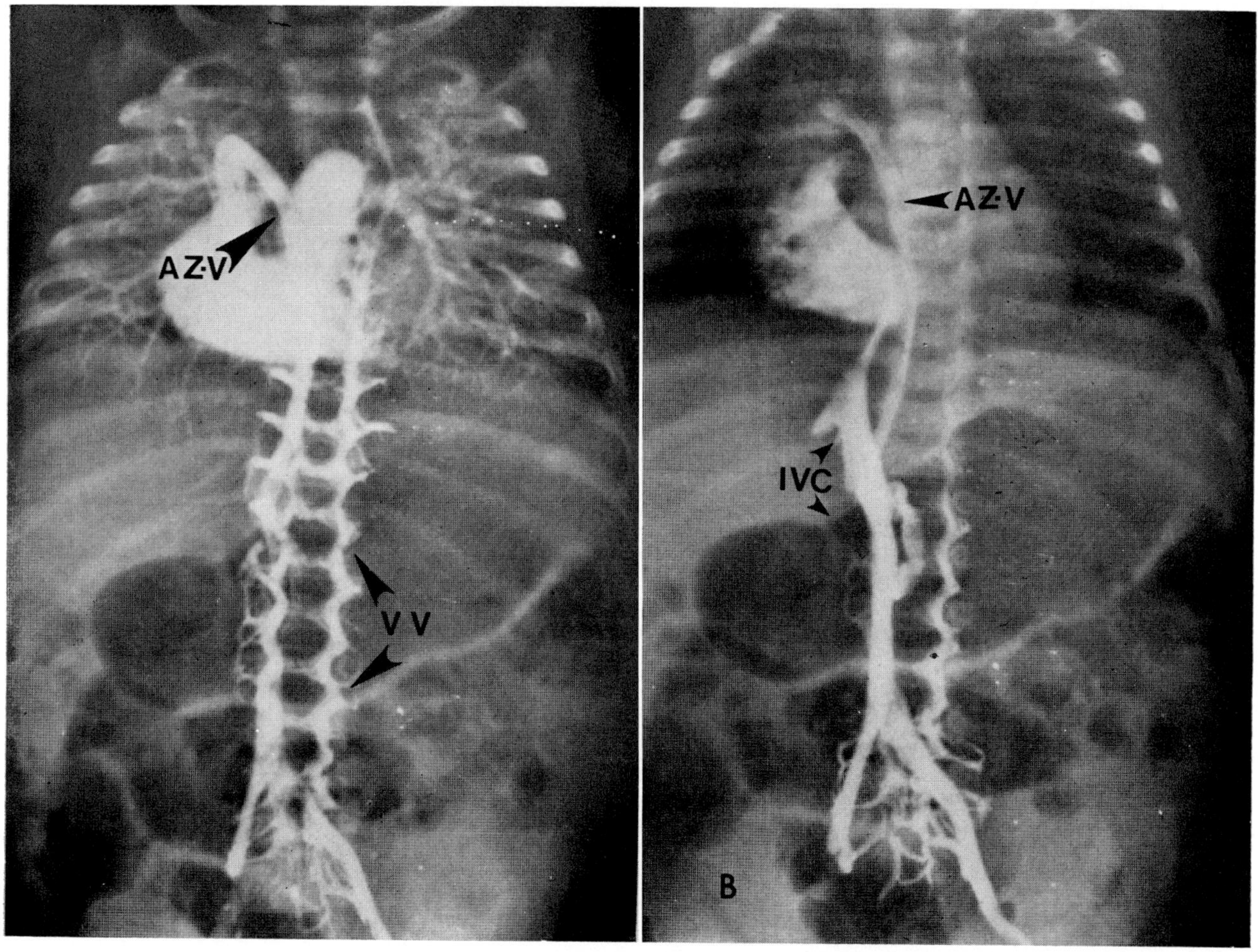

Figure 31.4. (A) Inferior vena cavagram: There is opacification of the vertebral venous system (V.V.) and the azygous venous system (AZ.V.). No opacification of the inferior vena cava occurs in a patient who was crying during the injection. (B) A repeat injection reveals good opacification of the inferior vena cava (I.V.C.). *Comment:* Diversion of the vena cava blood towards the vertebral venous plexus occurs during intentional or unintentional Valsalva maneuver.

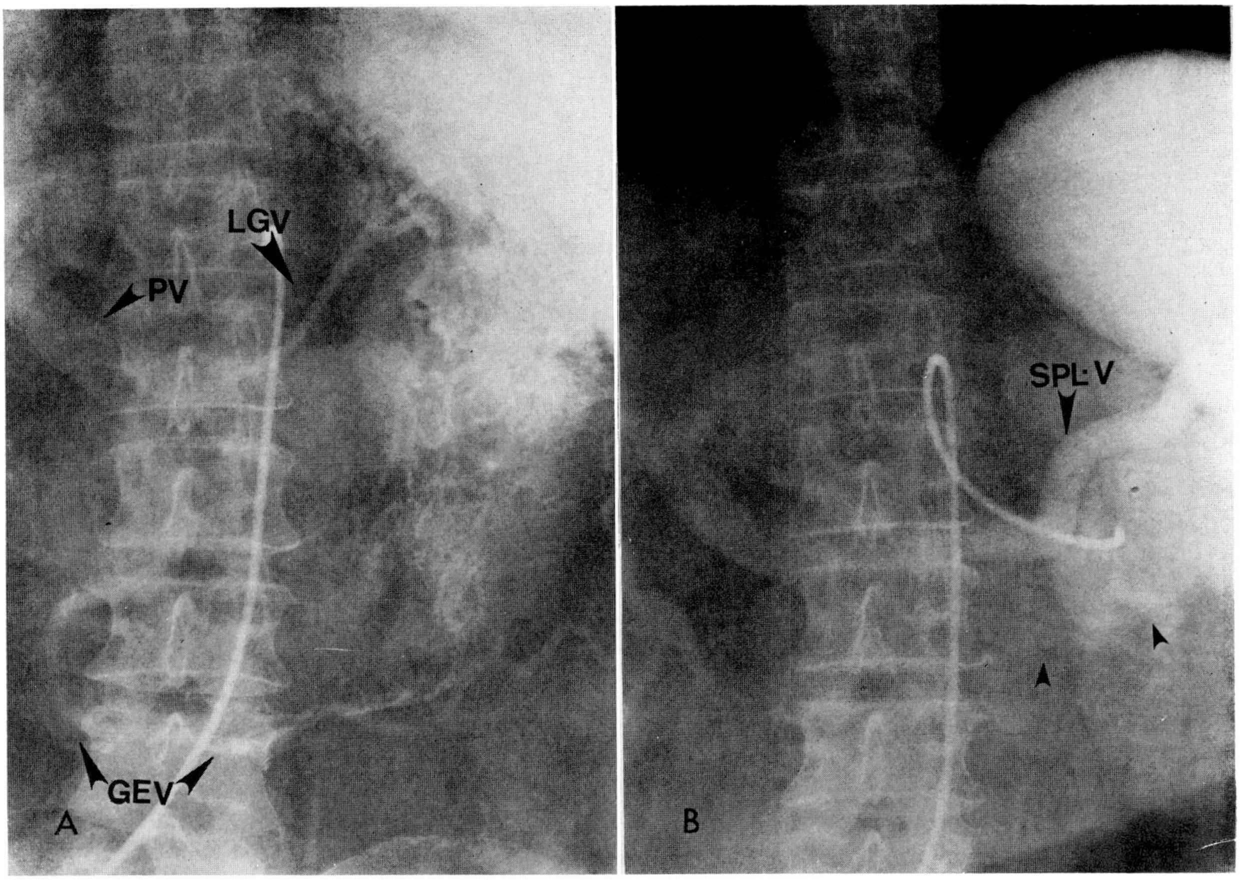

Figure 31.5. (A) Celiac angiogram—venous phase: Left gastric vein (L.G.V.), gastroepiploic vein (G.E.V.) and portal vein (P.V.). (B) Splenic arteriogram—venous phase: Splenic vein (Spl. V.). There is stain of the pancreas (Arrow). *Comment:* The normal splenoportal circulation is seen above. Filling of the left gastric vein during a celiac angiogram is normal, but filling of the left gastric vein during a splenic arteriogram may represent portal hypertension with reversal of flow in the left gastric vein.

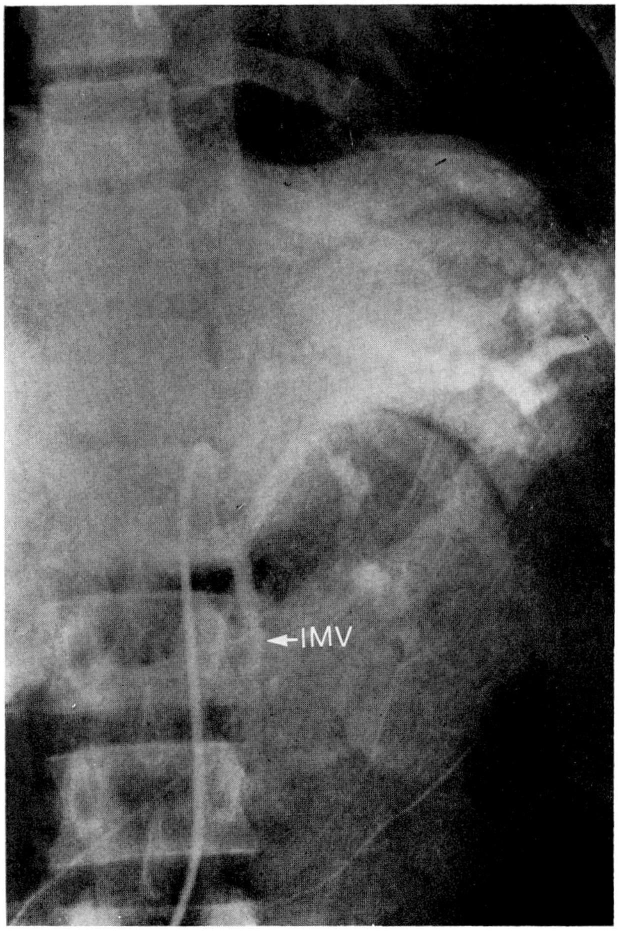

←

Figure 31.6. Celiac Arteriogram. The venous phase reveals good opacification of the splenic, portal and inferior mesenteric vein (I.M.V.). This twenty-year-old patient had no known diseases. *Comment:* Occasionally reflux into the inferior mesenteric vein may not be considered abnormal.

Figure 31.7. Lower Extremity Phlebogram. There is good filling of the deep veins and perfusion of the tortuous superficial vein via the perforating communicating vein. *Diagnosis:* Incompetency of the perforating veins with superficial varices.

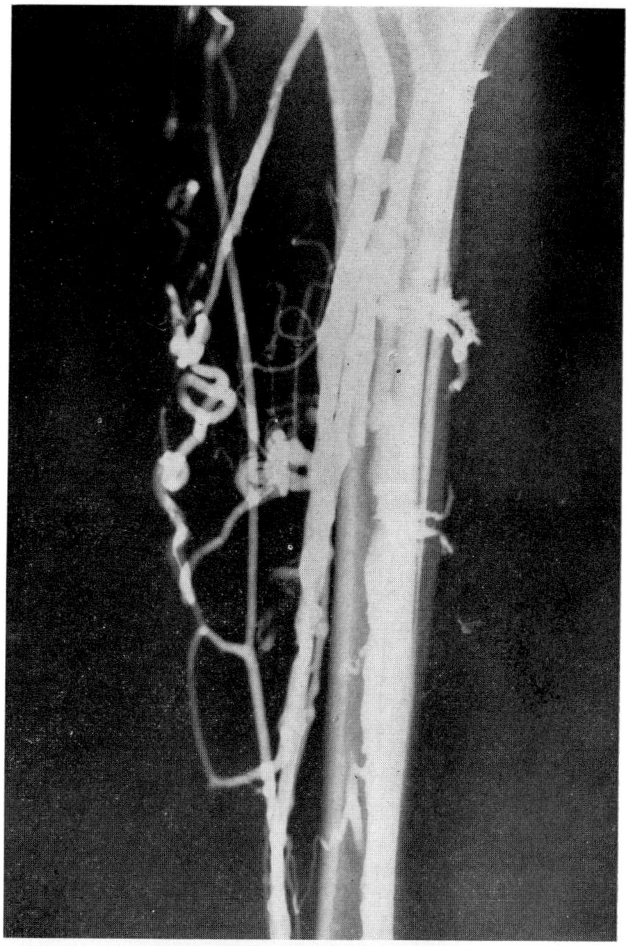

Figure 31.8. Hepatic arteriogram late phase demonstrates opacification of the portal vein (P.V.) and tortuous dilated veins (Arrow) in a patient who had alcoholic cirrhosis of the liver. *Diagnosis:* Reversal of flow in the portal vein due to severe degree of post sinusoidal obstruction caused by cirrhosis. *Comment:* Visualization of portal vein after a selective hepatic arteriogram is definitely abnormal. It indicates the presence of a severe degree of post sinusoidal obstruction, thereby converting the portal vein as an outflow tract. (Courtesy of Dr. Himmat T. Shah, Radiologist, Michael Reese Medical Center, Chicago, Illinois.)

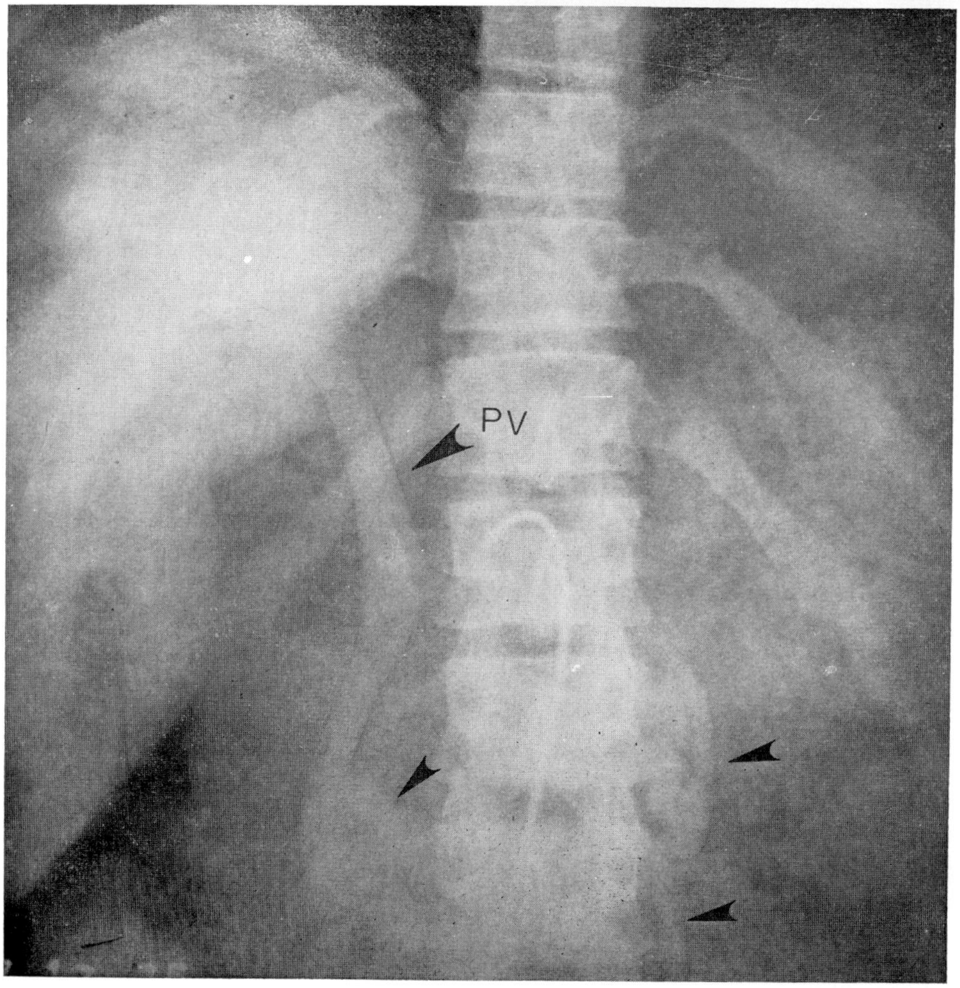

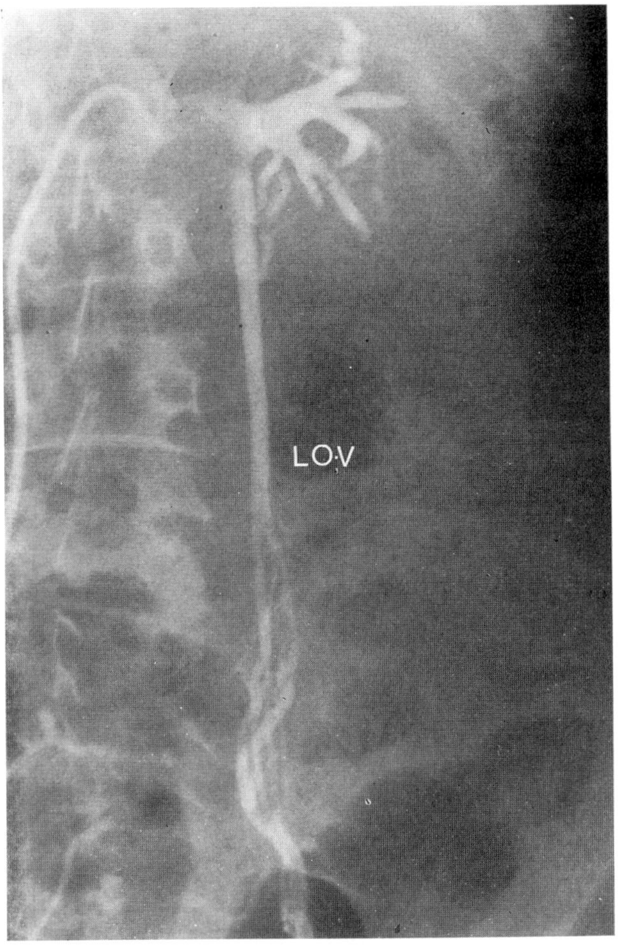

←

Figure 31.9. Left Renal Venogram. Very good opacification of the left ovarian vein all the way down to the pelvis is seen. *Comment:* Incompetent left ovarian vein (L.O.V.).

Figure 31.10. Wedge Hepatic Venogram. (A) There is a very good filling of the sinusoids without opacification of the portal vein branches. The pattern is consistent with normal or mildly restricted portal blood flow to the liver. (B) Retrograde flow is seen into the intrahepatic portal vein branches, but the flow in the portal vein is hepatopetal. This pattern indicates moderate increase in peripheral portal vascular resistance. (C) The contrast stagnates in the branches of the portal vein which is opacified in a retrograde manner. This pattern may be seen with advanced stages of liver cirrhosis and also in portal vein thrombosis. (D) Retrograde opacification of the portal vein occurs with a predominatingly hepatofugal flow in the portal vein. There is also opacification of its tributaries. These patients have spontaneous reversal of portal blood flow: Catheter (C.), hepatic vein (H.V.), coronary vein (C.V.), splenic vein (S.V.). (From Viamonte, M., Warren, W. D., Fomon, J. J., and Martinez, L. O. Angiographic investigations in portal hypertension. *Surg Gynecol Obstet, 130:*37, 1970. Courtesy of the authors and publishers.)

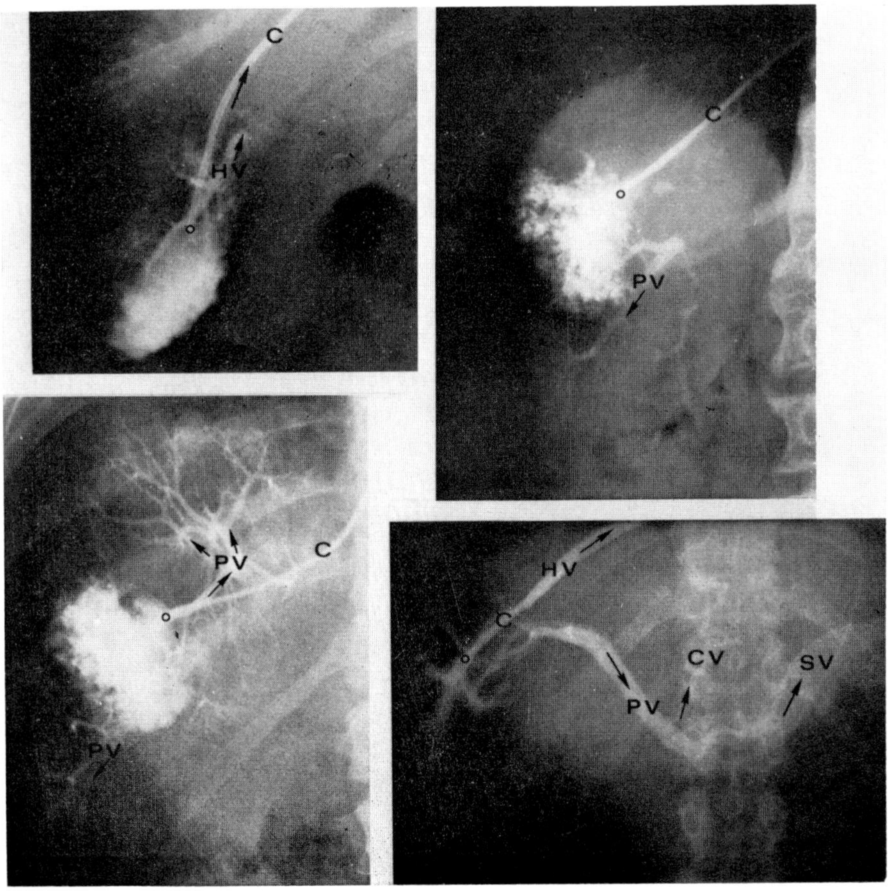

Figure 31.11. Wedge Hepatic Venogram. There is irregularity and narrowing of the hepatic venous branches (H.V.), sparseness of the venous arcade (Arrow) and visualization of the portal vein (P.V.) in a known alcoholic. *Diagnosis:* Alcoholic cirrhosis with minimal reversal of flow in the portal vein. *Comment:* Normally, wedge injections into the hepatic vein do not cause visualization of the portal vein unless excessive force or higher rate of injection of contrast material is used.

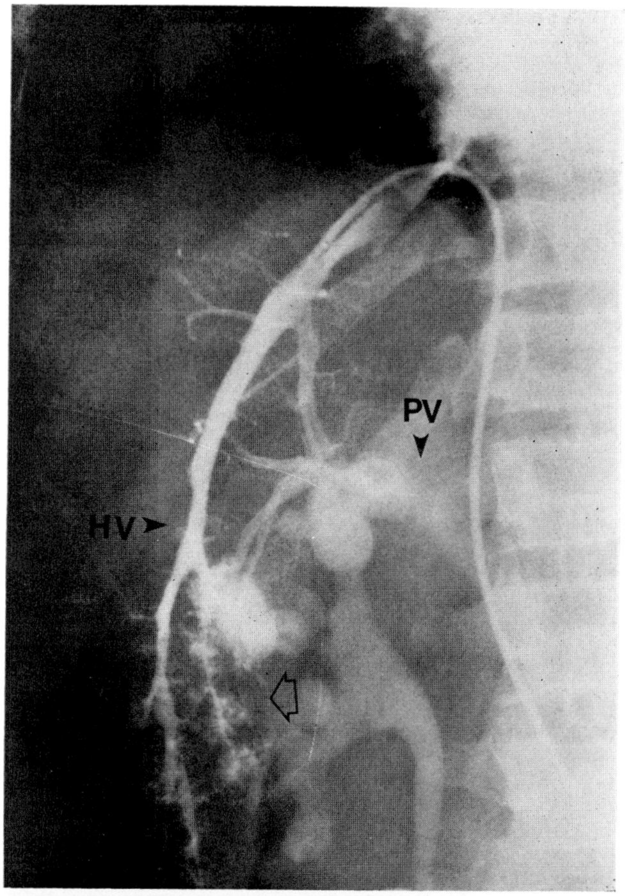

Figure 31.12. Venous Phase Celiac Angiogram. (A) After twenty-six seconds the splenic vein and a huge collateral "left gastric vein" (Arrow) are seen. There is no visualization of the portal vein. (B) The venous phase of a superior mesenteric angiogram reveals good filling of the portal vein (Arrow) in an individual with moderate portal hypertension. *Comment:* Nonfilling of the patent portal vein during celiac angiogram was probably due to draining of the contrast via left gastric vein. This case illustrates the advantage of doing both celiac and superior mesenteric angiograms for demonstration of the portal vein.

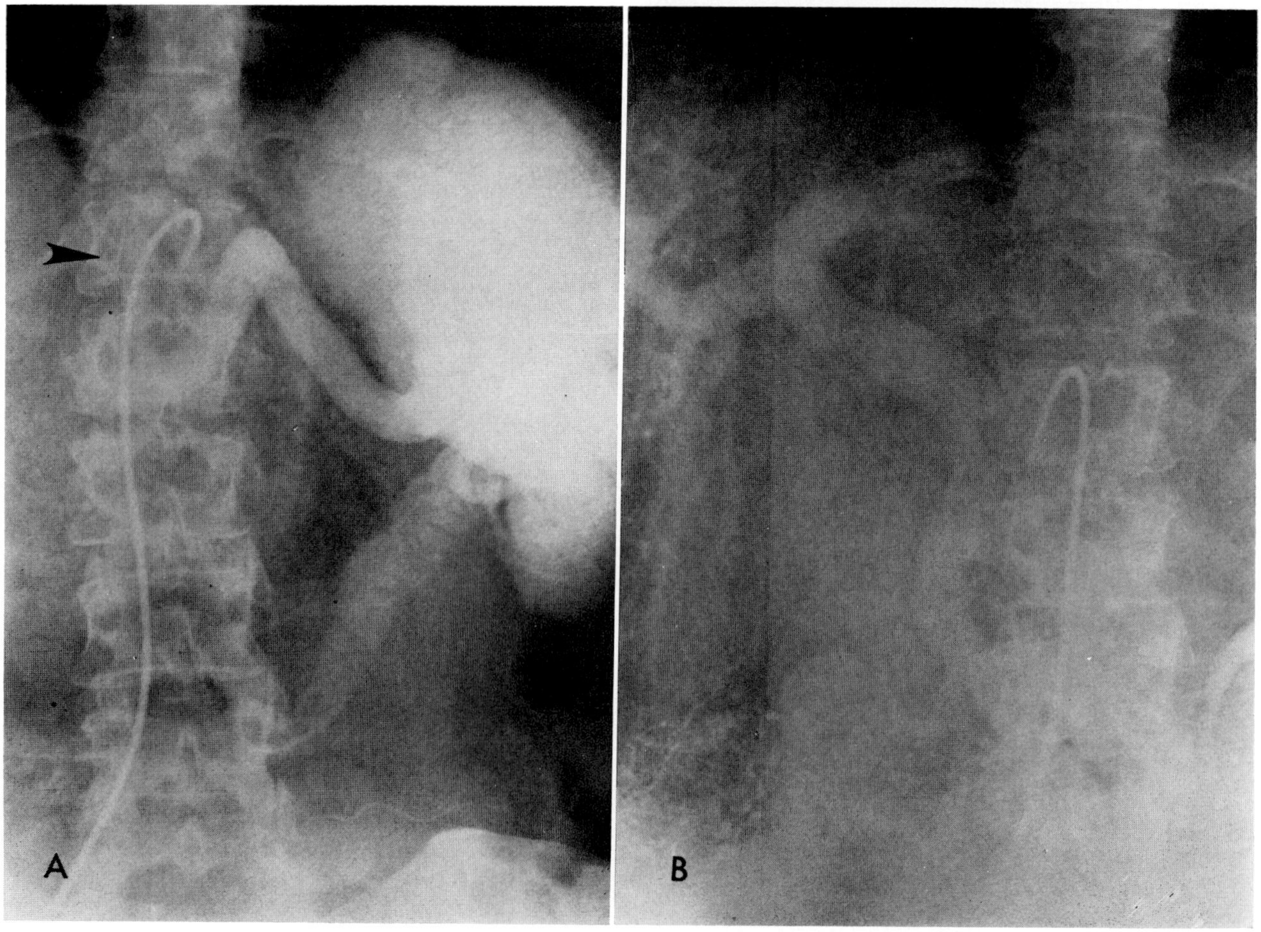

flow when there is excessive metabolic demand or decreased resistance as seen with tumors or arteriovenous fistula respectively. Increase in renal blood flow has been described with essential hypertension[1144] in some individuals.

DECREASED FLOW

Severe decrease in blood flow to the mesenteric, femoral and carotid circulations is a well-known clinical observation during *hemorrhagic shock.*[1143] A decrease, or even cessation, of blood flow to the outer two thirds of the renal cortex because of functional intrarenal redistribution of blood has also been described.[265, 1133, 1145] The decreased flow in the severe renal disease may drop to a rate of only 1 to 2 cc per second. Decreased flow is also noted in hepatic failure related to chronic liver disease.[1142]

Slow flow has been noted in collateral vessels. It has also been frequently observed in elderly individuals with or without congestive heart failure. Slow flow reaches its extreme as creeping circulation in dilated tortuous arteries, named *arteria dolicho et magna.* Extrinsic compression on the vessels in closed compartments may cause extremely slow flow in patent vessels. Thus, flow through the anterior tibial artery is diminished when there is a space-occupying lesion in this compartment.[294] Flow may be diminished when there is increased resistance in an organ; an example is that of a hydronephrotic kidney. Oscillating flow in the aorta in patients with aortic insufficiency is an interesting observation during angiography.

FLOW REVERSAL

This is most commonly seen in venous flow and is usually the result of distal obstruction to the normal antegrade flow of blood. Reversal of flow in the inferior vena cava may occur due to tricuspid insufficiency.[354] Reversal of flow in the gonadal veins[1147] or extremity veins may be due to incompetent valves.

In high grade obstructions at the hepatic sinusoidal level, as seen in cirrhosis there may be *reversal of flow within the portal vein*[1182] (Figs. 31-10 to 31-12). The veins draining an arteriovenous fistula may show reversal of flow due to communications with a high pressure system. Reversal of flow is also seen in the pulmonary artery when it is perfused from collaterals arising from the bronchial artery.[1181] Transient reversal of flow during injection of contrast into the aorta with a dissecting hematoma, or in an individual with aortic insufficiency[522] may occur. Besides the reversal of flow in the *vertebral artery* with occlusions of the subclavian artery (*subclavian steal syndrome),* reversal in that vertebral artery can occur even without occlusion of the subclavian or innominate arteries.[270, 457] A marked change in the direction of flow in the vertebral venous system due to change in body position is a very interesting observation.[403]

CHAPTER 32
HYPERTENSION

PORTAL HYPERTENSION

Most types of portal hypertension[302, 364] result from increased resistance to flow in the portal vein, sinusoids, hepatic veins, or inferior vena cava. In all, except a few varieties such as arteriovenous fistula, telangiectasia, or idiopathic, there is always an anatomic lesion either macroscopically or histologically. The levels of obstruction may either be pre- or postsinusoidal and either due to intra- or extrahepatic abnormalities (Fig. 32-1).

Portal Hypertension Due to Cirrhosis

The overall hemodynamic[1189] effect of cirrhosis is a postsinusoidal outflow obstruction causing an increase in the hepatic sinusoidal pressure. As the severity of the obstruction increases, the sinusoidal pressure exceeds that of the portal venous pressure and spontaneously converts the portal vein into an outflow tract. The mean hepatic blood flow in cirrhotic livers is diminished and there is a decrease in the total hepatic vascular bed.[1171] Diffuse fibrous scarring is almost invariably preceeded by fatty change. With progression of the disease, there is decrease in the fatty change and increase in the fibrous tissue reaction. Regeneration may occur at this time.

Angiographically, stretched or tortuous, distorted, abruptly angulated arteries, tiny portal venules, and distorted curled hepatic veins all tell the tale of a crumbling liver due to the repeated insults of fatty infiltration, connective tissue proliferation, and nodular regeneration. The greater the size of the regenerating nodules, the greater is the distortion of the vascular architecture of the liver.[479, 1167–1169, 1187] In the cirrhotic liver, anastomosis between the portal venules and hepatic arterial branches, or the portal and hepatic veins is not unusual.[1192] *Correlation of the angiographic appearance* of the hepatic vasculature with the stage of cirrhosis may be difficult to determine, as multiple processes may be occurring in the same liver at different areas at the same time.

Collateral Vessels

The presence of collateral veins[297, 302, 1188, 1190] implies portal hypertension (Figs. 25-37 and 25-45). However, portal hypertension may be present without collaterals, especially if the duration is of short interval. Portal venous stasis occurs not just with portal hypertension, but only after the formation of collaterals. As the extrahepatic collaterals become larger due to increase in the outflow obstruction, the flow through the collaterals increases and the inflow to the liver decreases. The blood diverted via collaterals may amount to as much as 87 percent of the total flow to the liver. This may not diminish the portal hypertension except in unusual situations where there is extensive formation of collateral vessels. As the venous flow to the liver decreases, the arterial flow increases in an attempt to compensate for the loss of blood, and at the same time to feed the regenerating nodules.[1191]

Portal and Systemic Venous Shunts

Patients with predominately *hepatofugal* circulation with slight or absent liver blush during the venous phase, large varices, and dilated hepatic arterial vessels probably constitute the *ideal candidates* for portocaval shunts. In such situations the surgically created anastomosis cannot further reduce the already decreased portal venous input to the liver. Individuals with predominately *hepatopetal* venous flow with intense staining of the hepatic parenchyma during the portal venous phase, may *not,*

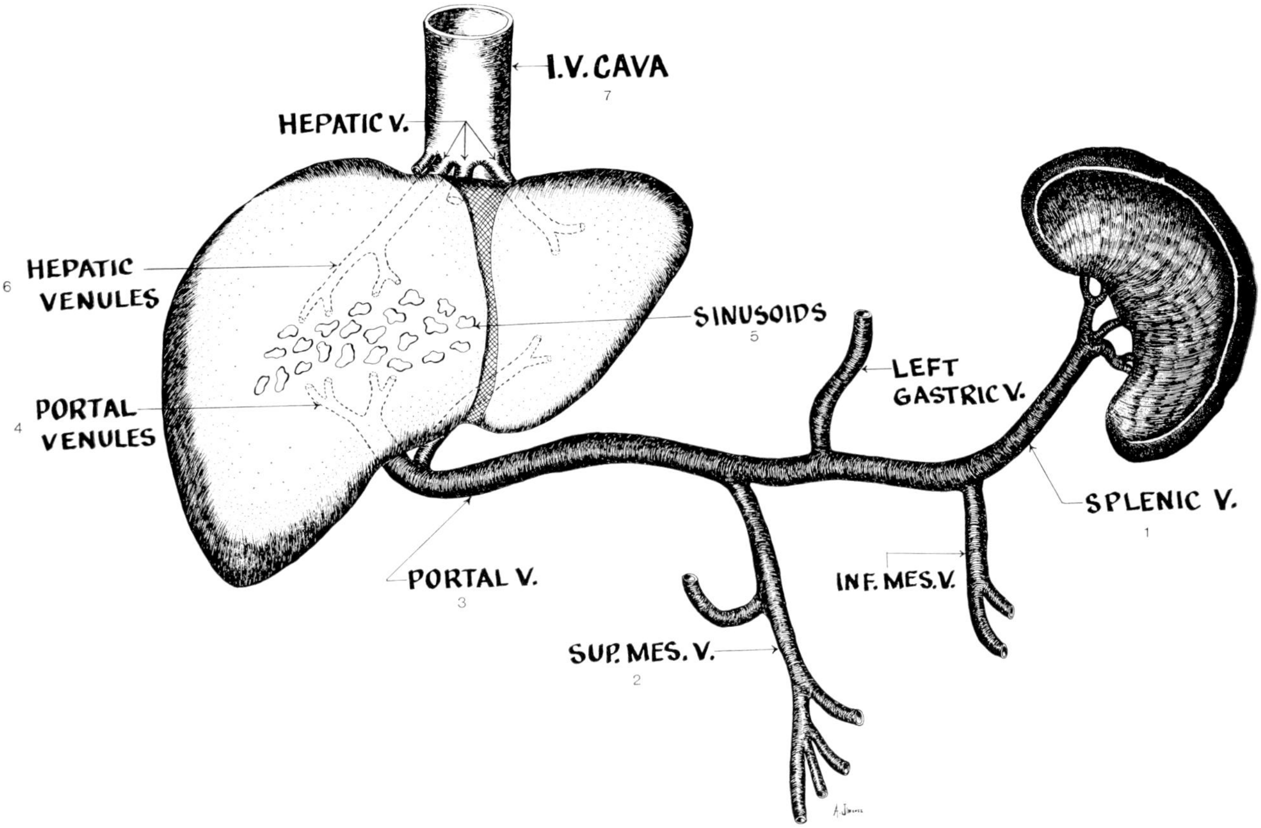

OBSTRUCTION OF PORTAL VENOUS SYSTEM

Figure 32.1. *Presinusoidal extrahepatic.* Occlusion of the splenic vein and superior mesenteric vein portal vein.

1. *Splenic vein:* (a) pancreatic lesions (pancreatitis, pseudocyst, benign and malignant tumors), (b) retroperitoneal masses, (c) gastric malignancies, (d) extension of the portal vein thrombus, (e) increased viscosity of the blood.

2. *Superior mesenteric vein:* (a) pancreatic lesions, (b) sepsis (colitis, pyelophlebitis), (c) increased viscosity.

3. *Portal vein main trunk:* (a) pancreatic lesions, (b) extension of thrombus from splenic vein or superior mesenteric vein, (c) stasis due to cirrhosis, (d) sepsis.

Presinusoidal Intrahepatic: Portal Vein Branches: Masses of varying etiologies.

4. *Portal venules:* (a) congenital hepatic fibrosis, (b) nutritional cirrhosis, (c) idiopathic sclerosis, (d) schistosomiasis, (e) metastatic tumor emboli, (f) infiltrative disorders (lymphoma, leukemia, granulomas, Gauchers, myeloproliferative disorders), (g) increased viscosity of the blood.[1184, 1185, 1186]

5. *Sinusoidal (Intrahepatic):* (a) acute fatty infiltration, (b) metastatic tumor emboli, (c) infiltrative disorders.

6. *Postsinusoidal intrahepatic:* (a) all types of cirrhosis, (b) fatty infiltration, (c) veno occlusive disease of hepatic venules, (d) infiltrative disorders, (e) metastatic tumor emboli, (f) masses (tumor, hematoma, abscess), (g) obstruction of the hepatic veins ostia.

7. *Postsinusoidal extrahepatic obstruction of the inferior vena cava:* (a) thrombosis, (b) tumors of inferior vena cava, (c) tumor thrombus (renal, adrenal, hepatic), (d) other masses in the vicinity, (e) constriction, diaphragms, membranes in the inferior vena cava, (f) congestive heart failure, (g) constrictive pericarditis.

Nonobstructive Causes: Arteriovenous fistulae in the splanchnic circulation.

however, prove *ideal candidates* for the surgical creation of a portocaval shunt. In reality this may actually cause further hepatic ischemia and hepatocellular damage due to increased diversion of blood away from the liver.[297–299]

End to side *portocaval shunts*[589] divert all of the portal venous blood away from the liver and do not allow hepatic arterial blood to escape from the liver without passing through the hepatic veins. This produces a great fall in portal venous pressure.[302] Side to side portal and systemic shunts (portocaval, mesocaval or splenorenal) may divert arterial blood from the liver, but are effective in relieving ascites. After an effective end to side anastomosis, the diameter of the hepatic artery branches increases. The increase in collateral supply from the superior mesenteric artery to the hepatic arterial circulation is also increased. The size of the liver and spleen diminish.[301, 1183]

RENOVASCULAR HYPERTENSION

Renovascular disease[1193, 1194] as a cause of hypertension may be seen in the following clinical situations: (1) recent onset of hypertension, (2) recent increase in the severity of existing hypertension, (3) onset of hypertension under twenty years of age or over fifty years of age, (4) no family history of hypertension, (5) recent flank pain or trauma followed by hypertension, (6) bruits in the epigastrium or flank, (7) disparity in renal size, (8) malignant hypertension arising without a preliminary period of essential hypertension, (9) hypertension in any age with rapid development of malignant hypertension, (10) vascular insufficiency of the extremities and an associated abdominal aortic aneurysm, (11) papilledema, or (12) hemorrhage or exudates in the fundi of the eye.

Causes[1211]

The lesion which is unable to damage the renal vasculature, parenchyma, or perinephric space is also probably unable to induce renovascular hypertension. Renal arterial causes[1195, 1196] include atherosclerotic narrowing usually in the proximal segment, fibromuscular diseases[633] which usually spares the proximal segment, aneurysms of the renal arteries,[1198] renal arteriovenous fistulae[1197] causing incomplete infarction, vasculitis,[1202] neurofibromatosis of the renal arteries,[1342] lateral extrinsic pressure from the diaphragmatic crura,[1085] arterial malformation,[1199] angiomas,[1200] dissecting hematomas of the aorta, masses compressing the renal artery such as hypernephroma[1201] and pheochromocytoma,[1315] recurrence after surgical correction[1208–1210] due to occlusion and narrowing of the graft or infarcts of the kidney due to thrombi at the anastomotic site, and intrarenal arteriolopathy.[277] *Venous causes* of renovascular hypertension relate to constriction of the renal vein.[278] *Parenchymal causes* include infarcts,[1052] atrophy, pyelonephritis,[1203] hypoplasia, renin secreting tumors,[32] and postradiation nephritis.[1205] Abnormalities of the draining apparatus producing hydronephrosis[1204, 1492] are also implicated in renovascular hypertension. *Subcapsular and perinephric processes* causing hypertension include subcapsular hematomas,[1206] perinephric hematomas,[580] pancreatic pseudocysts, and posttraumatic fibrous bands around the kidney.[1207] Extrarenal abnormalities causing hypertension include abdominal aortic coarctation,[808] superior mesenteric artery insufficiency,[280] and carcinoid tumors with associated previous renal disease.[1393]

Assessing a Renal Lesion

Not all lesions suggesting renovascular hypertension are curable. The *hemodynamic significance of the narrowing* as of now may be evaluated[1212] by noting the impairment of blood flow to the functional renal tissue, decreased pulsation of the renal tissue by stenosis or scarring, or demonstration of a pressure gradient or collateral circulation to the renal artery. Revascularization procedures[29, 30] may be indicated for an individual with collaterals and a renin ratio of 1:4 or greater, an individual without collaterals but with a renin ratio of 1:4 or greater, and finally an individual under fifty years of age with collaterals regardless of the renin ratio. The appearance of collaterals in young people may lower the renin ratio.

CHAPTER 33

HYPERVASCULARITY

GRANULATION TISSUE

ACTIVE GRANULATION tissue of inflammation or of an organizing hematoma of sufficient amount and duration will be nourished by dilated tortuous vessels. This may give rise to a florid, vascular pattern. The range of *hypervascularity* may vary from a *microscopic* to an *angiographic level.* The *microscopic* hypervascularity may present itself as a nebulous or sharply defined area of *increased staining.* To depend on such vague factors may lead to errors, as perfusion of a large amount of contrast into a normal small branch may give the same results. Inflammatory vasculature if any adjacent to a neoplasm may add to the confusion. Finally, the hypervascularity of an organizing hematoma or myositis ossificans may drive both the angiographer and the pathologist crazy.

DYSPLASTIC VASCULATURE

At the initial look, and sometimes even after many looks, *hamartomas, neurofibromas,* vessels of a *multicystic kidney, telangiectasia,* and elastic tissue disorders such as pseudoxanthoma elasticum with dysplastic vessels have a great resemblance to malignant neoplastic circulation. Histologically, though not angiographically, to a certain extent, these dysplastic vessels are different from the intrinsic neoplastic vessels of malignant tumors. Their *walls* may contain variable amounts of musculature and normal or abnormal elastic tissue, collagen and/or hyaline material. Such *dysplastic vessels* may dilate in certain areas, giving rise to *aneurysms* or form *cavernomatous malformations* which are probably *inherent* to that neoplasm. The amorphous, tortuous course of benign hyalinized or collagenized vessels may angiographically resemble malignant sinusoidal streams. In lesions containing dysplastic vessels there may be *lack of early arteriovenous shunting.* Because of the inherent bizarre angio-architecture of angiomyolipomas or neurofibromas, the *presence of malignant degeneration or their malignant counterparts may go unnoticed by the angiographer.*

NEOPLASTIC VASCULATURE

Benign

Since these tumors are provided with tortuous dilated feeding vessels, in some, perfusing a sinusoidal type of intrinsic neoplastic circulation, there may be a *method in their vascular madness.* Some benign tumors may have certain *organized patterns,* though chaotic, but having some regularity and discipline. This may be due to slow growth rate, encapsulation, or metabolic demands that are lower than malignant cells. There *may not be any* demonstrable *arteriovenous shunting in some* of these benign lesions. If the neovascularity is only at the *microscopic* level, then the angiographic reflections are those of an *intense, discrete* area of *staining. Chaotic vasculature* is the usual situation in the following benign tumors: vascular wall tumors, leiomyomas, pheochromocytomas, ganglioneuromas, cystadenomas, glomangiomas, angiofibromas, adenomas, chemodectomas, gastric and pulmonary carcinoids, hibernomas, mesenchymomas, or focal nodular hyperplasias. Because of such hypervascularity in many of these benign neoplastic lesions, it may be *difficult to differentiate them from their malignant counterparts,* particularly when malignant degeneration occurs in preexisting benign lesions. Occasionally a well-differentiated, comparatively *slow-growing malignant lesion* with pseudoencapsulation can have a circulatory pattern almost exactly resembling that of a benign mass.

Malignant

Dilated, elongated, tortuous feeding vessels in and around the mass, breaking up into a chaotic arborization; vessels lacking normal tapering with irregular segments of narrowing and dilatation leading into or communicating with islands of contrast collection and usually with early arteriovenous shunting characterize hypervascular malignant neoplastic circulation. These tumors have *madness in all their methods*. This *appropriated or newly created* abnormal circulation[85] consists of channels fitted against the adjacent cells of the neoplastic tissue. They are lined by either endothelium alone or by the adjacent neoplastic tissue with disorganized free and wide communications with other channels. Such bizarre patterns may not be seen in all malignant neoplasms, especially those with a very high degree of differentiation.

CHAPTER 34
STAINING

INCREASED ABNORMAL STAINING

PERSISTENT, INTENSE, prolonged staining of swollen parenchyma or of thickened bowel wall is the usual situation when there is an *exit problem* to the outflow of the injected contrast material. The intraarterially injected contrast material cannot escape if there is venous occlusion. Hemorrhagic infarcts are usually due to acute venous occlusion but rarely due to arterial ones. This can cause intense staining of the infarcted area, well exemplified in superior mesenteric venous occlusion.[1014–1016] Pulmonary artery emboli,[868] and on rare occasions renal arterial occlusions,[1483] may also cause hemorrhagic infarcts in their respective organs.

GRANULATION TISSUE

The wall of an *abscess* or of an *organizing*

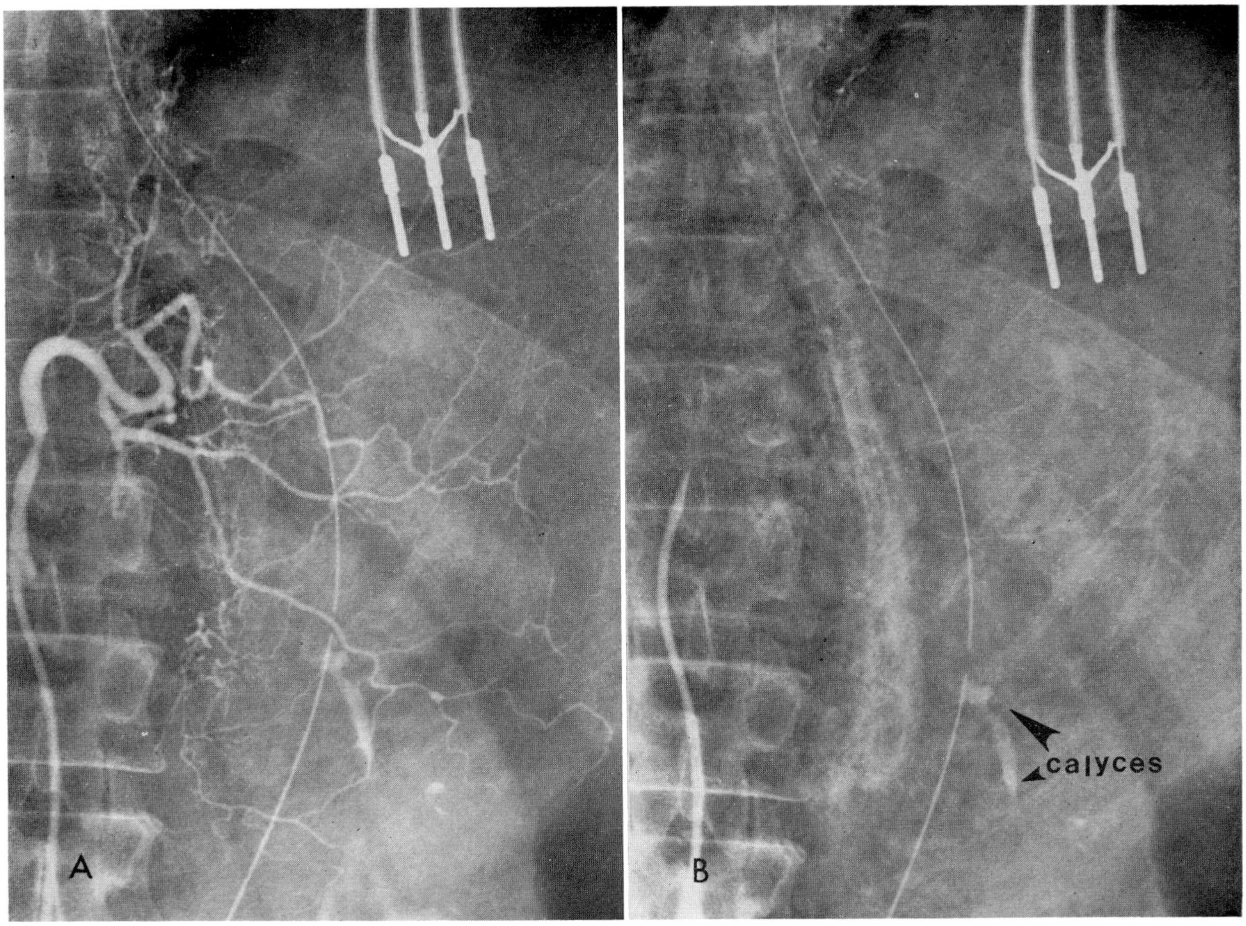

Figure 34.1. Left Gastric Arteriogram. (A) Arterial phase: There is no significant abnormality noted. (B) Late phase: There is increased staining of the gastric mucosa. This patient had hematemesis after excessive alcohol consumption and aspirin ingestion. *Diagnosis:* Probable hemorrhagic gastritis. This was confirmed at gastroscopy.

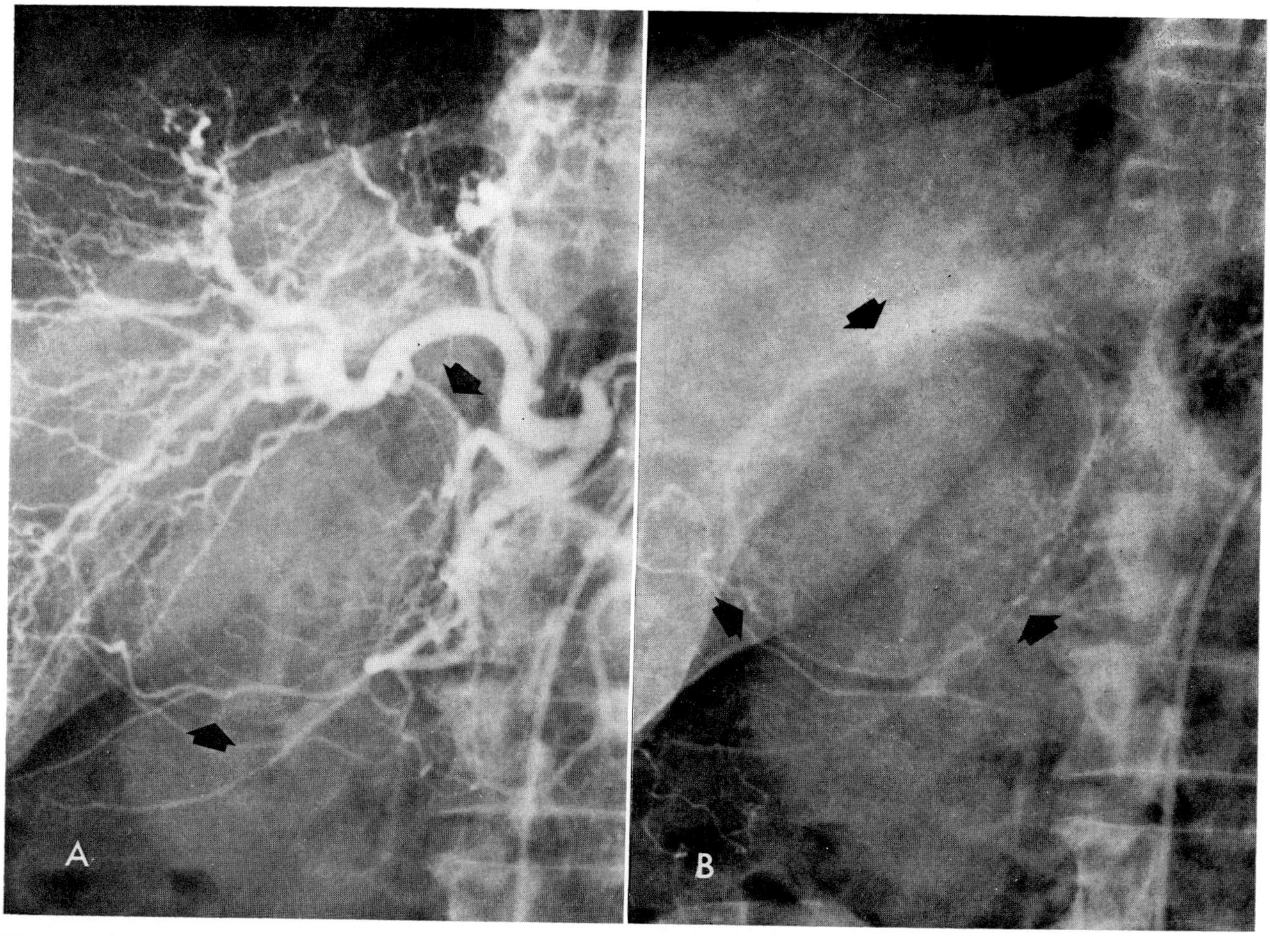

Figure 34.2. Hepatic Arteriogram. (A) The cystic artery branches (Arrow) are splayed. Incidentally seen is a corkscrew appearance of the intrahepatic branches. (B) Note the thin wall of a distended gallbladder. The patient was asymptomatic but had a palpable right upper quadrant mass. *Diagnosis:* Hydrops of the gallbladder (Arrow Head) and cirrhosis. No further information was obtained regarding the hepatic vasculature.

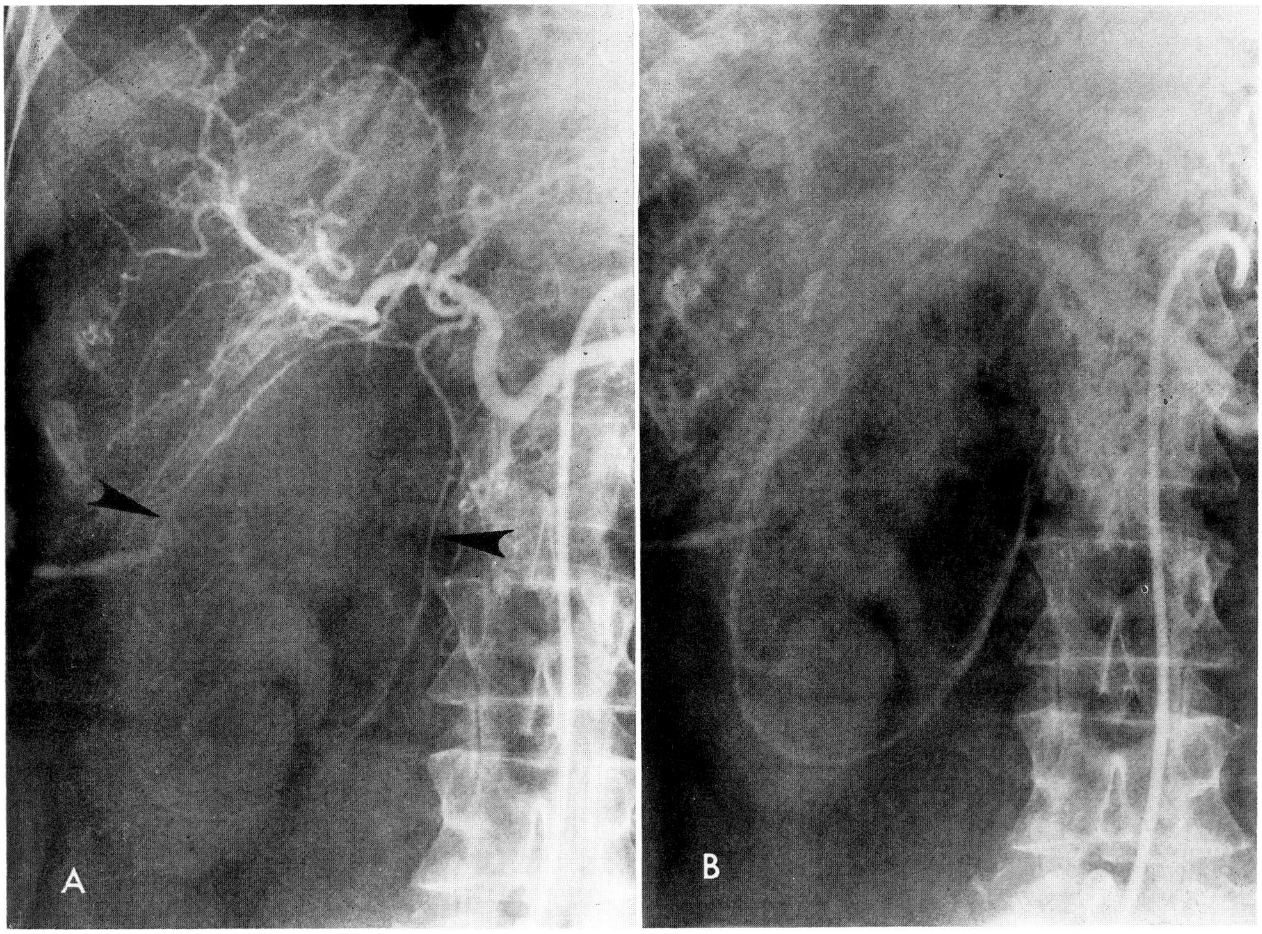

Figure 34.3. Celiac Arteriogram. (A) Arterial phase: A prominent cystic artery and its branches encircle a dilated gallbladder. (B) Late phase: A well-stained wall of an enlarged gallbladder is seen in a patient with a right upper quadrant mass and who is otherwise asymptomatic. *Diagnosis:* Hydrops of the gallbladder.

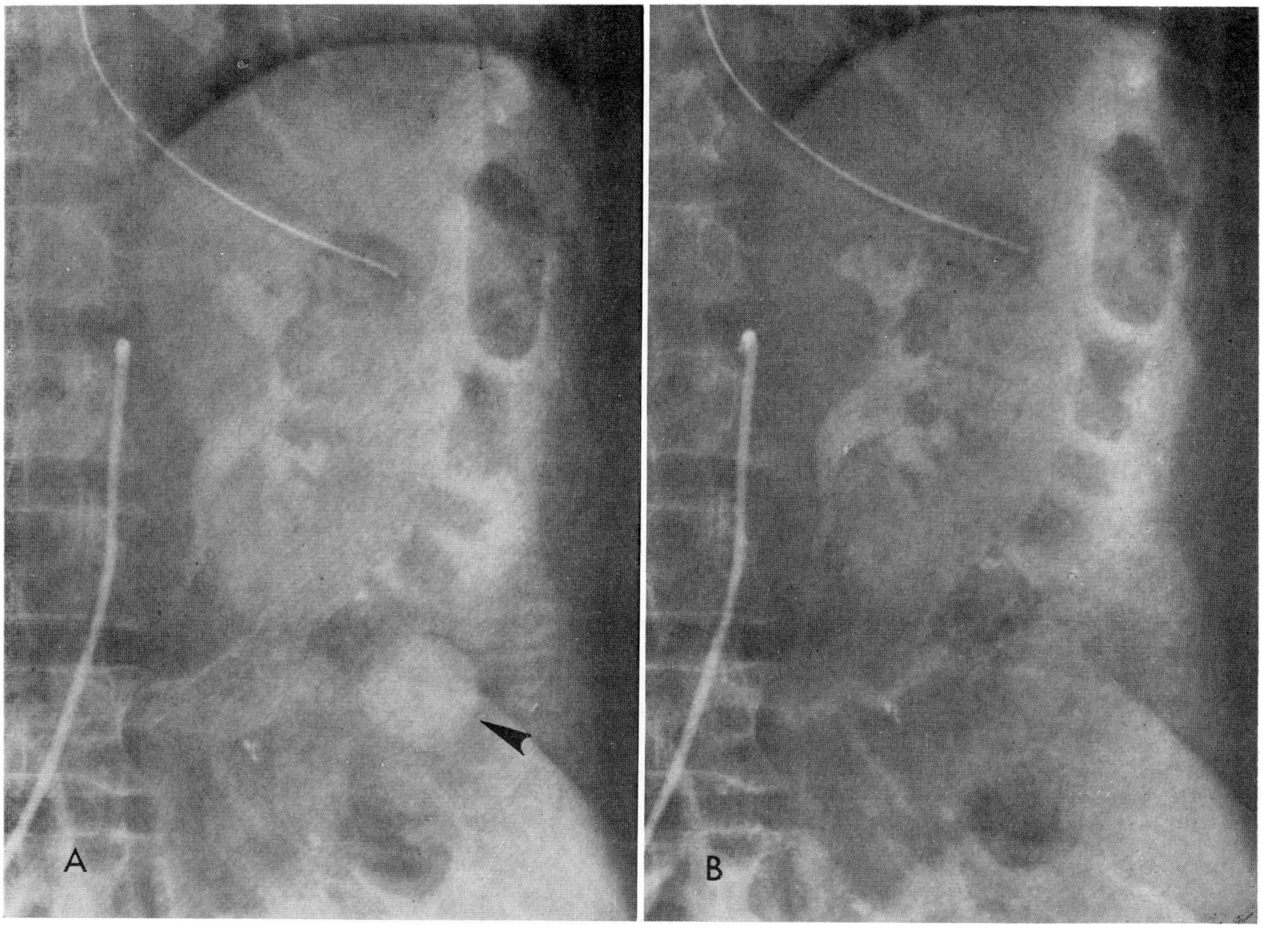

Figure 34.4. Superior Mesenteric Arteriogram. (A) A well-circumscribed, homogeneous stain is seen. (B) Later the stain disappears. *Comment:* End-on bowel with mucosal stain.

hematoma is provided with very vascular connective tissue.[111] The numerous capillaries perfused by contrast are revealed as increased *staining* of their *walls* of *variable thickness.* The intense staining of a granuloma also is not unusual as seen with tuberculous granulomas of the kidney.[1323]

STAIN OF THE WALL OF A VISCUS

The gallbladder wall[111, 1382, 1385] may be well-stained and *thick* in *acute cholecystitis.* A well-stained thin wall in a *distended gallbladder is seen in hydrops.* Lack of stain or *poor staining* of a *thick wall* due to fibrosis in a contracted, normal sized, or dilated gallbladder can be seen in *chronic cholecystitis.* The walls of the *ureter* may be thickened and stained in chronic hydronephrosis (Figs. 30-10, 34-2, 34-6).

STAIN OF THE WALLS OF CYSTIC STRUCTURES (TOTAL BODY OPACIFICATION)

Beside the staining of the wall of a cystic structure during angiography, opacification by rapid intravenous infusion of contrast material and body section radiography of the mass at the desired level may show staining of the walls of a hollow viscus or cystic mass. This technique is known as *total body opacification.*[1505]

The following cystic lesions may be demonstrated by angiography or total body opacification: the true fibrous wall of a simple cyst, the reactive host tissue of a parasitic cyst, the adventitious fibrous wall of a pancreatic or urinary pseudocyst, the granulation tissue of hemorrhagic cyst or abscess, the peripheral surviving layers of tumor tissue of a necrotic tumor or the tumoral walls of a cystadenoma.

CAPSULAR STAINING

The capsule of an organ is rarely seen unless it is thickened or there is increased capsular circulation. Examples include the thickened splenic capsule due to multiple infarcts[913] or due to increased capsular circulation in infiltrating processes such as leukemia[1484] (Fig. 29-47).

LOCALIZED STAINING DUE TO HYPERTROPHY OF THE PARENCHYMA

In some *regenerating nodules* of *cirrhotic livers,* intense staining almost resembling a malignant tumor such as a hepatoma may be seen. However, colloidal isotope scans reveal good concentration in the nodules suggesting normal functioning hepatic tissue, thus differentiating it from nonfunctioning tumor.[298, 1351, 1356] In the *kidneys,* staining of islands of compensatory hypertrophy of the parenchyma adjacent to scars is a frequent observation.[1485, 1486] Increased staining may also be seen in the kidney due to hypertrophy of the columns of Bertin. This is a product of developmental error with excessive infolding of the renal cortical tissue with or without hematuria.[1487, 1488] The hematuria is attributed to fibromuscular types of change in the microvasculature (Figs. 34-19 to 34-21).

TUMOR STAIN

Discrete, intense, persistent, homogeneous opacification extending beyond the venous phase is a usual angiographic observation in many parenchymal or nonparenchymal *benign tumors.* This is probably due to the extravascular collection of contrast which does not return to the vascular system until the plasma contrast level has fallen sufficiently to allow for back diffusion kinetics.[1489] This phenomenon is well exemplified in many benign tumors such as *adenomas* and *meningiomas,* and in very *well-differentiated malignant tumors.* A prolonged stain in a malignant tumor is not seen usually, probably because of comparatively rapid arteriovenous circulation. In parenchymal tumors the stain of the lesion may not be appreciated if the intensity of the stain is the same as that of the adjacent parenchyma, as seen in both benign and malignant tumors of the pancreas, liver, spleen and kidney. The homogeneity of the stain is obviously influenced by the presence or absence of hemorrhage or necrosis in the bulk of the tumor.

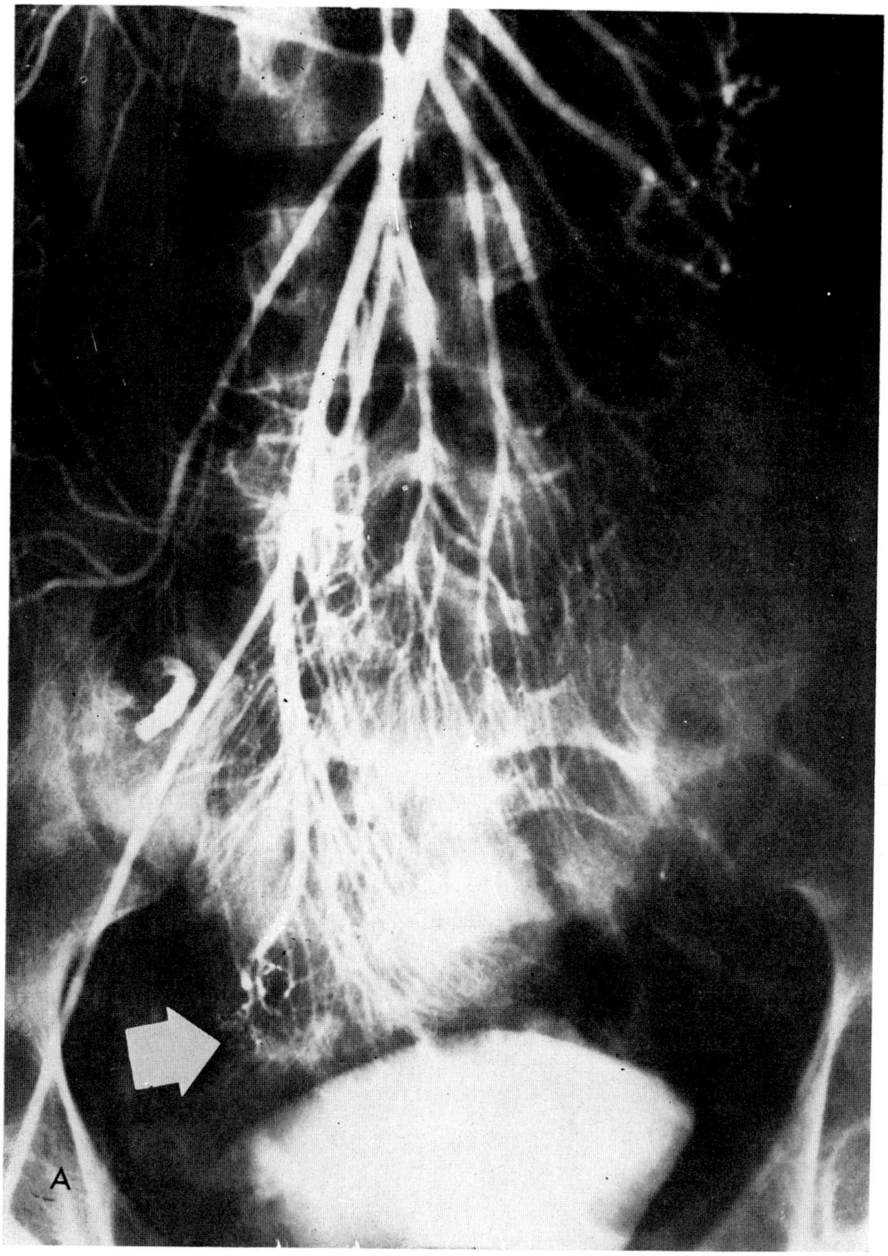

Figure 34.5A

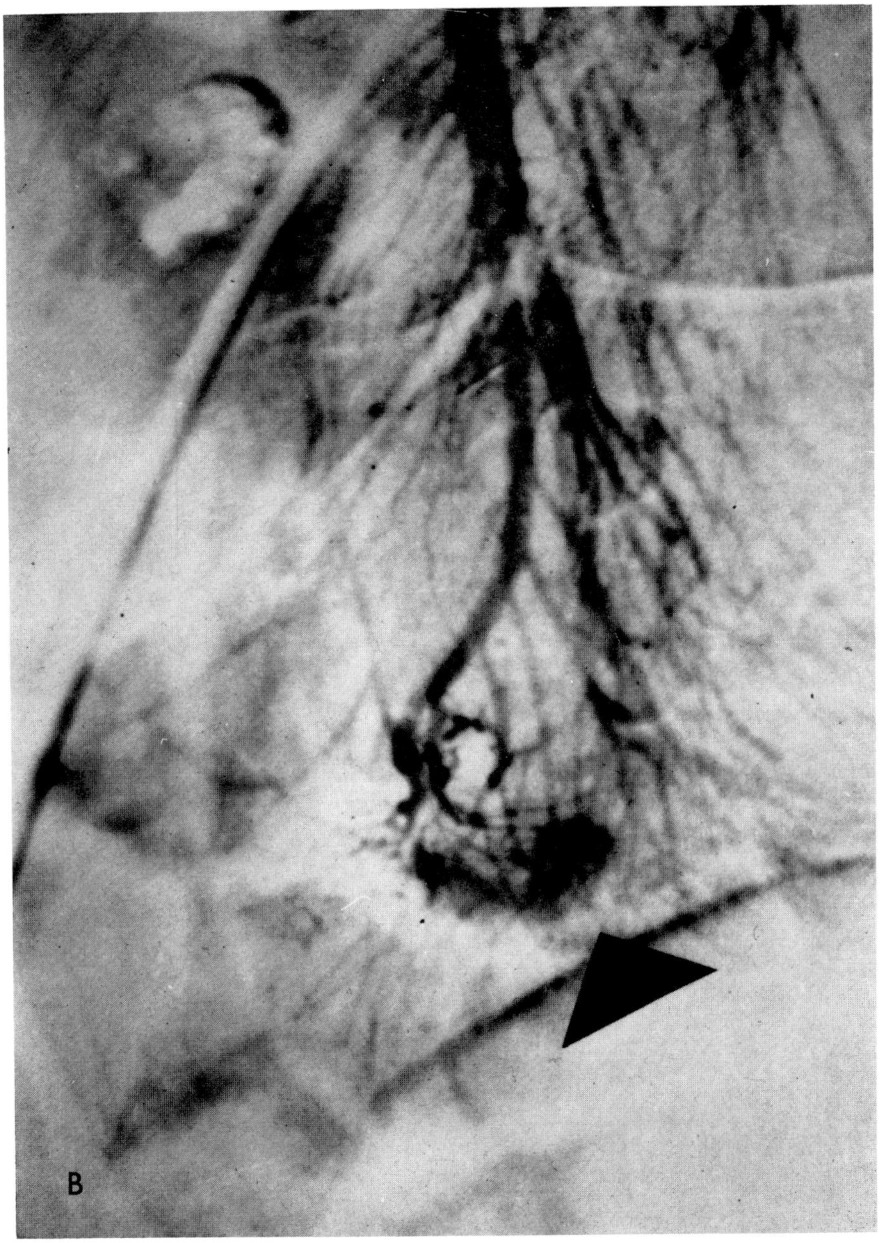

Figure 34.5. Superior Mesenteric Arteriogram. (A) There is a localized, irregular group of vessels (Arrow). (B) Subtracted image-close-up: Staining of the gastric mucosa in a Meckel's diverticulum is revealed. *Diagnosis:* Meckel's diverticulum. (From Farris, J. C., and Whitley, J. E. Angiographic demonstration of Meckel's diverticulum. *Radiol, 108*:285, 1973. Courtesy of the authors and publishers.)

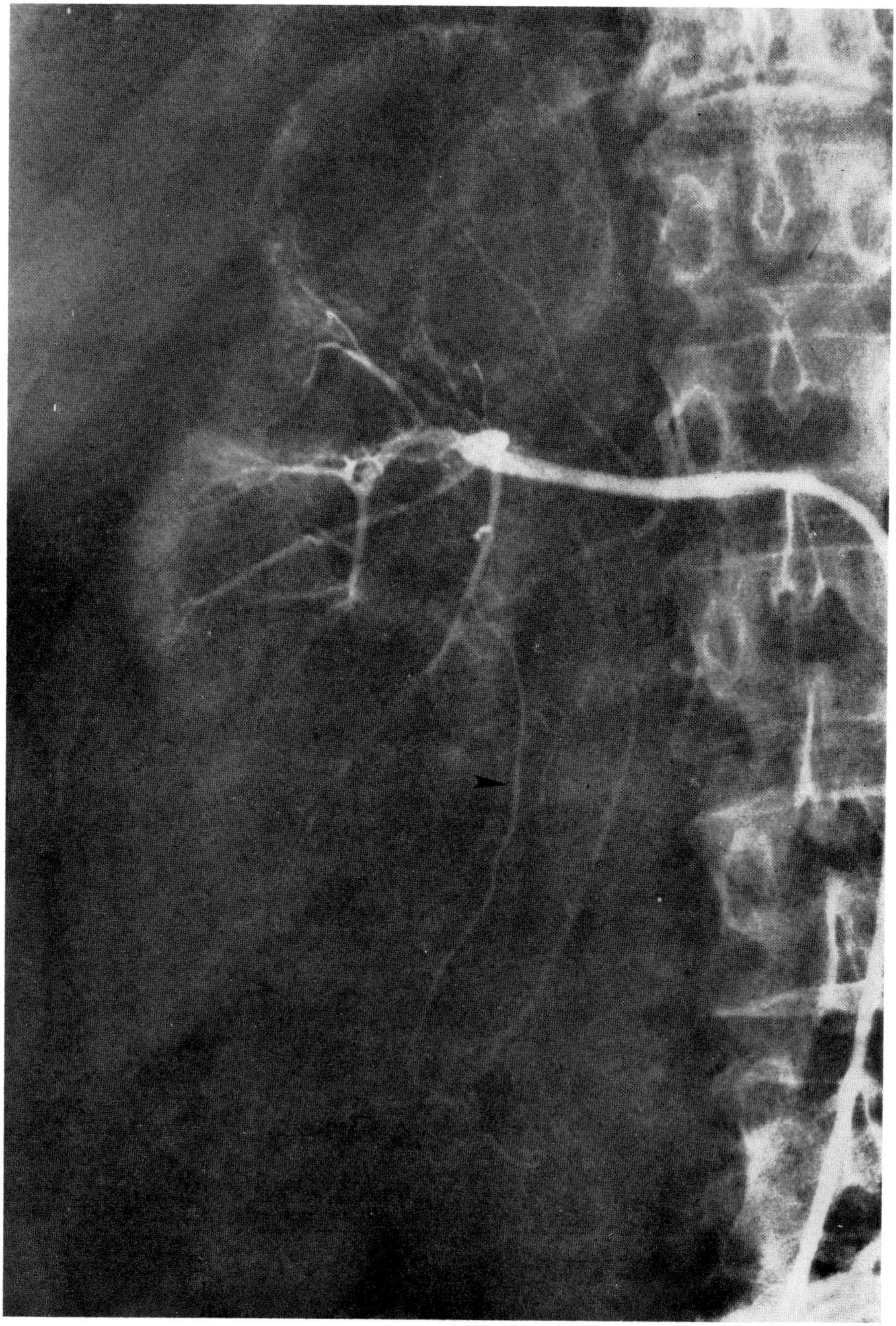

Figure 34.6A

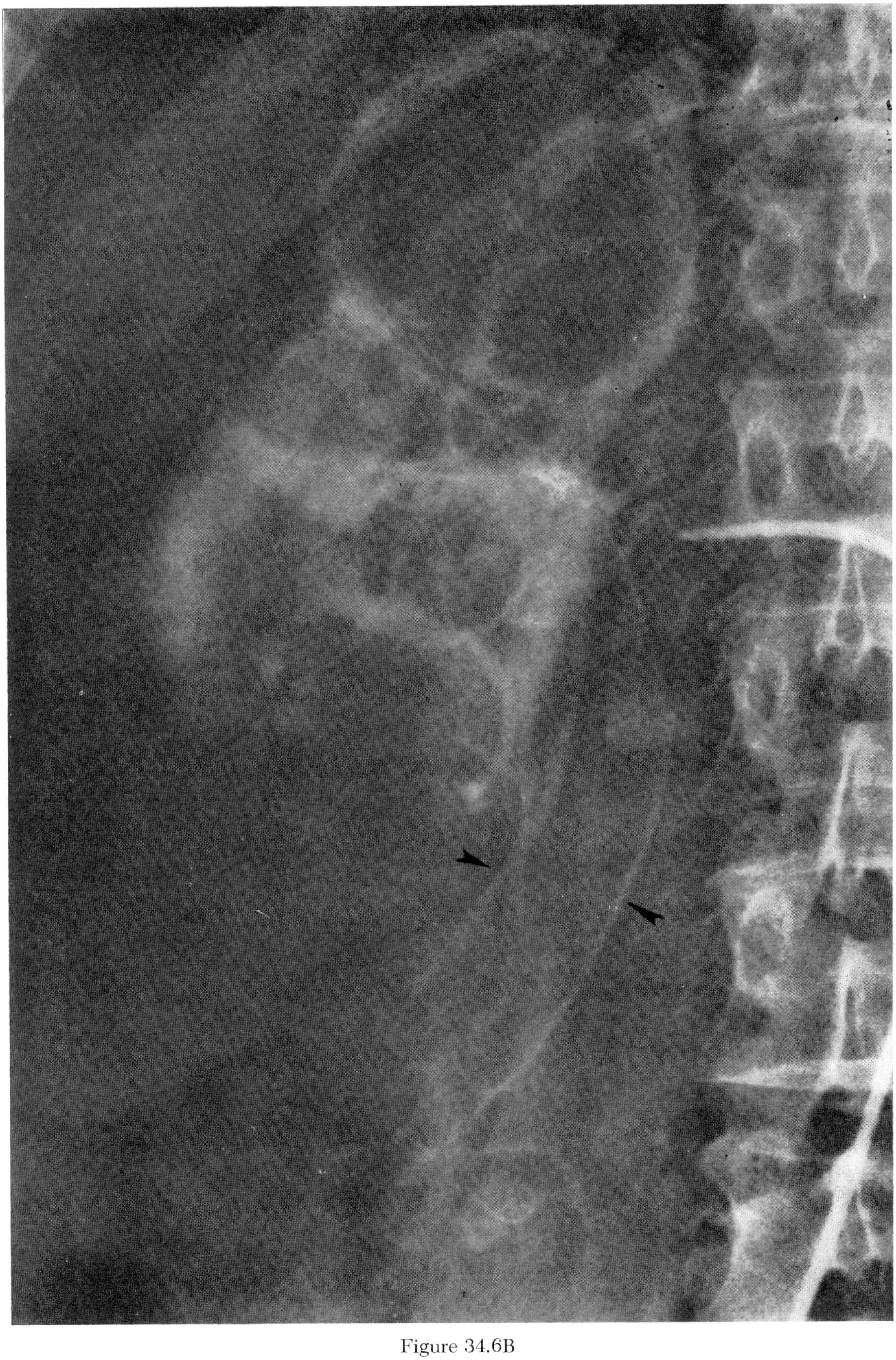

Figure 34.6B

Figure 34.6. Renal Arteriogram. Marked thinning of the right renal artery occurs with stretching and deviation of the intrarenal arterial branches. A very prominent pelviureteral branch gives rise to stain of the ureteric wall (Arrow). *Diagnosis:* Hydronephrosis with marked dilatation of the ureter and thickening of the ureter wall.

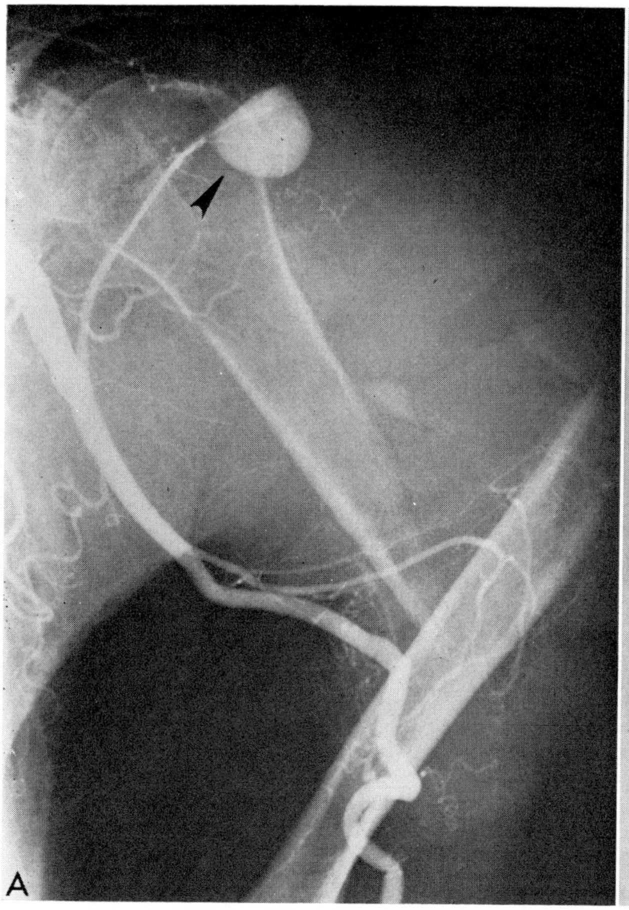

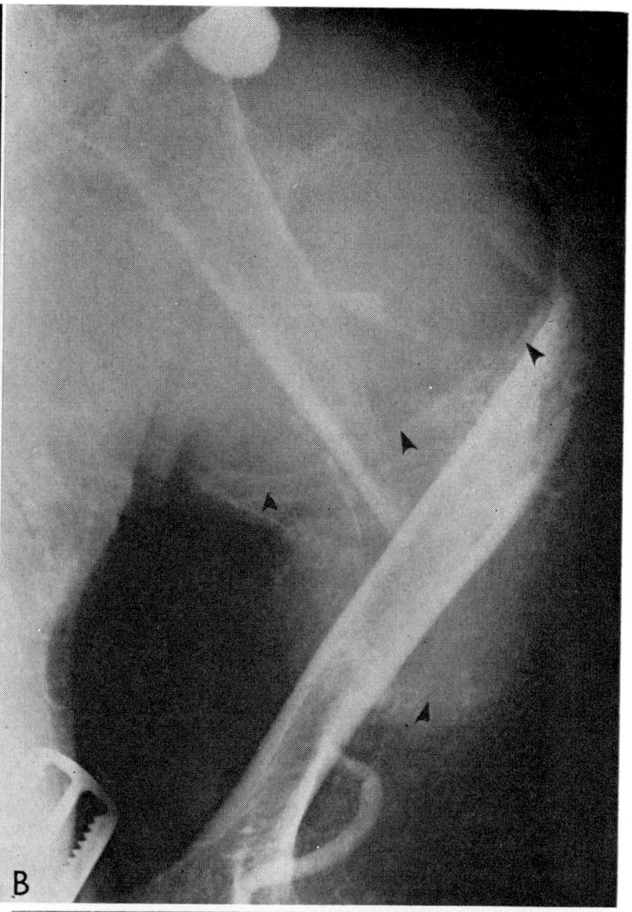

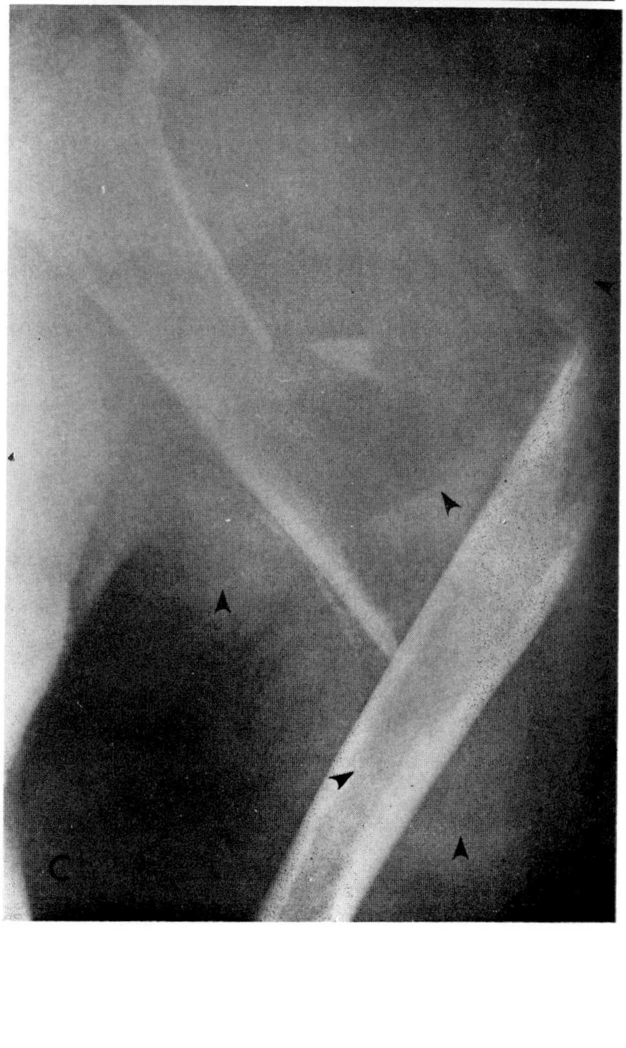

Figure 34.7. (A) Left axillary arteriogram: Note extravasation of the contrast material from the circumflex humeral branch of the axillary artery (Arrow). Marked deviation of the axillary arterial branches occurs around a huge soft tissue mass. (B) Late arterial phase: A uniformly lucent mass is delineated from the adjacent muscular stain (Arrow). Stasis of contrast in the extravasated area. (C) Sixty seconds after the arteriogram: A well-defined, huge lucent mass is in the upper part of the arm (Arrow) and another one is of a smaller size in the lower part of the arm (Arrow). This patient had a fracture three months prior to this examination which was suspected of being a pathological fracture. *Diagnosis:* Organized hematomas with a pseudoaneurysm from the circumflex humeral artery.

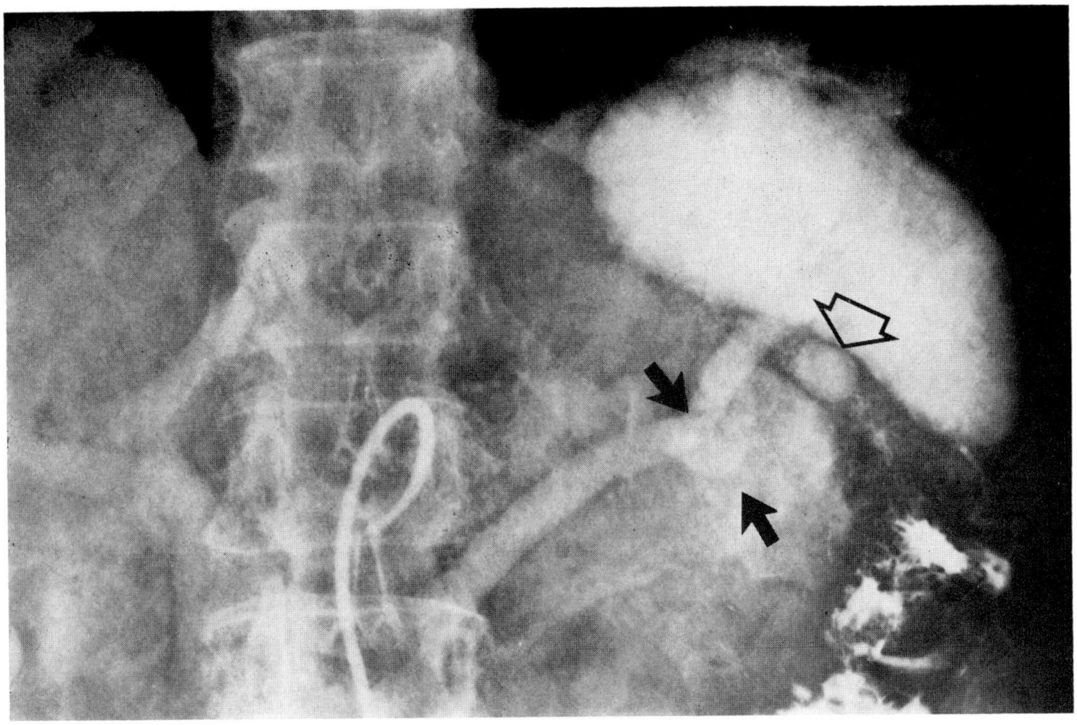

Figure 34.8. Celiac Arteriogram—venous phase. Notice the stain of an accessory spleen (Blank Arrow) and a discrete staining of an insulinoma (Arrows).

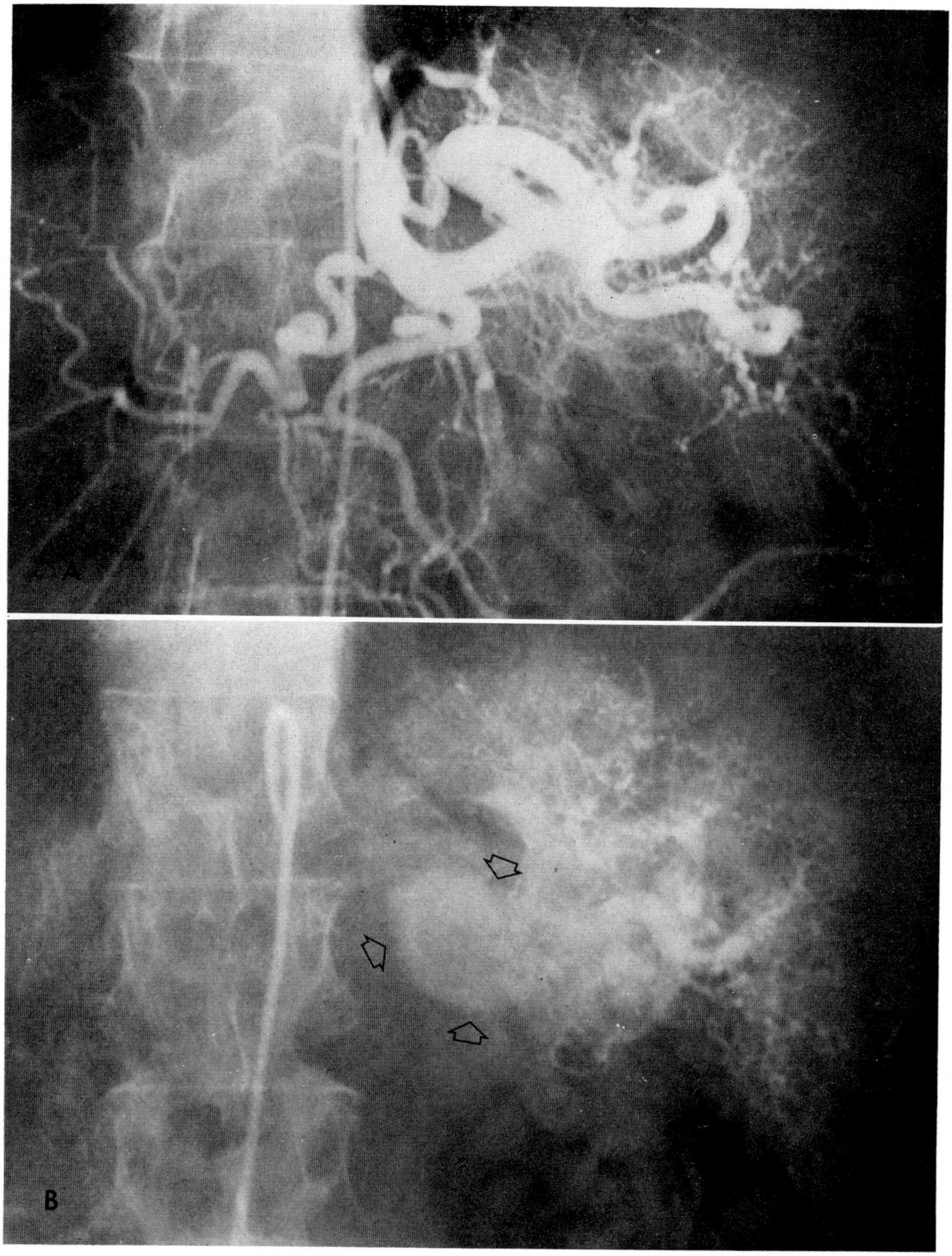

Figure 34.9. Splenic Arteriogram. (A) An increased number of pancreatic branches are seen to arise from the splenic artery. (B) There is discrete circumscribed stain at the tail of the pancreas. The patient had hypoglycemia. *Diagnosis:* Insulinoma. (Courtesy of Dr. F. J. Mulopulos, Chairman, Department of Radiology, Lutheran General Hospital, Park Ridge, Illinois.)

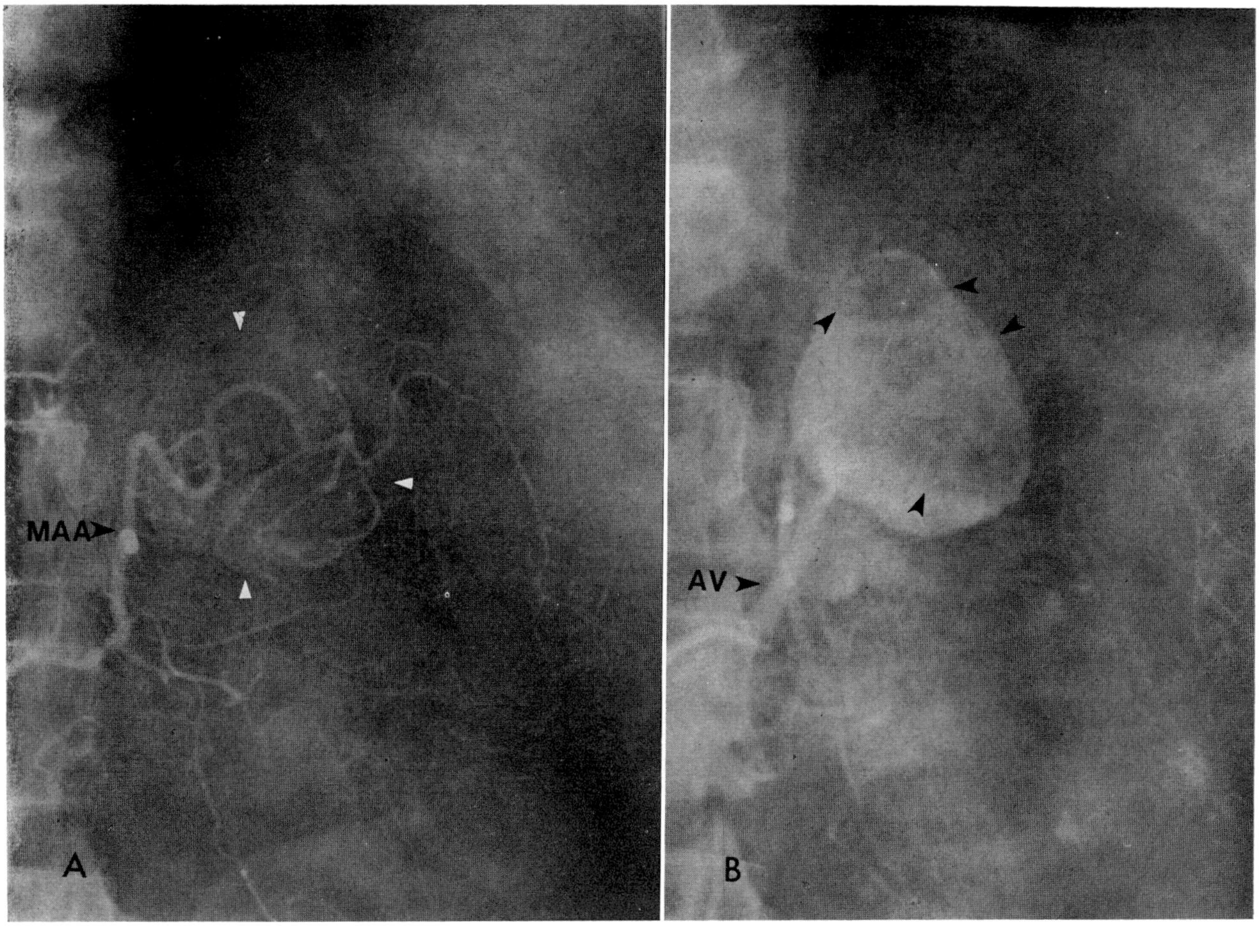

Figure 34.10. (A) Left middle adrenal arteriogram: A very prominent middle adrenal artery (M.A.A.) perfuses a mass in the adrenal gland. (B) Parenchymal phase: Intense staining of this well-defined mass with two lucent areas (Arrow) occurs. Notice the adrenal vein (A.V.). This patient had two attacks of left flank plain localized to this area. *Diagnosis:* Adrenal adenoma with recent and old hemorrhages. *Comment:* Reproduction of the same type of pain during test injections of contrast material in this particular patient was noteworthy.

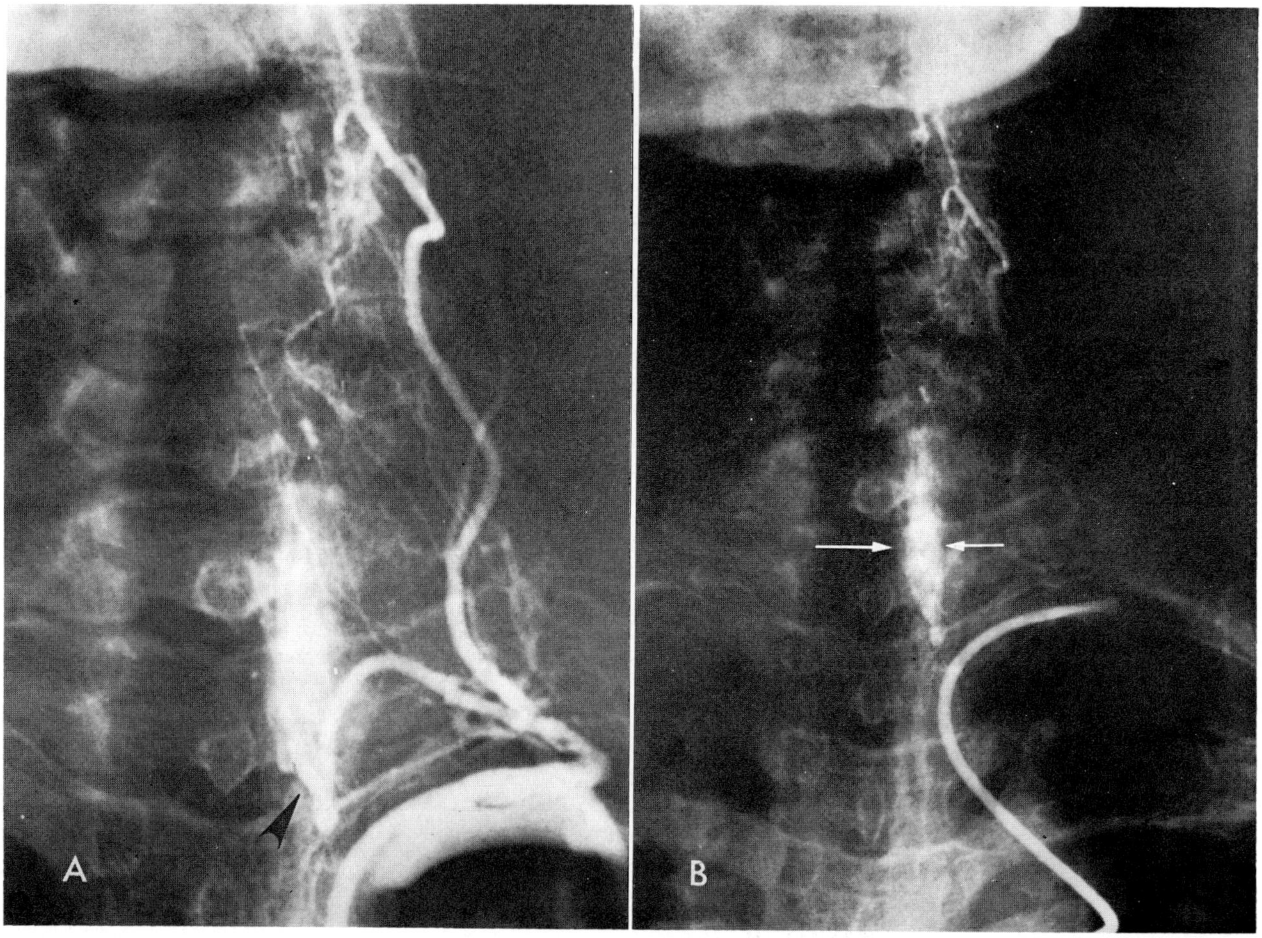

Figure 34.11. Left Thyrocervical Arteriogram. (A) Distortion and flattening of the "S" loop of the inferior thyroid artery. (B) Parenchymal phase: A well-circumscribed mass measuring 4 mm x 6 mm seen through the staining of the thyroid. *Diagnosis:* Parathyroid adenoma.

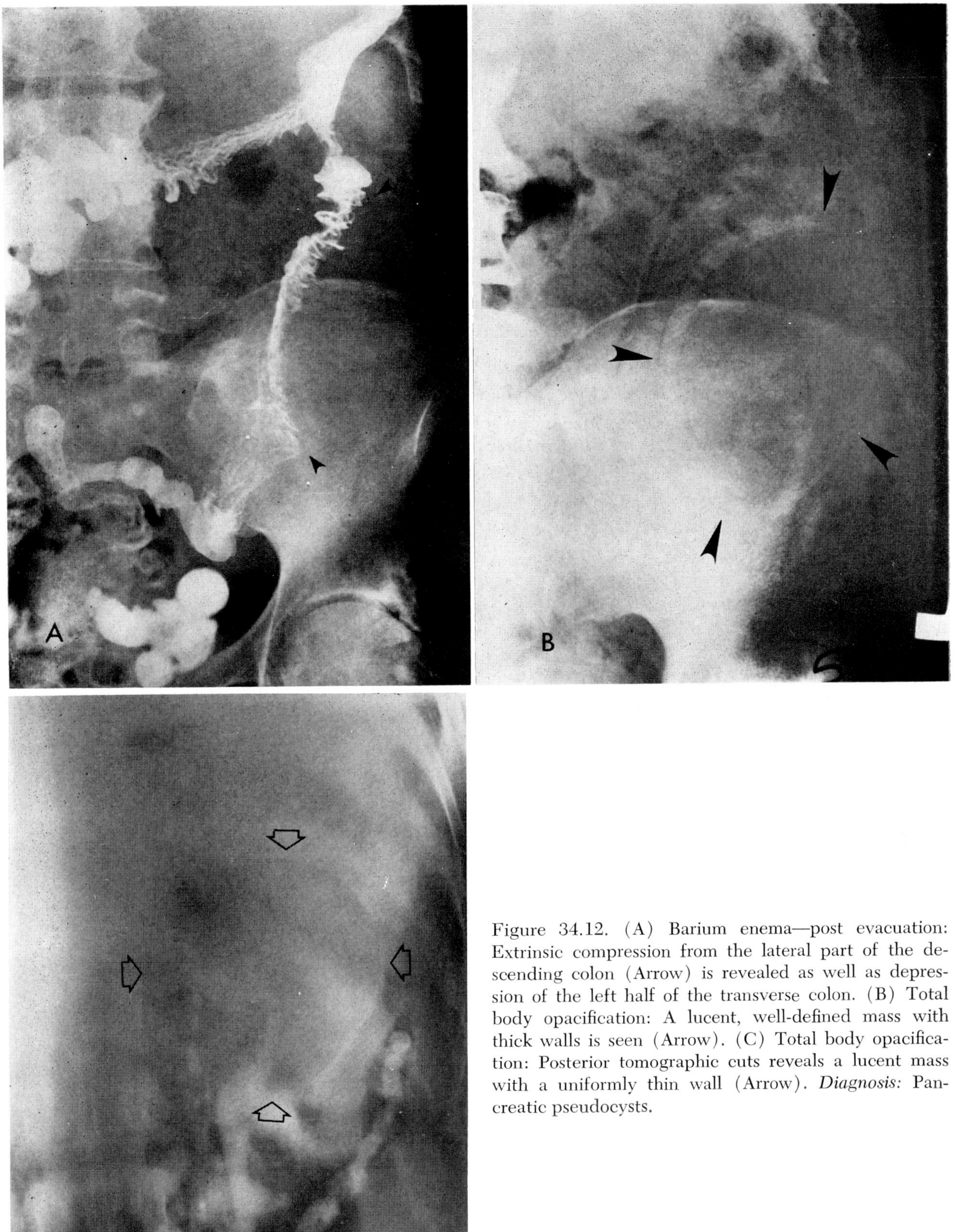

Figure 34.12. (A) Barium enema—post evacuation: Extrinsic compression from the lateral part of the descending colon (Arrow) is revealed as well as depression of the left half of the transverse colon. (B) Total body opacification: A lucent, well-defined mass with thick walls is seen (Arrow). (C) Total body opacification: Posterior tomographic cuts reveals a lucent mass with a uniformly thin wall (Arrow). *Diagnosis:* Pancreatic pseudocysts.

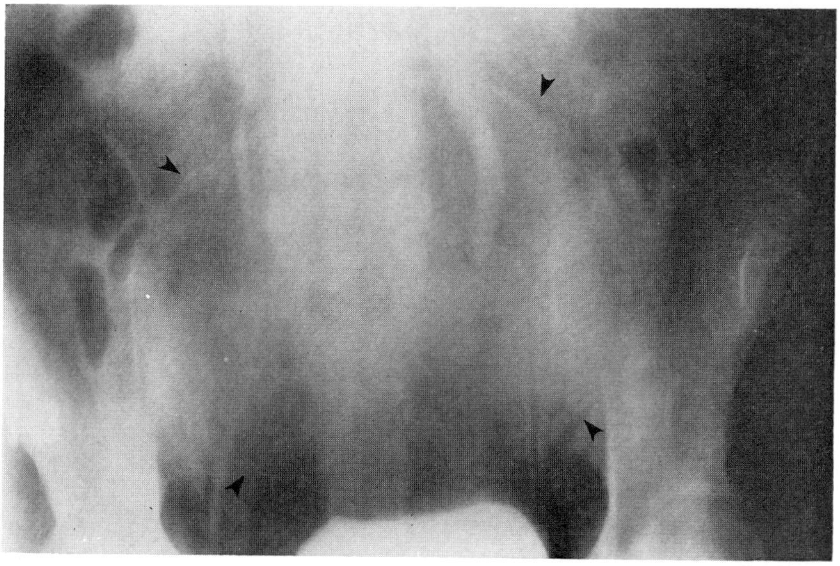

Figure 34.13. Total Body Opacification. A moderately sized lucent mass with a thin wall is seen in the lower abdomen. *Diagnosis:* Cystic mass arising from the ovary probably ovarian cyst or a cystadenoma. *Pathology:* Simple ovarian cyst.

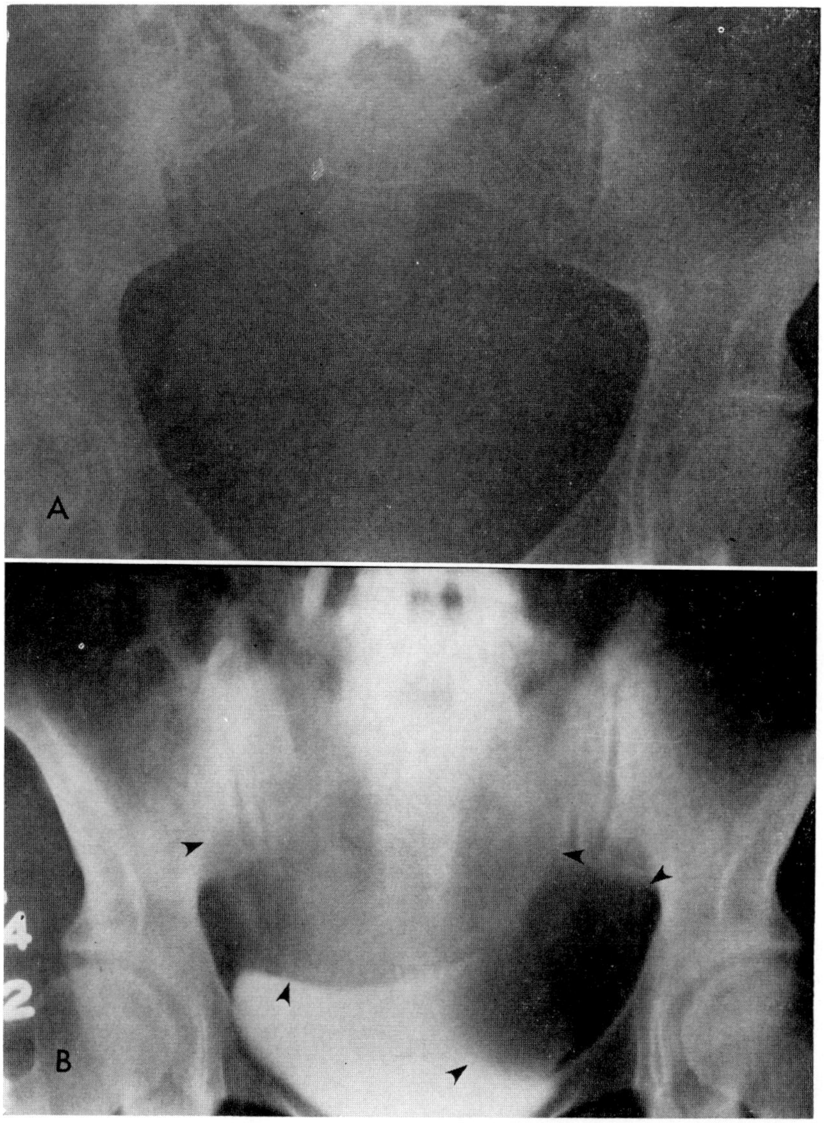

Figure 34.14. (A) Plain film of the abdomen: A water density mass is revealed in the true pelvis. (B) Total body opacification: Two lucent masses of different sizes lined by thin white walls are seen. *Diagnosis:* Cystic masses probably arising from the ovaries. *Pathology:* Ectopic **pregnancy.**

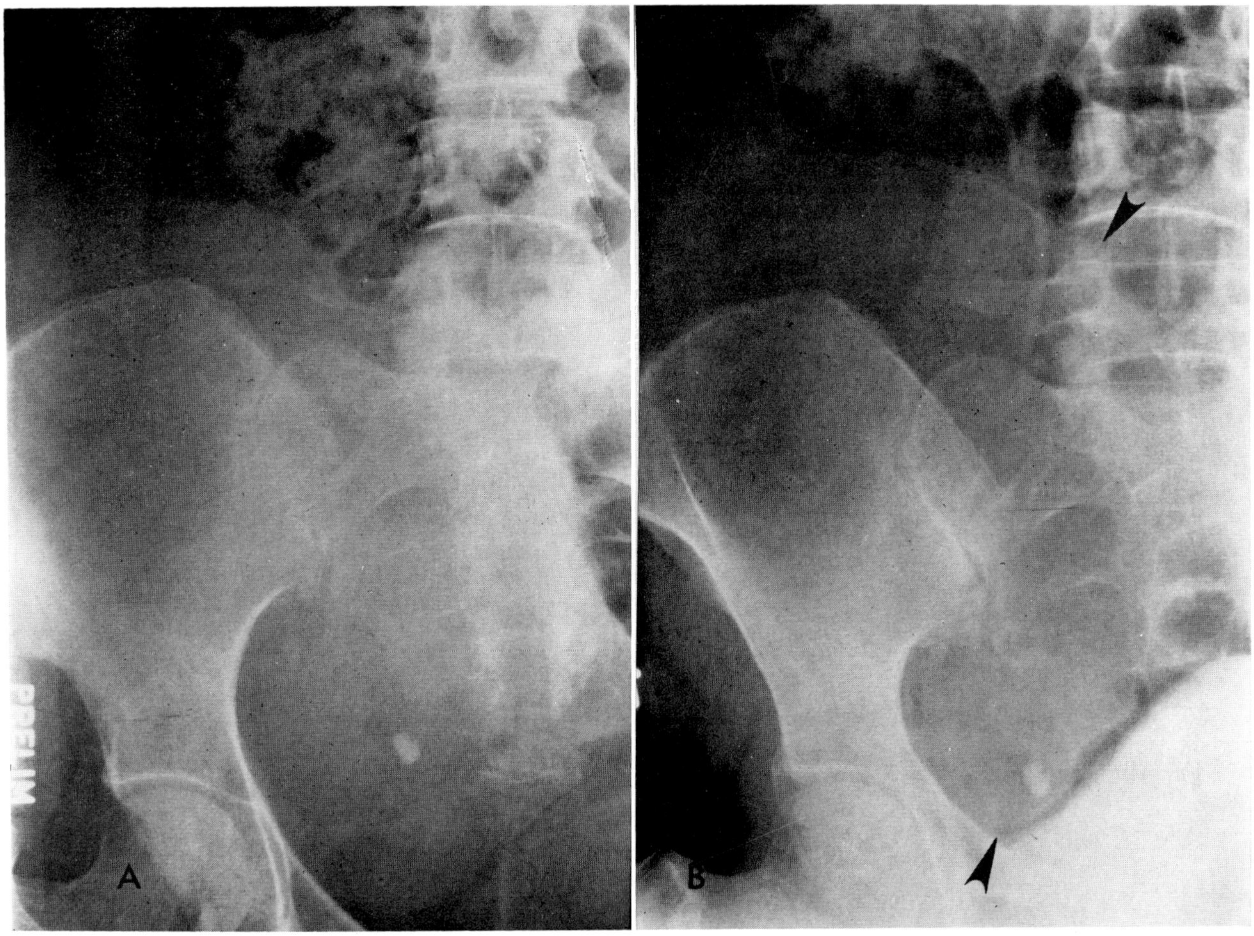

Figure 34.15. (A) Plain film of the abdomen: An irregularly shaped water density mass is in the right half of the pelvis extending to the right lower quadrant with occasional calcific parts within it. (B) Total body opacification: A comparatively lucent mass is seen. *Diagnosis:* Cystic ovarian mass probably cystadenoma in view of the calcification. *Pathology:* Loculated abscesses due to old pelvic inflammatory disease.

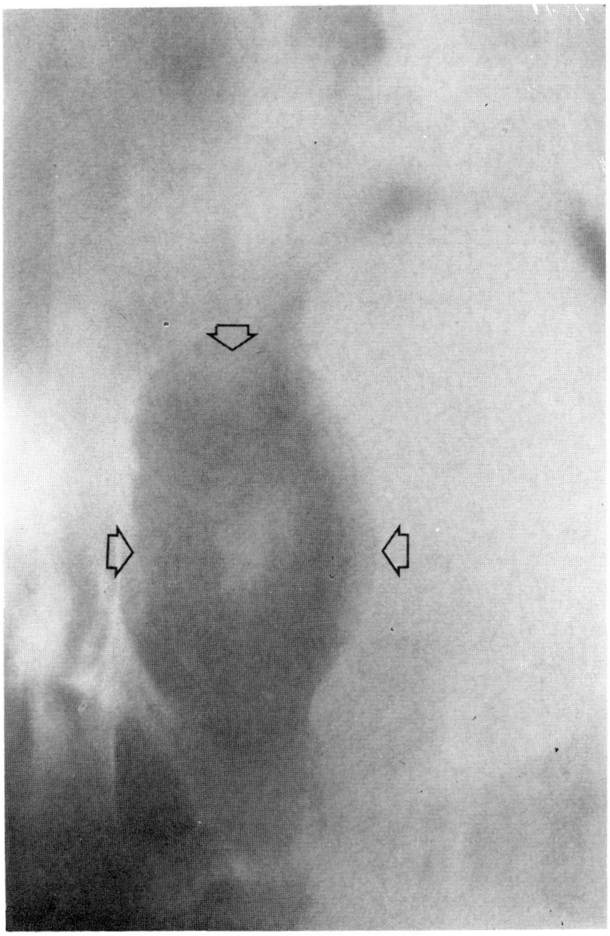

←

Figure 34.16. Total Body Opacification. A moderately sized, lucent mass with a thin wall displaces the contrast filled urinary bladder. Notice contrast in the lymph nodes from a lymphangiogram. *Diagnosis:* Cyst in the pelvis. *Pathology:* A lymphocyst.

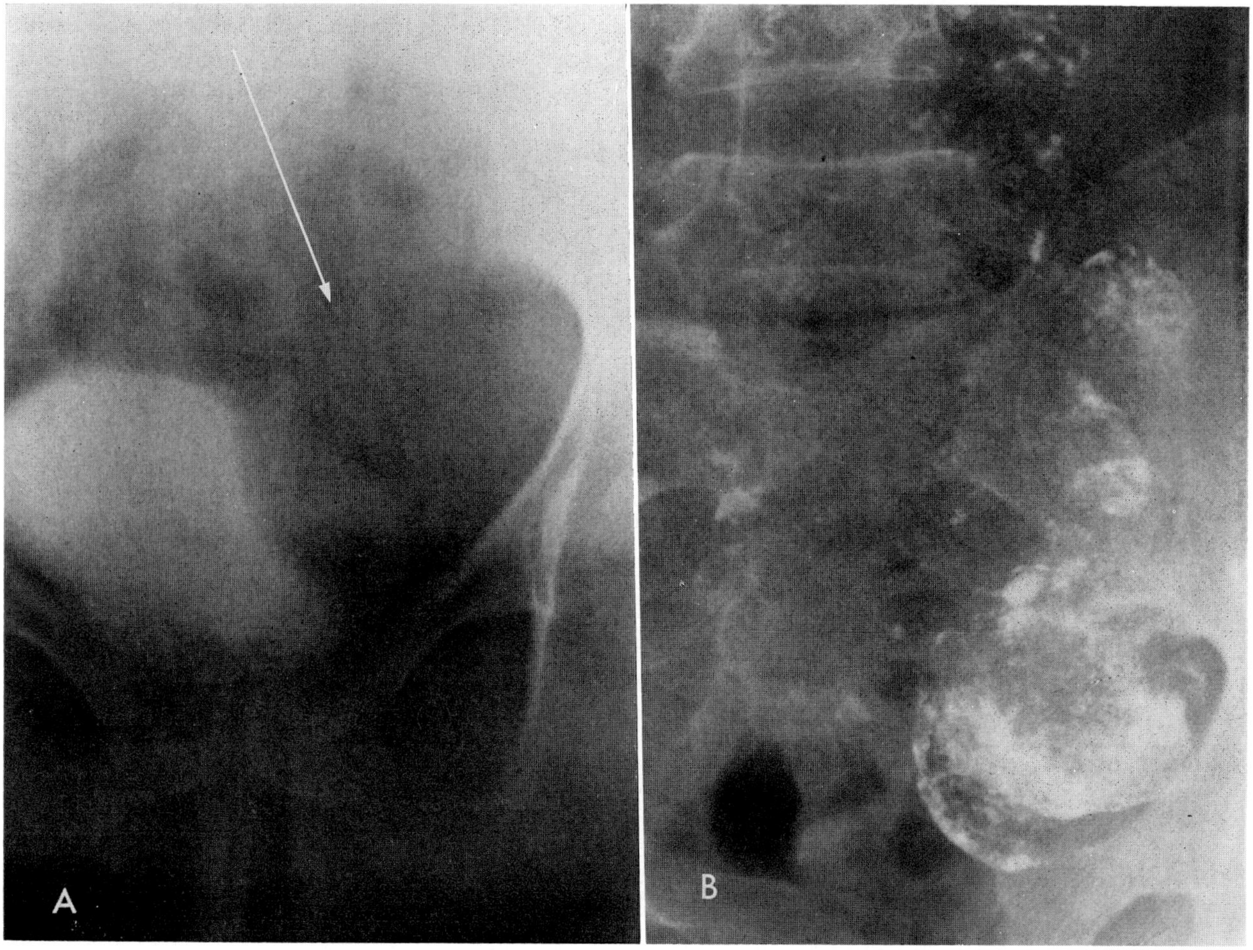

Figure 34.17. Total Body Opacification. (A) A oval-shaped, translucent mass secondarily compressing the urinary bladder (Arrow). (B) Lymphangiogram: huge lymph nodes with filling defects. *Diagnosis:* Lymphoma. *Pathology:* Tuberculous lymph nodes.

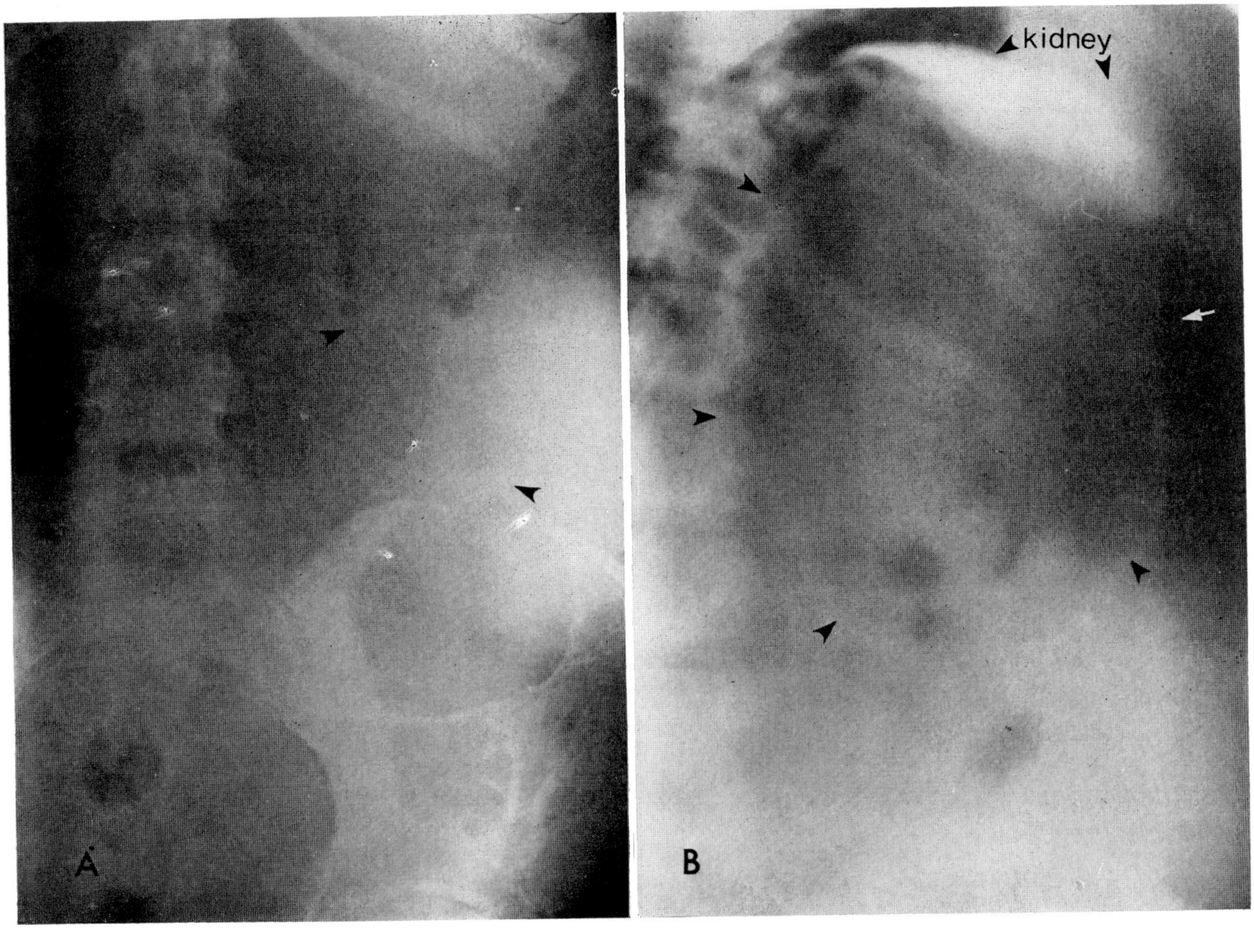

Figure 34.18. (A) Plain film of the abdomen: A huge mass density occupies the entire left hemiabdomen obliterating the left psoas margin. Areas of calcific density are noted in the soft tissue mass (Arrow). There is cystic destruction of the left iliac bone. (B) Total body opacification reveals a well-marginated, lucent mass (Arrow). Another water density mass is between the lucent mass and the iliac bone. This is a hemophiliac patient. *Diagnosis:* Retroperitoneal hematomas occurring at different times.

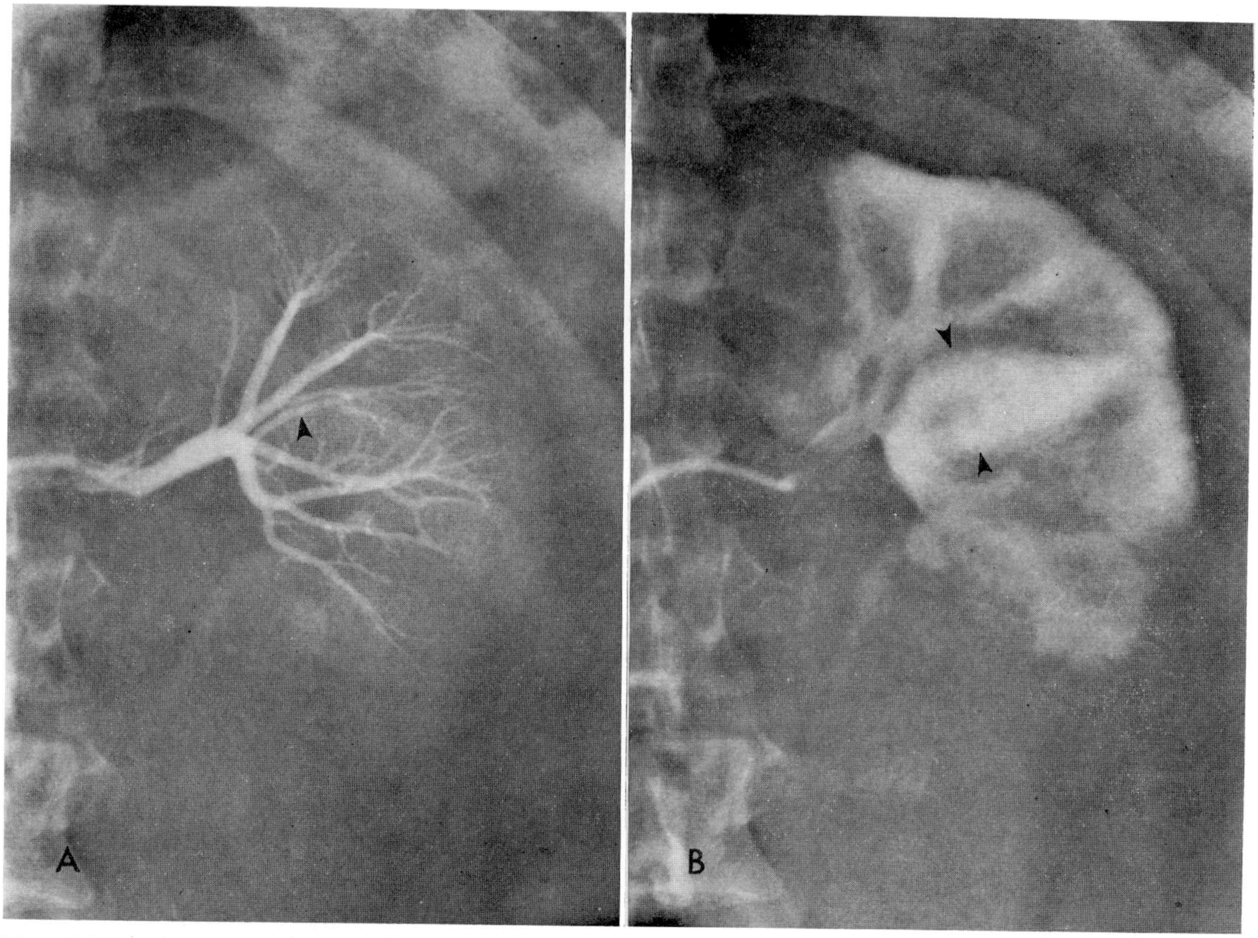

Figure 34.19. Renal Arteriogram. (A) Arterial phase: There is stretching and deviation of the midintrarenal arterial branches. (B) Parenchymal phase: There is staining of cortical invagination (Arrow). Incidentally, there were two separate aberrant arteries perfusing the lower and the upper poles. *Comment:* Duplicated kidneys with fusion of the cortices of the two duplicated segments of the renal buds.

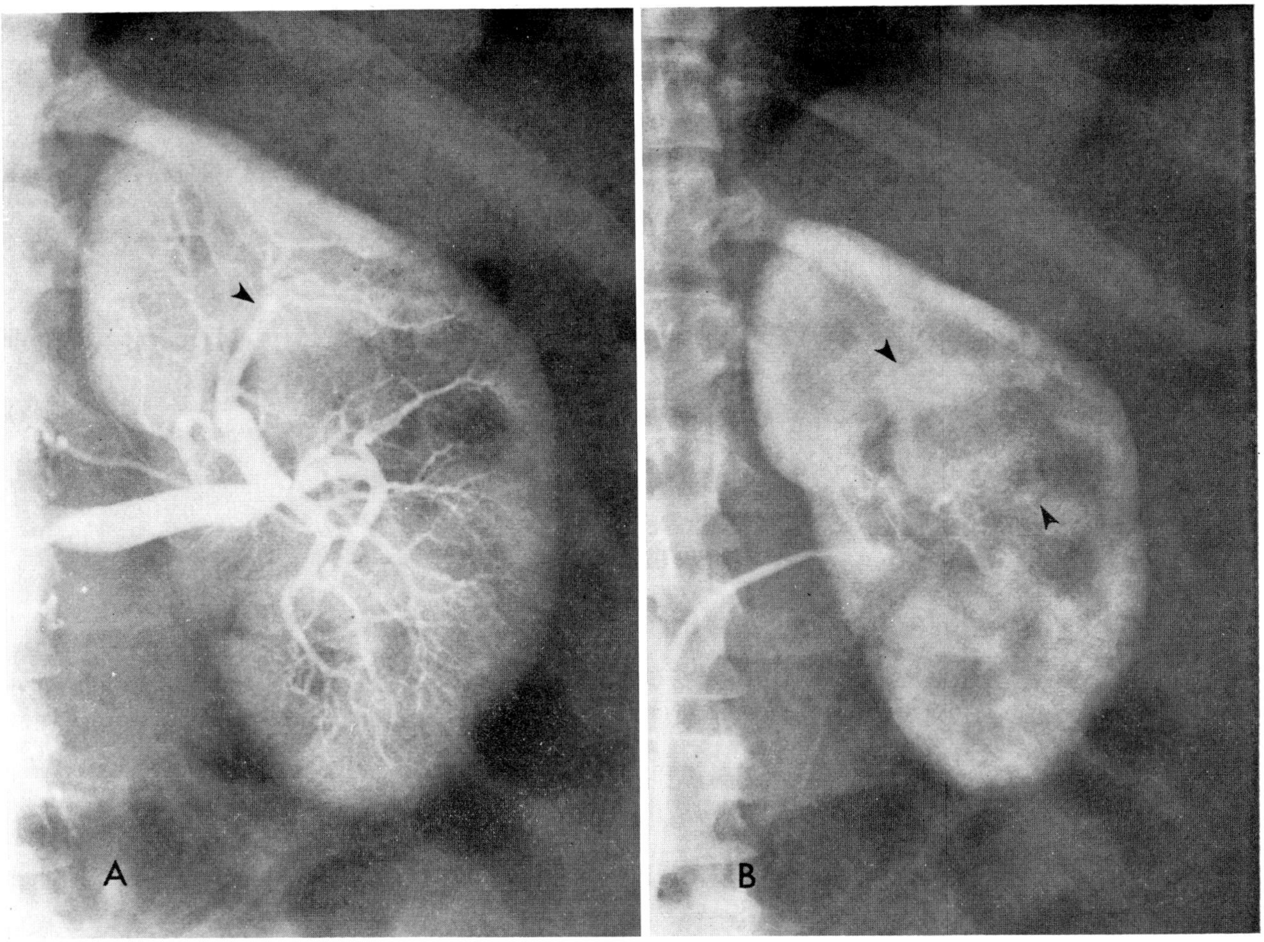

Figure 34.20. Renal Arteriogram. (A) Arterial phase: There is deviation of the major intrarenal branch with no apparent abnormal vascularity. (B) Parenchymal phase: No abnormal vascularity is seen. Normal staining of the cortex (Arrow) occurs. *Comment:* Normal renal arteriogram with cortical disorientation.

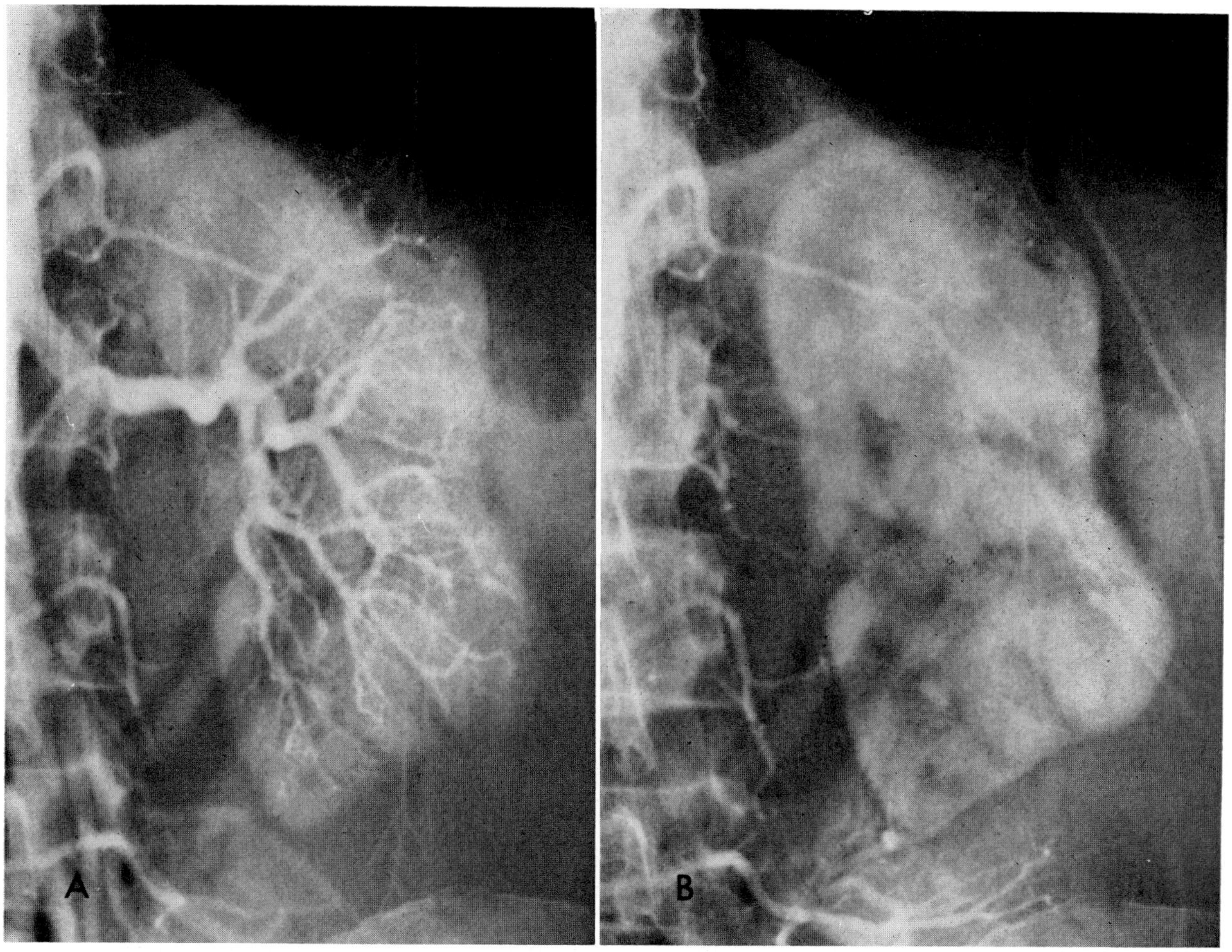

Figure 34.21. Flush Aortogram. (A) There is a bulbous configuration of the upper half of the left kidney and bulbous projection from the lateral part of the lower portion. (B) The same area is shown much better with no abnormal vascularity. A patient with repeated kidney infections. *Diagnosis:* Islands of hypertrophy and islands of scars due to pyelonephritis.

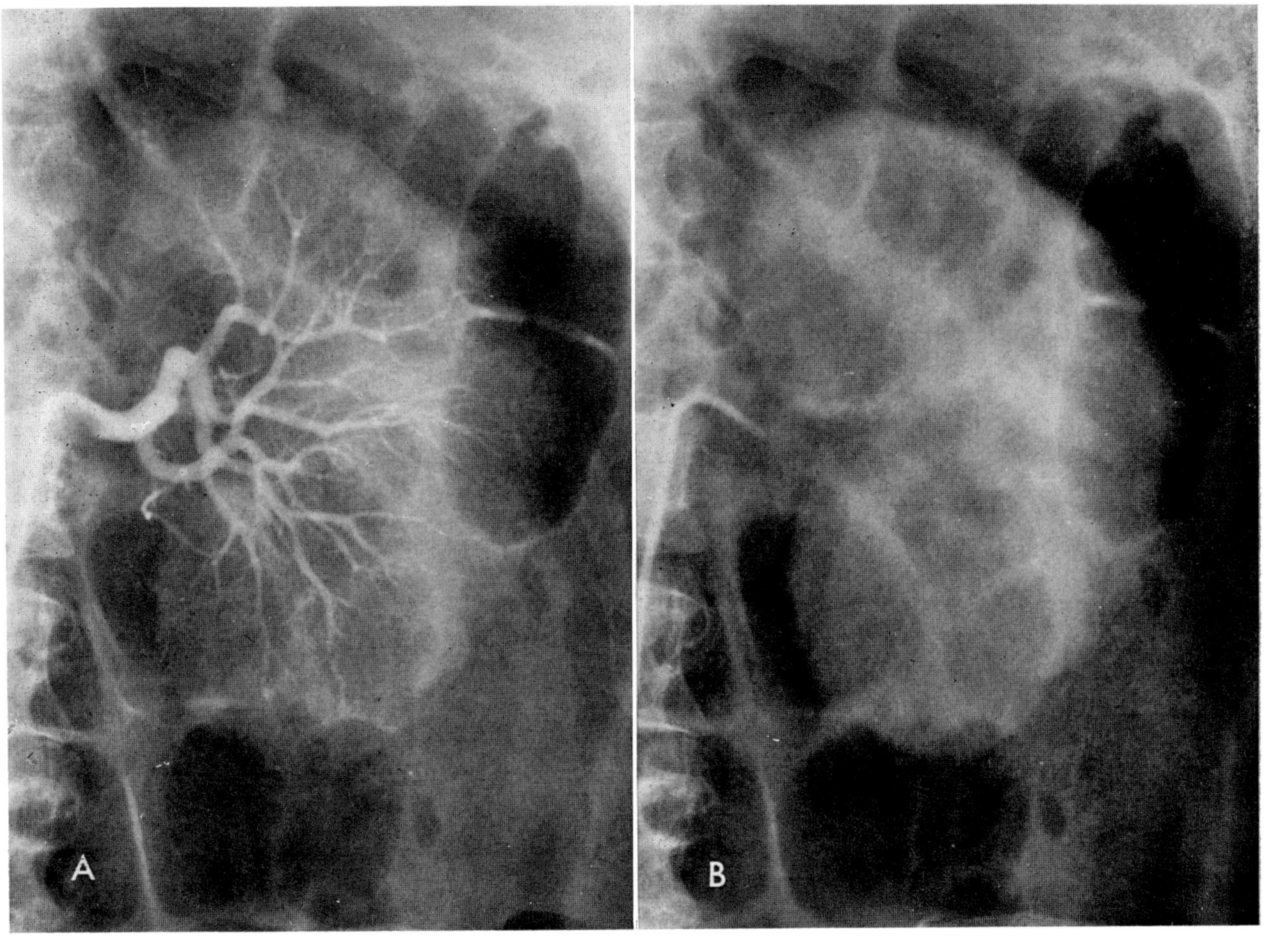

Figure 34.22. Renal Arteriogram. (A) Increase in size of the kidney is seen with diffuse stretching of the intrarenal branches. (B) Parenchymal phase: At twelve seconds intense staining of the renal parenchyma occurs with no cortical medullary landmarks and no visualization of the renal vein. *Diagnosis:* Edema of the kidney causing stretching of the intrarenal branches. Intense staining of the renal parenchyma due to renal vein thrombosis. Renal venogram (Fig. 24-31) confirmed the diagnosis.

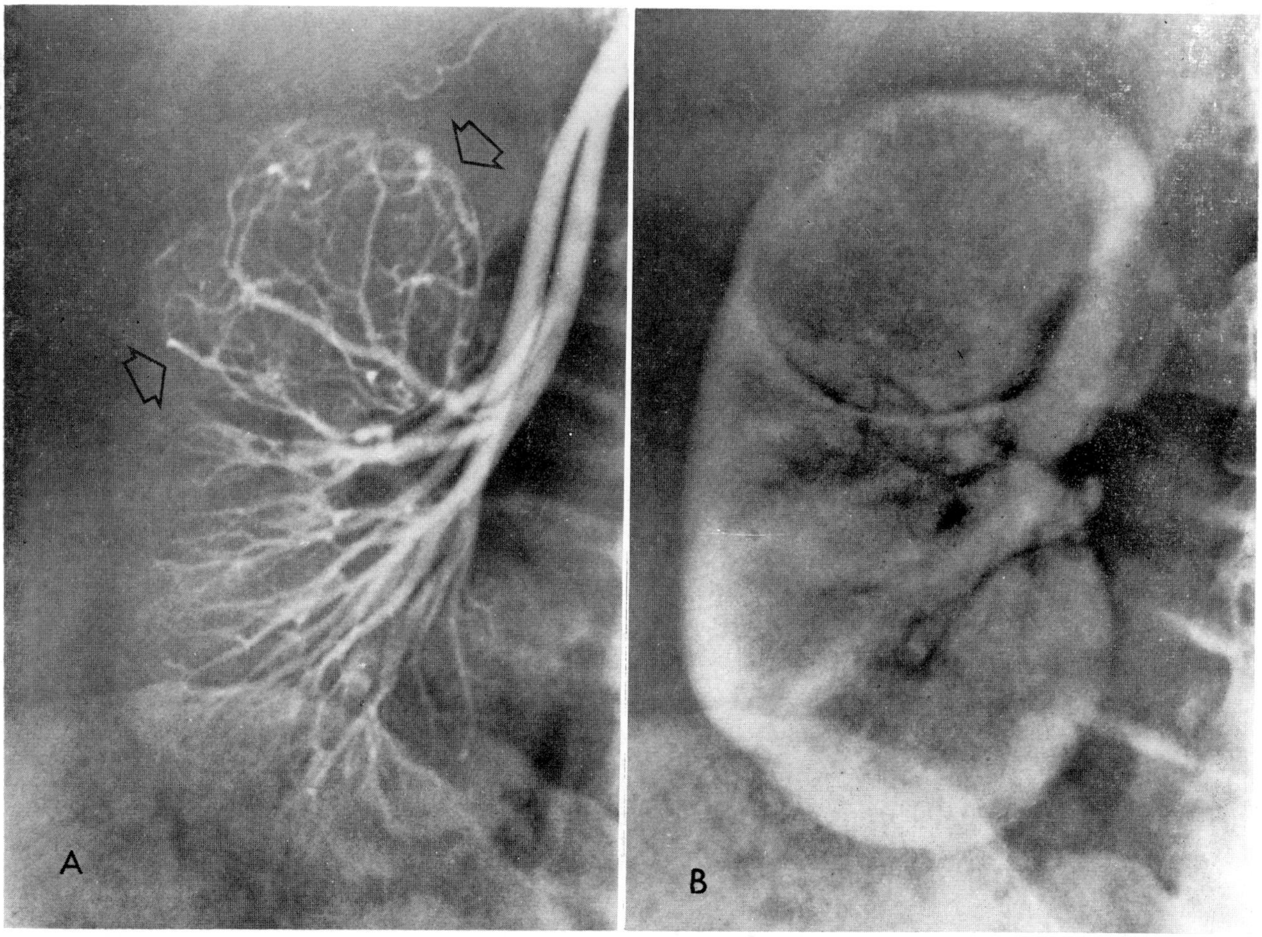

Figure 34.23. Renal Arteriogram. (A) Arterial phase: There is abnormal arborization of renal vessels around and within a mass in the upper pole of the kidney. (B) Smooth homogeneous stain of this well-defined, circumscribed mass occurs in a twenty-three-year-old girl who presented with hypertension. *Diagnosis:* Hypernephroma. A well-fed tumor with high degree of differentiation and an appearance of encapsulation.

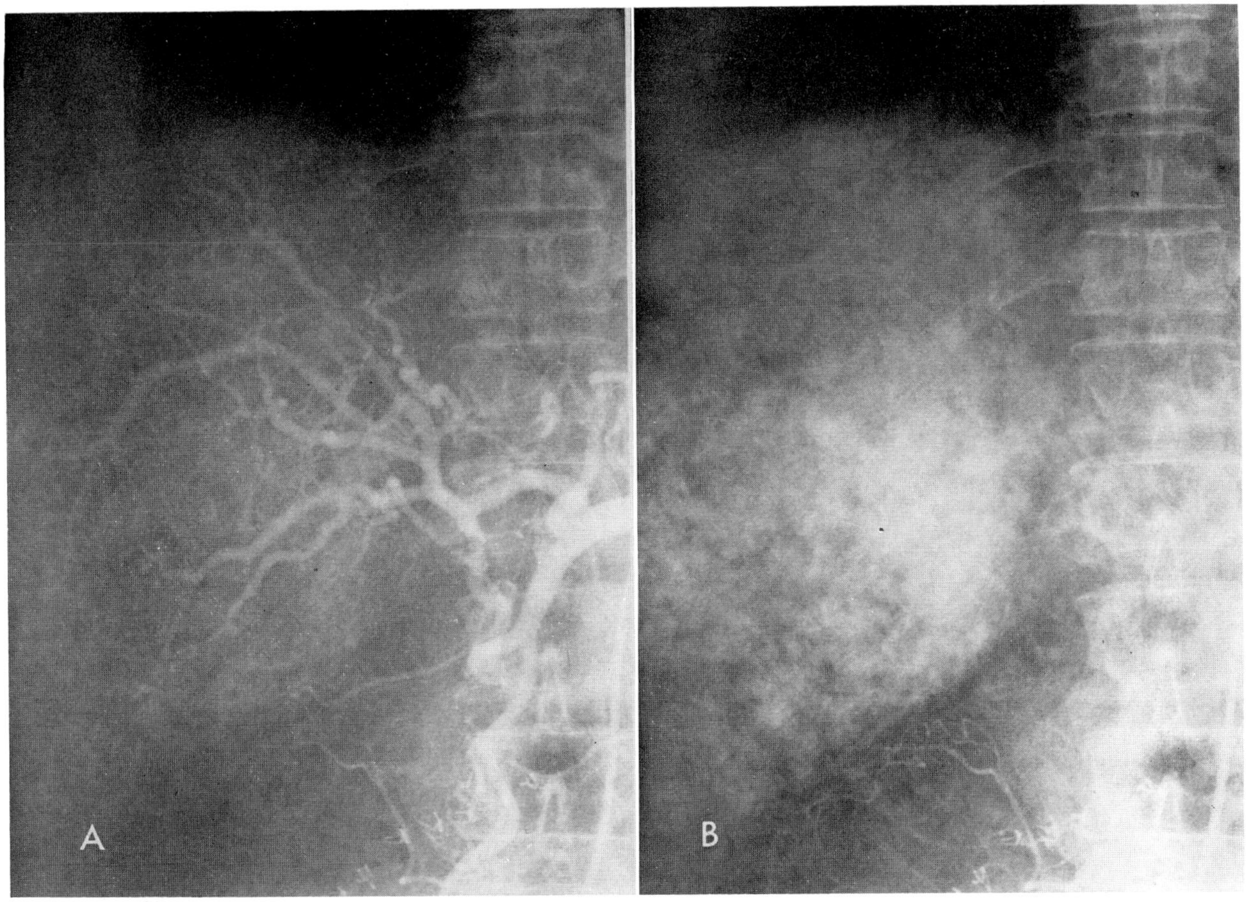

Figure 34.24. Celiac Arteriogram. (A) Arterial phase: There are prominent intrahepatic branches and abnormal arborization with stretching and deviation of the intrahepatic branches. (B) Parenchymal phase: multiple islands of increased density throughout the liver parenchyma are seen. This patient had carcinoma of the breast. *Diagnosis:* Liver metastases from a breast carcinoma.

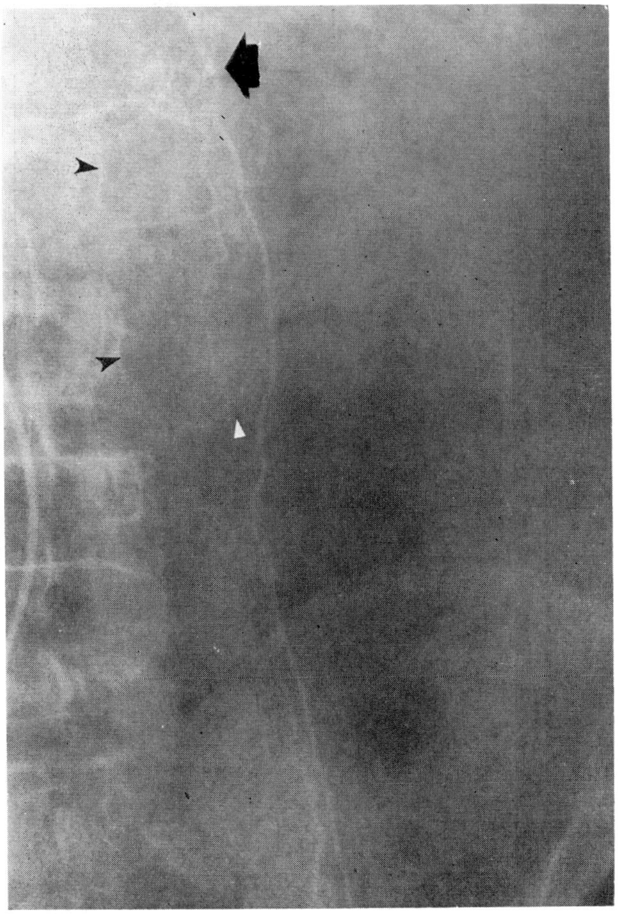

Figure 34.25. Left Gonadal Arteriogram. Abnormally prominent branches course towards the paravertebral area around a mass with slight staining of this mass (Arrow Head). Adrenal branches are given by the same gonadal artery (Arrow). This patient had a nonvisualized kidney on the left side and had no renal artery on the same side on a flush aortogram. *Diagnosis:* Possible embryological remnant of renal tissue with no function. *Pathology:* Lymphoma. Surgery confirmed the absence of left kidney.

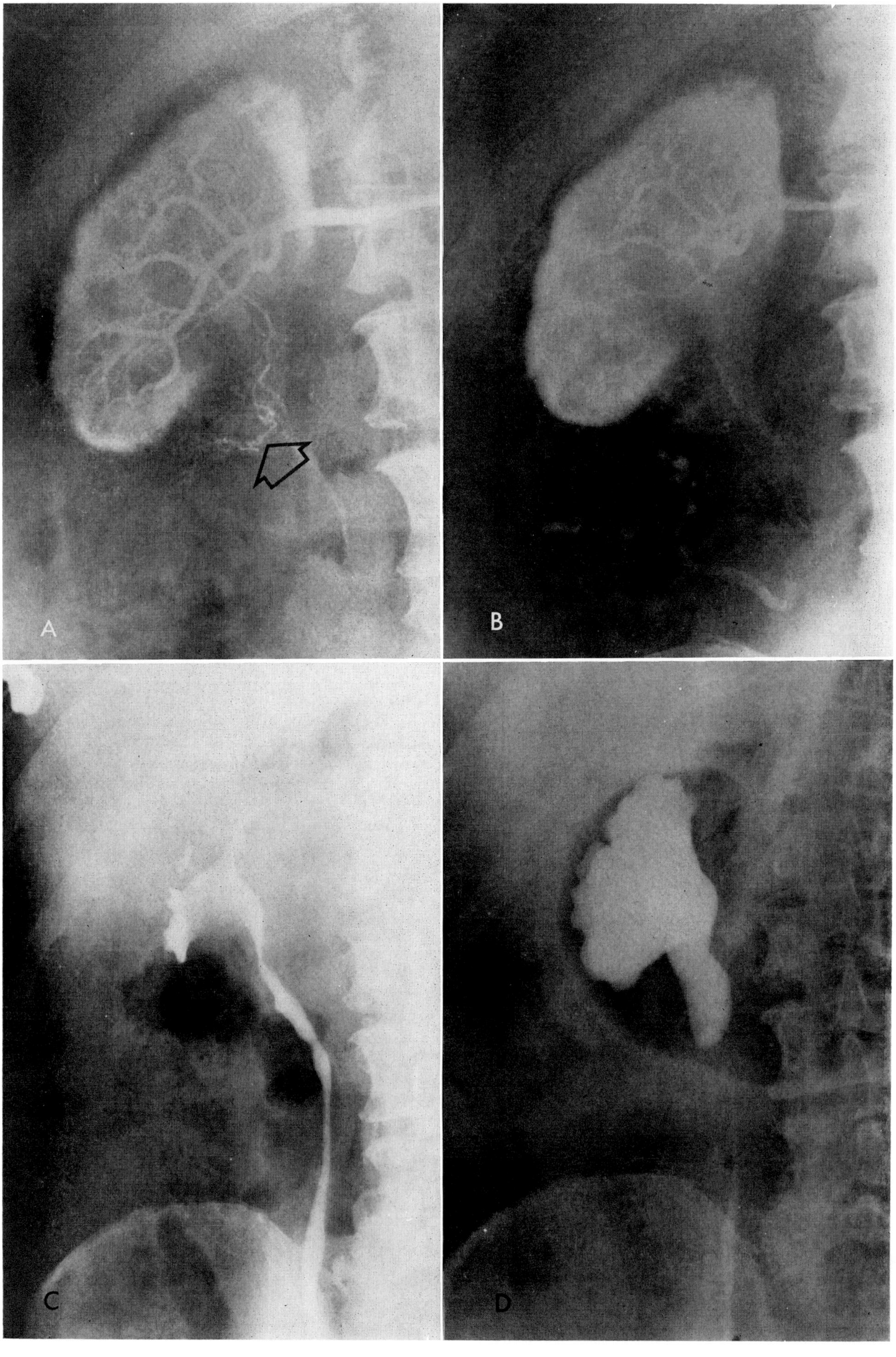
A
B
C
D

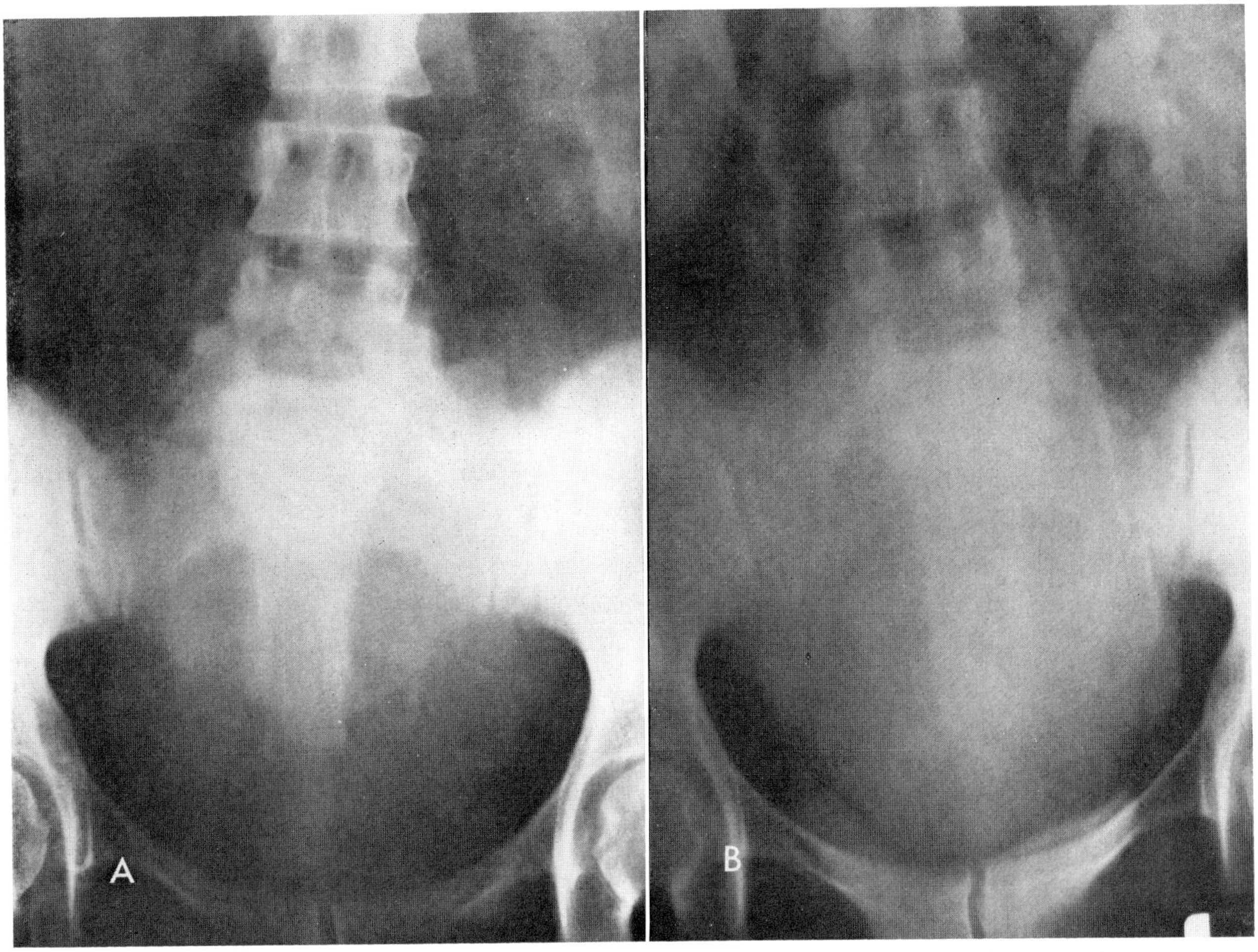

Figure 34.27. (A) Plain tomographic section of the abdomen. A water density mass is in the true pelvis. (B) Total body opacification: Intense staining of this solid mass is seen. *Diagnosis:* Solid mass probably arising from the uterus. May be fibroids of the uterus. *Pathology:* Fibroids of the uterus.

←

Figure 34.26. Renal Arteriogram. (A) Arterial phase: A very prominent pelviureteric branch is seen with a corkscrew course and multiple new vessels. Notice the intrarenal arterial stretching. (B) Increased homogeneous staining in the renal pelvic area and abnormal perinephric tortuous veins suggest increased perinephric activity. (C) A retrograde pyelogram on the same side reveals narrowing of the pelviureteric junction. (D) A retrograde pyelogram four years prior to the present studies reveals dilatation of the proximal ureter with abrupt change in caliber. Surgery four years earlier reveals fibrofatty tissue around the pelviureteric area. The patient recently presented with palpable lymph nodes. *Diagnosis:* Retroperitoneal fibrosis with lymphoma. *Comment:* The abnormal corkscrew vessels at the renal pelvic area with tortuous branches are supplying the fibrofatty mass.

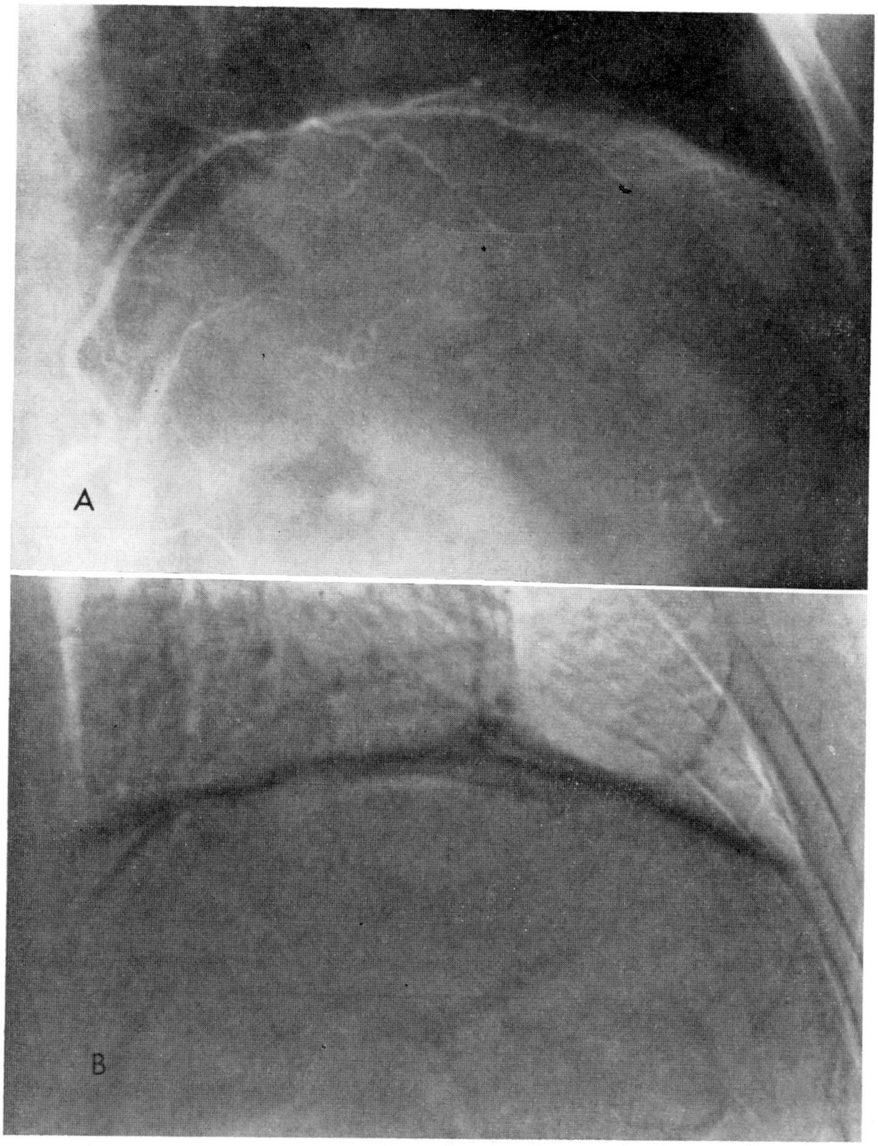

Figure 34.28. Inferior Phrenic Arteriogram. (A) Arterial phase: A prominent left inferior phrenic artery is seen with its anterior and posterior branches. (B) Parenchymal phase (subtraction film): There is staining of the diaphragm which is thicker. *Surgery:* This patient had sclerosing hemangioma (Cholesterol pneumonitis) of the left lower lobe with marked thickening of the diaphragmatic pleura.

CHAPTER 35

INFLAMMATION

HYPEREMIA

BLOOD VESSELS not only react to inflammation,[111, 1263–1267] but also dominate the process as well. Widening of the blood vessels, increased rate of flow and pressure, opening of preexisting or new capillaries, and arteriovenous shunting are all evident adjacent to inflammation, but not within it. The capillary dilatation and the new capillary formation occurs at about three days and reaches its peak by one week. After differentiating into arterioles and veins, they eventually recede to the stable vascular activity of connective tissue.[1261, 1262]

STAIN

Staining is due to increased *permeability* of

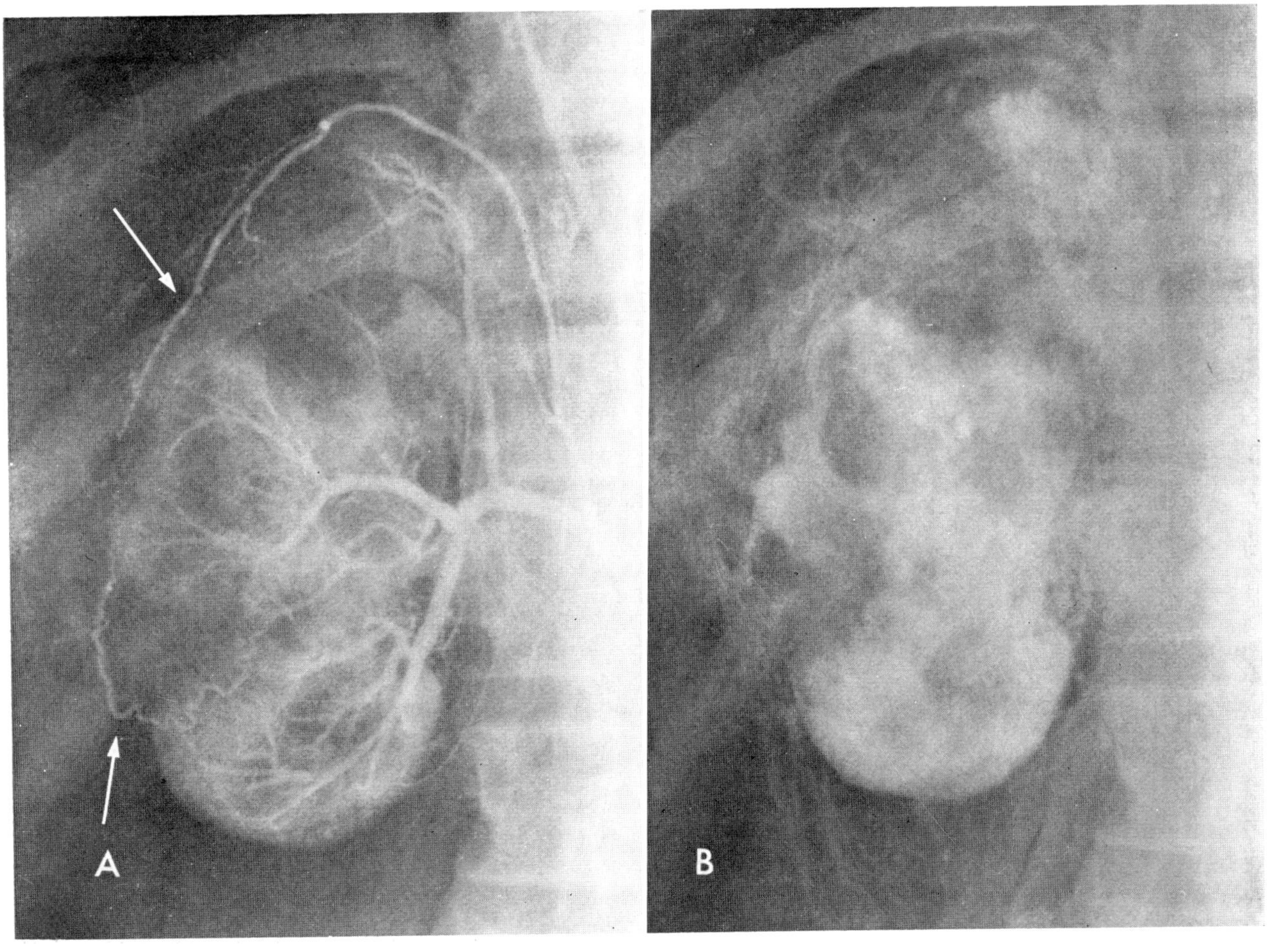

Figure 35.1. Renal Arteriogram. (A) Early phase: Very prominent capsular vessels (Arrows) terminate in the perinephric area with a corkscrew appearance. Islands of avascularity are noted in the renal parenchyma. (B) Late phase: Irregular filling defects and increased perinephric venous circulation are seen. *Diagnosis:* Pyohydronephrosis with perinephric extension.

abnormally fragile vessels with irregular gaps in their endothelial junctions and in the basement membrane. As the lesion progresses there is *genesis of a wall* consisting of new tissue, *granulation tissue*. This is comprised of actively proliferating new capillaries and fibroblasts. The proportion of the constituents of the wall varies, depending on the duration of the inflammatory process. In *subacute* inflammation there is an increase in the vascularity and number of fibroblasts. In *chronic* inflammatory process the tissue is principally proliferative with increase in the number of fibroblasts and decrease in the vascularity. In abscesses the walling off of the inflammation by a very highly vascularized connective tissue occurs with gradual expansion of the necrotic area.

Vascular granulation tissue accompanying the *organization of a hemorrhage* duplicates angiographically the pathologic findings of myositis ossificans[1276, 1277] and muscle rupture.[1278] This aids in obtaining a biopsy from the periphery of the lesion in instances of myositis ossificans circumscripta[1276] to establish a proper diagnosis. Hyperemias and increased stain, even arteriovenous shunting in inflammatory disease

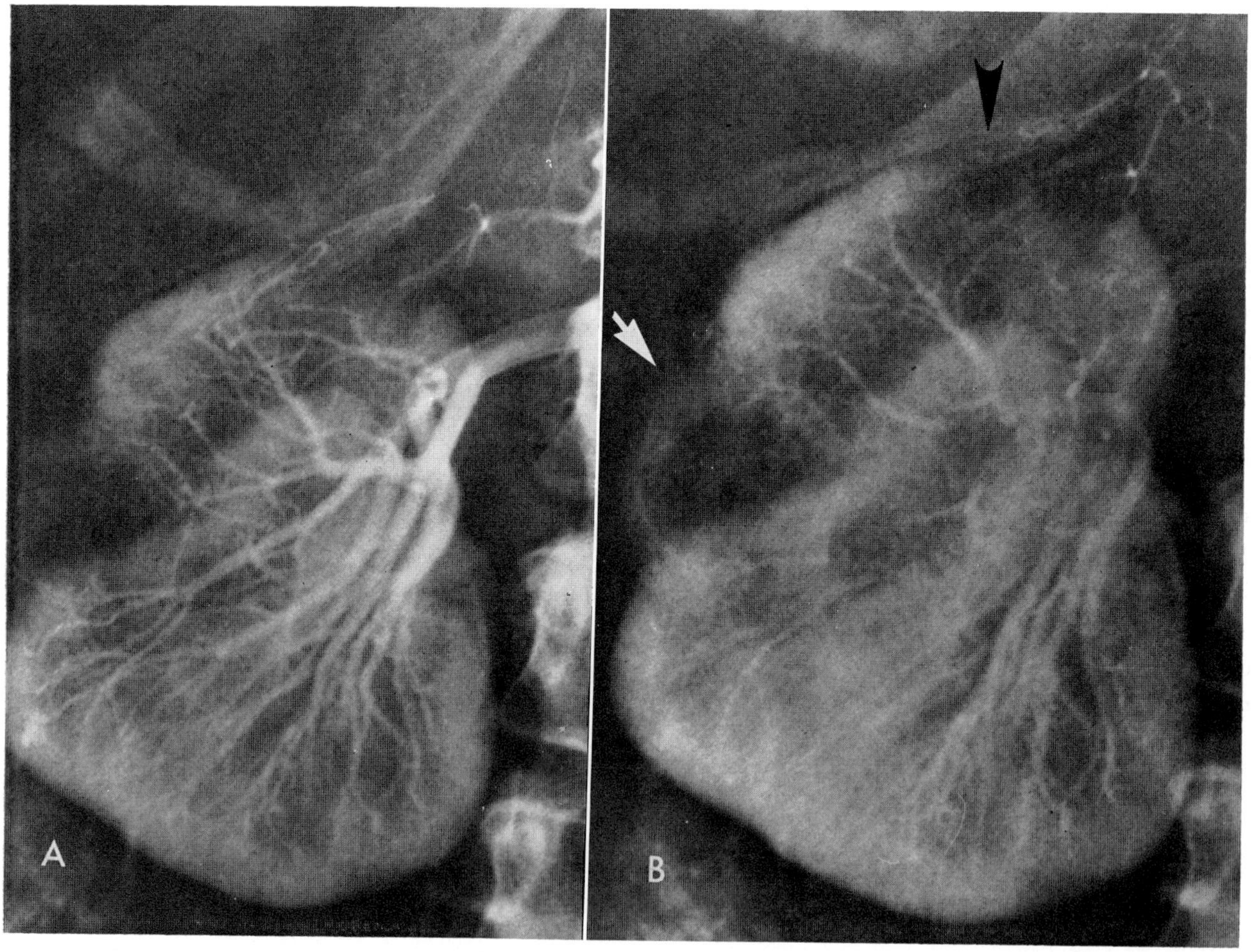

Figure 35.2. Renal Arteriogram. (A) Stretching and deviation of the intrarenal peripheral branches of the kidney with avascular areas are seen. Another avascular area is seen in the upper pole of the same kidney. Notice the surrounding increased vascularity. (B) The avascular lesions are well defined. *Diagnosis:* Abscesses in the kidney versus avascular hypernephromas. *Surgery:* Tuberculous abscesses of the kidney. (Courtesy of Dr. H. Katzen, Chairman, Department of Radiology, Chicago Osteopathic Hospital, Chicago.)

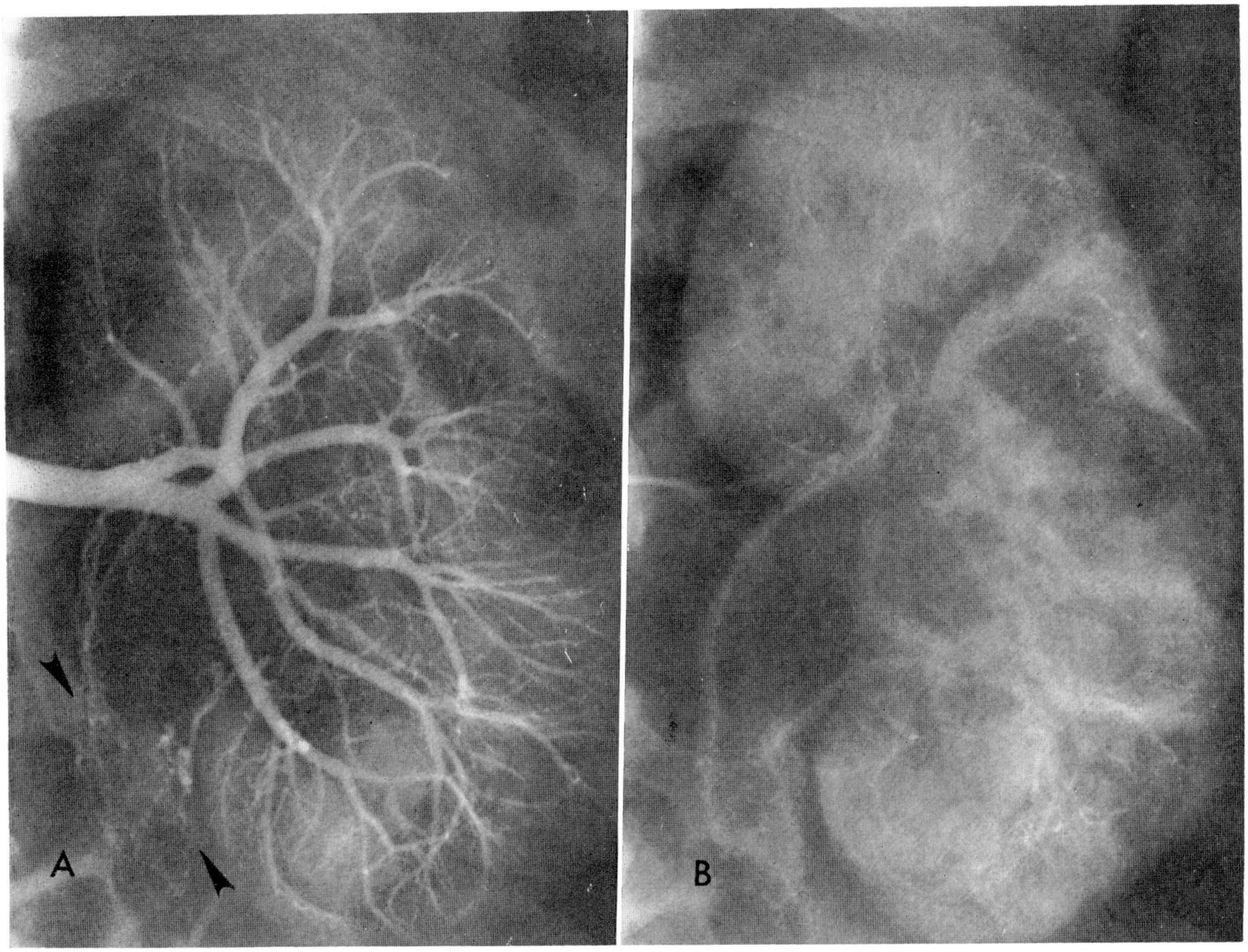

Figure 35.3. Renal Arteriogram. (A) The arterial phase reveals an enlarged kidney with diffuse stretching and deviation of the intrarenal branches. Very prominent pelvic and proximal ureteral vessels with a corkscrew appearance are also seen (Arrows). (B) The parenchymal phase reveals multiple intrarenal filling defects due to dilated calyces and a well-stained, dilated renal pelvis and proximal ureter. *Diagnosis:* Pyohydronephrosis.

of the G.I. tract,[1268–1273] pancreatitis,[1274] and alcoholic hepatitis[1275, 1276] are entities of academic interest. *Synovial hypervascularity* can range from subtle increases in rheumatoid arthritis,[111] synovial osteochondromatosis, neurotropic arthritis, or chronic osteoarthritis[1274] to an extreme degree as seen in pigmented villonodular tenosynovitis.[1275]

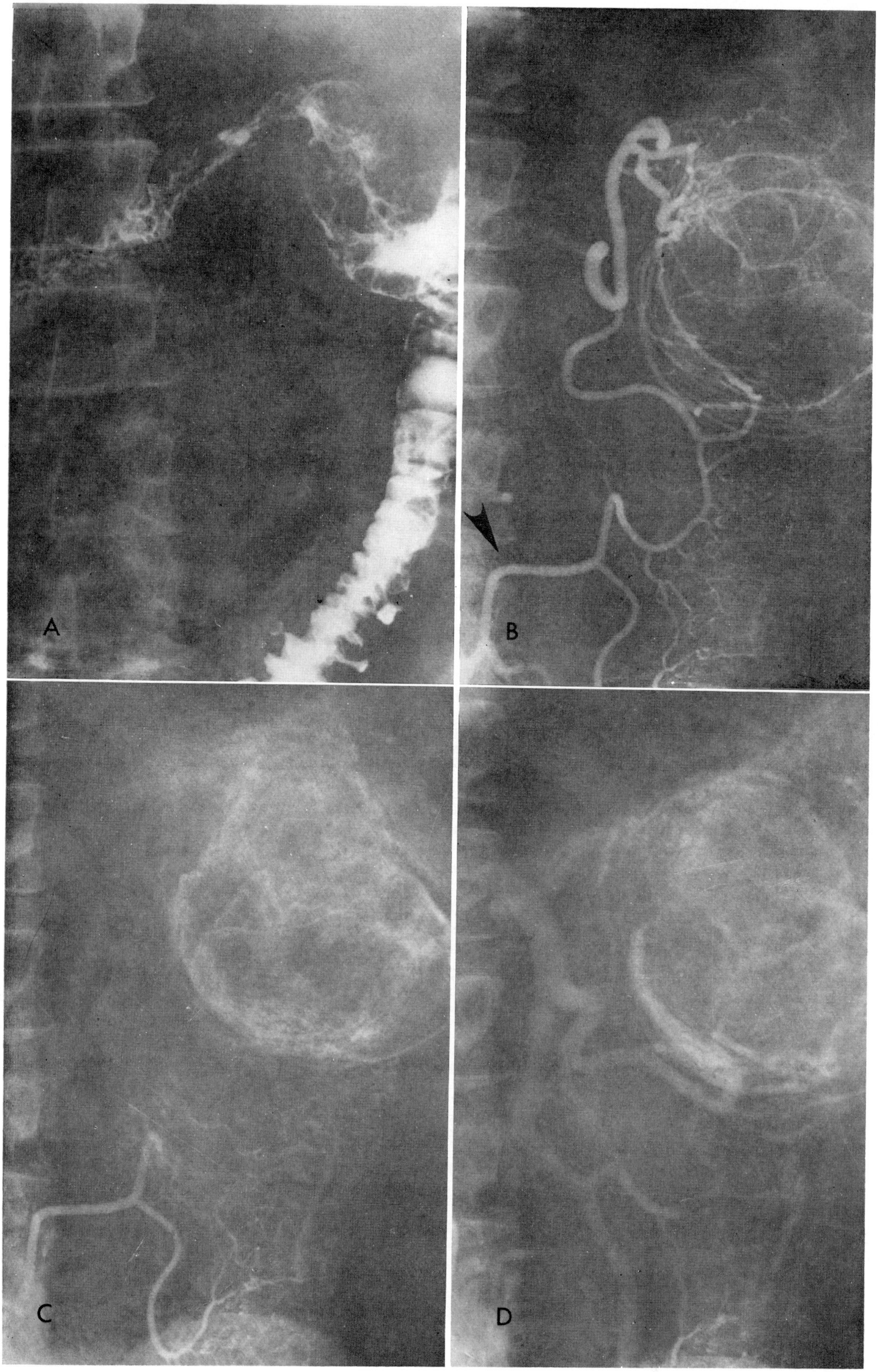
A
B
C
D

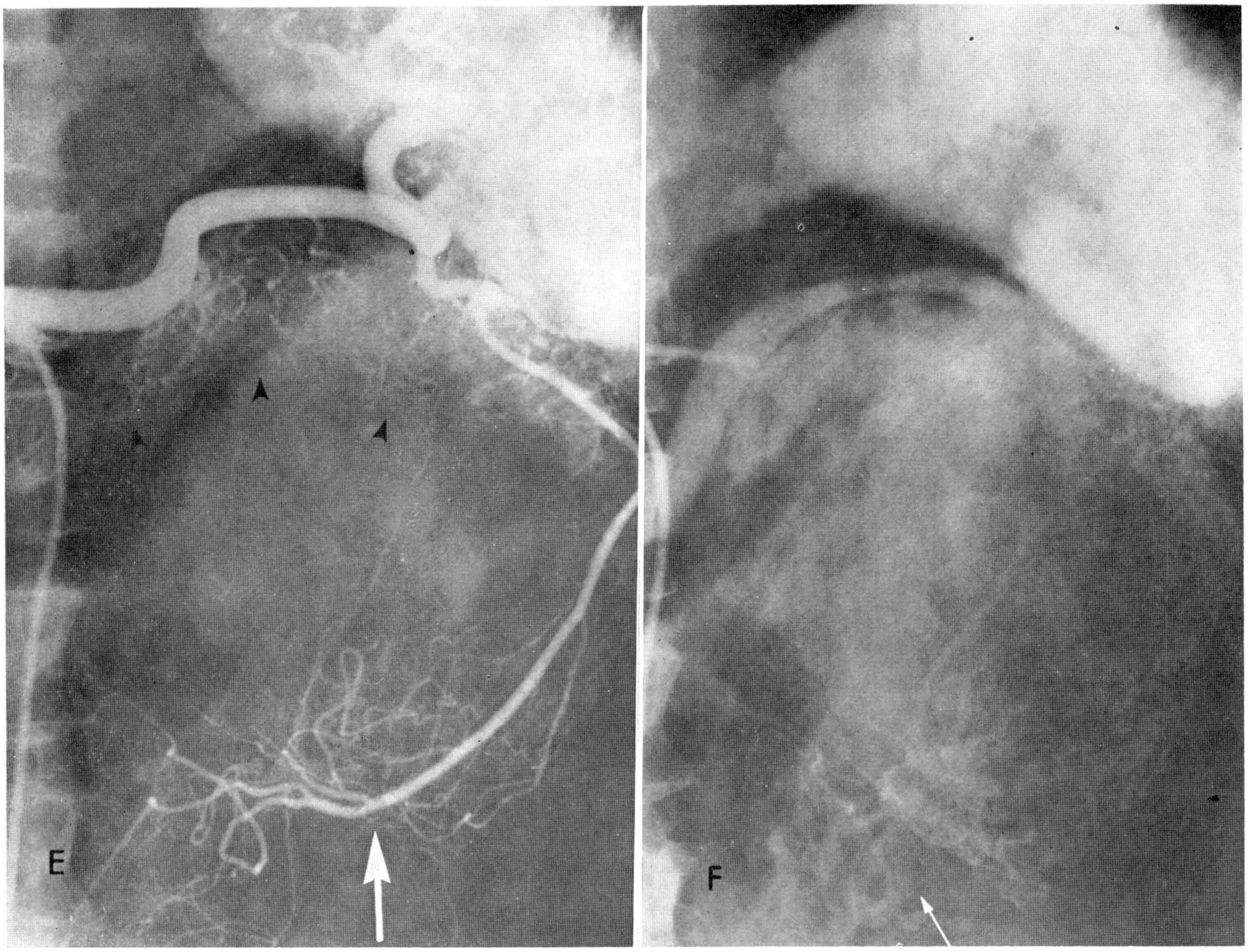

Figure 35.4. (A) Barium enema: A postevacuation film reveals an expansile mass at the splenic flexure level with destruction of the mucosa and a huge soft tissue mass associated with this colon lesion. (B) Inferior mesenteric arteriogram: Very prominent hypertrophied branches from the left colic artery encircle and perfuse this mass with vessels of abnormal caliber. (C) The late arterial phase reveals the dimensions of this mass with irregular staining within the mass as well as the wall of the mass. (D) Late venous phase: There is excessive venous drainage from the same mass towards the inferior mesenteric vein. (E) Splenic arteriogram: A very prominent and elongated omental vessel with numerous branches of normal caliber encircles as well as perfuses the mass (Arrow). Notice the compression of the pancreas by this mass (Arrow Head). (F) Splenic arteriogram venous phase: Peripheral increased staining of this mass and also very prominent veins along the contour of the mass (Arrow) as well as compression of the splenic vein are seen. *Diagnosis:* Carcinoma of the splenic flexure with a huge inflammatory mass adjacent to it.

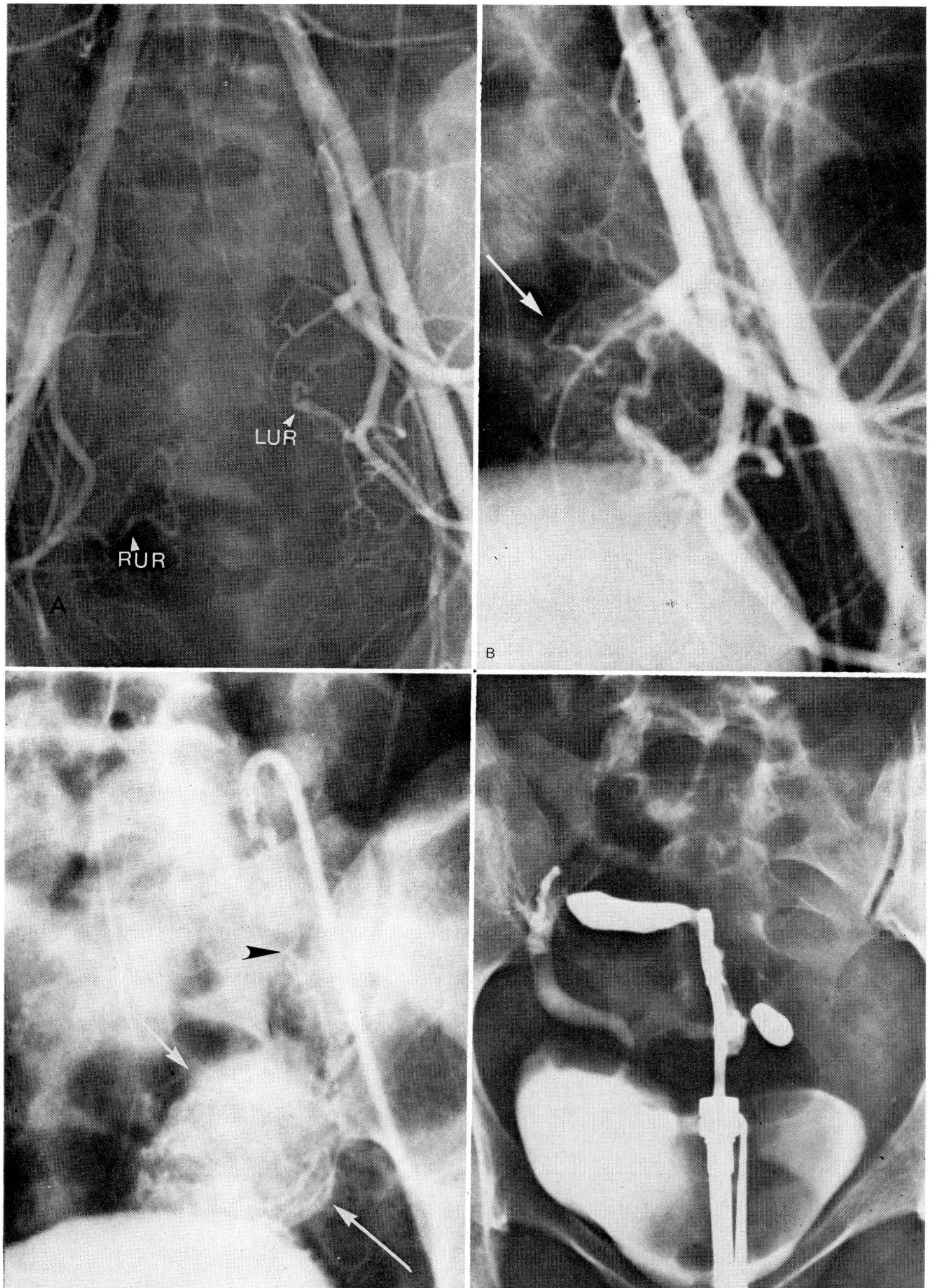
LUR
RUR
A
B
C
D

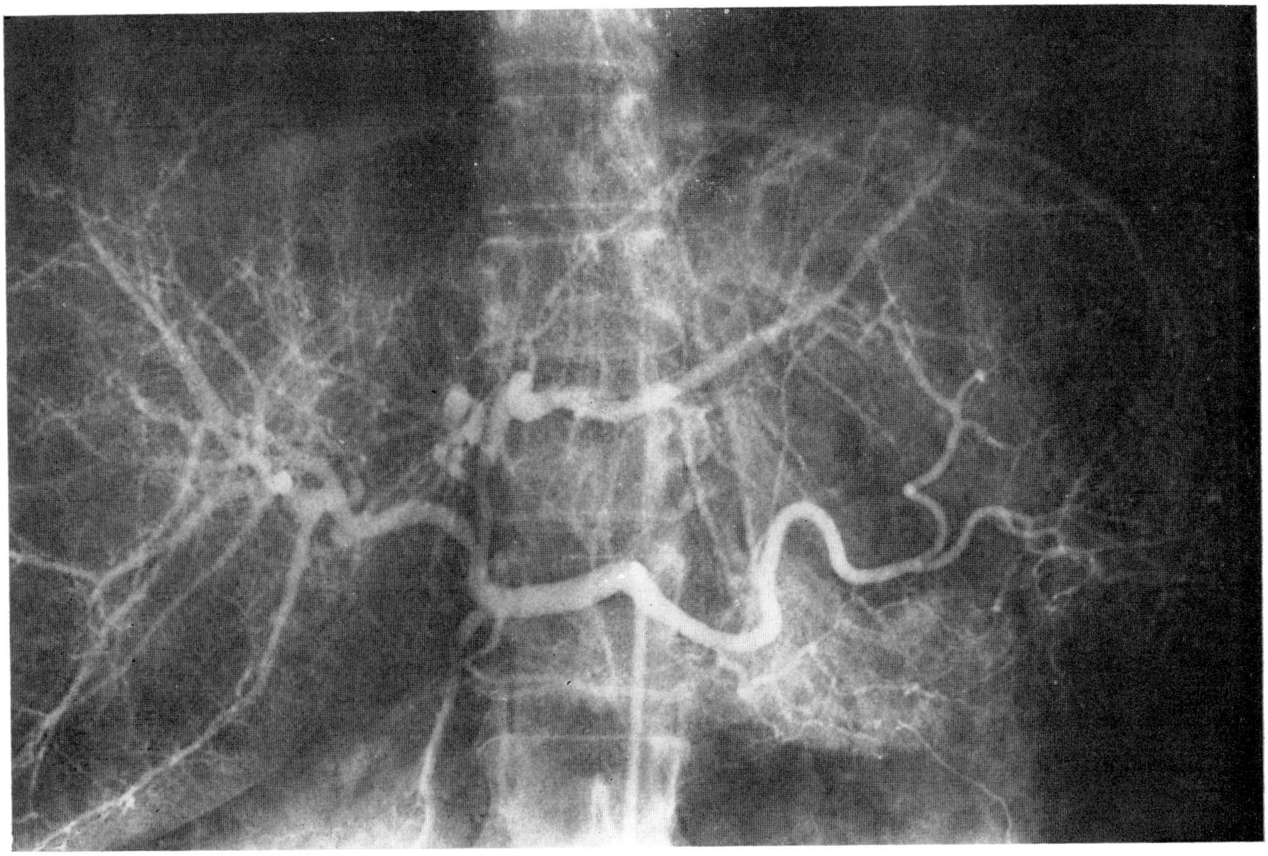

Figure 35.6. Celiac Arteriogram. There is an increased number of small vessels of the hepatic arcade as well as stretching of the intrahepatic vessels. The patient was a known alcoholic. *Diagnosis:* Alcoholic cirrhosis with alcoholic hepatitis.

←

Figure 35.5. (A) Pelvic arteriogram: An abnormal course of the left uterine artery (L.U.R.). The course of the uterine artery on the right side (R.U.R.) is normal. (B) Midarterial phase of internal iliac arteriogram on the left side. The uterine artery courses around a moderately sized hypervascular mass (Arrow). Minimal filling of the left ovarian artery (Arrow Head) can be seen. (C) Late arterial phase: A faint, homogeneous stain of this mass (Arrow) is present. (D) Hysterosalpingogram: A peculiarly shaped uterus without filling of the left salpinx is demonstrated. *Diagnosis:* Possible bicornuate uterus with an infected left component. *Surgery:* Double uterus with infection and pyometra.

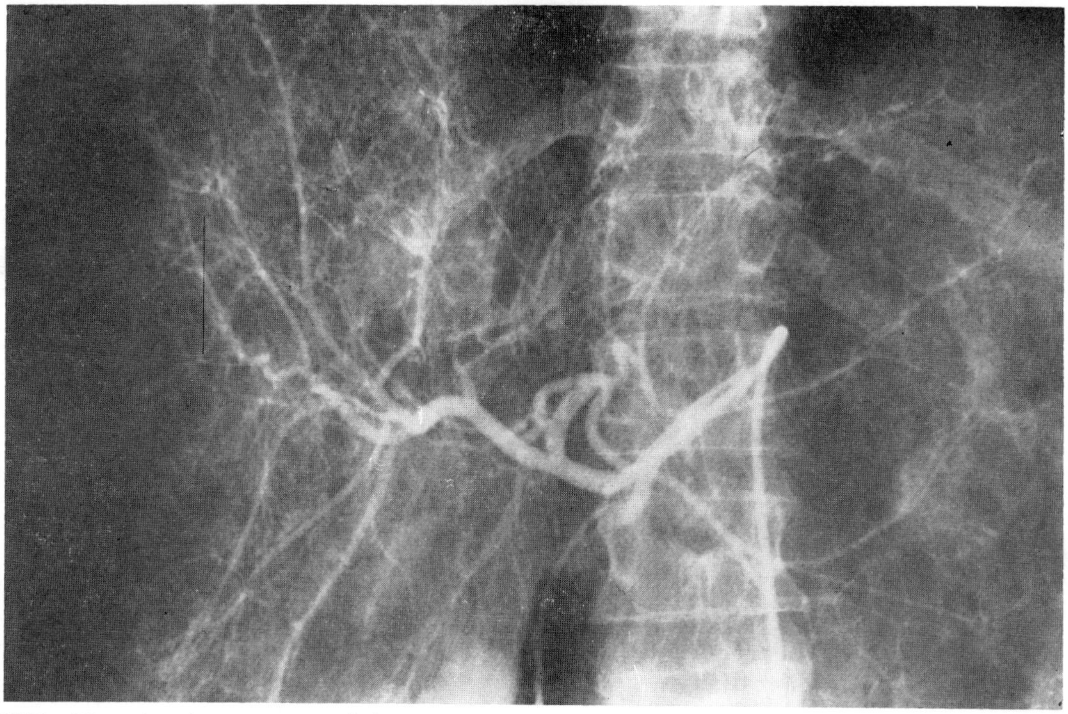

Figure 35.7. Hepatic Arteriogram. (A) There is stretching of the intrahepatic branches of the right lobe of the liver. Those to the left lobe (Arrows) are stretched and deviated. There is an increase in the number of small vessels. Radioisotope scan revealed normal uptake of radioactive material by the left lobe of the liver. *Diagnosis:* Advanced cirrhosis with regeneration of the left lobe of the liver.

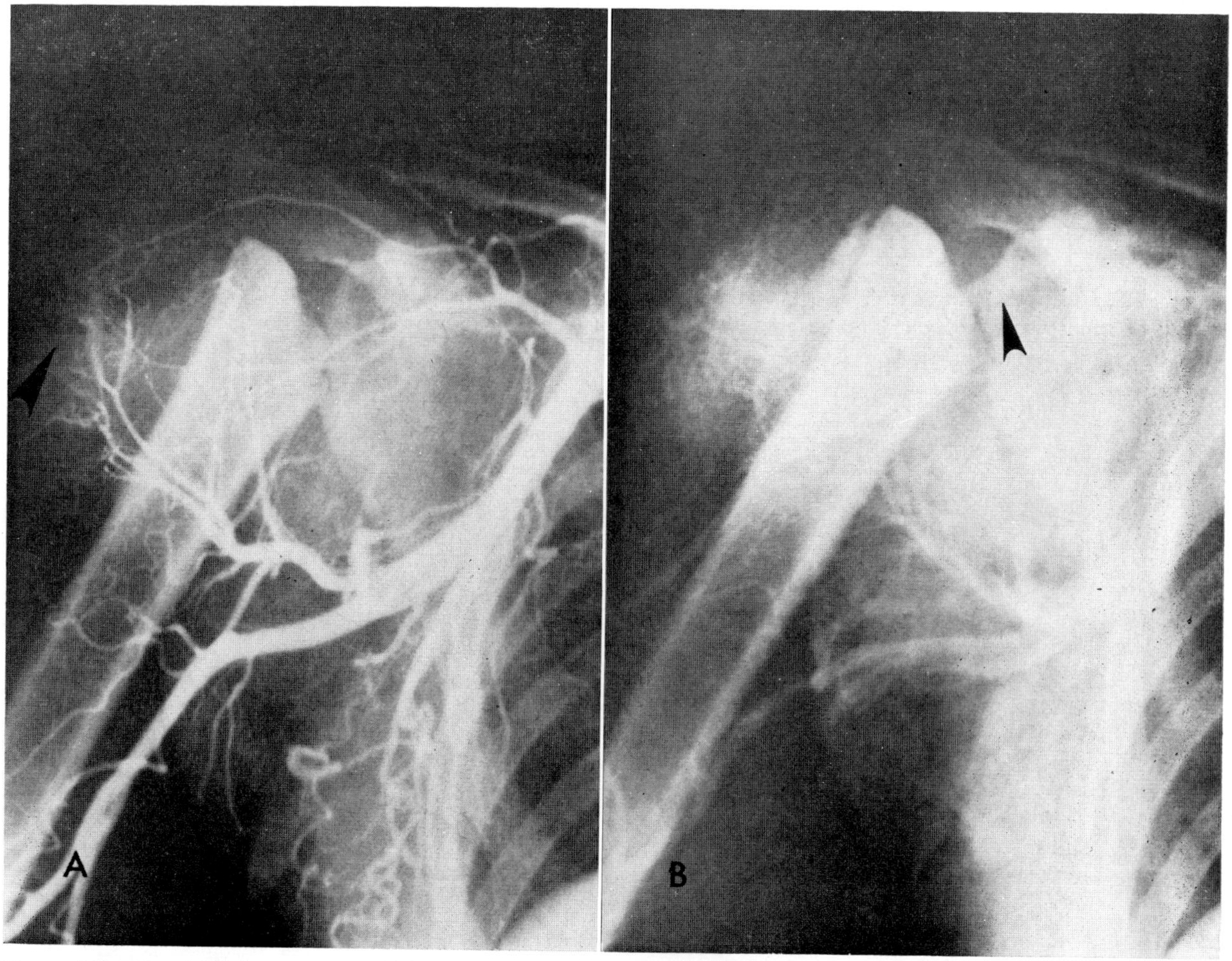

Figure 35.8. Brachial Arteriogram. (A) There is hypervascularity about the shoulder joint capsule (Arrow Head) and deviation of the axillary artery. (B) There is relatively early venous drainage. This patient had a swollen shoulder joint and the demonstrated osseous abnormalities. *Diagnosis:* Neurotrophic arthropathy with hyperemia and effusion into the disorganized joint.

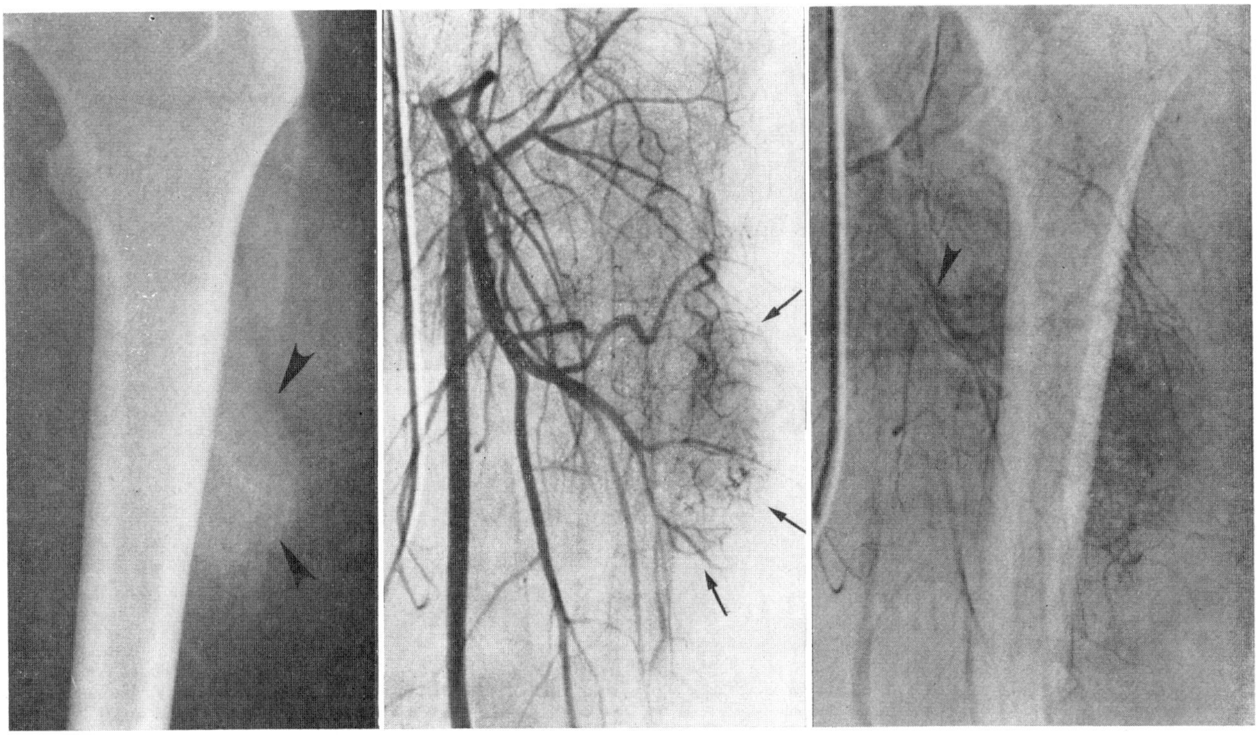

Figure 35.9. Femoral Arteriogram. (A) A plain film of the thigh reveals a well-defined mass with calcifications. (B) Early arterial phase: The same mass is perfused with irregular vessels with obvious hypervascularity. (C) Early A.V. Shunting is shown by opacification of the regional veins (Arrow). *Diagnosis:* Malignant tumor versus myositis ossificans. *Surgery:* Myositis ossificans. (From Probst, F. P. Angiography in juxtacortical osteosarcomas. *Acta Radiologica, 11*:49, 1971. Courtesy of the author and publishers.)

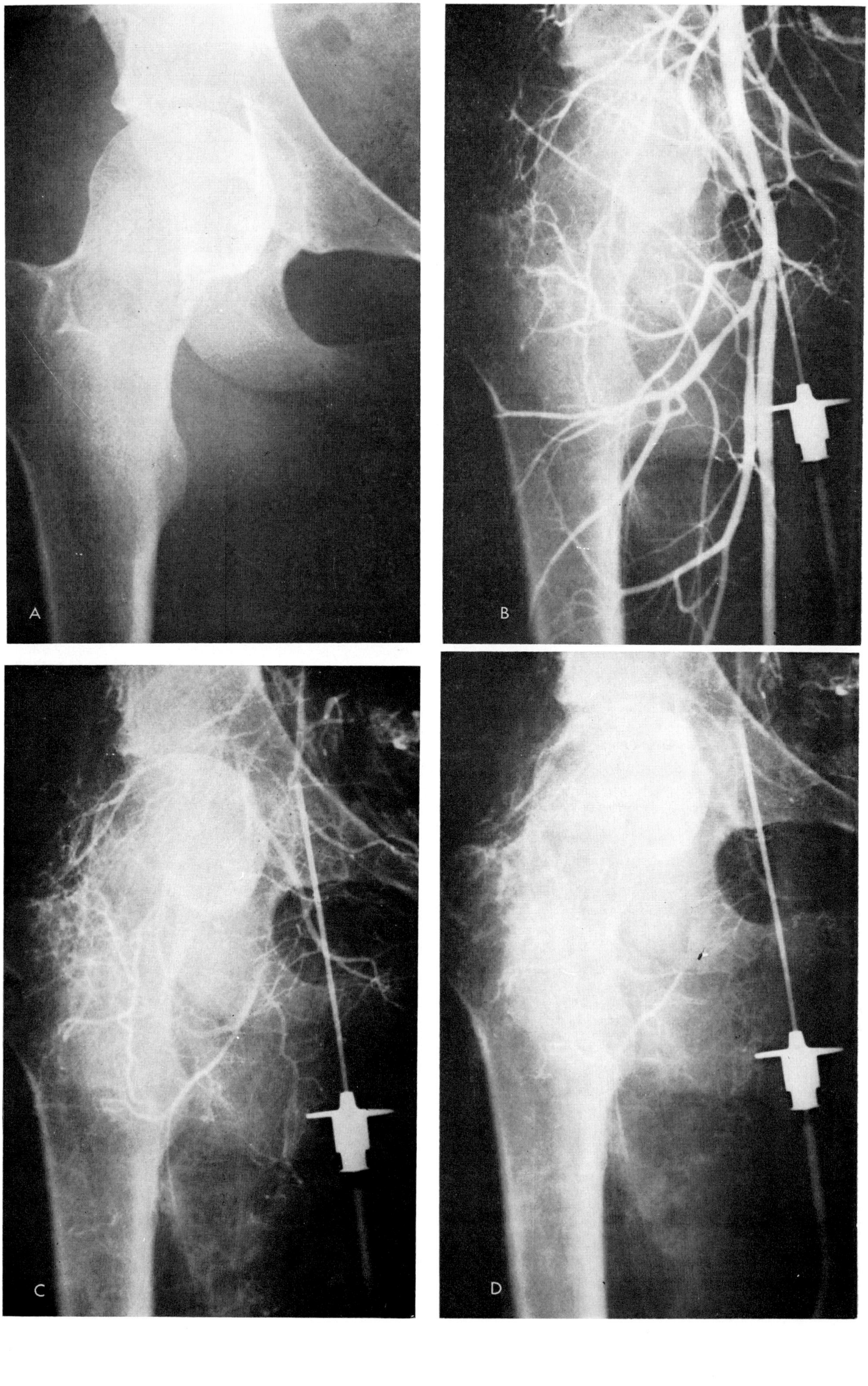
A
B
C
D

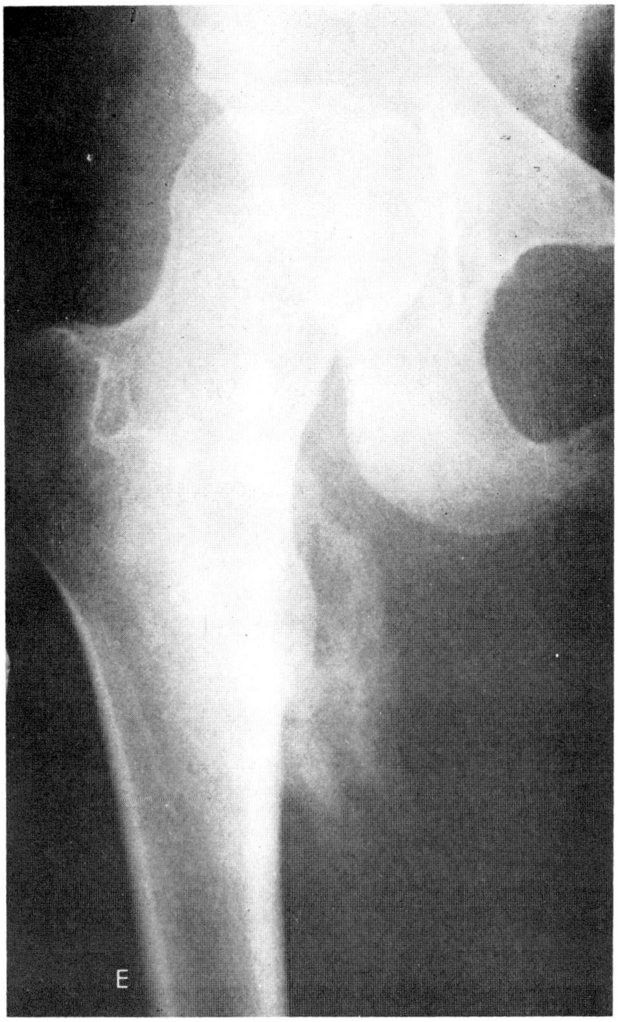

Figure 35.10. (A) A plain film reveals soft tissue mass adjacent to the lesser trochanter forty-two days after trauma. (B) Femoral arteriogram: Hypervascularity. (C) Late arterial phase: Again increased vascularity is seen without A.V. shunting. (D) Increased staining is seen in the same area. *Diagnosis:* Sarcoma. *Pathology:* Myositis ossificans. (E) Calcification in the mass sixty days after trauma. (From Hutcheson, J., Klatte, E. C., and Kremp, R. The angiographic appearance of myositis ossificans circumscripta. *Radiol, 102:*57, 1972. Courtesy of the authors and publishers.)

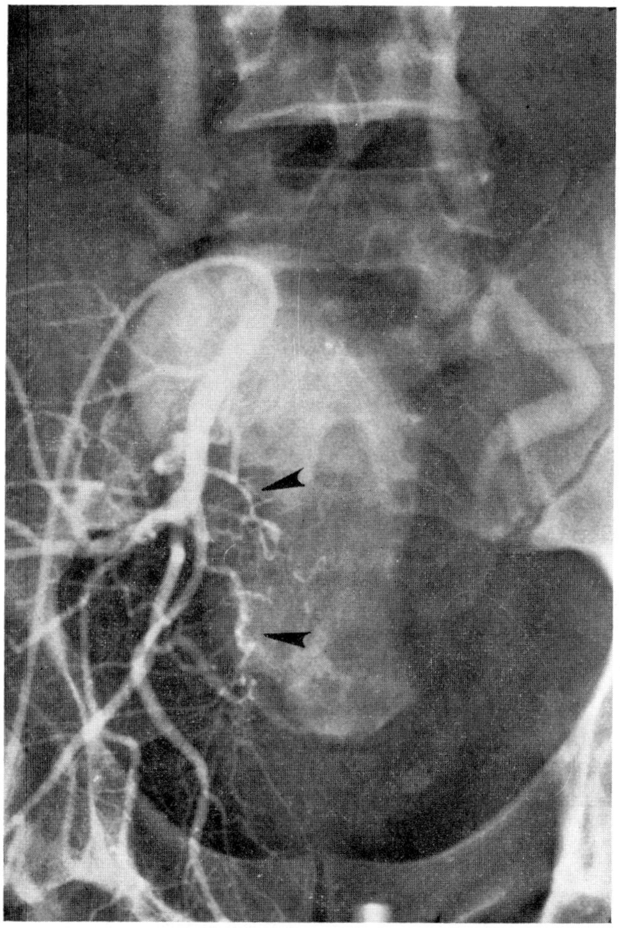

Figure 35.11. Right Internal Iliac Arteriogram. There is deviation of the parietal branches of the internal iliac artery with slightly increased vascularity (Arrow) and compression of the urinary bladder bilaterally with moderate hydronephrosis. *Diagnosis:* Pelvic lipomatosis. *Comment:* The plain films of the true pelvis revealed increased lucency. Surgery confirmed the diagnosis.

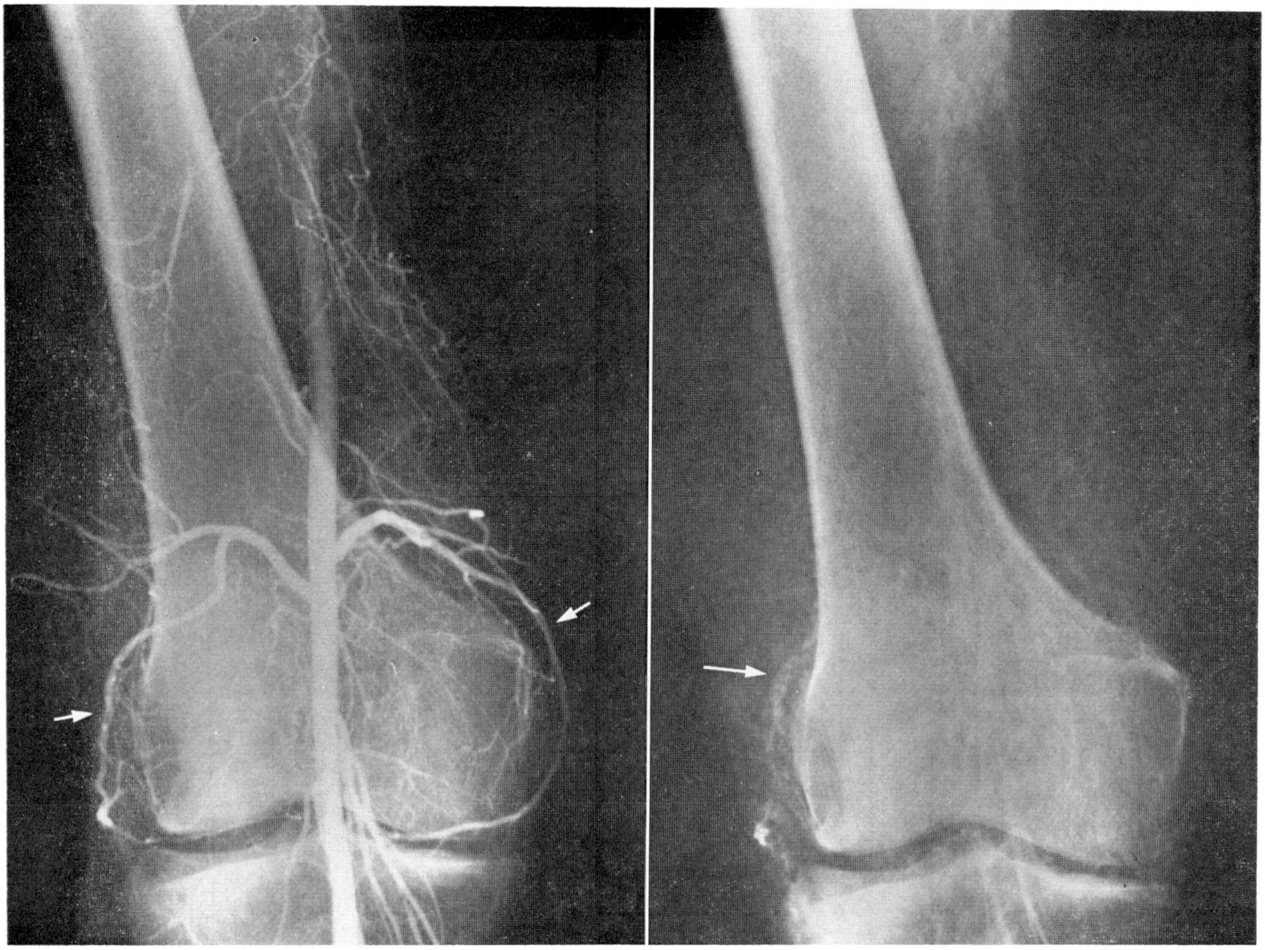

Figure 35.12. Femoral Arteriogram. (A) Arterial phase: There are very prominent branches perfusing the synovial membrane of the knee joint (Arrows). (B) Late phase: There is early venous opacification (Arrows) in a patient who had swelling of that knee. *Diagnosis:* Synovial hyperemia due to chronic synovitis? *Arthrogram and Surgery:* Revealed synovial chondromatosis.

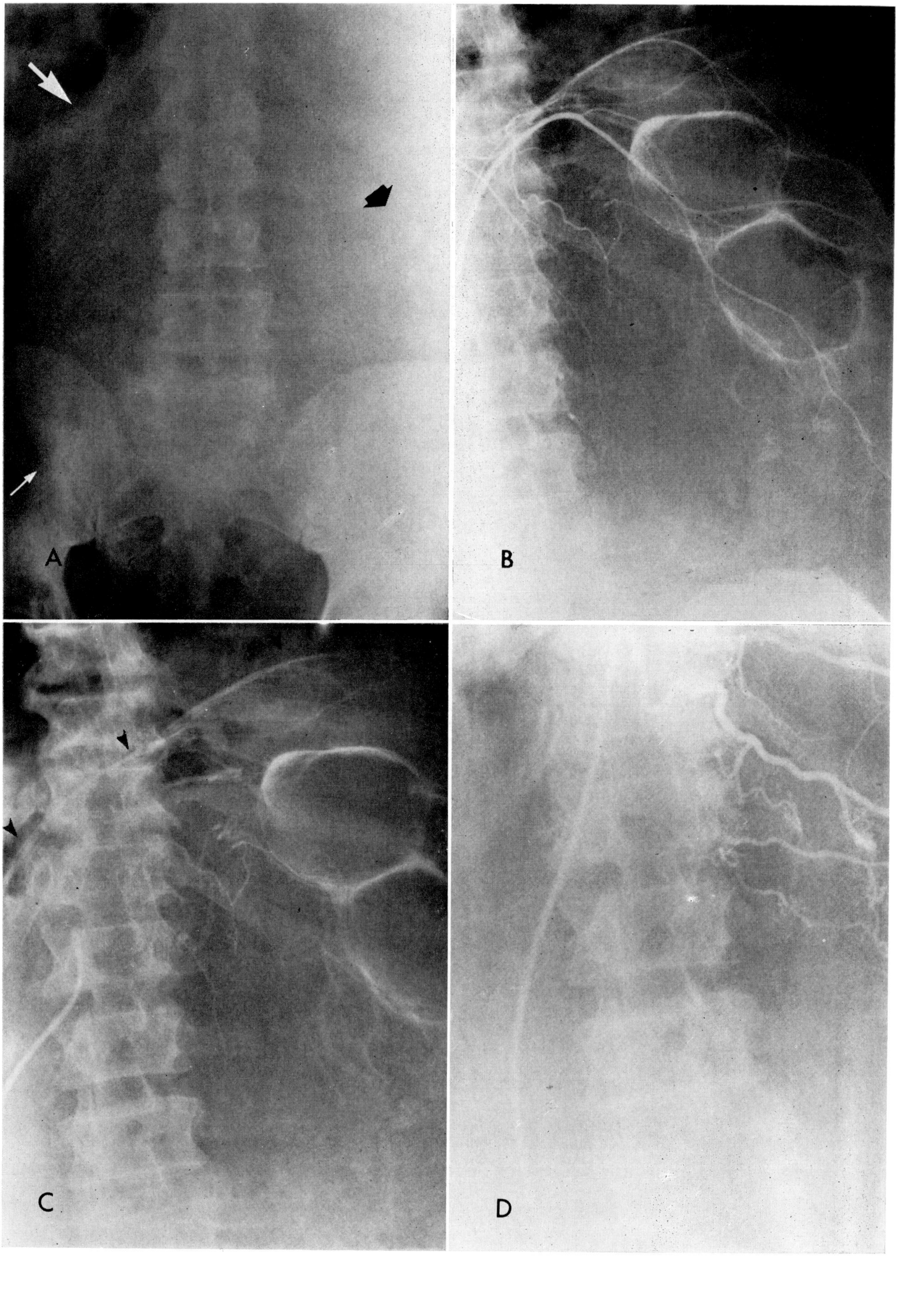
A
B
C
D

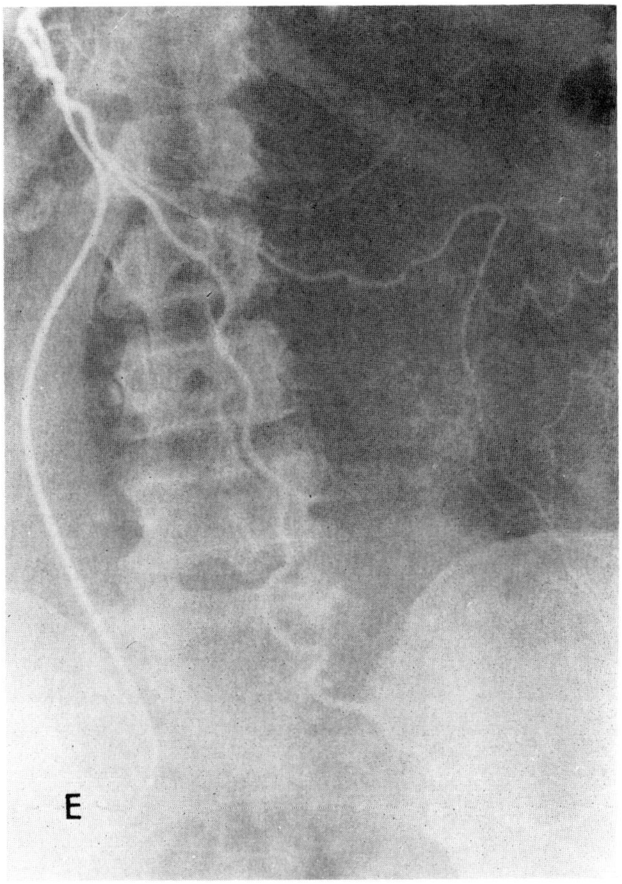

Figure 35.13. (A) Scout film of the abdomen reveals a huge mass and some calcific densities (Arrow). (B) Renal arteriogram reveals thinning and stretching of the main renal artery as well as renal hilar and intrarenal branches. (C) Late phase reveals hydronephrosis of the left kidney and opacification of a huge cystic structure which has a thin wall. (D) Lumbar arteriogram reveals marked hypervascularity. (E) Inferior phrenic arteriogram reveals its prominent branches arborizing on the surface of this thin-walled mass. *Diagnosis:* Cystadenomatoid tumor from the retroperitoneum or a necrotic tumor obtaining parasitic vascular supply. *Pathology:* Huge hydronephrosis. The enormous cystic structure was the dilated renal pelvis.

CHAPTER 36
TUMORS

VASCULAR WALL TUMORS

Hemangiomas

THESE ARE AUTONOMOUS new growths in which there is formation of new vessels or proliferation of the vessel walls.[1213, 1214] They may remain constant in size or may grow *pari passu* with the individual; the momentum of growth is uncertain and self-limited. The growth of the *vessels,* whether a *simple elongation* such as *capillary hemangiomas* or *sinusoidal pools in cavernous hemangiomas,* is accomplished by mechanical pressure of the circulation. Therefore, the growth and type of a hemangioma is somewhat influenced by its blood supply. These lesions are characterized by capillary and cavernous networks of irregular endothelial tubes of varying size lacking elastic tissue, arranged closely and branching repeatedly with tortuous curves supplied by a single artery and drained by a single vein.

Hemangiomas are usually of an indolent disposition and may continue to grow in proportion with the neighboring tissues. They may be well delineated or nondescript, totally arterial or totally venous, with or without variable components of fibrous tissue or fat within them.[1215, 1216] They may regress and become atrophied or fibrotic. In pregnant women and some children it is not unusual for these tumors to attain a large size rapidly and exsanguinate. Large hemangiomas can cause cardiac failure.[1222] If they occur in the portal circulation,[1223] they may cause portal hypertension or hematuria if they develop within the kidney.[1224] Synovial[1225] and skeletal muscle[1226] hemangiomas are of unusual angiographic and clinical interest. When a capillary hemangioma is transformed into a solid cellular mass by progressive proliferation of connective tissue, it is termed a *sclerosing hemangioma*[1213, 1214] which is obviously avascular angiographically.

Cavernous hemangiomas have blood vessels which are more dilated than those in capillary hemangiomas. This is due to an expanding connection between the general circulation and the feeding channels of the hemangioma. As a result, the capillaries become distended to form pools or sinuses. These cul-de-sacs are limited by thin septa and a *sluggish circulation.* Thrombosis and organization are not uncommon in these tumors. *Visceral hemangiomas are usually cavernous and seen most frequently in the liver.* Characteristic features *angiographically*[1217, 1218] are large feeding vessels and vascular spaces arranged in a ring-like shape or C-shape due to the fibrous obliteration of the center. A very slow washout of the contrast, characteristic of sinusoidal pools, is frequently seen in these cavernous spaces. The extent of avascularity depends on the amount of fibrosis present in the lesion. Extreme cases may be totally avascular resulting from complete obliteration of the hemangioma by fibrous tissue[1219] (renal[1227]) (Figs. 36-1 to 36-4 and 36-74).

Hemangioendothelioma[111, 642, 1220] is a true neoplasm of vascular origin arising from the endothelial cells. It is more cellular than a capillary hemangioma. Small blood-filled channels lined by single to multiple layers of endothelium characterize this lesion. A hemangioendothelioma is actually a grade of tumor falling between hemangiomas and hemangiosarcomas. On angiography, dilated tortuous vessels with *arteriovenous shunting* are seen, unlike hemangiomas or hemangiosarcomas. They are more common in children, and congestive heart failure may occur with tumors of sufficient size.[1221]

Angiosarcoma[642] is a rare tumor usually oc-

(Text continues on page 694)

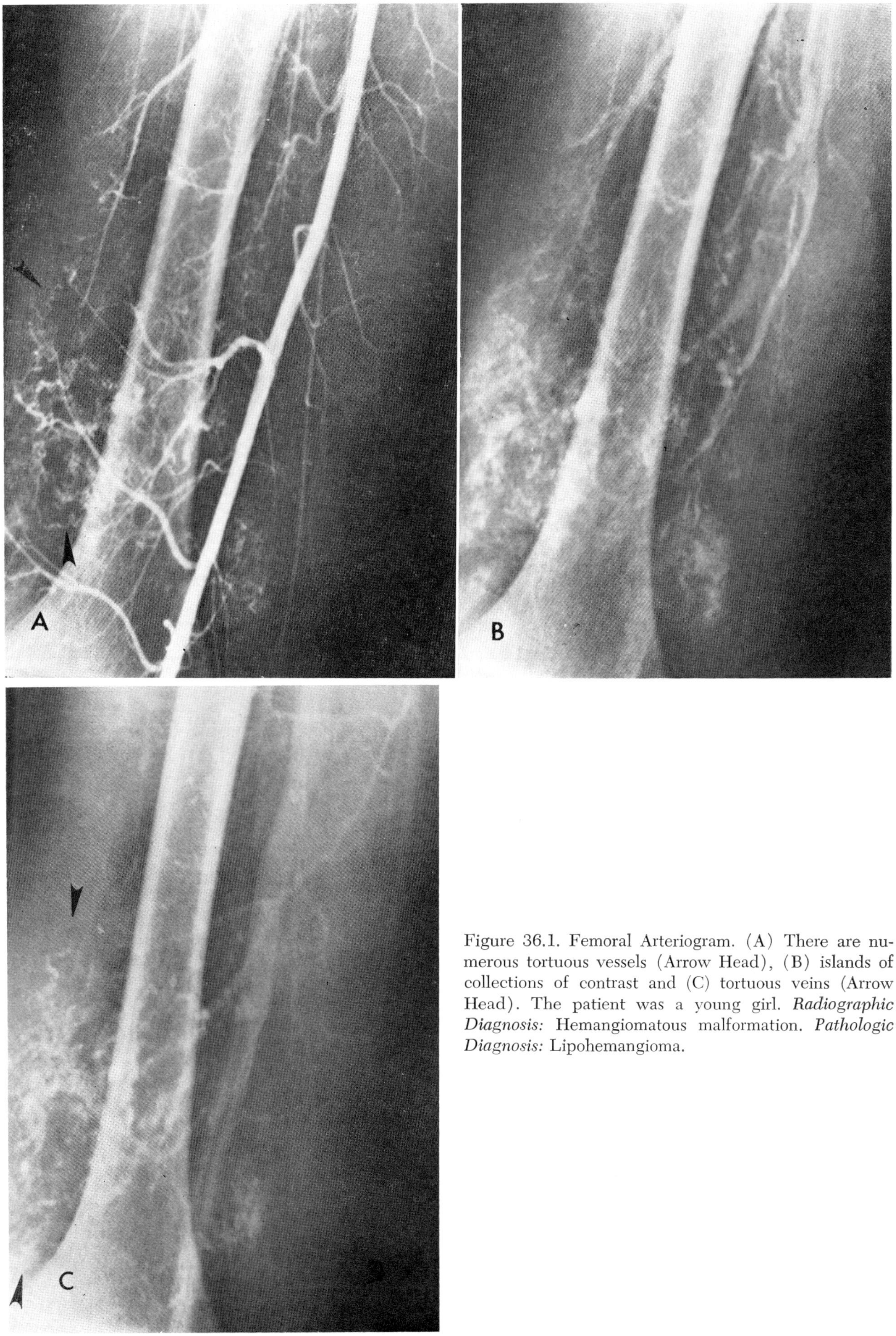

Figure 36.1. Femoral Arteriogram. (A) There are numerous tortuous vessels (Arrow Head), (B) islands of collections of contrast and (C) tortuous veins (Arrow Head). The patient was a young girl. *Radiographic Diagnosis:* Hemangiomatous malformation. *Pathologic Diagnosis:* Lipohemangioma.

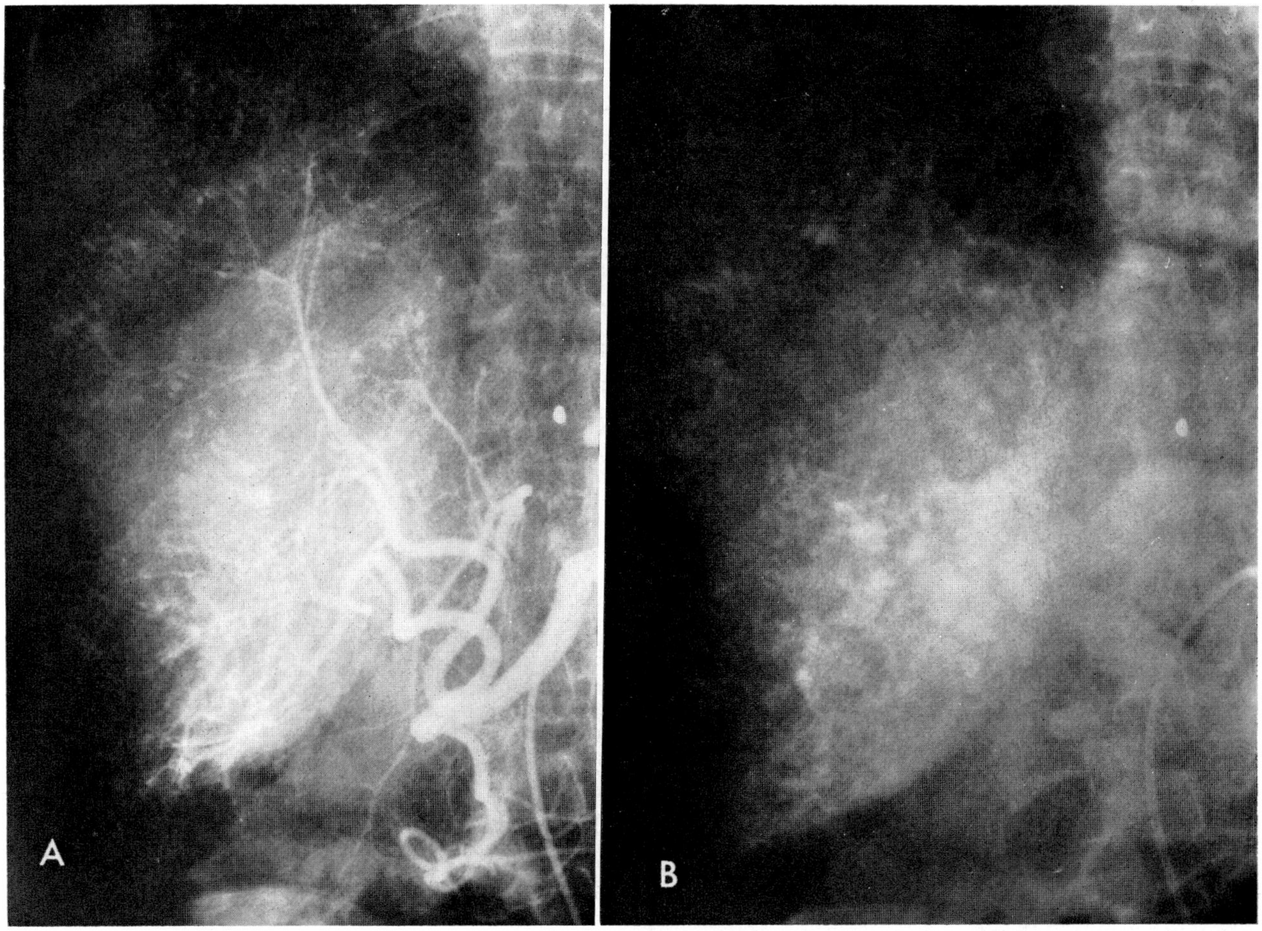

Figure 36.2. Celiac Arteriogram. (A) Arterial phase: Reveals abnormal collections of contrast material from the terminal branches of the intrahepatic branches. (B) Parenchymal phase: Reveals the same. *Diagnosis:* Hemangioma of the liver. (Courtesy of Dr. J. Petasnick, Associate Professor, Diagnostic Radiology, Rush Presbyterian Medical Center, Chicago.)

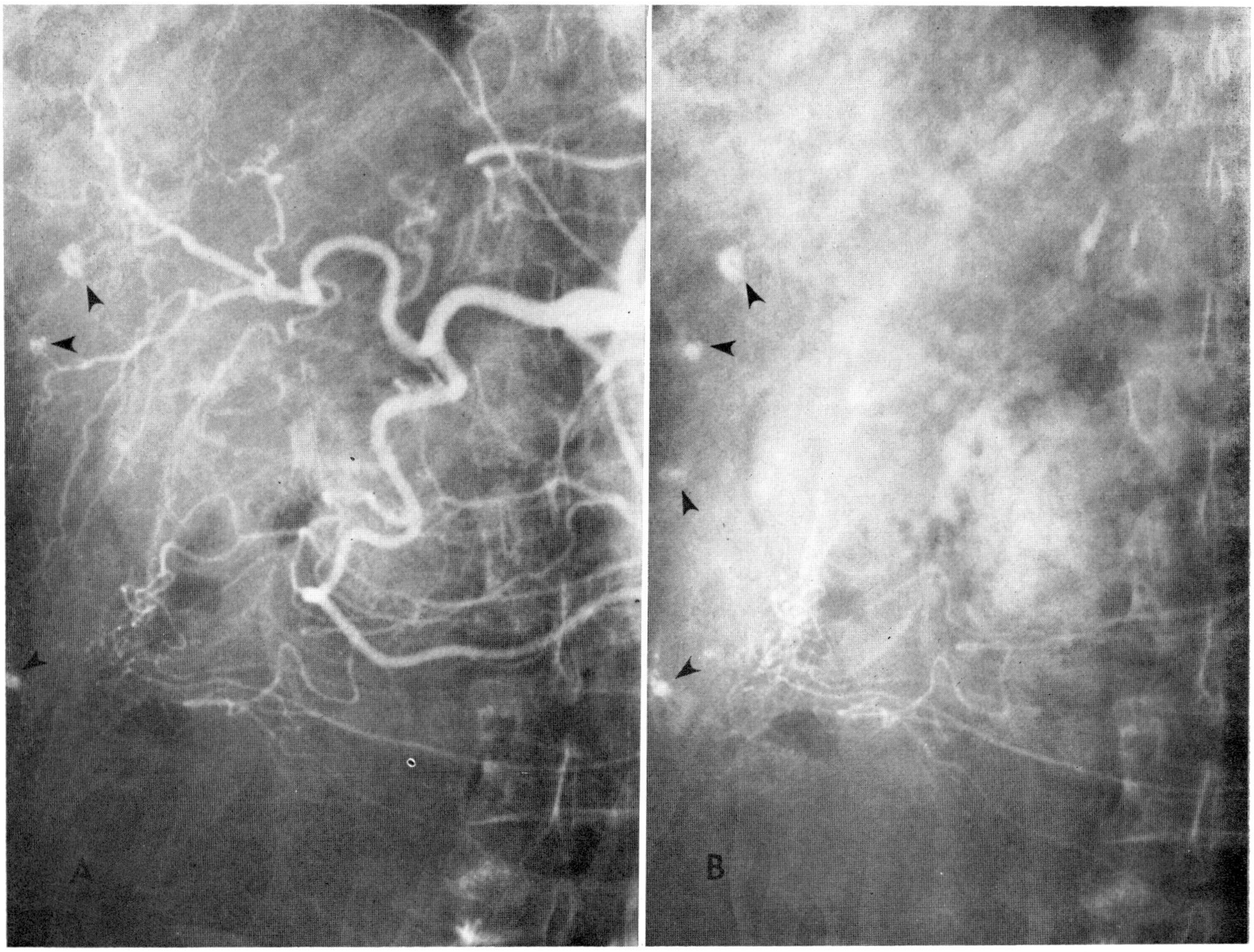

Figure 36.3. Celiac Arteriogram. (A) There are multiple, circumscribed, amorphous collections of contrast (Arrow). (B) There are central lucencies in these contrast collections and stasis. *Radiographic Diagnosis:* Cavernous hemangiomas. *Comment:* These common incidental lesions of the liver may be easily mistaken for hepatic metastasis, but the central lucency and prolonged stasis may help in making the proper diagnosis.

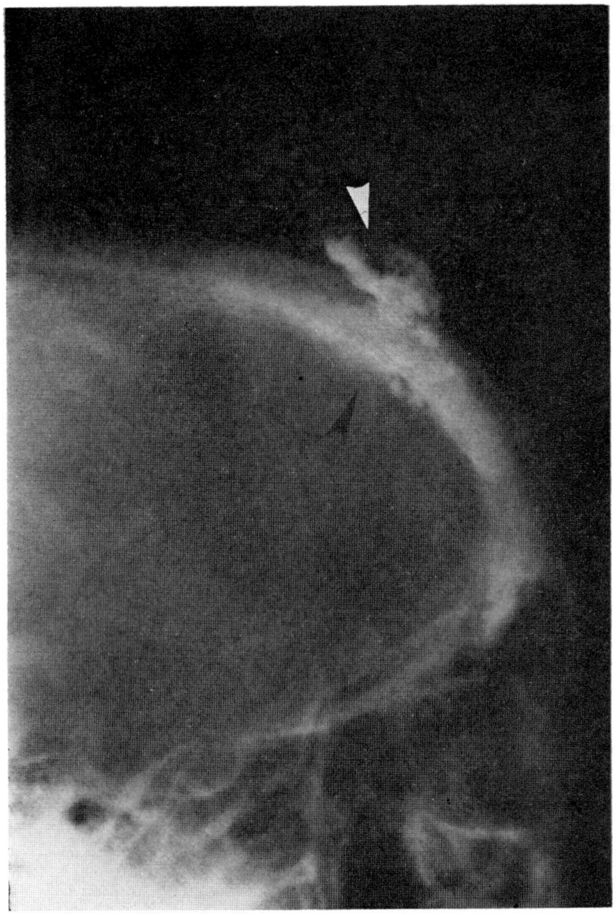

Figure 36.4. Lateral Projection. Injection into a scalp vein shows abnormal collection of contrast material in a conglomerate of venous channels with intracranial extension. This patient had a compressible scalp swelling which used to increase in size while he was tying his shoe laces. *Diagnosis:* Sinus pericranium.

curring in muscular or deep tissues in adults and older children. They are very vascular provided their lumen is not obliterated. *Angiographically* they resemble hemangioendotheliomas, but the vessels are infiltrated. Contrast material may pool in sinusoids for a long time.[1221]

Hemangiopericytoma[1228, 1229] arises from the pericytes of Zimmerman of the blood vessel walls and is a very vascular tumor. It is most common in the superficial soft tissues of the thigh, chest, retroperitoneum and mesentery. Its biologic behavior is unpredictable and requires long-term follow-up. On *angiography* hemangiopericytomas have very wide tortuous vessels feeding the tumor, and sinusoidal pools can be clearly demonstrated (Fig. 36-5).

Renin secreting tumors[32, 1249, 1250] are fascinating lesions which histologically may resemble hemangiopericytomas. They tend to cause hypertension and increase the plasma renin and aldosterone levels. These relatively lucent lesions may contain tortuous vessels.

Leiomyomas and leiomyosarcomas of the vessel wall may occur anywhere, but are usually seen in the inferior vena cava. They are very vascular tumors, and if the tumor is in the proximal portion of the inferior vena cava it may be well opacified by celiac angiography.[1114, 1230]

Angiofibroma[1234–1236] is a benign, unencapsulated, very vascular tumor restricted primarily to the *nasopharynx* of young boys and with a reputation for regression at puberty and with only occasional recurrence. It is not unusual for them to become completely fibrotic as the patient gets older. This fully developed angiomatous cavernous lesion with dense, cellular fibromatous change, ranges angiographically from a very vascular to an avascular tumor. The *degree of vascularity* depends upon the proportions of angiomatous to fibromatous compo-

(Text continues on page 703)

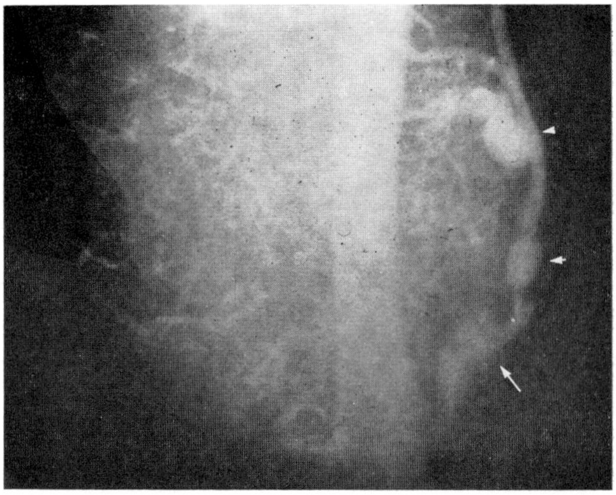

Figure 36.5. Femoral Arteriogram. Reveals dilated femoral artery with extensive abnormal vessels. Multiple dilated angiomatous areas are seen. *Diagnosis:* Vascular tumor arising from the wall of a vessel-like hemangiosarcoma. *Pathology:* Hemangiopericytoma.

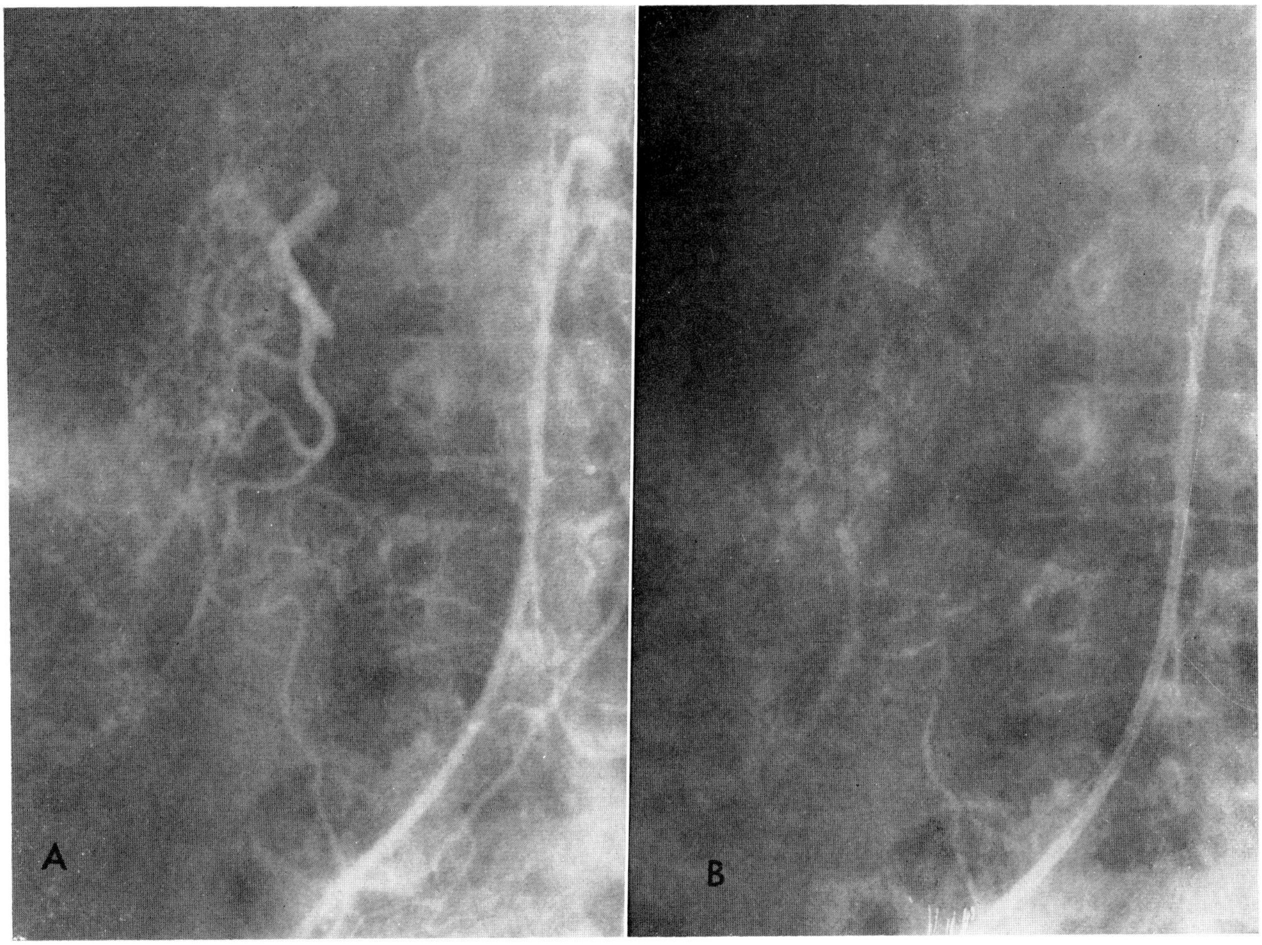

Figure 36.6. Superior Mesenteric Arteriogram. (A) There is abnormal arborization and caliber of the vessels to the entire ascending colon supplied by the right colic artery. (B) Late arterial phase: The same findings in these vessels are revelaed. Dysplastic telangiectatic vessels in a patient who was known to have hereditary hemorrhagic telangiectasia.

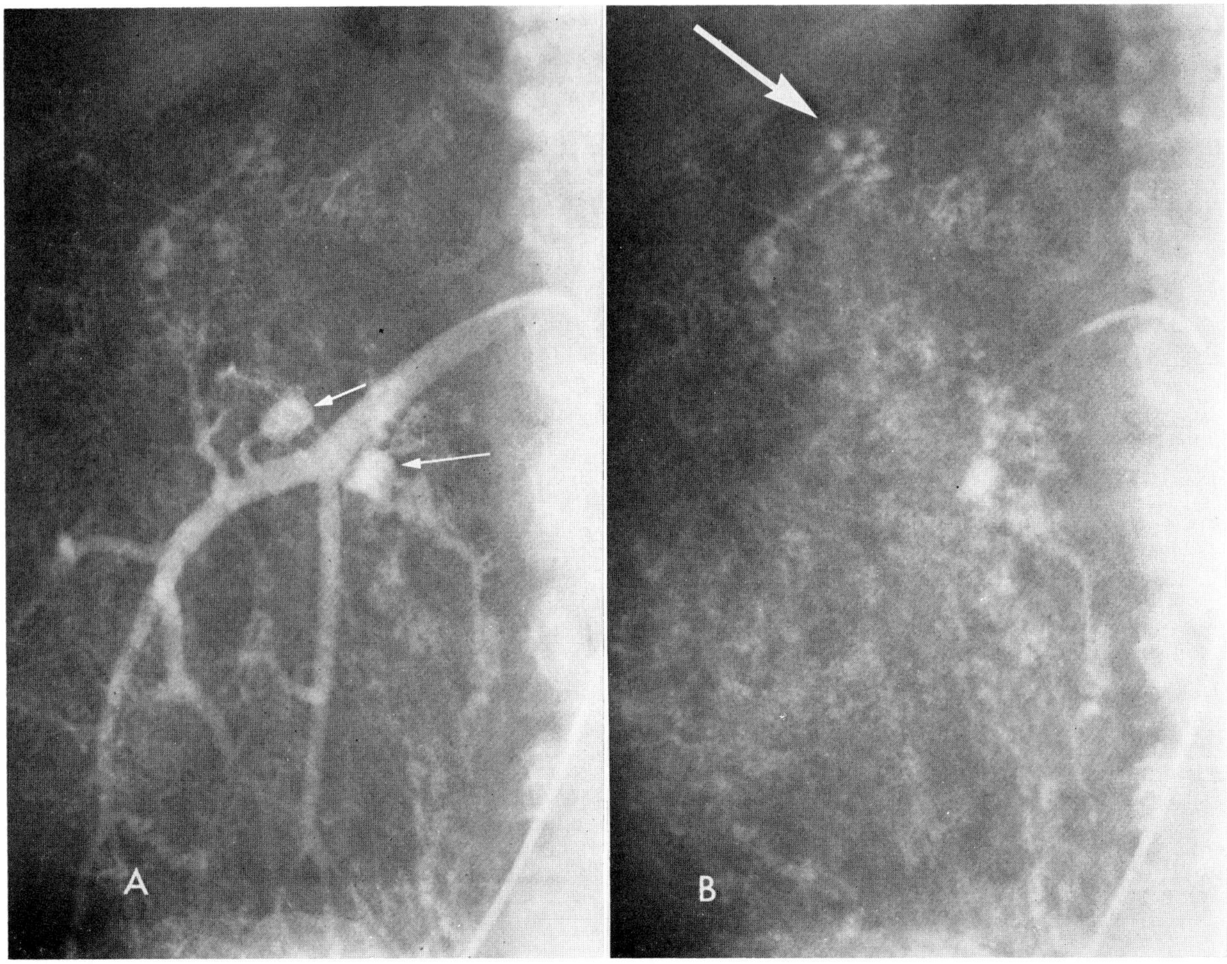

Figure 36.7. Renal Arteriogram. (A) Note increase in renal size. There is a very hypertrophied main renal artery and its branches, multiple circumscribed collections of contrast material (Arrow) and abnormal vessels with irregularly dilated branches and a tortuous course. (B) Late arterial phase: Again the saccular collections of contrast are noted in this huge mass arising from the kidney with abnormal small tortuous vessels. This was a patient with known tuberous sclerosis. *Diagnosis:* Angiomyolipoma with Berry aneurysms, angiomatous lacunae and dysplastic vessels.

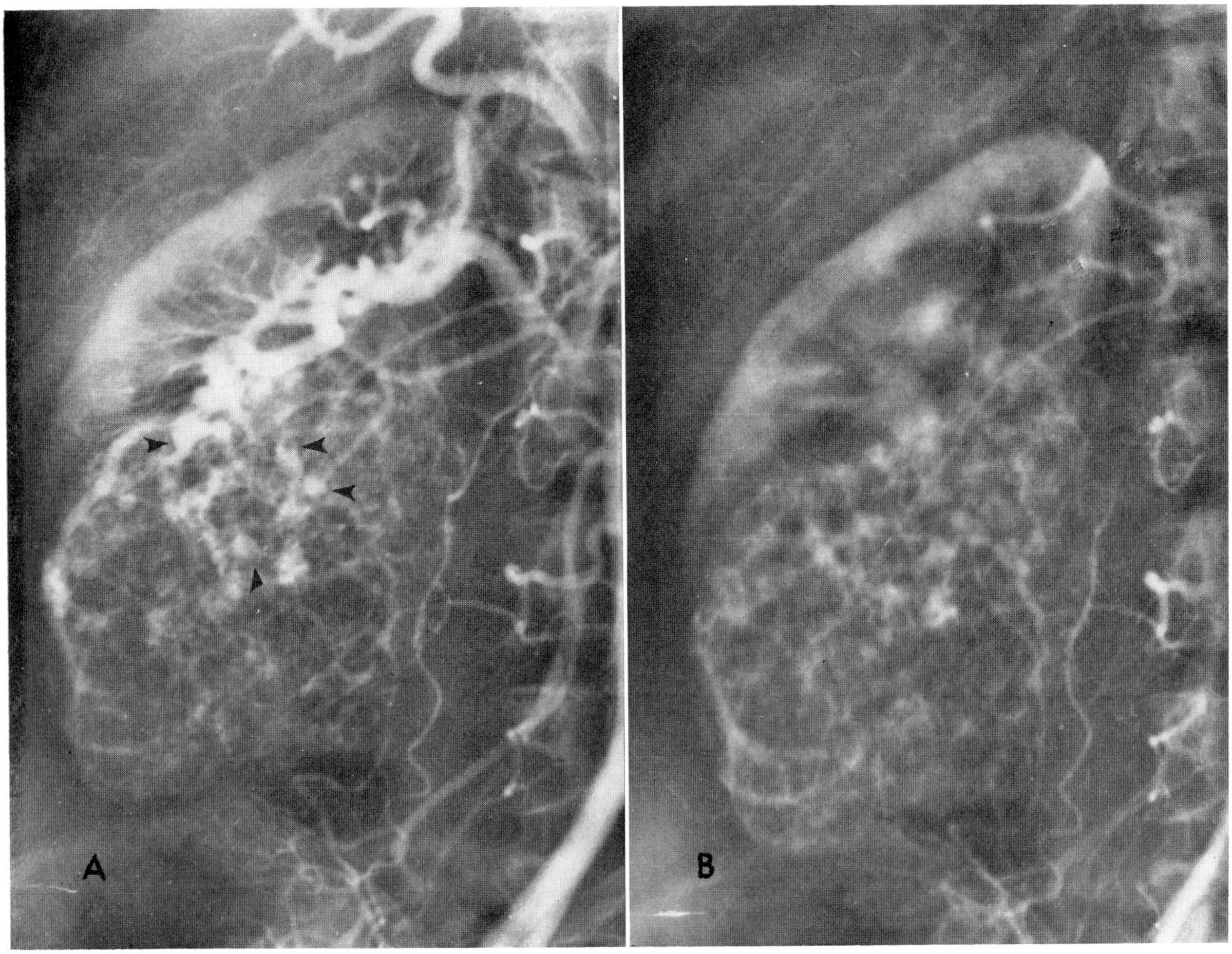

Figure 36.8. Flush Aortogram. (A) Right kidney: Very prominent intrarenal arterial branches with abnormal course and caliber supply an intrarenal mass. Aneurysmal collections of contrast material are found within this mass. (B) Late arterial phase: The tumor mass is well-defined with stasis of contrast in these aneurysmal dilatations. *Diagnosis:* Hypernephroma with tumor sinusoids or angiomyolipoma with angiomatous malformations and aneurysms. *Pathology:* Angiomyolipoma. (Courtesy of Dr. L. Love, Chairman, Department of Radiology, Loyola University Medical Center, Maywood, Illinois.)

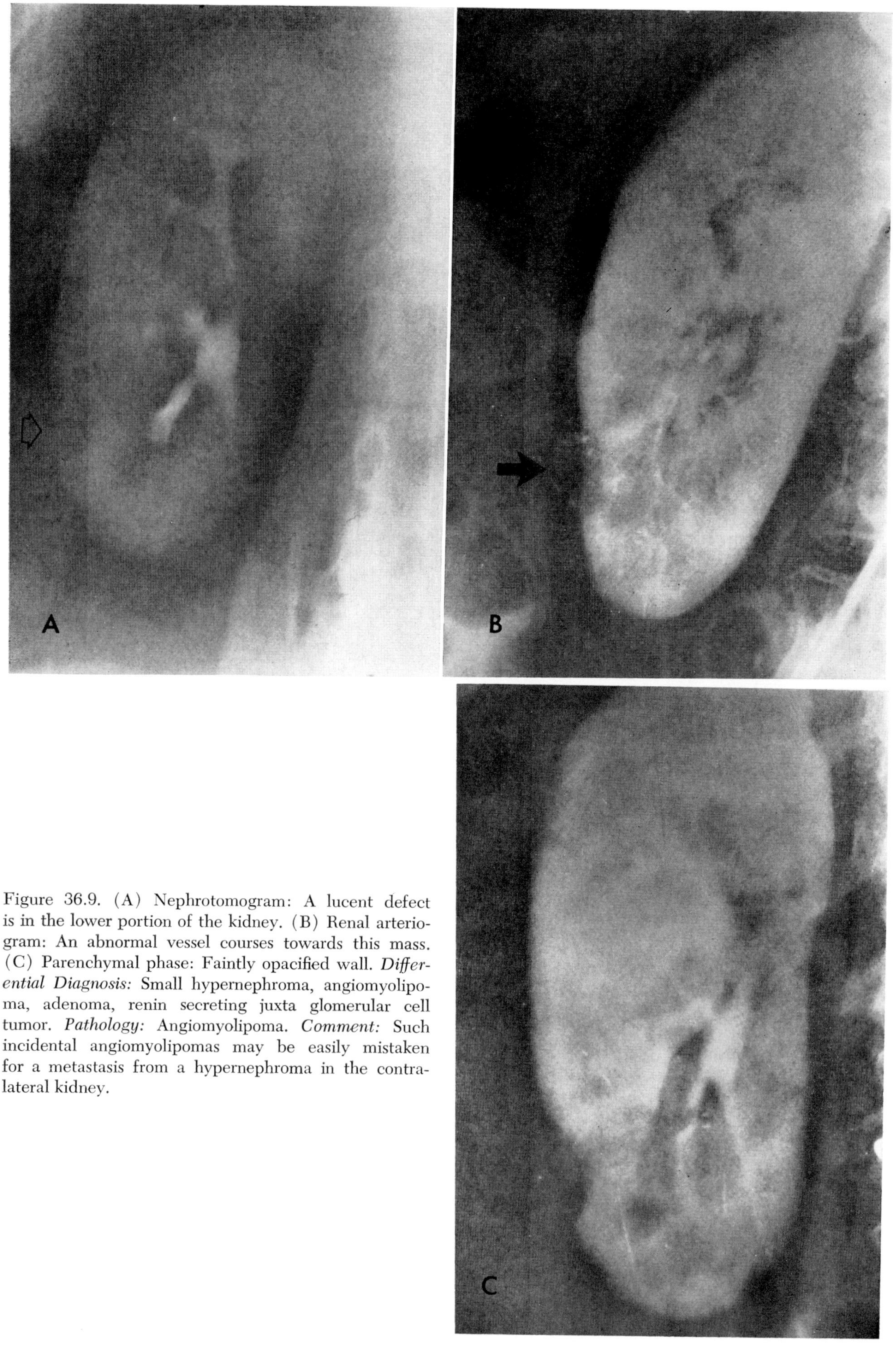

Figure 36.9. (A) Nephrotomogram: A lucent defect is in the lower portion of the kidney. (B) Renal arteriogram: An abnormal vessel courses towards this mass. (C) Parenchymal phase: Faintly opacified wall. *Differential Diagnosis:* Small hypernephroma, angiomyolipoma, adenoma, renin secreting juxta glomerular cell tumor. *Pathology:* Angiomyolipoma. *Comment:* Such incidental angiomyolipomas may be easily mistaken for a metastasis from a hypernephroma in the contralateral kidney.

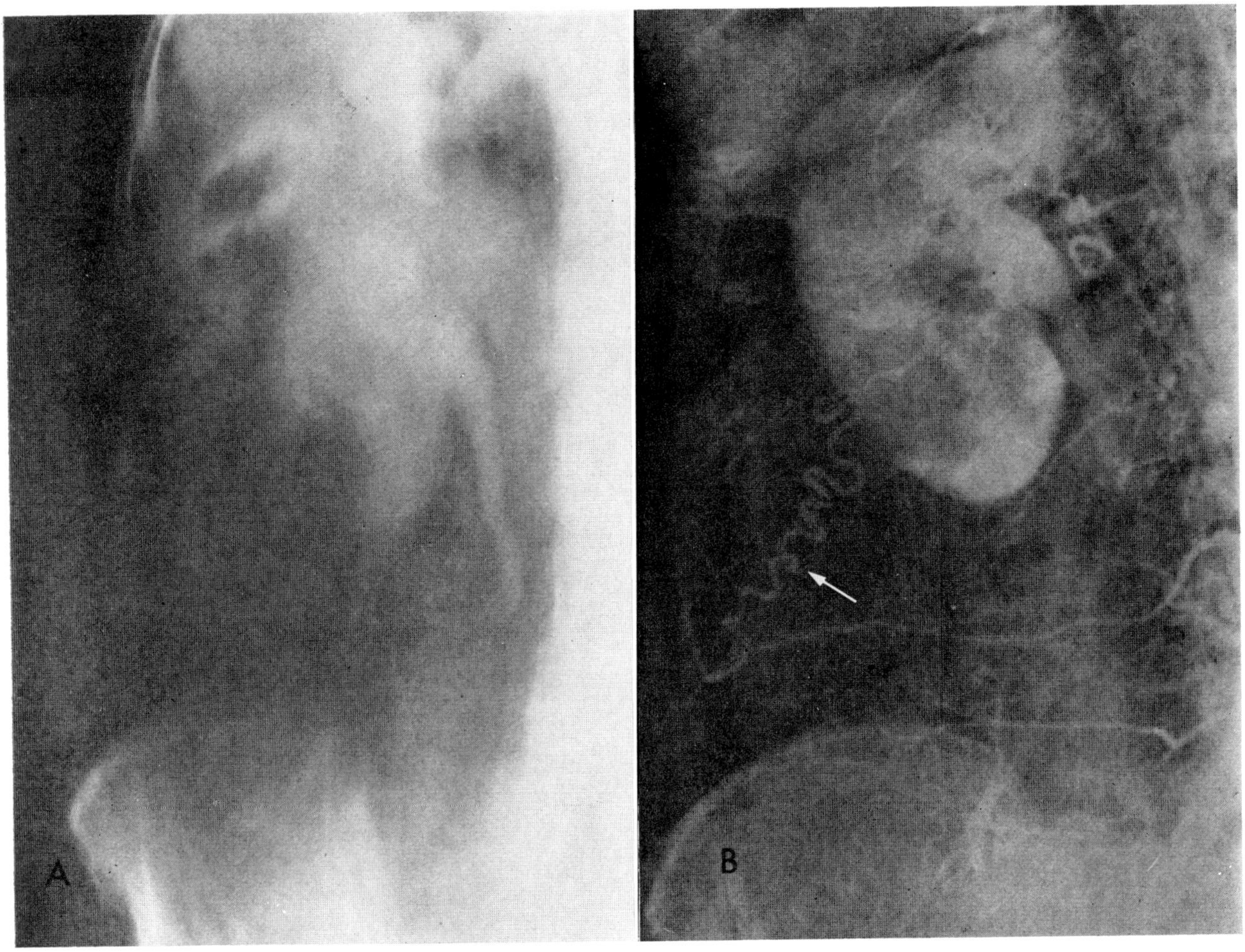

Figure 36.10. (A) Nephrotomogram: Note a huge lucent mass is in the lower pole of the kidney with multiple small loculations. (B) Flush aortogram: Note the very prominent capsular vessels supplying this lucent mass. *Diagnosis:* Angiomyolipoma. *Pathology:* Angiomyolipoma. *Comment:* The degree of vascularity depends on the proportions of angiomatous and lipomatous components present in the tumor.

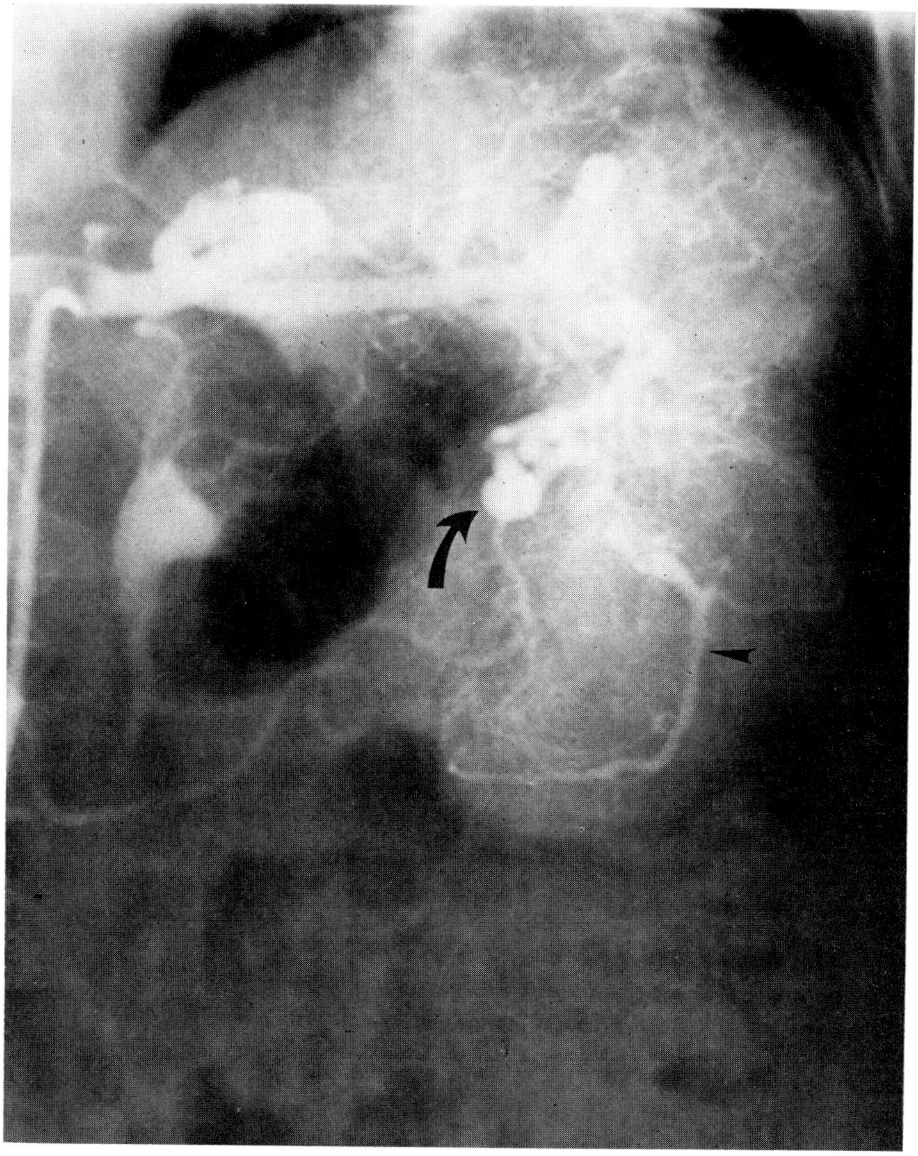

Figure 36.11A

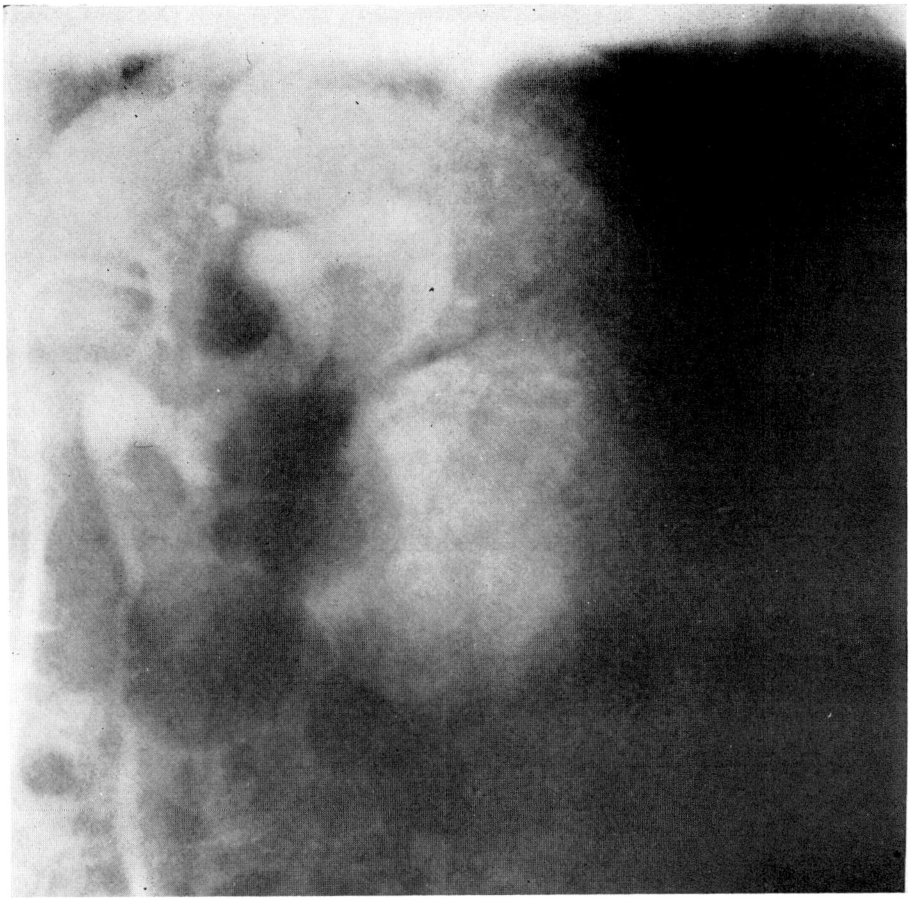

Figure 36.11B

Figure 36.11. Splenic Arteriogram. (A) Arterial phase: A neovascular mass is revealed in the lower half of the spleen fed by a prominent artery (Arrow Head). There is also aneurysmal dilatation (Arrow). (B) Parenchymal phase: This mass has a dense homogeneous stain. Isotope scan with Cr.51 labelled RBC revealed sequestration of RBC in this area suggesting the presence of splenic pulp in this mass. *Diagnosis:* Splenic Hamartoma. (Teates, C. D., Seale, D. L., and Allen, M. S. Hamartoma of the spleen, *Am J Roentgen, 116:*419, 1972. Courtesy of the authors and publishers.)

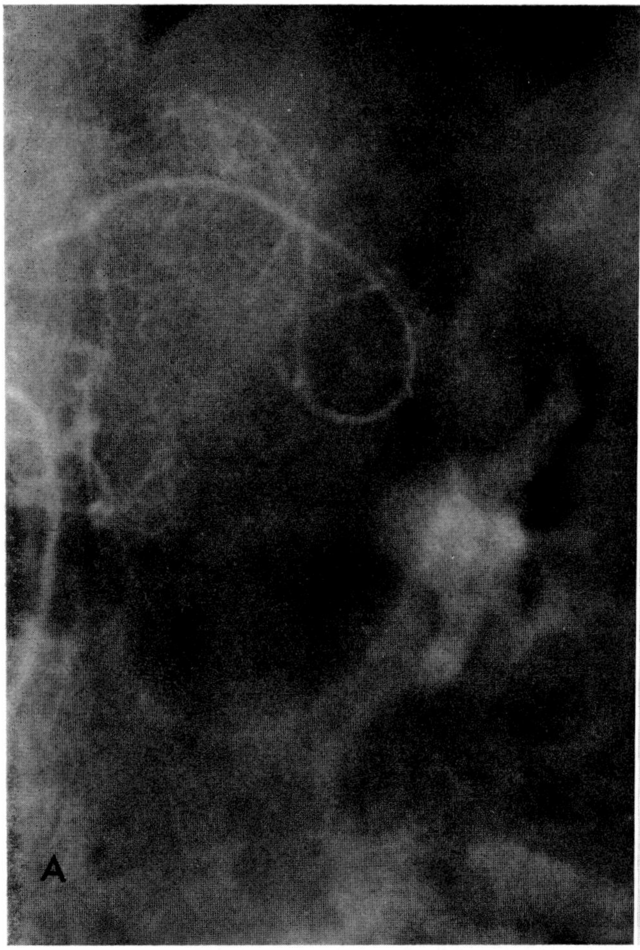

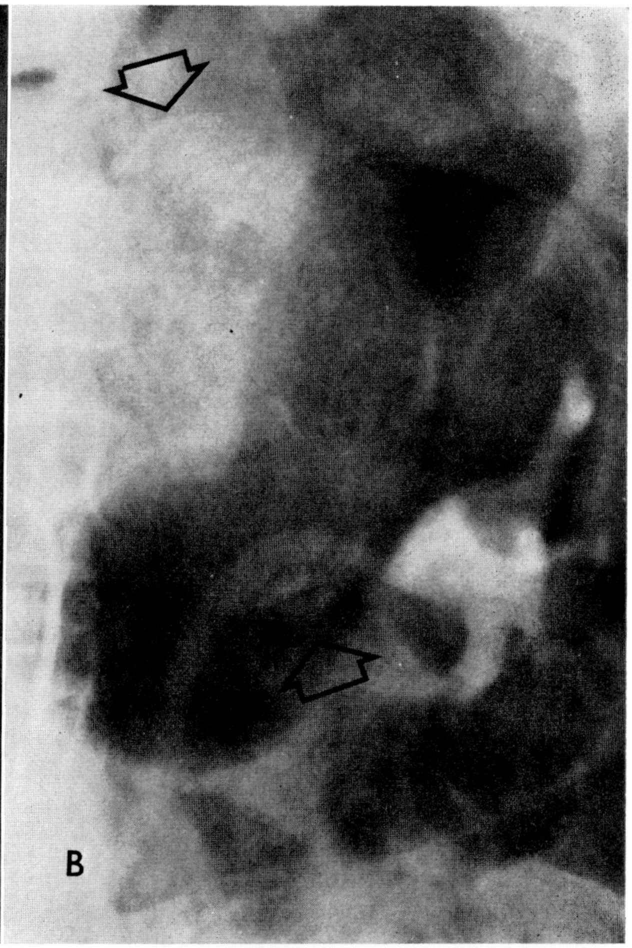

Figure 36.12. Lumbar Arteriogram. (A) There is a prominent left lumbar artery with change in its course and distortion around a mass with abnormal vessels coursing through the mass. (B) There is moderate staining of this well-circumscribed mass. *Diagnosis:* With the help of the other radiographic findings: neurofibroma. *Comment:* It is usual for tumors like neurofibroma and hamartoma to have dysplastic vessels.

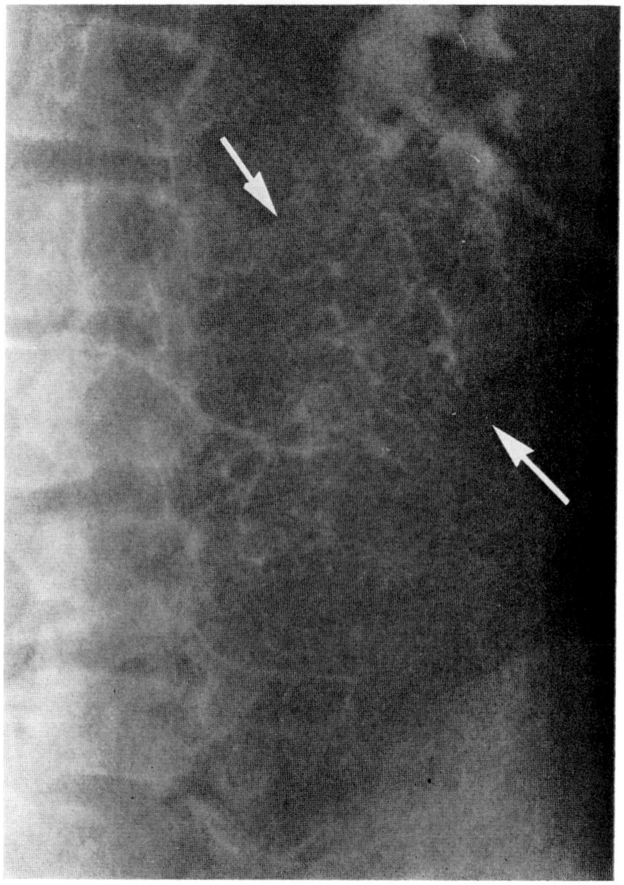

Figure 36.13. Selective Lumbar Arteriogram. A prominent lumbar artery with numerous abnormal vessels of irregular caliber and course, perfuse a moderately sized left, paravertebral mass. This patient had a known neurofibromatosis. *Diagnosis:* Neurofibroma. *Comment:* Notice the benign dysplastic vessels. Because of such vessels, the malignant counterpart of a neurofibroma may be difficult to diagnose angiographically.

nents in the mass. The absence of elastic fibers and paucity of smooth muscle in the tumor vessels causes the clinically alarming picture of profuse bleeding.[1232] Being in or *close to the mid-line* means that they have a luxurious blood supply from many of the regional vessels depending on its exact anatomical extent.[1233]

Glomangioma (angiomyoneuroma)[111, 1213] is a rare, fascinating, vascular tumor with very little connective tissue stroma. The tumor vessels lack smooth muscle and elastic tissue in certain areas, and thus have only an endothelial lining. Arteriovenous shunting may also be seen.[1237]

Kaposi's sarcoma[1214] is a vascular tumor with vasoformative tendencies. It is lined by endothelium which may be absent in certain areas and has a mixture of fibrosarcomatous elements. Arteriovenous shunting and an orderly leash of vessels supplying each nodule by a single branch is interesting angiographically.[1238]

Other rare tumors of the vascular wall include round cell tumors, endothelial sarcomas, and myxomas.[1114, 1123, 1124] Lesions such as telangiectasia, pseudoxanthoma elasticum,[1231] and the hepatic arterial branches in atrophic cirrhosis[1003] may also have an *angiomatoid* appearance.

HAMARTOMAS

Hamartomas are circumscribed overgrowth of normal mature cells of improper proportions found in an organ, or tissues composed of identical elements. Disorganization, overgrowth and encapsulation indicate the anomalous status of such masses. Their components may include varying amounts of blood vessels, muscle, fat, etc. They are common in the liver, spleen, kidney, lung and pancreas.[111, 1239] *Choristomas* are like hamartomas, but the composition of the tissues of this tumor is not similar to that present in the part of the body where the tumor occurs.[1239]

Hepatic hamartomas[1220, 1235] may be solid or cystic, and if solid they are very vascular. If they are cystic, rapid growth may occur because of rapid accumulation of fluid. Very vascular hamartomas may be found in the liver, kidneys and adrenal glands in individuals with *tuberous sclerosis.*[1252]

Splenic hamartomas[1241–1243] may be associated with tremendous erythropoiesis. Clinically they may present with anemia. The nodules are very vascular with vessels of varying caliber, early venous shunting, and a dense parenchymal blush.[1240] To aid in the diagnosis, a Cr^{51} labeled red blood scan may reveal sequestration of the red blood cells. A Tc^{99M} pertechnetate study may show increased flow and blood pooling[1240] (Fig. 36-11).

Renal hamartomas[96] are anomalies of development rather than neoplasms. They may be small or large, unilateral or bilateral, may occur in the renal cortex or in the medulla.[1241] Conglomerate tortuous vessels, some with thick, hyalinized walls lacking in musculature in some areas,[95] and others with thick musculature, are seen with interspersed aneurysms or angiomatous malformations depending on the extent of the dysplasia. The above findings are reflected *angiographically*[1246] with *berry-like aneurysms and angiomatous malformations, without early arteriovenous shunting* (Figs. 36-7 to 36-9). Some of them may resemble malignant types of tumor vasculature such as hypernephroma,[1245] and some may even be avascular.[97] The avascularity is probably related to the proportion of blood vessels, fat and muscle present in the hamartoma (Fig. 36-10). The malignant counterpart of angiomyolipoma is angiomyoliposarcoma.[1247] Bilateral hamartomas in the kidneys, along with hepatic and adrenal hamartomas, are not uncommon in *tuberus sclerosis.* Their association with polycystic renal disease is also very interesting.[1248] There may be no angiographic dissimilarity between an unencapsulated mesenchymal hamartoma in an infant and a Wilm's tumor.[1479]

NEURAL TUMORS

Neurofibroma

Neurofibromas are provided with very bizarre chaotic vessels of irregular caliber. These are also *dysplastic vessels* with excessive collagen or

(Text continues on page 707)

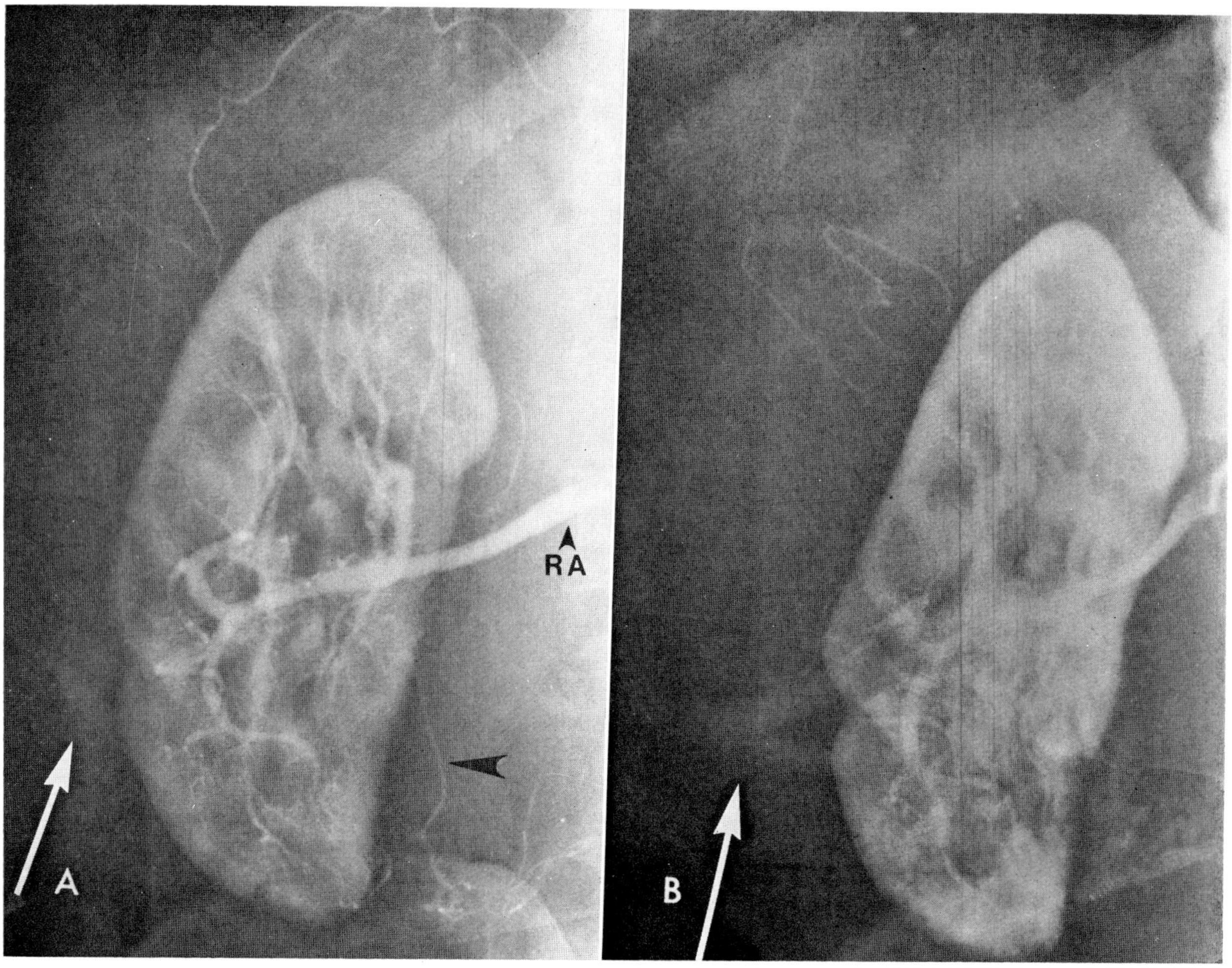

Figure 36.14 A and B

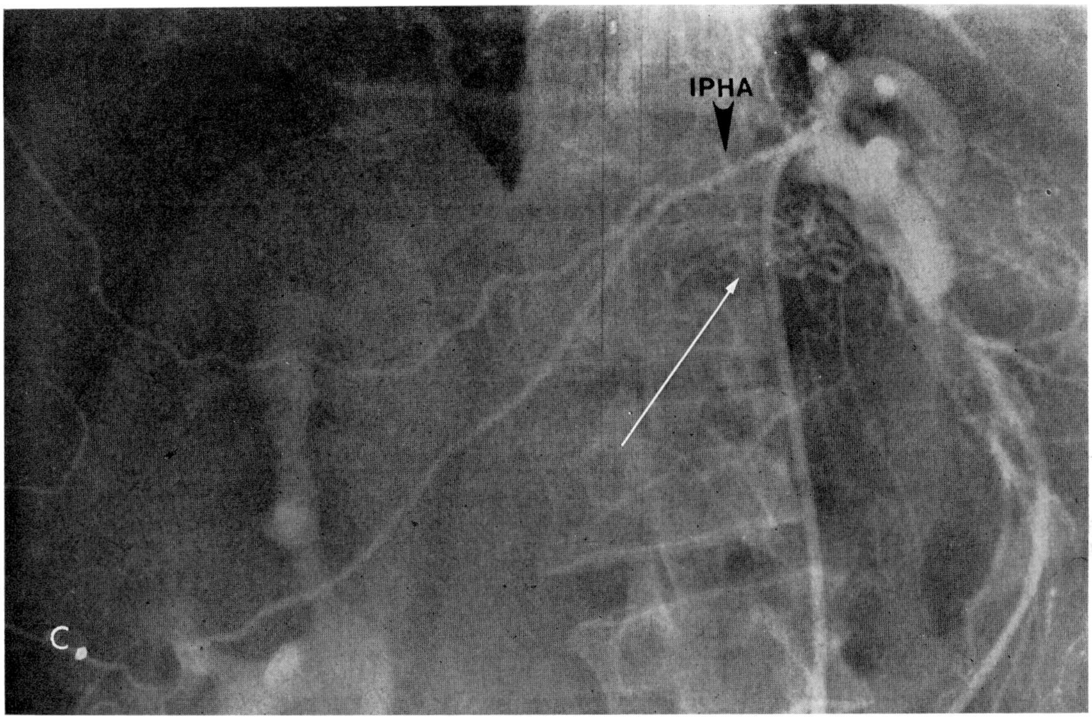

Figure 36.14. (A) Right renal arteriogram: The right renal artery is elongated and stretched (R.A.). Notice the change in axis of the right kidney. An abnormal perforating capsular vessel originates from the kidney (Arrow Head) with early opacification of a retroperitoneal vein (Arrow). (B) Late arterial phase—oblique projection: The same very prominent retroperitoneal vein (Arrow) is seen. (C) Inferior phrenic arteriogram: A prominent inferior phrenic artery and its distorted branches (I.P.H.A.) as well as abnormal small branches from the very proximal inferior phrenic artery (Arrow) are seen. This patient had a huge right upper quadrant mass but was otherwise asymptomatic. *Diagnosis:* Retroperitoneal mesenchymal tumor with blood supply from the perforating renal capsular and the inferior phrenic artery. *Pathology:* Chemodectoma. *Comment:* The parasitic blood supply from the inferior phrenic and the perforating renal capsular arteries is quite obvious.

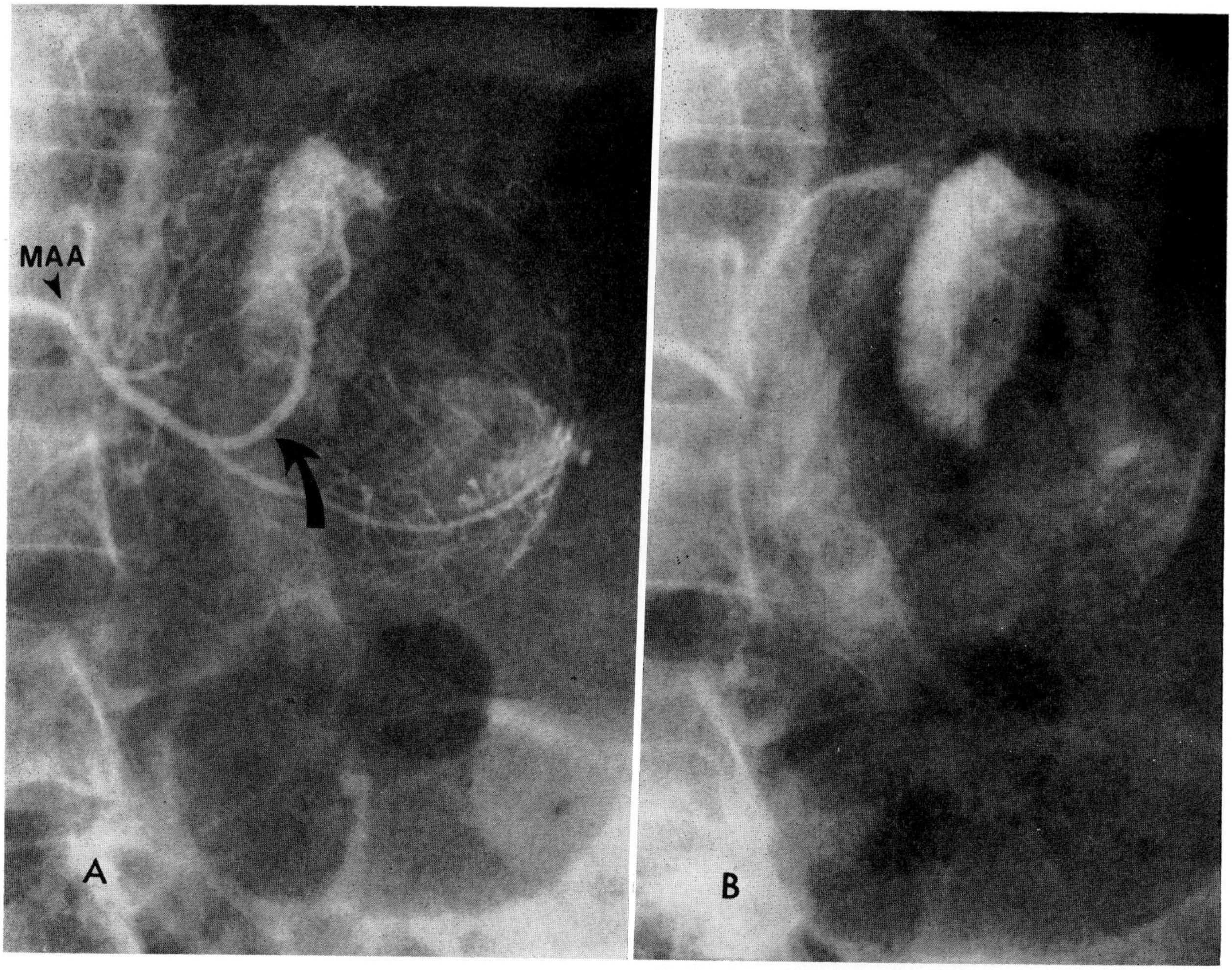

Figure 36.15. Left Middle Adrenal Arteriogram. (A) Early arterial phase: A very prominent elongated left middle adrenal artery supplies a moderately sized mass with abnormal vasculature (M.A.A.). Notice a branch from the same adrenal artery supplying the kidney (Arrow). (B) Late arterial phase: Opacification of this mass with a thick wall and central comparative lucency occurs. Notice the segmental nephrogram obtained by this upper pole vessel. A patient with periodic episodes of hypertensive crisis. *Diagnosis:* Partially necrotic left adrenal pheochromocytoma. Because of such abundant vascularity, the malignant counterpart of a benign pheochromocytoma may be difficult to diagnose angiographically.

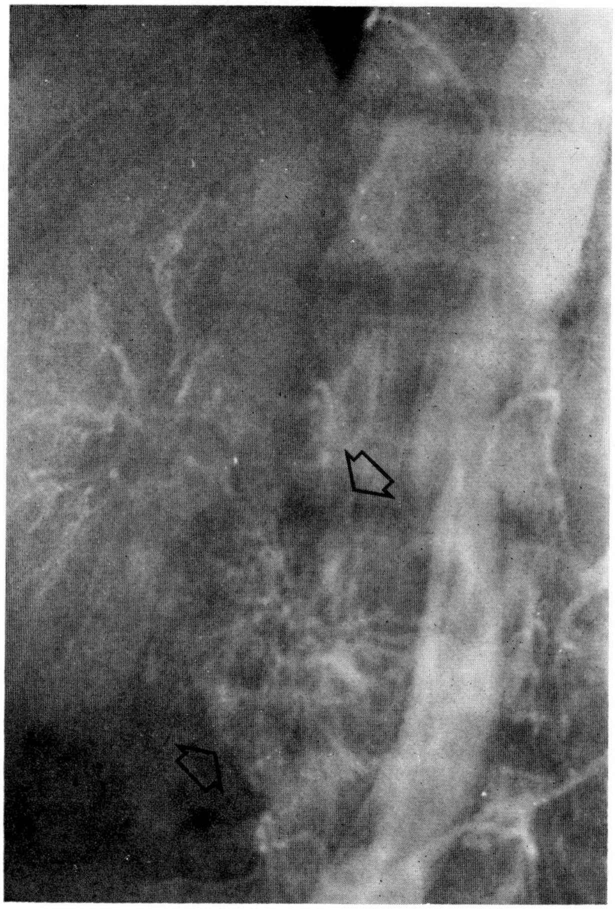

Figure 36.16. Flush Aortogram. A very hypervascular mass to the right of the abdominal aorta (Arrow) compresses that segment of the aorta. This young patient had repeated hypertensive episodes. *Diagnosis:* Extraadrenal pheochromocytoma.

hyalinization of the vessel walls, having variable amounts of smooth muscle in their vascular walls. Neurogenic tumors occurring at the bifurcation of the common carotid artery may be comparatively less vascular than chemodectomas[1251] (Figs. 36-12 and 36-13).

Paraganglionic Tumors

Collections of chromaffin tissue or neuroepithelial cells (paraganglia) are scattered throughout the body.[1235] The most conspicuous one is the adrenal medulla. The other significant areas of islands of chromaffin tissue are seen prominently along the thoraco-lumbar, and para-aortic areas. Apart from these, another paired collection is found at the origin of the inferior mesenteric artery. Known as the *organs of Zuckerkandl,* the main source of epinephrine in the fetus, they usually become fibrotic at birth, although they do not disappear completely.[1253]

Paraganglionic tissue may be chromaffin positive or negative. Paraganglia connected with the orthosympathetic chain are usually chromaffin positive, while those connected with the parasympathetic ones are chromaffin negative. Paraganglia related with the parasympathetic chain are concentrated mainly in the head, neck and mediastinum. *Tumors* of paraganglionic tissue may be chromaffin positive or negative.[1254] Functional chromaffin positive tissue may give rise to pheochromocytomas; functional chromaffin negative tissue may give rise to functioning chemodectomas; nonfunctioning chromaffin positive tissue gives rise to nonfunctioning pheochromocytomas; while nonfunctioning chromaffin negative tissue may give rise to nonfunctioning chemodectomas.

Pheochromocytomas[1316–1318] arise from collections of chromaffin positive tissue usually concentrated in the adrenal medulla, but in 10 percent of cases may also be found in other extra-adrenal sites. They may be unilateral, or in 10 percent of the cases, bilateral. While they are usually benign, 10 percent may be malignant. Although 90 percent of all cases are usually isolated, 10 percent may have a family history. Again, pheochromocytomas may be functional or nonfunctional. Their association with neurofibromatosis[1319] or with medullary carcinomas of the thyroid[1320] is of unusual interest. In addition to their usual locations, they may occur in the kidney,[1321] in the organ of Zuckerkandl,[1322] from the urinary bladder,[1323] or may even be intrathoracic.[1324] Boys are affected more than girls, while women are affected more than men. If the individual presents with a sustained, rather than a fluctuating, hypertension[52] or with only intermittent claudication,[1327] the well-known clinical manifestations[1325, 1326] may not always be present (Fig. 36-15 and 36-16).

Histologically these tumors have thin-walled sinuses and fibrous trabaculae, developing central necrosis and hemorrhage[111] when they become bulky. These findings are reflected *angiographically* with abnormal vessels, sinusoids, and avascular areas. At the other end of the spectrum is the totally avascular mass which can only be detected by adrenal venography.[26–28] As usual, medullary hyperplasia of the adrenal[22] with the identical clinical manifestations may go unnoticed if it were not for venous sampling from the adrenal veins and further assay studies. The malignant counterpart of this benign vascular tumor may not be easily detected by angiographic methods alone. Removal of the existing tumor does not guarantee against recurrence or occurrence of a new tumor.[1328]

Chemodectoma,[1257] whether occurring in the neck[1255] or in the retroperitoneal area,[1256] whether functional[1258] or not, is usually provided with extremely vascular stroma and a capsule. On rare occasions it may have comparatively increased fibrous stroma, making it avascular or minimally vascular.[1214] Locally infiltrative with little propensity for distal metastasis, this tumor is characterized by slow, steady growth with a potential malignant nature. It is more common in females and has a familial tendency. Chemodectomas may be bilateral when they occur in the carotid bodies. Late occurrence of a contralateral tumor at the carotid

(Text continues on page 712)

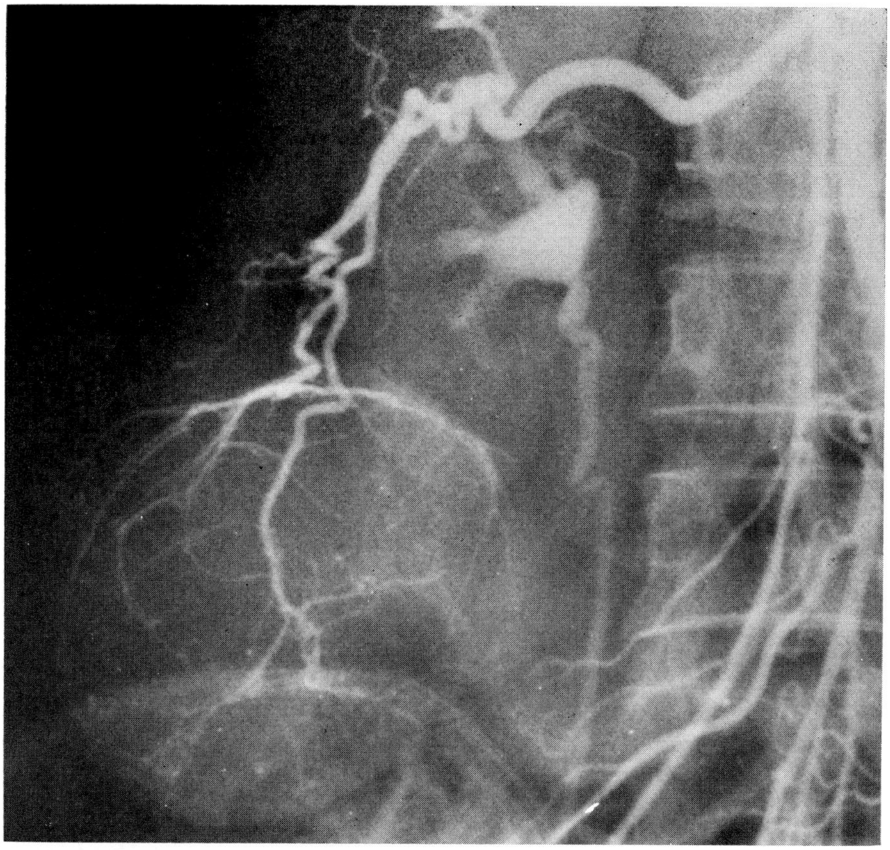

Figure 36.17A

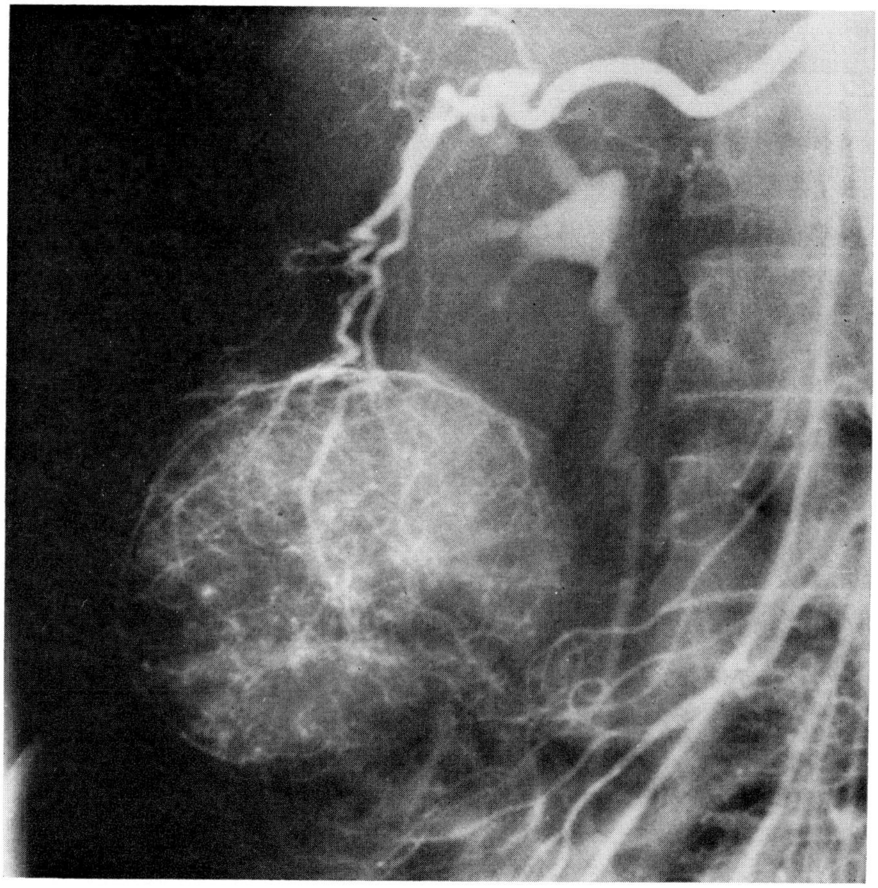

Figure 36.17B

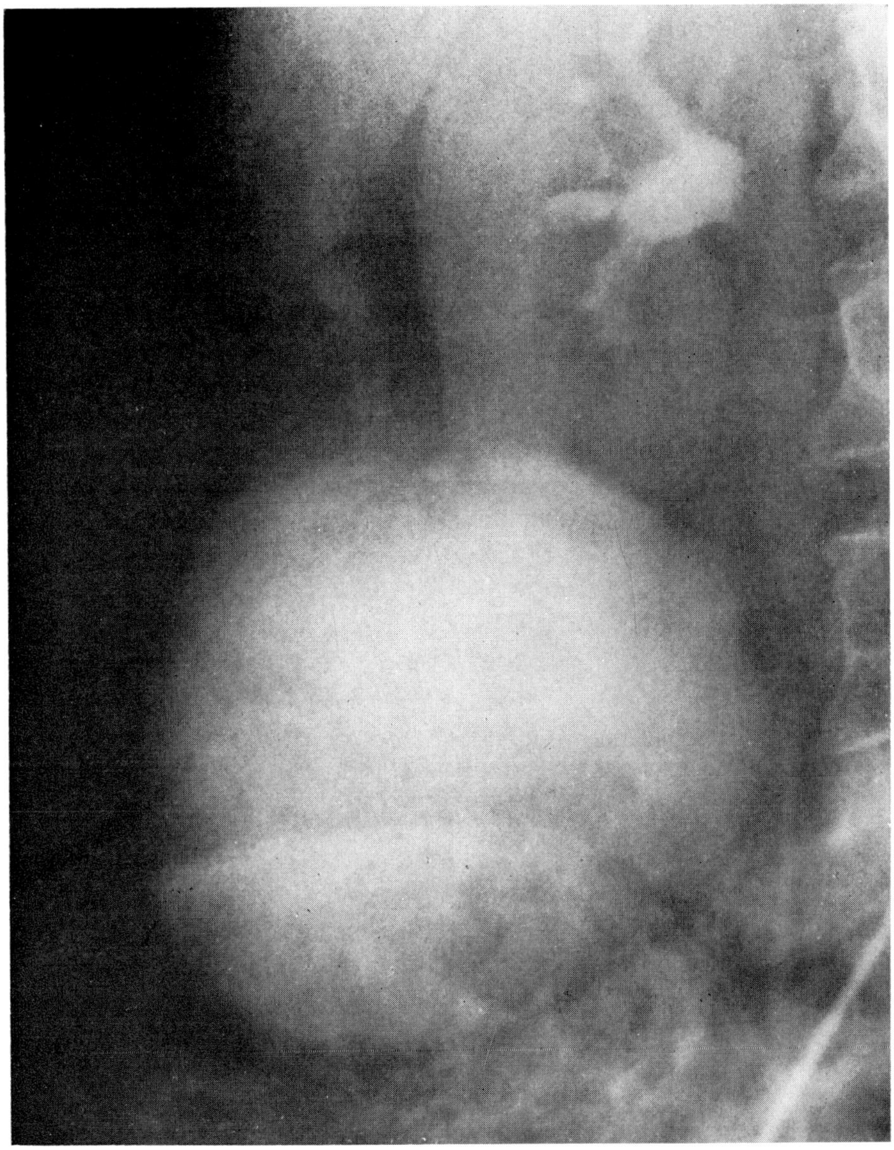

Figure 36.17C

Figure 36.17. Hepatic Arteriogram. A & B. Arterial phase: A very vascular mass is seen in the right lobe of the liver with circumferential vascular supply. C. Parenchymal phase: A well-stained and well-defined tumor is seen in a twenty-nine-year-old woman. *Diagnosis:* Adenoma of the liver. *Comment:* Such circumferential vascular supply may not be unusual in a hepatoma also.

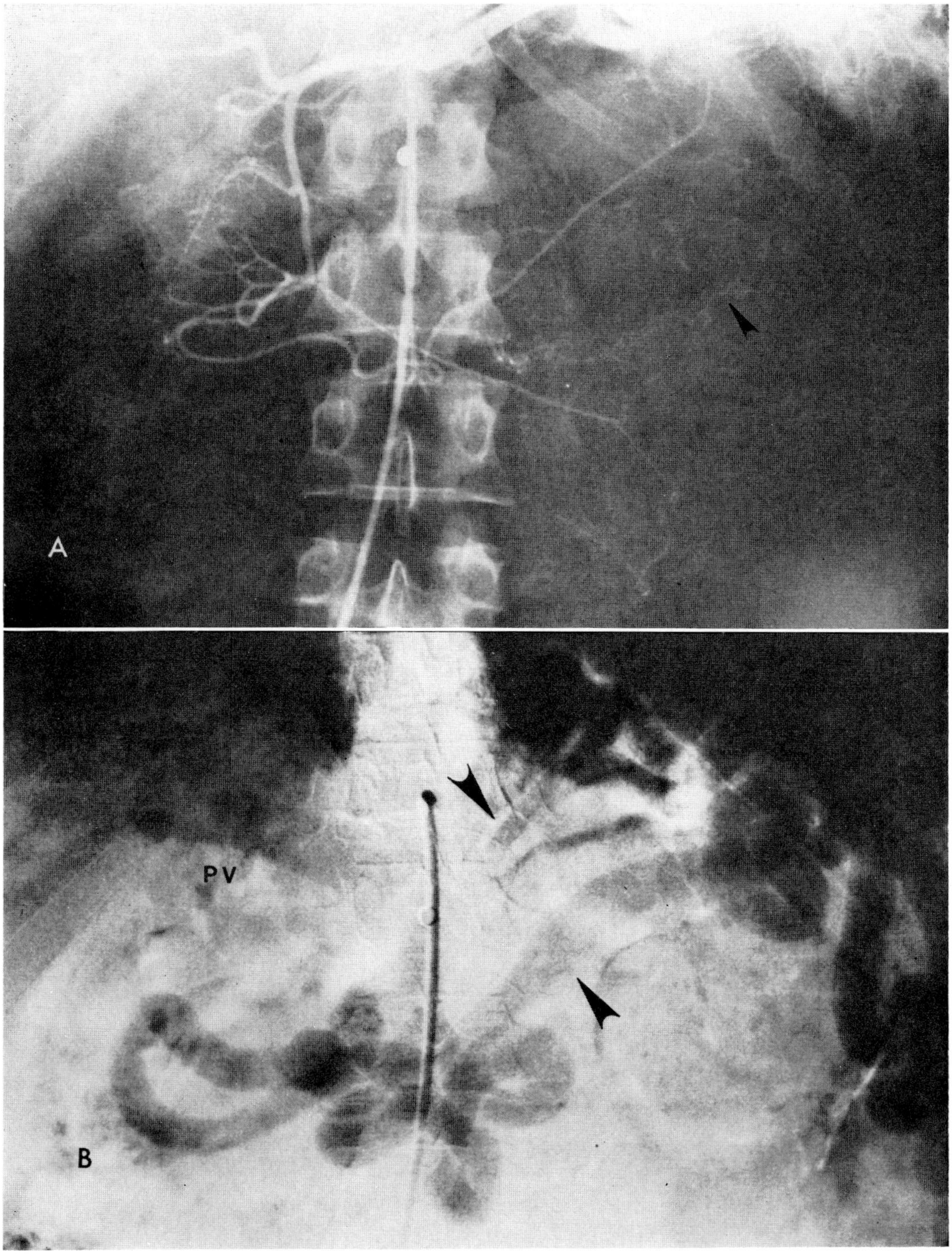

Figure 36.18. Celiac Arteriogram. (A) Early phase reveals stretching of the pancreatic vessels terminating in abnormal vessels on the surface of a mass. (B) Venous phase reveals no opacification of the splenic vein but huge collateral vein coursing along the lesser and greater curvatures of the stomach (Arrow) to opacify the portal vein (P.V.). *Diagnosis:* Pancreatic cystadenoma (benign) with splenic vein thrombosis. Dilated gastric veins by-passing the splenic vein occlusion. *Comment:* The degree of abnormal vascularity depends on the proportions of cystic and solid components in cystadenomatous tumors. (Courtesy of Dr. J. Petasnick, Associate Professor, Diagnostic Radiology, Rush Presbyterian-St. Luke Medical Center, Chicago.)

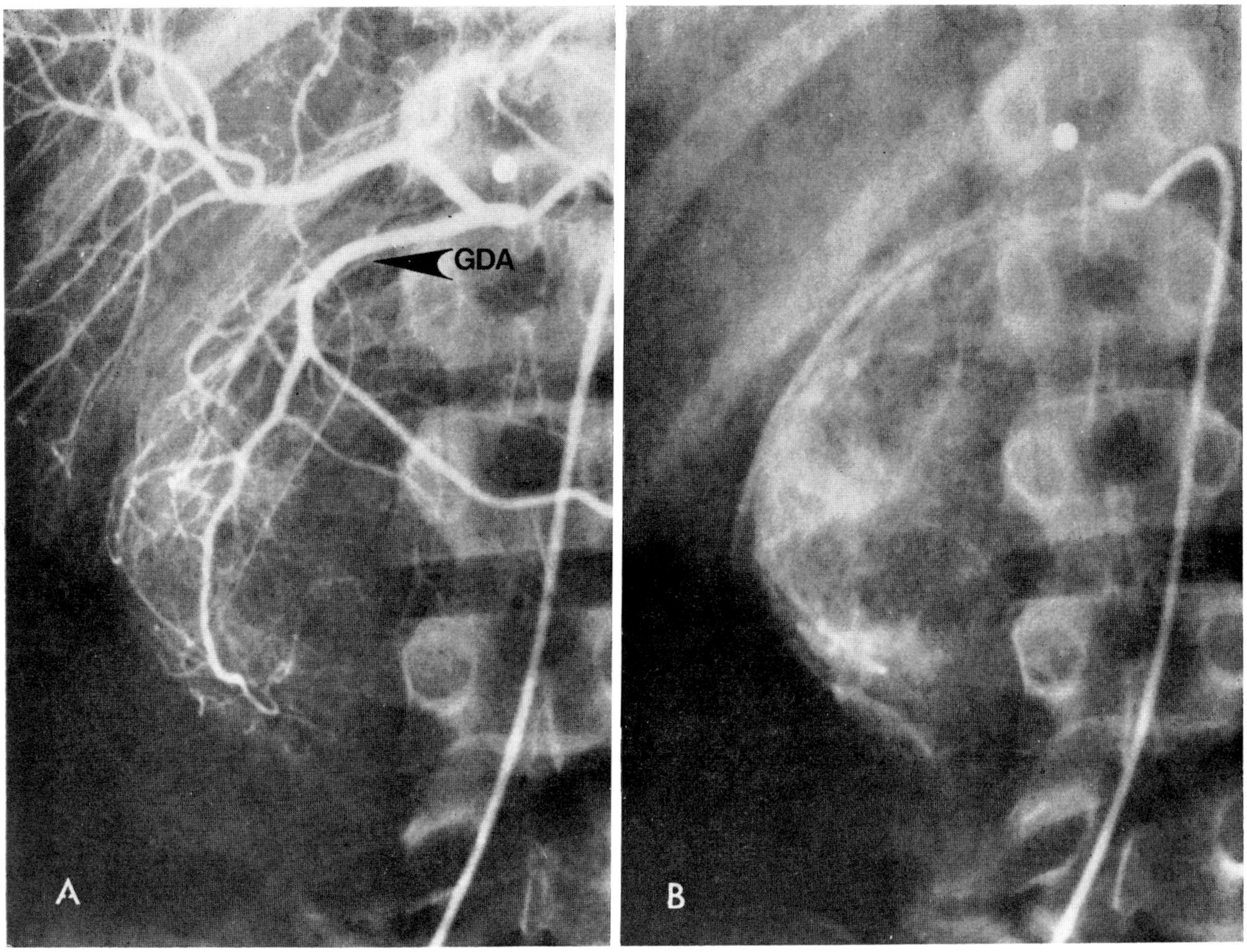

Figure 36.19. Hepatic Arteriogram. (A) Early phase reveals deviation and stretching of the gastroduodenal artery and its branches terminating in an abnormal mesh work of vessels supplying a pancreatic mass. This was a young patient. (B) Late phase reveals the mass with islands of lucencies and stains. *Diagnosis:* Malignant pancreatic tumor? *Pathology:* Islet cell tumor (Benign, nonfunctioning). *Comment:* Malignant counterparts of such vascular benign tumors may not be detected angiographically unless there are hepatic metastases. (Courtesy of Dr. J. Petasnick, Associate Professor, Diagnostic Radiology, Rush Presbyterian-St. Luke Medical Center, Chicago.)

bifurcation[1259] or small tumors on the opposite side are not unusual[1260] (Fig. 36-14).

Ganglioneuromas

These tumors arise from the sympathetic nervous system and may be located in the lumbar, pelvic, suprarenal, mediastinal, or cervical areas.[1348] They are well-encapsulated, circumscribed vascular tumors with a tendency to envelop the aorta or inferior vena cava. On occasion they may be avascular.[1349]

Tumors of the Sympathetic Neural Crest

Sympathatogonia may give rise to neuroblastoma, ganglioneuroblastoma or benign ganglioneuromas.[1254] They are usually seen in the adrenal medulla, but may also be seen in other heterotopic areas such as the mediastinum.[1235] Like other vascular neoplasms their angiographic presentation may be hypervascular or avascular.[222, 1491]

ADENOMAS

Adenomas are circumscribed aggregations or groups of benign cells, expansile in nature and encapsulated.[111, 1279] They often resemble the surrounding cells and are provided with a fibrous septum which sets them *discretely* apart from the compressed surrounding parenchyma. The amount of *vascularity* of these adenomas depends on the metabolic needs of the cells and their function. Some may have a rich vascular stroma containing thin-walled capillaries lacking endothelium within certain areas in their walls. In some, *obvious abnormal vessels* are present, and in others increased vascularity at the *microscopic level* is reflected angiographically as a *discrete area of increased stain.* The presence of cystic components and hemorrhage into the tumor parenchyma may alter the homogeneity of the stain. Some adenomas, particularly in the liver, have well-organized vasculature with the vessels arranged peripherally and circumferentially. This may be a reflection of slow steady growth of these encapsulated masses. In *endocrinal glands* there is very little correlation between the morphology of these adenomas and their functional status.

Pancreatic Adenomas

This group includes insulinomas (beta cell), glucagonomas (alpha cells, rare) and ulcerogenic (delta cells) adenomas.[111, 1214, 1298–1300] These expansile islet cell adenomas, with or without encapsulation, are located mainly in the body and tail of the pancreas.

Beta cells constitute the majority of adenomas with alpha and delta cells constituting the rest. They may be single or multiple and of varying size. The size is not related to their functional activity. *Angiographically,*[1301–1305] the three types have almost identical appearances.

Hypervascularity, discrete staining which persists for a comparatively long period of time, up to twenty seconds, are usually the finding in vascular lesions. Avascular lesions and localized hyperplasia causing the related clinical syndrome may go unnoticed. *The malignant counterpart of these benign lesions can be detected with confidence only when there is associated metastasis in the liver.* An aggressive search by an ambitious individual may be *misleading* if well-stained accessory spleens, hyperplastic lymph nodes, or focal pancreatitis project into the pancreatic area.[1306, 1307] (Figs. 34-8 and 34-9)

Renal Adenomas

This group also includes *renin secreting* juxtaglomerular cell adenoma. *Renal adenomas* are usually seen in patients over fifty years old with associated vascular disease such as nephrosclerosis or infarcted scarred kidneys. Hypernephromas may arise from a renal adenoma. If the so-called adenoma is less than 3 cm in size, metastasis is rarely seen. The diameter of the adenoma will not prove the prognostic or diagnostic significance of the lesion.[1244, 1295, 1296]

Renin secreting juxtaglomerular cell adenomas are important lesions which may cause hypertension with decrease in the serum potassium level and an increase in the plasma renin and aldosterone levels. This lesion has tortuous vessels feeding a relatively lucent mass.[1250]

Hepatic Adenoma

This encapsulated mass contains cords of he-

(Text continues on page 718)

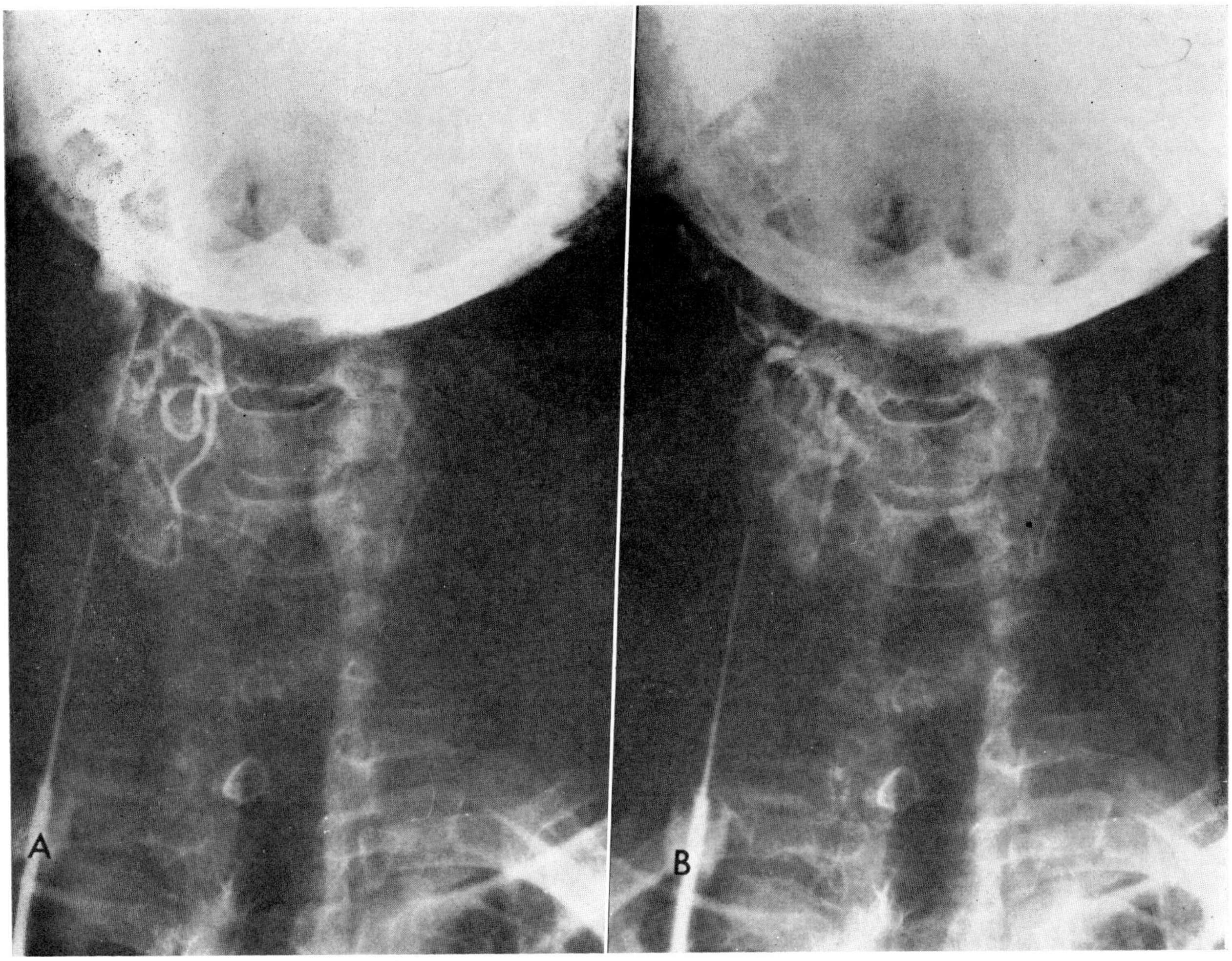

Figure 36.20. Common Carotid Arteriogram. (A) The superior thyroid artery is prominent and supplies a unilateral vascular thyroid mass. (B) The venous phase demonstrates homogeneous staining of the perfused area of the mass with multiple draining veins. *Diagnosis:* Thyroid adenoma. *Pathologic Diagnosis:* Hyperplastic normal thyroid tissue.

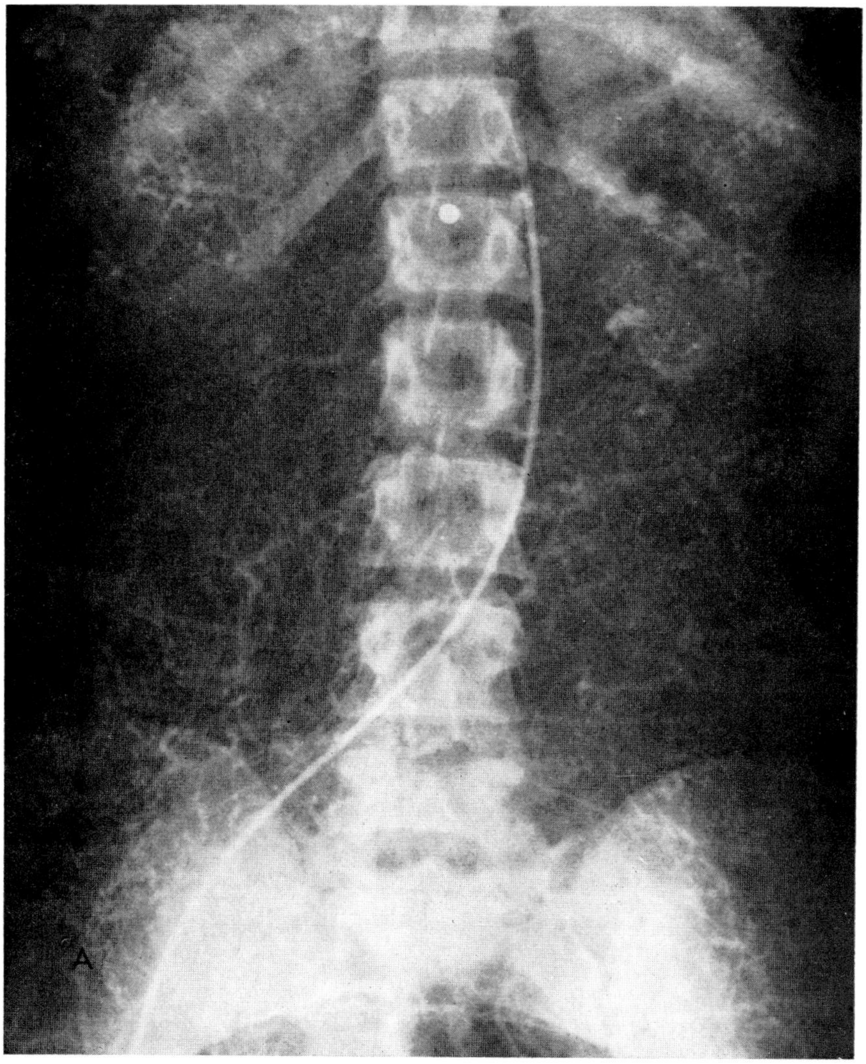

Figure 36.21A

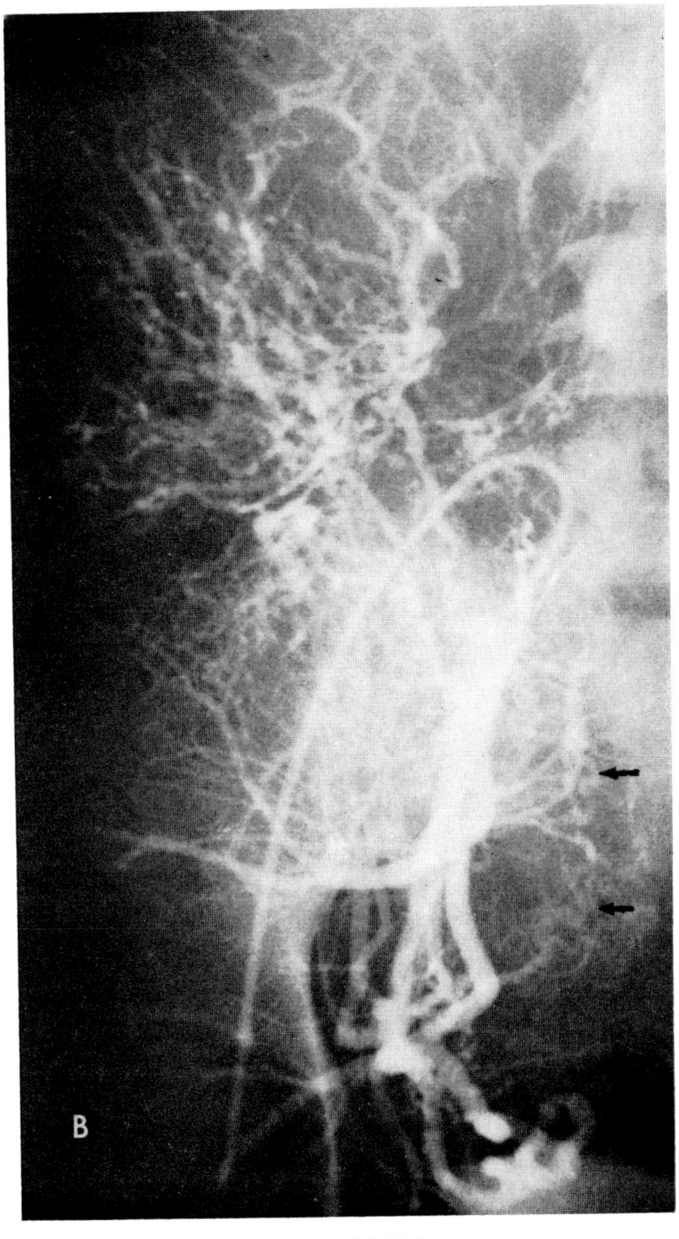

Figure 36.21B

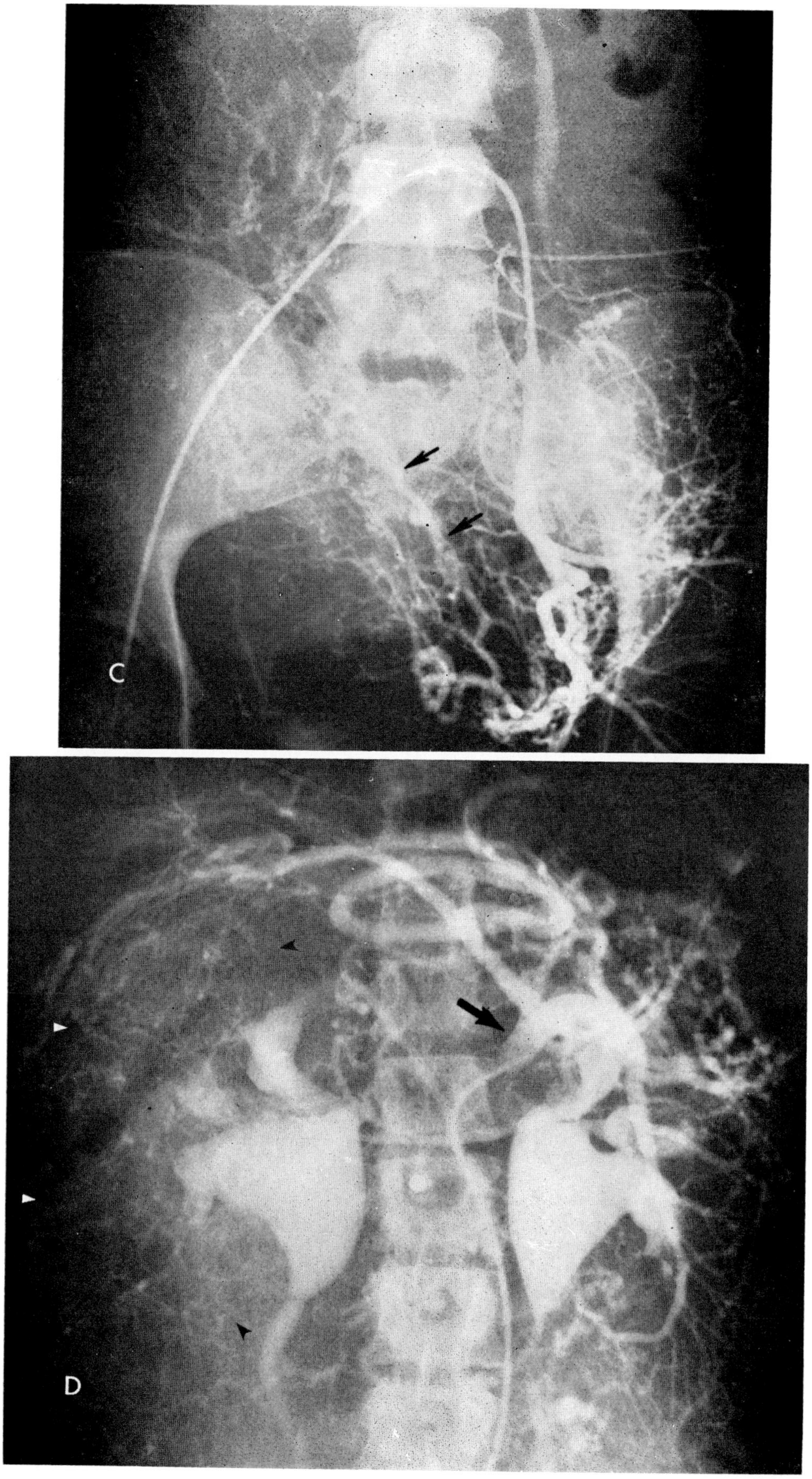

Figure 36.21 C and D

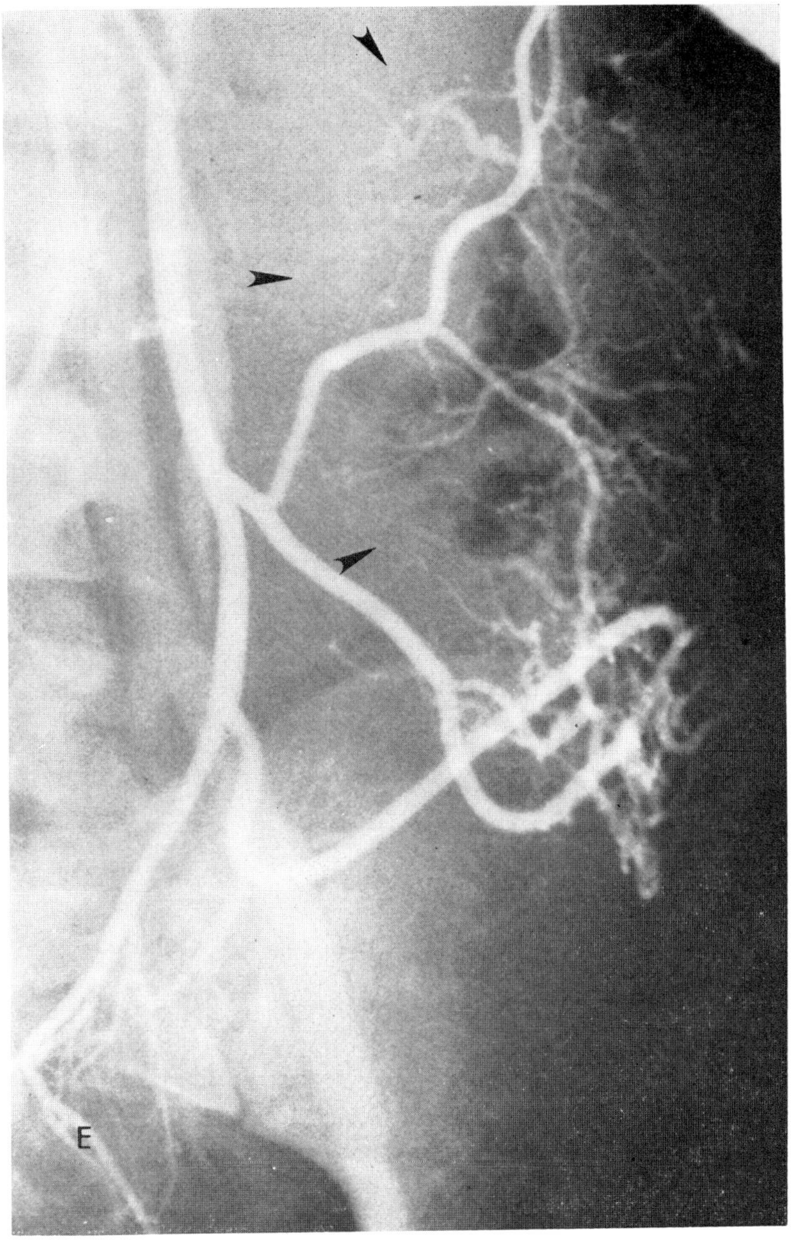

Figure 36.21. (A) Abdominal aortogram: The capillary phase reveals a hypervascular tumor occupying the entire abdominal cavity. (B, C) Right and left internal iliac arteriograms reveal marked hypervascularity and abnormal vessels. Note the tortuous dilated left uterine artery (Arrows) and the visceral branches of the right internal iliac artery supplying a portion of this mass (Arrows). (D) Celiac arteriogram: The celiac artery is distorted and deviated (Arrow) and supplies abnormal vessels and hypervascularity (Arrow Heads). (E) Inferior mesenteric arteriogram: Tumor vessels arise from the inferior mesenteric artery as well (Arrow Heads). This twenty-two-year-old woman had a progressively enlarging abdominal mass. *Diagnosis:* A pedunculated leiomyosarcoma or angiosarcoma. *Pathology:* Pedunculated leiomyoma of the uterus with no evidence of invasion of the mesentery or omentum. *Comment:* Though parasitic blood supply is associated with malignant invasion of the adjacent structures, it may also be seen in benign hypervascular lesions. (From Kurti, D. J., Patel, S. K., and Petasnick, J. P. Pedunculated uterine leiomyoma with parasitic blood supply from the superior and inferior mesenteric arteries. *Rush Presbyterian-St. Luke Medical Bulletin, 12:*269, 1973. Courtesy of authors and publishers.)

patic cells, bile ducts and fibrous tissues which usually develop in normal livers of young women.[1308, 1309] It may arise from hepatic or bile duct cells, or may be mixed; it can be *cystic or solid* in consistency. When the hepatic adenoma is solid in nature it is usually well defined with very prominent feeding vessels from the periphery, lacking arteriovenous shunting, lakes or venous invasion. If the tissues can pick up[1312] colloidal isotope material, it indicates benign functioning hepatic tissue and suggests the nonmalignant nature of this vascular mass. If the areas are cold[1310, 1311] after isotope administration, then the differential diagnosis of a hepatoma may still exist (Fig. 36-17).

Adrenal Adenoma

Hyperadrenalism may be caused by adenomas, adrenal hyperplasia, or carcinomas.[111, 142, 1235, 1331, 1332] Clinically these lesions may present as adrenogenital, Cushing's, or Conn's syndromes. The adrenogenital syndrome, if feminizing in men, is usually malignant; if virilizing in children is usually a congenital hyperplasia; and if virilizing in female adults is usually due to adenomas. Cushing's syndrome is usually related to carcinomas in girls, hyperplasias and adenomas in boys, and hyperplasia in adults. Conn's syndrome or aldosteronoma is usually an adenoma or hyperplasia (Fig. 34-10).

There is very little correlation between the morphology of the adrenal tumors, their histology, whether benign or malignant, and their function. Adenomas and carcinomas may be nonfunctional. Hyperplasias may be congenital or acquired, and in prolonged hyperplasias nodularity is not unusual. Adenomas and hyperplasias are not unusual in patients with essential hypertension.[1333]

Aldosteronomas[419, 1334–1336] may be single or multiple and are usually adenomas. On rare occasions aldosteronism may be related to bilateral hyperplasia. Small tumors may not be demonstrated angiographically, but venous samplings for hormonal assay may yield higher diagnostic results.

In the above abnormalities, adrenal venography[1329, 1330] may reveal stretching of veins in hyperplasia and stretching and deviation of the veins in long-standing hyperplasia with nodularity. If the veins are deviated and distorted then the diagnosis may include adenomas, cysts, malignancy or ganglioneuromas.

Parathyroid Adenomas

In order, primary hyperparathyroidism may be caused by an adenoma, hyperplasia or carcinoma.[1337] Apart from their usual location in the parathyroid glands, adenomas may also be found in the mediastinum.[1338] The blood supply to these ectopic lesions may come from the inferior thyroid, internal mammary, or anomalous arteries.[1339] They are usually demonstrated[1340, 1341] as well-defined discrete areas of stain, providing they are not cystic in nature. Angiography coupled with thyroid scan facilitates stronger and more confident diagnosis. Misleading stains of the thyroid or esophageal walls are not unusual (Fig. 34-11).

Cystadenomas

Are a combination of solid and cystic components of varying proportions enclosed in a capsule with or without papillary projections into the cystic cavities. The *angiographic presentation* depends on the proportion of solid and cystic elements within these lesions. The findings may range from totally hypervascular solid lesions to totally avascular cystic lesions or island of hypervascularity interspersed amidst lucent areas in mixed, solid and cystic lesions.[111, 1280, 1281]

Pancreatic cystadenomas,[1280, 1281] more common in the pancreatic body or tail, have a greater affinity for middle age women. Being a vascular tumor, recent and/or old hemorrhage into the mass is not unusual. They may be multilocular, cystic or solid with papillary projections. Whether benign or malignant they can be adherent to adjacent structures and may encase the vessels that come across. There may be bleeding into the gastrointestinal tract as well. Total avascularity should not be a surprise because of the associated cystic components.[1017,

(Text continues on page 725)

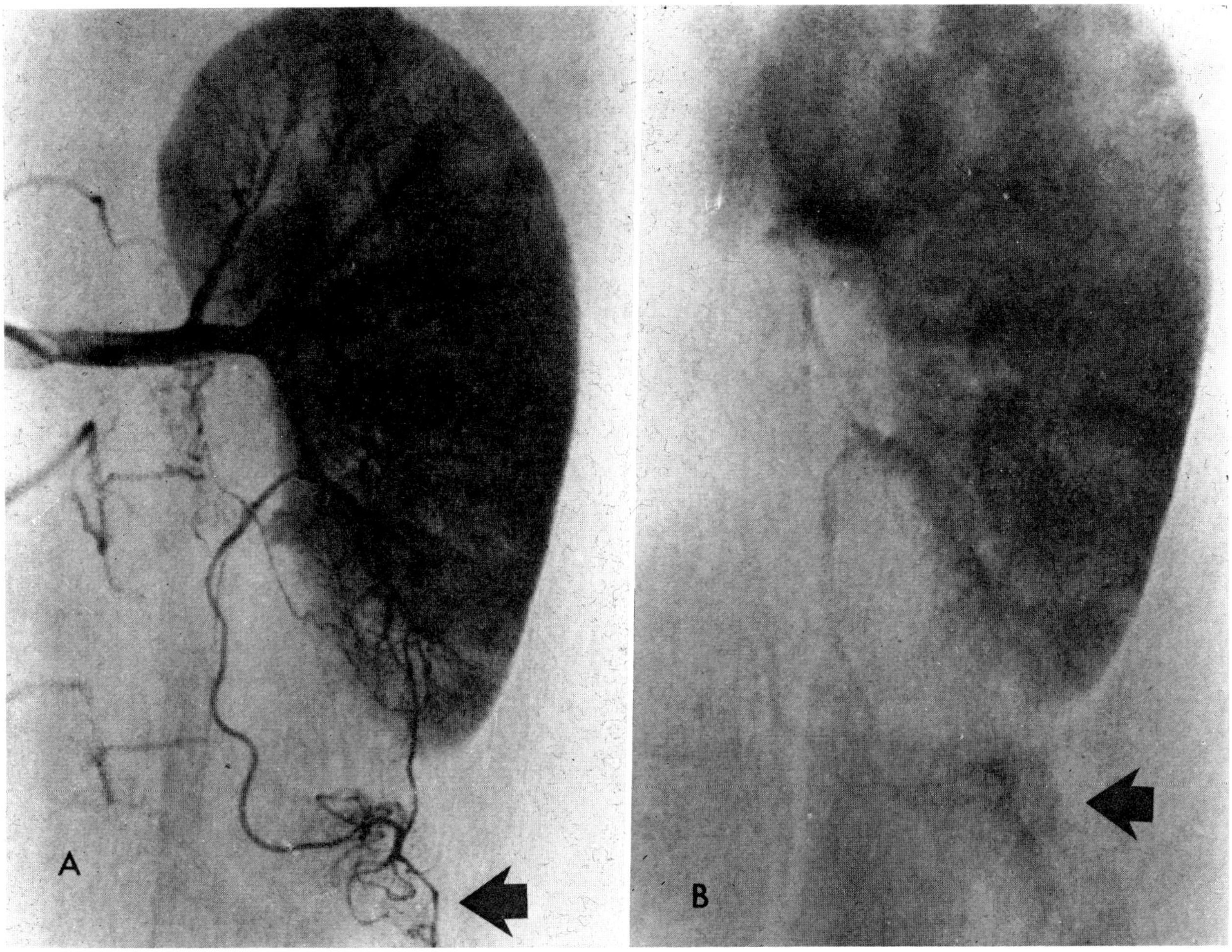

Figure 36.22. (A) Very prominent perforating capsular arteries feed a vascular lesion below the inferior pole of the kidney. (B) Moderate staining of the same lesion. This patient had an intrathoracic pheochromocytoma. *Diagnosis:* Hibernoma. *Differential Diagnosis:* Extraadrenal pheochromocytoma. (From English, J. T., Patel, S. K., and Flanagan, M. J., Association of phenochromocytomas with brown fat tumors. *Radiol, 107:*279, 1973. Courtesy of the authors and the publishers.)

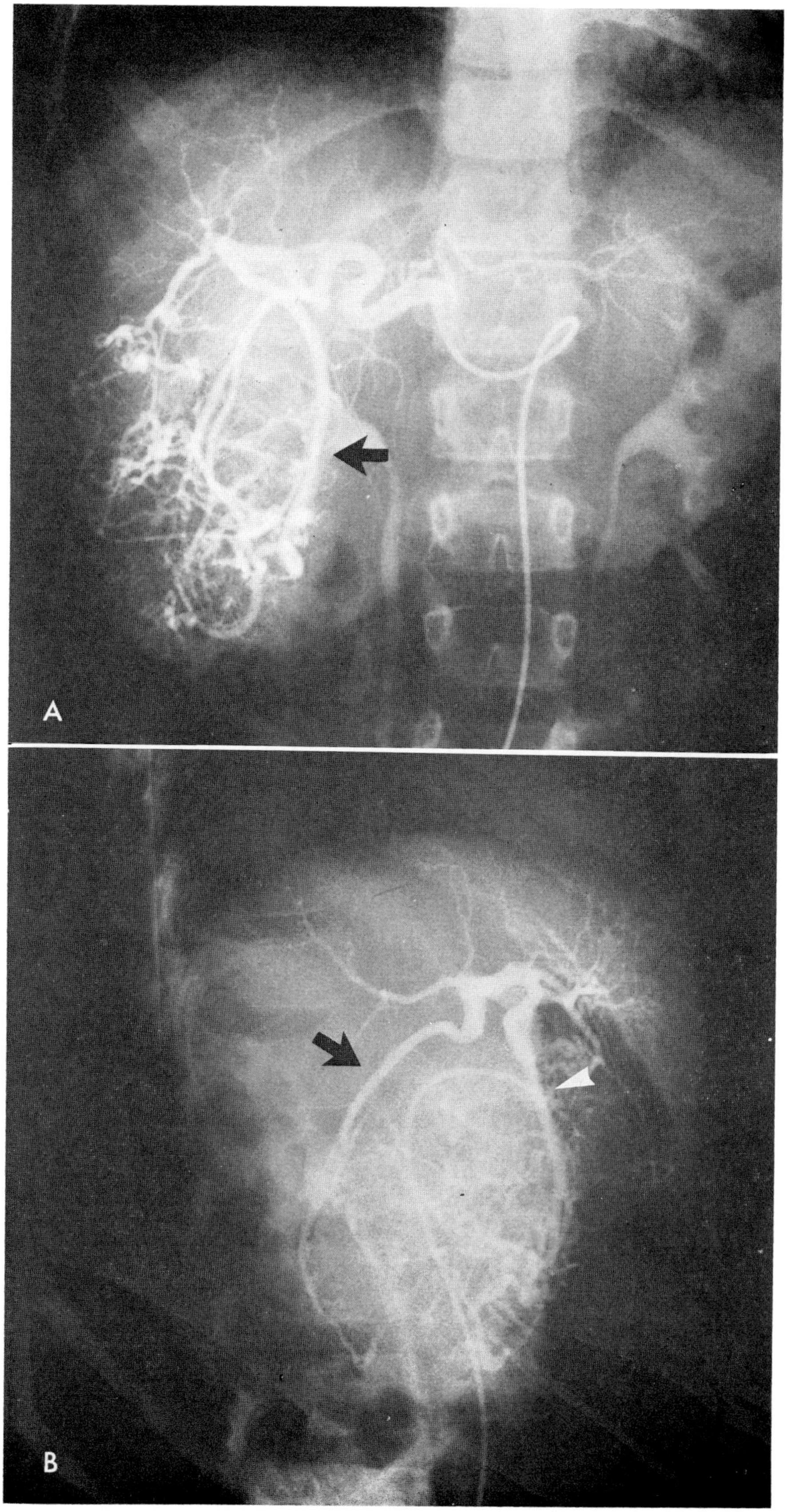
A
B

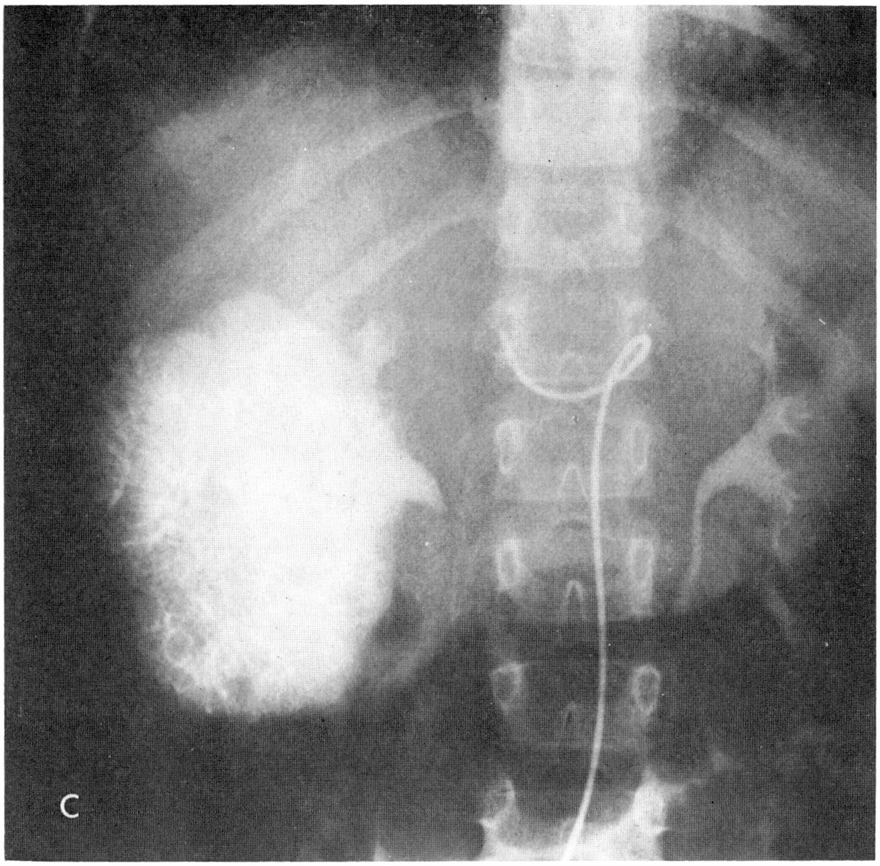

Figure 36.23. Selective Hepatic Arteriogram. (A) Frontal projection, (B) Lateral projection: Large feeding arteries circumferentially surrounding a very vascular mass are seen in the lower part of the right lobe of the liver. (C) Capillary phase: A large, well-defined, densely stained mass is seen. This patient is a nine-year-old girl. *Pathologic Diagnosis:* Focal nodular hyperplasia of the liver. (From McLoughlin, M. J., Colapinto, R. F., Gilday, D. L., Hobbs, B. B., Korobkin, M. J., McDonald, P., and Phillips, M. J. Focal nodular hyperplasia of the liver. *Radiol, 107*:257, 1973. Courtesy of the authors and publishers.)

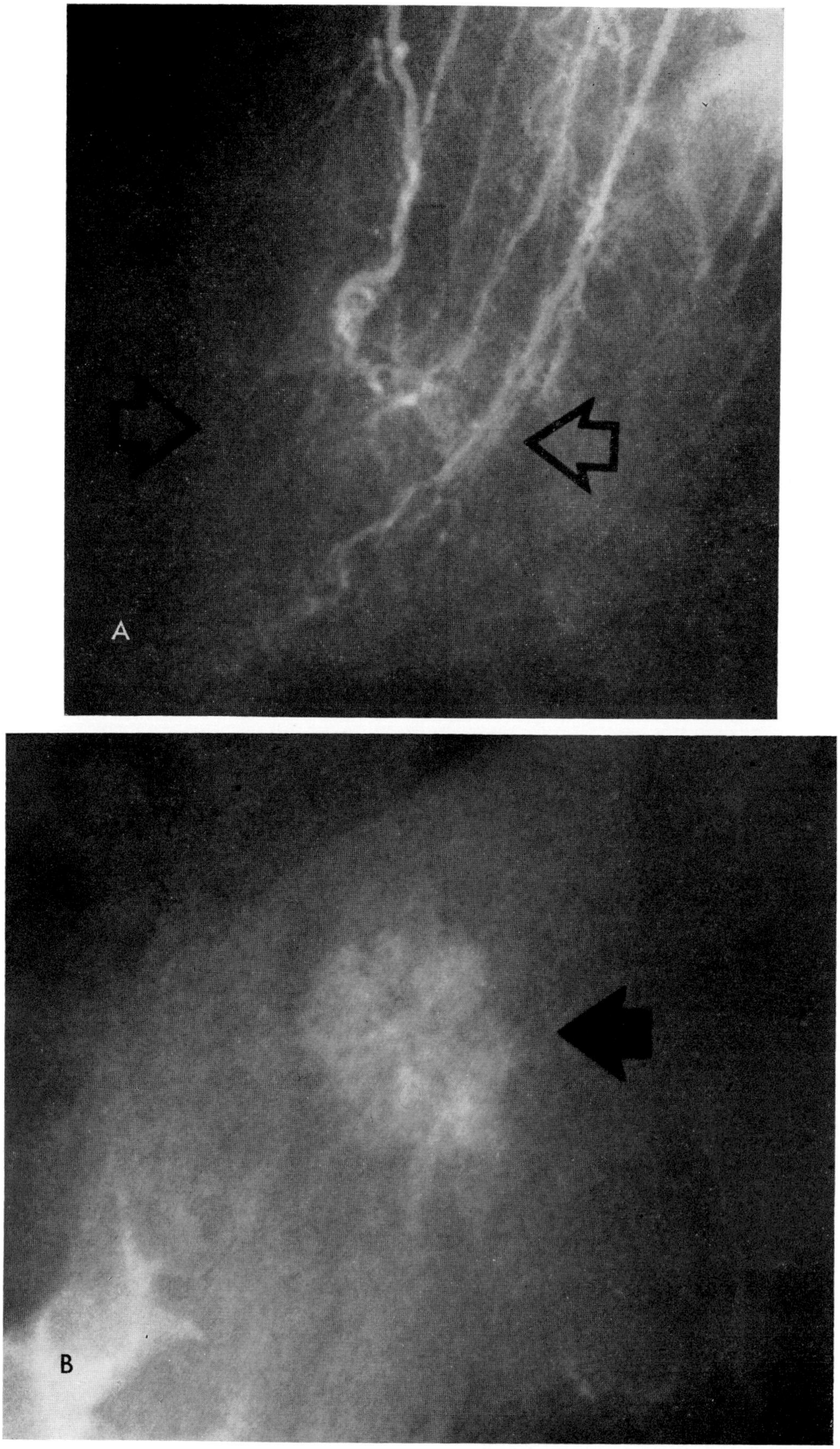

Figure 36.24. Hepatic Arteriogram (enlarged view of the right lobe, lower portion). (A) There is a very vascular lesion with abnormal vasculature. (B) Dense staining of this well-defined mass occurs in this twenty-six-year-old woman. *Pathologic Diagnosis:* Focal nodular hyperplasia. (From McLoughlin, M. J., Colapinto, R. F., Gilday, D. L., Hobbs, B. B., Korobkin, M. J., McDonald, P., and Phillips, M. J. Focal nodular hyperplasia of the liver. *Radiol, 107:*257, 1973. Courtesy of the authors and publishers.)

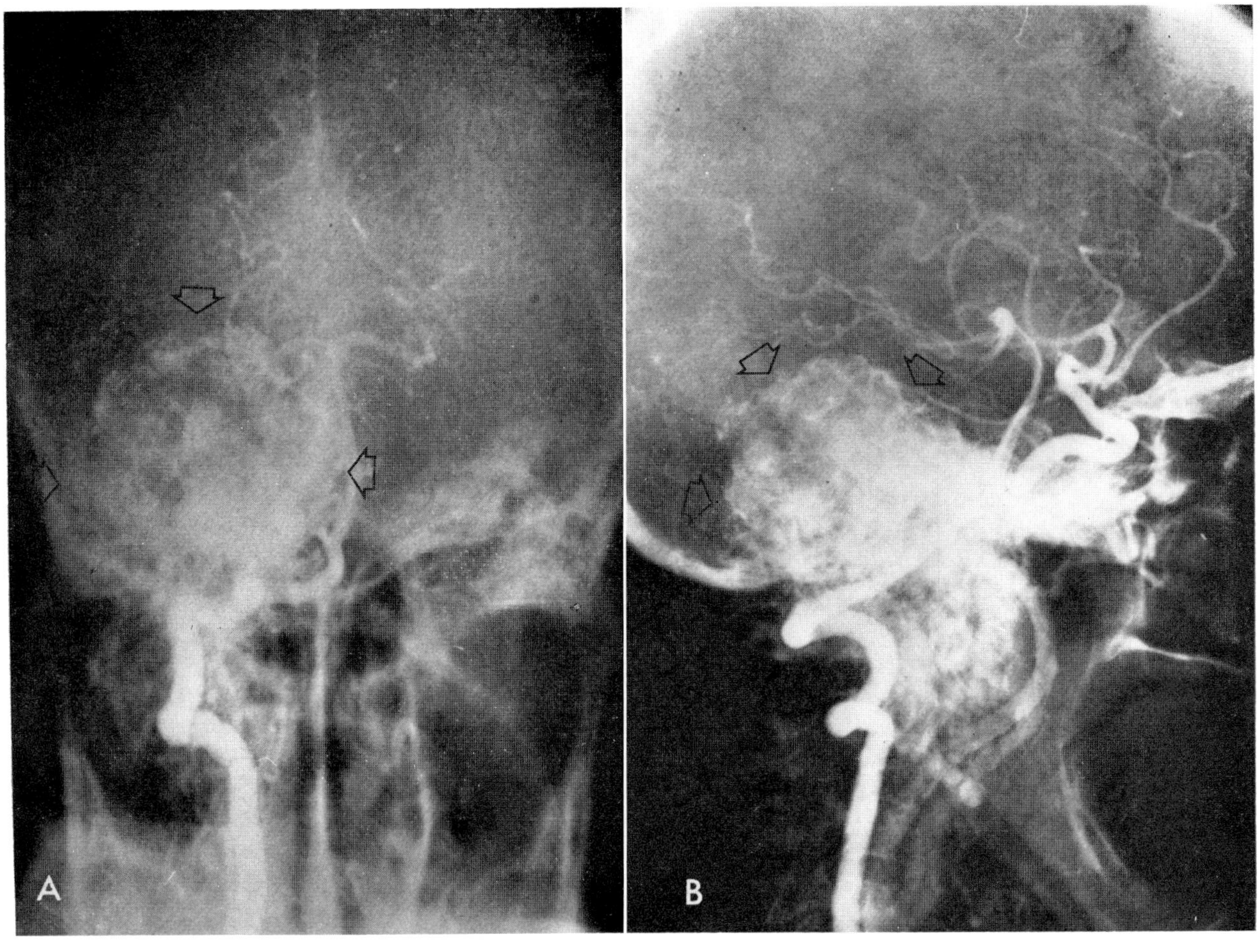

Figure 36.25. Brachial Arteriogram. An extremely vascular mass with pools of contrast material is seen in the posterior fossa. The patient clinically had signs and symptoms of a glomus jugulare tumor.

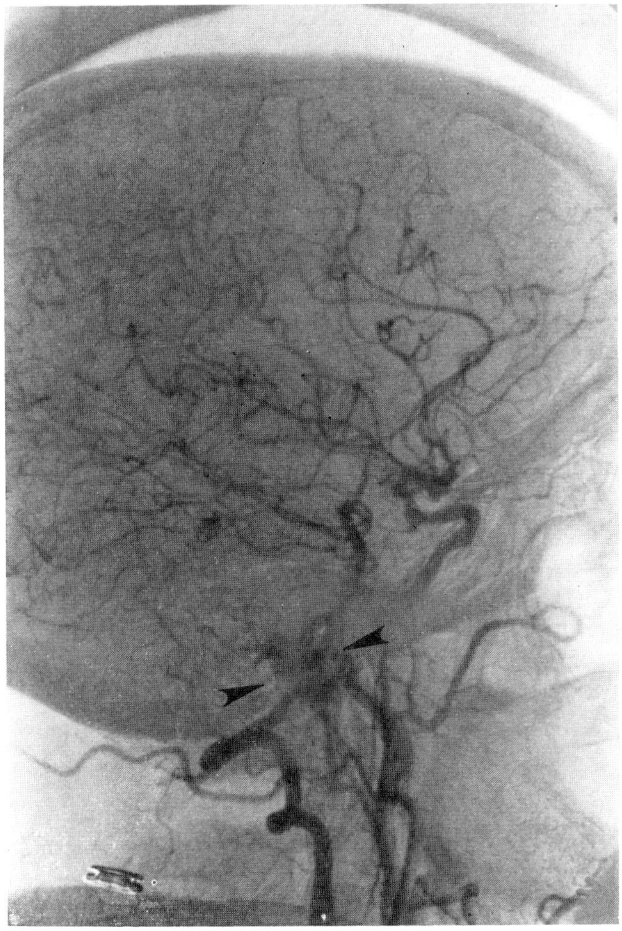

←

Figure 36.26. Brachial Arteriogram. An area of abnormal staining is revealed at the level of the jugular fossa in a patient with a known glomus jugulare tumor. (Courtesy of Dr. D. V. Patel, Michael Reese Medical Center, Chicago, Illinois.)

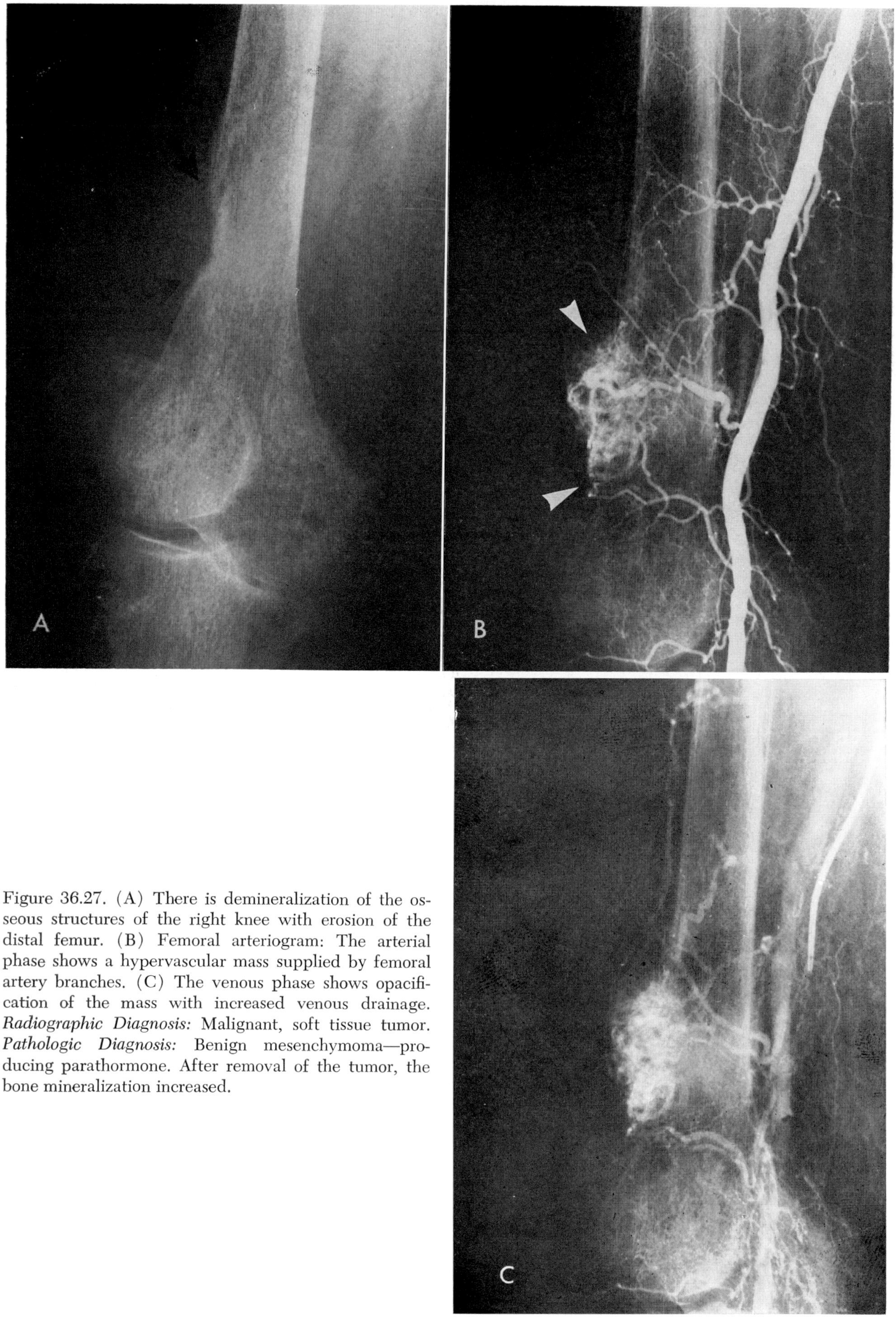

Figure 36.27. (A) There is demineralization of the osseous structures of the right knee with erosion of the distal femur. (B) Femoral arteriogram: The arterial phase shows a hypervascular mass supplied by femoral artery branches. (C) The venous phase shows opacification of the mass with increased venous drainage. *Radiographic Diagnosis:* Malignant, soft tissue tumor. *Pathologic Diagnosis:* Benign mesenchymoma—producing parathormone. After removal of the tumor, the bone mineralization increased.

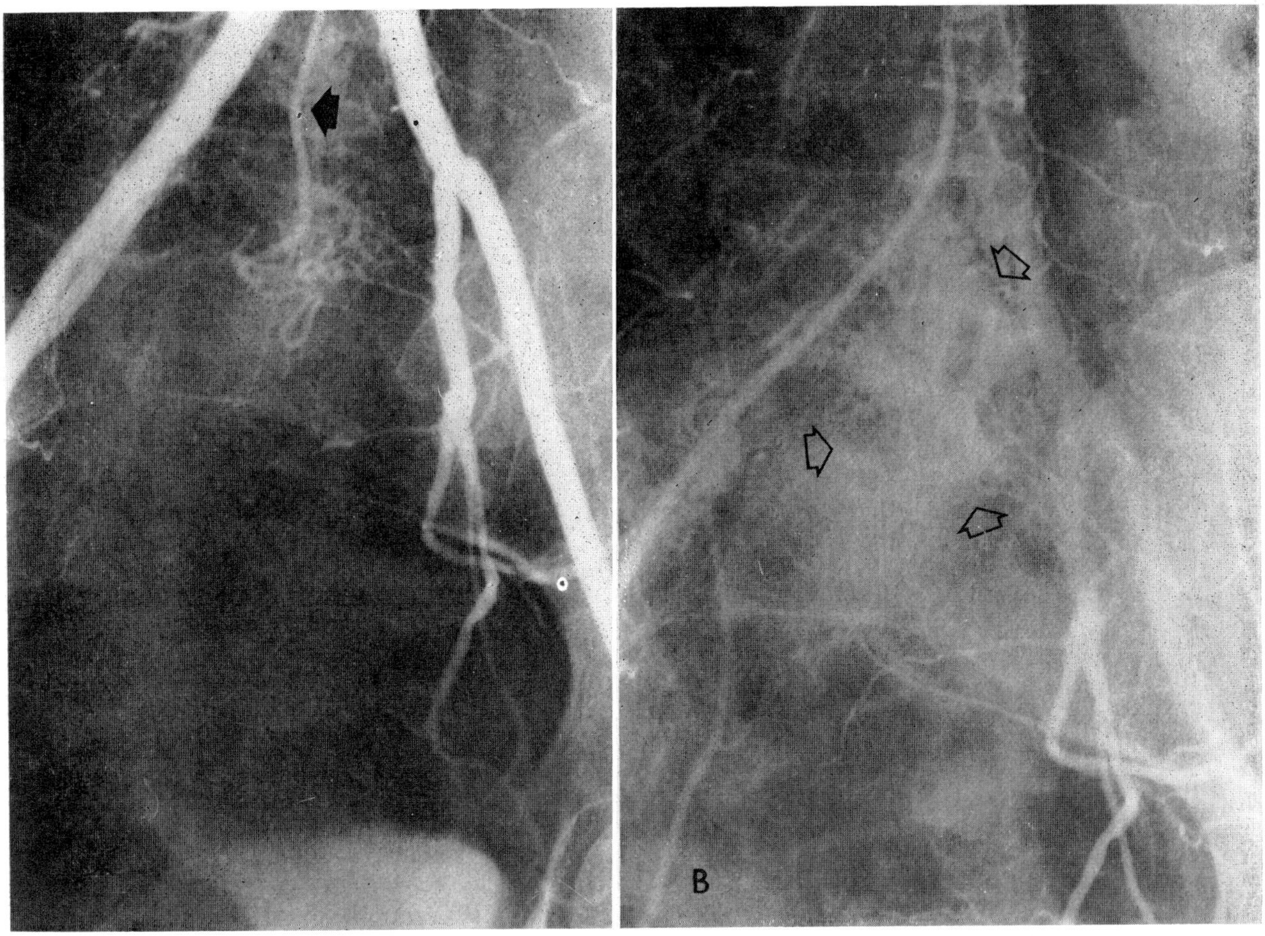

Figure 36.28. Pelvic Arteriogram. (A) A very prominent artery courses towards the sacrum (Arrow) probably the middle sacral artery with hypertrophic branches. (B) Late arterial phase: There is increased abnormal staining of a mass type of density (Arrow). A young female with hypertension. *Diagnosis:* Possible pheochromocytoma? *Pathology:* Vascular transformation of a lymph node.

[1239, 1297] *Angiographically* it would be very difficult to detect malignant counterparts, if any, in a benign cystadenoma unless associated metastasis is seen elsewhere, usually in the liver.

MISCELLANEOUS BENIGN TUMORS

Papillomas and Polyps

These masses have a delicate fibrovascular stroma with a few tumor vessels and staining of the solid components.[301, 1282, 1283]

Villous Tumors—Benign

These masses have irregular vessels with arteriovenous shunting.[1284]

Hibernomas

These represent residuals of infantile, reddish-brown fat seen usually between the scapulae in the paravertebral areas of the thoracic vertebral column and between the kidneys and the aorta.[1290, 1291] This richly vascularized fatty tissue has a functional relation to the adrenal and thyroid glands. It has a fascinating association with *pheochromocytomas.*[1292, 1293] Being extremely vascular, it is provided with irregular vessels and even has arteriovenous shunting.[1294]

Leiomyomas

Leiomyomas[1214] arise from the smooth mus-

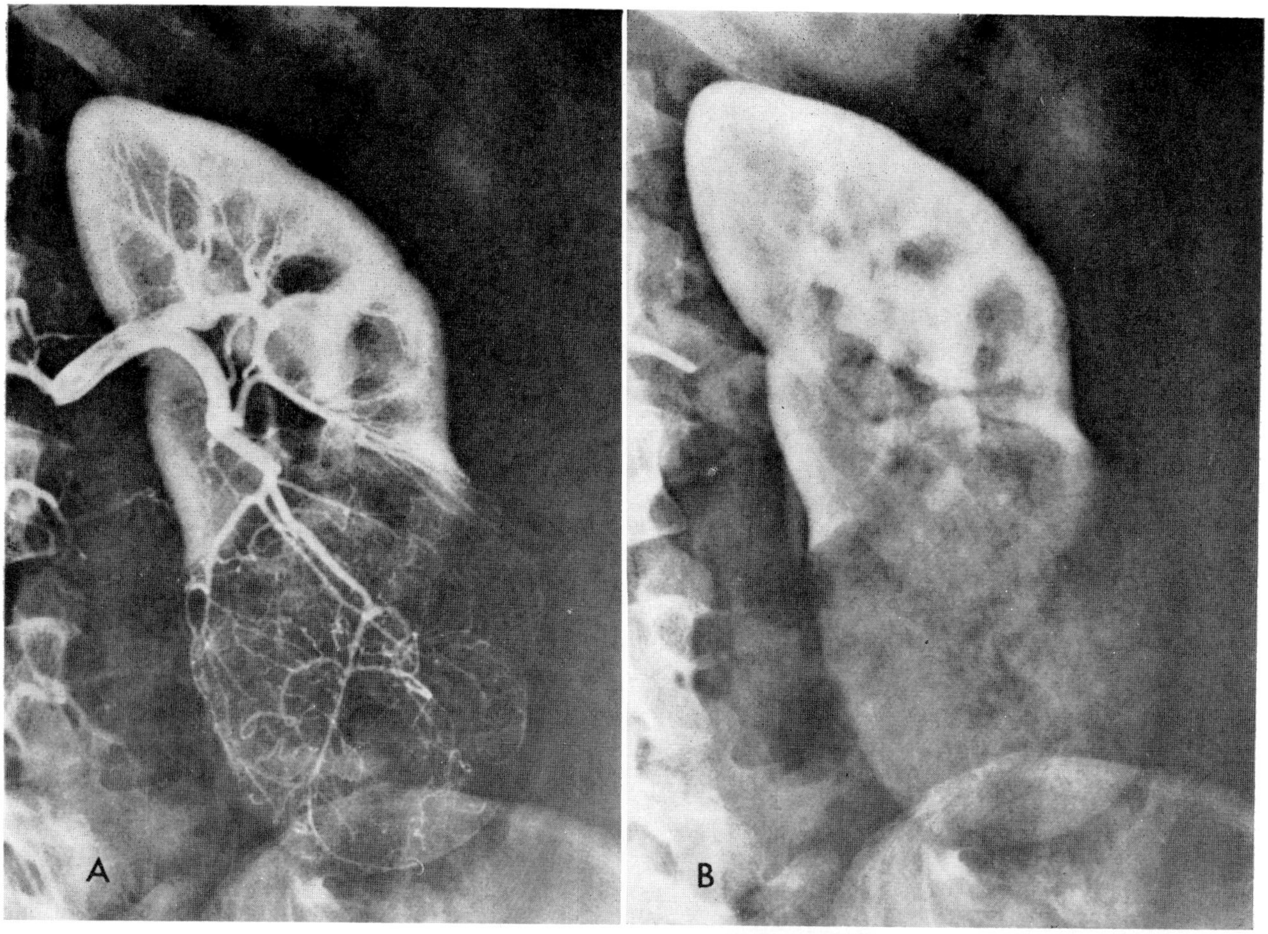

Figure 36.29. Renal Arteriogram. (A) Arterial phase: Abnormal arborization of the lower pole vessels within a mass is seen. (B) Parenchymal phase: Note the homogeneous smooth staining of this mass. *Diagnosis:* Hypernephroma. *Pathology:* Well-differentiated hypernephroma.

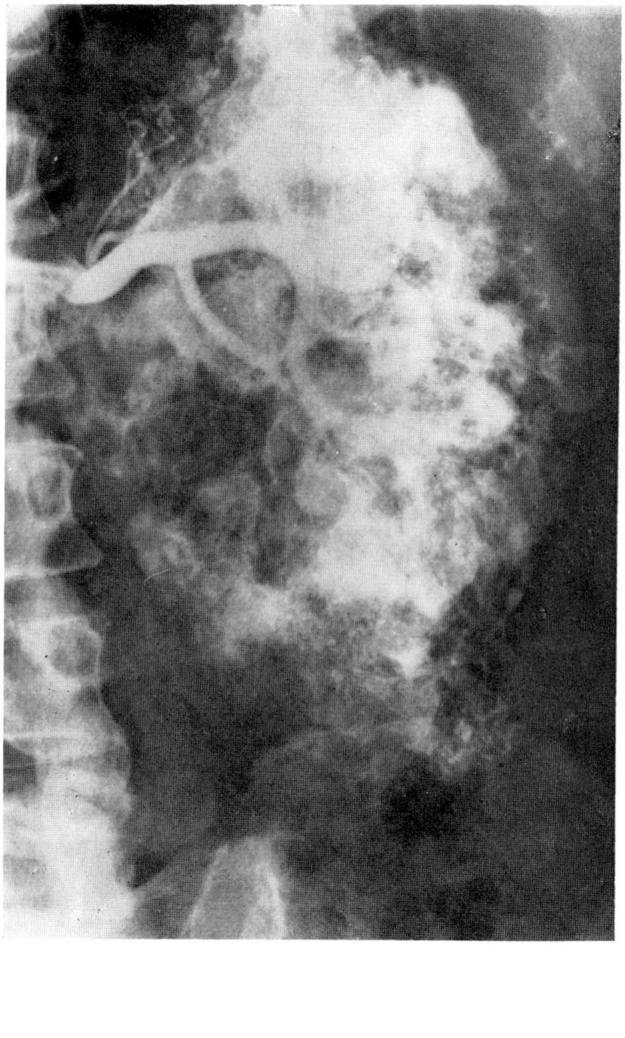

Figure 36.30. Renal Arteriogram. The normal anatomical landmarks of the kidney are lost with very vascular islands of masses having central translucencies and peripheral abnormal vasculature. Perinephric extension of this process is also shown. *Diagnosis:* Hemangioendotheliosarcoma of the kidney? *Pathology:* Anaplastic hypernephroma involving the entire kidney with perinephric extension.

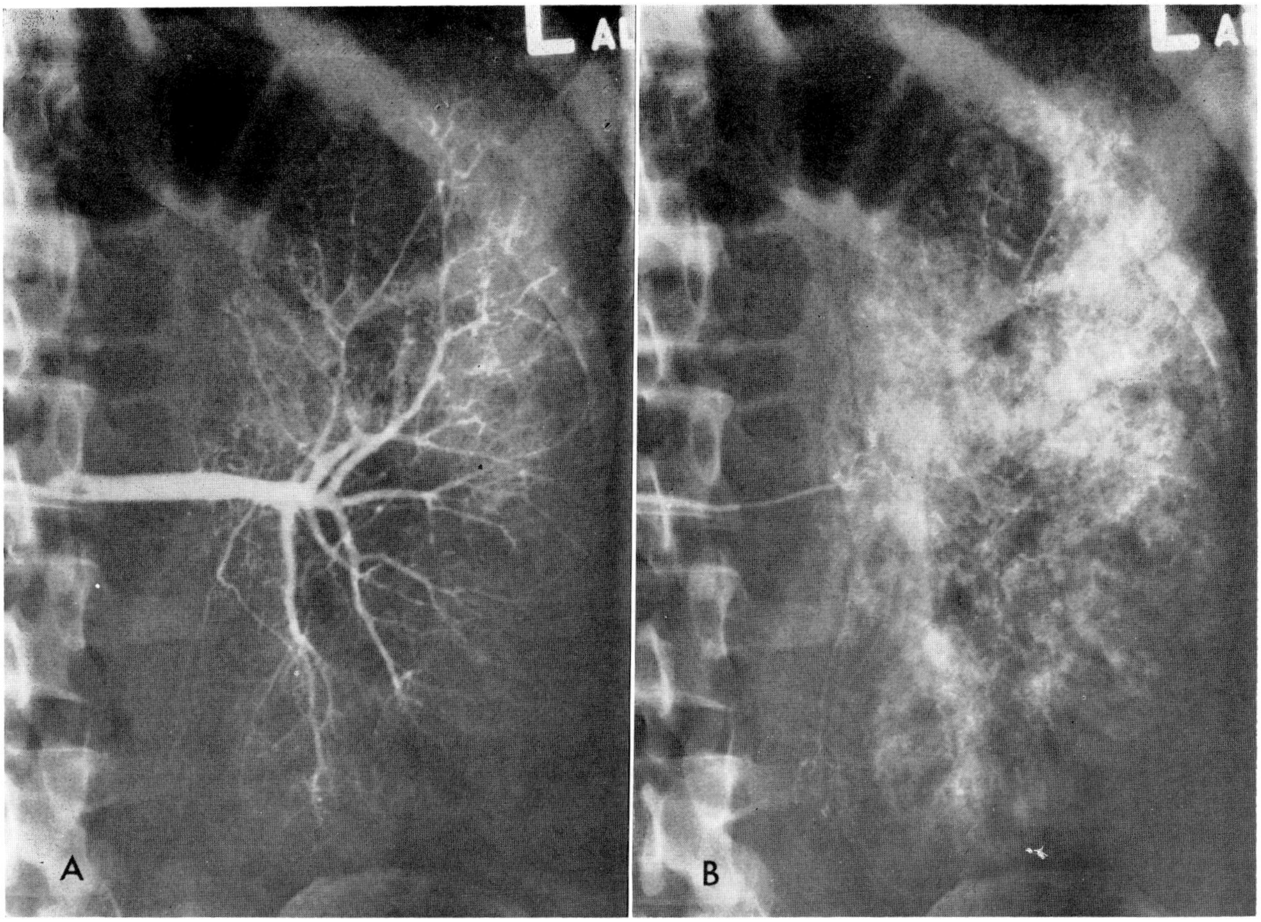

Figure 36.31. Renal Arteriogram. (A) Stretching of the main renal artery and of the intrarenal arterial branches occurs with abnormal terminations with multiple irregularities of these intrarenal branches. (B) There is retention of contrast in these irregularly dilated, small vessels. *Diagnosis:* Diffusely infiltrating hypernephroma. (Courtesy of Dr. F. J. Mulopulos, Chairman, Department of Radiology, Lutheran General Hospital, Park Ridge, Illinois.)

cle of the structure in concern or from the smooth muscles of vessels. They may develop wherever smooth muscle is found. These tumors are very vascular, thereby developing and hemorrhagic necrotic areas within the tumor mass. They are usually well circumscribed, very vascular, with lakes and puddles, and arteriovenous shunting. As usual, the malignant counterpart of these tumors may not be detected as a specific entity angiographically.[1346, 1347] Intestinal leiomyomas are comparatively more malignant than those found in the stomach. Gastric leiomyomas tend to be avascular[1346] (Fig. 36-21).

Focal Nodular Hyperplasia of the Liver

These lesions are formed by hepatocytes and biliary epithelial cells.[1309] They usually occur in normal livers, as well-circumscribed single or multiple lesions, and have a great affinity for younger women. They are very vascular lesions, provided with *dysplastic* tortuous irregular vessels, prolonged stain, and with or without demonstrable arteriovenous shunting.[1498] The vascular supply may be from the periphery, but may also be central with peripheral radiation[1350–1352] (Figs. 36-23 and 36-24).

If colloidal isotope material is concentrated

in the lesions then it probably represents the presence of functioning hepatic tissue. If not, the differential diagnosis of hepatoma still exists.[1353]

Hepatic Regeneration

Regenerating nodules which are accompaniments of cirrhotic livers may be micronodular in portal cirrhosis or macronodular in biliary cirrhosis. Again, they may be single or multiple lesions. The pressure exerted by their growth and expansion causes narrowing and obliteration of the small vessels against the rigid connective tissue of the cirrhotic liver at the postsinusoidal level.[302, 1354] They may receive their blood supply either from the portal vein[1355] or hepatic artery.[302] During angiography they may present as vascular,[298] hypovascular[1356] or even avascular[1351] lesions. The normal uptake of colloidal isotope by these lesions aids in revealing their true nature.[298, 1351, 1356]

MALIGNANT TUMORS

Malignant tumors consist of metabolically superior, proliferating, neoplastic cells either densely or scantily interspersed amidst their supporting stroma. The *stroma* is built of variable proportions of vascular, fibrous and lymphatic tissues. Some tumors are well differentiated with a well-defined architecture and decor, closely resembling the cell from which they originated, and even reproducing glandular patterns. Well-differentiated hepatoma cells may

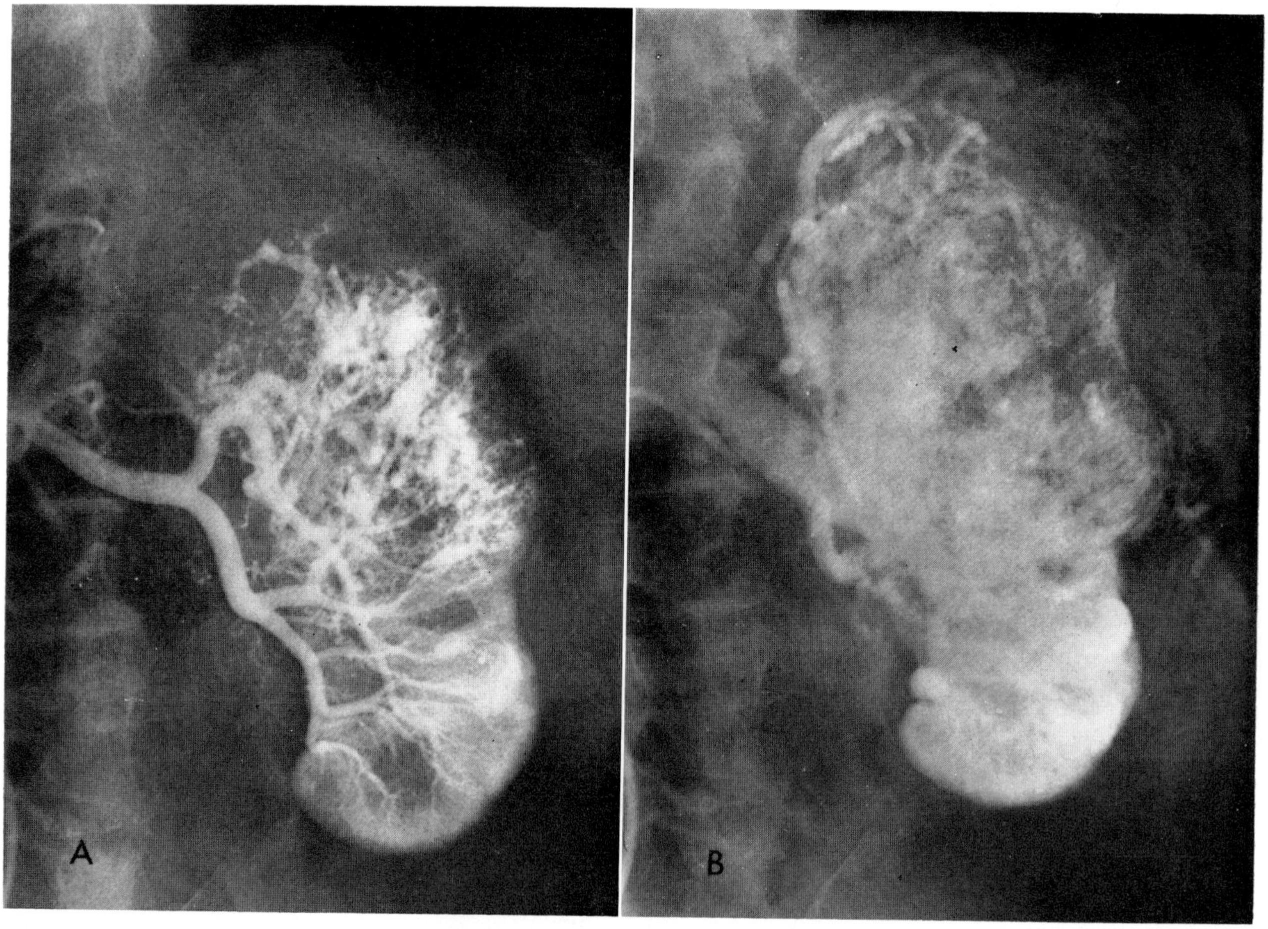

Figure 36.32. Renal Arteriogram. (A) Arterial phase: Very abnormally dilated irregularly calibered vessels lead into amorphous collections of contrast material in the upper half of the kidney. (B) A moderately sized mass with irregular islands of abnormal collections of contrast material is seen with very prominent perinephric veins. *Diagnosis:* Hypernephroma. Notice the patent renal vein.

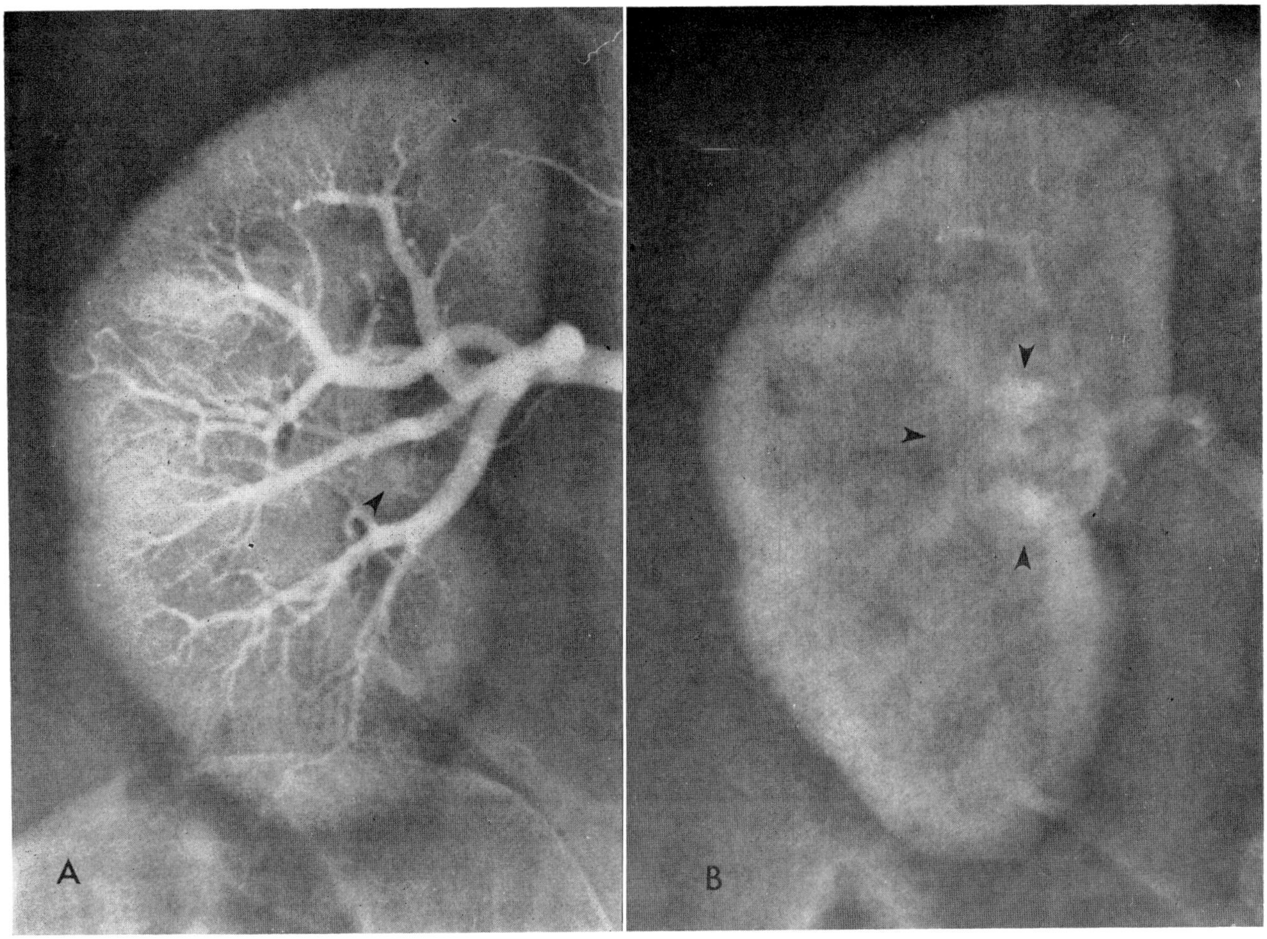

Figure 36.33. Renal Arteriogram. (A) Arterial phase: Slight increase in vasculature is seen in the renal hilar area. (B) A well-defined mass with increased stain is in the renal hilar area. *Diagnosis:* Hypernephroma.

be very similar to normal hepatocytes and their functions. Such tumors may be provided with a well-organized vascular pattern. On the contrary, some neoplasms have extremely deviant cells with a helter-skelter arrangement, deserving the name anaplastic or extremely undifferentiated cells. Obviously these lesions demand a luxurious blood supply for their survival and growth.

The richness of the *connective tissue stroma* decides the consistency of the tumor and also characterizes its angiographic presentation. Neoplasms with very *little fibrous stroma,* but densely packed cells, develop a rich vascular stroma. This is exemplified by sarcomas, medullary cancers, hepatomas and hypernephromas. At the other extreme are the *scirrhous neoplasms* with their monotonous fibrous background and almost negligible vascular mirage. Their islands of cancer cells are like a *lost caravan* amidst the desert. Adenocarcinomas of the pancreas and desmoplastic tumors in general are examples of this type of tumor. The same desmoplastic lesions, desmoid tumors, and fibromas become soft in consistency when they undergo sarcomatous degeneration and build up increased tumor vasculature.

The *stroma of neoplasms* is derived from the normal tissue. In a passive sense it is a part of the tumor. The fibrous tissue component of a neoplasm may be a part of the neoplastic proliferative phase as in carcinosarcoma, or it may be a response to the presence of a neoplasm as seen in a scirrhous carcinoma. The stroma

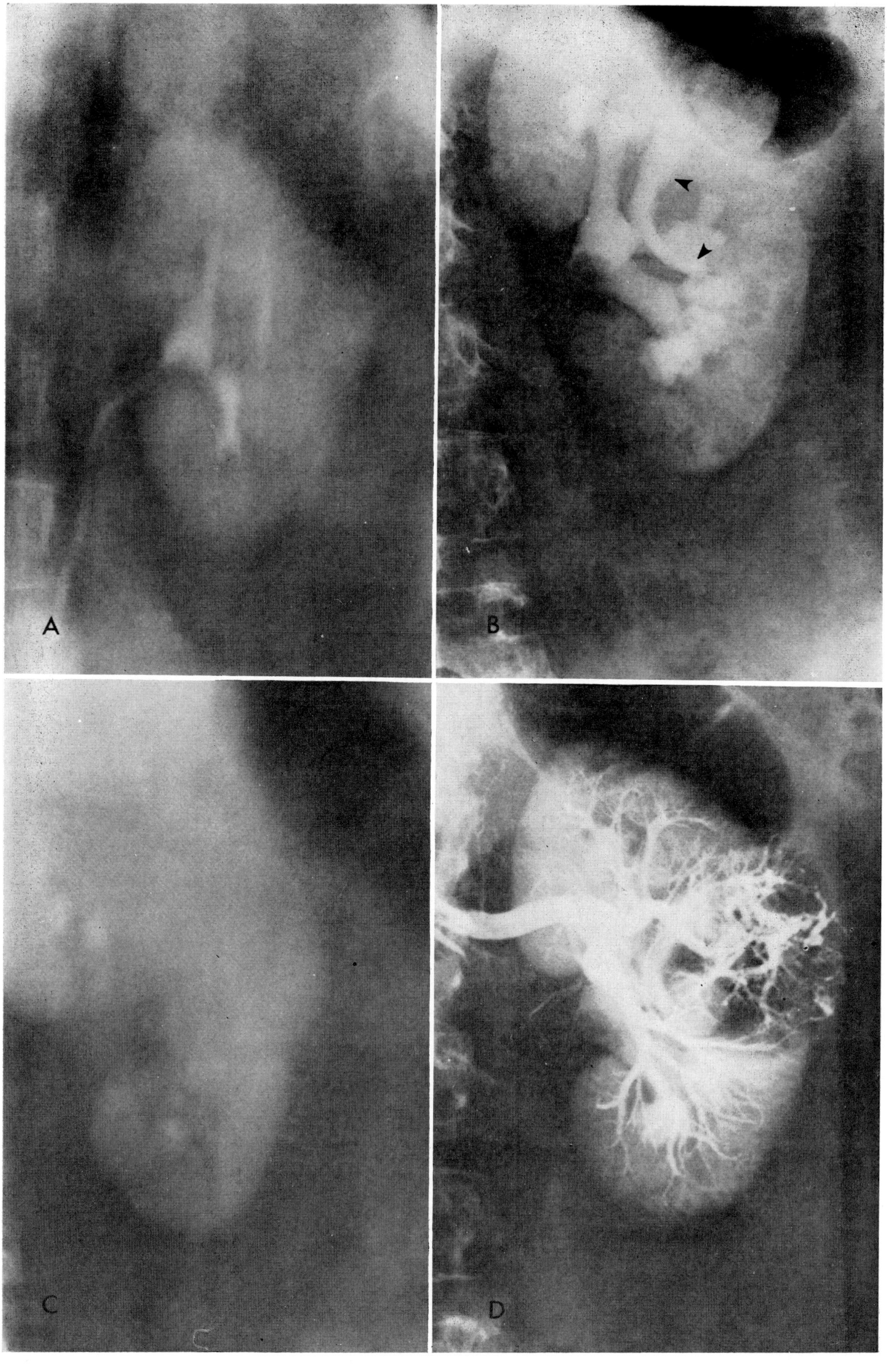
A
B
C
D

which is critical to the survival and growth of the tumor modifies its angiographic presentation, but not the histologic differentiation.[111]

Tumors virtually vascularize themselves by appropriation or by evocation of a fibrovascular response from the host. This helps build a new supply of blood vessels for the tumor.[85] The population of tumor cells and capillary endothelial cells within a neoplasm constitutes a highly integrated ecosystem. The mitotic index of the two cell populations depends on each other. Tumor *angiogenetic factor,* which is essential for angiogenesis, is absent in normal tissue except in the placenta.[1357] The difference between a malignant cell and the normal cell from which it arose may lie in the ability of the malignant cell to provoke a continuous vascular proliferation. This may be the underlying factor responsible for the autonomous growth inherent within tumor cells.[1358, 1359] The angioblastic and fibroblastic powers of a tumor comprise a delicate balance which is very vital to the growth of the tumor cells. Hemorrhage, necrosis or edema are not uncommon when the tumor is highly anaplastic. This is because of excessive metabolic demand and self-destruction if the tumor outgrows its blood supply. Too great a blood supply with an insufficient stroma is unfavorable to tumor growth because of the repeated hemorrhages into the tumor parenchyma.[1360] *Rapidly growing tumors,* which have an abundant vascular stroma with a meager connective tissue stroma, are vulnerable to repeated hemorrhage and pressure necrosis.

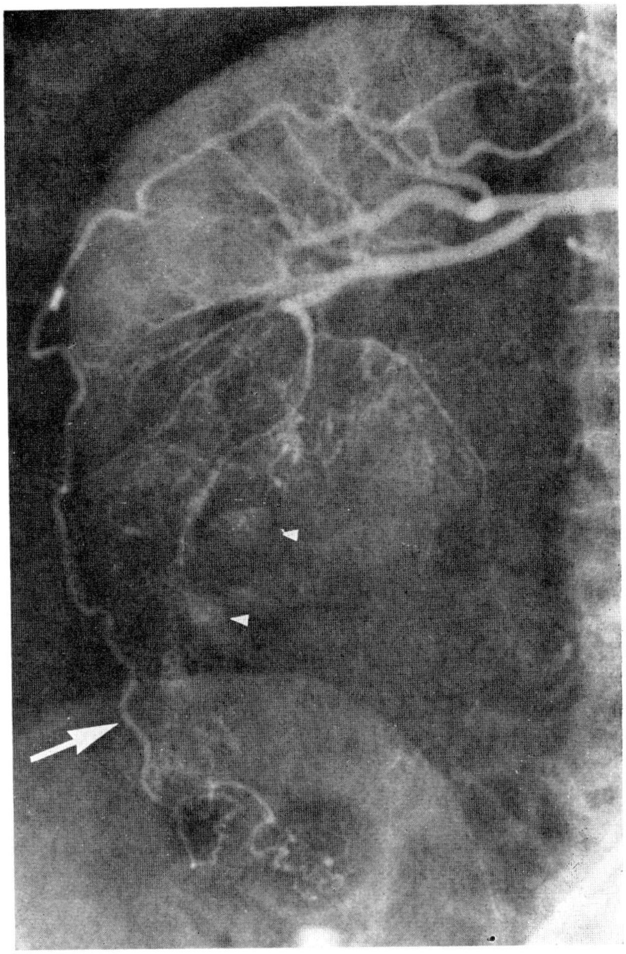

Figure 36.35. Renal Arteriogram. A very prominent, dilated, elongated, tortuous artery courses along the perinephric area with an abnormal termination (Arrow). Abnormal islands of contrast material (Arrow Head) and abnormally dilated irregularly arborizing vessels are present. *Diagnosis:* Hypernephroma of the lower half of the kidney with central necrosis and peripheral vascular supply.

←

Figure 36.34. (A) A nephrotomogram reveals prominent renal parenchyma with a hump. (B) Two years later the same patient presented with acute renal colic on the left side. Notice the extrinsic compression on the midrenal calyx (Arrow) and the filling defect in the renal pelviureteral area. (C) Nephrotomogram: At the second visit to the hospital the hump is becoming a bump! (D) Left renal arteriogram reveals abnormal arborization of the midportion vessels with irregular dilatation and lack of tapering in this same mass. *Diagnosis:* Hypernephroma presenting with renal colic. The first I.V.P. finding was felt to be due to dromedary hump.

Slowly growing tumors have a relatively less adequate blood supply with a more proportional balance in their constituents.[111] A well-differentiated malignant neoplasm may have an almost normal vascular architecture similar to that of a benign neoplasm.[1361]

When the tumor becomes too bulky, central necrosis develops because the tumor growth outpaces the blood supply. The periphery of the tumor, however, still has a tremendous capacity to elicit a vigorous vascular supply from the

(Text continues on page 740)

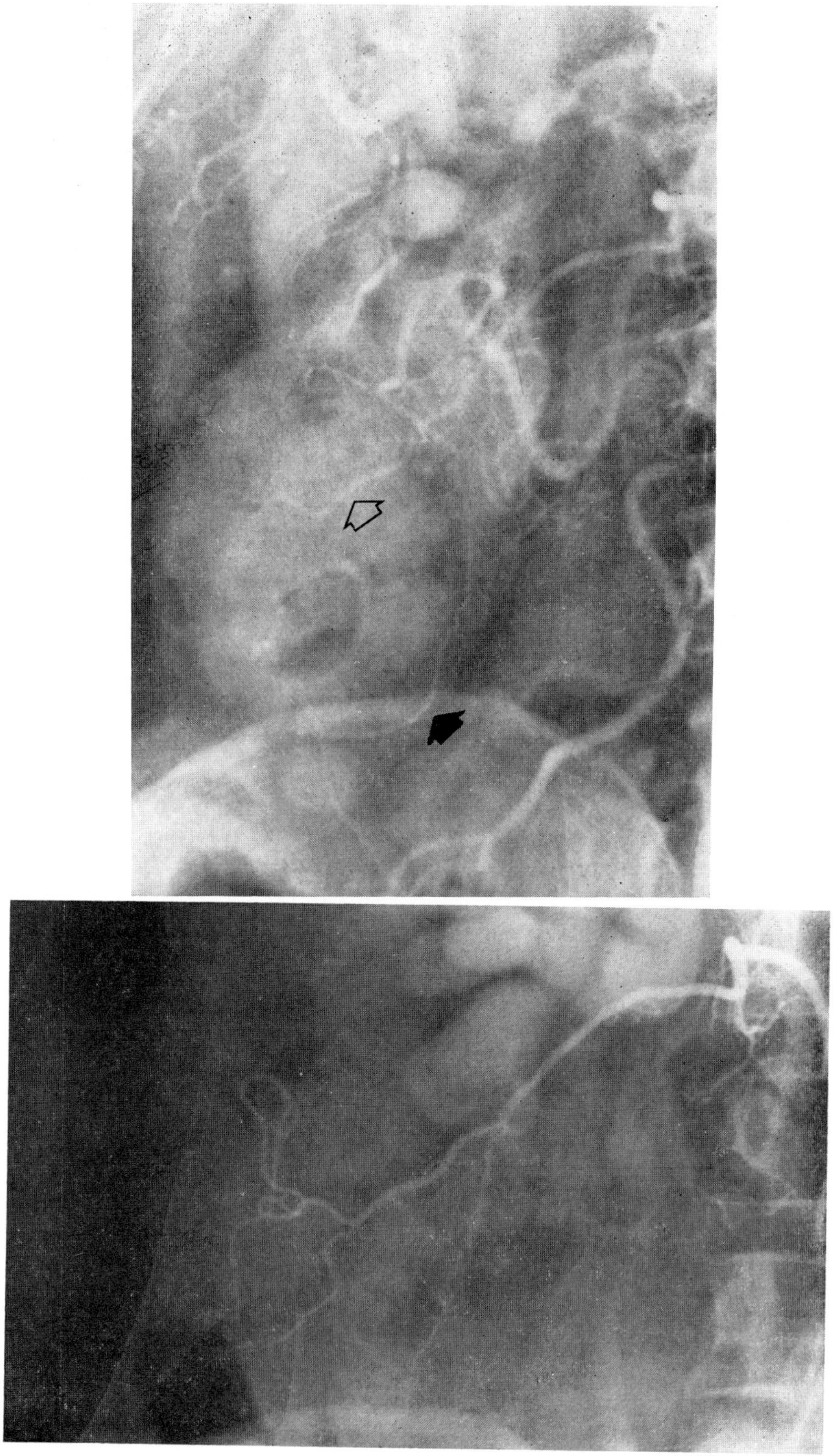

Figure 36.36. Flush Aortogram. (A) Small abnormal vessels course along a mass arising from the lower pole of the kidney. (B) Selective lumbar arteriogram at the same level. Notice the abnormal tortuous course of the distal branches of the lumbar artery with increased caliber of the vessels. *Diagnosis:* Hypernephroma of the kidney with central necrosis and peripheral vascular supply from adjacent vessels.

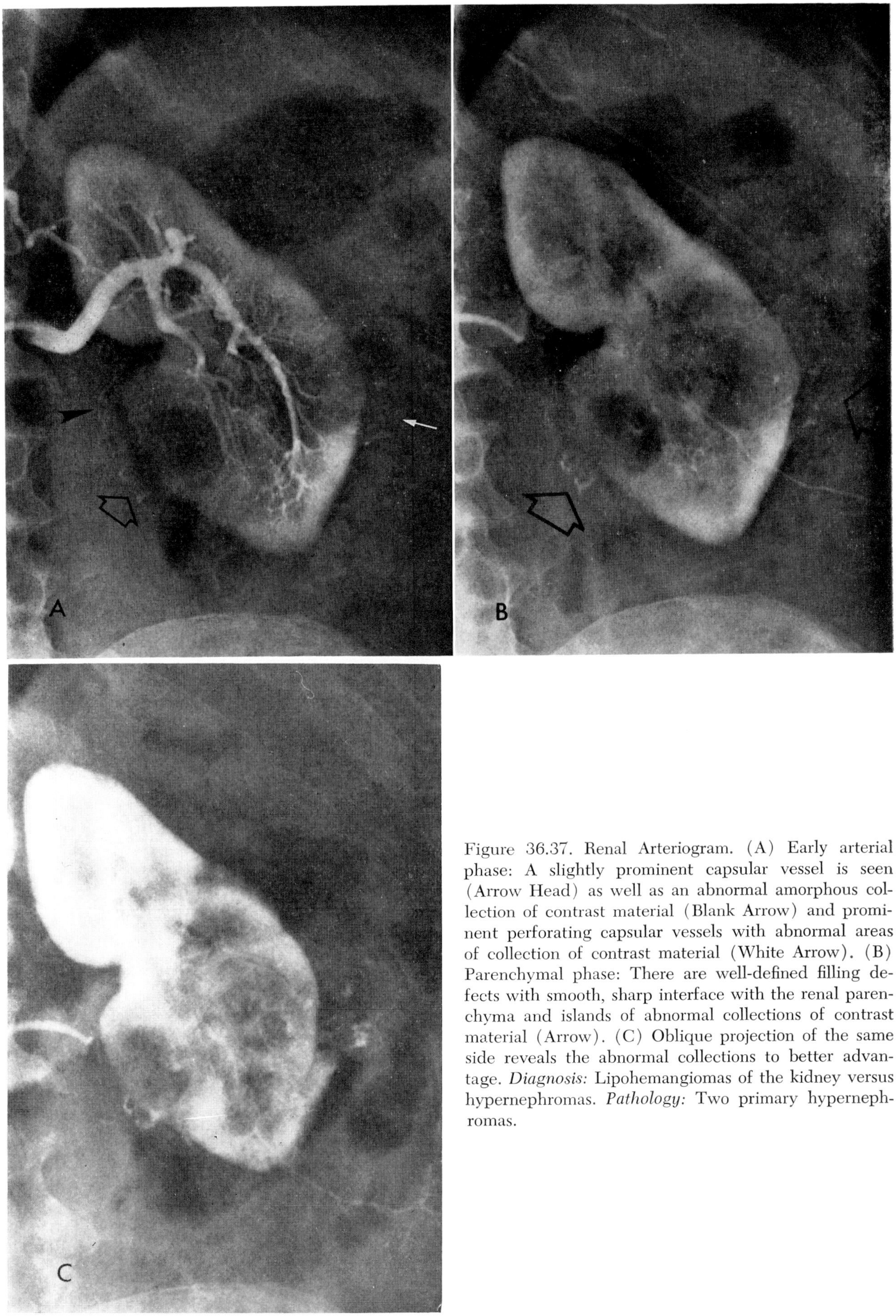

Figure 36.37. Renal Arteriogram. (A) Early arterial phase: A slightly prominent capsular vessel is seen (Arrow Head) as well as an abnormal amorphous collection of contrast material (Blank Arrow) and prominent perforating capsular vessels with abnormal areas of collection of contrast material (White Arrow). (B) Parenchymal phase: There are well-defined filling defects with smooth, sharp interface with the renal parenchyma and islands of abnormal collections of contrast material (Arrow). (C) Oblique projection of the same side reveals the abnormal collections to better advantage. *Diagnosis:* Lipohemangiomas of the kidney versus hypernephromas. *Pathology:* Two primary hypernephromas.

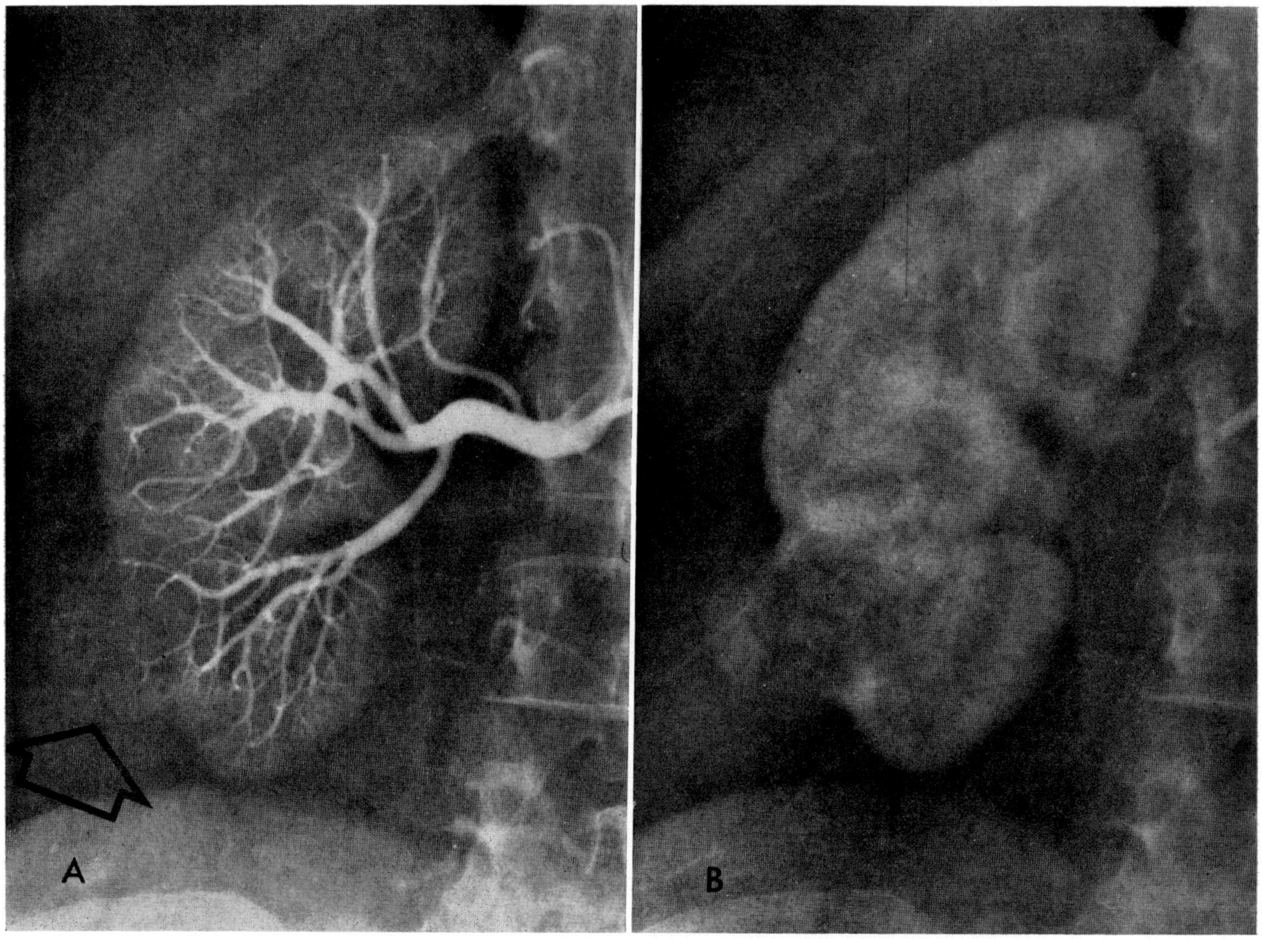

Figure 36.38. Renal Arteriogram. (A) Arterial phase: A soft tissue mass with increased vasculature is seen in the lateral contour of the kidney. (B) Parenchymal phase: Note the irregular staining of this mass. A patient who presented with intractable anemia. *Diagnosis:* In question. *Surgery:* Hypernephroma.

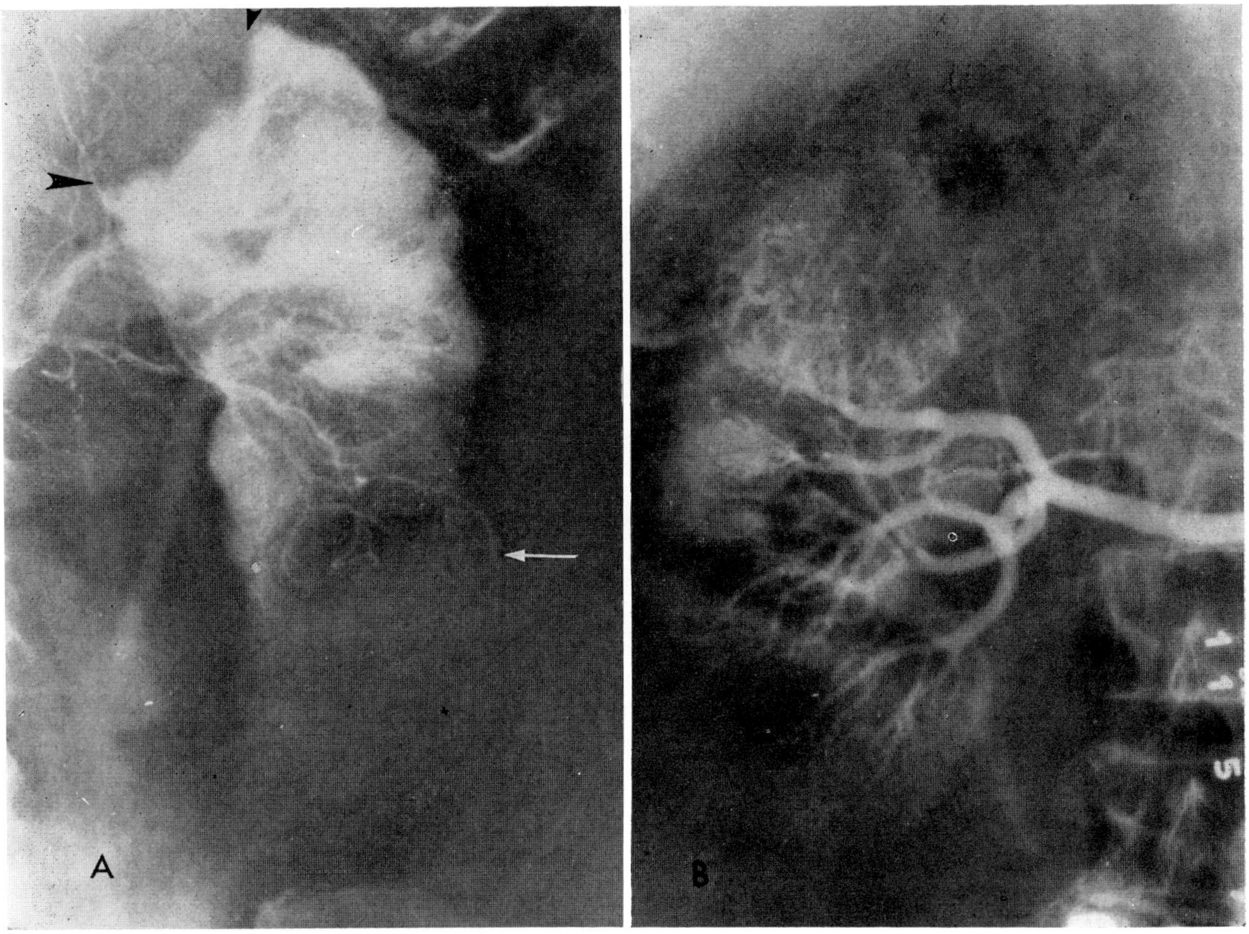

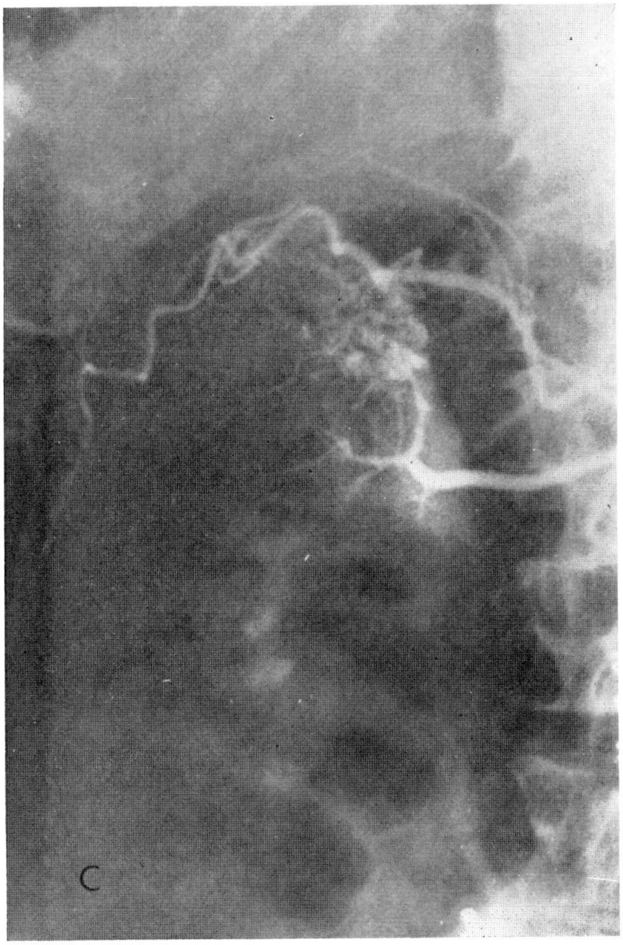

Figure 36.39. Renal Arteriogram. (A) Left renal arteriogram: A mass is in the lower pole of the kidney with very prominent vessels arborizing on its surface (Arrow). Another moderately well-defined defect is in the upper pole of the same kidney (Arrow Head). (B) The right renal arteriogram on the same patient reveals an abnormal vessel coursing through and around a mass in the upper pole of the right kidney. (C) Catheterization of the upper pole aberrant vessel reveals a very prominent capsular artery supplying the upper pole hypervascular mass with abnormal vascularity. *Diagnosis:* (1) Avascular hypernephroma left lower pole with aberrant artery to upper pole, (2) Very vascular hypernephroma rupturing the capsule on the right side.

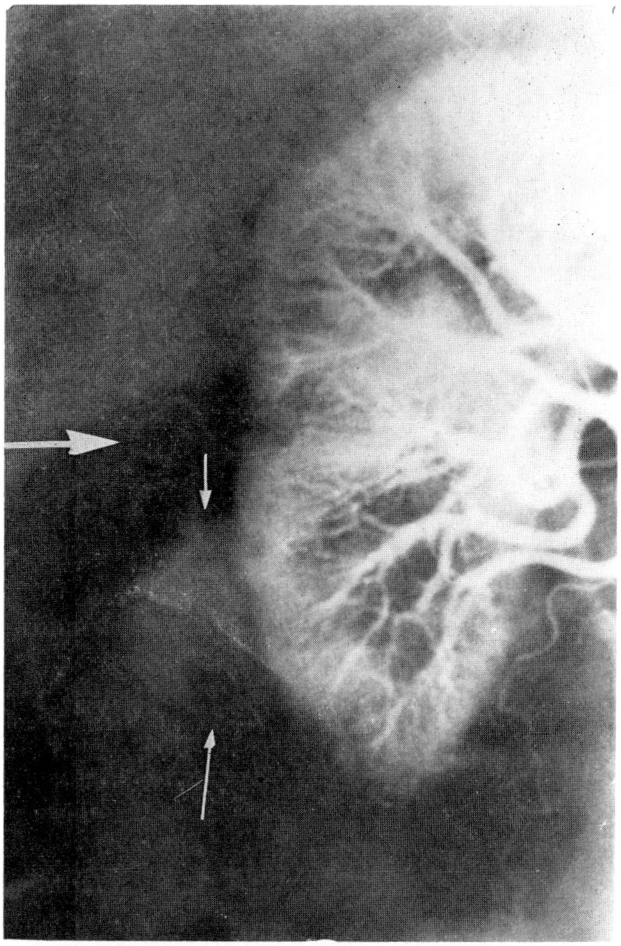

Figure 36.40. Renal Arteriogram. A soft tissue mass projects from the lateral part of the kidney (Small Arrow). A prominent perforating capsular vessel courses towards the mass (Large Arrow). *Diagnosis:* Avascular mass arising from the kidney. *Pathology:* Necrotic hypernephroma.

Figure 36.41. Renal Arteriogram. (A) Arterial phase: Very prominent perforating renal capsular branches course along a moderately sized mass with irregularly calibered vessels (Arrow Head) supplying hyperstaining islands of masses (Arrow). (B) Parenchymal phase: Intense staining of these masses occurs with very prominent venous drainage. *Diagnosis:* Hypernephromas arising in the wall of the cyst. *Pathology:* The fluid within the cystic cavity was urine colored. (The radiographic diagnosis was confirmed.)

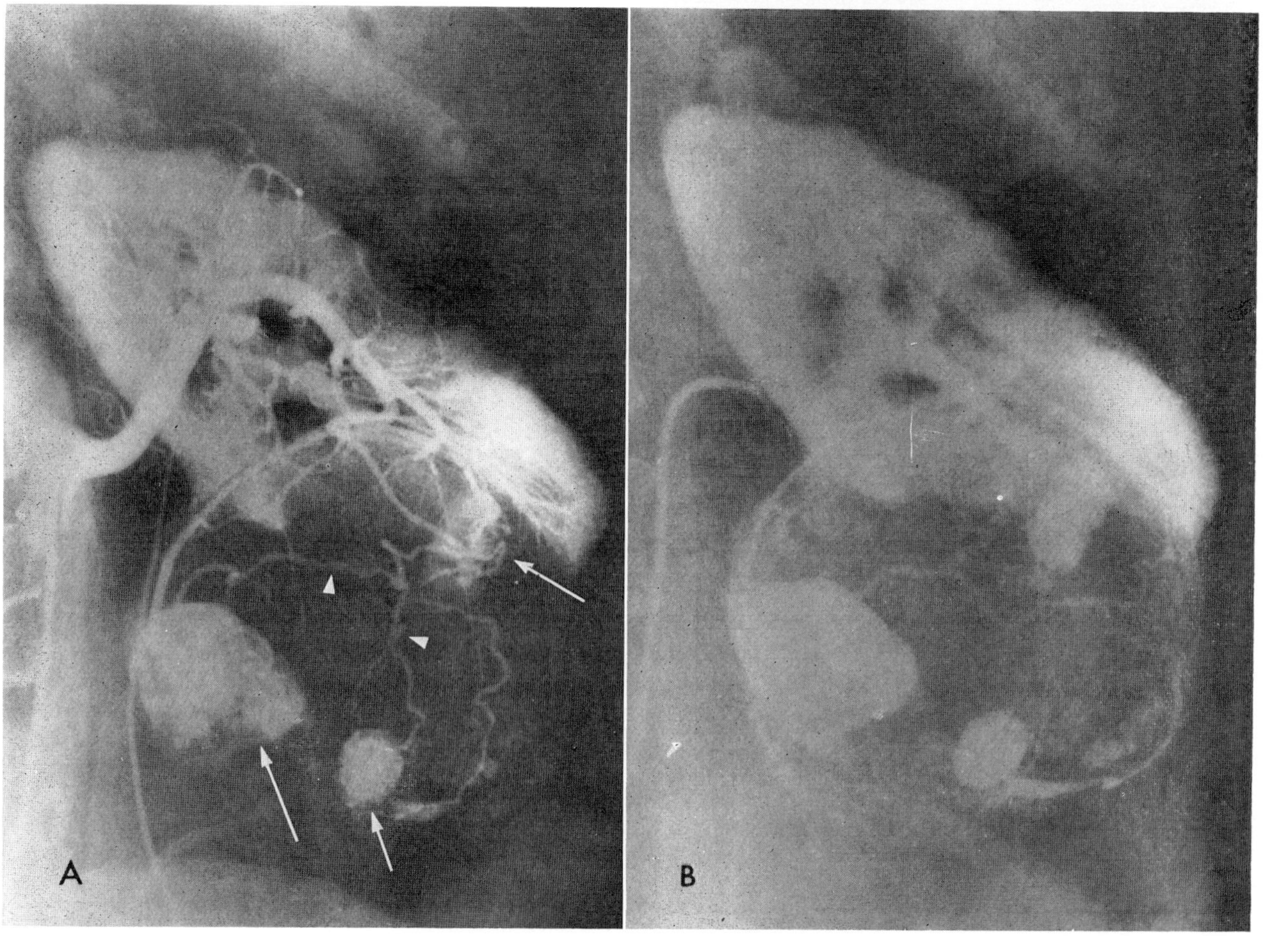

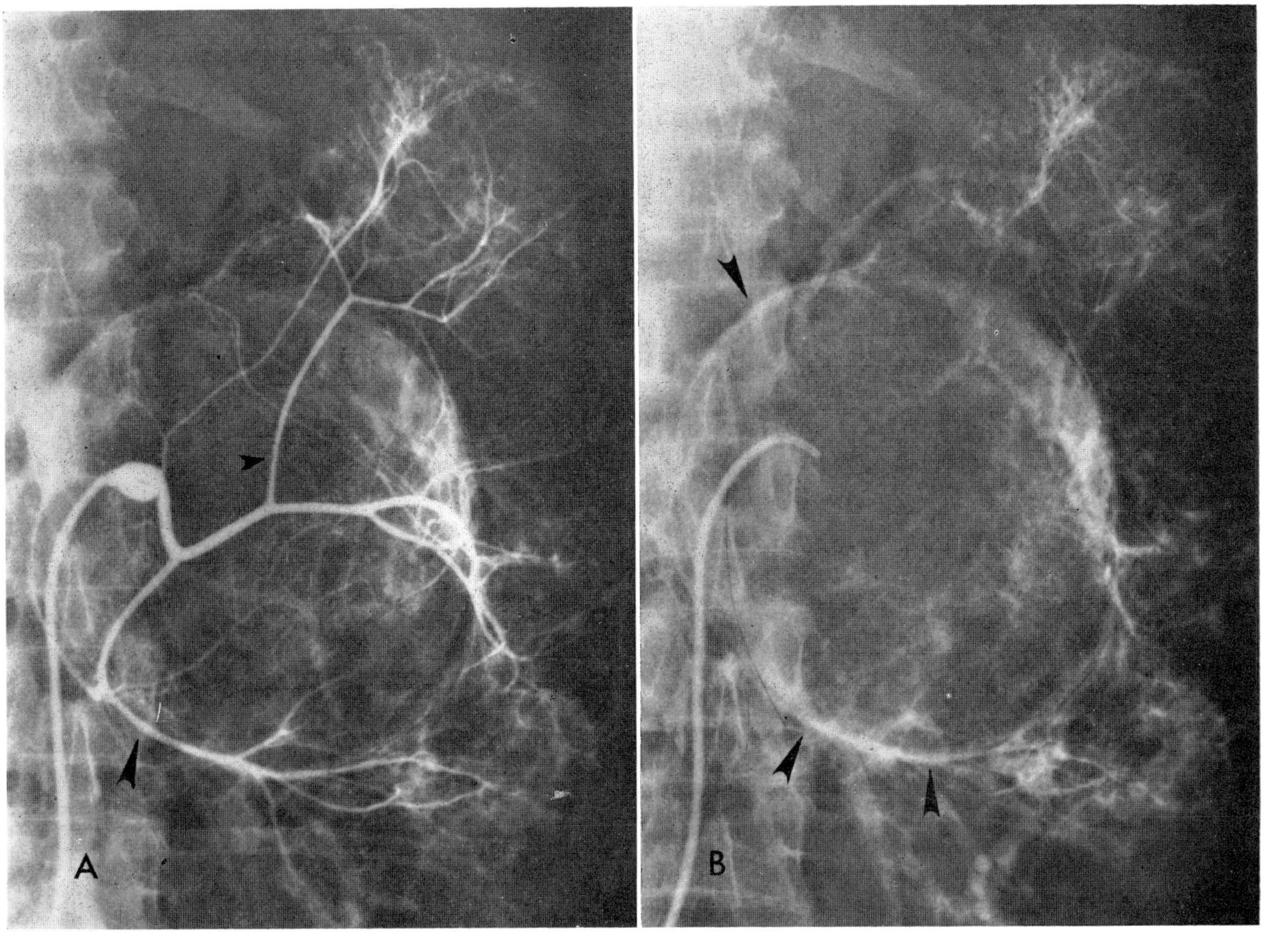

Figure 36.42. Renal Arteriogram. (A) Arterial phase: Stretching and deviation of the renal hilar branches (Arrow) and also of the intrarenal branches can be seen. Questionable abnormal corkscrew branches are within his hilar mass. (B) Parenchymal phase: The big mass in the renal hilar area is well-demonstrated with a thick wall (Arrow). The other lucent, well-defined defects in the renal parenchyma are demonstrated with thin walls. The patient had bilateral polycystic kidneys with left flank pain. *Diagnosis:* Complicated cyst either due to an abscess or due to a tumor. *Pathology:* Hypernephroma with hemorrhage into the avascular thick wall mass and two more small hypernephromas the size of 1 cm in the lower pole cyst.

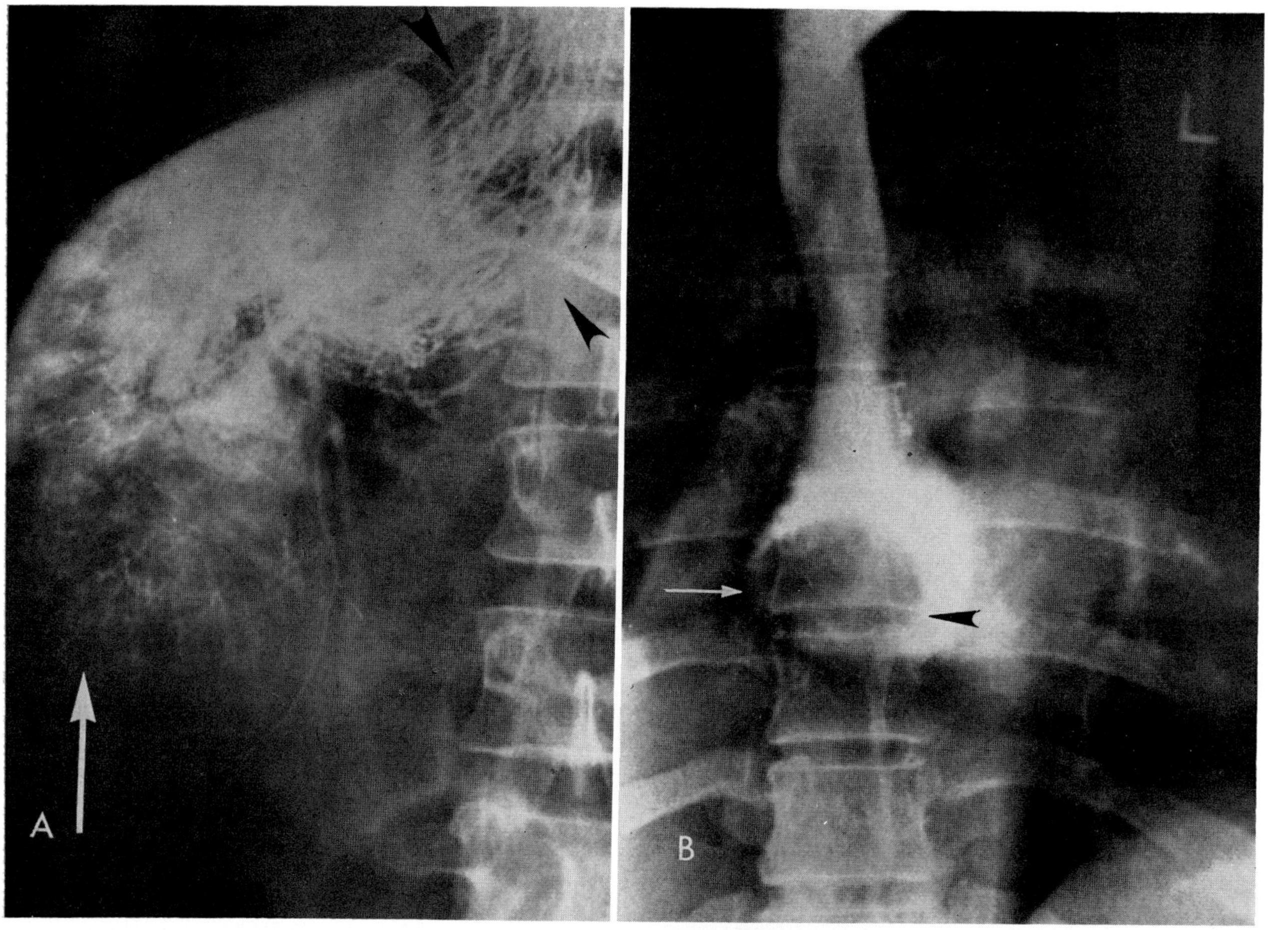

Figure 36.43. (A) Right renal arteriogram—midarterial phase: There are abnormal vessels in a right lower pole mass (Arrow) with very prominent abnormal vessels coursing along the path of the right renal vein ending near the right atrium (Arrow Head). (B) Superior vena cavogram via jugular vein: A moderately sized filling defect within the right atrium (Arrow) is seen. *Diagnosis:* Hypernephroma with the tumor thrombus growing all the way into the right atrium.

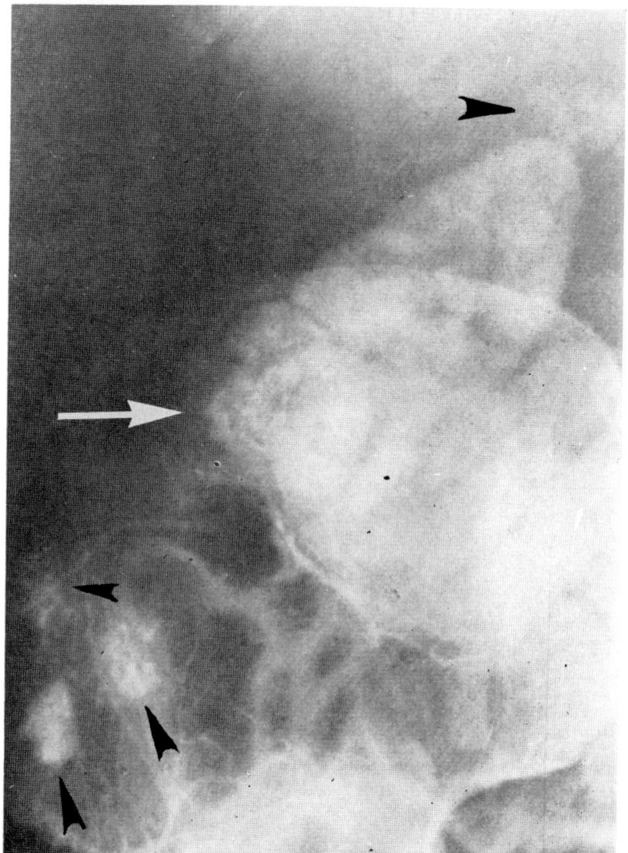

Figure 36.44. Flush Aortogram. Late phase: A mass is seen with increased stain in the lateral portion of the mid-kidney (Arrow). Increased staining of small masses in the retroperitoneal area (Arrow Head). *Diagnosis:* Retroperitoneal satellite metastases from a hypernephroma.

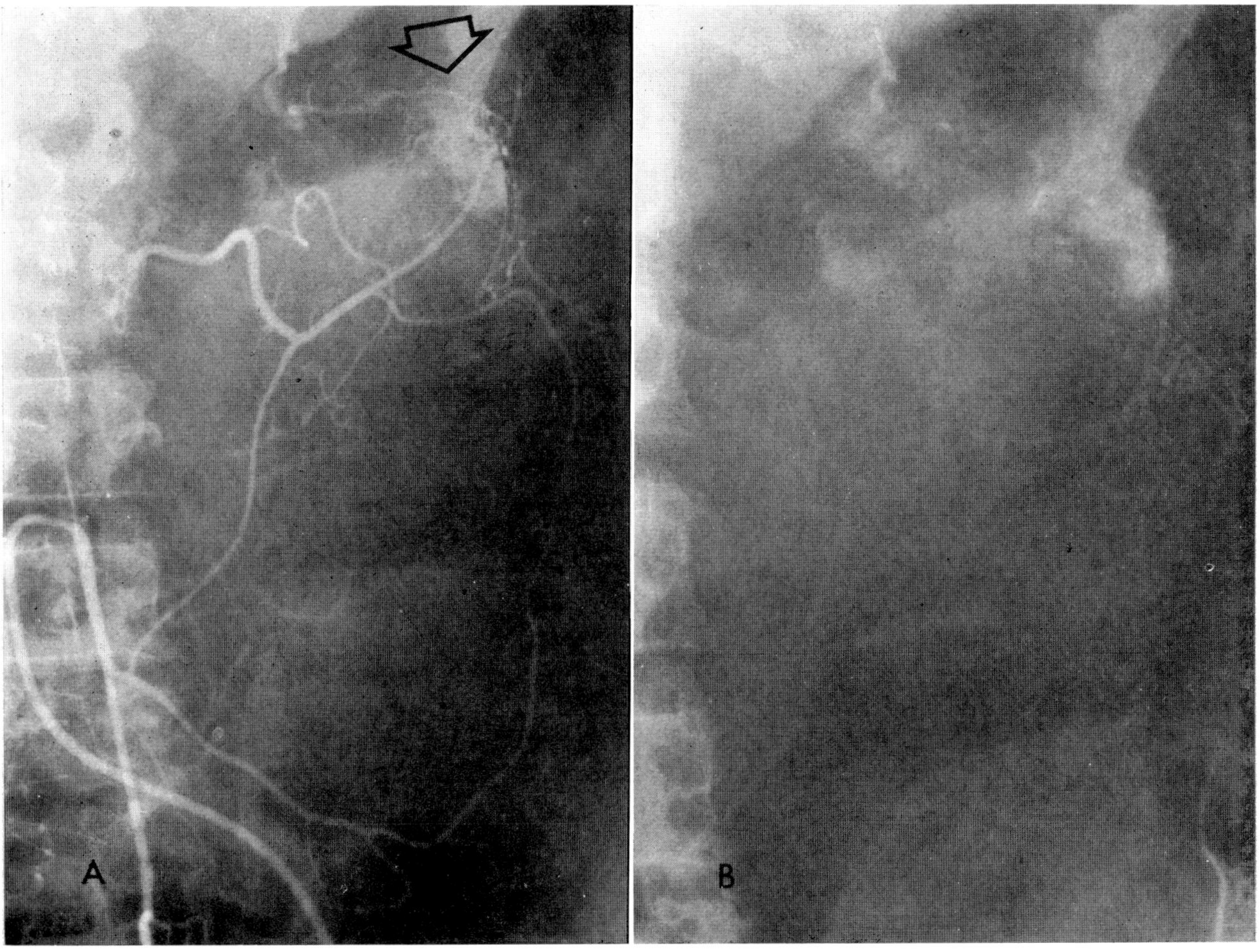

Figure 36.45. Inferior Mesenteric Arteriogram. (A) Early arterial phase: There is slight stretching and deviation of the vessels at the splenic flexure level. An amorphous collection of contrast material is in the same vicinity. (B) Late phase: The amorphous collection of contrast material is in the same vicinity. This is a patient with lower G.I. hemorrhage. *Diagnosis:* Mass with tumor stain in the vicinity of the splenic flexure. *Surgery:* Hypernephroma attached to the splenic flexure with ulceration of the mucosa and secondary bleeding into the lower G.I. tract.

host.[1358, 1359] Before the arterioles start supplying the tumor, an initial venous capillary bed is formed. Some of these vessels are sinusoids.[1362] In some areas, particularly the liver, very small tumors in the order of 1 to 2 mm may get their supply from the portal vein. After a gradual increase in size the venules are obliterated; lesions greater than 1 cm, whether primary or secondary, are exclusively supplied by the arterial tree. With some exceptions metastatic lesions, however, actually receive less blood supply.[1363–1365]

In normal organs nourished by one vessel, that vessel enters that organ through the hilum and branches into vessels of finer caliber. But in neoplasms, the arteries penetrate the tumors from all directions and break up into an irregular chaotic pattern without decorum or discipline. They lack normal proportions and end in amorphous spaces.[1367] Usually malignant neoplastic vessels are embryologic in nature, lacking contractile elements in their walls.[94] The high oxygen content in venous blood samples from tumors suggests a rapid blood flow through the tumors with arteriovenous shunting.[1367]

Malignant or benign masses, with or without *juxtaterritorial invasion,* may obtain perfusion from adjacent anatomically unrelated vessels.[1368, 1369] This type of anomalous supply depends on the availability of blood supply, metabolic needs of the tumor and invasion of adjacent structures. This added extravaganza may be due to preexisting anastomotic complexes between embryologically related or contiguous structures, associated inflammation or adhesions if any, siphonage due to arteriovenous shunting or luxurious vascularity with torrential blood flow, direct invasion of an adjacent structure, central necrosis with retention of a peripheral rind of tumor drawing blood supplies from neighboring vessels for its existence, or tumors situated at junctional zones of blood supply. If the anomalous artery leads into the malignant sinusoidal circulation without interposition of normal vasculature, then a juxtaterritorial extension of the tumor may be probable.

Malignant tumors are not encapsulated, although a slowly growing one may deceptively appear to be encapsulated by the stroma of the surrounding tissues. Progressive growth may result in gradual infiltration, invasion and destruction of neighboring tissues. The chance of angiographic demonstration of tumor vessels of a scirrhous neoplasm is obviously meager because of decreased perfusion, which is in proportion to the decreased metabolic needs of a scantily populated neoplastic cell group. These tumors, because of their invasive fibrous stroma, encase or even occlude vascular arcades when they come across them during their journey of invasion. Strangulation of their own vascular supply is a common feature in these scirrhous lesions, whether they are malignant such as adenocarcinoma of the pancreas, probably malignant such as ileocecal carcinoid tumors, or benign such as fibromatosis, retractile mesenteritis, pancreatitis, or ideopathic fibrosis.

In reality the *angiographic* demonstration of such *scirrhous* disorders is related to their secondary effect on intrinsic or extrinsic vasculature. This is in the form of seripigenous, sawtooth, serrated, or smooth encasement, including occlusion of the blood vessels. Occasionally, juxtaterritorial invasion of comparatively avascular infiltrating tumors may elicit an abundant vascular reaction from the neighboring tissues. This is seen in transitional cell carcinomas of the renal pelvis with extension into the renal parenchyma, or a cholangiocarcinoma extending into the liver.

It is probably logical to assume that the *so-called avascular* (but not scirrhous) or cystic (but not cystadenomatous) malignancies were originally solid tumors with an abundant vascularity which over the days became cystic or avascular because of increase in the metabolic needs, repeated bleeding into their own parenchyma, and tamponade causing ischemic as well as pressure necrosis. These changes produce a bulky necrotic tumor with a peripheral rind of

(Text continues on page 743)

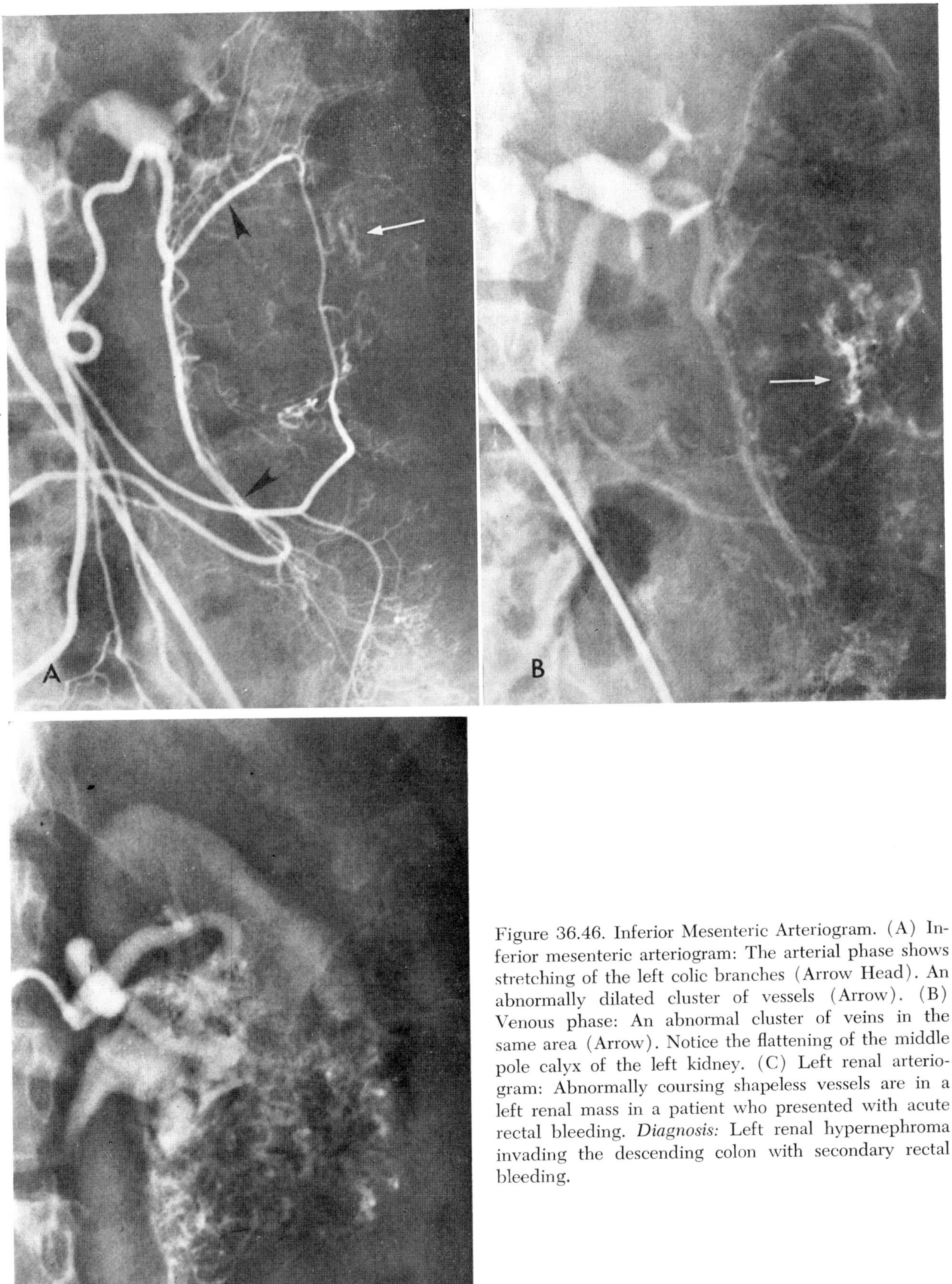

Figure 36.46. Inferior Mesenteric Arteriogram. (A) Inferior mesenteric arteriogram: The arterial phase shows stretching of the left colic branches (Arrow Head). An abnormally dilated cluster of vessels (Arrow). (B) Venous phase: An abnormal cluster of veins in the same area (Arrow). Notice the flattening of the middle pole calyx of the left kidney. (C) Left renal arteriogram: Abnormally coursing shapeless vessels are in a left renal mass in a patient who presented with acute rectal bleeding. *Diagnosis:* Left renal hypernephroma invading the descending colon with secondary rectal bleeding.

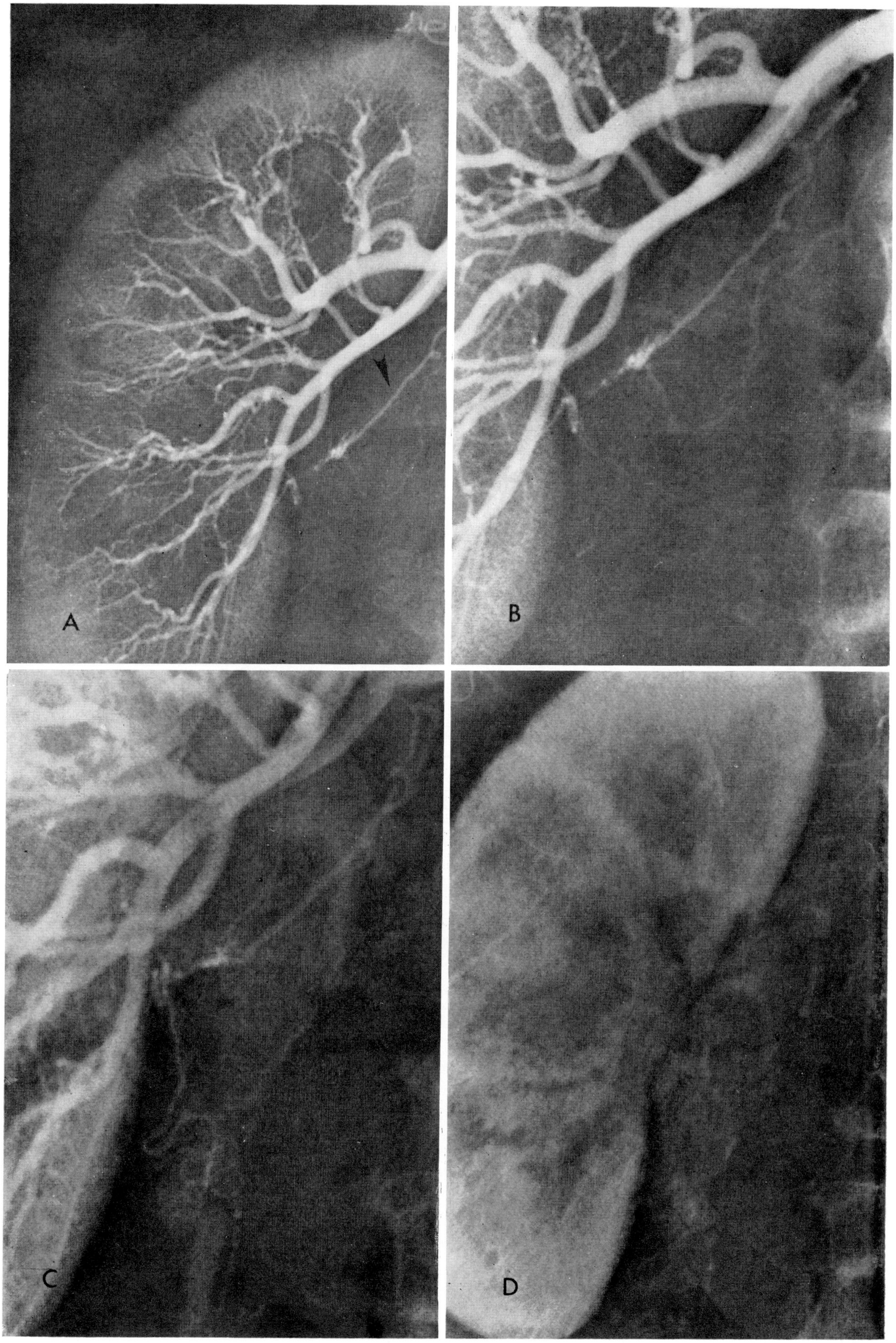
A
B
C
D

varying amounts of tumor tissue. Certain other tumors strangulate their own blood supply because of a severe desmoplastic reaction which they induce. Thus while carcinoids are vascular in the lung, stomach and liver, they are comparatively avascular or hypovascular in the ileocecal area. Finally, tumors may arise from the lining cells of an incidental simple cyst, like in renal, mesenteric[1098, 1099] and pancreatic cysts.[1092, 1093]

For various technical reasons *angiographic avascularity* may not always imply true pathologic avascularity. When insufficient amounts of contrast are used to opacify a luxurious vascular pool, avascularity may be suggested. Hemorrhage or edema may cause a tamponade effect on the tumor vessels. Superselective injections of contrast into smaller branches may give the appearance of avascularity, or an anatomically unrelated vessel may have been injected. Finally, central necrosis of the major bulk of the tumor may leave only a remaining peripheral layer which is nourished by accessible or inaccessible neighboring vessels.

Biological Peculiarities

It is very interesting to note the angiographic resemblance of tumors of draining systems of the liver and kidney and their effects on adjacent vessels. Thus cholangiocarcinomas from bile ducts and transitional cell or squamous cell carcinomas from renal pelvis cause encasement, infiltration and occlusion of adjacent vessels. At the same time, one notes the similar, extremely vascular stroma with scanty fibrous stroma of hepatomas and hypernephromas are apparent, as is the reflection of their secondary metastatic lesions in varying vascular beds. Whether this appearance is due to increased availability of blood supply or due to increased angiogenetic capacities of the cells of metastatic lesions is difficult to answer at present.

Some tissues may have an *identical end response* to different pathologic processes. In the *pancreas* an extreme scirrhous response is produced by both pancreatic carcinoma and pancreatitis. In the *bile ducts* both cholangiocarcinoma and sclerosing cholangitis[1370] produce the same end result. In the *mesentery,* fibroplastic reaction due to ileocecal carcinoid, retractile mesenteritis and fibromatosis may look identical. Such identical end responses may limit angiographic evaluation because of the same appearance, more or less, produced by the involved vessels. These responses are basically encasement or vascular occlusion.

The *biologic behavior* of a cancer is, however, unpredictable. Organs or tissues which usually tend to evoke a scirrhous response may on rare occasions respond with an extremely cellular and vascular stroma. For example, there are vascular medullary carcinomas of the pancreas and fungating carcinomas of the gallbladder or bile ducts. Contrarily, the same is true in organs such as the kidneys. At times, some of their malignant lesions may respond with very little vascular stroma: Like in renal infiltrating papillary adenocarcinomas which may appear avascular or hypovascular.

Renal Carcinomas

Hypernephromas are the most common malignant neoplasm of the adult kidney, although these tumors appear in the adolescent[1399] as well as in the elderly. Hypernephromas may occur in normal, horseshoe or polycystic kidneys or even arise from the lining of a simple benign cyst. Histologically, they range from very well differentiated to highly undifferentiated anaplastic lesions. Apart from the well-known manner of clinical presentation, patients may be totally asymptomatic or present with any one of the renal or nonrenal symptoms or signs: loss of weight, anemia, renal colic, lower ex-

←

Figure 36.47. Renal Arteriogram. (A) Early renal arterial phase: Prominent peripelvic vessel with an abnormal cluster of vessels is seen. (B) Close-up of the same. (C) There is slight increased staining of the same area with very fine tumor vessels. (D) Cluster of veins draining this mass. *Diagnosis:* Transitional cell tumor of the renal pelvis which is more expansile and less invasive in this instance.

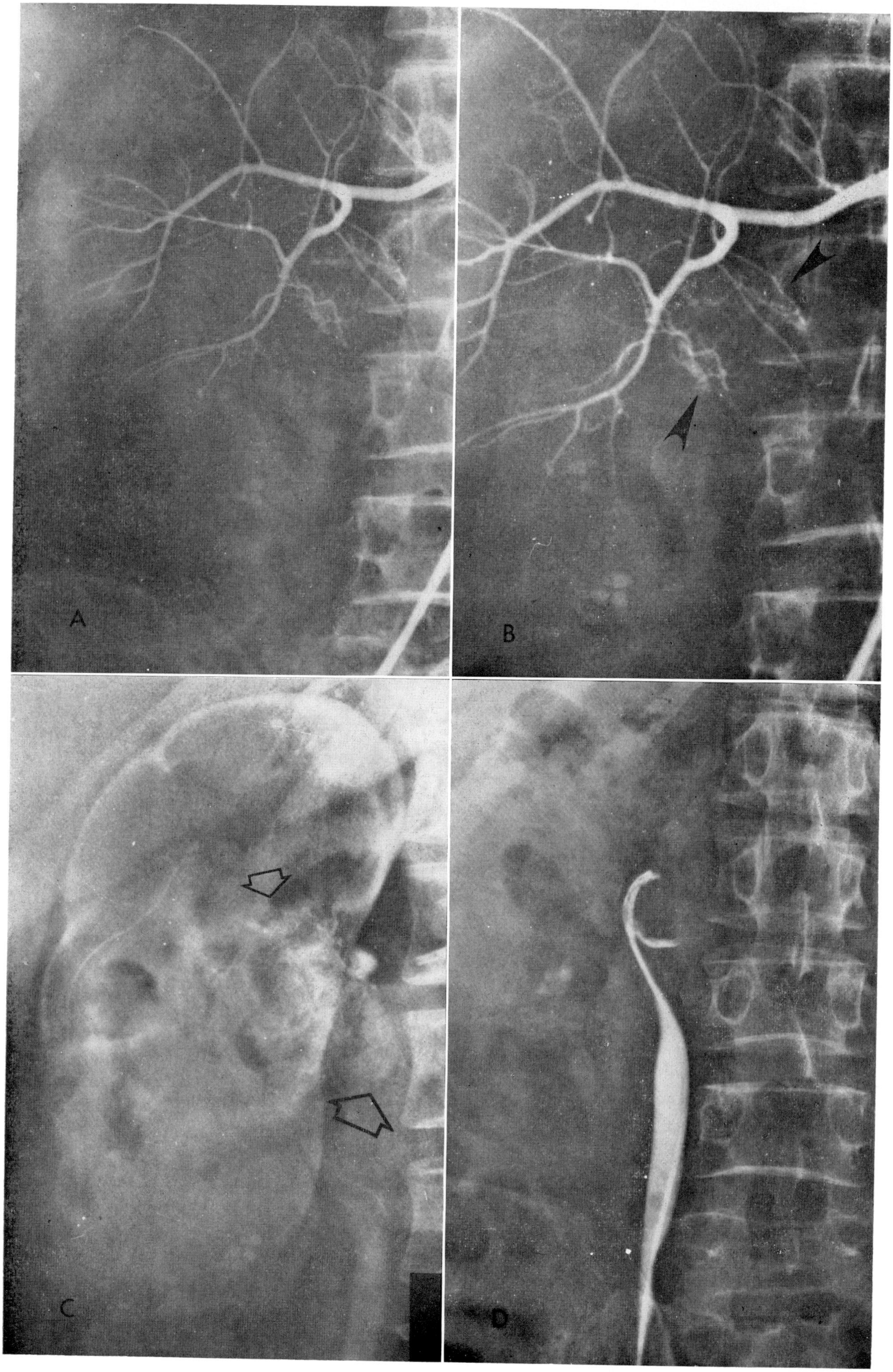
A
B
C
D

tremity edema, hypercalcemia, acute renal hemorrhage, shock due to excessive intrarenal or perirenal hemorrhage, soft tissue metastasis, hypertension or varicoceles on either the right or left sides.

Hypernephromas are usually provided with a rich vascular supply and meager supporting stroma. In addition to the main arterial supply, they may receive blood from all available retroperitoneal sources[1397, 1398] due to either increased need or extracapsular extension. The importance of the retroperitoneal sources increases when the peripheral layers of a centrally necrotic hypernephroma depend on them for survival.

At the same time, the renal and retroperitoneal veins aid in draining this torrential blood supply. If the renal vein is occluded by the neoplastic process, the entire burden of drainage is laid upon the retroperitoneal veins. The renal veins provide an easy path for the tumor to reach the right atrium via the inferior vena cava. The cost of being a very vascular lesion is the spontaneous occurrence of intrarenal or perirenal bleeding. Arteriovenous shunting in these tumors ranges from obvious clinical presentation to subtle angiographic demonstration.

The size of the tumor may not have a specific prognostic value. Because of their excessive metabolic needs, some may undergo complete necrosis with a totally avascular appearance at the time of clinical presentation. Some may be basically avascular. A high proportion of avascular tumors are either mixed, clear, and glandular cell carcinomas with papillary components.[1400, 1401] Cortical retraction, if present in an avascular hypernephroma, as a dimple which may aid in establishing the proper diagnosis.[1402] Instead of the usual expansile lesion, a hypernephroma may invade and infiltrate the normal renal parenchyma (Figs. 36-29 to 36-46).

Contralateral metastasis, though rare, creates a real problem for further management. The metastatic lesion of hypernephroma faithfully reproduce the angioarchitecture of the primary lesion.

Wilm's Tumor

The majority of these tumors[1213] occur in males under five years of age. Five to ten percent may be bilateral. This encapsulated lesion containing mesodermal tissues has a manner of growth in the kidneys which might suggest that the anlage of the tumor might have originated prior to the organic identity of the kidney. When these tumors are vascular they are usually provided with thick- and thin-wall vessels with corkscrew configuration and spider-leg like arborization with thin-walled sinusoids.[98, 1407] Angiographically they may be similar to mesenchymal hamartomas.[1479]

Other tumors of the kidney which can have neoplastic vasculature are lymphomas,[1408, 1409] plasmacytomas[1410] and leiomyosarcomas.[1411]

Hepatomas

These are the common primary malignant neoplasms of the liver and possess a great angiographic similarity to hypernephromas.[1412, 1413, 1416] Hepatomas may be nodular, single or multinodular. They do not spare infants or children,[1414, 1415] although it appears that cirrhotic livers provide an ideal soil for their growth. When they occur in cirrhotic livers they are usually multinodular. Like hypernephromas, they have an exuberant capillary stroma with negligible fibrous support. They have their choice of growing either through the portal or

←

Figure 36.48. Renal Arteriogram. (A) Early renal arterial phase: Numerous dilated hypertrophied vessels are in the renal pelvic area (Arrow). Amidst these vessels, some of them are abnormally dilated with amorphous collections of contrast material. The intrarenal branches are stretched and deviated. Incidental stones are in the left lower portion of the kidney. (B) Midarterial phase: The same abnormal vessels in the pelvic area are shown to better advantage. (C) Parenchymal phase: There is uniform thinning of the renal cortex with intrarenal filling defects. A faint homogeneous stain is seen at the renal pelvic area. (D) Retrograde pyelogram: A smooth, meniscus-like filling defect is revealed. *Diagnosis:* Transitional cell tumor of the right renal pelvis with tumor vasculature and secondary hydronephrosis.

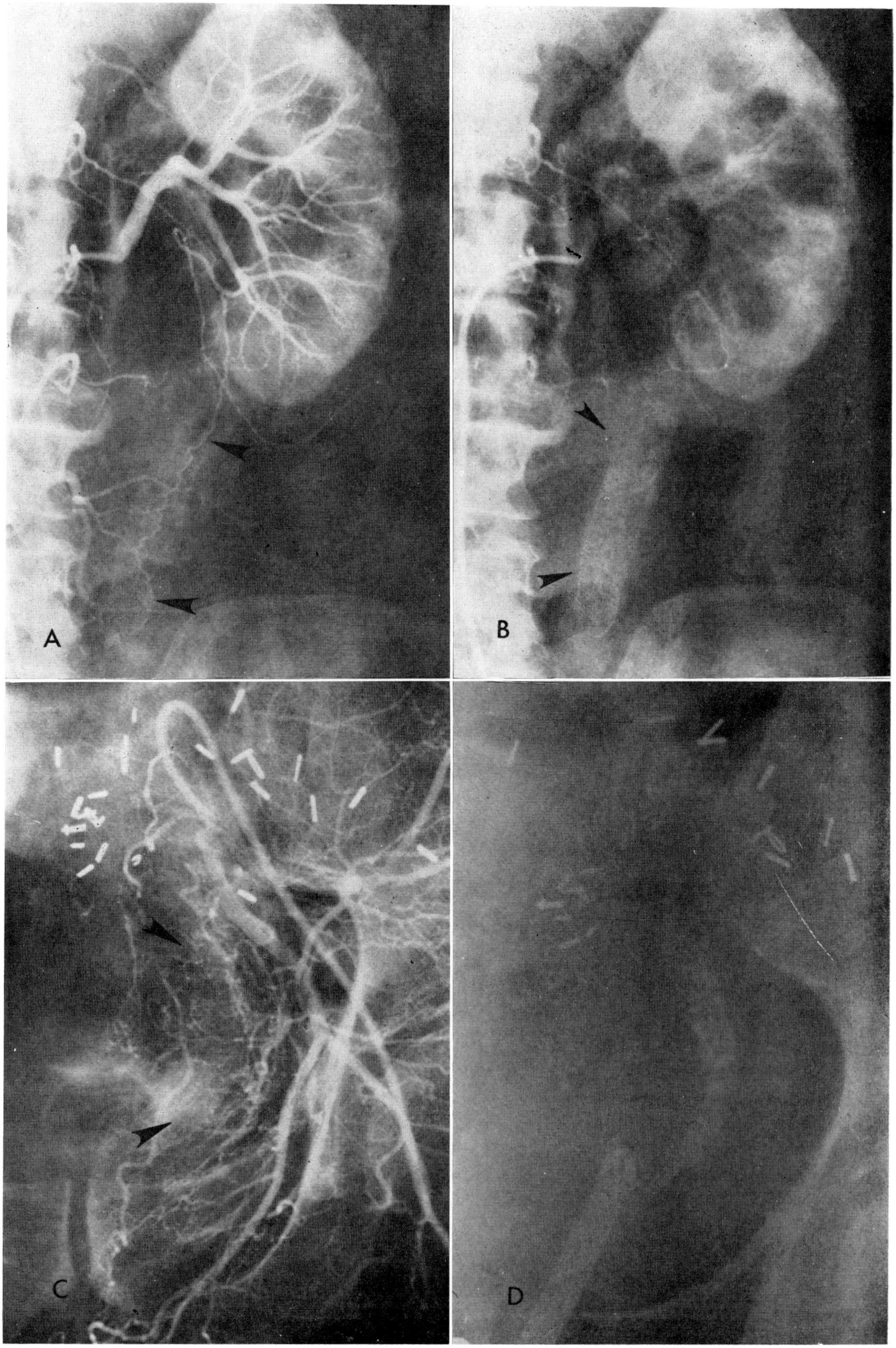
A
B
C
D

the hepatic veins. Just like any other hypervascular tumor, they are also prone to rupture and bleeding. Metastatic lesions from a hepatoma are faithful duplicators of the angioarchitecture of their parent primary lesions. Accidental biopsy of the soft tissue metastasis may lead to alarming bleeding.

Clinically, a hepatoma may present as a hemobilia, hematemesis, innocent abscess, or a Budd-Chiari syndrome.[1417] Avascular hepatomas are very rare and may be uncovered with the assistance of epinephrine.[1418] It may be extremely difficult to diagnose a diffuse hepatoma when it occurs in a cirrhotic liver[301] (Figs. 36-50 to 36-52).

Other vascular neoplasms of the liver include hemangiomas, hemangioendotheliomas and hemangioendotheliosarcomas.

Isotopes and Vascular Neoplastic Lesions of the Liver

Active uptake by a hepatic vascular mass[1501–1503] of either rose bengal^{131}, Au^{198}, or Tc^{99m} colloid materials suggests functioning liver tissue in that mass lesion. This may be seen with adenomas,[1312, 1351] focal nodular hyperplasia,[1350, 1353] or regenerating nodules.[1356] The absence of uptake of these isotopic materials does not necessarily imply that they are not benign lesions.[1310] On rare occasions a functioning hepatoma may concentrate the isotope masquerading as a benign lesion.[1503, 1504] Gallium^{67} citrate by actively concentrating may aid in detecting hematomas, hepatoma, or abscesses[1499, 1500] of the liver. Gallium is also useful in detecting hepatomas in cirrhotic patients.[1499]

Figure 36.49. (A) Renal arteriogram reveals very prominent ureteric branches supplying a dilated ureter. (B) Parenchymal phase demonstrates staining of the ureter as well as a mass within the ureter. (C) Pelvic arteriogram reveals dilated abnormal ureteric branches supplying the pelvic segment of the ureter. (D) Retrograde pyelogram demonstrates masses occupying the dilated ureter. *Diagnosis:* Transitional cell tumor of the ureter. *Pathology:* Metastatic adenocarcinoma from colon occupying the entire ureter.

Pancreas—Medullary or Anaplastic Tumors

These are bulky or fleshy cellular tumors with abundant vascular stroma.[1371] The primary as well as the secondary tumors, such as liver metastasis, are vascular and provided with typical neoplastic vasculature.

Sarcomas are rare tumors more frequent in young people. If they have not undergone necrosis, they are by nature vascular (Fig. 36-56).

Gallbladder

These are rare fungating types of tumors,[1214] but are usually more invasive than expansive. A dilated gallbladder due to secretions or tumor tissue is not uncommon. Neoplastic vessels are seen with these malignant neoplasms of the gallbladder (Fig. 36-54).

Splenic Tumors

Primary splenic malignant tumors, although rare, may arise from a variety of structures constituting the spleen.[1440–1442] Cellular tumors include lymphomas; connective tissue tumors include sarcomas; the vascular sinuses give rise to endotheliomas and angiosarcomas. Sarcomas[1443, 1444] are basically very vascular with meager supporting stroma, but repeated hemorrhage and necrosis may make them partially, or even totally avascular. On rare occasions a plasmacytoma may be very vascular.[1445] Reticulum cell sarcomas[1379, 1438, 1439] of the spleen vary in their vascularity, ranging from hypervascularity to an avascular filling defect. Some metastatic lesions also have variable vasculature. This includes melanoma,[1438] hemangiosarcoma[1439] and choriocarcinoma.[301]

Omental and Mesenteric Neoplasms

In addition to benign infiltrating fibrosing processes, these layers[1446] may be involved by lesions such as lipomas, leiomyomas, and leiomyosarcomas, hemangiopericytomas, mesotheliomas,[1447] neurofibromas, nonchromaffin paragangliomas,[1448] and last but not least, metastatic lesions. Angiographically[1447–1449] one may demonstrate hypertrophied omental vessels with abnormal branching and even staining.

(Text continues on page 751)

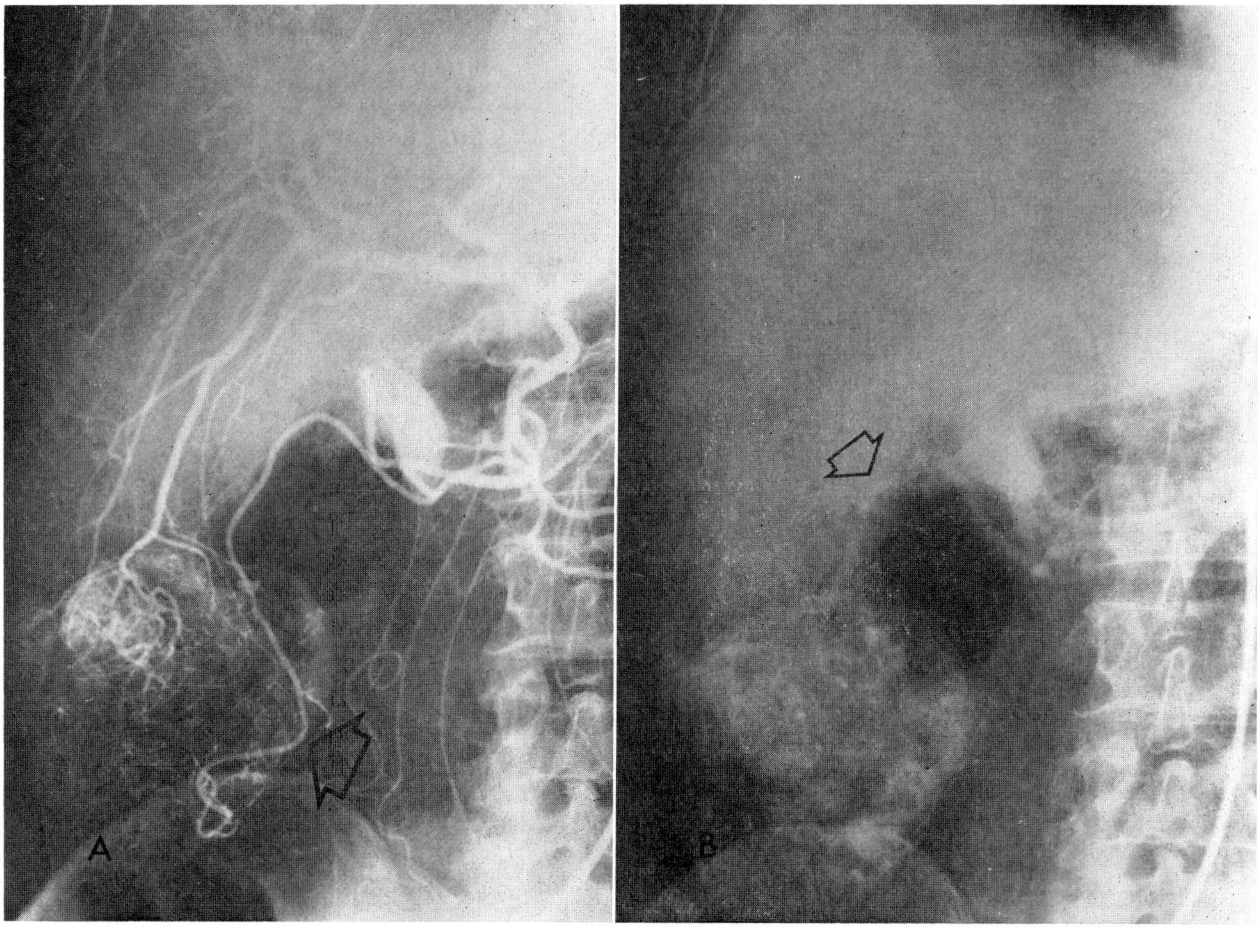

Figure 36.50. Hepatic Arteriogram. (A) Arterial phase: There is a prominent, inferior, lobar branch supplying a moderately sized mass with chaotic abnormal branches. A very prominent omental vessel is seen supplying the same area (Arrow). (B) Parenchymal phase: There is a well-stained, irregular mass with excellent opacification of the omental vein (Arrow). *Diagnosis:* Hepatoma or solitary metastasis. *Pathological Diagnosis:* Hepatoma. *Comment:* Apart from the main arterial supply there is parasitic blood supply from the omental vessel. (Courtesy of Dr. Himmat T. Shah, Radiologist, Michael Reese Medical Center, Chicago.)

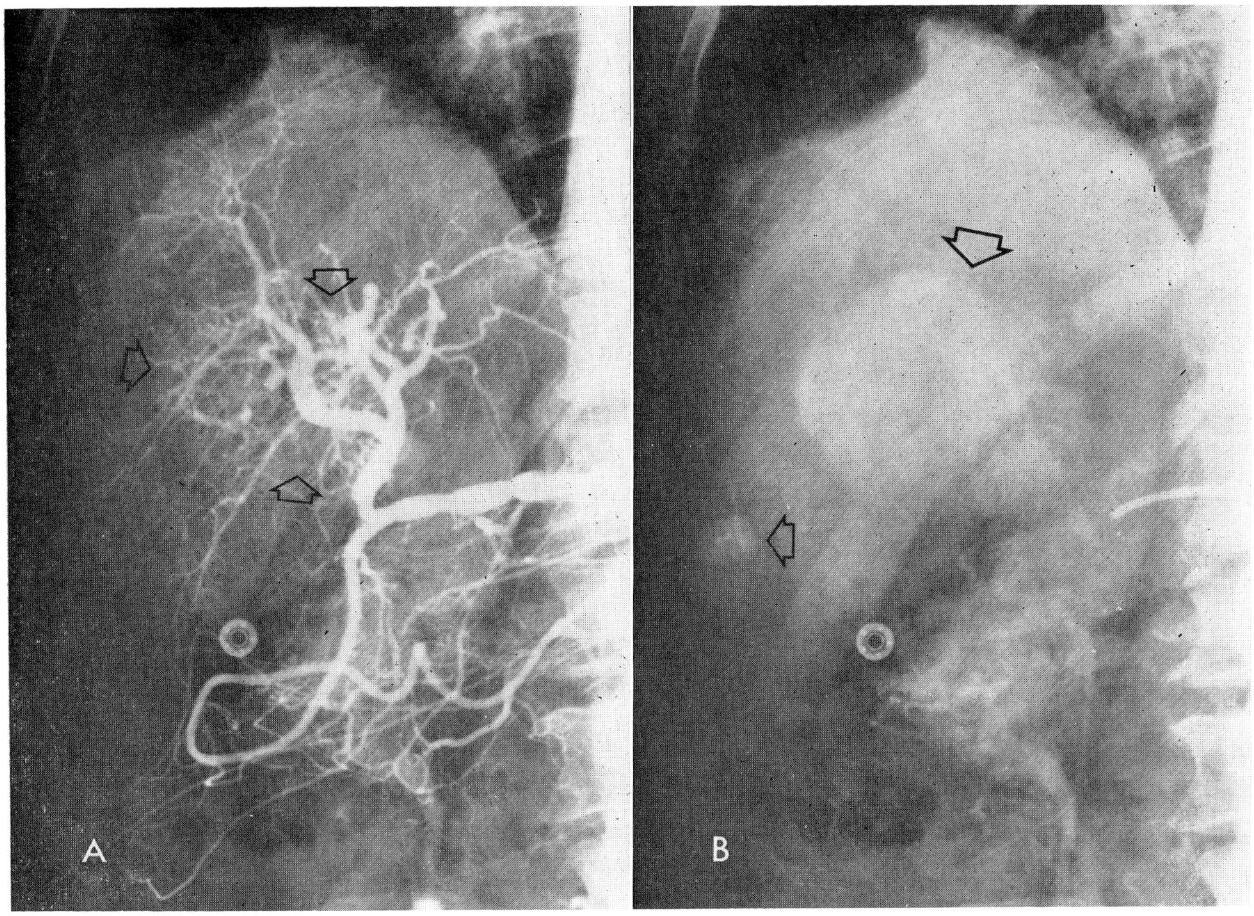

Figure 36.51. Hepatic Arteriogram. (A) Numerous, abnormal, tortuous, irregularly dilated vessels (Arrow). (B) Late arterial phase: Increased stain in two mass lesions in the liver of different sizes (Arrow) is seen. *Diagnosis:* Multiple metastases versus multinodular hepatoma. *Surgical Biopsy:* Hepatoma.

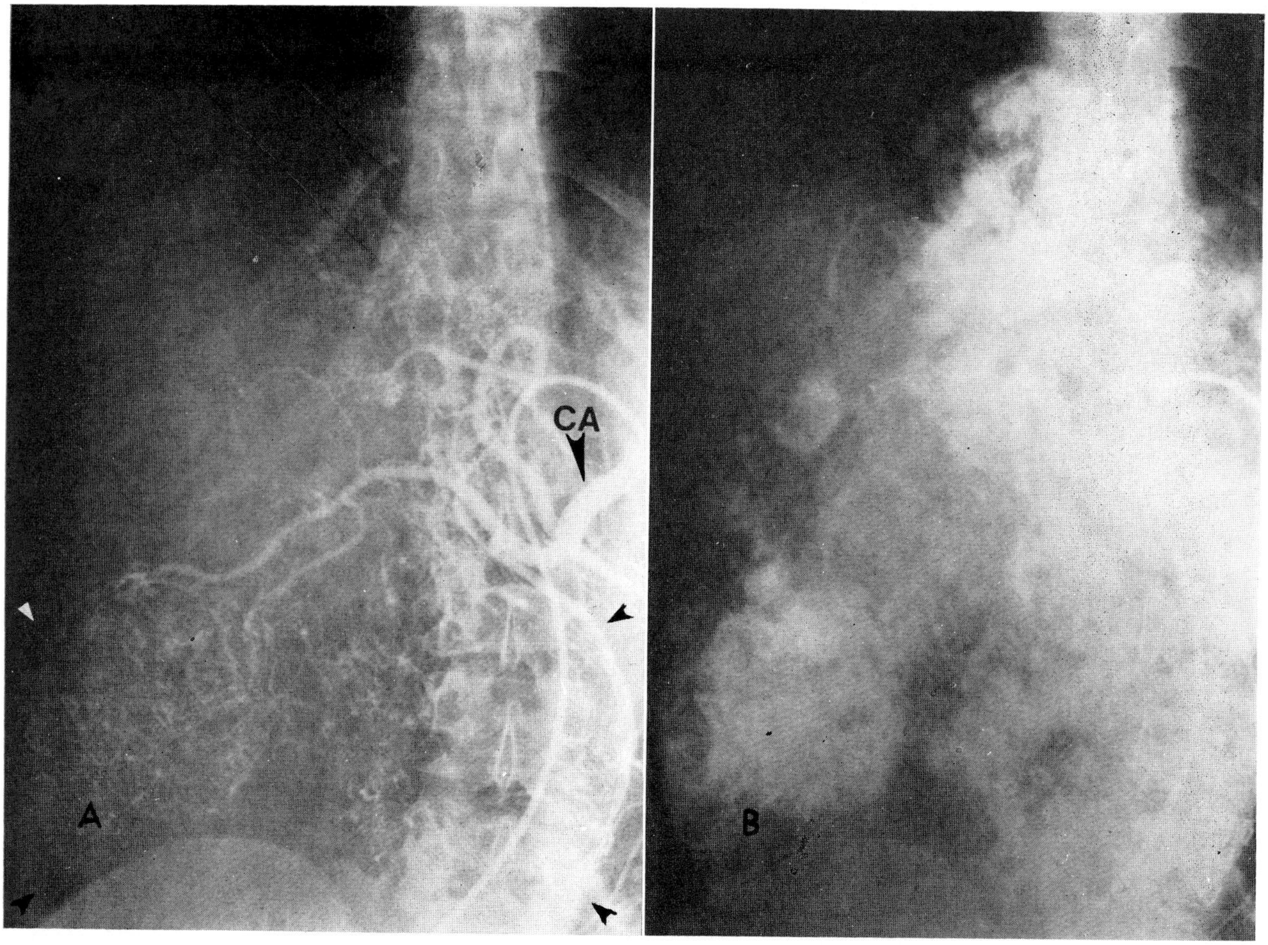

Figure 36.52. Celiac Arteriogram. (A) Arterial phase: The celiac axis is deviated towards the left (C.A.) with stretching and deviation of the intrahepatic branches around a huge mass within the liver (Arrow). There are very abnormal vessels of irregular caliber within this mass. (B) Parenchymal phase: Islands of intense staining are seen. *Diagnosis:* Multinodular hepatoma with necrosis or metastases to the liver. *Pathology:* Hepatoma.

Soft Tissue Tumors

Logistically or statistically, a vascular tumor in the kidney or liver usually is a hypernephroma or hepatoma, respectively, or hepatic metastasis. But it is not that simple in the soft tissues. Avascular or vascular soft tissue neoplasms make an angiographer humble, if he attempts to arrive at a histologic diagnosis. Therefore, it may be worthwhile to save the energy by merely *mapping the arterial anatomy, the extent of the lesion, and the amount of vascularity present.* Retroperitoneal[1235, 1450] soft tissue tumors may have the same angiographic pattern as other tumors. Tumors of the retroperitoneum include lipomas, liposarcomas, leiomyomas, leiomyosarcomas, rhabdomyosarcomas, histiocytomas, hemangiomas, and hemangiosarcomas, paragangliomas, mesenchymomas, undifferentiated sarcomas, ganglioneuromas, teratomas, chordomas and metastases. Common soft tissue tumors[1451] in the extremities and elsewhere, with the same angiographic appearance, include fibro- and liposarcomas, vascular wall tumors, synovial sarcomas,[1452] neurofibrosarcomas, plasmacytomas,[1453] histiocytomas, alveolar soft part sarcomas,[1235, 1454] and mesenchymomas (Figs. 36-61 to 36-67).

Malignant Osseous Lesions

While angiography is rarely used to diagnose primary bone lesions, it may help in evaluating the osseous, as well as soft tissue extent of the malignant process.[1288, 1455–1457] Apart from the primary malignant neoplasms of bones, secondary osteolytic lesions may be vascular provided they are not intramedullary and small. Osteoblastic lesions are usually avascular[1458] (Fig. 36-68).

Metastatic Neoplasms

The incidence of metastatic implants probably depends on the amount of blood flowing through that organ. Metastasis is less invasive than the primary tumor and may be comparatively more regular in cellular arrangement. It has a comparatively decreased incidence in skeletal muscle and spleen.[111, 1239]

In organs like the *liver*, metastatic lesions less than 1 cm in size have a unique arterial blood supply. Initially no alteration in the vascular architecture may be present. Lesions greater than 1 cm frequently have venous deformities such as compression and interruption.[1363–1365] If the primary is drained by the portal venous system, metastases are usually due to emboli; if the primary is drained by nonportal venous system such as the renal vein, then the metastatic implants occur via subcapsular lymphatics.[1363, 1364] No organ is immune from metastasis. However, some structures such as the liver, kidney,[1433, 1434] adrenal,[1435, 1436] and rarely the spleen[1437–1439] may be more frequently involved than others.

Hepatic Metastasis

It would be difficult to predict with great accuracy which metastatic lesions have the ability to initiate angiogenesis from the host bed. Some primary vascular neoplasms have the same angioarchitecture when they metastasize to other sites beside the liver. Examples include hypernephromas, sarcomas, anaplastic tumors, islet cell malignant tumors of the pancreas, leiomyosarcomas, choriocarcinomas, carcinoid tumors (Figs. 36-69 to 36-73).

Lakes, Pools and Puddles

The accumulation of pools of contrast material is not unusual in certain lesions and is related to the sinusoidal distribution of thin-walled vascular spaces. These pools may be seen in hemangiomas, aneurysmal bone cysts,[1285, 1286] giant cell tumors,[1287, 1288] or malignant lesions in general (Figs. 36-74 to 36-77). Occasionally the benign sinusoidal pools of a tumor may not be opacified by contrast (Giant Cell Tumor[1289]).

Angiographically, What Makes a Lesion Malignant?

Hypervascularity? Chaotic, bizarre patterns? Premature arteriovenous shunting? Encasement or occlusion of vessels? Can any of these angiographic signs be present in a benign process? The answer is "yes." Can none of these be seen in a malignant process? The answer is

(Text continues on page 754)

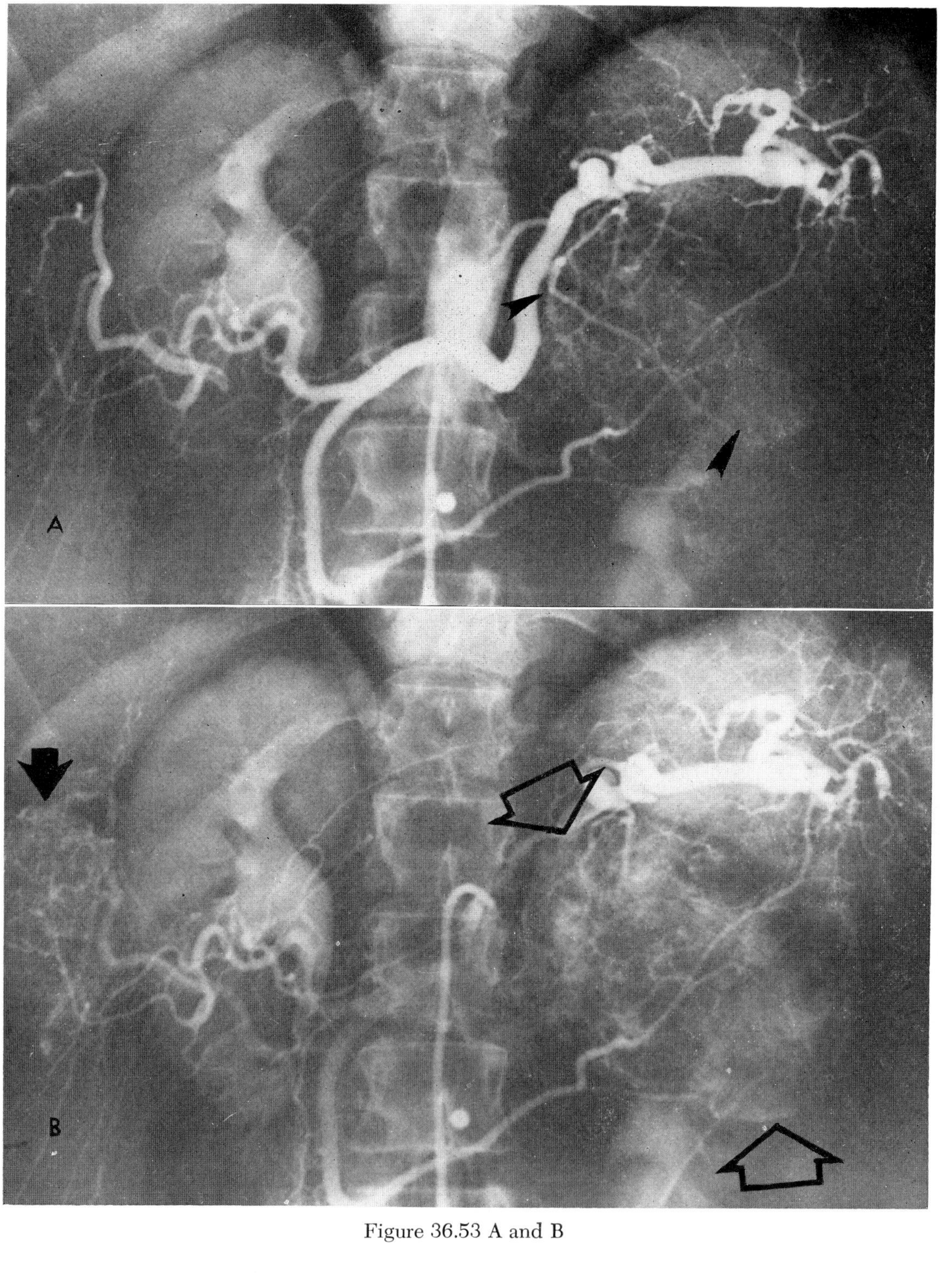

Figure 36.53 A and B

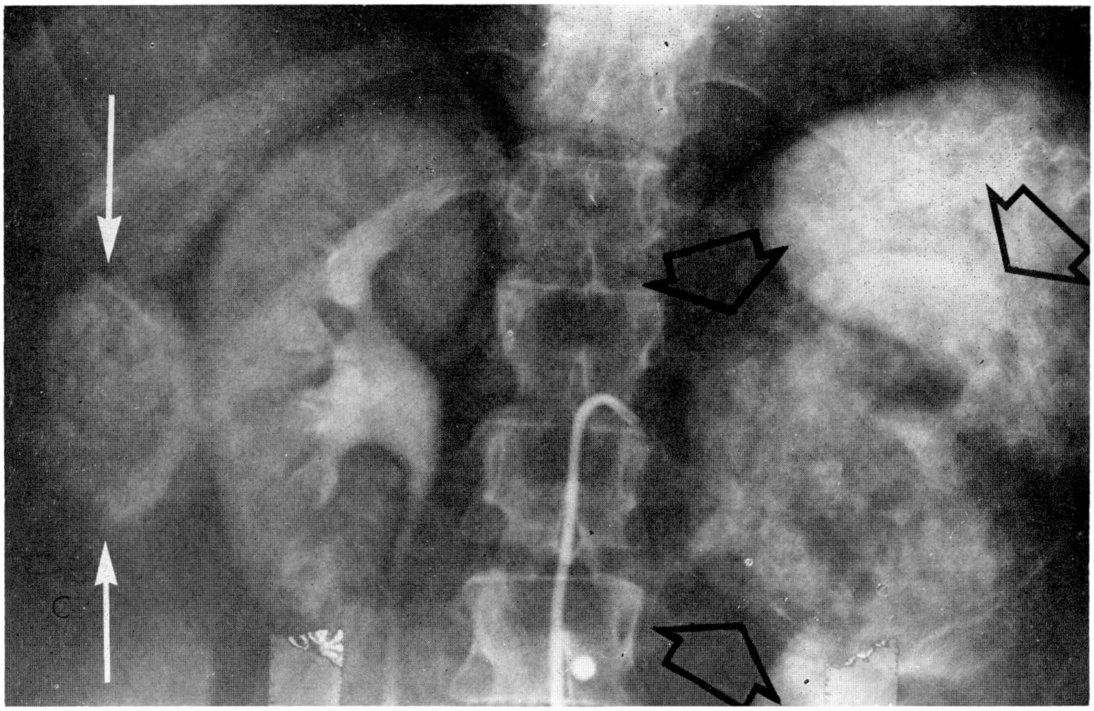

Figure 36.53. Celiac Arteriogram. (A) Arterial phase: There is elevation of the midportion of the splenic artery and stretching of the pancreatic branch arising from the splenic artery (Arrow). Numerous abnormal, irregularly dilated vessels are seen in the vicinity of the body and tail of the pancreas. (B) Late arterial phase: Increased abnormal vasculature in the body and tail of the pancreas with early amorphous collections of contrast material (Blank Arrow) are noted. Abnormal vasculature with irregular dilation is seen in a mass in the right lobe of the liver (Arrow). (C) A hyperstaining mass is seen in the right lobe of the liver and in the tail of the pancreas (Arrows). *Diagnosis:* Pancreatic carcinoma, probably anaplastic in nature, with hepatic metastases. Surgery confirmed the diagnosis. Angiographic differential diagnosis includes malignant islet cell tumors and cystadenocarcinomas.

"yes." Then how is a malignant lesion suspected angiographically? By its location? Circumstantial evidence (clinical correlation)? Statistics coupled with logistics? Inspiration, imagination or intuition?

On many occasions it is very easy to recognize a hypervascular mass in the kidney as a hypernephroma or in the liver as a hepatoma or metastatic neoplasm, and it is easy to recognize encasement of a vessel around the pancreas as a pancreatic carcinoma.

But without available clinical history, what name will a chemodectoma receive if it arises in the retroperitoneum instead of at the carotid bifurcation, or if a pheochromocytoma arises in the urinary bladder rather than above the kidney? If the angioarchitecture of a lesion were itself sufficient to establish a histologic diagnosis, irrespective of its location, age of the patient, or lack of any clinical information, it would be interesting to see the psychological reaction of a "neoplastic mass" toward the strange name it receives before the true pathology is revealed.

However, one should not be that disheartened since a good diagnostic batting average may be maintained because of the frequent and common occurrence of the same lesions in certain organs. This coupled with many angiographic signs, reinforced by clinical information, plus some imagination . . . some inspiration . . . and some intuition, should prevail in making the correct diagnosis. It should always be remembered, however, that we all win a few . . . and lose a few!

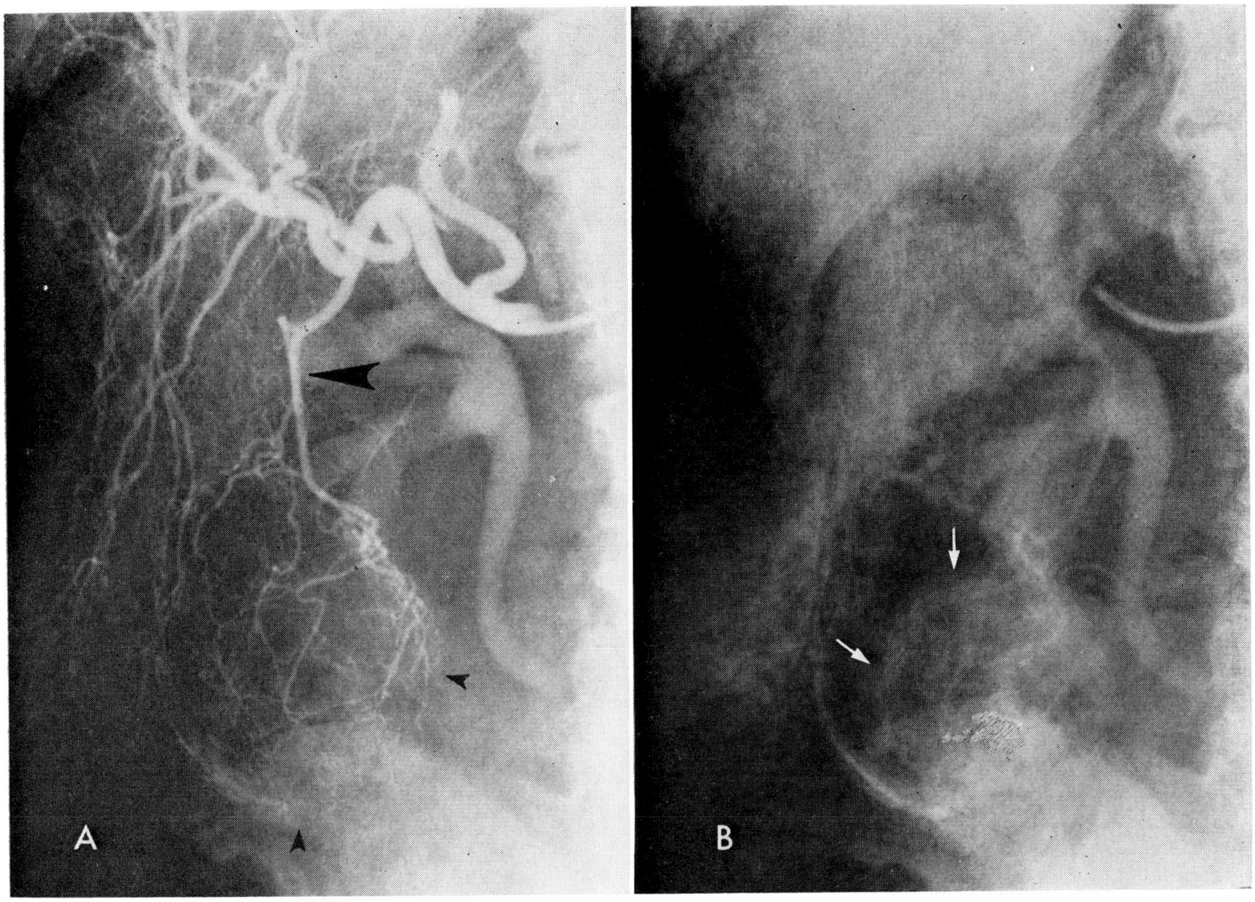

Figure 36.54. Hepatic Arteriogram. (A) Reveals a very prominent cystic artery giving rise to numerous abnormal branches supplying a distended gallbladder. (B) Venous phase reveals a huge gallbladder with suggestion of a mass within the gallbladder. *Diagnosis:* Fungating carcinoma of the gallbladder. *Pathology:* Confirmed the diagnosis.

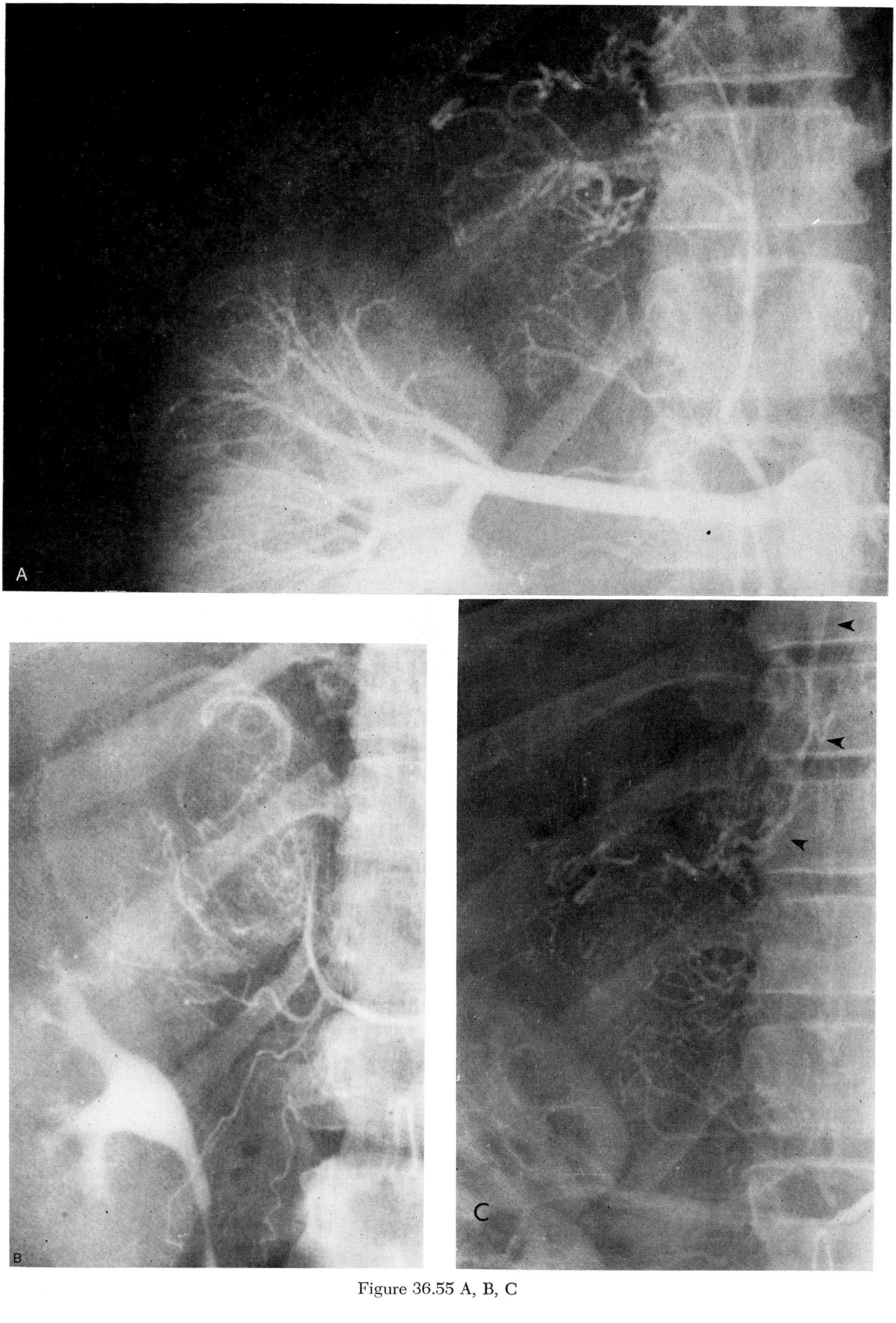

Figure 36.55 A, B, C

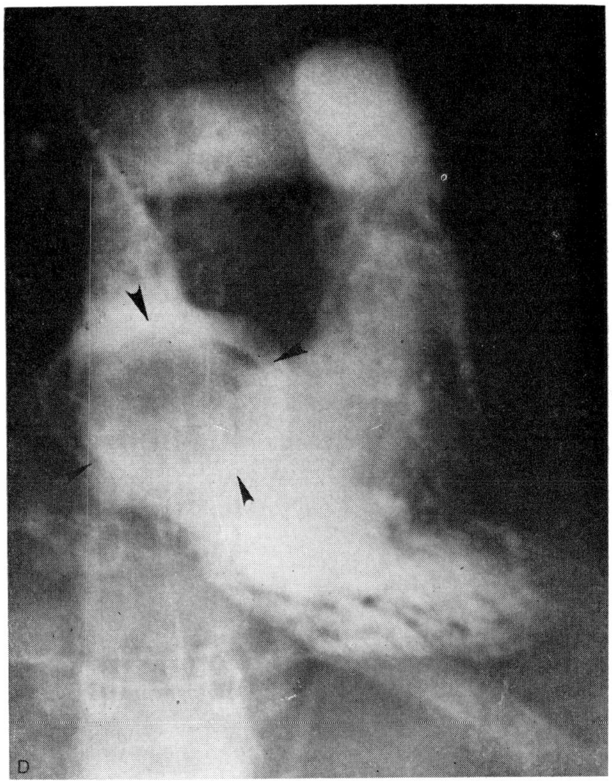

Figure 36.55. (A) Renal arteriogram—reveals a prominent inferior adrenal artery supplying a mass with abnormal vascularity. (B) Middle adrenal arteriogram—demonstrates a very prominent middle adrenal artery supplying the same mass. (C) Late arterial phase—irregular vessels course towards inferior vena cava and right atrium. (D) Angiocardiogram via jugular vein—a filling defect occupies the right atrial chamber. This patient presented with ascites and lower leg edema (Budd Chiari Syndrome). *Diagnosis:* Nonfunctioning right adrenal carcinoma growing through the adrenal vein into the right atrium via inferior vena cava.

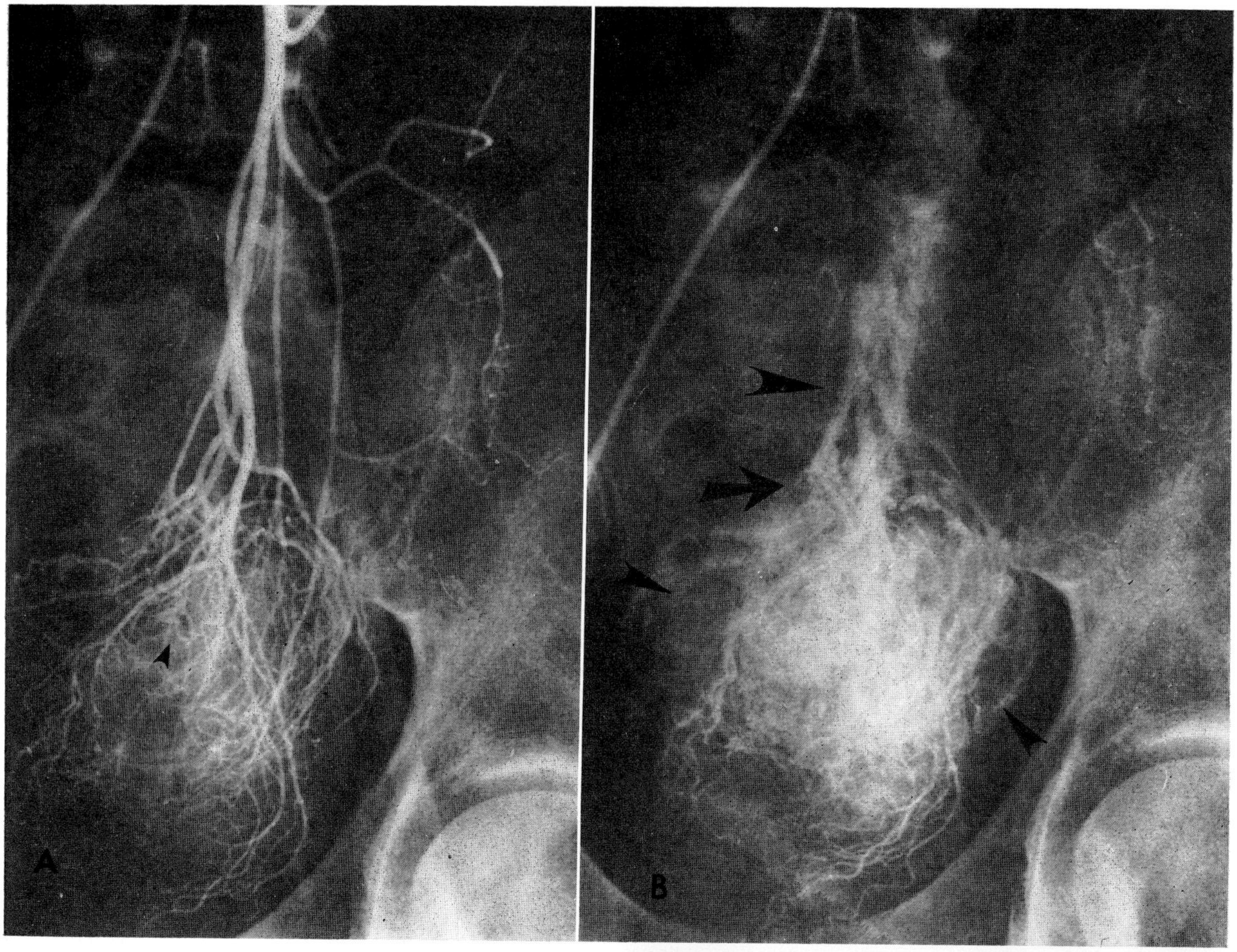

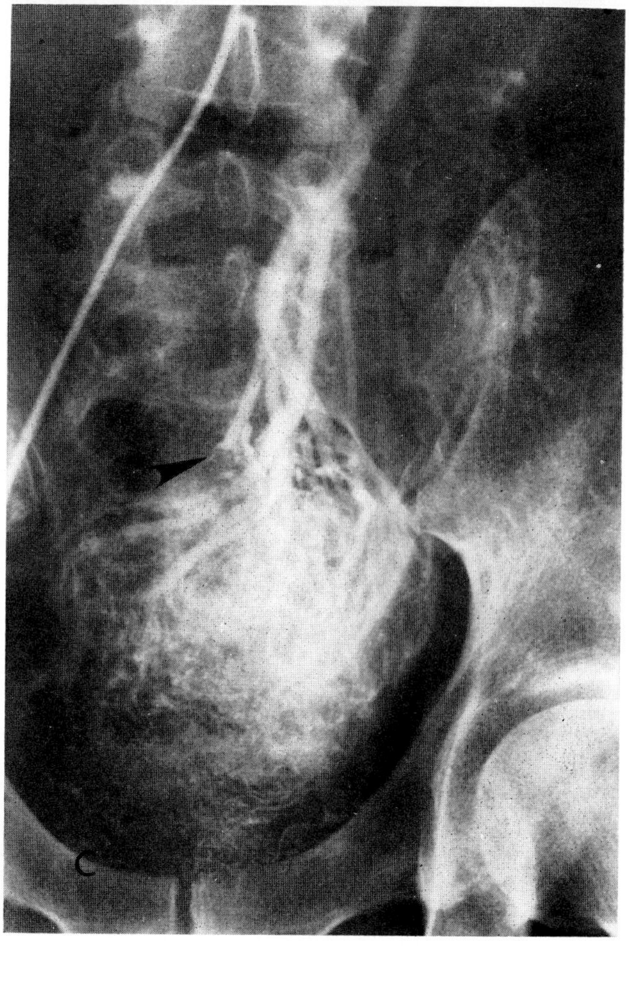

Figure 36.56. Inferior Mesenteric Arteriogram. (A) Early arterial phase: There is a marked increase in the vasculature of the rectal branches and abnormal angulations of a few branches. (B) Late arterial phase: Intense abnormal staining of this area with early venous opacification (Arrow Head) and occlusion of one of the rectal veins (Arrow) are seen. (C) The abnormal intense opacification of this mass and the occlusion of the rectal vein is shown to better advantage. This patient had a pelvic mass with irregularities of the right lateral wall of the rectum. *Proctoscopy and Biopsy:* Histologically lymphoid hyperplasia. *Angiographic Diagnosis:* Adenocarcinoma of the rectum with encasement of the arterial branches and occlusion of the rectal vein. *Surgical Pathology:* Adenocarcinoma of the rectum.

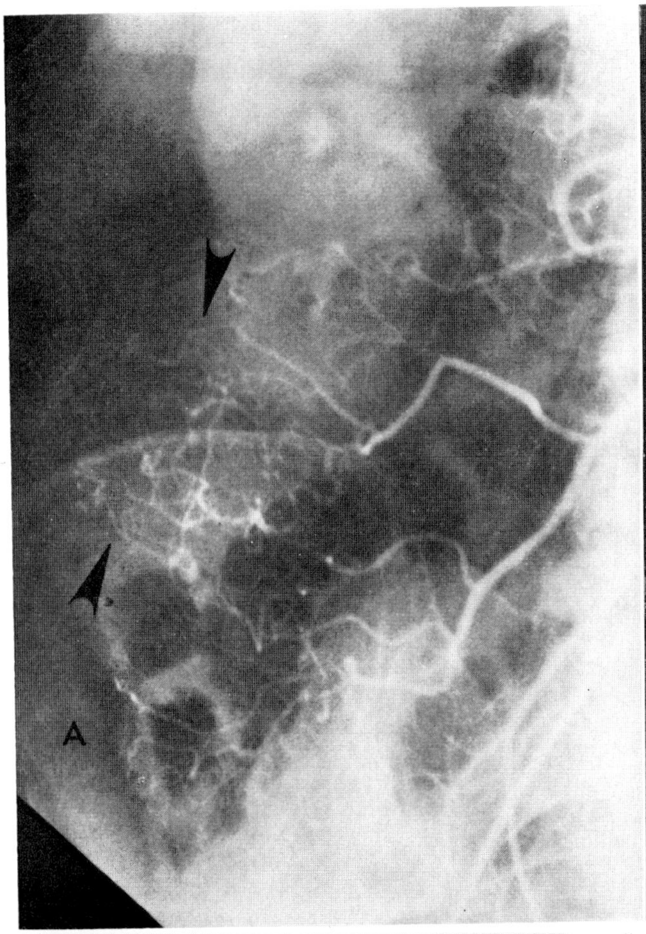

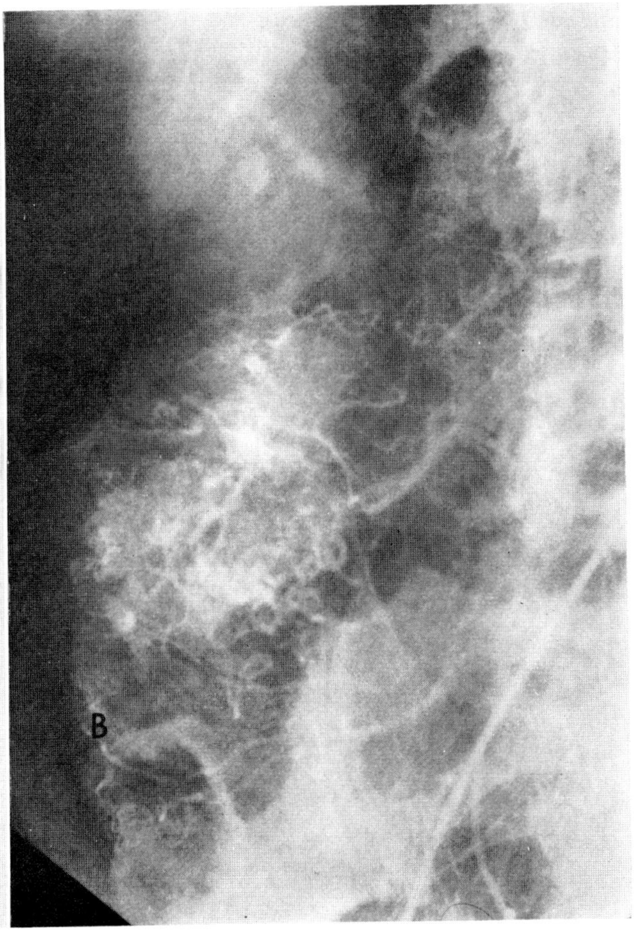

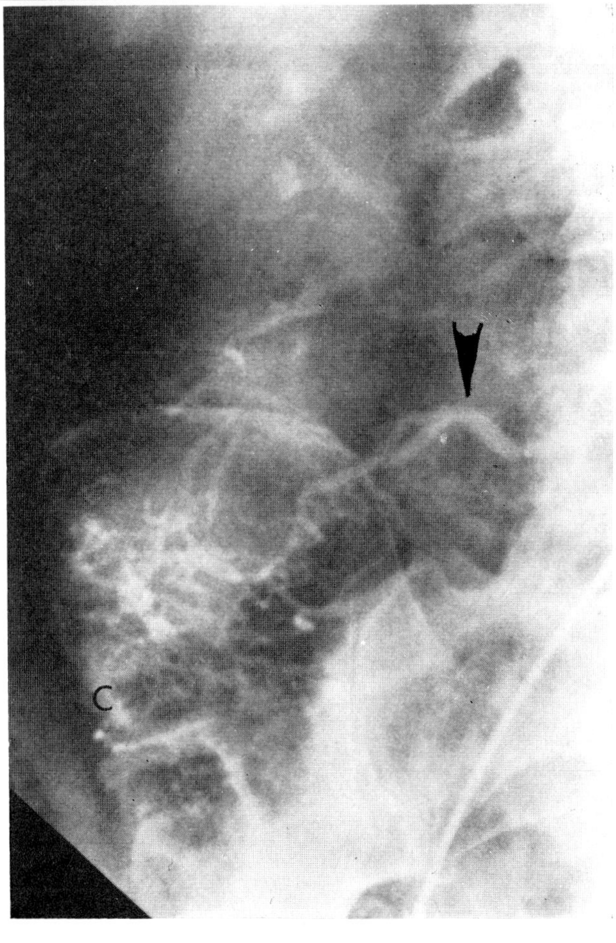

Figure 36.57. Superior Mesenteric Arteriogram. (A) Early phase reveals a cluster of abnormal vessels in the hepatic flexure level. (B) Midarterial phase reveals abnormal vascularity with staining of the mass. (C) Late arterial phase reveals localized early increased opacification of the veins in a patient who had an adenocarcinoma of that segment of the colon. (Courtesy of Dr. J. Petasnick, Associate Professor, Diagnostic Radiology, Rush Presbyterian-St. Luke Medical Center, Chicago.)

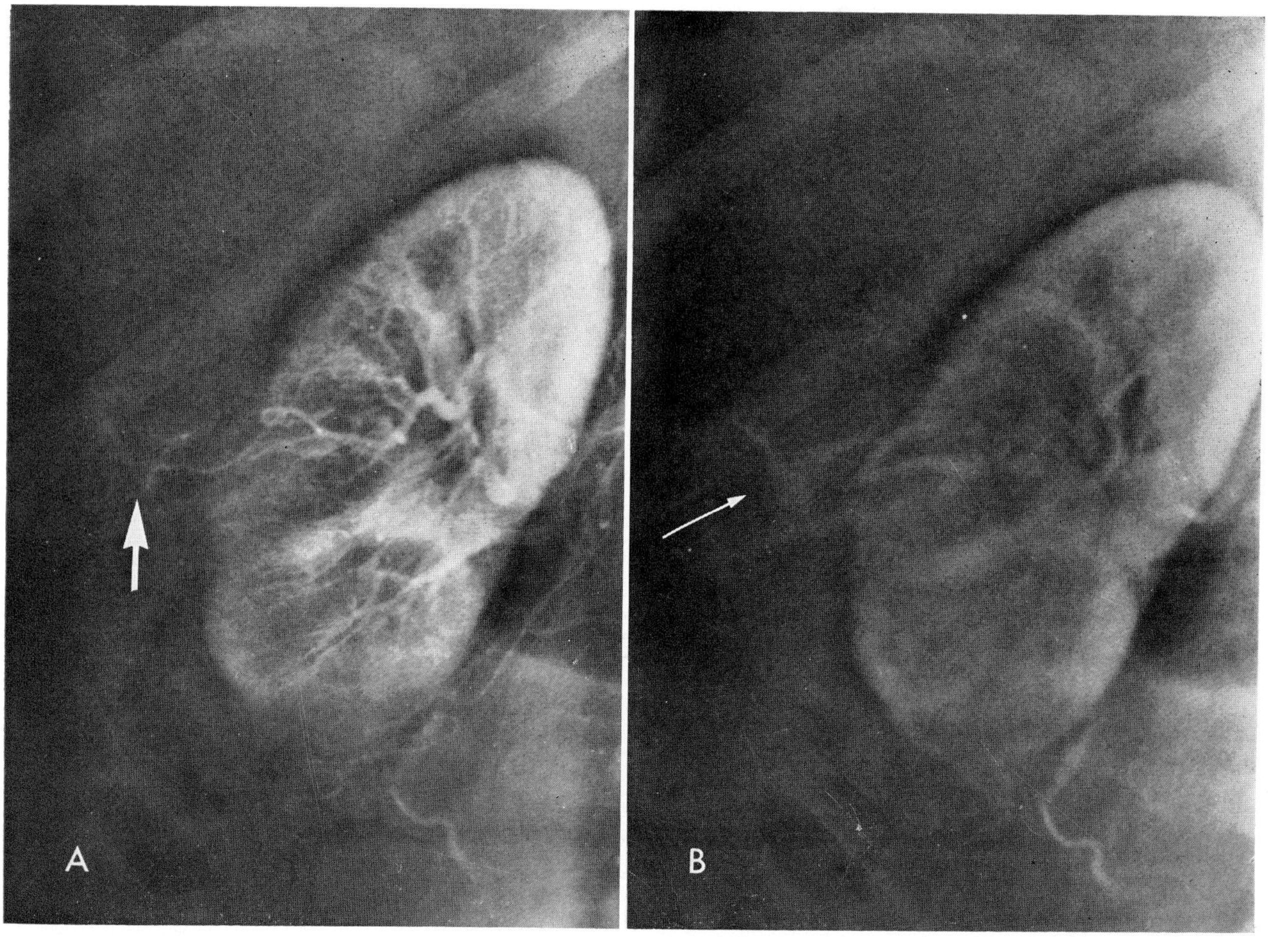

Figure 36.58. Renal Arteriogram. (A) Early arterial phase: A dilated perforating capsular artery terminates in abnormal arborization (Arrow). (B) Parenchymal phase: A faint abnormal stain is noted in the same vicinity (Arrow). A patient who had a known carcinoma of the colon in the same vicinity. *Pathology:* Carcinoma of the colon infiltrating into the renal capsule and to the renal cortex with blood supply from the perforating capsular artery.

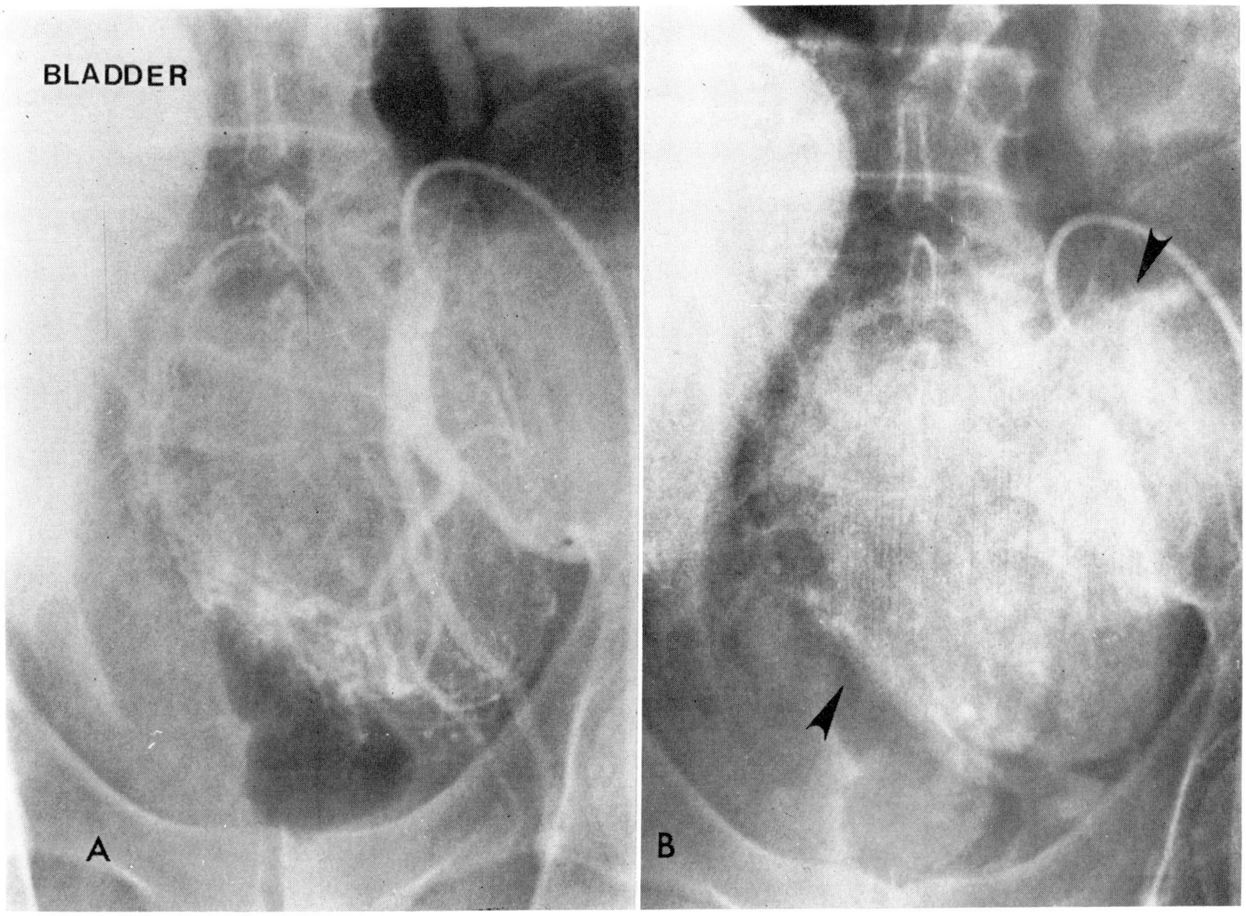

Figure 36.59. Internal Iliac Arteriogram. (A) Arterial phase: A dilated internal iliac artery with very prominent pelvic visceral branches with abnormal course and irregular dilatation supplies a moderate sized mass in the pelvis. This deviates the bladder toward the contralateral side. (B) Late phase: Diffuse homogeneous stain is revealed in this sixty-seven-year-old male. *Diagnosis:* Possible prostatic sarcoma. *Differential Diagnosis:* Smooth muscle tumors from the pelvis and other mesenchymal tumors from the pelvic connective tissues. *Pathology:* Prostatic adenocarcinoma.

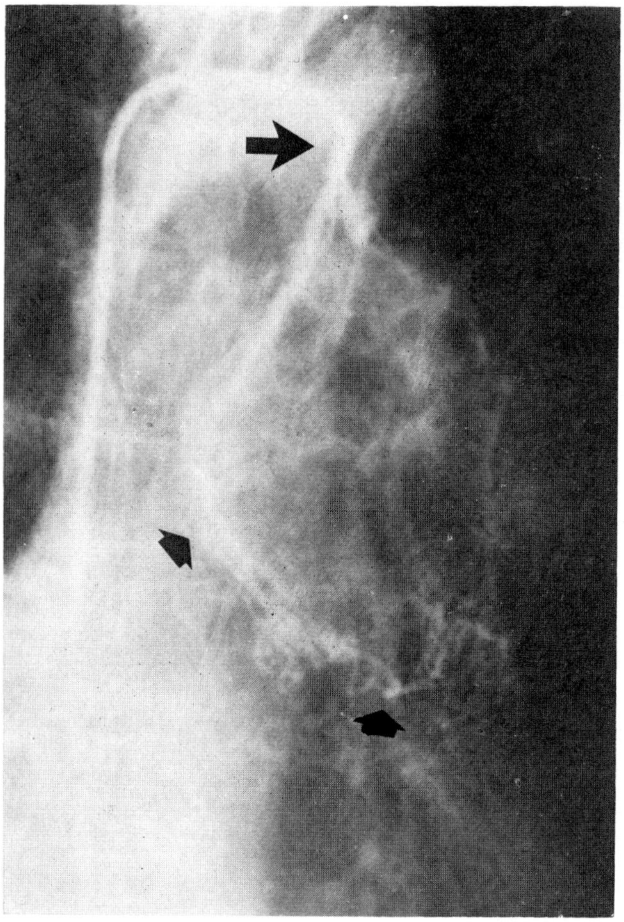

Figure 36.60. Thymic Venogram. Prominent thymic vein with multiple prominent branches encircles an anterior mediastinal mass. *Diagnosis:* A thymic mass probably thymoma. *Pathology:* Thymoma.

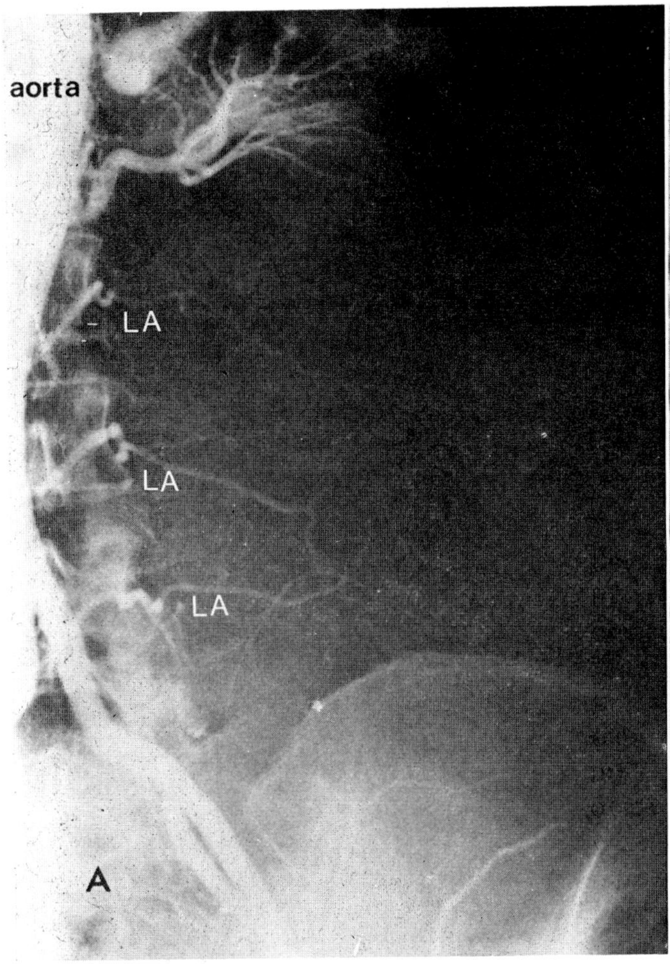

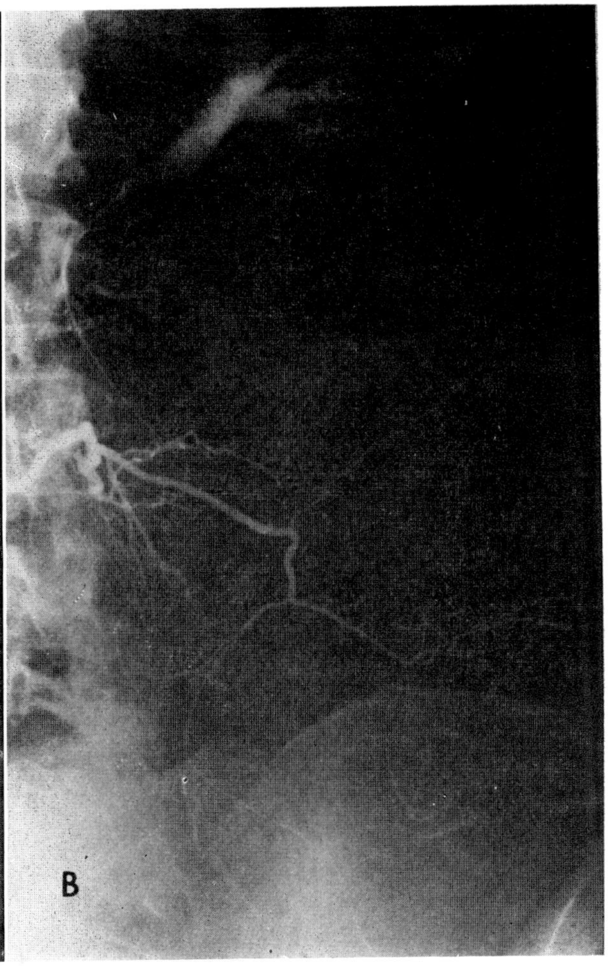

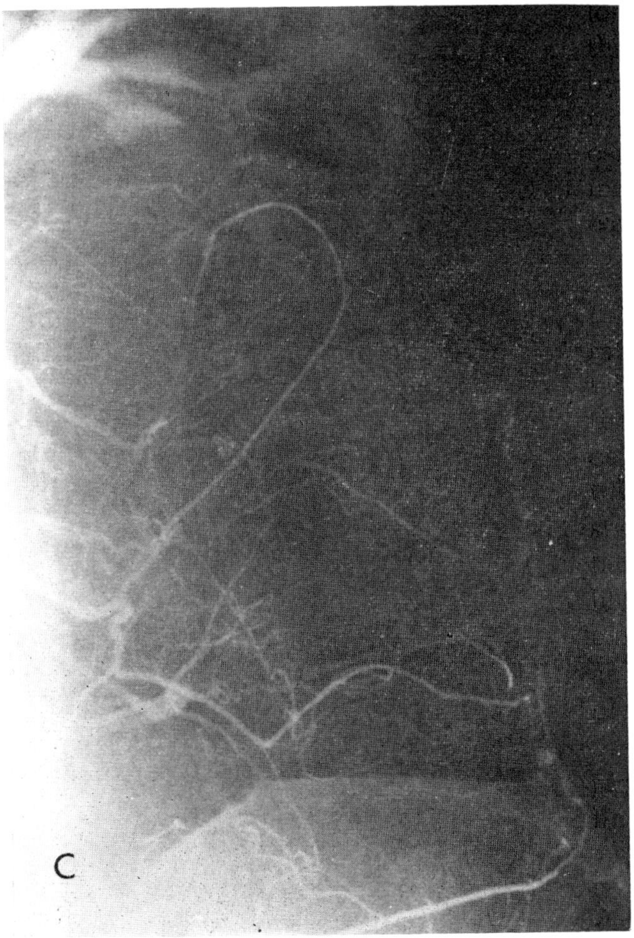

Figure 36.61. (A) Flush aortogram: The abdominal aorta is deviated to the right side (Aorta). Prominent second, third and fourth lumbar arteries with abnormal branches and a disoriented course (L.A.) are seen. (B) Selective lumbar arteriogram: Very prominent abnormal branches from the posterior branch of the lumbar artery encircle a huge retroperitoneal mass with vessels of irregular caliber. (C) Further abnormal peripheral vessels within this mass are opacified to better advantage. *Diagnosis:* Retroperitoneal malignant mesenchymal tumor. *Pathology:* Liposarcoma.

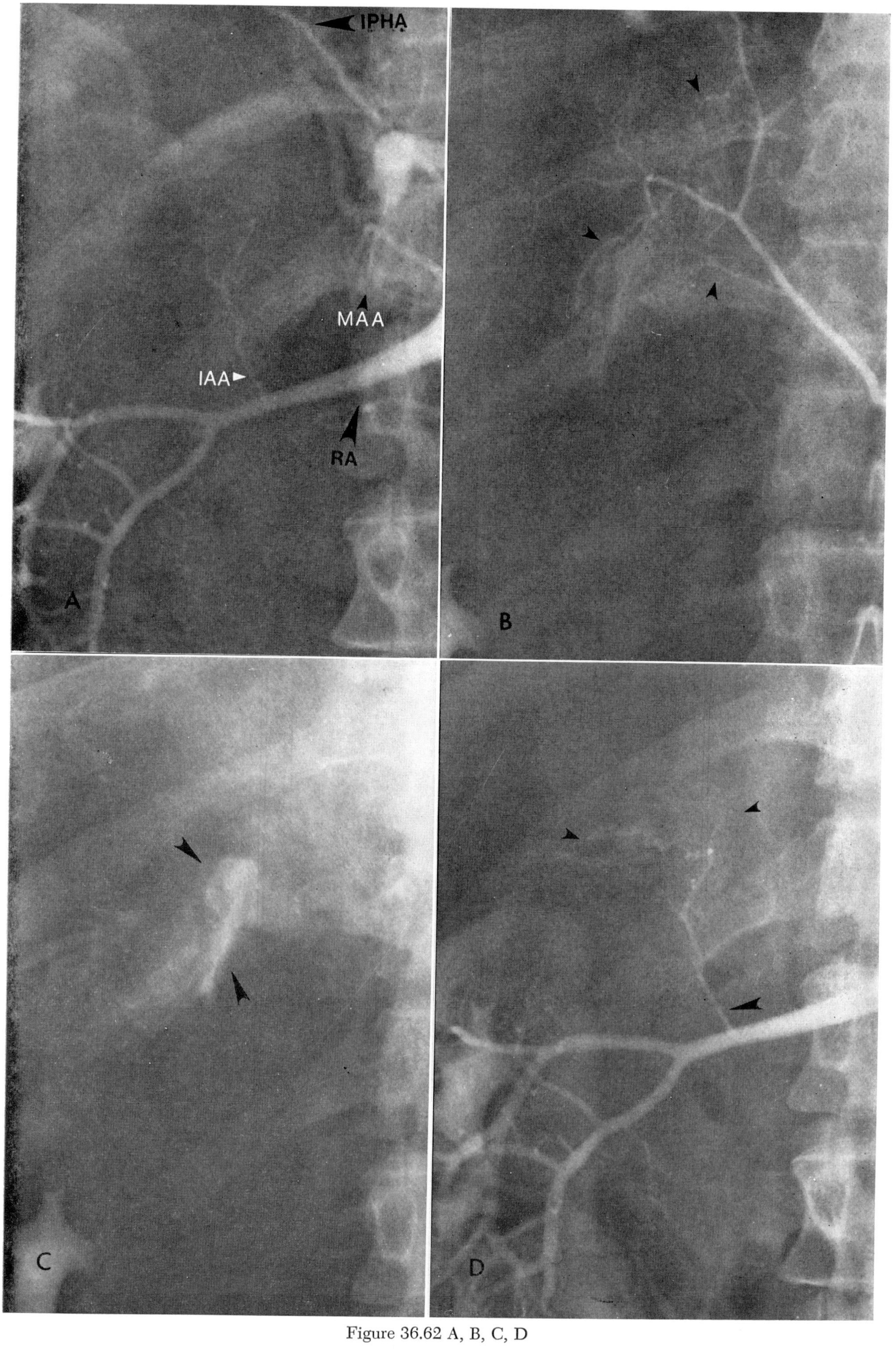

Figure 36.62 A, B, C, D

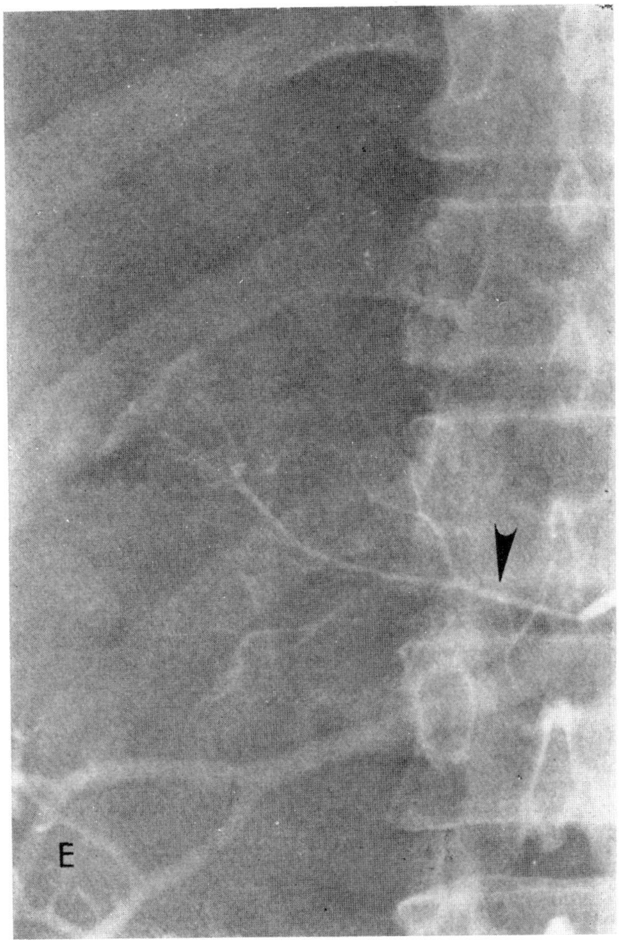

Figure 36.62. (A) Flush aortogram: Stretching of the right renal artery (R.A.). A prominent inferior adrenal artery (I.A.A.) visualization and stretching of the middle adrenal arteries (M.A.A.) and also the inferior phrenic artery (I.P.H.A.) are seen. (B) Selective inferior phrenic arteriogram: There are abnormal branches from the posterior ramification of the inferior phrenic artery (Arrow) and also an increased stain in the same area. (C) Increased staining in the retroperitoneal area. Notice the compressed and deformed adrenal stain (Arrow). (D) Renal arteriogram: There is a prominent inferior adrenal artery with abnormal ramification and early abnormal staining (Arrow). Incidentally, notice the change in the axis of the kidney. (E) Selective middle adrenal arteriogram: A large elongated middle adrenal artery (Arrow) with abnormal branches courses towards this retroperitoneal mass. This patient presented with right pleural effusion. *Diagnosis:* Extraadrenal paravertebral mass extending from the diaphragm to the level of the renal pedicle; possible lymphoma. *Pathology:* Reticulum cell sarcoma.

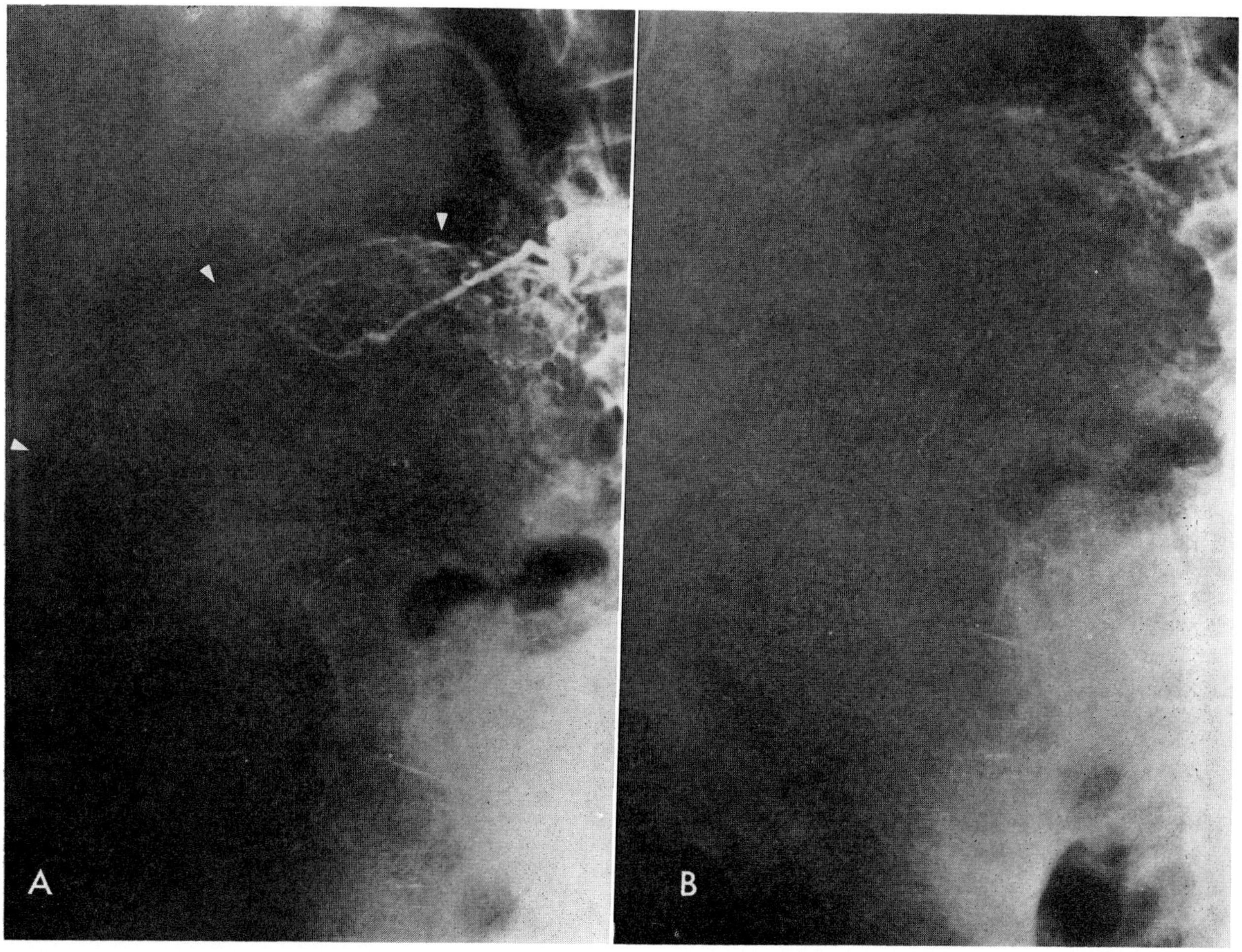

Figure 36.63. Lumbar Arteriogram. (A) Arterial phase: very prominent retroperitoneal branches from the lumbar artery with an abnormal course supply a huge mass in the right lower quadrant. (B) Late arterial phase: There is moderate staining of this portion of the mass supplied by the lumbar artery. *Diagnosis:* Retroperitoneal malignant mesenchymal tumor. *Pathology:* Undifferentiated retroperitoneal sarcoma.

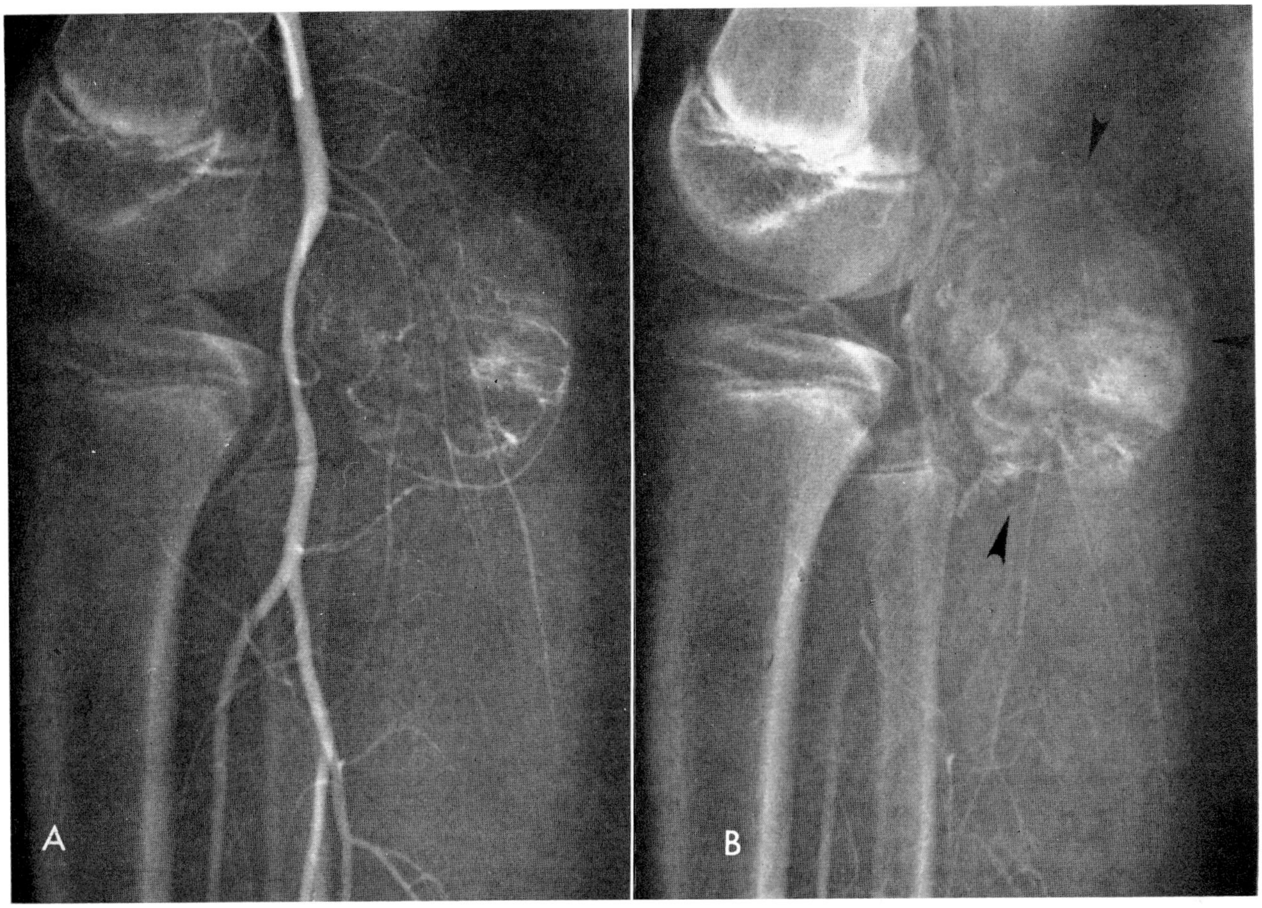

Figure 36.64. Femoral Arteriogram. (A) There is extrinsic compression on the popliteal artery which supplies neovasculature to a mass. (B) There are irregular areas of stain in the mass, with early venous opacification. The patient was fourteen years old. *Diagnosis:* Malignant neoplasm, synovial sarcoma? *Pathologic Diagnosis:* Synovial sarcoma.

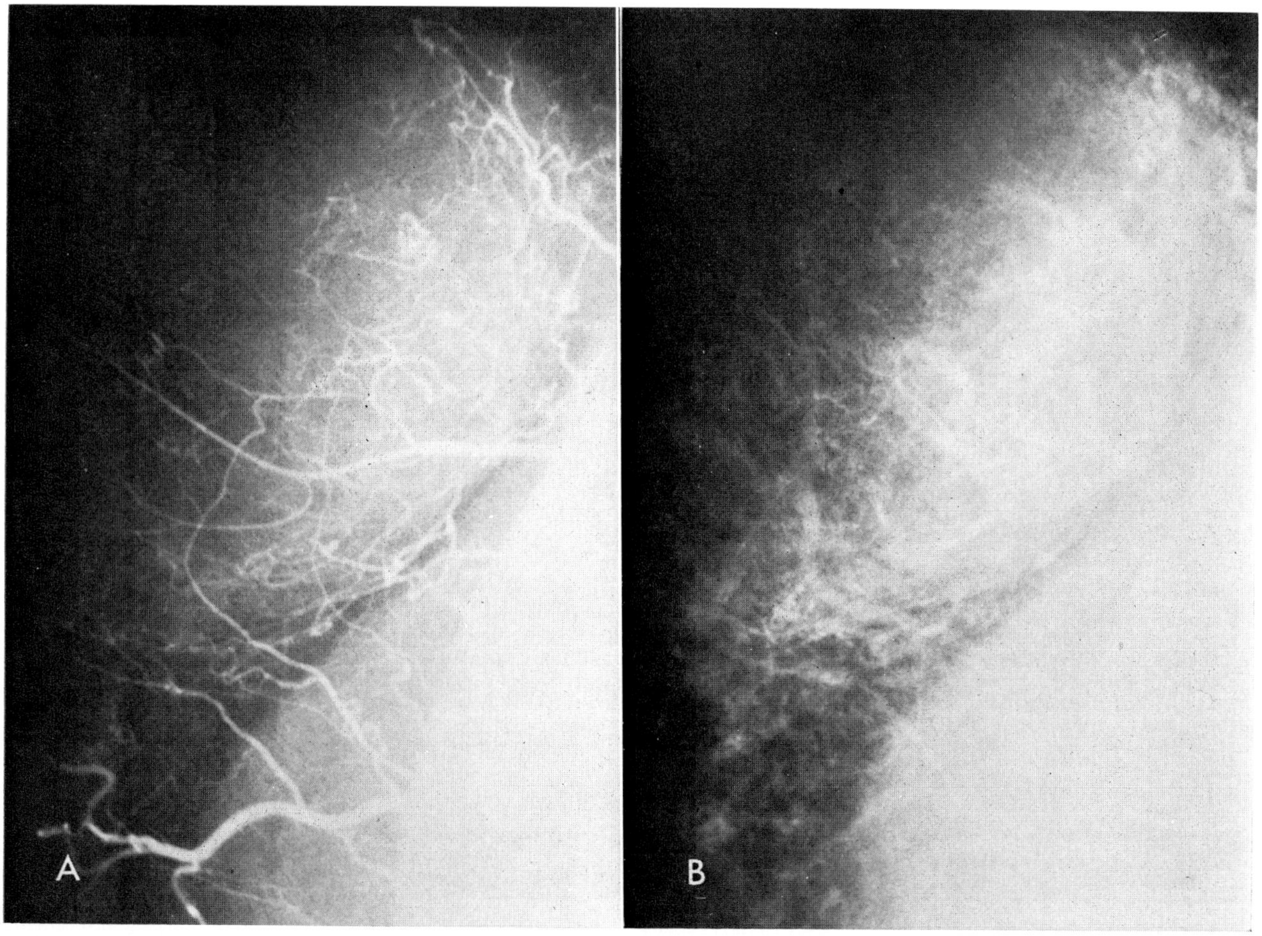

Figure 36.65. Internal Iliac Arteriogram—(tangenital view for the buttocks). (A) The arterial phase reveals a mass with a very abnormal vascularity. (B) The late phase reveals increased venous drainage and an island of avascularity. *Diagnosis:* Malignant tumor with necrosis. *Pathology:* Fibrosarcoma.

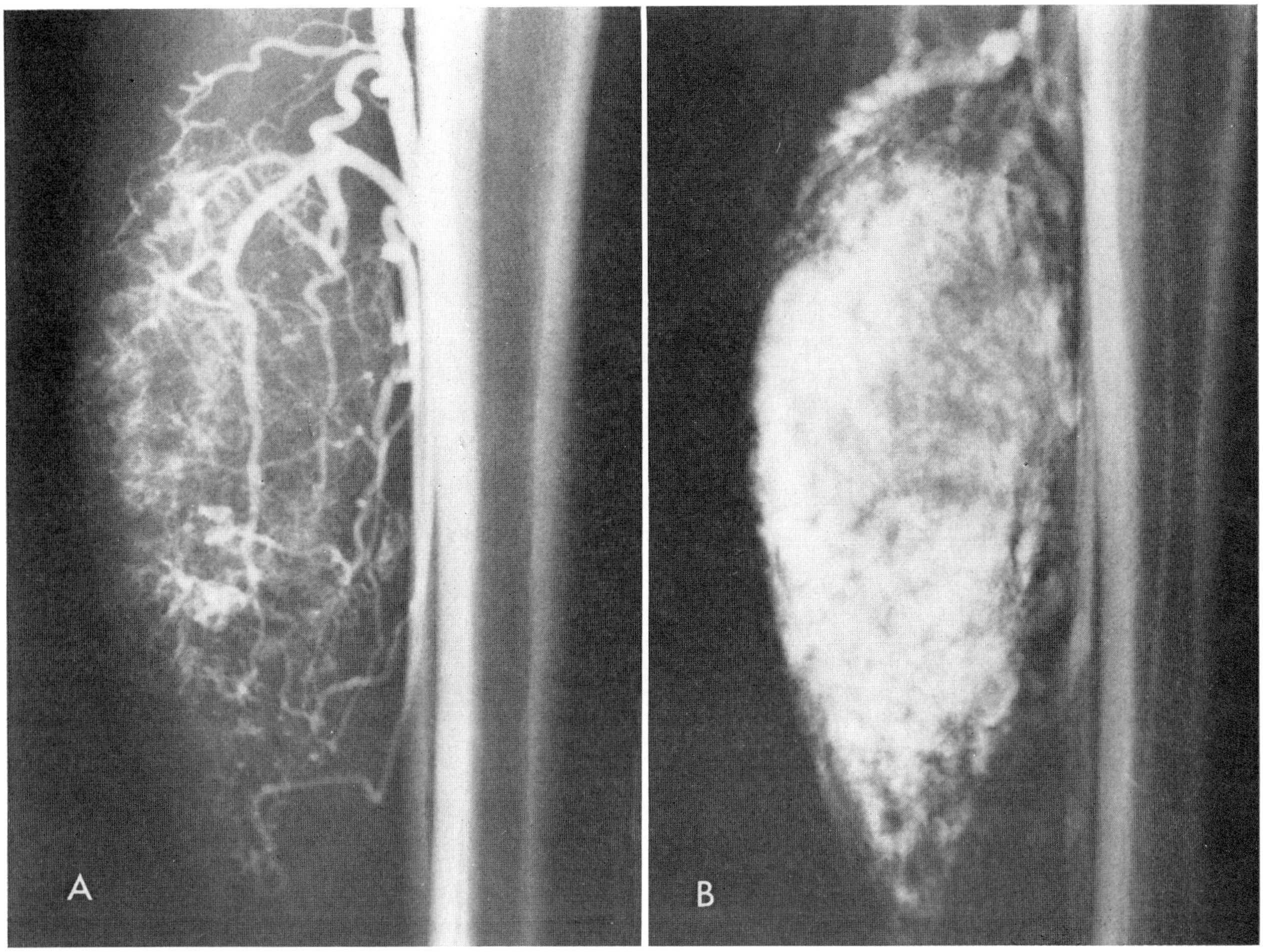

Figure 36.66. Femoral Arteriogram. (A) There is a highly vascularized tumor of the calf with irregular vessels. (B) The tumor mass is opacified with numerous dilated veins. *Angiographic Diagnosis:* Malignant tumor. *Pathologic Diagnosis:* Alveolar cell soft part tumor.

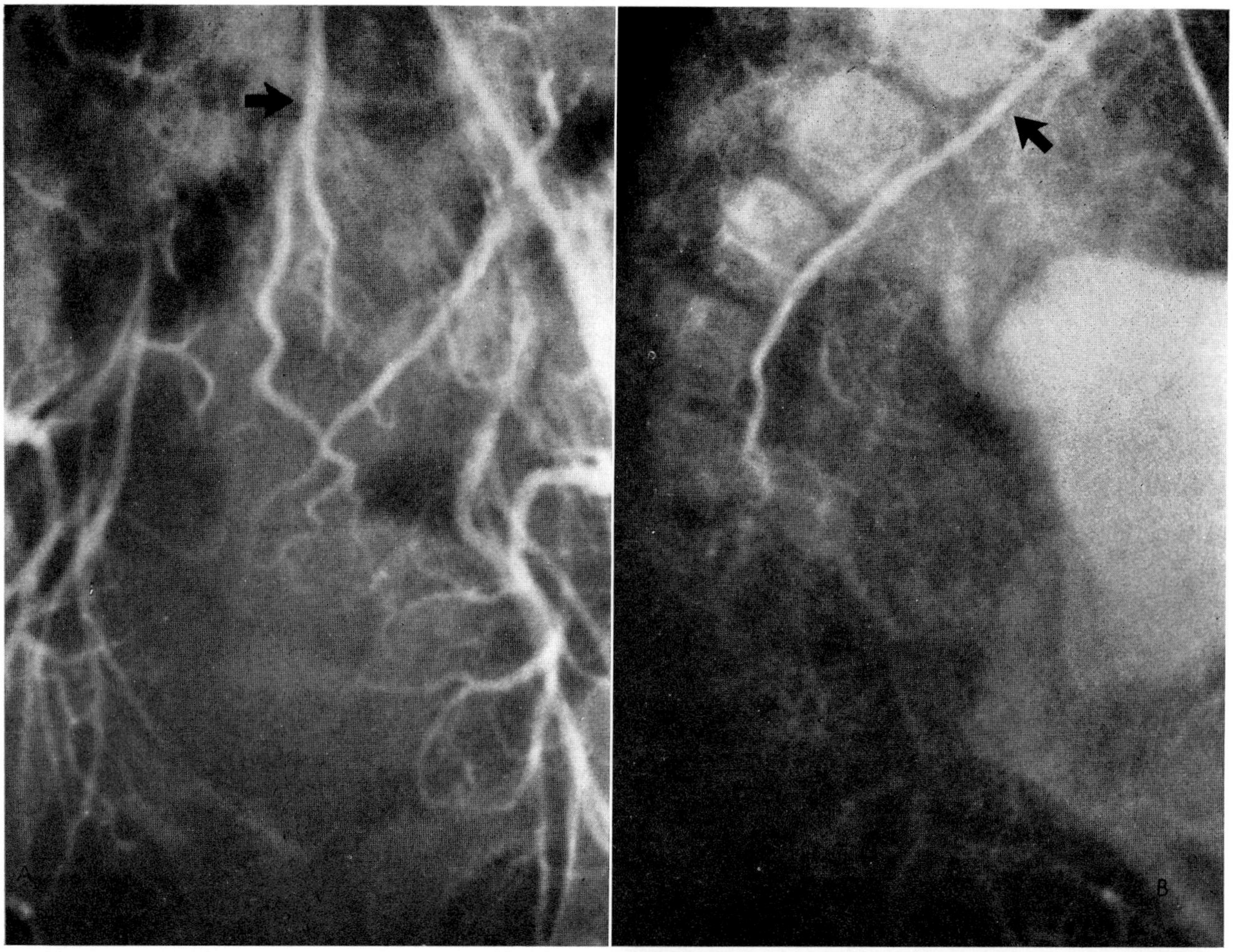

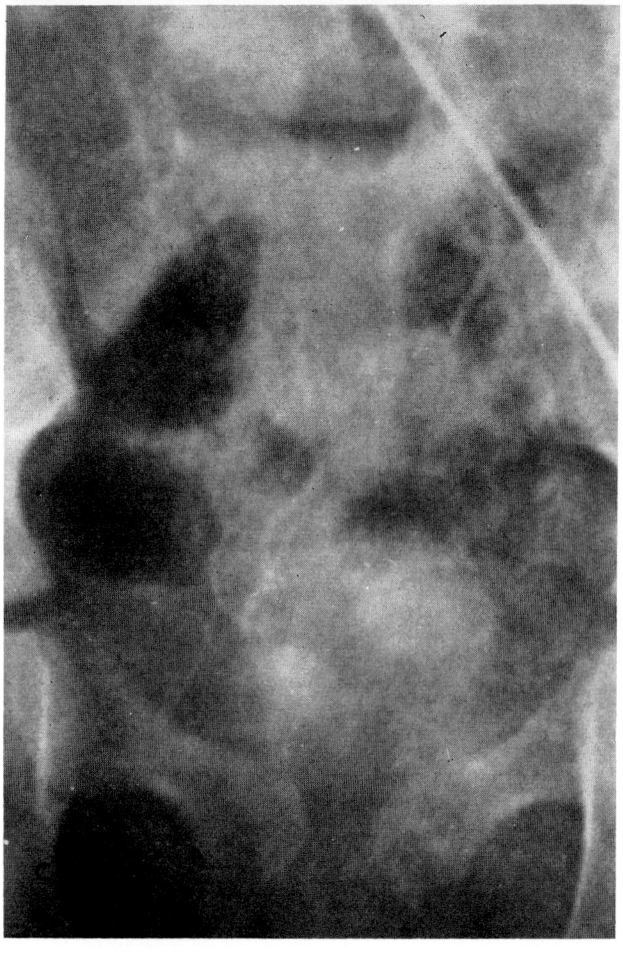

Figure 36.67. Pelvic Arteriogram. (A) Frontal projection. (B) Lateral projection: A very prominent middle sacral artery (Arrow) is seen supplying a tumor in the lower part of the pelvis along with the internal iliac artery branches. (C) Late arterial phase: Faint staining of the tumor mass is revealed. *Pathology:* Malignant sacrococcygeal teratoma. (From McDonald, P. Malignant sacrococcygeal teratoma. *Am J Roentgenol, 118:*444, 1973. Courtesy of the authors and publishers.)

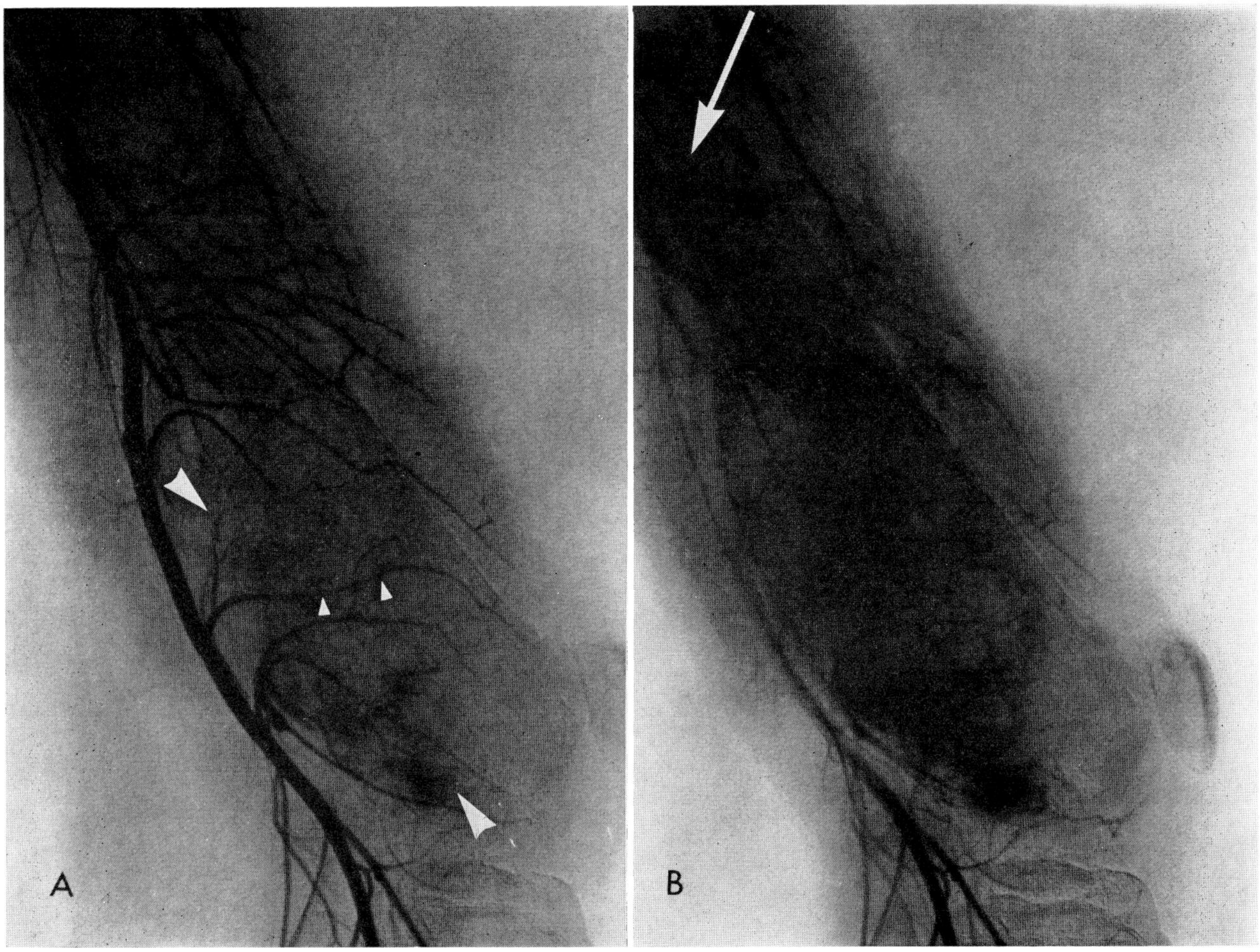

Figure 36.68. Femoral Arteriogram—subtraction films. (A) There are malignant neoplastic vessels (Large Arrow Head). One vessel is encased (Small Arrow Head). (B) Late arterial phase: There are islands of stain in the tumor parenchyma with early venous drainage (Arrow). *Diagnosis:* Malignant osseous tumor. *Pathologic Diagnosis:* Osteogenic sarcoma.

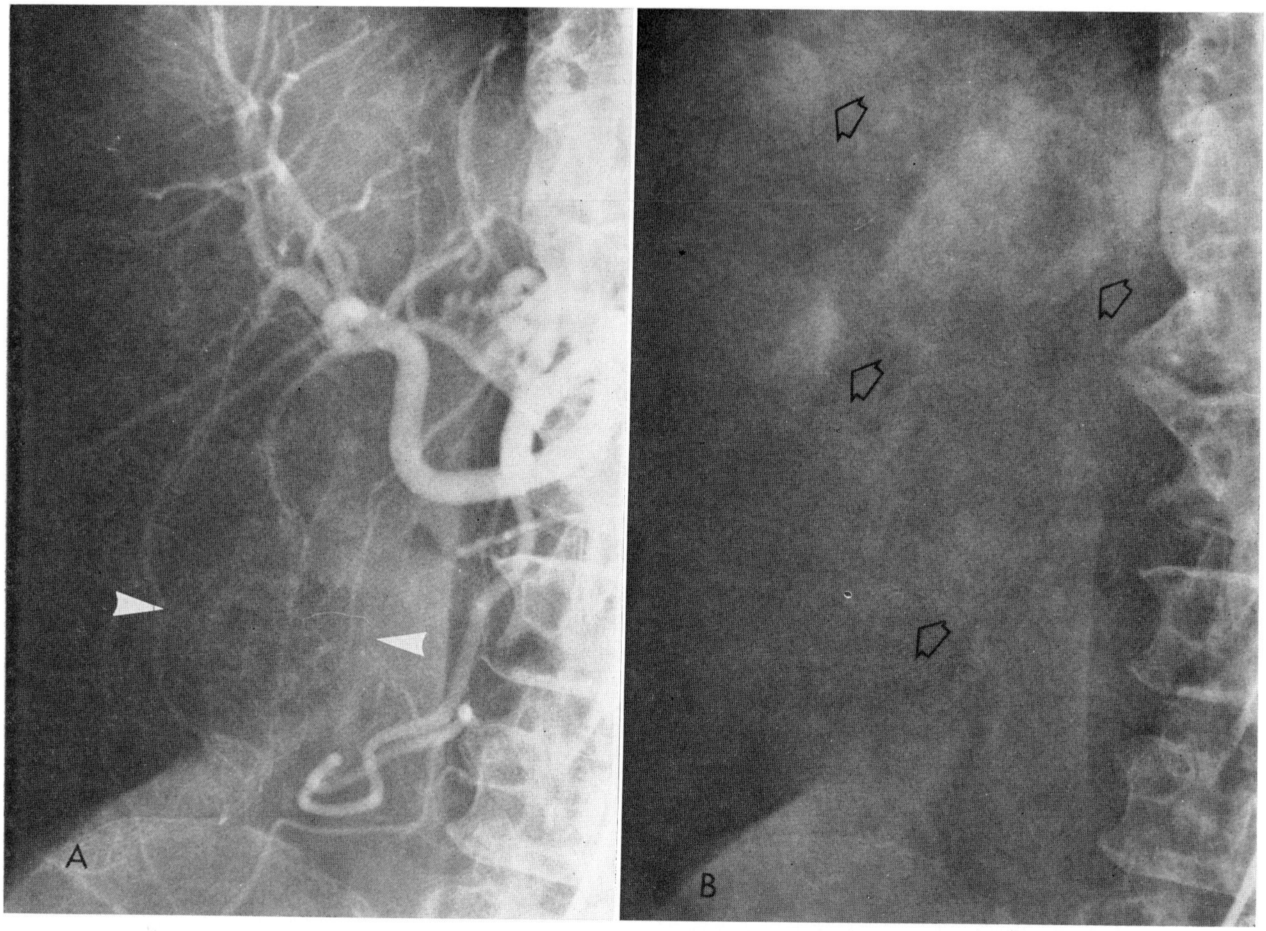

Figure 36.69. Celiac Arteriogram. (A) There is an increased number of abnormal vessels (Arrow) arising from the intrahepatic arteries. (B) There are multiple masses with increased stain seen. The patient had a carcinoid tumor of the ileocecal area. *Diagnosis:* Vascular metastasis.

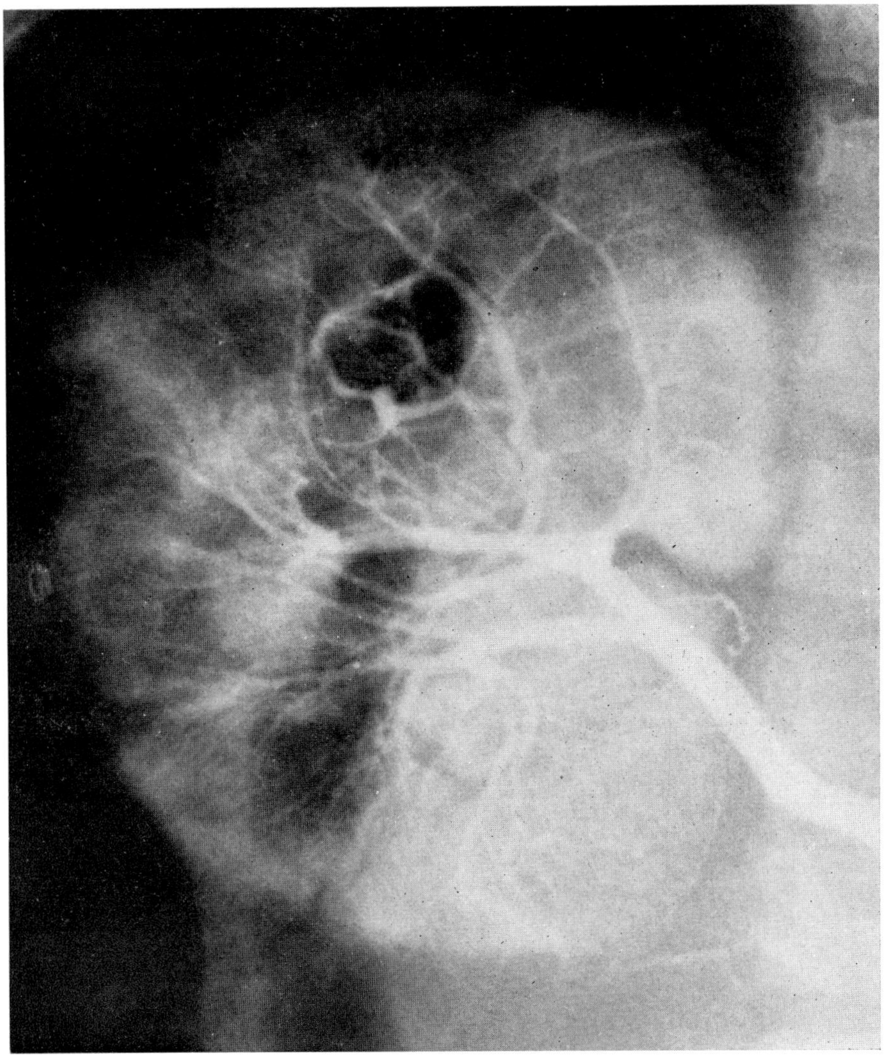

Figure 36.70. Renal arteriogram reveals malignant sinusoids within a mass in the upper portion of the kidney. This young boy has his right lobe of the liver resected, because of a hepatoblastoma. *Diagnosis:* Malignant tumor of the kidney, probably metastasis from the hepatoblastoma. *Pathology:* Metastasis from hepatoblastoma.

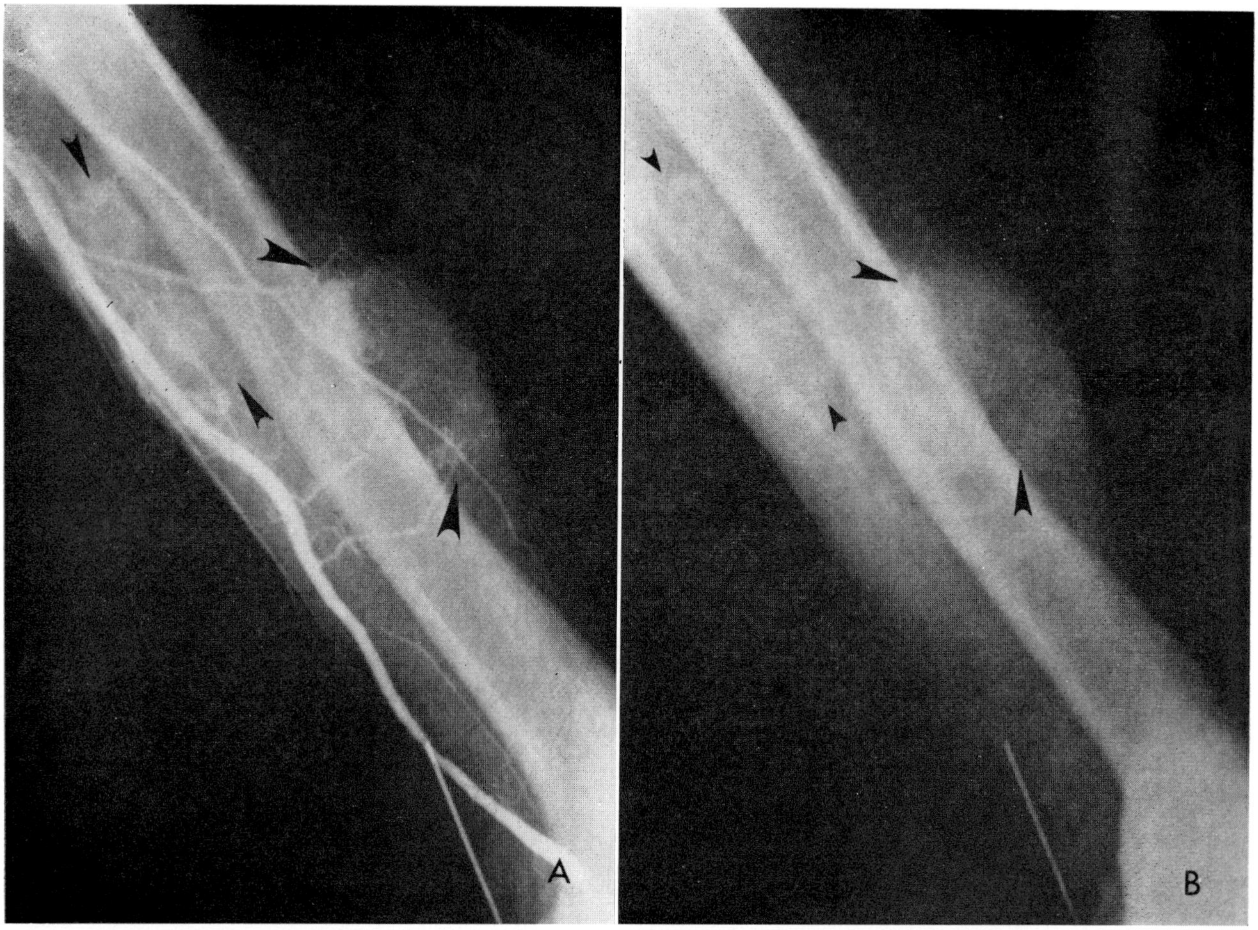

Figure 36.71. Brachial Arteriogram. (A) There is neovascularity arising from the muscular branches of the brachial artery (Arrow). (B) Three well-defined masses opacify in the arm muscles with early venous visualization. *Diagnosis:* Metastasis to the muscles from a known bronchogenic carcinoma.

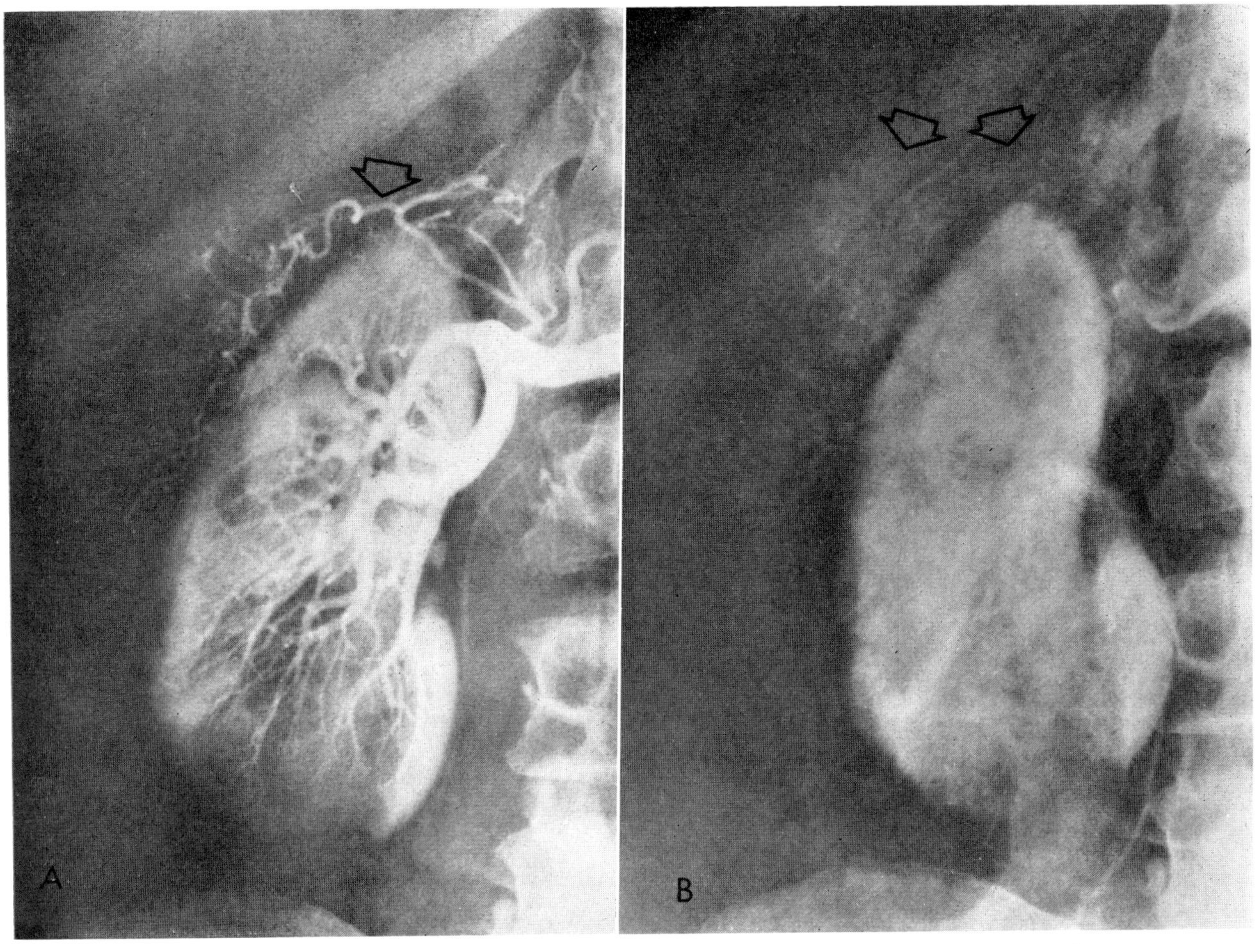

Figure 36.72. Renal Arteriogram. (A) Arterial phase: A very prominent capsular artery with increase in its caliber and length and multiple abnormal branches lead into an amorphous area (Arrow). Incidentally seen is lack of perfusion of the lower pole of the right kidney with stretching and deviation of the branches. (B) Parenchymal phase: An abnormal stain is noted around the upper pole and the upper lateral surface of the kidney (Arrow). A filling defect in the lower pole of the kidney is again noted with a smooth, sharp interface with the adjacent renal parenchyma. A patient whose hepatic arteriogram revealed very abnormal tumor vasculature. *Diagnosis:* Malignant tumor in the liver with blood supply from the renal capsular artery. Incidental cyst in the right lower pole of the kidney. *Pathology:* Cyst lower pole of the kidney. Anaplastic carcinomatous metastases in the liver breaking through the inferior surface of the liver. The primary site was unknown.

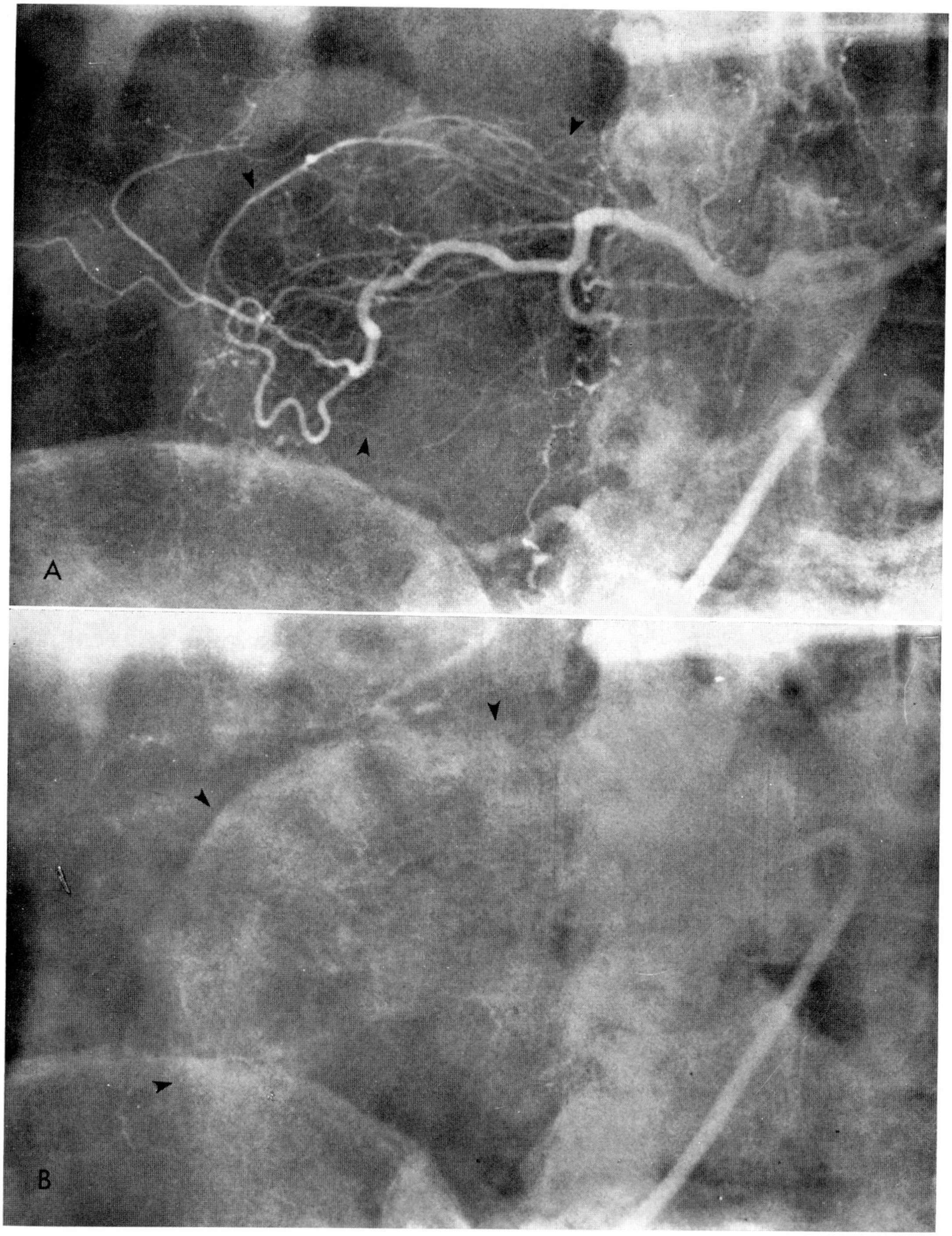

Figure 36.73. Lumbar Arteriogram. (A) Arterial phase: Very prominent retroperitoneal branches from the lumbar artery perfuse a mass in the paravertebral area (Arrow). Note the distortion of the lumbar arterial course. (B) Parenchymal phase: There is moderate staining of this mass. *Diagnosis:* Retroperitoneal mesenchymal malignant tumor. *Pathology:* Metastases from a pancreatic adenocarcinoma.

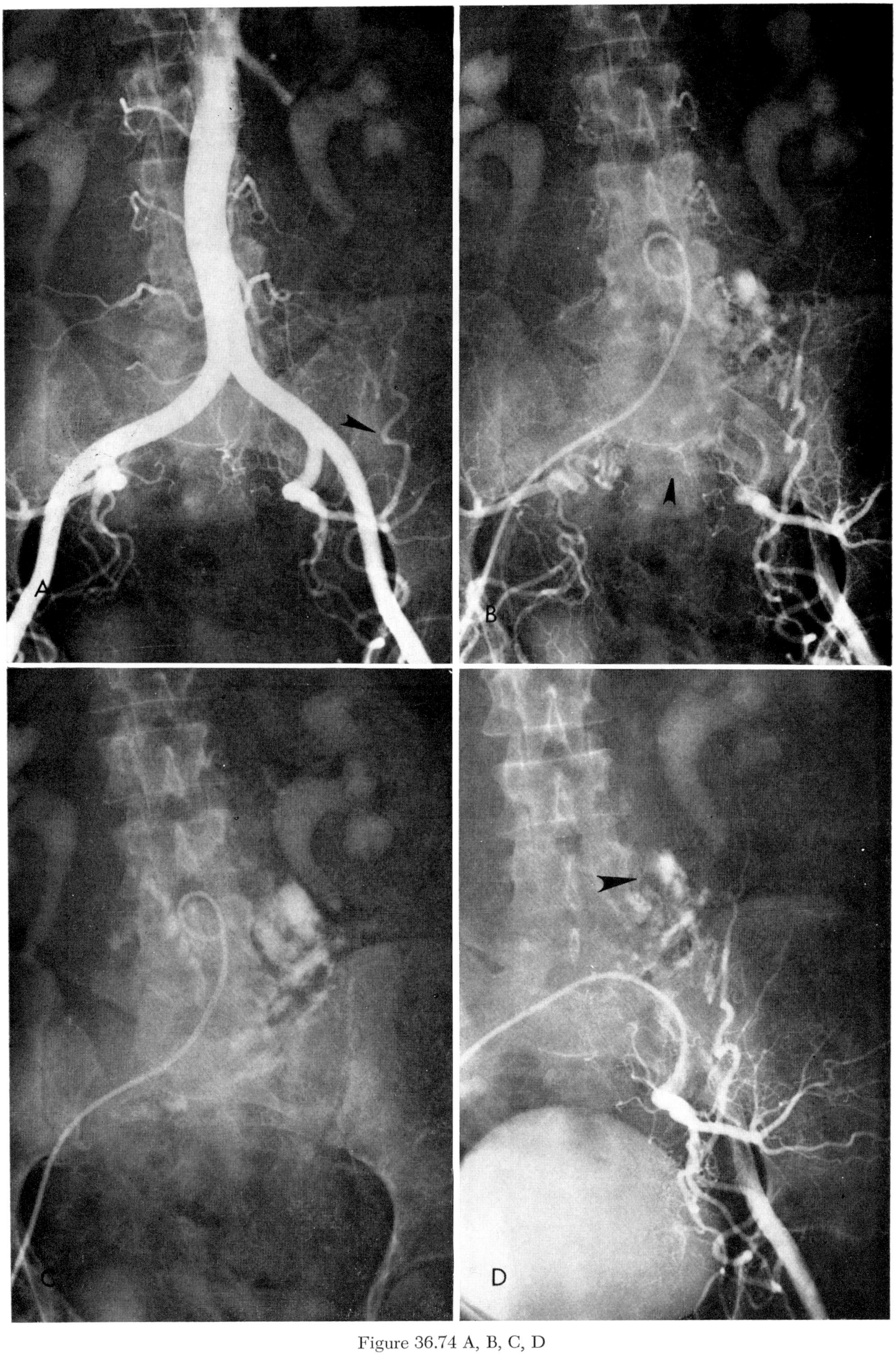

Figure 36.74 A, B, C, D

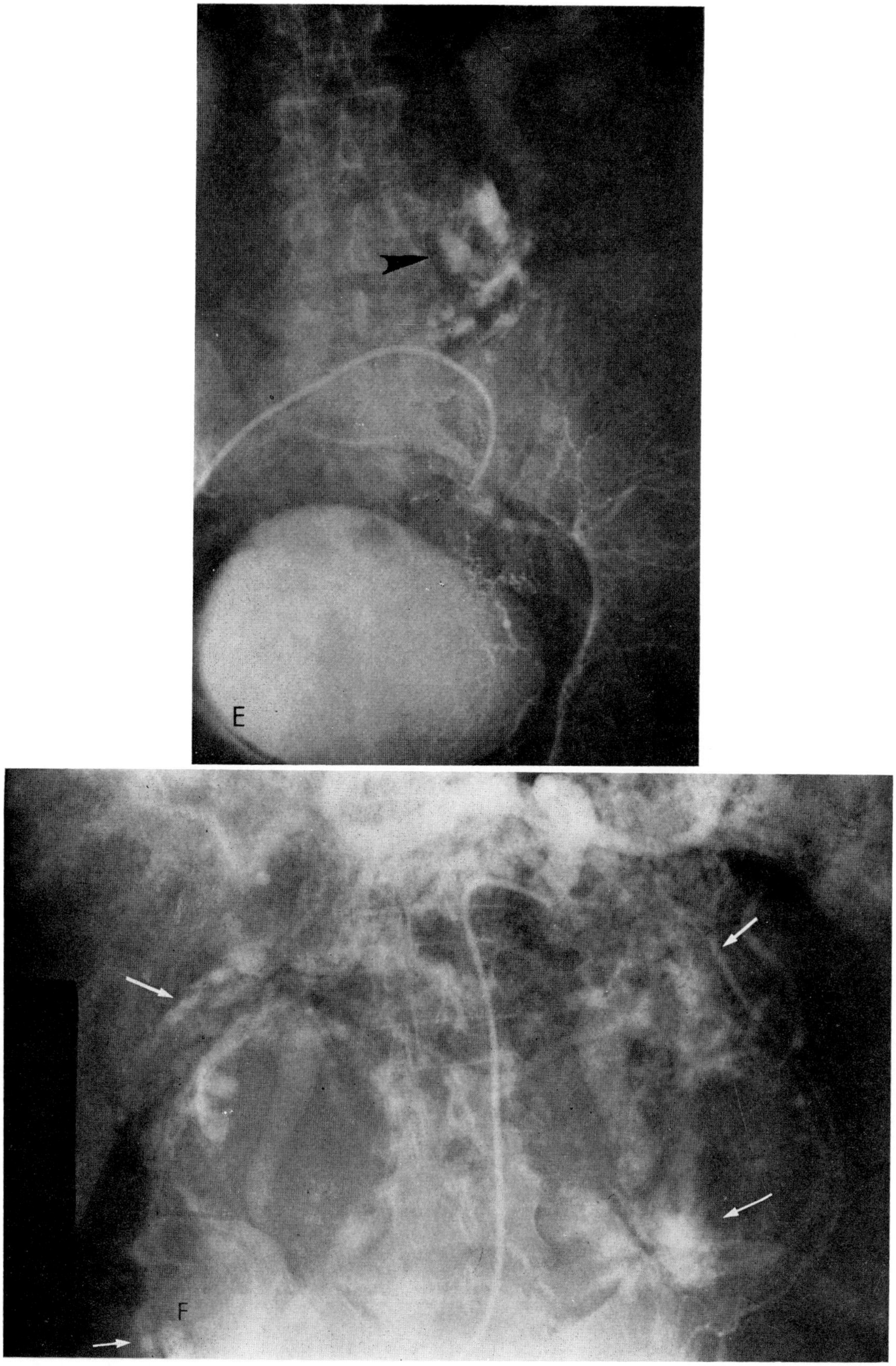

Figure 36.74 E and F

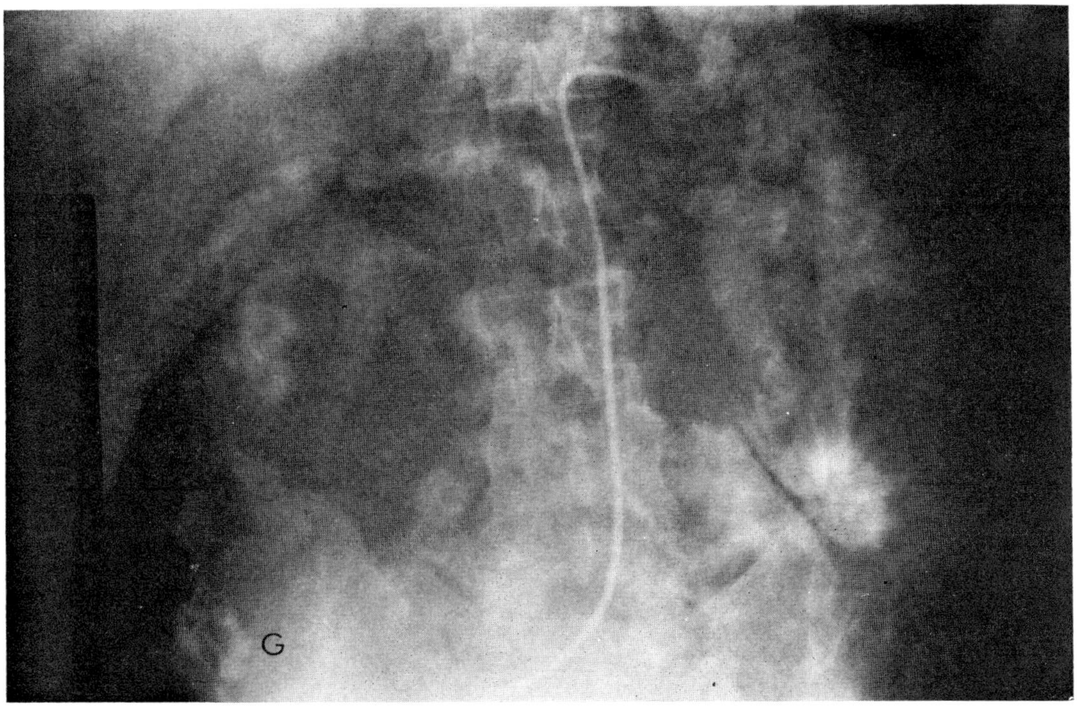

Figure 36.74. (A, B & C) Flush aortogram reveals prominent vessels from the internal iliac artery ending in sinusoidal pools. (D & E) Selective internal iliac arteriogram reveals the same sinusoids. (F & G) Celiac arteriogram demonstrates very prominent branches again opacifying some more sinusoidal pools of a huge mass in a middle aged female. *Diagnosis:* Probable uterine leiomyoma or mesenteric vascular tumor with parasitic blood supply. *Pathology:* Huge cavernous hemangioma of the liver. In retrospect, the dilated celiac branches opacifying these sinusoidal pools should have alerted us.

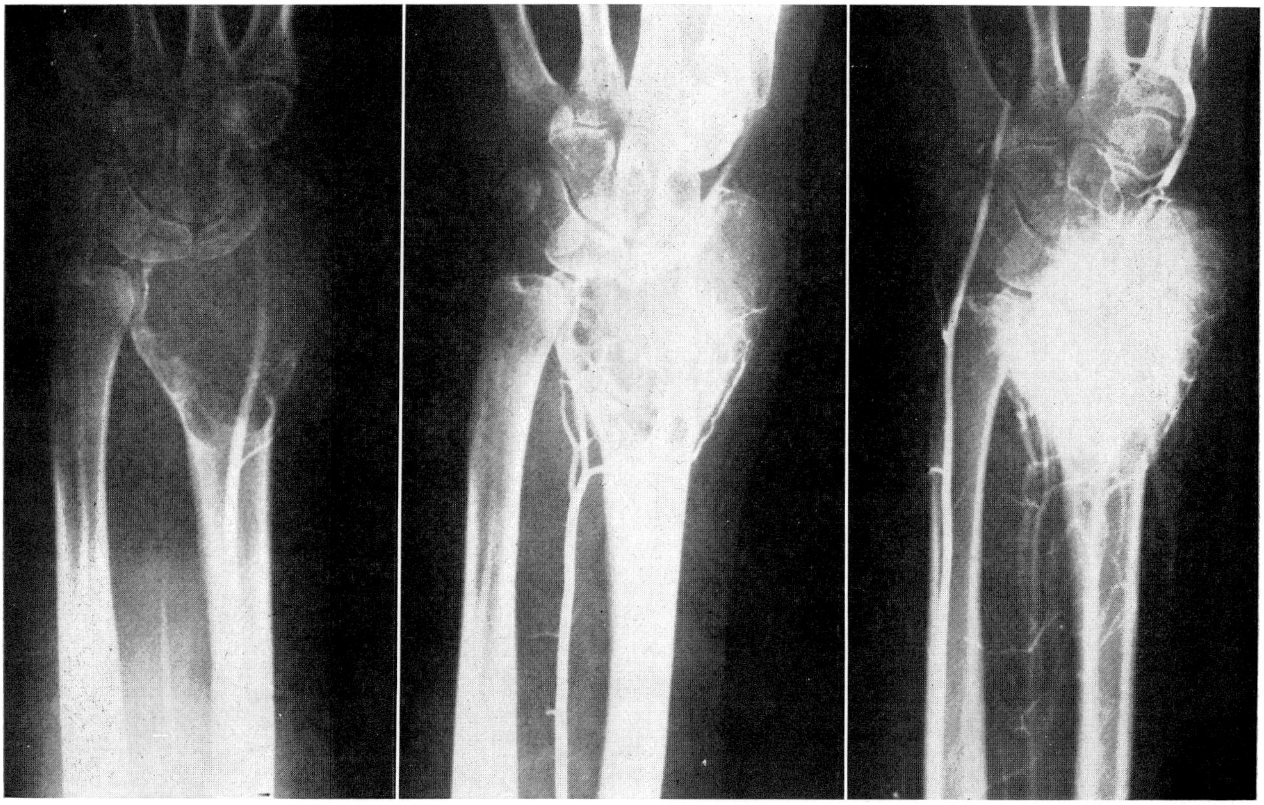

Figure 36.75. Brachial Arteriogram. (A) Early arterial phase: A lesion is revealed in the distal part of the radius. (B) Early arterial phase: Hypervascularity is seen in the same area. (C) Contrast material fills the bone lesion causing puddling. *Diagnosis:* Benign versus malignant lesion of the distal radius. *Pathology:* Benign giant cell tumor of the radius. (From Herzberg, D. L., and Schreiber, M. Angiography in the mass lesions of the extremities. *Am J Roentgenol, 111*:541, 1971. Courtesy of the authors and publishers.)

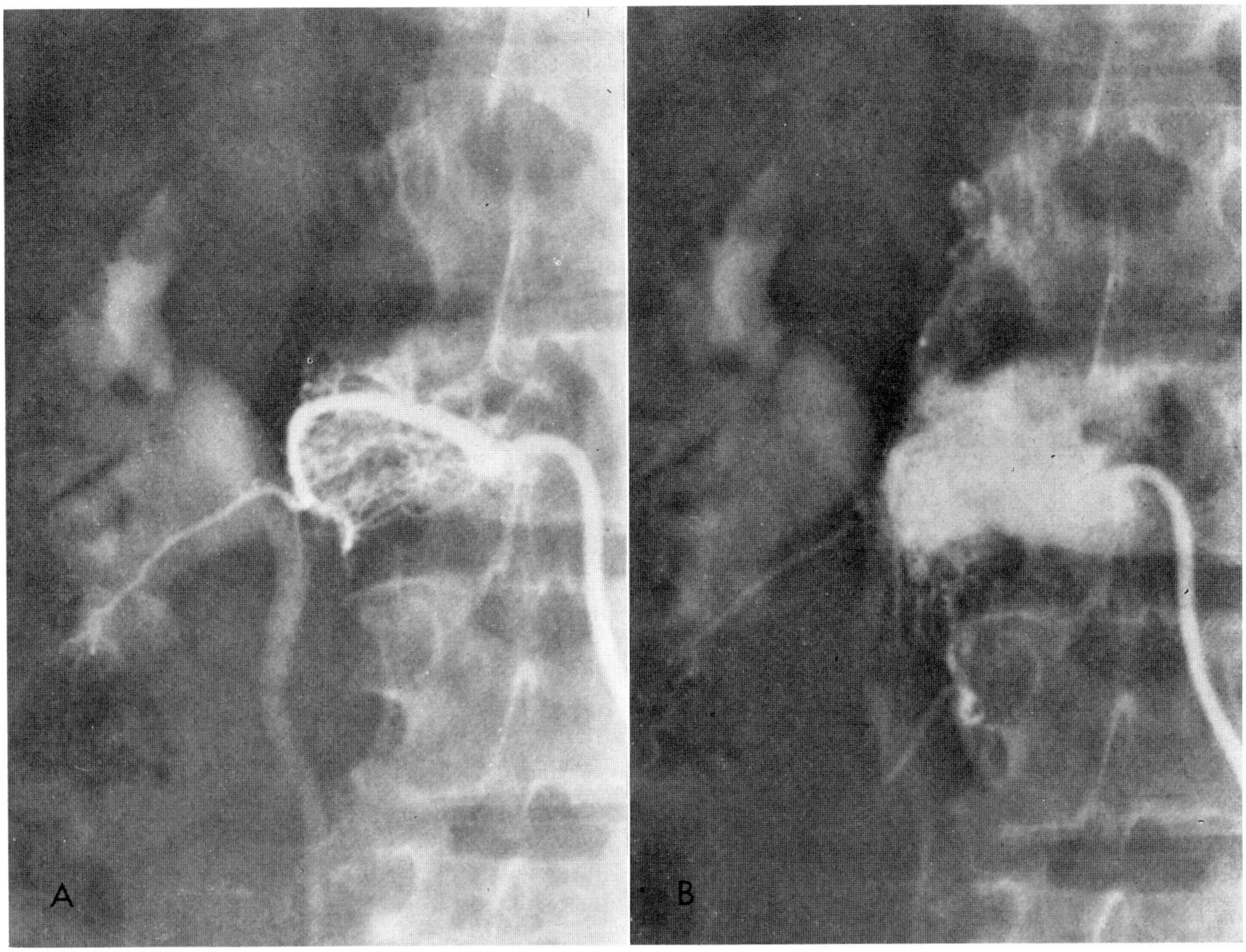

Figure 36.76. Lumbar Arteriogram. (A) Arterial phase: very prominent lumbar artery with abnormal prominent branches coursing towards the vertebral body. (B) A large amorphous collection of contrast material is in the same area. This patient had a known hypernephroma with destruction of the vertebral body. *Comment:* Metastases to the lumbar vertebral body with a big sinusoidal pool.

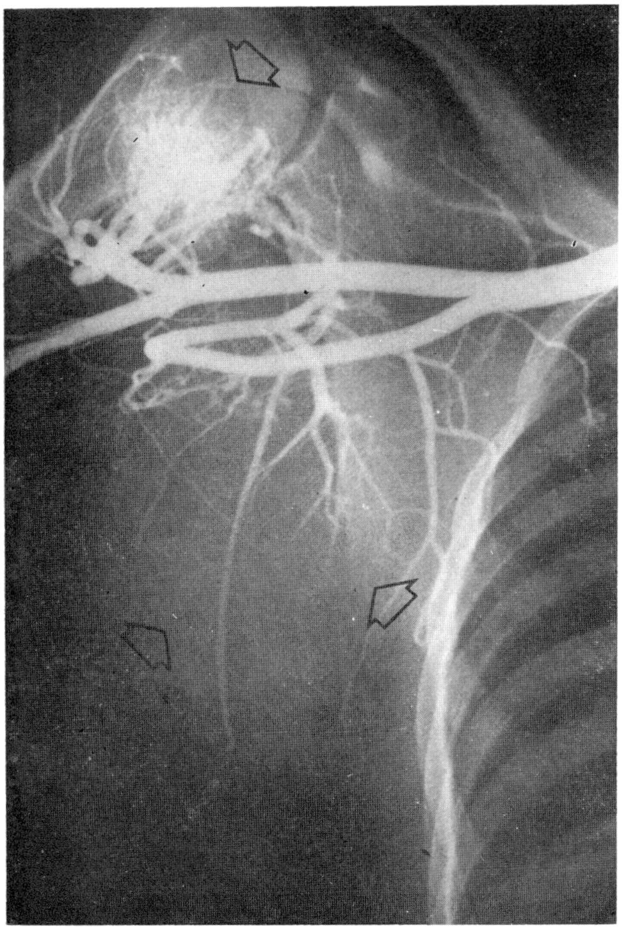

←

Figure 36.77. Subclavian Arteriogram. A soft tissue mass is seen with hypervascularity (Arrow) and amorphous collection of contrast material in the shape of a puddle. *Diagnosis:* Malignant neoplasm. *Pathologic Diagnosis:* Undifferentiated sarcoma.

CHAPTER 37
MISCELLANEOUS

OBSTETRICAL COMPLICATIONS AND ANGIOGRAPHY

GENERALIZED DILATATION of the uterine arteries and their myometrial branches reflect not only the normal physiologic response to pregnancy, but other disorders which increase the metabolic demands of the uterus.[111, 368, 1420, 1427] At the second month in a *normal pregnancy*, the uterine artery hypertrophies; by eight to twelve weeks the placental circulation may be shown.[1428] In a normal pregnancy both ovarian and uterine arteries are hypertrophied, while in an *ectopic pregnancy*, the vessel supplying that circulation is asymmetrically hypertrophied. However, in a *bicornuate uterus*, only the uterine artery supplying the cornua lodging the fetus, will be hypertrophied, while the contralateral uterine artery minds its own business.[1429] Were it not for the homogeneous round or oval stain of the *corpus luteum*, many early ectopic pregnancies with their irregular intervillous spaces would be mistaken for the corpus luteum.

Tubal Gestation

Visualization depends on the placental maturation and its continuity with the utero-placental circulation. If there is blood supply from the aorta or the ovarian arteries, the ectopic circulation may be demonstrated even after tubal rupture. The earliest period to demonstrate the intervillous space of the ectopic gestation ranges from five to seven weeks.[1430] Unlike a normal pregnancy, an abdominal pregnancy reveals ipsilateral dilatation of the ovarian artery and a normal size uterine artery supplying a uterus of small size in relation to the duration of gestation. Characteristically, the placental circulation is extrauterine and may lie anywhere in the abdomen. If it is a late abdominal pregnancy and if the product of conception is in the peritoneal cavity, the placenta may not opacify because of an imperfect or absent decidual layer. A missed abortion may have very subtle angiographic dissimilarities from a normal pregnancy. But opacification of the veins in the vicinity, if seen, may aid in diagnosing a suspected missed abortion. A missed abortion and a mole may have similar angiographic appearances.[1431]

Trophoblastic Tumors

Moles, chorioadenoma destruens, and choriocarcinomas are three complications of pregnancy with different stages in progression from benign proliferative to malignant invasive disease.[111, 1420] A mole represents hydropic swelling of chorionic villi with various size locules. It is demonstrated as overall avascularity of the uterus and its content with contour defects within or at the margins of opacified intervillous spaces. Chorioadenoma destruens is an invasive mole. Choriocarcinoma is an aggressive, purely epithelial neoplasm without villi which tends to invade the uterine muscle. Like any other malignant vascular tumor, abnormal neoplastic vessels and arteriovenous shunting are the frequent angiographic findings. From the angiographic point of view, however, it is not easy to differentiate choriocarcinoma from chorioadenomadestruens.[1421] Angiography is helpful to localize the primary lesion as well as secondary deposits of choriocarcinoma in the pelvis. Arteriographic regression of the disease during follow-up studies does not indicate clinical regression.[1422–1425]

Placenta Previa

The well-known placenta previa and its clinical manifestations probably do not need any

(Text continues on page 789)

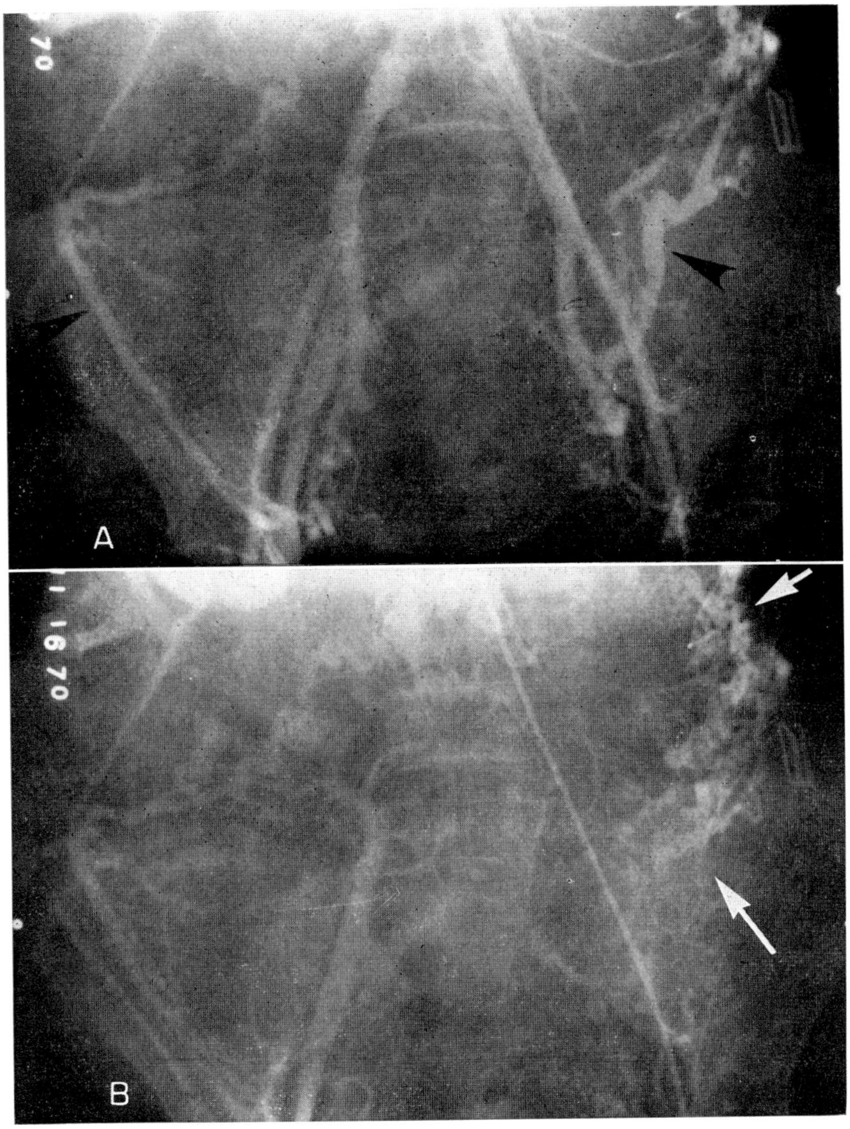

Figure 37.1. Pelvic Arteriogram. (A) Arterial phase: Note the very prominent uterine arteries. (B) Abnormal collections of contrast material representing the placental sinusoids (Arrows) can be seen. *Comment:* Normal location of placenta.

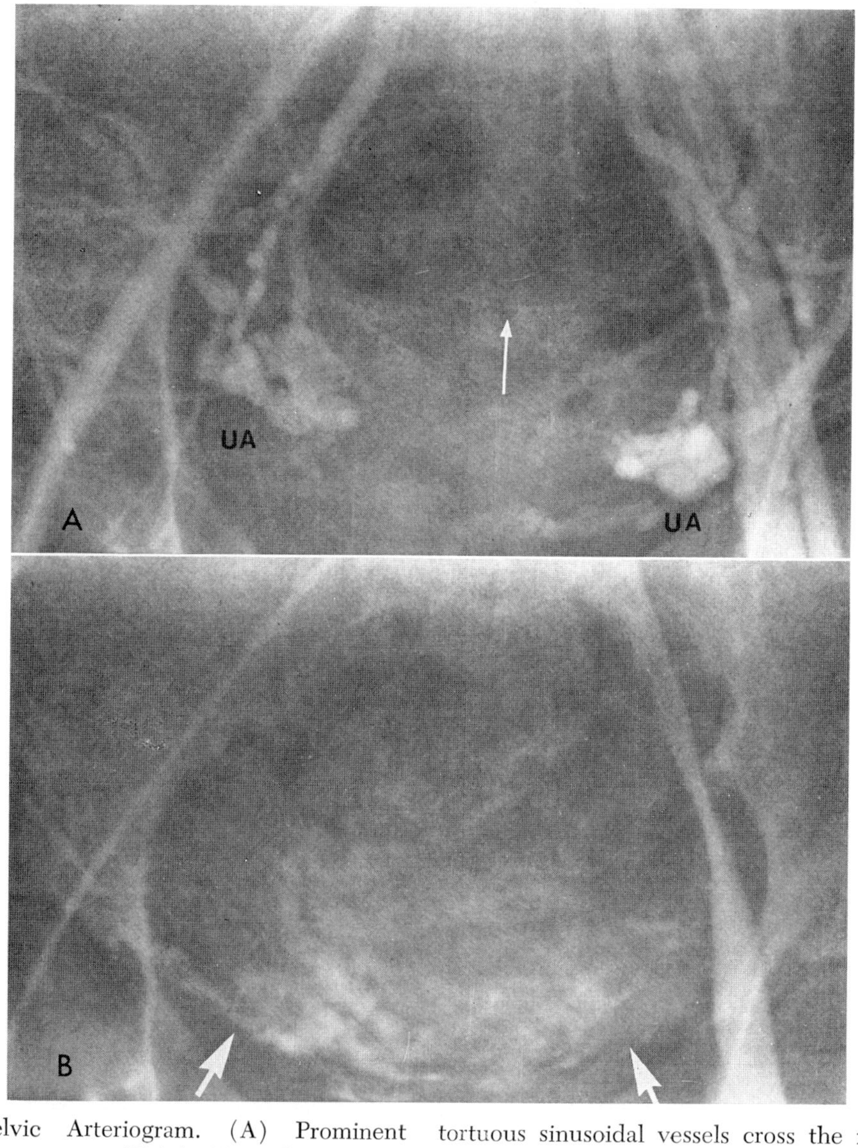

Figure 37.2. Pelvic Arteriogram. (A) Prominent uterine arteries are present (U.A.). Note the position of the fetal skull (Arrow). (B) Venous phase: Very tortuous sinusoidal vessels cross the midline (Arrow). *Diagnosis:* Placenta previa.

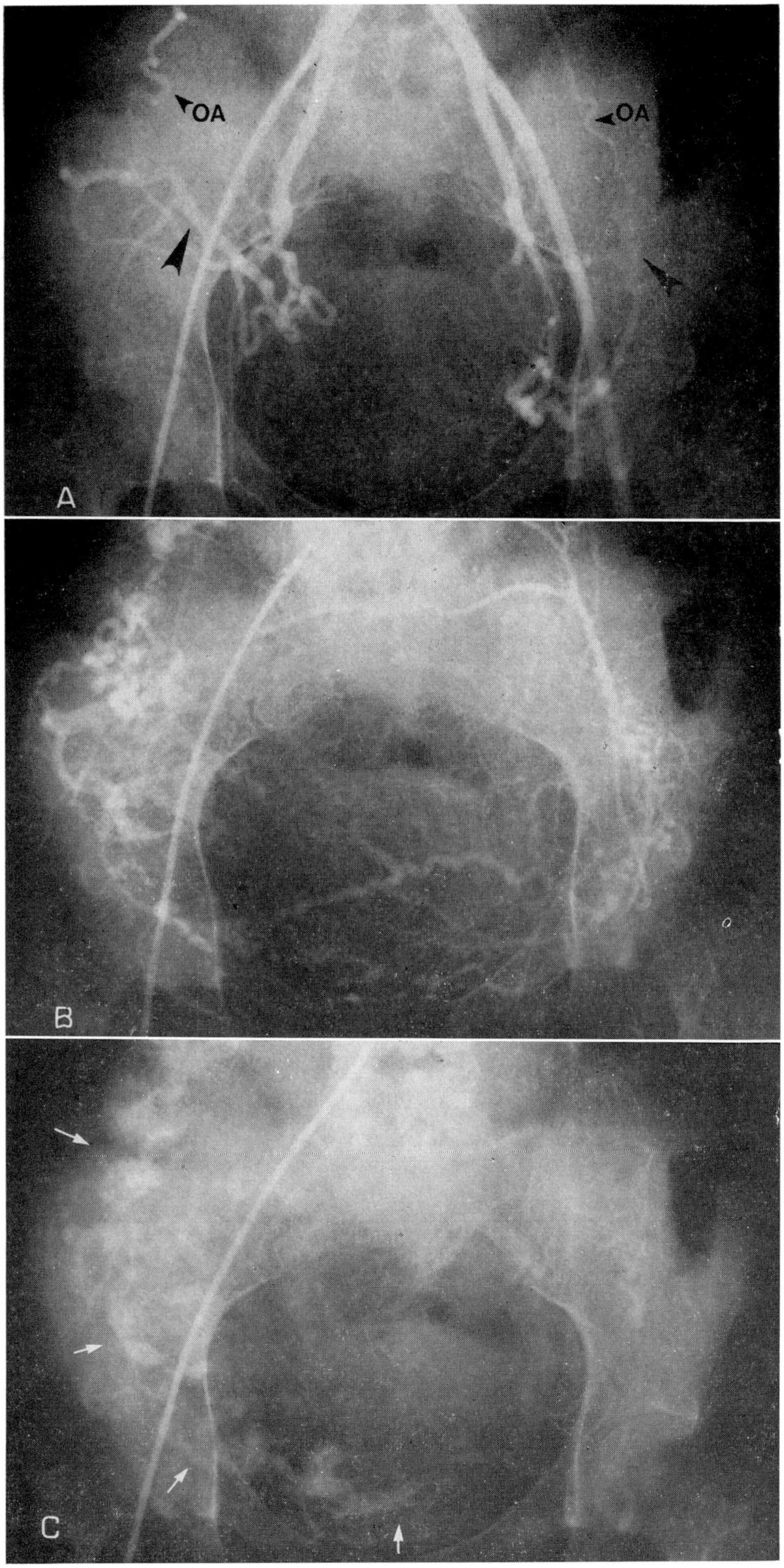

Figure 37.3. Pelvis Arteriogram. (A) Prominent uterine branches. (B) Very tortuous dilated right ovarian artery localized to the right side (O.A.). (C) Venous phase: Amorphous collections of contrast material are in the placental sinusoids and just crossing the midline. *Diagnosis:* Partial placenta previa.

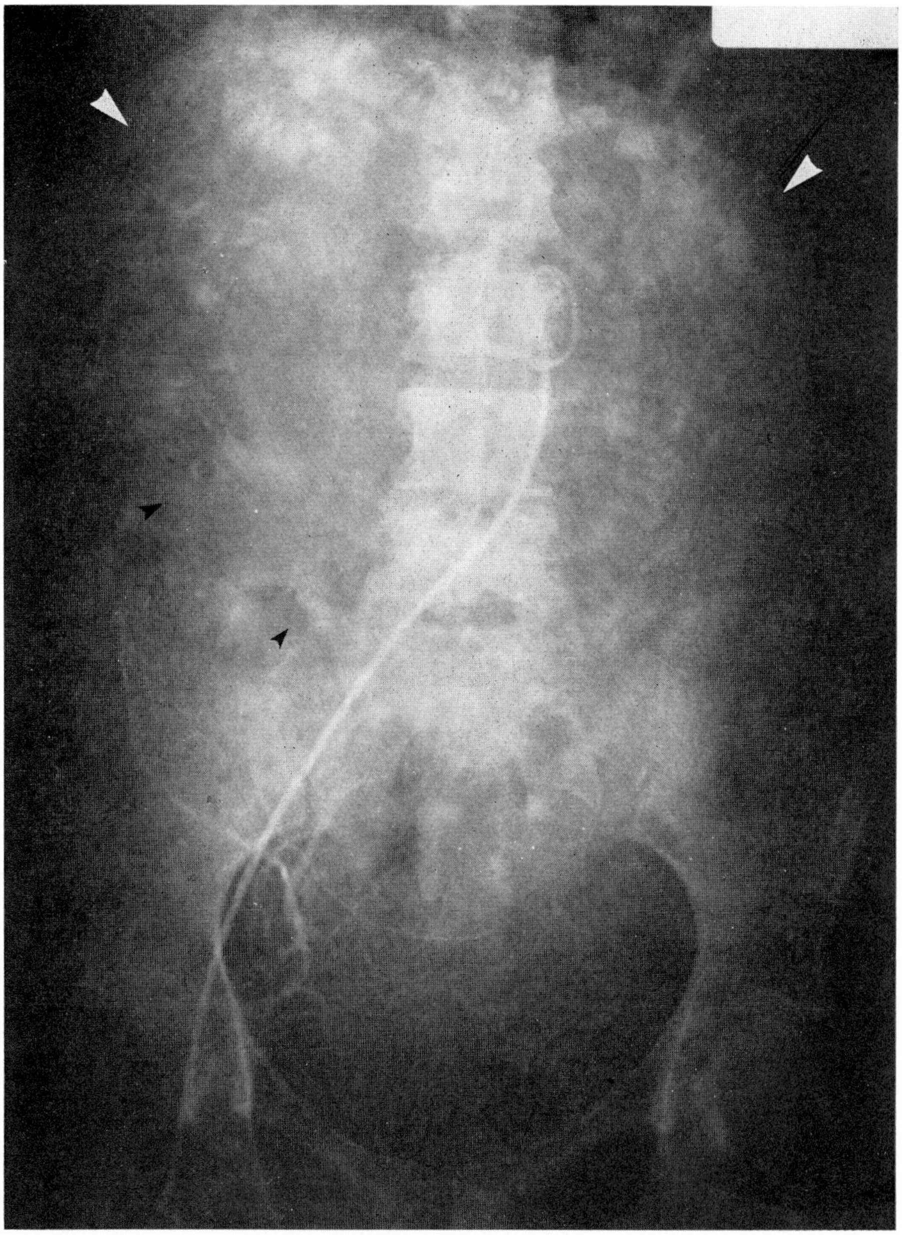

Figure 37.4. Arterial Placentogram. The bulk of the placenta is in the fundus of the uterus (White Arrow Heads) and does not have a defined margin. Opacified placental cotyledons are present throughout the uterine outline (Black Arrow Heads). *Diagnosis:* Placenta membranacea. (From Culp, W. C., Bryan, R. M., and Morettin, L. B. Placenta membranacea. *Radiol, 108:* 309, 1973. Courtesy of the authors and publishers.)

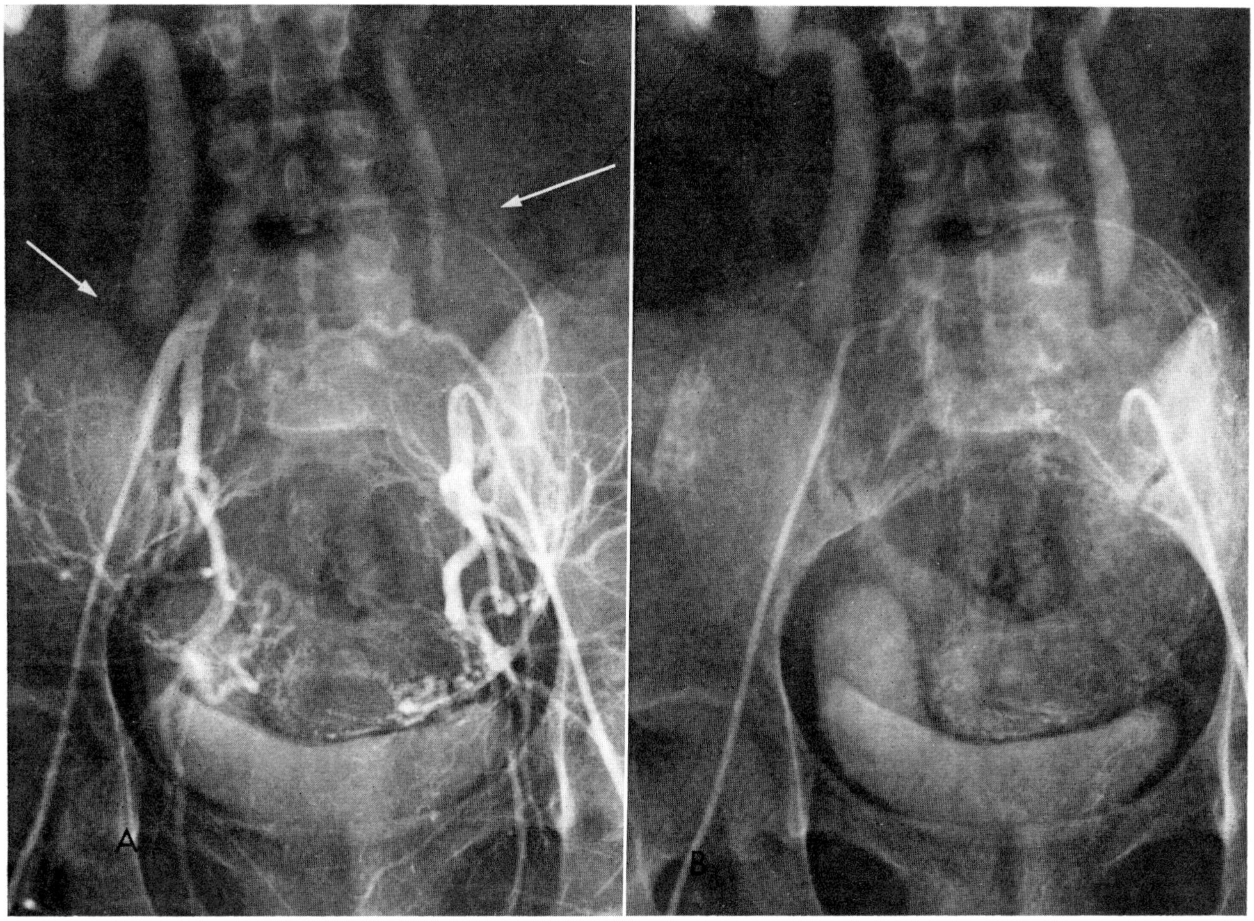

Figure 37.5. Bilateral Internal Iliac Arteriograms. Prominent uterine artery and myometrial branches. Two vessels course around a mass (Arrow). Late arterial phase: A moderately sized mass with marginal hypervascularity and filling defects is seen. This patient had marked increased chorionic gonadotrophins. *Diagnosis:* Hydatidiform mole.

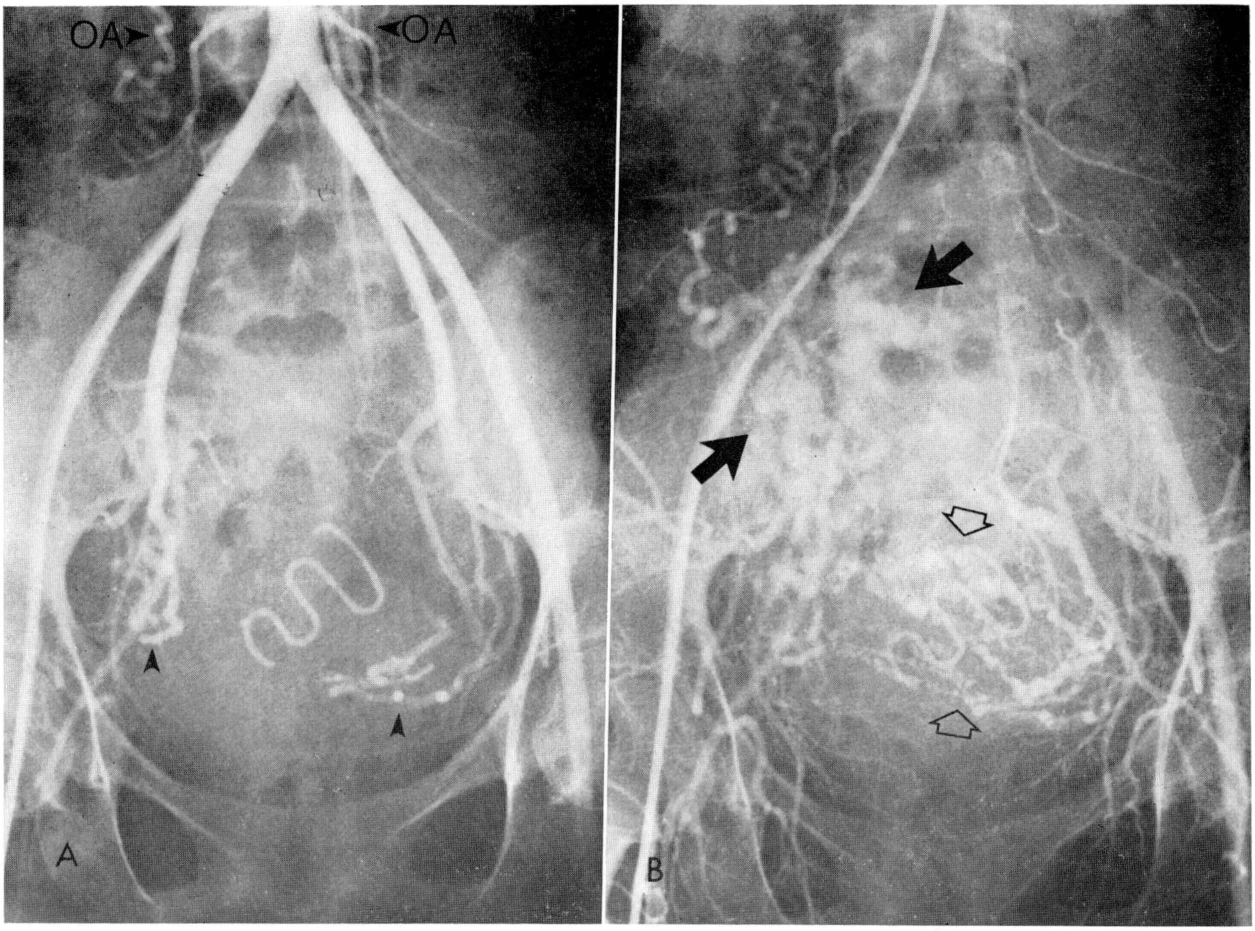

Figure 37.6. Pelvic Arteriogram. (A) Arterial phase: Prominent uterine arteries (Arrow) prominent right ovarian artery (O.A.) and normal sized left ovarian artery (O.A.). (B) Late arterial phase: Very dilated tortuous placental vessels in the right lower quadrant are supplied by the uterine artery (Arrow) as well as the hypertrophied right ovarian artery (O.A.). Myometrial branches are in the true pelvis (Arrow Head). This patient was thirty-four weeks pregnant. *Diagnosis:* Ectopic pregnancy. The ectopically located placenta is supplied by the hypertrophied right ovarian as well as the right uterine artery with a slightly enlarged uterus. The myometrial branches are confined to the true pelvis and the asymmetrical hypertrophy of the right ovarian artery and the location of the placental sinusoids beyond the confines of the uterus gives clues to the diagnosis. Incidentally, notice the intrauterine contraceptive device.

verbal description at this point. In the early part of pregnancy the placenta may lie in a low position and then change its position in a later part of pregnancy.[1432]

Placenta Membranacea

This is suspected when placenta previa is considered clinically and when ultra-sound and isotope studies do not contribute to the diagnosis. Then an angiogram will reveal a placenta without clearly defined boundaries but appearing to envelop the fetus. Placental cotyledons are seen all over the uterus. Thus the clinically suspected diagnosis is angiographically confirmed.[1426]

CONGENITAL ANOMALIES

Accessory Spleens

Ten percent of the population have from one to six accessory spleens[1459, 1460] ranging in size from 0.2 cm to 6.0 cm. The majority of these accessory spleens are located at the splenic hilus, and the rest are found at the tail of the pancreas, greater omentum, mesentery, adenexa, and in the scrotum.[1461] These accessory spleens may or may not be involved by diseases such as lymphoma, metastasis, etc. They may hypertrophy if left behind following splenectomy. Accessory spleens may be supplied by the inferior pancreatico-duodenal artery or the splenic artery, if found in the hilus of the spleen, and drain into the portal vein. They may be supplied by the inferior adrenal artery if they are in a perirenal position, or by the lumbar, inferior phrenic, or splenic arteries if they are retroperitoneal.[1462, 1463] In atypical locations Tc^{99m} sulphur colloid scan may aid in demonstrating them.[1462] They are obviously demonstrated because of their diffuse homogeneous stain, and on occasion may be mistaken for adrenal or pancreatic islet cell adenomas. Splenosis[1464] is an interesting entity caused by autotransplantation of splenic tissue which may possibly occur after injury to the spleen. The implants of the shattered spleen may develop anywhere, including the chest.

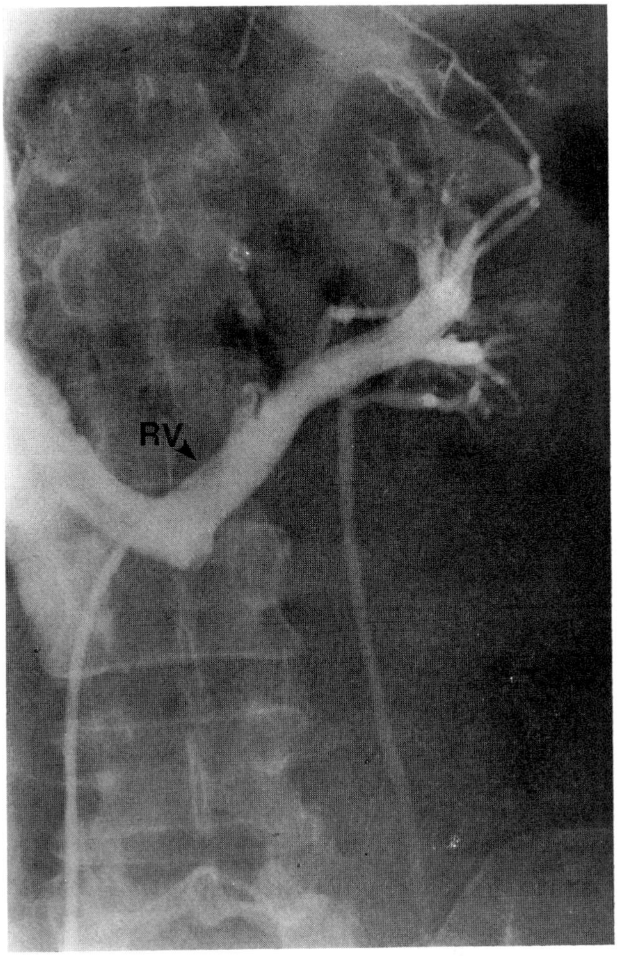

Figure 37.7. Left Renal Venogram. The course of the left renal vein is abnormal with abrupt angulation (R.V.). *Diagnosis:* Persistent right and left supracardinal veins (double inferior vena cava). This is a very unusual variation. The left inferior vena cava receives the left renal vein and drains cephalad to join the right inferior vena cava via the iliac anastomosis. (That we did not do the left common iliac venogram for confirmation is obvious—because we did not know that there was an entity like this.)

Accessory Lobe of the Liver

Accessory lobes of the liver[1464] may be intrathoracic[1465] or near the gallbladder[1466] and supplied by the hepatic artery. Riedel's lobe of the liver is usually well demonstrated by a vascular pedicle. If it is totally fibrotic it may mimic an avascular mass.[1467]

Anomalies of the Inferior Vena Cava

The hepatic, prerenal and postrenal segments

(Text continues on page 795)

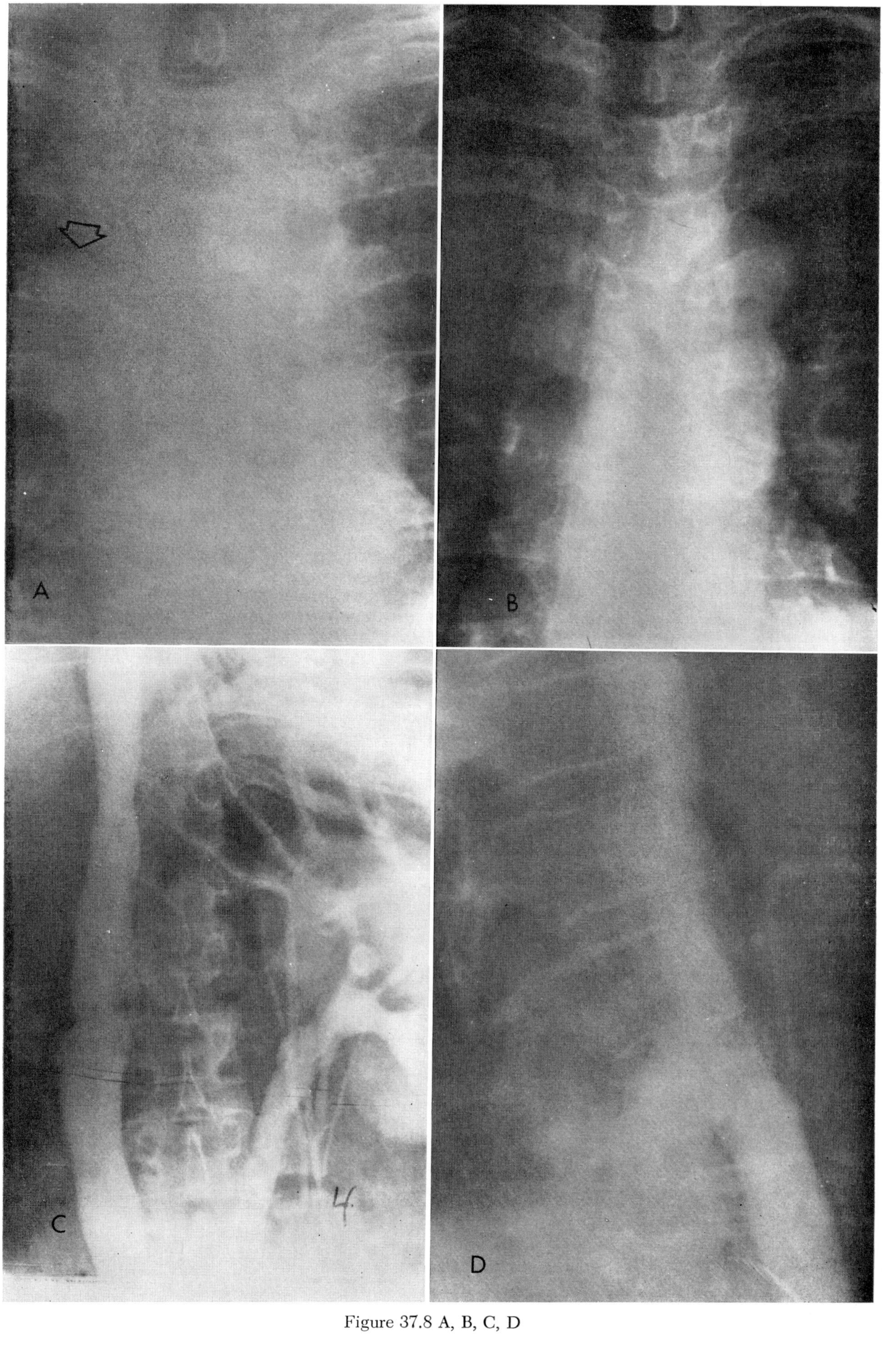

Figure 37.8 A, B, C, D

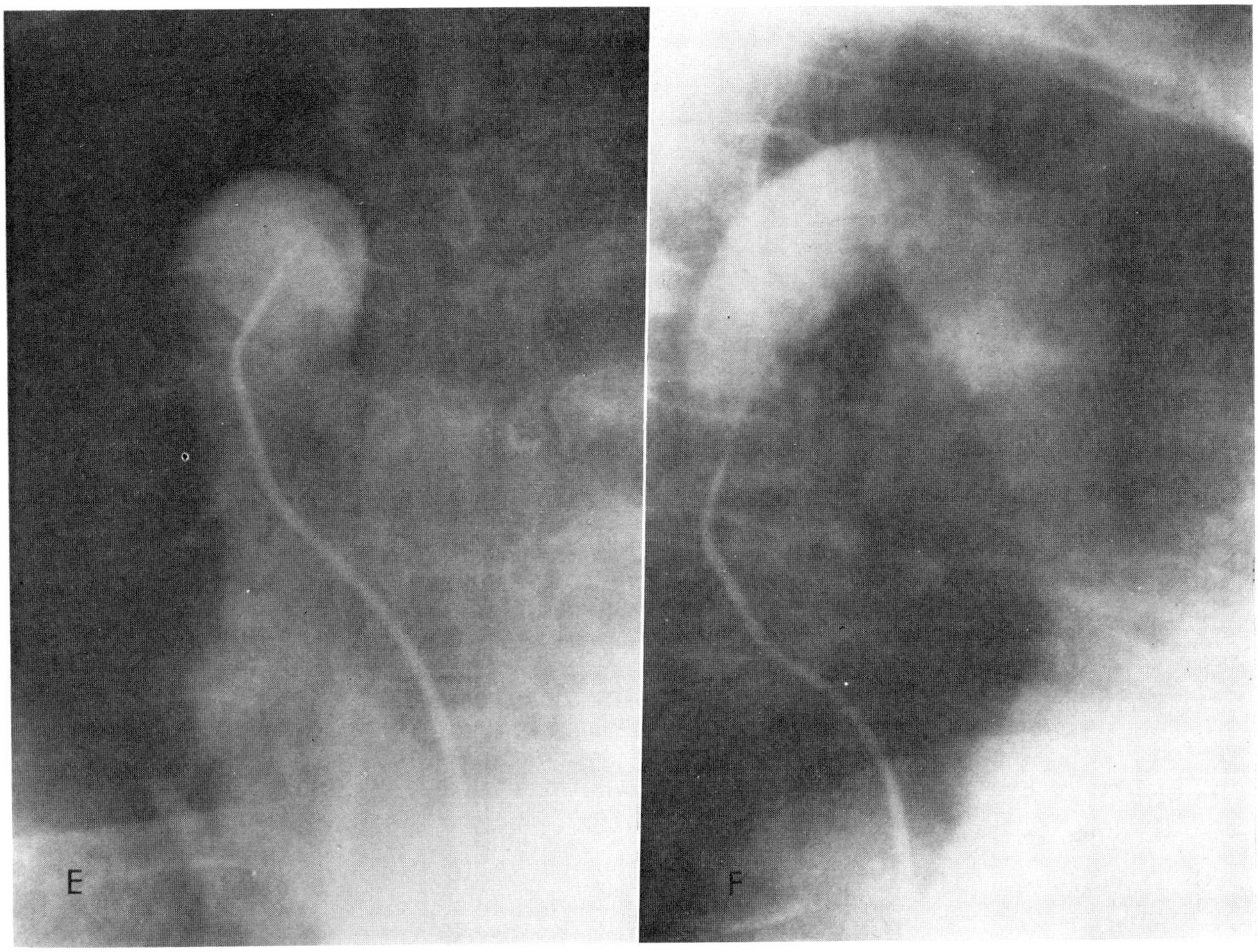

Figure 37.8. (A) A soft tissue mass is in the right tracheobronchial angle. (B) During a Valsalva maneuver the mass has disappeared suggesting that this is a compressible mass such as a vascular structure. (C) A.P.—inferior vena cavagram: The opacified venous structure continues beyond the right atrial level. (D) A lateral projection of the same. (E) Frontal projection: A huge azygous vein is opacified. (F) Lateral projection: A catheter was passed via the same vein into the azygous vein. *Diagnosis:* Hepatic interruption of the inferior vena cava, with azygous continuation.

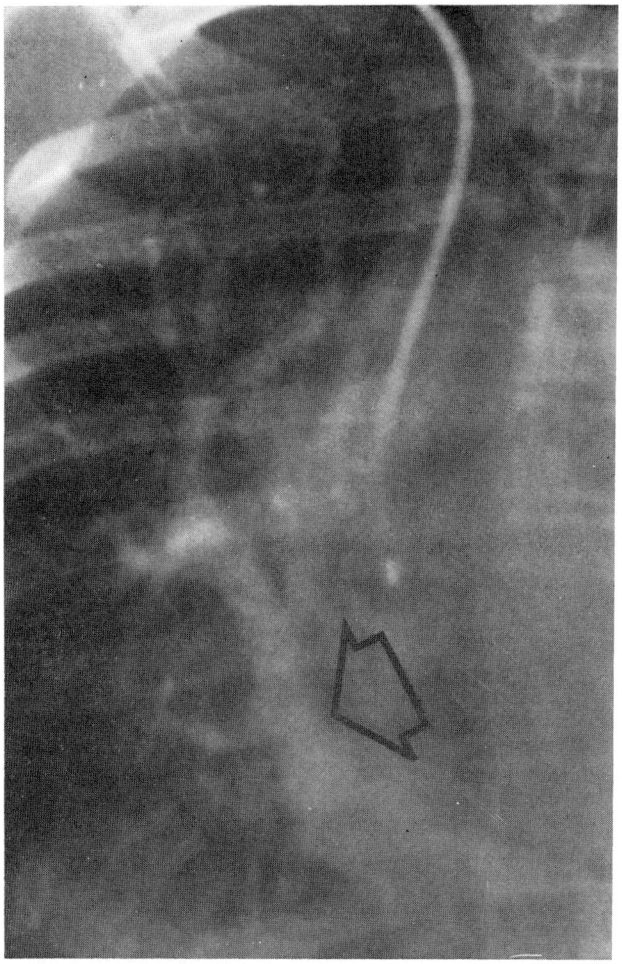

Figure 37.9. Basilic Vein Catheterization. The catheter tip is in the superior vena cava—pulmonary venous phase. Opacification of a venous channel with an abnormal course towards the junction of the inferior vena cava and the right atrium is seen. *Diagnosis:* Partial anomalous venous drainage of the right lung (Arrow). Scimitar syndrome.

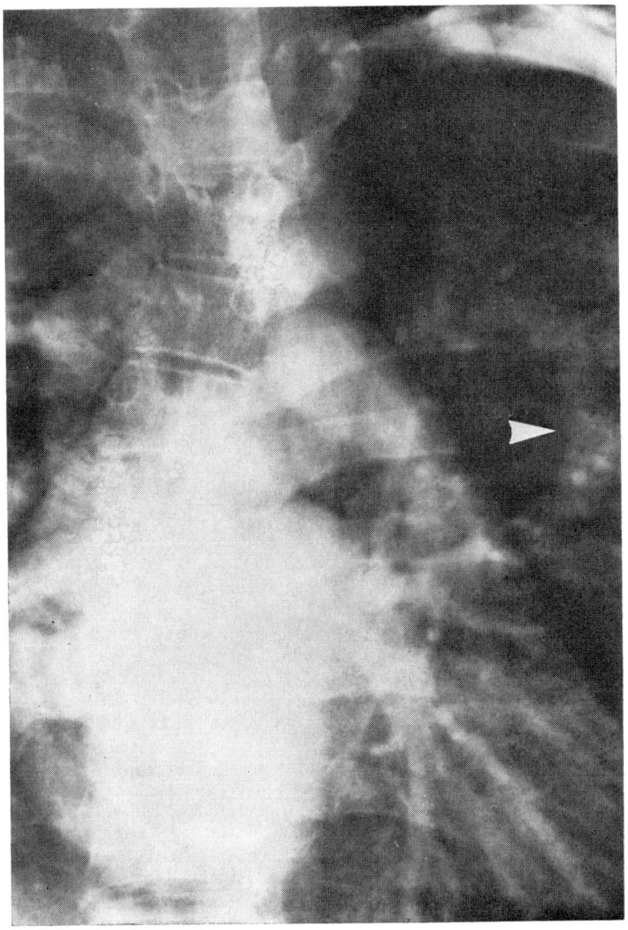

Figure 37.10. Intravenous Angiocardiogram. The pulmonary venous phase reveals an abnormal vein coursing towards the left atrium (Arrow). *Comment:* Note anomalous course of a segmental pulmonary vein into the left atrium.

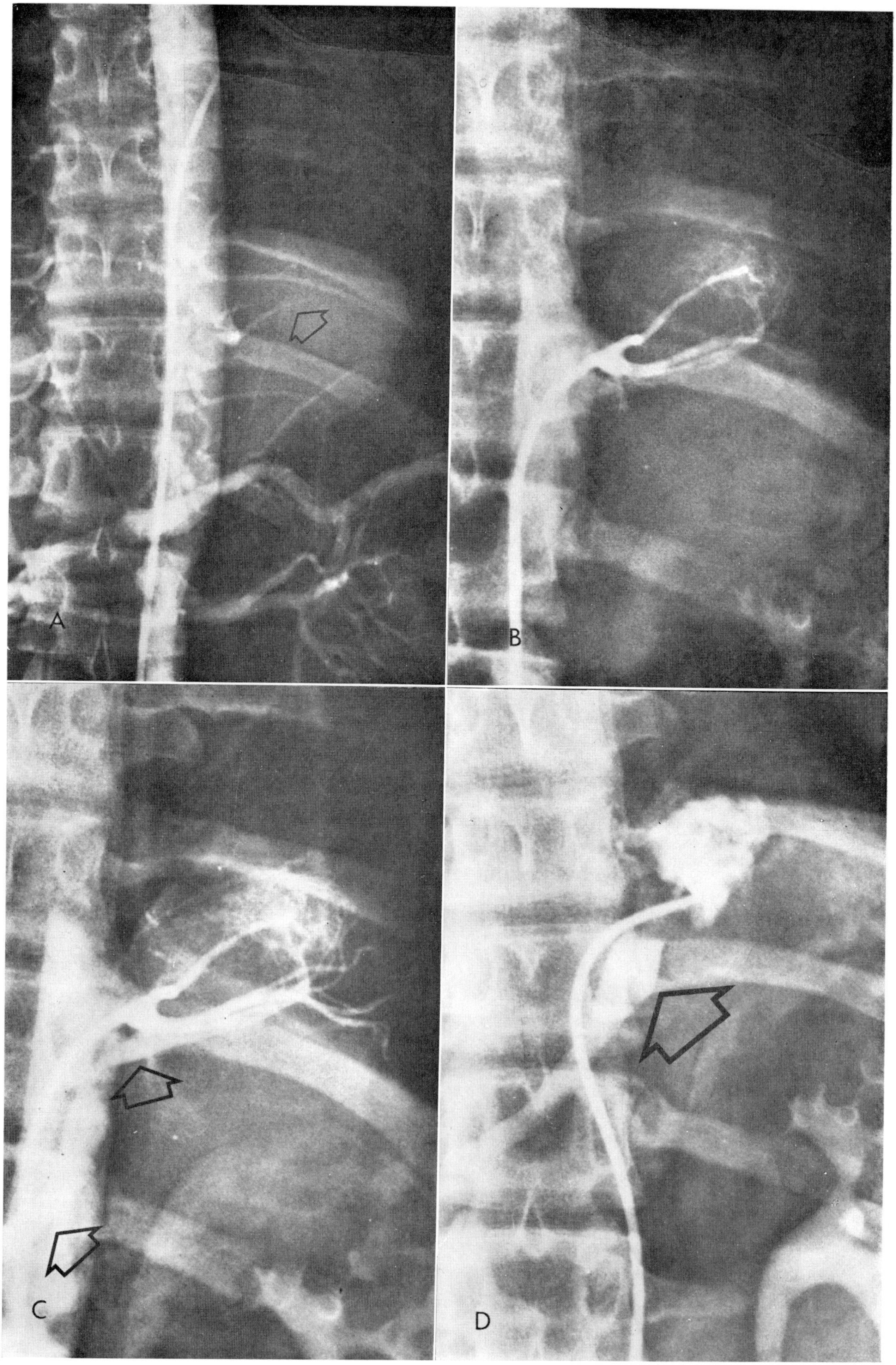
A
B
C
D

of the inferior vena cava have different embryological origins.[1468, 1469] The posterior cardinal veins are related to the development of the hepatic veins and inferior vena cava, while the renal veins develop from the subcardinal veins. *The complicated interplay between new growth and atrophy provides ample scope for numerous and various types of malformations.*[1470] Since the frequency of catheterization of renal veins has increased, more embryological anomalies of the inferior vena cava and renal veins have been explored angiographically.[1480] Some of the more common anomalies include double inferior vena cavae, circumaortic renal veins, and retroaortic single left renal vein.

Hepatic Interruption of the Inferior Vena Cava with Azygos Continuation

The lack of formation of effluent veins from the liver, necessary to the development of that portion of the inferior vena cava, forces the blood through the azygos vein.[1471] Sometimes this entity may be suspected on a P-A and lateral chest film. A prominent azygos venous shadow is seen in the P-A projection, while on the lateral projection the inferior vena caval shadow[1472] is absent. This anomaly may or may not be associated with abnormal positions of the heart and abdominal viscera[1473] or polysplenia.[1474] Ligation of such a vein which is draining the lower part of the body may result in death of the patient.[1475]

Anomalous Venous Drainage of the Right Lung to the Inferior Vena Cava

This abnormal pulmonary vein which receives blood from all or most of the existing lobes of the right lung descends parallel to the right heart border to join the inferior vena cava. It gives a characteristic shadow known as the "scimitar sign." It may be associated with some pulmonary abnormalities, congenital heart disease, or diaphragmatic defects.[1476, 1477]

Left-sided Vena Cava

In this situation there is usually an inferior vena cava on the right side as well.[1478] There may be associated malposition of the abdominal viscera and congenital heart disease. The left-sided vena cava usually drains into the right atrium through the coronary sinus.

THE PLASTIC KNIFE AND AVASCULAR SURGERY

The practical and potential powers of the plastic tube have been revealed through control of acute hemorrhage, transluminal angioplasty, and clot lysis with streptokinase, occlusive therapies using ferro-magnetic silicone, Gelfoam®, clots, and electro-coagulation; ablation of such organs as the adrenal glands and spleen, and last but not least, vascular endoscopy.[12, 13, 1490–1498]

You've come a long way . . . baby!

←

Figure 37.11. Thoracic and Abdominal Aortic Angiogram. (A) There are two unusual branches arising from the thoracic aorta (Blank Arrow). (B) Selective catheterization reveals a cluster of vessels supplying a mass-like density. (C) The midarterial phase demonstrates numerous small vessels supplying this density with opacification of a vein following an abnormal course (Blank Arrow). (D) The vein is better seen in its course towards the portal vein. This young boy had repeated left lower lobe infiltrates and infections. *Diagnosis:* Pulmonary sequestration with a systemic arterial supply and venous drainage into the portal system.

BIBLIOGRAPHY

BIBLIOGRAPHY

1. Forsmann, W.: *Klinwchnchr, 8:*2085, 1929.
2. Farinas, P. L.: *Am J Roentgenol Radium Ther Nucl Med, 46:*641, 1941.
3. Peirce, C. C., II: *Surg Gynecol Obstet, 93:*56, 1956.
4. Seldinger, S. I.: *Acta Radiol Diagn (Stockh), 39:*368, 1953.
5. Odman, P.: *Acta Radiol Diagn (Stockh), 45:*1, 1956.
6. Odman, P.: *Acta Radiol Diagn (Stockh), 45:* 117, 1956.
7. duPont, E. I., deNemours & Co., Inc.
8. Redman, H. C., et al.: *Invest Radiol, 4:*24, 1969.
9. Abrams, H. L.: *Radiology, 82:*217, 1964.
10. Olin, T. B., et al.: *Radiology, 85:*1036, 1965.
11. Viamonte, M., Jr., et al.: *Radiol Clin North Am, 8:*147, 1970.
12. Dotter, C. T., et al.: *Radiology, 84:*631, 1965.
13. Baum, S., et al.: *Surgery, 58:*797, 1965.
14. Hanafee, W., et al.: *Radiology, 88:*35, 1967.
15. Doppman, J. L., et al.: *Radiology, 95:*603, 1970.
16. Eisenberg, H., et al.: *Am J Med, 56:*810, 1974.
17. Hinck, V. C., et al.: *Radiology, 97:*688, 1970.
18. Meaney, T. F., et al.: *Radiology, 87:*309, 1966.
19. Friedlander, W. J.: In Eckert, C. (Ed.): *Emergency Room Care,* 2nd ed. Boston, Little, 1971.
20. Caldicott, W. J. H.: *Invest Radiol, 5:*539, 1970.
21. Effler, D. B., et al.: *JAMA, 146:*1321, 1951.
22. Montalbano, F. P., et al.: *JAMA, 182:*264, 1962.
23. Schecter, M. M.: *Acta Radiol Diagn (Stockh), 5:*488, 1966.
24. Nusbaum, M., et al.: *Arch Surg, 97:*1005, 1968.
25. Doppman, J.: Editorial. *Invest Radiol, 8:*425, 1973.
26. Baltaxe, H. A., et al.: *Am J Roentgenol Radium Ther Nucl Med, 119:*793, 1973.
27. Zelch, J. V.: *Radiology, 111:*279, 1974.
28. Gold, R. E., et al.: *Radiology, 102:*579, 1972.
29. Ernst, C. B., et al.: *Arch Surg, 104:*496, 1972.
30. Vaughn, E. D., Jr., et al.: *Am J Med, 55:*402, 1973.
31. Voneuler, U. S., et al.: *Circulation, 15:*5, 1957.
32. Robertson, P. W., et al.: *Am J Med, 43:*963, 1967.
33. Helmer, O. M., et al.: *Can Med Assoc J, 90:* 221, 1964.
34. O'Neal, L. W., et al.: *Cancer, 21:*1219, 1968.
35. USCI: United States Catheter and Instrument Corporation, Glens Falls, New York.
36. Beckton-Dickenson (B-D), Rutherford, New Jersey.
37. Cook Incorporated, Bloomington, Indiana.
38. Squibb, E. R., and Sons.
39. Picker XRay Corporation.
40. Nebesar, R. A., et al.: *Am J Roentgenol Radium Ther Nucl Med, 97:*508, 1966.
41. Rossi, P., et al.: *Am J Roentgenol Radium Ther Nucl Med, 97:*511, 1966.
42. Judkins, M. P., et al.: *Radiology, 88:*1127, 1967.
43. Amplatz, K.: *Invest Radiol, 6:*280, 1971.
44. Cramer, R.: *Radiology, 109:*585, 1973.
45. Cordis Corporation, Miami, Florida.
46. Susman, N., et al.: *Radiology, 92:*843, 1969.
47. Bove, A., et al.: *Invest Radiol, 3:*159, 1968.
48. Desilets, D. T., et al.: *Radiology, 85:*147, 1965.
49. Mannila, T. O., et al.: *Invest Radiol, 2:*176, 1967.
50. Brodey, A., et al.: *Radiology, 110:*711, 1974.
51. Odman, P.: *Acta Radiol Diagn (Stockh), 52:* 51, 1959.
52. Guyton, A. C.: *Textbook of Medical Physiology,* 3rd ed. Philadelphia, Saunders.
53. Komar, N., et al.: *Radiology, 90:*981, 1968.
54. Viamonte, M., Jr., et al.: *Invest Radiol, 2:*262, 1967.
55. Viamonte, Hobbs Injector Barber-Colman Electro-Mechanical Products, Rockford, Illinois.
56. Amplatz, K.: In Abrams, H. L. (Ed.): *Angiography,* 2nd ed. Philadelphia, Lippincott, 1971, vol. I.
57. Baum, S., et al.: *Am J Surg, 117:*170, 1969.
58. Bookstein, J. J., et al.: *Radiology, 98:*23, 1971.
59. Goodman, L. S., and Gilman, A.: *The Pharmacological Basis of Therapeutics,* 4th ed. New York, Macmillan, 1970.
60. Meditech, 372 Main Street, Watertown, Massachusetts.
61. Electro Catheter Corporation, Rahway, New Jersey.
62. Hilal, S. K.: *Invest Radiol, 5:*458, 1970.
63. Ansell, G.: *Invest Radiol, 5:*374, 1970.
64. Cattell, W. R.: *Invest Radiol, 5:*473, 1970.
65. Hansson, R., et al.: *Acta Med Scand, 174:*611, 1963.
66. Kaufman, H. J., et al.: *Ann Radiol (Paris), 9:* 311, 1966.

67. Davidson, A. J., et al.: *Radiology, 96:*249, 1970.
68. Stage, P., et al.: *Acta Radiol Diagn (Stockh), 11:*337, 1971.
69. Becker, J. A., et al.: *Radiology, 93:*1301, 1969.
70. Becker, J. A., et al.: *Radiology, 107:*37, 1973.
71. Editorial. *Pharmaco/Angiography Radiology, 91:* 583, 1968.
72. Melville, K. I., et al.: In Abramson, D. I. (Ed.): *Blood Vessels and Lymphatics.* New York, Acad Pr, 1962.
73. Abrams, H. L., et al.: *Radiology, 79:*911, 1962.
74. Kahn, P. C., et al.: *Radiology, 85:*301, 1965.
75. Abrams, H. L.: *Curr Probl Radiol, 1:*1, 1971.
76. Redman, H. C., et al.: *Invest Radiol, 1:*458, 1966.
77. Olin, T. B., et al.: *Radiology, 85:*1036, 1965.
78. Bookstein, J. J.: *Radiology, 108:*55, 1973.
79. Doppman, J. L., et al.: *Radiology, 93:*57, 1969.
80. Bierman, H. R., et al.: *J Natl Can Inst, 12:*107, 1951.
81. Natadze, T. G.: *Probl Oncol, 5:*14, 1959.
82. Abram, H. L.: *Nature, 201:*167, 1964.
83. Viamonte, M., Jr., et al.: *Radiology, 106:*59, 1973.
84. Palmisano, P. J.: *Radiology, 88:*249, 1967.
85. Day, E. G.: *Prog Exp Tumor Res, 4:*57, 1964.
86. Castellino, R. A.: *Radiology, 97:*607, 1970.
87. Rockoff, S. D., et al.: *Invest Radiol, 1:*205, 1966.
88. Shield, P. N.: *Radiology, 95:*657, 1970.
89. Lecky, J. W.: *Selective Angiography, Section 18, Golden's Diagnostic Radiology.* Baltimore, Williams & Wilkins, 1972.
90. Ross, L. S.: *Am J Roentgenol Radium Ther Nucl Med, 112:*600, 1971.
91. Kahn, P. C., et al.: *Radiology, 89:*1062, 1967.
92. Caro, G., et al.: *Radiology, 92:*1262, 1969.
93. Kahn, P. C., et al.: *J Urol, 99:*133, 1968.
94. Billings, L.: *Acta Radiol (Stockh), 25:*625, 1944.
95. Silbiger, M. L., et al.: *J Urol, 106:*363, 1971.
96. Klapproth, H. J., et al.: *Arch Pathol, 67:*400, 1959.
97. Clark, R. E., et al.: *Am J Roentgenol Radium Ther Nucl Med, 114:*715, 1972.
98. Cremin, B. J., et al.: *Br J Roentgenol, 45:*415, 1972.
99. Stein, H. L.: *Radiology, 93:*367, 1969.
100. Boijsen, E., et al.: *Invest Radiol, 2:*184, 1967.
101. Coffman, J. D.: *Circulation (Suppl), 3:*62, 1964.
102. Baum, S., et al.: *Radiology, 98:*497, 1971.
103. Conn, H. O., et al.: *Am J Roentgenol Radium Ther Nucl Med, 119:*102, 1973.
104. Frolich, E. D., et al.: *Clin Res, 11:*183, 1963.
105. Nusbaum, M., et al.: *Surgery, 62:*299, 1967.
106. Siegelman, S. S., et al.: *Invest Radiol, 6:*340, 1971.
107. Carlsson, B., et al.: *Am J Roentgenol Radium Ther Nucl Med, 109:*161, 1970.
108. Baum, S., et al.: *Advances in Surgery.* Chicago, Yearbk Med, 1973, vol. VII.
109. Mortray, G. J., et al.: *Ann Surg, 178:*648, 1973.
110. Renert, W. A., et al.: *Radiology, 102:*299, 1972.
111. Robbins, S. L.: *Pathologic Basis of Disease.* Philadelphia, Saunders, 1974.
112. Ekelund, L., et al.: *Radiology, 110:*533, 1974.
113. Kaplan, J. H., et al.: *Radiology, 105:*33, 1972.
114. Redman, H. C., et al.: *Invest Radiol, 4:*24, 1969.
115. Jacobs, J. B., et al.: *Radiology, 88:*957, 1967.
116. Hawkins, I. F., Jr.: *Radiology, 110:*541, 1974.
117. Bron, K. M., et al.: *Radiology, 99:*295, 1971.
118. Widrich, W. C., et al.: *Am J Roentgenol Radium Ther Nucl Med, 121:*374, 1974.
119. Merrill, S. L., et al.: *Fed Proc, 21:*200, 1962.
120. Darle, N., et al.: *Acta Chir Scand, 140:*217, 1974.
121. Danford, R. O.: *Am J Roentgenol Radium Ther Nucl Med, 108:*665, 1970.
122. Redman, H. C.: *Invest Radiol, 9:*199, 1974.
123. Danford, R. O., et al.: *Radiology, 93:*173, 1969.
124. Tibbin, S., et al.: *Arch Surg, 100:*84, 1970.
125. Harvey, R. B., et al.: *Fed Proc, 26:*437, 1967.
126. Murphy, G. A., et al.: *J Surg Res, 5:*525, 1965.
127. Harvey, R. B.: *Am J Phys, 211:*487, 1966.
128. Hollenberg: In Hilal, S. K. (Ed.): *Small Vessel Angiography.* St. Louis, Mosby, 1973.
129. Freed, T. A.: *Am J Roentgenol Radium Ther Nucl Med, 104:*312, 1968.
130. Swift, M. R., et al.: *Lancet, 1:*513, 1966.
131. Dollery, C. T., et al.: *Clin Sci, 29:*433, 1965.
132. Siegelman, S. S., et al.: *Radiology, 112:*533, 1974.
133. Uden, R.: *Acta Radiol Diagn (Stockh), 12:*363, 1962.
134. Eisenberg, H.: In Hilal, S. K. (Ed.): *Small Vessel Angiography.* St. Louis, Mosby, 1973.
135. Menguy, R.: *Am J Dig Dis, 7:*383, 1962.
136. Taylor, D. A., et al.: *Radiology, 84:*351, 1965.
137. Taylor, D. A., et al.: *Radiology, 86:*707, 1966.
138. Finck, E. J., et al.: *Radiology, 101:*79, 1971.
139. Lunderquist, A., et al.: *Am J Roentgenol Radium Ther Nucl Med, 107:*191, 1969.
140. Ferrer, I. M., et al.: *Circulation, 32:*524, 1965.
141. Shanbour, L. L., et al.: *Am J Dig Dis, 17:*826, 1972.
142. Nichols, J.: In Bloodworth, J. M. B., Jr. (Ed.): *Endocrinic Pathology.* Baltimore, Williams & Wilkins, 1968.
143. Dean, R. E., et al.: *JAMA, 187:*27, 1964.
144. Knisley, M. H., et al.: *Science, 106:*431, 1947.
145. Read, R. C., et al.: *Circ Res, 8:*538, 1960.
146. Almen, T., et al.: *Invest Radiol, 4:*63, 1969.
147. O'Connor, J. F., et al.: *Radiology, 89:*20, 1967.

148. Harrington, G. J., et al.: *Radiology, 84:*1108, 1965.
149. Bjork, L.: *Acta Radiol Diagn (Stockh), 6:*459, 1967.
150. Meyer, M. W., et al.: *Radiology, 82:*630, 1964.
151. Hilal, S. K.: In Hilal, S. K. (Ed.): *Small Vessel Angiography.* St. Louis, Mosby, 1973.
152. Garber, G. L., et al.: *Proc Soc Exp Biol Med, 107:*165, 1961.
153. Read, R. C.: *J Thorac Cardiovasc Surg, 38:*685, 1969.
154. Hilal, S. K.: *Radiology, 86:*615, 1966.
155. Fischer, H. W.: *Radiology, 91:*66, 1968.
156. Foda, M. J., et al.: *Am J Med Sci, 250:*390, 1965.
157. Bernstein, E. F.: *Radiology, 84:*670, 1965.
158. Lasser, E. C., et al.: *Invest Radiol, 1:*237, 1966.
159. Lasser, E. C.: *Invest Radiol,* 5(no. 6): , 1970.
160. Kormano, M., et al.: *Invest Radiol, 8:*68, 1973.
161. Barnhard, H. J.: *Radiol Clin North Am, 3:*51, 1965.
162. Siegelman, S. S., et al.: *Radiology, 96:*101, 1970.
163. Lin, J. P., et al.: *Radiology, 83:*640, 1964.
164. Fischer, H. W.: *Radiology, 91:*66, 1968.
165. Roberts, P. N.: *Lancet, 1:*985, 1967.
166. Krovetz, L. J., et al.: *Am Heart J, 74:*453, 1967.
167. Gonzalez, L. L., et al.: *Radiology, 86:*1070, 1966.
168. Efsan, F., et al.: *Invest Radiol, 3:*6, 1968.
169. Rosenbaum, E. H., et al.: *Radiology, 86:*515, 1966.
170. Kutt, H., et al.: *J Lab Clin Med, 59:*118, 1962.
171. Talner, L. B., et al.: *Invest Radiol, 7:*311, 1972.
172. Davidson, A. J., et al.: *Radiology, 85:*1043, 1965.
173. Kirkland, J. A., et al.: *Lancet, 1:*693, 1961.
174. Cunningham, J. J., et al.: *Radiology, 111:*85, 1974.
175. Moss, A. A., et al.: *Radiology, 108:*279, 1973.
176. Redman, H. C., et al.: *Invest Radiol, 2:*123, 1967.
177. Sutherland, G. R., et al.: *Clin Radiol, 18:*200, 1967.
178. Cooley, R. N., et al.: *Angiology, 15:*107, 1964.
179. Goldstein, H. M., et al.: *Radiology, 111:*293, 1974.
180. Bonakdarpour, A., et al.: *Radiology, 108:*291, 1973.
181. Witten, D. M., et al.: *Am J Roentgenol Radium Ther Nucl Med, 119:*832, 1973.
182. Green, H. D.: In Glasser, O. (Ed.): *Medical Physics.* Chicago, Yearbk Med, 1944.
183. Mann, M. R.: *Proc R Soc Med, 54:*473, 1961.
184 Peacock, L. B., et al.: *Ann Surg, 15:*158, 1967.
185. Rockoff, S. D., et al.: *Invest Radiol, 7:*403, 1972.
186. Lasser, E. C., et al.: *Radiology, 110:*49, 1974.
187. Rushmer, R. F.: *Cardiovascular Dynamics,* 2nd ed. Philadelphia, Saunders,
188. Dichiro, G.: *Radiology, 112:*231, 1974.
189. Kardjiev, V., et al.: *Radiology, 112:*81, 1974.
190. Head, R. M., et al.: *Radiology, 102:*307, 1972.
191. Adams, D. F., et al.: *Radiology, 84:*678, 1965.
192. Takahashi, M., et al.: *Acta Radiol Diagn (Stockh), 25, 30:*494, 1967.
193. Howland, W. J., et al.: *Radiology, 83:*428, 1964.
194. Judkins, M. P., et al.: *Radiology, 83:*433, 1964.
195. Rhea, W. G., Jr., et al.: *Surgery, 55:*831, 1964.
196. Fiegelson, H. H., et al.: *Radiology, 85:*663, 1965.
197. Killen, D. A., et al.: *Surgery, 59:*969, 1966.
198. Brodey, P. A., et al.: *Radiology, 111:*711, 1964.
199. Kott, E., et al.: *Vasc Dis, 3:*398, 1966.
200. Berdon, W. E., et al.: *Radiology, 92:*714, 1969.
201. Cohen, L. S., et al.: *Radiology, 92:*329, 1969.
202. Spence, H. M., et al.: *Urol Survey, 22:*131, 1972.
203. Lonni, Y. G. W., et al.: *Radiology, 93:*63, 1969.
204. Kovnat, P. J., et al.: *Radiology, 108:*541, 1973.
205. Jacobsson, B., et al.: *Scand J Hematol, 6:*386, 1969.
206. Deykin, D.: *N Engl J Med, 276:*622, 1967.
207. Jacobsson, B.: *Acta Radiol Diagn (Stockh), 8:* 289, 1969.
208. Jacobsson, B.: *Acta Chir (Suppl), 387:*103, 1968.
209. Formanek, G., et al.: *Circulation, 41:*833, 1970.
210. Skouborg, F., et al.: *Lancet, 1:*129, 1966.
211. Meyer, G. A.: *Circulation (Suppl), 3:111:*21, 1964.
212. Burris, M. B., et al.: *Surg Clin North Am, 33:* 1023, 1953.
213. Gormsen, J.: *Acta Med Scand, 148:*61, 1954.
214. Eisenberg, G.: *Circulation, 30:*686, 1964.
215. Gore, I., et al.: *Arch Intern Med, 113:*323, 1964.
216. Pechet, L., et al.: *N Engl J Med, 265:*1093, 1961.
217. Behar, D.: *Invest Radiol, 5:*493, 1970.
218. Ashford, T. P., et al.: *Am J Phys, 50:*257, 1967.
219. Hoshal, V. L., Jr., et al.: *Arch Surg, 102:*353, 1971.
220. Fries, E. D., et al.: *Circulation, 28:*723, 1963.
221. Jacobsson, B., et al.: *Acta Radiol Diagn (Stockh), 8:*221, 1969.
222. McDonald, P.: *Am J Roentgenol Radium Ther Nucl Med, 112:*167, 1971.
223. Glancy, J. J., et al.: *Am J Roentgenol Radium Ther Nucl Med, 108:*716, 1970.
224. Morreels, C. L., Jr., et al.: *Radiology, 90:*1150, 1968.
225. Williams, H. J., et al.: *Am J Roentgenol Radium Ther Nucl Med, 116:*475, 1972.

226. Ritchie, W. G. M., et al.: *Invest Radiol, 8:*279, 1973.
227. Thomas, L.: *Br J Radiol, 43:*528, 1970.
228. Levine, H. S., et al.: *Radiology, 88:*253, 1967.
229. Schiantarelli, P., et al.: *Invest Radiol, 8:*199, 1973.
230. Gelin, L. E.: *Acta Chir Scand Suppl (Stockh),* 210: , 1956.
231. Bernstein, E. F., et al.: *Radiology, 76:*260, 1961.
232. Weidman, M. P.: *Am J Roentgenol Radium Ther Nucl Med, 92:*682, 1964.
233. Bygdeman, S.: *Acta Chir Scan Supp, 387:*44, 1967.
234. Reuter, S., et al.: *Radiology, 105:*573, 1972.
235. Bergentz, S. E., et al.: *Acta Chir Scand, 122:* 343, 1967.
236. Morgan, T. O., et al.: *Br Med J, 2:*737, 1966.
237. Bergeron, R. T., et al.: *Radiology, 98:*689, 1971.
238. Bove, A. A., et al.: *Invest Radiol, 3:*159, 1968.
239. Bailey, H.: *J Intl Coll Surg, 25:*675, 1956.
240. Birkin, B. B., et al.: *Am J Roentgenol Radium Ther Nucl Med, 116:*487, 1972.
241. Gilbert, G. J., et al.: *Radiology, 85:*306, 1965.
242. Rowe, G. J., et al.: *JAMA, 192:*947, 1965.
243. Bousvaros, G. A., et al.: *Can Med Assoc J, 872:* 286, 1962.
244. Weinberg, D. I., et al.: *Circ Res, 11:*1004, 1962.
245. Lang, E. K.: *Radiology, 88:*950, 1967.
246. McAfee, J.: *Radiology, 68:*825, 1957.
247. DeNosaquo, N.: *Radiology, 91:*92, 1968.
248. Baum, S., et al.: *Radiology, 86:*835, 1966.
249. Crawford, T.: *J Pathol Bact, 72:*547, 1956.
250. Crinic, D. M., et al.: *Radiology, 108:*295, 1973.
251. Doumanian, H. O., et al.: *Am J Roentgenol Radium Ther Nucl Med, 100:*344, 1967.
252. Molnar, W., et al.: *Radiology, 104:*269, 1972.
253. Dudrick, S., et al.: *Radiology, 88:*271, 1967.
254. Siegelman, S. S., et al.: *Radiology, 91:*251, 1968.
255. Jacobbson, B., et al.: *Acta Radiol Diagn (Stockh), 8:*97, 1969.
256. Bassett, F. H., et al.: *South Med J, 61:*1013, 1968.
257. Jeffery, R. F.: *Radiology, 103:*573, 1972.
258. Buxton, D., et al.: *Radiology, 111:*39, 1974.
259. Bayliss, R. I. S., et al.: *Br J Radiol, 43:*531, 1970.
260. Bookstein, J. J., et al.: *Radiology, 90:*778, 1968.
261. Egan, R. T., et al.: *JAMA, 215:*115, 1971.
262. Lynch, P. R., et al.: *Am J Physiol, 199:*1139, 1960.
263. Barnhard, H. J., et al.: *Radiology, 91:*74, 1968.
264. Daniel, P. M., et al.: *Q J Exp Physiol, 36:*199, 1951.
265. Trueta, J.: *Studies of the Renal Circulation.* Springfield, Thomas, 1947.
266. Davidson, A. J.: In Hilal, S. K. (Ed.): *Small Vessel Angiography.* St. Louis, Mosby, 1973.
267. Sherwood, T., et al.: *Lancet, 1:*784, 1967.
268. Edling, N. P. G., et al.: *Acta Radiol Diagn (Stockh), 51:*17, 1959.
269. Khademi: *Radiology, 113:*51, 1974.
270. Gonzalez, L. L.: *Arch Surg, 91:*185, 1965.
271. Gupta, J. M., et al.: *Arch Dis Child, 43:*382, 1968.
272. Robb, G. P., et al.: *Am J Roentgenol Radium Ther Nucl Med, 41:*1, 1939.
273. Steinberg, I., et al.: *Am J Roentgenol Radium Ther Nucl Med, 89:*294, 1963.
274. Fenwal Laboratories, Morton Grove, Illinois.
275. Palubinskas, A. J.: *Radiology, 82:*40, 1964.
276. Abrams, H. L., et al.: *Radiology, 83:*597, 1964.
277. McAllister, R. G., et al.: *JAMA, 221:*865, 1972.
278. Derrick, J. R., et al.: *Ann Surg, 160:*589, 1964.
279. Blalock, A., et al.: *J Exp Med, 69:*833, 1969.
280. Schwartz, D. T.: *N Engl J Med, 272:*1318, 1965.
281. Onnis, M., et al.: *Ann Surg, 157:*56, 1963.
282. Alfidi, R. J., et al.: *Radiology, 102:*545, 1972.
283. Wirtamen, G. W.: *Radiology, 108:*51, 1973.
284. Reuter, S., et al.: *Radiology, 105:*573, 1972.
285. Emmanouilides, G. C., et al.: *Radiology, 82:*447, 1964.
286. Nebesar, R., et al.: *Am J Roentgenol Radium Ther Nucl Med, 106:*81, 1969.
287. Sagel, S. S., et al.: *Radiology, 91:*797, 1968.
288. Martin, P., et al.: *Surgery, 71:*182, 1972.
289. Boijsen, E., et al.: *Acta Radiol Diagn (Stockh),* 3:543, 1965.
290. Kahn, P. C., et al.: *Radiology, 90:*975, 1968.
291. Beales, J. S. M., et al.: *Br J Radiol, 44:*854, 1971.
292. Reich, S. B., et al.: *Radiology, 104:*291, 1972.
293. Arkoff, R. S., et al.: *Radiology, 90:*66, 1968.
294. Greenbaum, E. J., et al.: *Radiology, 93:*373, 1969.
295. Rossi, P., et al.: *JAMA, 205:*547, 1968.
296. Viamonte, M., Jr., et al.: *Radiology, 96:*539 1970.
297. Warren, W. D., et al.: *Surg Gynecol Obstet, 126:*315, 1968.
298. Viamonte, M., Jr., et al.: *Surg Gynecol Obstet, 130:*37, 1970.
299. Warren, W. D., et al.: *Ann Surg, 165:*999, 1967.
300. Wexler, L.: *Circ Res, 23:*349, 1968.
301. Reuters, S., and Redman, H. C.: *Gastro Intestinal Angiography.* Philadelphia, Saunders, 1972.
302. Sherlock, S.: *Diseases of the Liver,* 4th ed. Philadelphia, Davis, 1900.
303. Greenspan, R., et al.: *Radiology, 78:*248, 1962.

304. Schlant, R. C., et al.: *Am J Med, 35:*343, 1963.
305. Lang, E. K.: *Radiology, 109:*257, 1973.
306. Laufman, H., et al.: *Ann Surg, 152:*621, 1960.
307. Kelly and Burnam: *Diseases of the Kidney, Ureters and Bladder.* New York, Appleton, 1914.
308. Falconer, C. W. A., et al.: *Br J Surg, 37:*334, 1950.
309. Pierson, J. M.: *Surg Gynecol Obstet, 77:*426, 1943.
310. Olsen, L. L., et al.: *Surg Gynecol Obstet, 99:* 713, 1954.
311. Michels, N. A.: *Am J Anat, 70:*21, 1942.
312. Kupic, E. A., et al.: *Invest Radiol, 2:*70, 1967.
313. Blaustein, A.: *The Spleen.* New York, McGraw, 1963.
314. Frates, R. E.: *Radiology, 92:*1014, 1969.
315. Herman, P. G.: *Radiology, 92:*1073, 1969.
316. Orkin, L. A.: *Trauma to the Ureter.* Philadelphia, Davis, 1964.
317. Lindner, H. H., et al.: *Arch Surg, 103:*600, 1971.
318. Michels, N. A.: *Ann Surg, 133:*503, 1951.
319. Tandler, J.: *Anat Hefte, 25:*472, 1904.
320. Healey, J. E., Jr., et al.: *J Intl Coll Surg, 20:*133, 1953.
321. Healey, J. E., Jr., et al.: *J Intl Coll Surg, 22:*542, 1954.
322. Michels, N. A.: *Am J Surg, 112:*337, 1966.
323. Schultz, R. D.: In Strandness, D. E., Jr. (Ed.): *Collateral Circulation in Clinical Surgery.* Philadelphia, Saunders, 1969.
324. George, R. J.: *Anatomy, 69:*196, 1935.
325. Boijsen, E.: In Abrams, H. L. (Ed.): *Angiography,* 11th ed. Boston, Little, 1971.
326. Beaton, L. E., et al.: *Q Bull Northwest Med, 16:* 114, 1942.
327. Minot, C. S.: *Proc Boston Soc Nat History, 29:* 189, 1900.
328. Brodel, M.: *Johns Hopkins Med J, 12:*10, 1901.
329. Boatman, D. L.: *Am J Roentgenol, 113:*447, 1971.
330. Graves, F. T.: *Arterial Anatomy of the Kidney.* Baltimore, Williams & Wilkins, 1971.
331. Anson, B. J., et al.: *J Urol, 60:*714, 1948.
332. Boijsen, E.: *Acta Radiol Suppl,* No. 183, 1959.
333. Odman, P., et al.: *Am J Roentgenol Radium Ther Nucl Med, 104:*283, 1968.
334. Sabagh, A., et al.: *Vasc Dis, 4:*19, 1970.
335. Jeffery, R. F.: *Radiology, 102:*309, 1972.
336. Guggemos, E., et al.: *Ann Surg, 156:*940, 1962.
337. Morris: In Anson, B. J. (Ed.): *Human Anatomy.* New York, McGraw, 1966.
338. Basmajian, J. V.: *Surg Gynecol Obstet, 101:*585, 1955.
339. Kegaries, D. L.: *Mayo Clin Proc, 8:*160, 1933.
340. Kegaries, D. L.: *Surg Gynecol Obstet, 58:*46, 1934.
341. Gardner, E., et al.: *Anatomy.* Philadelphia, Saunders, 1960.
342. Sonneland, J., et al.: *Surg Gynecol Obstet, 106:* 385, 1958.
343. Griffiths, J. D.: *Ann R Coll Surg Engl, 191:*241, 1956.
344. Falla, A., et al.: *Surg Gynecol Obstet, 116:*405, 1963.
345. Nathan, H.: *Thorax, 15:*229, 1960.
346. Seib, G. A.: *Am J Physiol Anthropol, 19:*39, 1934.
347. McDonald, J. J., et al.: *Am J Physiol Anthropol, 27:*91, 1940.
348. Degaris, C. F., et al.: *J Anat, 67:*599, 1933.
349. Bardsley, J. L., et al.: *Radiology, 94:*581, 1970.
350. Keen, J. A.: *Am J Anat, 108:*245, 1961.
351. Sackler, J. P., et al.: *Angiology, 19:*67, 1968.
352. Braithwaite, J. L.: *J Anat, 86:*423, 1952.
353. Doumanian, A. V., et al.: *Arch Surg, 91:*604, 1965.
354. Hipona, F.: In Ferris, Hipona and Kahn (Ed.): *Venography of the Inferior Venacava and Its Branches.* Baltimore, Williams & Wilkins, 1969.
355. Daesler, E. H., et al.: *Surg Gynecol Obstet, 108:* 149, 1959.
356. Halstead, W. S., et al.: *Ann Surg, 46:*489, 1907.
357. Sutton, D.: In Abrams, H. L. (Ed.): *Angiography,* 2nd ed. Boston, Little, 1971, vol. II.
358. Huelke, D. F.: *Anat Rec, 135:*33, 1959.
359. McCormack, L. J., et al.: *Surg Gynecol Obstet, 96:*43, 1953.
360. Chatrapathi, D. N.: *Indian Med Sci, 18:*462, 1964.
361. Mitra, S. K.: *J Anat, 100:*651, 1966.
362. Wakin, K. J.: *Am J Med, 16:*256, 1964.
363. Marks, C.: *Am J Surg, 117:*671, 1969.
364. Reynolds, T. F.: In Schiff, L. (Ed.): *Diseases of the Liver.* Philadelphia, Lippincott, 1972.
365. Michels, N. A.: *Cancer, 6:*708, 1953.
366. Doppman, J., et al.: *Br J Radiol, 41:*40, 1968.
367. Doppman, J., et al.: *JAMA, 204:*174, 1968.
368. Borell, U., et al.: *Acta Radiol Diagn (Stockh), 40:*561, 1953.
369. Borell, U.: In Abrams, H. L. (Ed.): *Angiography.* Boston, Little, 1971.
370. Merklin, R. J., et al.: *J Intl Coll Surg, 29:*41, 1958.
371. Pick, J. W., et al.: *Anat Rec, 78:*413, 1940.
372. Greig, H. W., et al.: *Q Bull Northwest U, 25:* 345, 1951.
373. Kahn, P. C., et al.: *Am J Roentgenol Radium Ther Nucl Med, 102:*407, 1968.
374. Gagnon, R.: *Rev Can Biol, 14:*350, 1956.

375. Gagnon, R.: *Rev Can Biol, 16:*421, 1957.
376. Gagnon, R.: *Rev Can Biol, 23:*461, 1964.
377. Clark, K.: *J R Coll Surg Engl, 4:*257, 1958.
378. Anson, B. J., et al.: *Surg Gynecol Obstet, 112:* 439, 1961.
379. McLachlan, M. S. F., et al.: *Br J Radiol, 44:*664, 1971.
380. Cope, C., et al.: *Radiology, 90:*1105, 1968.
381. Purtilo, D. T.: *JAMA, 215:*1329, 1971.
382. Johnstone, F. R. C.: *Am J Surg, 94:*615, 1957.
383. Field, S., et al.: *Br J Radiol, 47:*219, 1974.
384. Jacobs, J. B.: *Radiology, 92:*885, 1969.
385. Ahlberg, N. E., et al.: *Acta Radiol, 4:*517, 1966.
386. Shimkin, P. M., et al.: *Am J Roentgenol Radium Ther Nucl Med, 118:*654, 1973.
387. Anson, B. J., et al.: *Surg Gynecol Obstet, 100:* 157, 1955.
388. Odgers, P. N. B.: *J Anat, 66:*98, 1931.
389. Davis, C. J., Jr., et al.: *Am J Clin Pathol, 50:* 700, 1968.
390. Cope, C., et al.: *Radiology, 92:*867, 1969.
391. Baston, O. V.: *Am J Roentgenol Radium Ther Nucl Med, 48:*715, 1942.
392. Batson, O. V.: *Ann Surg, 112:*138, 1940.
393. Abrams, H. L.: *Radiology, 69:*508, 1957.
394. Bergstrand, I., et al.: *Acta Radiol Diagn (Stockh), 2:*1, 1964.
395. Banner, R. L., et al.: *Cancer, 11:*22, 1958.
396. Douglas, B. E., et al.: *Surg Gynecol Obstet, 91:* 562, 1950.
397. Doehner, G. A., et al.: *Radiology, 64:*675, 1955.
398. Grietz, T.: *Acta Radiol Diagn (Stockh), 44:*1, 1955.
399. Edwards, E. A., et al.: *Surg Gynecol Obstet, 85:* 547, 1947.
400. Kampmeier, O. F.: *Am J Anat, 38:*451, 1922.
401. Rodboard, S.: *Ann Intern Med, 50:*1339, 1959.
402. Powell, J., et al.: *Surg Gynecol Obstet, 94:*453, 1951.
403. Dilenge, D., et al.: *Radiology, 108:*333, 1973.
404. Ahlberg, N. E., et al.: *Acta Radiol Diagn (Stockh), 7:*431, 1968.
405. Sylwanowicz, W.: *Assoc Anat, 26:*503, 1931.
406. Sutherland, D. L., et al.: *Surgery, 38:*320, 1955.
407. Nordenstrom, B., et al.: *Acta Radiol Diagn (Stockh), 6:*65, 1967.
408. Edwards, E. A., et al.: *Surg Gynecol Obstet, 65:* 310, 1937.
409. Gunderson, J.: *Vasc Dis, 3:*273, 1966.
410. Barry and Patten: In Gould, S. E. (Ed.): *Pathology of the Heart,* 2nd ed. Springfield, Thomas, 1960.
411. Cornell, S. H.: *Radiology, 86:*421, 1966.
412. Edwards, J. E., et al.: *Congenital Heart Disease.* Philadelphia, Saunders, 1965, vol. II.
413. Friedenberg, M. J., et al.: *Am J Roentgenol Radium Ther Nucl Med, 97:*428, 1966.
414. Masoni, A.: *Acta Med Scand, 159:*225, 1957.
415. Bucht, H.: *Scand J Clin Lab Invest Suppl, 64* (14):27, 1962.
416. Starer, F.: *Br J Radiol, 38:*675, 1965.
417. Reuter, S. R., et al.: *Radiology, 89:*805, 1967.
418. Kahn, P. C.: *Radiol Clin North Am, 5:*221, 1967.
419. Melby, T. C., et al.: *N Engl J Med, 277:*1050, 1967.
420. Lang, E. K.: *Radiology, 84:*296, 1965.
421. McKenzie, A. D., et al.: *Ann Surg, 148:*139, 1958.
422. Edwards, E. A.: *Surg Gynecol Obstet, 107:*183, 1958.
423. Smith, G. W., et al.: *Arch Surg, 83:*702, 1961.
424. Templeton, A. W.: *Am J Roentgenol Radium Ther Nucl Med, 95:*383, 1965.
425. Strandness, D. E., Jr.: In Strandness, D. E., Jr. (Ed.): *Collateral Circulation in Clinical Surgery.* Philadelphia, Saunders, 1969.
426. Longland, C. J.: *Ann R Coll Surg Engl, 13:*161, 1953.
427. Edwards, E. A.: *Surg Gynecol Obstet, 97:*87, 1953.
428. Bookstein, J. J.: *Invest Radiol, 1:*281, 1966.
429. Holman, E.: *Surgery, 26:*889, 1949.
430. Longenecker, C. G., et al.: *Surg Forum, 11:*166, 1960.
431. Reid, M. R.: *Arch Surg, 11:*25, 1925.
432. Takahasi, M., et al.: *Invest Radiol, 3:*108, 1968.
433. Callow, A. D., et al.: *Surgery, 49:*26, 1961.
434. Edwards, E. A.: *Arch Intern Med, 88:*137, 1951.
435. Edwards, J. E., et al.: *Mayo Clin Proc, 23:*433, 1948.
436. Bramwell, C., et al.: *Br Heart J, 3:*205, 1941.
437. Siekert, R. G., et al.: *Ann Intern Med, 61:*64, 1964.
438. Gerber, N.: *Am J Dis Child, 113:*709, 1967.
439. Dardik, H., et al.: *Ann Surg, 164:*171, 1966.
440. Rojas, R. H., et al.: *J Thorac Cardiovasc Surg, 51:*113, 1966.
441. Folger, G. M.: *Circulation, 31:*241, 1965.
442. Agee, O. F.: *Am J Roentgenol Radium Ther Nucl Med, 97:*497, 1966.
443. Lochaya, S., et al.: *Am Heart J, 73:*369, 1967.
444. Shuford, W. H., et al.: *Am J Roentgenol Radium Ther Nucl Med, 109:*75, 1970.
445. Coder, D. M., et al.: *Mayo Clin Proc, 40:*473, 1965.
446. Antia, A. V., et al.: *Am J Cardiol, 18:*599, 1966.
447. Patel, A.: *Medicine (Baltimore), 44:*289, 1965.
448. Piccone, V. A., et al.: *Angiology, 21:*240, 1970.
449. Newton, T. H., et al.: *Am J Roentgenol Radium Ther Nucl Med, 91:*394, 1964.

450. Bosniak, M. A.: *Am J Roentgenol Radium Ther Nucl Med, 91:*1232, 1964.
451. Handa, J., et al.: *Surgery, 58:*703, 1965.
452. Eklof, B.: *Surgery, 68:*431, 1970.
453. Gonzalez, L. L., et al.: *Arch Surg, 91:*185, 1965.
454. Reivich, M., et al.: *N Engl J Med, 265:*878, 1961.
455. Santischi, D. R., et al.: *J Thorac Cardiovasc Surg, 51:*103, 1966.
456. Killen, D. A., et al.: *Arch Surg, 51:*539, 1966.
457. Scatliff, J. H., et al.: *Radiology, 88:*64, 1967.
458. Pratesi, F., et al.: *Vasc Dis, 5:*214, 1968.
459. Mozerski, D. J., et al.: *Ann Surg, 178:*123, 1973.
460. Young, J. R., et al.: *Arch Surg, 86:*51, 1963.
461. Connally, J. E., et al.: *Am J Surg, 126:*197, 1973.
462. Sugarbaker, E. V., et al.: *Arch Surg, 104:*213, 1972.
463. Brolin, I.: *Acta Radiol Diagn (Stockh), 6:*401, 1967.
464. Engell, H. C.: *Ann Surg, 171:*533, 1970.
465. Bookstein, J. J.: *Radiology, 90:*1073, 1968.
466. Love, L., et al.: *Am J Roentgenol Radium Ther Nucl Med, 104:*296, 1968.
467. Meng, C. H., et al.: *Radiology, 109:*59, 1973.
468. Abrams, H. L.: *Semin Roentgenol, 2:*157, 1967.
469. Paul, R. E., Jr., et al.: *Radiology, 84:*1013, 1965.
470. Reiner, L., et al.: *Surgery, 45:*820, 1959.
471. Griffiths, J. D.: *Br Med J, 1:*323, 1961.
472. Chiene: *J Anat, 3:*65, 1869.
473. Matz, E. M., et al.: *Vasc Dis, 5:*130, 1968.
474. Popovsky, J.: *Arch Surg, 92:*202, 1966.
475. Glauser, F.: *Surgery, 33:*333, 1953.
476. Seagall, H. N.: *Surg Gynecol Obstet, 37:*152, 1953.
477. Bengmark, S., et al.: *Am J Surg, 119:*620, 1970.
478. Wall, J. K.: *Vasc Dis, 3:*351, 1966.
479. McIndoe, A. H.: *Arch Pathol, 5:*23, 1928.
480. Bergstrand: *Acta Radiol Diagn (Stockh), 45:*1, 1957.
481. Lore, J. M., Jr., et al.: *Cancer, 11:*24, 1958.
482. Salam, A. A., et al.: *Surgery, 74:*961, 1973.
483. Yale, C. E., et al.: *JAMA, 217:*317, 1971.
484. Deutsch, V., et al.: *Am J Roentgenol Radium Ther Nucl Med, 116:*430, 1972.
485. Kreel, L., et al.: *Br J Radiol, 40:*755, 1967.
486. Pleasants, J. H.: *Johns Hopkins Bull, 16:*363, 1911.
487. Ferris, J., et al.: *Radiology, 89:*1, 1967.
488. Filler, R. M., et al.: *Arch Surg, 84:*10, 1962.
489. Missal, M. E., et al.: *Ann Intern Med, 62:*133, 1965.
490. Mavor, G. E., et al.: *Surg Gynecol Obstet, 125:* 561, 1967.
491. Okay, N., et al.: *Radiology, 92:*1493, 1969.
492. Hollinshead, W. H., et al.: *Surg Gynecol Obstet, 97:*213, 1963.
493. Klien, L. J., et al.: *Am J Med, 37:*263, 1964.
494. Doppman, J.: *Invest Radiol, 2:*332, 1967.
495. Ridley, D.: *J Pathol Bacteriol, 63:*17, 1951.
496. Candel, S., et al.: *Am J Med, 15:*307, 1953.
497. Carter, S. A., et al.: *Circulation, 33:*343, 1966.
498. Smith, G. T., et al.: *Surg Gynecol Obstet, 115:* 682, 1962.
499. Ramsay, G. C., et al.: *Radiology, 90:*716, 1968.
500. Ruzicka, F. F., Jr., et al.: *Radiology, 102:*253, 1972.
501. Shennan, T.: *Med Res Counc Spec Rep Ser (Lond), 193,* 1934.
502. Dotter, C. T.: *Semin Roentgenol, 5* (no. 3), 1970.
503. Meehan, J. J., et al.: *Circulation, 16:*615, 1957.
504. Gore, I., et al.: *Arch Surg, 53:*121 and 142, 1952.
505. Burman, S. O., et al.: *Ann Surg, 147:*511, 1958.
506. DeBakey, M. E., et al.: *J Thorac Cardiovasc Surg, 49:*130, 1965.
507. Hirst, A. E., et al.: *Medicine, 37:*217, 1958.
508. Hufnagel, C. A., et al.: *Surgery, 51:*84, 1962.
509. Wheat, M. W., Jr., et al.: *J Thorac Cardiovasc Surg, 58:*344, 1969.
510. Dinsmore, R. E., et al.: *Radiology, 105:*567, 1973.
511. Jones, A. M., et al.: *Br Heart J, 8:*191, 1946.
512. Drury, R. A. B.: *Br Med J, 2:*1114, 1955.
513. Prior, J. J., et al.: *J Thorac Cardiovas Surg, 33:* 213, 1957.
514. Johns, T. N. P.: *Ann Surg, 137:*232, 1953.
515. Erdheim, V. J.: *Virchows Arch Pathol Anat, 276:*187, 1930.
516. McKusick, V. A.: *Circulation, 11:*321, 1955.
517. Beaven, D. W., et al.: *Br Med J, 1:*77, 1956.
518. Elliott, D. P.: *J Thorac Cardiovasc Surg, 50:* 357, 1965.
519. Garret: *Am J Clin Pathol, 38:*406, 1962.
520. Marshall, T. R.: *J Clin Pathol, 11:*36, 1958.
521. Cambell, D. K., et al.: *Radiology, 92:*123, 1969.
522. Eyler, W. R., et al.: *Radiology, 85:*1047, 1965.
523. Soto, B., et al.: *Am J Roentgenol, 116:*146, 1972.
524. Shuford, W. H., et al.: *N Engl J Med, 280:*225, 1969.
525. Price, J. E., et al.: *Am J Roentgenol Radium Ther Nucl Med, 113:*710, 1971.
526. Siegelman, S. S.: *Radiology, 95:*73, 1970.
527. Watson, A. J.: *J Pathol Bacteriol, 72:*439, 1956.
528. Movitz, D.: *Surgery, 45:*834, 1959.
529. Dvorak, A., et al.: *Ann Surg, 109:*425, 1969.
530. Hare, W. S. C., et al.: *Radiology, 96:*255, 1970.
531. Englund, S. W.: *Am J Clin Pathol, 45:*472, 1966.
532. DeBakey, M. E., et al.: *Am J Surg, 109:*134, 1965.
533. New, P. F. J., et al.: *Radiology, 93:*41, 1969.

534. Brown, O. L., et al.: *Am J Roentgenol Radium Ther Nucl Med, 118:*648, 1973.
535. Patehefsky, A. S., et al.: *Arch Pathol, 83:*1141, 1967.
536. Ouchi, H., et al.: *Vasc Dis, 2:*340, 1965.
537. Mandelbaum, I., et al.: *Surgery, 45:*786, 1959.
538. McFarland, W., et al.: *N Engl J Med, 271:*1309, 1964.
539. Shepard, D., et al.: *Ann Surg, 153:*1029, 1961.
540. Mortorell, R.: *Ann Surg, 157:*292, 1963.
541. Carlsson, E., et al.: *Acta Chir, 125:*294, 1963.
542. Fraser, G. A.: *Ann Surg, 161:*539, 1965.
543. Lewin, J. R.: *Vasc Dis, 3:*332, 1966.
544. Kerr, W. S., Jr., et al.: *J Urol, 109:*479, 1973.
545. Olsen, W. R., et al.: *Arch Surg, 92:*123, 1966.
546. Stoney, R. J., et al.: *Am J Surg, 110:*153, 1965.
547. Ello, F. V.: *Surgery, 74:*460, 1973.
548. Thio, R. T.: *Am J Surg, 123:*604, 1972.
549. Parmley, L. F., et al.: *Circulation, 17:*1086, 1958.
550. Herber, G.: *J Cardiovasc Surg, 12:*115, 1971.
551. Hass, G. M.: *J Aviation Med, 15:*77, 1944.
552. Sandborn, J. C., et al.: *Radiology, 95:*293, 1970.
553. Bennett, D. E., et al.: *Surgery, 61:*516, 1967.
554. Zak, F. G., et al.: *N Engl J Med, 258:*824, 1958.
555. Peyton, R. W.: *Ann Surg, 162:*1069, 1965.
556. Fiessinger, N., et al.: *Rev Gastroenterol, 5:*383, 1938.
557. Zederfelt, Z.: *Acta Chir Suppl, 133:*165, 1967.
558. Angres, G. A., et al.: *JAMA, 228:*1026, 1974.
559. Christopher, F., et al.: *Surgery, 24:*864, 1948.
560. Sandblom, P.: *Hemobilia.* Springfield, Thomas, 1972.
561. Boijsen, E., et al.: *Radiology, 93:*781, 1969.
562. Mallory, G. K., et al.: *Am J Med Sci, 178:*506, 1929.
563. Freeark, R. J., et al.: *Arch Surg, 88:*882, 1964.
564. Katz, A. M.: *Ann Intern Med, 51:*212, 1959.
565. Baum, S., et al.: *Radiology, 95:*597, 1970.
566. Farris, J. C., et al.: *Radiology, 108:*285, 1973.
567. Bree, R. L.: *Radiology, 108:*287, 1973.
568. White, A. F., et al.: *Am J Roentgenol Radium Ther Nucl Med, 118:*86, 1973.
569. Paget, E. T., et al.: *Arch Surg, 104:*397, 1972.
570. Nordenloft, E. L., et al.: *Acta Chir Suppl, 133:* 256, 1967.
571. Kelley, D. J.: *Am J Surg, 100:*597, 1960.
572. Garrett, H. E., et al.: *Am J Surg, 105:*6, 1963.
573. Earley, C. M., Jr.: *Surg Gynecol Obstet, 104:*49, 1959.
574. Meyer, M.: *Invest Radiol, 8:*289, 1973.
575. Foster, J. H., et al.: *JAMA, 215:*636, 1971.
576. Sutherland, D., et al.: *Surgery, 71:*290, 1972.
577. Shiffman, M. A., et al.: *Arch Surg, 94:*771, 1967.
578. Koehler, P. R., et al.: *Radiology, 106:*537, 1973.
579. Galloway, S. J., et al.: *Radiology, 113:*11, 1974.
580. Sos, T. A., et al.: *Clin Radiol, 24:*464, 1973.
581. Athanasolis, C. A., et al.: *Radiology, 113:*37, 1974.
582. Schwartz, S. I.: In Schwartz, S. I. (Ed.): *Principles of Surgery.* New York, McGraw, 1969.
583. Coe, J. D.: *Arch Surg, 88:*888, 1964.
584. Lee, H. C., et al.: *Ann Surg, 147:*714, 1958.
585. Hardt, L. L., et al.: *Gastroenterol, 28:*70, 1955.
586. Whitcomb, F. F., Jr., et al.: *Ann Intern Med, 56:*834, 1962.
587. Bardsley, J. L., et al.: *Radiology, 93:*559, 1969.
588. Schoenbaum, S. W., et al.: *Am J Roentgenol, 119:*277, 1973.
589. Welch, C. E., et al.: *Adv Surg, 7:*94, 1973.
590. Enquist, I. F., et al.: *Surg Gynecol Obstet, 106:* 153, 1958.
591. Lipp, W. F., et al.: *Gastroenterol, 22:*181, 1952.
592. White, R. I., et al.: *Radiology, 111:*549, 1974.
593. Rosch, J., et al.: *Am J Roentgenol Radium Ther Nucl Med, 116:*279, 1972.
594. Nusbaum, M., et al.: *Surg Forum, 14:*374, 1963.
595. Nusbaum, M., et al.: *Ann Surg, 170:*506, 1970.
596. Sovak, M., et al.: *Invest Radiol, 8:*100, 1973.
597. Stadler, H., et al.: *Am J Med, 55:*99, 1973.
598. Coel, M. N., et al.: *Am J Roentgenol Radium Ther Nucl Med, 116:*37, 1972.
599. Sokoloff, J., et al.: *Radiology, 111:*285, 1974.
600. Janon, E. A.: *Radiology, 97:*385, 1970.
601. Schecter, M. M., et al.: *Radiology, 86:*686, 1966.
602. Pollack, M. M., et al.: *Radiology, 110:*1, 1974.
603. Uson, A. C., et al.: *J Urol, 81:*388, 1959.
604. Marshall, W. A., Jr., et al.: *Radiology, 101:*561, 1971.
605. McIndoe, A. H.: *Br J Surg, 20:*249, 1932.
606. Presman, D., et al.: *Am J Surg, 102:*586, 1961.
607. Gronner, A. T.: *Radiology, 103:*309, 1972.
608. Zeek, P. M.: *N Engl J Med, 248:*764, 1954.
609. Segovia, D. A., et al.: *Mayo Clin Proc, 39:*205, 1964.
610. Rodnan, G. D., et al.: *JAMA, 224:*722, 1973.
611. Fisher, E.: In Abramson, D. I. (Ed.): *Blood Vessels and Lymphatics.* New York, Acad Pr, 1962.
612. Halpern, M., et al.: *Am J Roentgenol Radium Ther Nucl Med, 111:*663, 1971.
613. Citron, B. P., et al.: *N Engl J Med, 283:*1003, 1970.
614. Louria, D. P., et al.: *Ann Intern Med, 67:*1, 1967.
615. Phillips, J., et al.: *JAMA, 206:*1569, 1968.
616. Hines, E. A., et al.: *JAMA, 174:*848, 1960.
617. Mays, E. T., et al.: *Arch Surg, 91:*58, 1965.
618. Nakao, K., et al.: *Circulation, 35:*1141, 1967.
619. Kozuka, T.: *Acta Radiol Diagn (Stockh), 4:*497, 1966.
620. Kozuka, T., et al.: *Acta Radiol Diagn (Stockh), 8:*49, 1969.

621. Judge, R. D., et al.: *Am J Med, 32:*379, 1962.
622. Thompson, J. R., et al.: *Radiology, 101:*591, 1971.
623. Rossrussell, R. W.: *Q J Med, 28:*471, 1959.
624. Danaraj, T. J., et al.: *Br Heart J, 25:*153, 1963.
625. Gotsman, M. S., et al.: *Radiology, 88:*232, 1967.
626. Schrire, V., et al.: *Q J Med, 33:*439, 1964.
627. Grollman, J. H., Jr.: *Radiology, 83:*387, 1964.
628. Harrison, E. J., et al.: *Am J Med, 43:*97, 1967.
629. Fisher, E. R., et al.: *Arch Intern Med, 89:*343, 1952.
630. Wylie, E. J., et al.: *Am J Surg, 112:*149, 1966.
631. Houser, O. W., et al.: *Radiology, 101:*605, 1971.
632. McCormick, L. J., et al.: *Am Heart J, 72:*188, 1966.
633. McCormick, L. J., et al.: *Am Heart J, 73:*602, 1967.
634. Hunt, J. C., et al.: *Mayo Clin Proc, 32:*181, 1962.
635. Meaney, T. F., et al.: *Radiology, 91:*881, 1968.
636. Schmidt, D. M., et al.: *Am J Clin Pathol, 44:* 546, 1965.
637. Schwartz, C. T., et al.: *Circ Res, 11:*63, 1962.
638. Crawford, T.: *Proc Roy Soc Med (Lond), 53:*9, 1960.
639. Rogers, W. H., et al.: *Arch Surg, 103:*93, 1971.
640. Derrick, J. R., et al.: *Ann Surg, 149:*684, 1959.
641. Mavor, G. E.: *Br J Surg, 43:*352, 1956.
642. Gore, I.: In Anderson, W. A. D. (Ed.): *Pathology,* 5th ed. St. Louis, Mosby,
643. Wagner, M.: *Angiology, 17:*574, 1966.
644. Lindbom, A.: *Acta Radiol Diagn (Stockh), 80:*1950.
645. Haimovici, H.: *Arch Surg, 95:*918, 1967.
646. Coran, A. G., et al.: *N Engl J Med, 274:*643, 1966.
647. Holman, E.: *Surg Gynecol Obstet, 100:*599, 1955.
648. Garland, H. G.: *J Pathol Bacteriol, 35:*333, 1932.
649. Estes, J. E., Jr.: *Circulation, 2:*258, 1950.
650. Szylagi, D. E., et al.: *Arch Surg, 85:*395, 1961.
651. Morris, G. C., Jr., et al.: *Am J Cardiol, 12:*303, 1963.
652. Bergan, J. J., et al.: *Basic Surgical Physiology.* Chicago, Yearbk Med, 1969.
653. Malcolm, J. E.: *Blood Pressure, Sounds and Their Meaning.* London, Heinemann, 1957.
654. Crawford, E. S., et al.: *Surg Clin North Am, 46:* 963, 1960.
655. Benjamin, H. B., et al.: *Surg Gynecol Obstet, 125:*1307, 1967.
656. Pirker, E., et al.: *Acta Radiol (Stockh), 25-30:* 425, 1967.
657. Hardy, J. D., et al.: *Ann Surg, 173:*945, 1971.
658. Darling, P. C.: *Am J Surg, 119:*397, 1970.
659. Sommerville, R. L., et al.: *Medicine (Baltimore), 38:*207, 1959.
660. Eastcott, H. H. G.: In Eastcott, H. H. G. (Ed.): *Arterial Surgery.* Philadelphia, Lippincott, 1969.
661. Smith, R. F., et al.: *Arch Surg, 86:*825, 1963.
662. Smith, J. W.: *Am J Surg, 104:*7, 1962.
663. Heggelveit, H. A., et al.: *Am J Clin Pathol, 42:* 69, 1964.
664. Sutton, D.: *Arteriography.* Edinburgh, Livingstone, 1962.
665. Abbott, W. M.: *Am J Surg, 125:*515, 1973.
666. Bennet, D. E., et al.: *Am J Surg, 113:*321, 1967.
667. Blum, L., et al.: *JAMA, 188:*505, 1964.
668. Rob, C. J., et al.: *Br Med J, 1:*378, 1955.
669. Hara, M., et al.: *J Thorac Cardiovasc Surg, 46:* 256, 1963.
670. Steinberg, I., et al.: *Radiology, 84:*626, 1964.
671. Kaufmann, S. L., et al.: *Circulation, 35:*90, 1967.
672. Ranniger, K., et al.: *Radiology, 90:*507, 1968.
673. Vitek, J. J.: *Radiology, 106:*101, 1973.
674. Longstreth, P. L., et al.: *Radiology, 113:*65, 1974.
675. Bron, K. M., et al.: *Arch Intern Med, 116:*450, 1955.
676. Herschman, A., et al.: *Radiology, 94:*147, 1970.
677. Chudacek, Z.: *Br J Radiol, 40:*864, 1967.
678. Gostigian, J., et al.: *Am J Surg, 105:*267, 1963.
679. Steinberg, I., et al.: *Ann Intern Med, 43:*120, 1955.
680. Kraft, R. O., et al.: *Surg Gynecol Obstet, 117:* 563, 1963.
681. McKusick, V. A.: *Circulation, 30:*326, 1964.
682. Imahaii, S., et al.: *Am J Med, 47:*967, 1969.
683. Halpern, M., et al.: *Radiology, 90:*1143, 1968.
684. Bird, R. M., et al.: *N Engl J Med, 260:*597, 1959.
685. Sherlock, S. P. V., et al.: *Br J Radiol, 30:*151, 1942.
686. Feldman, M.: *Am J Dig Dis, 22:*48, 1955.
687. Jones, E. L., et al.: *Arch Surg, 97:*640, 1968.
688. Boijsen, E., et al.: *Acta Radiol Diagn (Stockh), 8:*29, 1969.
689. Boijsen, E., et al.: *Acta Radiol Diagn (Stockh), 6:*487, 1967.
690. Pedowitz, P., et al.: *Am J Gynecol Obstet, 73:* 720, 1957.
691. Olin, T. B., et al.: *Vasc Dis, 3:*269, 1966.
692. Baird, R. J., et al.: *Surgery, 59:*911, 1966.
693. Shucksmith, H. S.: *Br Med J, 1:*918, 1966.
694. Leading Article. *Br Med J, 1:*625, 1966.
695. Abeshouse, B. S.: *Urol Cutan Rev, 55:*451, 1951.
696. Hug, H.: *Am J Surg, 102:*859, 1961.
697. Reuter, S. R., et al.: *Arch Surg, 97:*497, 1968.

698. Thomford, N. R., et al.: *Ann Surg, 168:*294, 1968.
699. Hoehn, J. G., et al.: *Am J Surg, 115:*832, 1968.
700. Boijsen, E., et al.: *Radiology, 93:*781, 1969.
701. Filly, R. A., et al.: *Radiology, 97:*629, 1970.
702. Wagenvoort, C. A., et al.: *Pediatrics, 32:*861, 1963.
703. Jofte, N.: *Clin Radiol, 15:*286, 1964.
704. Hershey, F. B., et al.: *Arch Surg, 86:*836, 1963.
705. Sawyers, J. L., et al.: *Arch Surg, 95:*802, 1967.
706. Pataro, V. F., et al.: *J Cardiovasc Surg, 2:*3, 1961.
707. Okay, N. H., et al.: *Radiology, 95:*629, 1970.
708. Abbott, O. A.: *Ann Surg, 131:*259, 1950.
709. Walker, W. A.: *Am J Roentgenol Radium Ther Nucl Med, 90:*575, 1963.
710. Sproul, G.: *Surgery, 58:*1027, 1965.
711. Thomas, T. V.: *Surgery, 61:*550, 1967.
712. Steinberg, I.: *Am J Roentgenol Radium Ther Nucl Med, 101:*947, 1967.
713. Hipona, F., et al.: *Circulation, 35:*471, 1967.
714. Thomas, M. L., et al.: *Am J Roentgenol Radium Ther Nucl Med, 113:*722, 1971.
715. Malan, E., et al.: *J Cardiovasc Surg, 6:*255, 1965.
716. Calem, W. S., et al.: *Arch Surg, 86:*571, 1973.
717. Chidkel, N., et al.: *Acta Radiol Diagn (Stockh), 7:*193, 1968.
718. Dixon, J. A., et al.: *Surg Gynecol Obstet, 131:* 458, 1970.
719. Helander, C. G., et al.: *Acta Radiol (Stockh), 53:*97, 1960.
720. McMillan, G. C.: In Abramson, D. I. (Ed.): *Blood Vessels and Lymphatics.* New York, Acad Pr, 1962.
721. Castellino, R. A., et al.: *N Engl J Med, 278:* 1087, 1968.
722. McDonald, C. J., et al.: *Radiology, 96:*533, 1970.
723. Otto, D. L., et al.: *Am J Roentgenol Radium Ther Nucl Med, 92:*1000, 1964.
724. Mikkelson, W. J.: *Radiology, 81:*945, 1963.
725. Schoenfield, M. R., et al.: *Am J Med, 50:*845, 1971.
726. Brill, D. R., et al.: *Am J Dig Dis, 14:*801, 1969.
727. Karr, S., et al.: *N Engl J Med, 263:*665, 1970.
728. Rothschild, J. J., et al.: *N Engl J Med, 278:*97, 1968.
729. Conn, H. O., et al.: *Surgery, 71:*828, 1972.
730. Miller, D., et al.: *Br J Surg, 44:*396, 1956-57.
731. Mathe, C. P.: *J Urol, 82:*412, 1959.
732. Holman, E.: In Holman, E. (Ed.): *Abnormal AV Communication.* Springfield, Thomas, 1968.
733. Sabin: *Contrib Embryol Carnegie Inst, 6:*7, 1917.
734. Woolard, H. H.: *Contrib Embryol Carnegie Inst, 14:*139, 1922.
735. Stricht, J. V.: *J Cardiovasc Surg, 13:*502, 1972.
736. Haimovici, H., et al.: *Ann Surg, 164:*990, 1964.
737. Clark, E. R., et al.: *Am J Anat, 54:*229, 1934.
738. Farrell, R., et al.: *Radiology, 102:*279, 1972.
739. Baum, S.: In Hilal, S. K. (Ed.): *Small Vessel Angiography.* St. Louis, Mosby, 1973.
740. Barlow, T. E., et al.: *Surg Gynecol Obstet, 93:* 657, 1951.
741. Prinzmetal, M., et al.: *Am J Physiol, 152:*48, 1948.
742. Sherman, J. L., Jr.: *Medicine (Baltimore), 42:* 247, 1963.
743. Elkin, D. C., et al.: *JAMA, 134:*1524, 1967.
744. Holman, E.: *Am J Surg, 108:*1101, 1955.
745. Holman, E.: *Circulation, 32:*1001, 1965.
746. Sumner, D. S.: In Strandness, D. E., Jr. (Ed.): *Collateral Circulation in Clinical Surgery.* Philadelphia, Saunders, 1969.
747. Matas, R.: *Surgery, 5:*290, 1909.
748. Matas, R.: *Ann Surg, 71:*403, 1920.
749. Rossi, P., et al.: *Radiology, 111:*47, 1974.
750. Creech, O., Jr., et al.: *Ann Surg, 161:*908, 1965.
751. Morgan, J., et al.: *Can Med Assoc J, 91:*920, 1964.
752. Lurus, A. G., et al.: *Radiology, 92:*1296, 1969.
753. Anthopoulos, L. P., et al.: *Angiology, 16:*89, 1965.
754. Gaspard, G. T., et al.: *Arch Surg, 105:*90, 1972.
755. Morley, G. W., et al.: *Obstet Gynecol, 31:*722, 1968.
756. Wheeler, G. W.: *Am J Roentgenol Radium Ther Nucl Med, 119:*619, 1973.
757. DeBakey, M. E., et al.: *Ann Surg, 147:*646, 1958.
758. Kazmier, F. J., et al.: *Am J Med, 55:*175, 1973.
759. Foster, J. H.: *Ann Surg, 154:*300, 1961.
760. Franklin, R. B., et al.: *Medicine (Baltimore), 34:*97, 1955.
761. McGregor, J. K., et al.: *Am J Surg, 108:*416, 1964.
762. Green, J. D., et al.: *Radiology, 108:*67, 1973.
763. Crawford, S., et al.: *Circulation, 27:*416, 1963.
764. Maldanado, J. E., et al.: *Am J Med, 29:*849, 1970.
765. Meng, C., et al.: *Radiology, 100:*335, 1971.
766. Ekelund, L., et al.: *Acta Radiol Diagn (Stockh), 11:*38, 1971.
767. Ekelund, L., et al.: *Acta Radiol Diagn (Stockh), 11:*289, 1971.
768. Spellman, M. W., et al.: *Ann Surg, 165:*458, 1967.
769. Vanway, C. M., III, et al.: *Surgery, 70:*876, 1971.
770. Brunner, J. H., et al.: *JAMA, 223:*316, 1973.

771. Martin, L. W., et al.: *Ann Surg, 161:*209, 1965.
772. Murray, M. J., et al.: *Am J Med, 29:*849, 1970.
773. Genant, H. K., et al.: *Am J Roentgenol Radium Ther Nucl Med, 115:*349, 1972.
774. Alfidi, R. J., et al.: *Ann Surg, 174:*573, 1971.
775. Baum, S., et al.: In Boley, S. J. (Ed.): *Vascular Disorders of the Small Intestine.* New York, Appleton, 1971.
776. Steinberg, I.: *Am J Med, 19:*549, 1955.
777. Hodgson, C. H., et al.: *Chest, 43:*449, 1963.
778. Pierce, J. A., et al.: *N Engl J Med, 260:*901, 1959.
779. Thompson, N. W., et al.: *Ann Surg, 170:*852, 1970.
780. Kinmonth, J. B.: *Br Med J, 1:*59, 1952.
781. Kinmonth, J. B., et al.: *Br J Surg, 44:*164, 1956-57.
782. Mustard, W. J., et al.: *Ann Surg, 155:*339, 1962.
783. Cohen, S. M.: *Lancet, 1:*1, 1944.
784. Wickbom, I., et al.: *Acta Radiol (Stockh), 47:*433, 1957.
785. Lindbom, A.: *Acta Radiol (Stockh), 47:*449, 1957.
786. Amplatz: *Radiology, 91:*392, 1968.
787. Haimovici, H.: *Circulation, 1:*225, 1950.
788. Sutton, M.: *Br Med J, 2:*859, 1952.
789. Manzie, M. W., et al.: *Vasc Dis, 1:*276, 1964.
790. Hardway, R. M., et al.: *Arch Surg, 83:*173, 1961.
791. Laplace, E.: *Penn Med J, 16:*699, 1913.
792. Burton, A. C., et al.: *J Appl Physiol, 4:*329, 1951.
793. Corday, E., et al.: *Am J Med, 33:*365, 1962.
794. Britt, L. G., et al.: *Ann Surg, 169:*704, 1969.
795. Laufman, H., et al.: *Surg Gynecol Obstet, 87:*641, 1948.
796. Corday, E., et al.: *Dis Chest, 56:*200, 1969.
797. Aakhus, T., et al.: *Acta Radiol Diagn (Stockh), 6:*1, 1967.
798. Shanbour, L. L., et al.: *Am J Dig Dis, 17:*826, 1972.
799. Buenger, R. E., et al.: *JAMA, 198:*559, 1966.
800. Pader, E.: *Vasc Dis, 4:*380, 1967.
801. Kramer, R., et al.: *Radiology, 84:*308, 1965.
802. Conley, J. E., et al.: *JAMA, 198:*808, 1966.
803. Richter, A. M., et al.: *Radiology, 106:*339, 1973.
804. Bland, J. E., et al.: *Am Surg, 166:*987, 1967.
805. Amirjahed, A. K.: *Surg Gynecol Obstet, 127:*609, 1968.
806. Gifford, R. W., Jr.: *Circulation, 27:*970, 1963.
807. Rogoff, S. M., et al.: In Abrams, H. L. (Ed.): *Angiography.* Boston, Little, 1971, vol. II.
808. DeBakey, M. E., et al.: *Ann Surg, 165:*830, 1967.
809. Hipona, F. A., et al.: *Am J Roentgenol Radium Ther Nucl Med, 110:*515, 1970.
810. Schuster, E. R.: *Ann Surg, 158:*1012, 1963.
811. Wood, C., et al.: *Arch Intern Med, 112:*79, 1963.
812. Schmidt, D. M., et al.: *Am J Clin Pathol, 44:*546, 1965.
813. Palma, E. C.: *Am J Surg, 83:*723, 1952.
814. Colquhon: *Radiology, 86:*454, 1966.
815. Tracy, G. D., et al.: *Vasc Dis, 3:*10, 1969.
816. Halpern, M., et al.: *N Engl J Med, 273:*248, 1965.
817. Fleming, M. P., et al.: *Am J Roentgenol Radium Ther Nucl Med, 113:*452, 1971.
818. Mena, E., et al.: *Am J Roentgenol Radium Ther Nucl Med, 118:*39, 1973.
819. Carillo, F. J., et al.: *Am J Roentgenol Radium Ther Nucl Med, 115:*396, 1972.
820. Simpson, R. D., et al.: *Cancer, 17:*526, 1964.
821. Gold, R. E., et al.: *Radiology, 103:*85, 1972.
822. Handelsman, J. C., et al.: *Arch Surg, 91:*842, 1965.
823. Reuter, S. R., et al.: *Radiology, 94:*271, 1970.
824. Danaraj, T., et al.: *Circulation, 20:*856, 1960.
825. McKusick, V. A., et al.: *JAMA, 181:*5, 1962.
826. Lambeth, J. T., et al.: *Am J Roentgenol Radium Ther Nucl Med, 109:*553, 1970.
827. Gilkes, R., et al.: *Br J Radiol, 46:*110, 1973.
828. Husner, E., et al.: *Mayo Clin Proc, 15:*7, 1940.
829. Nelson, R. M., et al.: *Ann Thorac Surg, 8:*437, 1969.
830. Dick, R., et al.: *Am J Roentgenol Radium Ther Nucl Med, 110:*141, 1970.
831. DeVillers, J. C.: *Br Med J, 2:*140, 1966.
832. Husni, E. A., et al.: *Angiology, 18:*106, 1967.
833. Powers, S. R., Jr.: *Surgery, 49:*257, 1961.
834. Hardin, C. A., et al.: *Ann Surg, 158:*133, 1963.
835. Love, J. W., et al.: *Am J Surg, 109:*620, 1965.
836. Haimovici, H., et al.: *Surgery, 72:*789, 1972.
837. Villanueva, A., et al.: *J Cardiovasc Surg, 13:*617, 1972.
838. Hinsman, G., et al.: *Invest Radiol, 6:*341, 1971.
839. Reuter, S. R.: *Radiology, 98:*561, 1971.
840. Colopinto, R. F., et al.: *Radiology, 103:*557, 1972.
841. Lord, R. S. A., et al.: *Lancet, 2:*795, 1968.
842. Harjola, P. J., et al.: *Am J Surg, 115:*864, 1968.
843. Marable, S. A., et al.: *Am J Surg, 115:*97, 1968.
844. Curl, J. H., et al.: *Ann Surg, 173:*314, 1971.
845. Dunbar, J. D., et al.: *Am J Roentgenol Radium Ther Nucl Med, 95:*731, 1965.
846. Cornell, S. H.: *Radiology, 99:*311, 1971.
847. Szilagyi, D. E., et al.: *Surgery, 72:*849, 1972.
848. Rob, C.: *Arch Surg, 93:*21, 1966.
849. Snyder, M. A., et al.: *Surgery, 61:*372, 1967.
850. Ottesen, O. E., et al.: *Radiology, 84:*430, 1966.
851. Boley, S. J., et al.: In Boley, S. J. (Ed.): *Vascular Disorders of the Small Intestine.* New York, Appleton, 1971.

852. Mann, F. C., et al.: *Surgery, 4:*249, 1938.
853. May, A. G., et al.: *Surgery, 53:*513, 1963.
854. May, A. G., et al.: *Surgery, 54:*250, 1963.
855. Fiddian, R. V., et al.: *Arch Surg, 88:*83, 1964.
856. Oberez, I., et al.: *Radiology, 104:*545, 1972.
857. Holey, K. E., et al.: *Am J Med, 37:*14, 1964.
858. Vertes, V., et al.: *N Engl J Med, 270:*656, 1964.
859. Thal, A. P.: *Circulation, 27:*36, 1963.
860. Abrams, H. L:. *Invest Radiol, 7:*249, 1972.
861. Tillotson, P. M., et al.: *Radiology, 80:*261, 1963.
862. Reiner, L., et al.: In Boley, S. J. (Ed.): *Vascular Disorders of the Small Intestine.* New York, Appleton, 1971.
863. Fry, W. G., et al.: *Surg Gynecol Obstet, 117:* 417, 1963.
864. Morris, G. C., Jr., et al.: *Surg Clin North Am, 46:*919, 1966.
865. Keeley, F. X., et al.: *Gastroenterol, 37:*480, 1959.
866. Drapanas, T.: *Am J Surg, 115:*101, 1968.
867. Gardner, B., et al.: *Ann Surg, 153:*23, 1961.
868. Bookstein, J. J.: *Radiology, 93:*1007, 1969.
869. Calnon, J., et al.: *Lancet, 2:*537, 1962.
870. Adams, J. T., et al.: *Surgery, 63:*147, 1968.
871. Bedsole, D. O., et al.: *Ann Surg, 158:*1039, 1963.
872. McCleery, R. S., et al.: *Ann Surg, 133:*588, 1951.
873. Fred, H. L., et al.: *Circulation, 29:*758, 1964.
874. Theander, G.: *Acta Radiol Diagn (Stockh), 2:* 100, 1964.
875. Gullmo, A.: *Acta Radiol (Stockh), 47:*119, 1957.
876. Doppman, J., et al.: *Am J Roentgenol Radium Ther Nucl Med, 100:*411, 1967.
877. Kerr, M. G., et al.: *Br Med J, 1:*532, 1964.
878. Rubinson, R. M., et al.: *Arch Surg, 94:*766, 1967.
879. Bergstrand, I., et al.: *Acta Radiol Diagn (Stockh), 2:*1, 1964.
880. Peterson, O.: *Acta Radiol (Stockh), 55:*97, 1961.
881. Nordenstrom, B., et al.: *Acta Radiol Diagn (Stockh), 6:*65, 1967.
882. Lam, C. R., et al.: *Circulation (Suppl), 1:*31, 188, 1965.
883. Watkins, E., Jr., et al.: *Ann Surg, 159:*536, 1964.
884. Peck, M. E.: *Ann Surg, 146:*619, 1957.
885. Schrire, V., et al.: *Q J Med, 33:*439, 1964.
886. Widen, J.: *Acta Radiol Suppl (Stockh), 162:* , 1958.
887. Hinman, F., et al.: *Surg Gynecol Obstet, 42:* 209, 1926.
888. Idbohrn, H., et al.: *Acta Physiol Scand, 38:*200, 1956.
889. Holman, E.: *Surgery, 36:*3, 1954.
890. Robicsek, F., et al.: *Ann Surg, 147:*835, 1958.
891. Holman, E.: *Surg Gynecol Obstet, 100:*599, 1955.
892. Rodboard, S., et al.: *Angiology, 18:*349, 1966.
893. Roach, M., et al.: *Invest Rad, 5,* No. 5, 1970.
894. Edwards, B. F., et al.: *Surgery, 52:*444, 1962.
895. Kitteridge, R. D., et al.: *Radiology, 79:*799, 1962.
896. Morreels, C. L., Jr., et al.: *Radiology, 90:*1150, 1968.
897. Lehrer, H.: *Radiology, 89:*11, 1967.
898. Mayall, G. F.: *Clin Rad, 15:*355, 1964.
899. Theander, G.: *Acta Radiol (Stockh), 53:*417, 1960.
900. Amato, J. J., et al.: *J Cardiovasc Surg, 13:*147, 1972.
901. Wilson, L. B.: *Milit Surg, 49:*249, 1921.
902. Black, A. N., et al.: *Br Med J, 2:*872, 1941.
903. Gerwig, W. H., et al.: *Surgery, 59:*1065, 1966.
904. Whitaker, W. G., Jr., et al.: *Surg Gynecol Obstet, 99:*129, 1954.
905. Zilkha, R.: *Radiology, 97:*543, 1970.
906. Makin, G. S., et al.: *Circulation Suppl, 111:*120, 1964.
907. Stone, H. H., et al.: *Am Surg, 36:*869, 1968.
908. Margolies, M. N., et al.: *New Eng J Med, 283:* 317, 1972.
909. Janon, E. A.: *Radiology, 96:*55, 1970.
910. Bassett, F. H., et al.: *Arch Surg, 92:*13, 1966.
911. Murray, D. S.: *Br J Surg, 44:*556, 1957.
912. Collins, H. A., et al.: *J Bone Joint Surg, 43:*193, 1961.
913. Rosch, J.: *Roentgenology of the Spleen and Pancreas.* Springfield, Thomas, 1967.
914. Little, R. D., et al.: *Ann Int Med, 37:*197, 1952.
915. Stiles, P. J.: *J Bone Joint Surg, 47B:*507, 1965.
916. Moore, T. C.: *Ann Surg, 148:*111, 1958.
917. Shuck, J. M., et al.: *J Trauma, 12:*481, 1972.
918. Robicsek, F., et al.: *Angiology, 16:*18, 1965.
919. Fogerty, T. J., et al.: *Surg Gynecol Obstet, 121:* 1295, 1965.
920. McGarity, W. C., et al.: *Surg Gynecol Obstet, 106:*399, 1958.
921. Shumacker, H. B., Jr., et al.: *Ann Surg, 145:* 145, 1957.
922. Wessler, S., et al.: *Circulation, 7:*641, 1953.
923. Warren, S., et al.: *Ann Surg, 140:*311, 1954.
924. Lowenberg, E. L.: *South Med J, 51:*35, 1958.
925. Baird, R. J.: *Ann Surg, 160:*905, 1964.
926. Metcalfe, W. J.: *Ann Royal Coll Surg, 27:*407, 1960.
927. Miles, R. M., et al.: *Ann Surg, 160:*801, 1968.
928. Flory, C. M.: *Am J Pathol, 21:*549, 1945.
929. Kazmier, J. J.: *Vas Dis, 3:*12, 1966.
930. Handler, F. P.: *Am J Med, 20:*366, 1950.
931. Sieniewicz, D. J.: *Radiology, 92:*1231, 1969.
932. Eliot, R. S., et al.: *Circulation, 30:*611, 1964.

933. Maddison, F. E., et al.: *Am J Roentgenol Radium Ther Nucl Med, 107:*530, 1969.
934. Wood, E. H., et al.: *Acta Radiol (Stockh), 25-30:*520, 1967.
935. Bookstein, J. J.: *Radiology, 110:*25, 1974.
936. Mathur, V., et al.: *Invest Rad, 2:*304, 1967.
937. Björk, L., et al.: *Acta Radiol (Stockh), 3:*129, 1965.
938. Fleischner, F. G.: *Radiology, 87:*705, 1966.
939. Bookstein, J. J., et al.: *Radiology, 93:*1007, 1969.
940. Josephson, S., et al.: *Invest Rad, 5:*220, 1970.
941. Williams, H. J., et al.: *Am J Roentgenol Radium Ther Nucl Med, 116:*475, 1972.
942. DeMuth, W. E., Jr.: *JAMA, 179:*130, 1962.
943. Reiner, L., et al.: *Arch Pathol, 73:*461, 1962.
944. Reiner, L., et al.: *Gastroenterology, 39:*747, 1960.
945. Laufman, H., et al.: *Arch Surg, 88:*1021, 1964.
946. Fry, W. J.: In Strandness, D. E., Jr. (Ed.): *Collateral Circulation in Clinical Surgery.* Philadelphia, Saunders, 1969.
947. Marston, A.: *Ann Royal Coll Surg, 35:*150, 1964.
948. Ratner, I. A., et al.: *New Eng J Med, 263:*1122, 1960.
949. Carter, R., et al.: *Am J Surg, 98:*271, 1959.
950. DeMos, N. J., et al.: *Ann Surg, 155:*599, 1962.
951. Donahoe, P. K., et al.: *Ann Surg, 178:*138, 1973.
952. Madden, J. L.: *Arch Surg, 97:*853, 1968.
953. Kassirer, J. P.: *New Eng J Med, 280:*812, 1969.
954. Thurlbeck, W. T., et al.: *New Eng J Med, 257:* 442, 1957.
955. Fortner, J. G., et al.: *Ann Surg, 178:*162, 1972.
956. Lucas, R. J., et al.: *Ann Surg, 173:*238, 1971.
957. Thorley, L. G., et al.: *Radiology, 85:*56, 1965.
958. Loeffler, L.: *Arch Pathol, 21:*496, 1936.
959. Tsapogas, M. J., et al.: *Ann Surg, 178:*179, 1973.
960. Sjödahal, R., et al.: *Acta Chir Scand, 140:*77, 1964.
961. Eastland, M. W., III: *Am J Surg, 122:*558, 1971.
962. Stoane, L., et al.: *Radiology, 87:*262, 1966.
963. Winkelmann, R. K., et al.: *Am J Med, 51:*692, 1971.
964. Vanway, C. W., III, et al.: *Am J Surg, 117:*745, 1969.
965. Christeus, N., et al.: *Am J Surg, 115:*673, 1968.
966. Derrick, J. R.: *Surgery, 52:*309, 1962.
967. Dible, J. H.: *J Pathol Bact, 75:*1, 1958.
968. Filshie, I., et al.: *J Pathol Bact, 76:*71, 1958.
969. Cox, J. S. T.: *Surg Gynecol Obstet, 116:*593, 1963.
970. Greenstone, S. M., et al.: *Vas Dis, 3:*162, 1966.
971. Nilsson, I. M.: *Acta Chir Scand Suppl, 387:*15, 1967.
972. Virchow: Cited in R. Fontaine, et al., *Surgery, 41:*6, 1957.
973. Abeshouse, B. S.: *Urol Cutan Rev, 49:*661, 1945.
974. McCarthy, L. J., et al.: *Ann Int Med, 58:*837, 1963.
975. Pollack, V. E., et al.: *Post Grad Med, 40:*282, 1966.
976. Pollack, V. E., et al.: *Am J Med, 21:*496, 1956.
977. Harrison, D. V., et al.: *Q J Med, 25:*285, 1956.
978. Wagner, G. P.: JAMA, 209:*1661, 1969.*
979. Koehler, P. R., et al.: *Radiology, 86:*851, 1966.
980. Hipona, F. A., et al.: *Am J Roentgenol Radium Ther Nucl Med, 98:*122, 1966.
981. Chiat, A., et al.: *Radiology, 90:*886, 1968.
982. Zygliczynsk, et al.: *Polskiprezeglad Radiologii Medycyny Nuklearnej, 30:*1, 1966.
983. Parker, R. G. F.: *Medicine, 38:*369, 1959.
984. Gore, D. O., et al.: *Surgery, 49:*334, 1961.
985. Szur, L., et al.: *Br Med J, 2:*1273, 1956.
986. Calkins, E. A.: *Dis Chest, 30:*404, 1956.
987. Cha, E. M., et al.: *Radiology, 102:*605, 1972.
988. Wertheimer, M., et al.: *JAMA, 224:*1172, 1973.
989. Hansen, K. F.: *Radiology, 85:*433, 1965.
990. Smith, R. A., et al.: *Am J Surg, 96:*353, 1958.
991. Steinberg, I., et al.: *Arch Surg, 64:*10, 1952.
992. Maruyama, Y., et al.: *Radiology, 79:*617, 1962.
993. Steinberg, I.: *New Eng J Med, 264:*686, 1961.
994. Adams, J. T.: *Arch Surg, 91:*29, 1965.
995. Gallagher: *Angiology, 17:*377, 1966.
996. Russo, P. E., et al.: *South Med J, 47:*430, 1954.
997. Child, C. G., III: *Hepatic Circulation and Portal Circulation.* Philadelphia, Saunders, 1954.
998. Clatworthy, H. W., Jr., et al.: *Ann Surg, 150:* 371, 1959.
999. Clatworthy, H. W., Jr., et al.: *Ann Surg, 150:* 371, 1959.
1000. Benz, E. J., et al.: *Proc Staff Mayo Clin, 28:* 232, 1953.
1001. Lerman, B., et al.: *Ann Surg, 155:*441, 1962.
1002. Scherl, N. D., et al.: *Am J Gastroenterol, 53:* 164, 1970.
1003. Rosch, J., et al.: *Am J Roentgenol Radium Ther Nucl Med, 112:*143, 1971.
1004. Koop, C. E., et al.: *Ann Surg, 147:*17, 1958.
1005. Hewitt, R. L.: *New Eng J Med, 279:*595, 1968.
1006. Hughes, E. S. R.: *Br J Surg, 36:*155, 1948.
1007. Cucii, C. E., et al.: *Circulation, 27:*275, 1963.
1008. Wilder, J. R., et al.: *Surgery, 55:*214, 1964.
1009. Johnson, C., et al.: *Proc Staff Mayo Clin, 24:* 649, 1949.
1010. Warren, S., et al.: *Surg Gynecol Obstet, 61:*102, 1935.
1011. Duncan, R. D., et al.: *Am J Surg, 83:*205, 1952.
1012. Partington, P. F.: *Am J Surg, 101:*239, 1961.
1013. Ellis, D. L., et al.: *Am J Surg, 125:*641, 1973.

1014. Friedenberg, M. J., et al.: *Radiology, 85:*38, 1965.
1015. Polk, H. C., Jr.: *Ann Surg, 163:*432, 1966.
1016. Bosniak, M. A.: In Boley, S. J. (Ed.): *Vascular Disorders of the Small Intestine.* New York, Appleton, 1971.
1017. Pressman, B. D., et al.: *Am J Roentgenol Radium Ther Nucl Med, 119:*115-73, 1971.
1018. Navarra, V. G., et al.: *JAMA, 226:*1466, 1973.
1019. Womack, N. A., et al.: *Ann Surg, 153:*1006, 1961.
1020. Bindeglass, et al.: *Ann Int Med, 48:*876, 1958.
1021. Berdon, W. E., et al.: *Radiology, 88:*111, 1967.
1022. Nylander, G.: *Acta Chir Scand Supply, 387:*30, 1967.
1023. Brodelius, A., et al.: *Am J Roentgenol Radium Ther Nucl Med, 111:*794, 1971.
1024. Thomas, Lea M., et al.: *Radiology, 99:*37, 1971.
1025. Almén, T., et al.: *Acta Radiol (Diag) (Stockh), 2:*345, 1964.
1026. Arkoff, R. S., et al.: *Radiology, 90:*66, 1968.
1027. Bors, E., et al.: *Surg Gynecol Obstet, 99:*451, 1954.
1028. Cope, C., et al.: *Radiology, 109:*581, 1973.
1029. Brodelius, A., et al.: *Radiology, 101:*297, 1971.
1030. Von Dangen, R. J. A. M.: *Photographic Atlas of Reconstructive Arterial Surgery.* New York, Springer-Verlag.
1031. DeBakey, M. E., et al.: *Ann Surg, 154:*698, 1961.
1032. DeBakey, M. E., et al.: *Ann Surg, 149:*690, 1959.
1033. Widmer, L. K., et al.: *Circulation, 30:*836, 1964.
1034. Leriche, R., et al.: *Ann Surg, 127:*193, 1948.
1035. Wyatt, J. M., et al.: *Radiology, 69:*676, 1957.
1036. Starrer, F., et al.: *Br Med J, 2:*644, 1960.
1037. Cherry, J. K., Maj., et al.: *Arch Surg, 93:*671, 1966.
1038. Robb, D.: *Br J Surg, 48:*221, 1960-61.
1039. Gitlitz, G. F.: *Vas Dis, 2:*121, 1965.
1040. Calem, W. S., et al.: *Surgery, 52:*612, 1962.
1041. Perlow, S.: *Am J Surg, 105:*285, 1963.
1042. Hiertonn, T., et al.: *Br J Surg, 44:*348, 1956-57.
1043. Gross, L., et al.: *Radiology, 93:*664, 1969.
1044. Burchmore, J. W., et al.: *Lancet, 2:*1008, 1962.
1045. Chavez, C. M., et al.: *Arch Surg, 93:*667, 1966.
1046. Massachusetts General Hospital, C. P. C.: *New Eng J Med, 279:*1279, 1968.
1047. Scotti, T. M.: In Anderson, W. A. D. (Ed.): *Pathology,* 5th ed. St. Louis, Mosby, 1966.
1048. Seagall, H. N.: *Surg Gynecol Obstet, 37:*152, 1923.
1049. Wooling, K., et al.: *Proc Staff Mayo Clin, 28:* 239, 1953.
1050. Foa, P.: *Anat UZ Allg Pathol, 5:*275, 1889.
1051. Oliva, D., et al.: *Am J Roentgenol Radium Ther Nucl Med, 98:*70, 1966.
1052. Asher, S. B.: *Ann Int Med, 23:*431, 1945.
1053. Scatliff, J. H., et al.: *Am J Roentgenol Radium Ther Nucl Med, 108:*674, 1970.
1054. Regan, F. C., et al.: *J Urol, 59:*981, 1948.
1055. Sweet, E. I., et al.: *Radiology, 92:*849, 1969.
1056. Vance, B. M.: *Arch Surg, 16:*631, 1928.
1057. Hardy, K. J., et al.: *Surg Gyn Obstet, 134:*39, 1972.
1058. Clarke, R.: *Lancet, 267:*877, 1954.
1059. Solheim, K.: *Acta Chir Scand, 126:*579, 1963.
1060. Parsons, L., et al.: *Ann Surg, 147:*214, 1958.
1061. Whitesell, F. B., Jr.: *Surg Gynecol Obstet, 110:* 750, 1960.
1062. Upadhyaya, P., et al.: *Surg Gynecol Obstet, 126:*781, 1968.
1063. Love, L., et al.: *Radiology, 91:*96, 1968.
1064. Gold, R. E., et al.: *Am J Roentgenol Radium Ther Nucl Med, 116:*413, 1972.
1065. Norell, H. G.: *Acta Rad (Stockh), 48:*445, 1957.
1066. Mills, R. H. B.: *Gut, 2:*267, 1961.
1067. Sandblom: *Surgery, 24:*57, 1948.
1068. Vasko, J. S., et al.: *Ann Surg, 163:*144, 1966.
1069. Markgraf, W. H., et al.: *Arch Surg, 81:*860, 1960.
1070. Boijsen, E., et al.: *Acta Radiol (Diag) (Stockh), 11:*363, 1971.
1071. Levin, D. C., et al.: *Am J Roentgenol Radium Ther Nucl Med, 119:*95, 1973.
1072. Nahum, H., et al.: *Radiology, 109:*557, 1973.
1073. Opit, L. J.: *Br J Surg, 48:*240, 1960-61.
1074. Sargeant, J. C., et al.: *J Urol, 63:*1, 1950.
1075. Forsythe, W. E., et al.: *Am J Surg, 97:*558, 1959.
1076. Elkin, M., et al.: *Am J Roentgenol Radium Ther Nucl Med, 98:*1, 1966.
1077. Waugh, W. H., et al.: *Circulation Res, 6:*116, 1958.
1078. Page, I. H.: *Science, 89:*273, 1939.
1079. Thompson, R. J., et al.: *Ann Surg, 163:*153, 1966.
1080. Cullota, R. J., et al.: *Surgery, 40:*320, 1956.
1081. Howell, J. F., et al.: *J Trauma, 1:*32, 1961.
1082. Stone, H. H., et al.: *Arch Surg, 85:*525, 1962.
1083. Haertel, M., et al.: *Br J Radiol, 47:*641, 1974.
1084. Hepler, A. B.: *Surg Gynecol Obstet, 50:*668, 1930.
1085. Martin, D. C.: *Am J Surg, 121:*351, 1971.
1086. Oppenheimer, G. D.: *Ann Surg, 100:*1130, 1964.
1087. Wright, F. W., et al.: *Clin Radiol, 25:*27, 1974.
1088. Ivemark, B. I., et al.: *Acta Chir Scand, 115:*100, 1958.
1089. Zuckner, J.: *Arch Pathol, 50:*468, 1950.

1090. Gregorie, H. B., Jr., et al.: *Surgery, 52:*860, 1962.
1091. Cerise, E. J., et al.: *Surgery, 63:*903, 1968.
1092. Becker, W. F., et al.: *Ann Surg, 161:*845, 1965.
1093. Warren, K. W., et al.: *Ann Surg, 163:*886, 1966.
1094. Judd, E. S., et al.: *Arch Surg, 22:*838, 1931.
1095. Greenstein, A., et al:. *Surgery, 69:*56, 1971.
1096. Zeller, M., et al.: *JAMA, 195:*869, 1966.
1097. Warshaw, A. L., et al.: *New Eng J Med, 287:* 72, 1972.
1098. Lahey, F. H., et al.: *Ann Surg, 100:*231, 1934.
1099. Walker, A. R., et al.: *Ann Surg, 178:*13, 1973.
1100. Fowler, R. H.: *Ann Surg, 57:*638, 1913.
1101. King, M. C., et al.: *Surg Gynecol Obstet, 127:* 509, 1968.
1102. Shanser, J. D., et al.: *Am J Roentgenol Radium Ther Nucl Med, 119:*166, 1973.
1103. Henson, S. W., Jr., et al.: *Surg Gynecol Obstet, 103:*607, 1956.
1104. Henson, S. W., Jr., et al.: *Surg Gynecol Obstet, 104:*63, 302, 551, 1957.
1105. Baltaxe, H. A., et al.: *Radiology, 97:*599, 1970.
1106. Garti, I., et al.: *Clin Radiol, 22:*466, 1971.
1107. McNulty, J.: *Am J Roentgenol Radium Ther Nucl Med, 102:*380, 1968.
1108. Rizk, G. K., et al.: *Radiology, 99:*303, 1971.
1109. McLoughlin, M. J., et al.: *Clin Radiol, 23:*377, 1972.
1110. Longmire, W. P., Jr., et al.: *Ann Surg, 174:*711, 1971.
1111. Ferris, E.: *Venography of the Inferior Venacava and Its Branches.* Baltimore, Williams & Wilkins, 1969.
1112. Lagergren, C., et al.: *Acta Radiol (Stockh), 52:* 401, 1959.
1113. Marshall, J. F.: *Ann Surg, 149:*126, 1959.
1114. Light, H. G., et al.: *Cancer, 13:*816, 1960.
1115. Meyers, M. A.: *Radiology, 89:*483, 1967.
1116. Takeuchi, J., et al.: *Am J Med, 51:*11, 1971.
1117. Kimura, C., et al.: *J Cardio Vas Surg, 4:*87, 1963.
1118. Kimura, C.: *Surgery, 72:*551, 1972.
1119. Schaffner, F., et al.: *Am J Med, 42:*838, 1967.
1120. Rossall, R. E., et al.: *J Clin Pathol, 10:*40, 1957.
1121. Negus, D., et al.: *Br J Surg, 55:*369, 1968.
1122. Stevenson, J. E., et al.: *Am J Med, 51:*553, 1971.
1123. Silverman, J. F., et al.: *Radiology, 102:*581, 1972.
1124. Moffat, R. E., et al.: *Radiology, 104:*283, 1972.
1125. Schoene, R. H.; *Ohio State Med J, 59:*695, 1963.
1126. Gibson, T. E.: *J Urol, 60:*838, 1948.
1127. Richmond, J., et al.: *Am J Med, 32:*184, 1962.
1128. Chuang, V. P., et al.: *Radiology, 111:*53, 1974.
1129. Jonutis, A. J.: *Clin Radiol, 24:*468, 1973.
1130. Castellino, R. A., et al.: *Am J Roentgenol Radium Ther Nucl Med, 114:*574, 1972.
1131. Ahmann, D. L., et al.: *Cancer, 19:*461, 1966.
1132. Bosniak, M. A.: *Radiology, 84:*692, 1965.
1133. Siegelman, S. S., et al.: *Radiology, 90:*1084, 1968.
1134. Steinberg, I.: *Am J Cardiol, 7:*33, 1961.
1135. Bryk, D., et al.: *Radiology, 93:*273, 1969.
1136. Dinsmore, et al.: *Radiology, 86:*425, 1966.
1137. Spitz, H. B., et al.: *Radiology, 103:*69, 1972.
1138. Meyers, M. A.: *Radiology, 92:*1035, 1969.
1139. Lunderquist, A., et al.: *Am J Roentgenol Radium Ther Nucl Med, 103:*354, 1968.
1140. Chang, T. T., et al.: *Am J Roentgenol Radium Ther Nucl Med, 117:*317, 1973.
1141. Buranasiri, S. I., et al.: *Radiology, 109:*555, 1973.
1142. Cohn, J. H., et al.: *Am J Med, 53:*704, 1972.
1143. Hinshaw, D. B.: *Am J Surg, 102:*224, 1961.
1144. Hollenberg, N. K., et al.: *Am J Med Science, 261:*233, 1971.
1145. Daniel, P. M.: *Q J Exper Physiol, 37:*11, 1952.
1146. Beuren, A. J.: *Circulation, 39:*109, 1969.
1147. Ertrugral, A.: *Circulation, 36:*400, 1967.
1148. Rabinov, K., et al.: *Vas Dis, 3:*122, 1966.
1149. Staple, T. W., et al.: *Acta Radiol (Stockh), 4:* 293, 1966.
1150. Davidson, A. J.: *Invest Radiol, 8:*363, 1973.
1151. Asken, M. H.: *Ann Roy Coll Surg, 40:*82, 1967.
1152. Baehr, G., et al.: *Arch Pathol, 7:*458, 1929.
1153. Hollenberg, N. K., et al.: *Am J Med, 47:*845, 1969.
1154. Davidson, A. J., et al.: *Radiology, 92:*975, 1969.
1155. Foster, R. S., et al.: *Am J Roentgenol Radium Ther Nucl Med, 95:*291, 1965.
1156. Graham, R. S.: *Am J Pathol, 4:*17, 1928.
1157. Jill, W. M., Jr., et al.: *Radiology, 96:*81, 1970.
1158. Ljungquist, A.: *J Pathol Bact, 84:*313, 1962.
1159. Greenblatt, M.: *Lab Invest, 12:*1271, 1963.
1160. Mena, E., et al.: *Radiology, 108:*523, 1973.
1161. Hodson, C. J.: *Radiology, 88:*857, 1967.
1162. Scanlon, G. T.: *Radiology, 94:*401, 1970.
1163. Lester, P. D., et al.: *Radiology, 99:*517, 1971.
1164. Pirani, C. L.: In Abramson, D. I. (Ed.): *Blood Vessels and Lymphatics.* New York, Academic, 1962.
1165. Lagergren, C., et al.: *Virch Arch Pathol, 335:* 584, 1962.
1166. Nebesar, R., et al.: *Am J Roentgenol Radium Ther Nucl Med, 106:*81, 1969.
1167. Mann, J. D., et al.: *Gastroenterol, 25:*540, 1953.
1168. Mann, J. D., et al.: *Proc Staff Mayo Clin, 28:* 227, 1953.
1169. Fuchs, W. A., et al.: *Invest Radiol, 7:*369, 1972.
1170. Pollard, J. J., et al.: *Radiology, 86:*276, 1966.
1171. Bradley, S. E.: *Circulation, 5:*419, 1952.
1172. Johnson, A. G., et al.: *Br J Radiol, 42:*937, 1969.
1173. Dencker, H., et al:. *Am J Roentgenol Radium Ther Nucl Med, 114:*476, 1972.

1174. Guglielmo, L. D., et al.: *Acta Radiol (Stockh), 44:*121, 1955.
1175. Hagstrom, J. W. C., et al.: *Circulation, 26:*726, 1962.
1176. Dungan, W. T., et al.: *Am J Dis Child, 119:* 401, 1970.
1177. Steinberg, I., et al.: *Am J Roentgenol Radium Ther Nucl Med, 106:*1, 1969.
1178. Boström, K., et al.: *Acta Radiol (Diag) (Stockh), 6:*105, 1967.
1179. Robicsek, et al.: *Vas Dis, 4:*101, 1970.
1180. Derrick, J. R., et al.: *Surgery, 58:*381, 1965.
1181. Alley, R. D., et al.: *Clin Res, 6:*41, 1958.
1182. Burchell, A. R., et al.: *Ann Surg, 162:*981, 1965.
1183. Bookstein, J. J., et al.: *Invest Radiol, 6:*101, 1971.
1184. Aishi, N., et al.: *Arch Surg, 81:*80, 1960.
1185. Rosenberg, J. C.: *Surgery, 69:*294, 1971.
1186. Shaldon, S., et al.: *Am J Med, 32:*758, 1962.
1187. Rappaport, A. M., et al.: *Gastroenterol, 46:*115, 1964.
1188. Atkinson, M., et al.: *Q J Med, 24:*77, 1955.
1189. Warren, W. D., et al.: *Ann Surg, 150:*413, 1959.
1190. Rousselot, L. M., et al.: *Ann Surg, 150:*384, 1959.
1191. Viamonte, M.: Radiological Society of North America. Chicago, 1973.
1192. Popper, H., et al.: *Am J Clin Pathol, 22:*717, 1952.
1193. Perloff, D., et al.: *Am J Surgery, 107:*97, 1964.
1194. Page, I. H., et al.: *Ann Int Med, 51:*196, 1959.
1195. Poutasse: *Am J Surg, 107:*97, 1964.
1196. Stamey, T. A., et al.: *Medicine, 40:*347, 1961.
1197. Maldanado, J. E., et al.: *Am J Med, 37:*499, 1964.
1198. Barry, W. F., Jr., et al.: *Am J Roentgenol Radium Ther Nucl Med, 98:*132, 1966.
1199. White, A. A., et al.: *Radiology, 95:*139, 1970.
1200. Karani, S., et al.: *Clin Radiol, 13:*287, 1962.
1201. Lampe, W. T., II: *Angiology, 16:*677, 1965.
1202. Clayman, A. S., et al.: *Radiology, 108:*107, 1973.
1203. Hickler, R. B.: *Am J Surg, 109:*715, 1965.
1204. Nemoy, N. J., et al.: *JAMA, 225:*512, 1973.
1205. Crummy, A. B., Jr., et al.: *Radiology, 84:*104, 1965.
1206. Engel, W. J., et al.: *J Urol, 73:*735, 1955.
1207. Zimmerman, S. J.: *New Eng J Med, 264:*238, 1961.
1208. Cornell, S. H.: *Radiology, 92:*880, 1969.
1209. Klatte, E. C., et al.: *Am J Roentgenol Radium Ther Nucl Med, 114:*696, 1972.
1210. Lang, E. K.: *Radiology, 92:*984, 1969.
1211. DeCamp, P. T.: *Surgery, 43:*134, 1958.
1212. Amplatz, K.; *Radiology, 83:*816, 1964.
1213. Pack, G. T., and Ariel, I. M.: *Tumors of the Soft Somatic Tissues.* New York, Hoeber & Harper, 1958.
1214. Evans, R. W.: *Histological Appearances of Tumors.* Edinburgh, London, E&S Livingstone, 1956.
1215. Jenkins, H. P., et al.: *Surg Gynecol Obstet, 55:* 466, 1932.
1216. Bartley, O., et al.: *Acta Radiol (Stockh), 51:*81, 1959.
1217. McLoughlin, M. J.; *Am J Roentgenol Radium Ther Nucl Med, 113:*50, 1971.
1218. Abrams, R. M., et al.: *Radiology, 92:*308, 1969.
1219. Henson, S. W., Jr., et al.: *Surg Gynecol Obstet, 103:*327, 1956.
1220. Edmondson, H. A.: *Am J Dis Child, 91:*168, 1956.
1221. Moss, A. A., et al.: *Am J Roentgenol Radium Ther Nucl Med, 113:*61, 1967.
1222. Berdon, W. E., et al.: *Radiology, 92:*1523, 1969.
1223. Tada, S., et al.: *Radiology, 104:*603, 1972.
1224. Anderson, J. B.: *Acta Radiol (Diag) (Stockh), 2:*201, 1964.
1225. Mahadevan, H., et al.: *Radiology, 106:*627, 1973.
1226. Angervall: *Acta Radiol (Diag) (Stockh), 7:*65, 1968.
1227. Peterson, N. E., et al.: *J Urol, 105:*27, 1971.
1228. Kaufman, S. L.: *Cancer, 13:*695, 1960.
1229. Stout, A. P.: *Cancer, 2:*1027, 1949.
1230. Wray, R. C., Jr., et al.: *Ann Surg, 174:*1009, 1971.
1231. Rösch, J.: *Selective Angiography, Section 18, Golden's Diagnostic Radiology.* Baltimore, Williams & Wilkins, 1972.
1232. Conley, J., et al.: *Surg Gynecol Obstet, 126:* 825, 1968.
1233. Wilson, G. H., et al.: *Radiology, 92:*279, 1969.
1234. Martin, H., et al.: *Ann Surg, 127:*513, 1948.
1235. Ackerman, L. V.: *Surgical Pathology,* 5th ed. St. Louis, Mosby, 1974.
1236. Schiff, M.: *Laryngoscope, 69:*981, 1959.
1237. Bergström, K. E.: *Acta Radiol (Stockh), 42:*33, 1954.
1238. Haylock, A.: *Clin Radiol, 14:*304, 1963.
1239. Warren, S.: In Anderson, W. A. O. (Ed.): *Pathology,* 5th ed. St. Louis, Mosby, 1966.
1240. Teates, C. D., et al.: *Am J Roentgenol Radium Ther Nucl Med, 116:*419, 1972.
1241. Coe, J. I., et al.: *Am J Physiol, 28:*663, 1952.
1242. Wesler, L., et al.: *Am J Roentgenol Radium Ther Nucl Med, 92:*1150, 1964.
1243. Schrijver, H., et al.: *Acta Med Scand, 158:*235, 1957.
1244. Anderson, W. A. D. (Ed.): *Pathology,* 5th ed. St. Louis, Mosby, 1966.
1245. Love, L., et al.: *Am J Roentgenol Radium Ther Nucl Med, 95:*406, 1965.

1246. Viamonte, M., Jr., et al.: *Am J Roentgenol Radium Ther Nucl Med, 98:*723, 1966.
1247. Berg, J. W.: *Cancer, 8:*759, 1955.
1248. Wright, F. W., et al.: *Clin Radiol, 25:*27, 1974.
1249. Schamblem, M., et al.: *Am J Med, 55:*87, 1973.
1250. Conn, J. W., et al.: *Radiology, 106:*543, 1973.
1251. Skucas, J., et al.: *Surg Gynecol Obstet, 137:*35, 1973.
1252. Compton, W. R., et al.: Radiological Society of North America. Chicago, 1974.
1253. Arey, L. B.: *Developmental Anatomy Textbook of LAB Manual and Embryology.* Philadelphia, W. B. Saunders, 1954.
1254. Abell, M. R., et al.: *Human Pathol, 1:*503, 1970.
1255. Palacios, E.: *Am J Roentgenol Radium Ther Nucl Med, 110:*129, 1970.
1256. Olson, J. R., et al.: *Cancer, 23:*1358, 1969.
1257. Cordell, A. R., et al.: *Ann Surg, 165:*880, 1967.
1258. Spitzer, R., et al.: *Radiology, 98:*577, 1971.
1259. Wychulis, A. R., et al.: *Arch Surg, 91:*690, 1965.
1260. Schecter, M. M.: *Acta Radiol (Diag) (Stockh), 5:*488, 1966.
1261. Algire, G. H., et al.: *J Nat Can Inst, 6:*73, 1945.
1262. Myers, M. B., et al.: *Arch Surg, 102:*49, 1971.
1263. Menkin, V.: *Science, 123:*527, 1956.
1264. Donnellan, W.: In Preston, F. W. and Beal, J. M. (Eds.): *Basic Surgical Physiology.* Chicago, Yearbook Med., 1969.
1265. Schoeft, G. I.: *Virch Arch Pathol, 337:*97, 1963.
1266. Clark, E. R., et al.: *Anat Rec, 50:*129, 1931.
1267. Lagergren, C., et al.: *Acta Radiol (Stockh), 49:*441, 1958.
1268. Pinto, R. S., et al.: *Am J Roentgenol Radium Ther Nucl Med, 110:*808, 1970.
1269. Kinkhabwala, M., et al.: *Radiology, 109:*553, 1973.
1270. Schobinger, R.: *Acta Radiol (Stockh), 52:*28, 1959.
1271. Lunderquist, A., et al.: *Am J Roentgenol Radium Ther Nucl Med, 101:*338, 1967.
1272. Boijsen, E., et al.: *Radiology, 87:*1028, 1966.
1273. McAlister, W. H., et al.: *Radiology, 79:*769, 1962.
1274. Müsbichler, H.: *Radiology, 107:*21, 1973.
1275. Steinbach, H., et al.: In Abrams, H. L. (Ed.): *Angiography.* Boston, Little, 1971.
1276. Hutcheson, J., et al.: *Radiology, 102:*57, 1972.
1277. Probst, F. P.: *Acta Radiol (Diag) (Stockh), 11:*55, 1971.
1278. Stener, B., et al.: *Acta Radiol (Diag) (Stockh), 4:*169, 1966.
1279. Golden, A.: In Bloodworth, J. M. B., Jr. (Ed.): *Endocrine Pathology.* Baltimore, Williams & Wilkins, 1968.
1280. Benson, R. E., et al.: *Surgery, 21:*353, 1947.
1281. Campbell, J. A., et al.: *J Clin Pathol, 15:*432, 1962.
1282. McAlister, W. H., et al.: *Radiology, 79:*769, 1962.
1283. Margulis, A. R., et al.: *Am J Roentgenol Radium Ther Nucl Med, 86:*103, 1961.
1284. Riba, P. O., et al.: *Am J Roentgenol Radium Ther Nucl Med, 117:*287, 1973.
1285. Billings, K.: *Radiology, 104:*19, 1972.
1286. Hanafee, W., et al.: *Selective Angiography, Section 18, Golden's Diagnostic Radiology.* Baltimore, Williams & Wilkins, 1972.
1287. Herzberg, D. L., et al.: *Am J Roentgenol Radium Ther Nucl Med, 111:*541, 1971.
1288. Dossantos, R.: *J Bone Joint Surg, 32B:*17, 1950.
1289. Strickland, B.: *Br J Radiol, 32:*705, 1959.
1290. Cramer, W.: *Br J Exper Pathol, 1:*184, 1920.
1291. Brines, O. A., et al.: *Am J Physiol, 25:*467, 1949.
1292. Melicow, M. M.: *Arch Pathol, 63:*367, 1967.
1293. English, J. T., et al.: *Radiology, 107:*279, 1973.
1294. Angervall, L., et al.: *Cancer, 17:*685, 1964.
1295. Murphy, G. P., et al.: *J Urol, 103:*31, 1970.
1296. Trinkle, A. J.: *Am J Cancer, 27:*676, 1936.
1297. Abrams, R. M., et al.: *Radiology, 89:*1028, 1967.
1298. Singleton, A. O., Jr., et al.: *Ann Surg, 155:*663, 1962.
1299. Zollinger, R. M., et al.: *Am J Med, 29:*761, 1960.
1300. Lacy, P. E.: In Bloodworth, J. M. B., Jr. (Ed.): *Endocrinic Pathology.* Baltimore, Williams & Wilkins.
1301. Bookstein, J. J., et al.: *Radiology, 86:*682, 1966.
1302. Auerbach, R. C., et al.: *Am J Roentgenol Radium Ther Nucl Med, 119:*133, 1973.
1303. Robins, J. M., et al.: *Radiology, 106:*525, 1973.
1304. Gray, R. K., et al.: *Radiology, 96:*39, 1970.
1305. Yamagata, F. S., et al.: *Am J Roentgenol Radium Ther Nucl Med, 120:*634, 1974.
1306. Korobkin, M. T., et al.: *Radiology, 100:*319, 1971.
1307. Deutsch, V., et al.: *Am J Roentgenol Radium Ther Nucl Med, 119:*121, 1973.
1308. Henson, S. W., Jr., et al.: *Surg Gynecol Obstet, 103:*23, 1956.
1309. Edmondson, H. A.: Tumors of the Liver and the Intrahepatic Bile Ducts. Atlas: *Tumor Pathology.* Armed Forces Inst Pathology (Fascicle 25), Washington, D.C. (1958).
1310. Palubinskas, A. J.: *Radiology, 89:*444, 1967.
1311. Danais, S., et al.: *Am J Roentgenol Radium Ther Nucl Med, 118:*836, 1973.
1312. Sackett, J. F., et al.: *Am J Roentgenol Radium Ther Nucl Med, 113:*56, 1971.
1314. Goldstein, H. M., et al.: *Radiology, 111:*339, 1974.
1315. Straube, K. R., et al.: *Am J Roentgenol Radium Ther Nucl Med, 98:*222, 1966.
1316. Priestley, J. T., et al.: *Arch Surg, 86:*778, 1963.
1317. Stackpole, R. H., et al.: *J Pediatr, 63:*315, 1963.

1318. Scott, H. W., Jr., et al.: *Surg Gynecol Obstet, 120:*707, 1965.
1319. Hume, D. M.: *Am J Surg, 99:*458, 1960.
1320. Schimke, R. N., et al.: *New Eng J Med, 279:*1, 1968.
1321. Moore, T.: *Br J Urol, 35:*384, 1963.
1322. Malter, I.: *Radiology, 97:*56, 1970.
1323. Lecky, J. W.: *Selective Angiography, Section 18, Golden's Diagnostic Radiology.* Baltimore, Williams & Wilkins, 1972.
1324. Maier, H. C., et al.: *J Thor Cardiovasc Surg, 36:*625, 1958.
1325. Greer, W. E. R., et al.: *Am J Surg, 107:*192, 1964.
1326. Gifford, R. W., et al.: *Proc Staff Meet Mayo Clin, 39:*281, 1964.
1327. Scharf, Y., et al.: *JAMA, 215:*1323, 1971.
1328. McGuire, L. B.: *Ann Int Med, 60:*125, 1964.
1329. Reuter, S. R., et al.: *Radiology, 89:*805, 1967.
1330. Mikaelsson, C. G.: *Acta Radiol (Diag) (Stockh), 8:*129, 1969.
1331. Danowski, T. S.: *Clinical Endocrinology.* Baltimore, Williams & Wilkins, 1962.
1332. Dix, V. W.: *Br J Urol, 35:*355, 1963.
1333. Russell, R. P., et al.: *Am J Med, 54:*44, 1973.
1334. Conn, J. W., et al.: *Am J Surg, 107:*159, 1964.
1335. Smithwick, R. H., et al.: *Am J Surg, 107:*178, 1964.
1336. Kahn, P. C., et al.: *Radiology, 101:*71, 1971.
1337. Krementz, E. T., et al.: *Ann Surg, 173:*872, 1971.
1338. Nathaniels, E. K., et al.: *Ann Surg, 171:*165, 1970.
1339. Dodds, W. J., et al.: *Radiology, 91:*923, 1968.
1340. Kuntz, C. H., et al.: *Radiology, 102:*21, 1972.
1341. Doppman, J. L., et al.: *Radiology, 90:*527, 1969.
1342. Salyer, W. R., et al.: *Angiology, 25:*510, 1974.
1343. Ormond, J. K.: *JAMA, 174:*41, 1960.
1344. Morgoles, J. S., et al.: *Arch Surg, 81:*660, 1960.
1345. Neistadt, A., et al.: *Surgery, 59:*950, 1966.
1346. Reuter, S. R., et al.: *Radiology, 94:*271, 1970.
1347. Ramer, M., et al.: *Am J Roentgenol Radium Ther Nucl Med, 113:*263, 1971.
1348. Stout, A. P.: *Surg Gynecol Obstet, 84:*100, 1947.
1349. McDonald, P.: In Abrams, H. L. (Ed.): *Angiography.* Boston, Little, 1971.
1350. McLoughlin, M. J., et al.: *Radiology, 107:*257, 1973.
1351. McLoughlin, M. J., et al.: *Clin Radiol, 23:*377, 1972.
1352. Goldstein, H. M., et al.: *Radiology, 111:*339, 1974.
1353. McMullen, C. T., et al.: *Am J Roentgenol Radium Ther Nucl Med, 117:*380, 1973.
1354. Kelty, R. H., et al.: *Gastroenterol, 15:*285, 1950.
1355. Wright, R. D.: *J Pathol Bact, 45:*405, 1937.
1356. Rabinovitz, J. G., et al.: *Am J Roentgenol Radium Ther Nucl Med, 121:*401, 1974.
1357. Folkman, J.: *New Eng J Med, 285:*1182, 1971.
1358. Algire, G. H., et al.: *J Nat Cancer Inst, 6:*73, 1945.
1359. Algire, G. H., et al.: *J Nat Cancer Inst, 8:*53, 1947.
1360. Gierke, E.: *Sci Rep Imp Cancer: Res Fund, 3:*115, 1908.
1361. Spjut, H. J., et al.: *Am J Roentgenol Radium Ther Nucl Med, 92:*1173, 1964.
1362. Kligerman, M. M., et al.: *Radiology, 76:*810, 1961.
1363. Breedi, C., et al.: *Fed Proc, 8:*351, 1949.
1364. Breedi, C., et al.: *Am J Physiol, 30:*969, 1954.
1365. Pinet, F., et al.: *Ann Radiol, 15:*437, 1972.
1366. Stulberg, H. J., et al.: *Radiology, 85:*46, 1965.
1367. Bierman, H. R., et al.: *J Nat Cancer Inst, 12:*701, 1952.
1368. Ruzicka, F. F., Jr., et al.: *Radiology, 96:*261, 1970.
1369. Sprayregen, S.: *Radiology, 106:*529, 1973.
1370. Glenn, F., et al.: *Surg Gynecol Obstet, 123:*1037, 1966.
1371. Clifton, E. F.: *Am J Med, 21:*760, 1956.
1372. Crohn, B. B.: *Am J Med Sci, 148:*839, 1914.
1373. Reuter, S. R., et al.: *Radiology, 96:*93, 1970.
1374. Nebesar, R. A., et al.: *Radiology, 89:*1017, 1967.
1375. Bookstein, J. J., et al.: *Radiology, 93:*757, 1969.
1376. Rösch, J., et al.: *Am J Roentgenol Radium Ther Nucl Med, 94:*182, 1965.
1377. Eisenberg, H.: In Hilal, H. K. (Ed.): *Small Vessel Angiography.* St. Louis, Mosby, 1973.
1378. Pollack, O. J.: *Ann N Y Acad Sci, 149:*928, 1968.
1379. Bron, K. M., et al.: *N Y State J Med, 67:*1875, 1967.
1380. Baron, M. G., et al.: *Am J Roentgenol Radium Ther Nucl Med, 101:*649, 1967.
1381. Glenn, F., et al.: *Ann Surg, 159:*945, 1964.
1382. Deutsch, V.: *Am J Roentgenol Radium Ther Nucl Med, 101:*608, 1967.
1383. Reuter, S. R., et al.: *Br J Radiol, 44:*636, 1971.
1384. Sprayregen, S., et al.: *Am J Roentgenol Radium Ther Nucl Med, 116:*382, 1972.
1385. Abrams, R. M., et al.: *Radiology, 94:*277, 1970.
1386. Kaude, J., et al.: *Radiology, 100:*573, 1971.
1387. Moertel, C. G., et al.: *Cancer, 14:*901, 1961.
1388. Pearson, C. M.: *Cancer, 2:*1005, 1949.
1389. Ostermiller, W. E., et al.: *Arch Surg, 93:*616, 1966.
1390. Horsley, B. L., et al.: *Am Surg, 36:*676, 1970.
1391. Morin, L. J., et al.: *JAMA, 216:*1647, 1971.
1392. Boijsen, E., et al.: *Acta Radiol (Diag) (Stockh), 15:*65, 1974.
1393. Schwartz, D. T.: *Angiology, 21:*569, 1970.
1394. Baum, S.: In Stein, G. N., and Finkelstein,

A. K. (Eds.): *Tumor Atlas of the GI Tract, Duodenum, Small Intestine and Colon.* Chicago, Yearbook Med., 1973.
1395. Mojab: Cook County Hospital, Chicago (Personal communication).
1396. Sjoerdsma, A., et al.: *Am J Med, 20:*520, 1956.
1397. Buist, T. A. S.: *Am J Roentgenol Radium Ther Nucl Med, 120:*653, 1974.
1398. Brindle, M. J.: *Clin Rad, 23:*321, 1972.
1399. Love, L., et al.: *Radiology, 92:*855, 1969.
1400. Becker, J. A., et al.: *Radiology, 88:*691, 1967.
1401. Watson, R. C., et al.: *Radiology, 91:*888, 1968.
1402. Baltaxe, H. A., et al.: *Am J Roentgenol Radium Ther Nucl Med, 120:*648, 1974.
1403. Foot, N. C., et al.: *J Urol, 61:*477, 1949.
1404. Boijsen, E., et al.: *Acta Radiol (Stockh), 56:*81, 1961.
1405. Rabinovitz, J. G.: *Radiology, 102:*551, 1972.
1406. Lagergren, C., et al.: *Acta Chir Scand, 130:*321, 1965.
1407. Clark, E. R., et al.: *Am J Roentgenol Radium Ther Nucl Med, 113:*476, 1971.
1408. Kyaw, M., et al.: *Radiology, 93:*1055, 1969.
1409. White, A. A., et al.: *Radiology, 96:*551, 1970.
1410. Solomito, V. L., et al.: *Radiology, 102:*559, 1972.
1411. Ziter, F. M. H., et al.: *J Urol, 105:*776, 1971.
1412. Ervasti, J.: *Acta Chir Scand Suppl, 334,* 1964.
1413. Tull, J. C.: *J Pathol Bact, 35:*557, 1932.
1414. Ishak, K. G., et al.: *Cancer, 20:*396, 1967.
1415. Shorter, R. G., et al.: *Pediatrics, 25:*191, 1960.
1416. Warvi, W. N.: *Arch Surg, 37:*367, 1944.
1417. Brenner, E. J., et al.: *Ann Int Med, 54:*620, 1961.
1418. Viamonte, M.: Radiological Society of North America. Chicago, 1973.
1419. Ong, G. D., et al.: *Br J Surg, 52:*123, 1965.
1420. Altemus, R.: *Rad Clin North Am,* April, 1974.
1421. Takahashi, M., et al.: *Am J Roentgenol Radium Ther Nucl Med, 112:*779, 1971.
1422. Bagshawe, K. D.: *Proc R Soc Med, 60:*241, 1967.
1423. Cockshott, P., et al.: *Clin Rad, 15:*1, 1964.
1424. Borell, U., et al.: *Acta Radiol (Stockh), 44:*378, 1955.
1425. Shimkin, P. M., et al.: *Am J Roentgenol Radium Ther Nucl Med, 111:*535, 1971.
1426. Culp, W. C., et al.: *Radiology, 108:*309, 1973.
1427. Cockshott, W. P., et al.: *Radiology, 103:*21, 1972.
1428. Borell, U., et al.: *Acta Radiol (Stockh), 38:*247, 1952.
1429. Solish, G. F.: *Am J Obstet Gynecol, 81:*57, 1961.
1430. Ozarus, H.: *Acta Radiol (Stockh), 51:*257, 1959.
1431. Borell, U.: *Acta Radiol (Stockh), 56:*113, 1961.
1432. Schrieber, M. M.: Radiological Society of North America. Chicago, 1973.
1433. Klinger, M. E.: *J Urol, 65:*144, 1951.
1434. Shimkin, P. M., et al.: *Acta Radiol (Diag) (Stockh), 12:*387, 1972.
1435. Alderte, J. S., et al.: *Am Surg, 33:*174, 1967.
1436. Reuter, S. R.: *New Eng J Med, 278:*1423, 1968.
1437. Abrams, H. L.: *Calif Med, 74:*281, 1952.
1438. Gould, H. R., et al.: *Am J Roentgenol Radium Ther Nucl Med, 109:*775, 1970.
1439. Rösch, J.: *Clin Rad, 17:*183, 1966.
1440. Rousselot, L. M., et al.: *Surg Clin North Am.*
1441. Lazarus, J. A., et al.: *Am J Surg, 71:*479, 1940.
1442. Dasgupta, T.: *Surg Gynecol Obstet, 120:*947, 1965.
1443. Story, P., et al.: *Br Med J, 1:*990, 1952.
1444. Morissette, J. J., et al.: *Radiology, 106:*549, 1973.
1445. Hanson, R. B.: *Am J Roentgenol Radium Ther Nucl Med, 117:*81, 1973.
1446. Yannopoulos, K., et al.: *Cancer, 16:*914, 1963.
1447. Lazarus, H., et al.: *Am J Roentgenol Radium Ther Nucl Med, 113:*171, 1971.
1448. Aréan, V. M., et al.: *Ann Surg, 144:*133, 1956.
1449. Deutsch, V., et al.: *Am J Roentgenol Radium Ther Nucl Med, 113:*174, 1971.
1450. Hastings, N., et al.: *Arch Surg, 82:*188, 1961.
1451. Schriber, W., et al.: *Surgery, 52:*295, 1962.
1452. Cadman, N. L., et al.: *Cancer, 18:*613, 1965.
1453. Sayre, R. W., et al.: *Radiology, 99:*329, 1971.
1454. Bateson, E. M.: *Clin Rad, 19:*389, 1968.
1455. Lagergren, C., et al.: *Acta Radiol (Stockh), 55:* 321, 1961.
1456. Lagergren, C., et al.: *Acta Radiol (Stockh), 55:* 161, 1961.
1457. Kitteridge, R.: *Radiology, 97:*609, 1970.
1458. Schobinger, R.: *Cancer, 11:*1264, 1958.
1459. Halpert, B., et al.: *Am J Clin Pathol, 32:*165, 1959.
1460. Curtis, G. M., et al.: *Ann Surg, 123:*276, 1946.
1461. Daniel, D. S.: *Ann Surg, 145:*960, 1957.
1462. Clark, R. E., et al.: *Radiology, 102:*41, 1972.
1463. Rosenkrantz, W., et al.: *Br J Rad,* 42:939, 1969.
1464. Cullen, T. S.: *Arch Surg, 11:*718, 1925.
1465. Hansbrough, E. T., et al.: *Ann Surg, 145:*564, 1957.
1466. Fraser, C. G.: *Ann Surg, 135:*127, 1952.
1467. Lipchik, E. O., et al.: *Radiology, 88:*48, 1967.
1468. McClure, C. F. W., et al.: *Am J Anat, 35:*331, 1925.
1469. Gladstone, R. J.: *J Anat, 64:*70, 1929.
1470. Kjellberg, S. R., et al.: *Diagnosis of Congenital Heart Disease.* Chicago, Yearbook Med., 1955.
1471. Milledge, R. D.: *Radiology, 85:*860, 1965.

1472. Heller, R. M., et al.: *Radiology, 101:*519, 1971.
1473. Anderson, R. C., et al.: *J Pediatr, 59:*370, 1961.
1474. Berdon, W. E.: *Am J Roentgenol Radium Ther Nucl Med, 104:*452, 1968.
1475. Effler, D. B., et al.: *JAMA, 146:*1321, 1951.
1476. Dotter, C. T., et al.: *Am J Med Sci, 218:*31, 1949.
1477. Kiley, B., et al.: *Am J Cardiol, 20:*102, 1967.
1478. Campbell, M., et al.: *Br Heart J, 164:*423, 1954.
1479. Berdon, W. E., et al.: *Am J Roentgenol Radium Ther Nucl Med, 118:*18, 1973.
1480. Chaung, V. P., et al.: *Br J Rad, 17:*206, 1974.
1481. McChesney, E. W., et al.: *Am J Roentgenol Radium Ther Nucl Med, 78:*137, 1957.
1482. Cavina, C., et al.: *Am J Roentgenol Radium Ther Nucl Med, 113:*486, 1971.
1483. Ranniger, K., et al.: *Radiology, 92:*343, 1969.
1484. Abrams, H. L.: *Angiography.* Boston, Little, 1971.
1485. Felson, B.: *Am J Roentgenol Radium Ther Nucl Med, 107:*720, 1969.
1486. King, M. C., et al.: *Radiology, 91:*217, 1968.
1487. Giltes, R. F., et al.: *J Urol, 109:*14, 1973.
1488. Flynn, V. F., et al.: *J Urol, 108:*54, 1972.
1489. Lasser, E. C.: *Dynamic Factors in Roentgen Diagnosis.* Baltimore, Williams & Wilkins, 1967.
1490. Dotter, C. T.: *Radiology, 111:*31, 1974.
1491. McDonald, P.: In Abrams, H. L. (Ed.): *Angiography,* 2nd ed. Boston, Little, 1971.
1492. Belman, B. A., et al.: *New Eng J Med, 278:*1133, 1968.
1493. Gerson, D. E., et al.: *Invest Rad, 9:*328, 1974.
1494. Cuttino, J. T., Jr., et al.: *Invest Rad, 9:*328, 1974.
1495. Kelly, K. M., et al.: *Invest Rad, 9:*327, 1974.
1496. Baum, S., et al.: *Invest Rad, 9:*327, 1974.
1497. Fisher, C. H., et al.: *Invest Rad, 9:*318, 1974.
1498. Aronsen, K. F., et al.: *Scand J Gastroenterol, 3:*58, 1968.
1499. Lomas, F., et al.: *New Eng J Med, 286:*1323, 1972.
1500. Hayes, R. L., et al.: *Science, 167:*289, 1970.
1501. Bonte, F. J., et al.: *Am J Roentgenol Radium Ther Nucl Med, 88:*275, 1962.
1502. Johnson, P. M., et al.: *Radiology, 84:*868, 1955.
1503. Gollin, F. F., et al.: *JAMA, 187:*111, 1964.
1504. Shoop, J. D.: *Am J Roentgenol Radium Ther Nucl Med, 107:*51, 1969.
1505. O'Connor, J. J., et al.: *Am J Roentgenol Radium Ther Nucl Med, 90:*63, 1963.
1506. Danto, L. A., et al.: *Arch Surg, 104:*569, 1972.
1507. Rabinov, K., et al.: *Arch Surg, 104:*134, 1972.

FIGURE INDEX*

* A figure index has been provided for the reader's quick reference of figures in this book.

G

H

L

M

N

O

S

SUBJECT INDEX*

---

* Please supplement this with the provided figure index.

B

D

E

O

P

T

W

Z